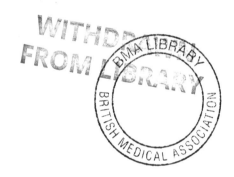
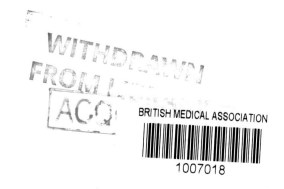

Walter and Miller's

TEXTBOOK OF
RADIOTHERAPY

Walter and Miller's

TEXTBOOK OF RADIOTHERAPY

Radiation Physics, Therapy and Oncology

EIGHTH EDITION

Edited by

Paul Symonds TD MD FRCP FRCR

Emeritus Professor of Clinical Oncology, University of Leicester, Leicester, UK; Honorary Consultant Oncologist, University Hospitals of Leicester, Leicester, UK

John A. Mills PhD MIPEM CPhys

Physicist, MACS-Quality Control Provider, James Watt House, Hinckley, UK

Angela Duxbury FCR TDCR MSc

Emeritus Professor of Therapeutic Radiography, Sheffield Hallam University, Sheffield, UK

ELSEVIER

ELSEVIER

First edition 1950
Second edition 1959
Third edition 1979
Fourth edition 1979
Fifth edition 1993
Sixth edition 2003
Seventh edition 2012

Notices

Practitioners and researchers must always rely on their own experience and knowledge in evaluating and using any information, methods, compounds or experiments described herein. Because of rapid advances in the medical sciences, in particular, independent verification of diagnoses and drug dosages should be made. To the fullest extent of the law, no responsibility is assumed by Elsevier, authors, editors or contributors for any injury and/or damage to persons or property as a matter of products liability, negligence or otherwise, or from any use or operation of any methods, products, instructions, or ideas contained in the material herein.

ISBN: 978-0-7020-7485-1

Content Strategist: Poppy Garraway Smith/Serena Castelnovo
Content Development Specialist: Veronika Watkins
Project Manager: Manchu Mohan
Design: Bridget Hoette
Illustration Manager: Narayanan Ramakrishnan

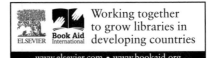

Printed in Scotland
Last digit is the print number: 9 8 7 6 5 4 3 2 1

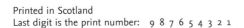

CONTENTS

CONTRIBUTORS

The editor(s) would like to acknowledge and offer grateful thanks for the input of all previous editions' contributors, without whom this new edition would not have been possible.

Matthew Ahearne, MBChB, MD, MRCP, FRCPath
Department of Haematology
University Hospitals of Leicester NHS Trust,
Leicester,
UK

Thankamma V. Ajithkumar, MBBS, MD, FRCR, FRCP, MBA
Consultant Clinical Oncologist
Department of oncology
Cambridge University Hospitals,
Cambridge,
UK

Matthew Aldridge, MSc, PhD
Radiotherapy Physics/Nuclear Medicine
University College London Hospital,
London,
UK

Richard A. Amos, BSc(Hons), MSc, CPhys, CSci, FIPEM
Associate Professor of Proton Therapy
Medical Physics and Biomedical
    Engineering
University College London,
London,
UK

Maria Mania Aspradakis, PhD
Head of Radiotherapy Physics
Department of Radiation Oncology
Kantonsspital Graubünden,
Chur,
SWZ

Helen Baines, BSc(Hons), MSc
Radiotherapy Physicist
Medical Physics and Engineering
St James's University Hospital,
Leeds,
UK

Laura Beaton, MBBS, BSc, MRCP, FRCR
Clinical Research Fellow
Research Department of Oncology
University College London Cancer Institute,
London,
UK

Neil G. Burnet, MA, MB BChir, MD, FRCS, FRCR
Professor
Manchester Cancer Research Centre
University of Manchester and Christie
    Hospital NHS Foundation Trust,
Manchester,
UK

Robert Coleman, MD, FRCP, FRCPE
Yorkshire Cancer Research Professor of
    Medical Oncology
Weston Park Hospital,
Sheffield,
UK

Mike Dunn, BSc, MSc
Retired Head of Radiation Protection
Medical Physics Department
University Hospitals of Leicester NHS Trust,
Leicester,
UK

Angela Duxbury, FCR, TDCR, MSc
Emeritus Professor of Therapeutic
    Radiography
Sheffield Hallam University
Sheffield,
UK

Jill Emmerson, DCR (T), HDCR (T)
QA Radiographer
Arden Cancer Centre
UHCW NHS Trust,
Coventry,
UK

Claire Fletcher, MSc, MIPEM
Principal Clinical Scientist,
Radiotherapy Physics,
UHCW NHS Trust
Coventry,
UK

Jenny Gains, MBBS, MRCP, FRCR, MD
Consultant Clinical Oncologist
Department of Radiotherapy
University College London Hospitals NHS
    Foundation Trust,
London,
UK

Pinelopi Gkogkou, MD, MSc, MA, PhD
Oncology Department
Norfolk and Norwich University Hospital,
Norwich,
UK

John R. Goepel, MB, ChB, FRCpath
Clinical Associate Professor and Honorary
Consultant Histopathologist
University of Nottingham and Nottingham
    University Hospitals NHS Trust,
Royal Hallamshire Hospital
Sheffield,
UK

Adrian Harnett, MBBS, MRCP, FRCR
Department of Clinical Oncology
Norfolk and Norwich University Hospital,
Norwich,
UK

Maria Hawkins, MD, FRCR, MRCP
MRC group leader
Department of Oncology
Oxford Institute of Radiation Oncology,
Oxford,
UK

Paul Hinton, BSc, MSc, CPhys, CSci, MInstP, MIPEM
Medical Physics - Nuclear Medicine
Royal Surrey County Hospital,
Guildford,
Surrey,
UK

David Hole, PhD (deceased)
Late Professor of Epidemiology and
    Biostatistics
University of Glasgow,
Glasgow,
Scotland

Shakardokht Jafari, PhD
Medical Physics Clinical Scientist,
Associate Tutor and Visiting Reasearch
    Fellow,
University of Surrey,
Guildford,
UK

Sarah J. Jefferies, BSc, MBBS, FRCP, FRCR, PhD
Oncology Department
Addenbrooke's Hospital,
Cambridge,
UK

George D.D. Jones, PhD, MScm, BSc
Professor of Cancer Radiation Research
Leicester Cancer Research Centre
University of Leicester,
Leicester,
UK

Andrzej Kacperek, BSc, PhD, FIPEM
Head of Eye Proton Therapy Service
The National Eye Proton Therapy Centre
The Clatterbridge Cancer Centre,
Bebington,
Merseyside,
UK

Charles Kelly, MBChB, MSc, FRCP, FRCR
Consultant Clinical Oncologist
Northern Centre for Cancer Care
Freeman Hospital,
Newcastle upon Tyne,
UK

Christopher Kent, MBChB, MRCP, MSc, FRCR
Consultant Clinical Oncologist
University Hospitals of Leicester
Infirmary Square
Leicester,
UK

Ian Kunkler, MA, MB Chir DMRT, FRCR, FRCPE
Professor
Institute of Genetic and Molecular Medicine
University of Edinburgh,
Edinburgh,
UK

Cliff Lawrence, MD, FRCP
Consultant Dermatologist
Royal Victoria Infirmary
Newcastle upon Tyne,
UK

Duncan B. McLaren, MBBS, BSc (Hons), FRCP (Ed), FRCR
Consultant Clinical Oncologist
Edinburgh Cancer Centre
Western General Hospital,
Edinburgh,
UK

Sofia Michopoulou, PhD, MIPEM
Principal Clinical Scientist
Imaging Physics
University Hospital Southampton NHS Foundation Trust,
Southampton,
UK

John A. Mills, PhD, MIPEM, CPhys
Physicist,
MACS- Quality Control Provider,
James Watt House,
Hinckley,
UK

Eva Morris, BSc, PhD
Professor of Cancer Epidemiology
Leeds Institute of Data Analytics
University of Leeds
Leeds,
UK

Abhik Mukherjee, MBBS, DMRT, MSc, PhD, FRCPath
Clinical Associate Professor
Department of Histopathology,
Division of Cancer and Stem Cells,
School of Medicine
University of Nottingham,
Nottingham,
UK

Somnath Mukherjee, FRCR, FRCP
Associate Professor
Department of Oncology
Oxford Institute of Radiation Oncology,
Oxford,
UK

Elizabeth M. Parvin, BSc, PhD
Honorary Associate
School of Physical Sciences
Open University,
Milton Keynes,
England,
UK

Andrew Penny, BSc, MSc, MIPEM
Radiotherapy Physicist
GenesisCare
Birmingham,
UK

Andrew Poynter, MSc, FIPEM, CSi
Operational Lead, Proton Physics,
Radiotherapy Physics
UCLH,
London,
UK

Andrew Rogers, FBIR
Lead Interventional Medical Physics Expert
Medical Physics & Clinical Engineering
Nottingham University Hospitals NHS Trust,
Nottingham,
UK

Tom Roques, BM BCh, MRCP, FRCR
Department of Clinical Oncology
Norfolk and Norwich University Hospital,
Norwich,
UK

John Sage, BSc, MSc, PhD
Head of Radiotherapy Physics
Clinical Physics and Biomedical Engineering
University Hospitals of Coventry and Warwickshire,
Coventry,
UK

Christopher D. Scrase, MA, MB, FRCP, FRCR
Department of Oncology
Ipswich Hospital NHS Trust,
Ipswich,
UK

Ricky A. Sharma, MA, MBBChir, FRCP, FRCR, PhD
Chair of Radiation Oncology
UCL Cancer Institute
University College London,
London,
UK

Phil Sharpe, MSc, MIPEM
Principal Clinical Scientist
Radiotherapy Physics
UHCW NHS Trust,
Coventry,
UK

Michael Snee, MBBS, FRCR, DM
Former Consultant in Clinical Oncology
St James' Institute of Oncology
Leeds,
West Yorkshire,
UK

Lesley Speed, MBChB, MSc, MRCP
Oncology Department
University Hospitals of Leicester NHS Trust,
Leicester,
UK

Katie Spencer, MB BChir, MA, FRCR
Leeds Institute of Data Analytics
University of Leeds,
Leeds,
UK

Aravindhan Sundaramurthy, MBBS, MRCP, FRCR
Consultant Clinical Oncologist
Edinburgh Cancer Centre
Western General Hospital,
Edinburgh,
UK

Paul Symonds, TD, MD, FRCP, FRCR
Emeritus Professor of Clinical Oncology
University of Leicester,
Leicester
UK;
Honorary Consultant Oncologist
University Hospitals of Leicester,
Leicester,
UK

Roger E. Taylor, MA, FRCP, FRCR
Professor
Clinical Oncology
Swansea University,
Swansea,
UK

Anne Thomas, BM, PhD, FRCP
Professor of Cancer Therapeutics
Leicester Cancer Research Centre
University of Leicester,
Leicester,
UK

Carl Tiivas, BSc, MSc
Lead Vascular Scientist
Vascular Laboratory
University Hospital Coventry,
Coventry,
Warwickshire,
UK

Karen Waite, DCR(T)
Advanced Practitioner Quality
Management, Governance & Paediatrics
The Nottingham Radiotherapy Centre
Nottingham University Hospitals NHS
Trust,
Nottingham,
UK

Harriet S. Walter, MBChB, MSc
Associate Professor of Medical Oncology
Leicester Cancer Research Centre
University of Leicester,
Leicester,
UK

Sarah Wayte, Bsc, PhD
Lead MR Physicist
Radiology Physics
Department of Clinical Physics &
Bioengineering
University Hospitals Coventry &
Warwickshire,
Coventry,
UK

Lorraine Webster, BSc(Hons), DCR(T), DipCouns
Macmillan Information Support Radiographer and Counsellor
Radiotherapy Department
The Beatson West of Scotland Cancer
Centre,
Glasgow,
UK

Michael Wynne-Jones, MSc, MIPEM
Head of Radiation Protection and
Radiology Physics,
Lincoln County Hospital
Lincoln,
UK

INTERNATIONAL SYSTEM OF UNITS AND PREFIXES FOR PHYSICAL QUANTITIES

There are seven international system (SI) base units:

Physical quantity	Unit	Symbol for unit
length	metre	m
mass	kilogram	kg
time	second	s
electric current	ampere	A
temperature	kelvin	K
amount of substance	mole	mol
luminous intensity	candela	cd

There is also a large number of derived units, some of which are listed here

Quantity	Derived Unit	Conversion
speed	$m\ s^{-1}$	—
acceleration	$m\ s^{-2}$	—
angular frequency	s^{-1}	—
angular speed	$rad\ s^{-1}$	—
angular acceleration	$rad\ s^{-2}$	—
linear momentum	$kg\ m\ s^{-1}$	—
angular momentum	$kg\ m^2\ s^{-1}$	—
force	newton (N)	$1\ N = 1\ kg\ m\ s^{-2}$
energy	joule (J)	$1\ J = 1\ N\ m = 1\ kg\ m^2\ s^{-2}$
torque	N m	—
power	watt (W)	$1\ W = 1\ J\ s^{-1}$
pressure	pascal (Pa)	$1\ Pa = 1\ N\ m^{-2}$
frequency	hertz (Hz)	$1\ Hz = 1\ s^{-1}$
charge	coulomb (C)	$1\ C = 1\ A\ s$
potential difference	volt (V)	$1\ V = 1\ J\ C^{-1}$
electric field	$N\ C^{-1}$	$1\ N\ C^{-1} = 1\ V\ m^{-1}$
radioactivity	Becquerel (Bq)	$1\ Bq = 1\ s^{-1}$
resistance	ohm (Ω)	$1\ \Omega = 1\ V\ A^{-1}$
capacitance	farad (F)	$1\ F = 1\ A\ s\ V^{-1}$
inductance	henry (H)	$1\ H = 1\ V\ s\ A^{-1}$
magnetic field	tesla (T)	$1\ T = 1\ N\ s\ m^{-1}\ C^{-1} = 1\ kg\ s^{-2}\ A^{-1}$
physical dose	gray (Gy) see Chapter 2	$1\ Gy = 1\ J\ kg^{-1}$
biological dose	sievert (Sv) see Chapter 4	$1\ Sv = 1\ J\ kg^{-1}$

The most common multiples and submultiples

Multiple	Prefix	Symbol for prefix
10^{12}	tera	T
10^{9}	giga	G
10^{6}	mega	M
10^{3}	kilo	k
10^{0}	—	—
10^{-3}	milli	m
10^{-6}	micro	μ
10^{-9}	nano	n
10^{-12}	pico	p
10^{-15}	femto	f

Online references : http://www.npl.co.uk/reference/measurement-units/

SECTION 1

1

Atoms, Nuclei and Radioactivity

Elizabeth M. Parvin

CHAPTER OUTLINE

INTRODUCTION

The aim of this first chapter is to lay some of the foundations of the physics of radiotherapy. It starts, in the section titled Atomic Structure, by looking at the main subatomic particles and the forces that hold them together in the atom. This leads on to an examination of the different types of nuclei, with an emphasis on some of the important ones used in medical physics. The behaviour of charged particles in electric and magnetic fields, central to much of the physics of radiotherapy, is covered in section titled Particles in Electric and Magnetic Fields. Waves, including the electromagnetic spectrum, and the basics of radioactive decay are introduced in the following sections.

For some readers, this chapter will be a reminder of previous knowledge, for others it will be new territory. For the latter, the references should provide some more in-depth material that it has not been possible to include here. For convenience, SI units are listed in the Physical Units and Constants Section.

ATOMIC STRUCTURE

Particles

Most readers will be familiar with the idea that molecules are composed of atoms chemically bonded together. Perhaps the most familiar example is the water molecule, which consists of two hydrogen atoms bonded to one oxygen atom to give the well-known molecular formula H_2O. In radiotherapy, we are often more interested in the particles that make up the atom—these are known as *subatomic particles*.

Table 1.1 lists the properties of the sub-atomic particles of most relevance to radiotherapy; the *proton, neutron, electron, positron, neutrino* and *antineutrino*. Strictly, only the electron, positron and neutrinos are

fundamental particles; the protons and neutrons are composed of *quarks*. Charges are, as is customary in physics, given as multiples of the electronic charge, *e*, which is 1.602×10^{-19} C. The proton and positron have charges of $+e$ and the electron has a charge of $-e$; all the other particles listed are neutral. The fourth column gives the masses in kilograms, but in nuclear physics, it is common practice to express the mass of a particle not in kilograms but in terms of its *rest mass energy*. This is based on Einstein's famous equation, which gives the equivalence of mass and energy:

$$E = mc^2 \qquad \textbf{1.1}$$

where *m* is the mass of the particle, *c* is the speed of light in a vacuum (2.998×10^8 m s^{-1}) and *E* is the energy. For an electron, the rest mass energy associated with a mass of 9.109×10^{-31} kg is 8.187×10^{-14} joules (J). It is more convenient to express this very small magnitude of energy in units of the *electron-volt* (eV), where

$$1\,eV = 1.602 \times 10^{-19}\,J \qquad \textbf{1.2}$$

The electron volt is the amount of energy acquired by an electron when it is accelerated through a voltage of 1 volt (see the section titled Electric Fields), hence the name *electron volt*. Using this conversion, we arrive at the values given in column 5 of Table 1.1. Note that the proton and neutron (known collectively as *nucleons*) are very much more massive than the electron and positron, and that the neutrino has almost zero mass—the exact value is still the subject of experiment.

The positron is the antiparticle of the electron, having the same mass but the opposite charge; it is emitted during β^+ decay (see the section titled Beta Decay) and is important in positron emission tomography (PET) (see Chapter 6). Neutrinos play a role in β decay (see the section titled Beta Decay). The photon is the particle associated with electromagnetic radiation (see the section titled Waves).

The Atom and the Nucleus

The *atom* is the smallest identifiable amount of an element. Each atom consists of a central *nucleus*, made up of protons and neutrons, which is surrounded by a 'cloud' of electrons. The diameter of an atom and nucleus are typically 10^{-10} m and 10^{-14} m, respectively. To put these dimensions into a more accessible perspective, if the atomic nucleus is represented by the point of a pencil (diameter approximately 0.5 mm) held in the centre of a medium-sized room (say 5 m × 5 m), then the electron cloud surrounding the nucleus would extend to the walls of the room.

It is the number of protons in a nucleus that determines the type of element. Because the protons in the nucleus are positively charged and the electrons are negatively charged, a neutral atom must contain equal numbers of protons and electrons. It is the electrons, which surround the nucleus and are often described as orbiting it, that interact with electrons from other atoms, thereby determining the chemical behaviour of the atom.

For example, a hydrogen atom has one proton in the nucleus, helium has two, carbon has six and so on. This number is known as the *atomic number, Z*, of the element. The elements listed in order of increasing atomic number form the periodic table of the elements [1].

As shown in Table 1.1, the neutrons in the nucleus carry no charge but do have a similar mass to the protons. The electrons have a very small mass, so the mass of an atom is almost entirely due to from the mass of the protons and neutrons. The sum of the number of neutrons (N) and protons in a nucleus is known as the *atomic mass number, A* and $A = Z + N$. Because both A and Z are needed to identify a nucleus, the notation used is of the form

$$^{A}_{Z}\text{X} \qquad\qquad 1.3$$

The symbol shown here as X is the chemical symbol for the element—H for hydrogen, He for helium, C for carbon and so on—and A and Z are the mass and atomic numbers. Because Z determines the chemistry and therefore the element, strictly speaking, it is not necessary to have the value of Z shown. For example, $^{12}_{6}\text{C}$ represents a carbon nucleus with six protons and six neutrons, but it could be written simply as ^{12}C, or even as carbon-12 because carbon always has six protons. However, to avoid confusion, it is often easier to include both atomic and mass numbers.

For any one element, the number of protons is always the same, but the number of neutrons, and hence A, can vary. For example, carbon can exist as, $^{11}_{6}\text{C}$, $^{12}_{6}\text{C}$, $^{13}_{6}\text{C}$ or $^{14}_{6}\text{C}$. These have 5, 6, 7 and 8 neutrons respectively and are known as *isotopes* of carbon. For many elements, some of the isotopes are radioactive (see the section titled Radioactive Decay) and this fact can be very useful in clinical investigations because the chemical behaviour of all the isotopes is the same. For example, radioactive $^{15}_{8}\text{O}$ is taken up by the body in the same way as the stable (i.e. nonradioactive) isotope, $^{16}_{8}\text{O}$, and can be used in PET; the radioactive iodine isotope $^{131}_{58}\text{I}$ is taken up by the thyroid gland in the same way as the stable isotope $^{127}_{58}\text{I}$, so can be used to treat thyroid cancer.

The Forces

The next point to address is the question of what holds the atoms together. The protons in the nucleus are positively charged, and the electrons surrounding the nucleus are negatively charged, so there is an attractive force between them. This electrostatic or *Coulomb force* depends on the product of the charges and is inversely proportional to the square of the distance between them. For one electron (charge $-e$) and a nucleus (charge Z), the magnitude of the force (F_{el}) is given by the equation

$$F_{\text{el}} = k\frac{Ze^2}{r^2} \qquad\qquad 1.4$$

where k is a constant and r is the distance between the electron and the nucleus. This inverse-square relationship is analogous to the gravitational force between two masses and we could use the rules of classical physics to calculate the orbits of the electrons around the nucleus (analogous to the orbits of the planets around the Sun). However, there is one big difference between the planetary orbits and the orbits of the electrons around the nucleus; in the planetary case, it is possible to have any value of the radius (and therefore energy), whereas, in the atomic case, quantum theory only allows certain permitted orbits. This gives rise to *electron energy levels* (or shells), which are the subject of the section titled Electron Energy Levels.

For like charges, the Coulomb force is repulsive, so, because the protons in the nucleus are all positively charged, it might be expected that the Coulomb force would cause the nucleus to fly apart. However, there is another force that acts on both protons and neutrons: the *strong force*. This force acts on protons and neutrons and other heavy particles called *hadrons*; it is independent of charge and is always attractive, but only at very short range. Fig. 1.1 shows the way in which the energy of a proton varies depending on how far away from the nucleus it is. As a proton approaches the nucleus, it experiences a repulsive force but, if it has enough energy to overcome this 'Coulomb barrier' and gets within

TABLE 1.1 Properties of the Subatomic Particles of Most Relevance to Radiotherapy

Particle	Symbol	Charge, e^{a}	Mass (kg)	Rest Mass Energy (MeV)
Proton	p	+1	1.673×10^{-27}	938
Neutron	n	0	1.675×10^{-27}	940
Electron	e^{-}	−1	9.109×10^{-31}	0.511
Positron	e	+1	9.109×10^{-31}	0.511
Neutrino	ν_e	0	>0	>0
Antineutrino	$\bar{\nu}_e$	0	>0	>0
Photon	γ	0	0	

^{a}e is charge on an electron.

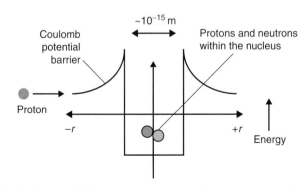

Fig. 1.1 Schematic illustration of the energy of a proton as a function of its distance, r, from the centre of the nucleus. As the proton approaches the nucleus, the repulsive Coulomb force increases, but close to the nucleus, this repulsion is overcome by the attractive strong force so the energy is reduced and the nucleons are held together in the nucleus.

the range at which the strong force works, then it has a much lower energy in the nucleus and stays there. An energy diagram like this is known as a *potential well*.

Electron Energy Levels

As mentioned in the section titled The Forces, planetary orbits around the Sun and electron orbits around the nucleus differ in that, in the case of the electrons, quantum theory predicts that only certain orbits are allowed. This means that only certain orbit energies can occur—these different values of energy are referred to as *energy levels* or shells and were first hypothesised by Niels Bohr in 1913.

A free electron, which is outside the nucleus, is said to have zero energy; any electrons in levels closer to the nucleus have a lower, and therefore negative energy. Fig. 1.2 shows the possible energy levels for

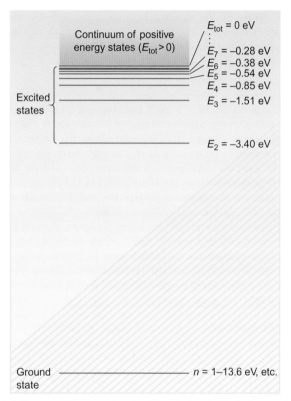

Fig.1.2 The possible energy levels of the electron in the hydrogen atom. Note that when the electron is bound in the atom, the energy is negative and can only take certain values. Outside the atom, the energy of the unbound electron is zero. The energy levels are numbered, $n = 1, 2$ and so on from the inside outwards.

the simplest element, hydrogen. No energy is lost or gained while an electron occupies a particular shell, and only discrete amounts of energy can be gained or lost by electrons when they move between shells. You can see from Fig. 1.2 that the lowest energy state for hydrogen has an energy of -13.6 eV. Therefore the amount of energy that would be required to remove this electron from the atom is 13.6 eV. This is the *ionisation energy* of the hydrogen atom. The energy required to raise an electron from the lowest energy state to the second lowest energy state is equal to the difference between the energies of the two states, that is, $(13.6 - 3.40) = 10.2$ eV, and so on for all other pairs of energy levels.

Large atoms have more complicated arrangements of electron energy levels; the energy levels are numbered according to the *principal quantum number, n* ($n = 1, 2, 3$ etc.) and are subdivided into other energy levels, sometimes known as *sub-orbitals*, with more quantum numbers relating to angular momentum and spin. These quantum numbers also dictate the number of electrons which can be in each shell. Historically, the principal quantum number may also be represented by the letters K ($n = 1$), L ($n = 2$), M ($n = 3$) etc., so the shells are often referred to as the *K, L, M shells* etc. If all the electrons in an atom are in the lowest possible energy states allowed by the rules, then the atom is said to be in the *ground state*. For example, a hydrogen atom in the ground state has the electron in the state with energy -13.6 eV.

Band Theory of Solids

In individual atoms, outer electrons occupy specific energy levels. When atoms are brought together, as occurs in solid materials, interactions between atoms broaden these specific energy levels into 'energy bands'. Electrons may occupy energy states only within these bands, between which are forbidden zones that normally do not have energy states for electrons to occupy, as illustrated in Fig. 1.3.

The outermost energy bands within the solid material are termed the *valence band* and the *conduction band*. Electrons within the valence band are considered as linked to the chemical bonds between individual atoms and are therefore bound in place, although the term *bound* is used loosely because at normal temperatures such bonds may be continually being broken and reformed. At an energy level slightly above the valence band is the conduction band. Electrons within this band are surplus to any requirements for chemical bonding. At normal temperatures, these electrons are not associated with specific atoms and chemical bonds, but migrate readily through the material. In some materials, there are insufficient electrons to fill the available energy levels of the valence band, so the conduction band is empty. Where a large forbidden zone exists, these materials are classed as nonconductors or insulators (see Fig. 1.3A). Other materials may have more outer electrons than the valence band can accommodate, so that the lower levels of the conduction band are also occupied. In these materials, the conduction band

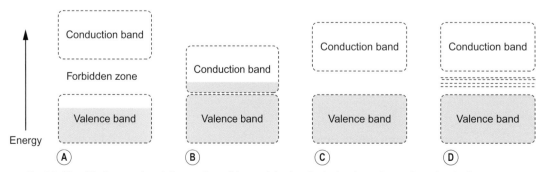

Fig.1.3 Simplified energy level diagram for solid materials: the shaded regions shows those levels that are normally occupied by electrons for (A) an insulator; (B) a conductor; (C) a semiconductor (undoped); (D) material with impurity levels within the forbidden zone.

overlaps with the valence band and the forbidden zone disappears, as shown in Fig. 1.3B. These materials will generally be good conductors of electricity. There are some materials in which the valence band is just filled, but the conduction band is effectively empty, and a small but significant forbidden zone exists. These materials are classed as *semiconductors*, illustrated in Fig. 1.3C. Any charges injected into a semiconductor will be free to travel through the material. It is to be stressed that this description is overly simplistic but serves as a basis for understanding the principles of solid-state dosimeters discussed in Chapter 3.

Impurity Bands

The introduction of impurities at low concentrations can alter the structure of the energy bands and may create energy bands that are located between the valence and conduction bands, within the forbidden zone as shown in Fig. 1.3D. The properties of the material so formed will depend upon whether these extra bands are normally occupied or empty of electrons, and their actual energy levels. The addition of impurities is critical to the formation of active semiconductor devices (see Chapter 3) and to the development and functioning of both scintillator and thermoluminescent materials (see Chapter 3).

PARTICLES IN ELECTRIC AND MAGNETIC FIELDS

Electric Fields

As already explained, a single charge exerts either an attractive or a repulsive force on another charge. A collection of charges will also exert a force on another charged particle. This force can be written as

$$F = qE \qquad 1.5$$

where F is the force on the charge q and the quantity E is known as the *electric field* (caused by other charges in the vicinity). The direction of the electric field is the direction in which a free positive charge would move; a free negative charge would move in the opposite direction, so the force on a particle in an electric field is always parallel or antiparallel to the field.

Magnetic Fields

The force on a charged particle in a magnetic field is more complicated. There is no force at all if the particle is not moving; if it is moving then the force is, like the force in an electric field, dependent on the charge, q, but it is perpendicular to the direction of both the magnetic field, B, and the velocity, v, of the particle and depends on the angle between them. Fig. 1.4 shows some examples.

The largest force occurs when the velocity of the particle is perpendicular to the magnetic field. As the angle θ between B and v decreases, the force decreases; when the velocity and field are parallel $\theta = 0$ and there is no force. In fact, the magnitude of the force is given by

$$F = q\,v\,B\,\sin(\theta) \qquad 1.6$$

So, when v and B are perpendicular, $\theta = 90^\circ$ and $F = q\,v\,B$.

The Lorentz Equation

The forces on a moving charged particle, which is subject to both an electric and a magnetic field, are complicated and are best dealt with using the mathematics of vectors, which is beyond the scope of this book. However, for the simple case where the magnetic field is perpendicular to the velocity of the charged particle, we can write

$$F = (qE + qvB) \qquad 1.7$$

The electric component of the force (qE) and the magnetic component (qvB) are not necessarily in the same direction. This equation is known as *the Lorentz equation* after the Dutch physicist Hendrik A. Lorentz, and is an extremely important equation in many areas of physics. In radiotherapy, it is useful when considering the behaviour of electrons in a linear accelerator and of charged particles in a cyclotron or synchrotron.

WAVES

Transverse and Longitudinal Waves

Energy, in the form of light, heat or sound, may be transmitted from place to place by waves. The direction of propagation of a wave is the direction in which the energy is transported; however, the particles in the medium do not change their overall position; they simply vibrate about an average position. We can distinguish two types of wave: *longitudinal* and *transverse*.

In a transverse wave (Fig. 1.5A), the oscillations are perpendicular to the direction of propagation of the wave. Water waves, or waves on a string, are good examples of transverse waves.

In the case of longitudinal waves (Fig. 1.5B), the particles in the medium move backwards and forwards in a direction parallel to the direction of propagation, although their mean position stays the same. A good example is a sound wave; the particles of the medium (e.g. air) oscillate parallel to the direction of the sound wave and this gives rise to changes in pressure along the wave.

Fig. 1.5 shows the *wavelength*, λ, of the wave—the distance between two adjacent peaks (or two adjacent troughs). Another important parameter is the *frequency, f*, which is the number of peaks that pass a point per second. In all cases, the speed of the wave, c, is related to the wavelength and frequency by the equation

$$c = f\lambda \qquad 1.8$$

This means that for a wave with constant speed, a larger wavelength corresponds to a lower frequency and vice versa. Wavelength is measured in units of metres (m) and frequency in hertz (Hz).

Longitudinal sound waves are important in ultrasound imaging (see Chapter 5), but for radiotherapy applications we are mostly concerned with the transverse waves of *electromagnetic radiation* and these are the subject of the next section.

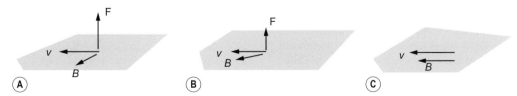

Fig.1.4 The force on a moving charge (positive in this case) in a magnetic field depends on the relative directions of the velocity (*v*) and the magnetic field (*B*). *(a)* *v* and *B* are perpendicular to each other. The force (*F*) is large and perpendicular to both *v* and *B*. *(b)* The angle between *v* and *B* is less than 90 degrees and the force is less but still perpendicular to both. *(c)* *v* and *B* are parallel: there is no force.

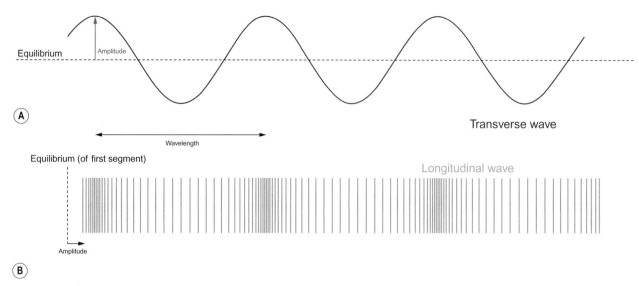

Fig.1.5 (A) Transverse and (B) longitudinal waves. Note the wavelength is the distance between two maxima.

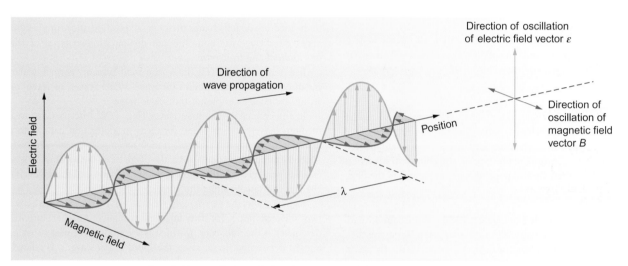

Fig.1.6 The oscillations of electric and magnetic fields in an electromagnetic wave.

Electromagnetic Radiation

Electromagnetic radiation is so called because it can be described as waves in which the quantities that oscillate are electric and magnetic fields. Fig. 1.6 shows how the fields in these electromagnetic waves oscillate at right angles to each other.

Because electromagnetic waves depend only on electric and magnetic fields, they can travel through any medium, including a vacuum. In a vacuum, all electromagnetic waves travel at a speed of approximately 3×10^8 m s^{-1} (often known rather loosely as *the speed of light in a vacuum*) but the properties of the radiation vary greatly with wavelength and frequency. Fig. 1.7 shows the vast range of the electromagnetic spectrum; note that as the frequency increases, the wavelength decreases, according to Equation 1.8. Radiotherapy physics is mostly concerned with the high frequency/small wavelength end of the spectrum, although radio waves are important in radiotherapy as they are used to accelerate the electron beam in a linear accelerator.

By the end of the 19th century, physicists were aware that all the different types of radiation shown in Fig. 1.7 were electromagnetic

waves and they could be explained in terms of wave physics. However, the beginning of the 20th century saw the development of quantum physics. Several key experiments, including the investigation of Compton scattering, an important process in radiotherapy, described in Chapter 2, showed that, when electromagnetic radiation interacts with matter, wave physics does not always predict the correct result. Instead the radiation behaves as particles known as *photons*. A photon is a small 'packet' or quantum of energy and each one has an energy given by

$$E = hf \qquad \qquad \textbf{1.9}$$

where E is the energy, f is the frequency of the electromagnetic wave and h is a constant, known as *Planck's constant* and equal to 6.626×10^{-34} J s.

As with the masses in the section titled Atomic Structure it is more usual to give these energy values in electron volts (eV) where 1 eV $= 1.602 \times 10^{-19}$ J. This has the advantage of allowing an easy comparison between the energy of a photon and the mass energy of a particle and is especially useful when considering the transfer of energy between a photon and particle or the conversion of a particle into radiation, annihilation radiation or radiation into particles, pair production (see Chapter 2). Fig. 1.7 shows the energies in eV in addition to the wavelengths and frequencies.

Continuous Spectra and Characteristic Radiation

In the section titled Electron Energy Levels we described the way in which the electrons in atoms can only be in specific energy states, defined by their quantum numbers. The energies of these states are different for each element; for example, Fig. 1.8 shows the main energy levels for tungsten, which is an element commonly used for the Target in x-ray production, such as x-ray tubes (see Chapters 4 and 8), and machines, such as linear accelerators (see Chapter 9).

As previously described, to raise an electron from one energy level to another, the energy required is equal to the difference in energy of the two states. If an atom is excited above its ground state by absorbing energy from incoming particles (e.g. photons or electrons) then some electrons can be moved up into allowable, but normally empty, energy levels. This happens, for example, in an x-ray tube (see Chapters 5 and 8). This leaves the atom in an excited state, that is, with a higher total energy than in the ground state. After a period of time, the atom will return to the ground state as the excited electrons drop from the higher levels back to vacant lower energy states. When this happens, the excess electron energy is carried away as a photon of electromagnetic radiation. Thus if we have two states with energies E_1 and E_2 then the energy of the photon (E_γ) is the difference between E_1 and E_2. Using Equation 1.9 to relate the energy of the photon to its frequency, we arrive at:

$$E_1 - E_2 = E_\gamma = hf \qquad \textbf{1.10}$$

The energy of photons produced is therefore dictated by the differences in energy between electron shells of the particular atom from which they are emitted. The spectrum of photons produced by an element is termed the *characteristic radiation* and will be different for each

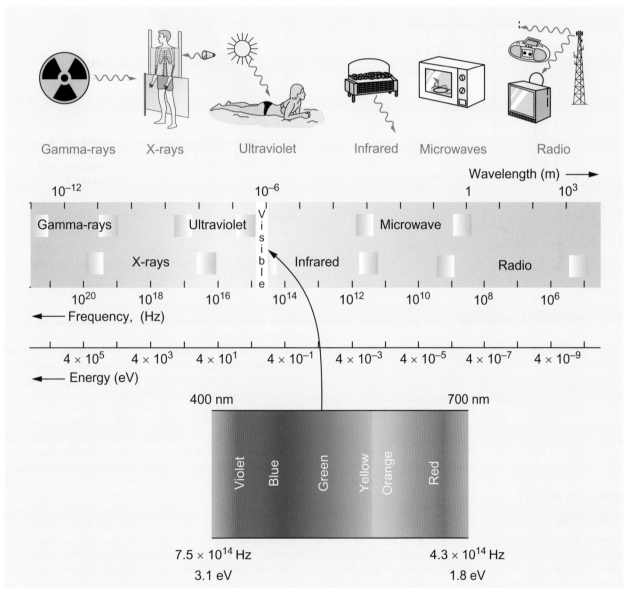

Fig.1.7 The different types of radiation that form the electromagnetic spectrum. The visible spectrum covers a very small range of wavelength values and is expanded below the spectrum.

element. Fig. 1.8 shows the possible electron transitions leading to the production of characteristic photons for tungsten. Distinction is made between electron transitions originating from different shells to the same destination shell by denoting the transition (and characteristic photon) with the final shell letter (K, L and so on) and adding a Greek letter suffix to indicate the originating shell, as shown in Fig. 1.8.

If the electrons in tungsten are excited, as in an x-ray tube, then the emitted photons will be a mixture of the continuous background spectrum (see Chapter 2) and the characteristic radiation from the tungsten atoms. This is shown in Fig. 1.9. The energy differences between the levels in heavy elements tend to be much larger than for lighter elements: note that for tungsten (see Fig. 1.8) the photon energies of the two main spectral lines are in the x-ray region at around 60 keV, which is in the x-ray range. They correspond to the L to K transition and the free electron to K transition. Contrast this with the energy of the largest possible transition in hydrogen, which is 13.6 eV, and in the ultraviolet region (see Fig. 1.7).

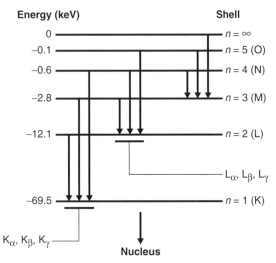

Fig.1.8 Electron energy levels and transitions leading to characteristic photons for tungsten. The main transitions into each shell are marked.

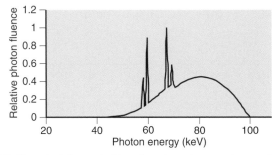

Fig.1.9 Characteristic spectral lines from tungsten superimposed on the continuous spectrum.

RADIOACTIVE DECAY

Stable and Unstable Isotopes

In the section titled The Atom and the Nucleus we explained that although the atomic number, Z, of a particular element is always the same, atomic mass number, A, can vary so that each element can have several different isotopes. Some of them will be stable: that is to say they will not decay; others will be unstable and will undergo radioactive decay. It is instructive to plot a graph which shows the number of

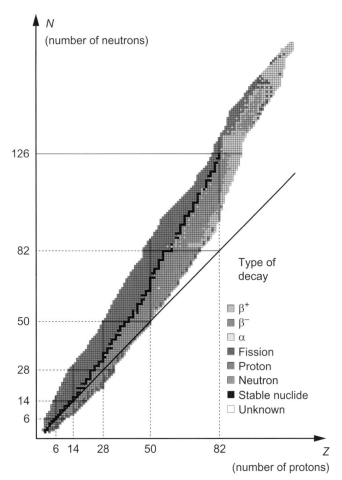

Fig.1.10 A graph of neutron number ($A–Z$) plotted against proton number (Z). The stable isotopes are shown in black and the solid line represents equal numbers of protons and neutrons.

neutrons ($A–Z$) against the number of protons (Z) for stable and unstable nuclei (Fig. 1.10). This figure shows the stable nuclei in black, which is known as the *stability line*. It also shows the solid line corresponding to equal numbers of protons and neutrons. We see that for low atomic number nuclei, an equal number of protons and neutrons is favoured, whereas a greater proportion of neutrons to provide stability for large nuclei. This may be explained by considering the increasing electrostatic force of repulsion between protons in the nucleus as the number of protons is increased. For a more detailed, interactive, diagram which allows you to look up individual nuclei [2].

Evidence suggests that protons and neutrons within a nucleus adopt a shell-like structure analogous to electron orbits and show particular stability when the number of protons or neutrons, or both, corresponds to a *magic number* (2, 8, 20, 28, 50, 82, 126). The strength of the strong force that holds the nucleons together is associated with a *nuclear binding energy* that must be overcome to break the nucleus apart. Essentially the mass of a given nucleus is less than the sum of its constituent protons and neutrons; this is known as the *mass defect*. Representing this in terms of energy, using $E = mc^2$, gives the nuclear binding energy. Nuclei with an even number of protons or an even number of neutrons are more stable than those with an odd number of one or both.

A nucleus lying off the stability line shown in Fig. 1.10 is unstable and decays by rearranging its nucleon numbers. This is achieved by releasing particles, changing a proton to a neutron or vice versa, or by absorbing nearby particles. The activity of an unstable, or radioactive, isotope is the rate at which its nuclei decay, expressed in *Becquerels* (Bq). One Becquerel corresponds to one decay or disintegration per second. The Becquerel is a very small unit so the activity of sources used in medicine is generally represented in MBq (1×10^6 disintegrations per second) or GBq (1×10^9 disintegrations per second). (You may also occasionally come across the old unit of activity, the curie (Ci); 1 Ci = 37 000 MBq.) Nuclei that undergo radioactive decay are known as *radionuclides*.

In the construction of practical radioactive sources, we are also interested in the amount of material that is needed to manufacture a source with a required activity, determined by the *specific activity*, the activity per unit mass (MBq kg^{-1}).

Half-life

Radionuclides decay at very different rates so it is important to have some way of quantifying the rate of decay. If we have a collection of identical nuclei, it is impossible to know exactly which one will decay next; one can only predict the probability of decay. The number of nuclei, dN, which decay in a short time dt will depend on two factors: the decay constant, λ, which is essentially the probability of decay, and N, the number of nuclei present at the start. This is expressed by the equation

$$dN = -\lambda N dt \qquad \textbf{1.11}$$

This equation can be rearranged and integrated to give

$$N(t) = N_o e^{-\lambda t} \qquad \textbf{1.12}$$

where N_o is the number of nuclei present at $t = 0$ and $N(t)$ is the number of nuclei present at time t. e is the exponential function. A graph of $N(t)$ plotted against time gives an exponential decay curve similar to that shown in Fig. 1.11.

The interesting thing about an exponential decay is that the length of time it takes for the number of undecayed nuclei to halve is always the same. In Fig. 1.11, this time is shown as 2 (arbitrary) time units. This time is known as the *half-life*, $T_{\frac{1}{2}}$, and it is related to the decay constant, λ, by the equation

$$T_{1/2} = \frac{\ln 2}{\lambda} = \frac{0.693}{\lambda} \qquad \textbf{(1.13)}$$

The term ln where the term ln represents the logarithm to base e; if $y = e^x$ then $x = \ln y$.

Half-lives can vary enormously—for example, the half-life of uranium-238 (not used for medical purposes!) is approximately the same as the age of the Earth, 4.5 billion years; the half-life of krypton-81, used in nuclear medicine, is 13s, and others are even shorter. The length of the half-life is an important consideration when choosing a radionuclide for medical use; if the half-life is too long, then the patient may be radioactive for the rest of their life; if it is too short then the activity will decay too fast for it to be useful.

When radioactivity was first discovered at the end of the 19th century, three different types of emitted particle were identified and were labelled alpha (α), beta (β) and gamma (γ) radiation. These names have remained, although there are now a few variants of them; the next four sections will cover these different types of decay.

Alpha Decay

Alpha (α) decay occurs most often from the unstable nuclei of heavy elements, such as uranium, radium or plutonium. The nucleus emits an alpha particle, which is actually a nucleus of helium, $^4_2$He. Having an equal number of protons and neutrons (both of which are magic numbers) the helium nucleus is very stable. The *parent* nucleus (X) decreases its atomic number by 2 and its mass number by 4 so the general equation is:

$$^A_Z X \rightarrow ^{A-4}_{Z-2} Y + ^4_2 He \qquad \textbf{1.14}$$

where Y is the *daughter* nucleus. For example, radium ($^{226}_{88}$Ra) decays to radon ($^{222}_{86}$Rn) and an alpha particle. Energy must be conserved in the transformation, so any difference, Q between the nuclear binding energies of the parent and daughter nuclei is shared between the emitted alpha particle, in the form of kinetic energy and any photons that are produced (see the section titled Gamma Decay). Alpha particles are typically emitted with kinetic energies of the order of several MeV.

Being relatively heavy (approximately $4 \times$ the mass of a proton) and highly charged (containing two protons), α particles are readily stopped in matter. For example, the 4.79 MeV α particle emitted from radium has a range of less than 4 cm in air, or less than 0.04 mm in tissue. This means that alpha particles can be very useful for radiotherapy, but only

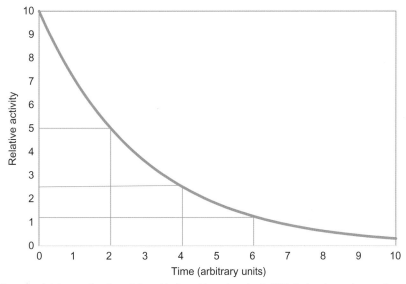

Fig.1.11 Exponential decay of radioactivity with time. Note that the half-life is the time taken to drop to one-half of the original value and is the same as the time taken to halve again to one-fourth and again to one-eighth.

if they can be released very close to the tumour tissue. Radium-226 was used in some very early external radiotherapy treatments but has the big disadvantage that the daughter product, radon, is a radioactive gas. More recently, Radium-223 is being trialled as an unsealed source of treatment for bone metastases.

Beta Decay

There are now known to be two types of beta decay. Beta minus (β^-) decay occurs frequently in naturally occurring radionuclides and involves the emission of an electron; beta plus (β^+) decay occurs mainly in artificially produced radionuclides and the particle emitted is a positron.

A nucleus lying above the stability line in Fig. 1.10, is neutron-rich and, by emitting an electron, can convert a neutron to a proton, thereby approaching the stability line. An example is iodine-131, which undergoes beta minus decay to become xenon-131:

$$^{131}_{53}I \rightarrow {}^{131}_{54}Xe \qquad \qquad \textbf{1.15}$$

Note that, because the total number of nucleons has not changed, the mass number stays the same, but because a neutron has been converted into a proton, the atomic number increases by one. The emitted β^- particle is a high-energy electron from the nucleus, not to be confused with the orbiting electrons in the atom.

By contrast, a nucleus lying below the stability line of Fig. 1.10, is proton-rich and therefore decays by converting a proton into a neutron. As with β^- decay the mass number does not change, but in this case, since a proton is converted into a neutron, the atomic number decreases by one. The emitted β^+ particle is a positron, the antimatter equivalent of the electron. A good example, which is widely used in PET imaging, is fluorine-18:

$$^{18}_{9}F \rightarrow {}^{18}_{8}O \qquad \qquad \textbf{1.16}$$

Observation that the β particles produced display a spectrum of kinetic energies, rather than the discrete energy difference between parent and daughter nuclei, indicates that a further particle must be involved. For β^+ decay, this particle is the neutrino, ν_e; for β^- decay, it is its antiparticle, $\bar{\nu}_e$. The processes for iodine-131 and fluorine-18 are therefore:

$$^{131}_{53}I \rightarrow {}^{131}_{54}Xe + {}^{0}_{-1}\beta + \bar{\nu}$$

and

$$^{18}_{9}F \rightarrow {}^{18}_{8}O + {}^{0}_{+1}\beta + \nu \qquad \qquad \textbf{1.17}$$

The energy arising from the difference in masses of the initial and final particles is carried away as kinetic energy of beta particle and the neutrino.

The range of a β^- particle is larger than that of an α particle as it is much lighter. However, whereas the heavy alpha particles will travel along a straight path, the beta particles will follow a much more erratic path as they interact with atomic electrons. The range of a beta particle in tissue is only of the order of a few millimetres and will depend on the energy with which it was emitted.

An emitted positron (β^+) travels through matter, rapidly losing kinetic energy through interactions with atomic electrons. When it collides with an electron, its antiparticle, both particles are annihilated and their energy converted into electromagnetic radiation. Using Einstein's mass-energy equivalence equation, $E = mc^2$, the total energy of the radiation must be 2×0.511 MeV (see Table 1.1). Conservation of momentum demands that two photons, each with energy 0.511 MeV are produced in opposite directions. This is the basis of PET (see Chapter 6).

Depending on its energy, a positron will be stopped within a very short distance of the site of emission in tissue. The annihilation photons, on the other hand, at 0.511 MeV, each can pass relatively easily through tissue. Detection of these coincident photons following administration of a positron-emitting radionuclide, such as fluorine-18 to a patient, therefore reveals where the annihilation event occurred and hence where the radionuclide was taken up within the body.

Gamma Decay

In the section titled Electron Energy Levels we showed that the electrons in atoms could only occupy certain allowed energy levels. In an analogous way, each nucleus can only have certain discrete energies and transitions between two levels involve the emission or absorption of photons of electromagnetic radiation. As with electron transitions, the energy values of the levels are different for different elements; however, in the nuclear case, the differences are much larger so the photons produced are generally of much higher energy. Following an α or β decay, the daughter nucleus is often left in an excited state. It will then reach its ground state by emitting a photon with an energy corresponding to the difference between the two energy levels. These photons are known as *gamma (γ) rays*. Fig. 1.12 shows the decay scheme for cobalt-60, which is an isotope formerly widely used for external beam therapy and now used in the Gamma Knife (see Chapter 8).

In most cases, the emission of gamma rays occurs immediately after the alpha or beta decay, however occasionally, the nucleus remains in an excited state and decays with a measurable half-life. Such an excited state is known as a *metastable* energy state and is denoted by the addition of an 'm' to the mass number. There is no change in Z or A during the transition from the excited state of the metastable nucleus to the ground state, so this is known as an *isomeric transition*. One important example, widely used in nuclear medicine, is technetium-99m (Fig. 1.13). This is a useful radionuclide because it produces only gamma rays, with an energy of 140 keV, which can be used for imaging, and no short range α or β particles, which would only damage tissue.

Note that both γ rays and x-rays are electromagnetic radiation at the top end of the spectrum (see Fig. 1.7); the energy ranges overlap and indeed both are used in radiotherapy. They are only distinguished by their origin: gamma rays coming from the nucleus and x-rays from the atomic electrons (see Chapter 2).

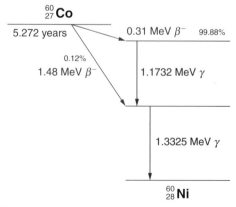

Fig.1.12 Cobalt-60 decays via beta decay to give nickel-60. The nickel nucleus is in an excited state and decays via the scheme shown, giving gamma rays with energies 1.1732 and 1.3325 MeV.

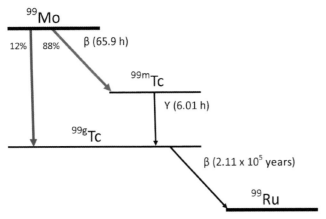

Fig.1.13 Technetium-99m is produced from molybdenum-99 by beta decay and then decays to the ground state (Tc-99g) via an isomeric transition with a half-life of 6 hours. The ground state technetium eventually decays to stable ruthenium-99 but with an extremely long half-life and therefore very low activity.

Electron Capture and Internal Conversion

As an alternative to positron emission (β⁺ decay), the nucleus of a proton-rich atom may capture one of its own inner shell electrons, via *electron capture* (EC). The captured electron combines with a proton in the nucleus to produce a neutron and neutrino, the latter being emitted from the nucleus carrying kinetic energy equal to the difference in nuclear binding energy between the parent and daughter nuclei. As with β⁺ decay, the mass number does not change but the atomic number decreases by 1. Nuclei that decay by this method can be useful because there is no particulate emission. An example of a nuclide that decays by EC is iodine-125; it emits gamma rays of up to 35 keV, which can be used for brachytherapy (see Chapter 8).

Another possible mode of decay is *internal conversion* (IC). An excited nucleus may de-excite by emitting a single photon, which interacts with the inner shell electron so that the electron is ejected from the atom. In contrast to beta decay, the emitted electron will have a single kinetic energy equal to the excitation energy of the nucleus minus the electron binding energy. The vacancy in the atomic shells left by the emitted electron will be filled by outer electrons, giving rise to characteristic radiation (see the section titled Continuous Spectra and Characteristic Radiation).

Radioactive Decay Series

There are many cases of radioactive nuclei that decay to give daughter nuclei, which are themselves radioactive and so on. This gives rise to a decay series. Fig. 1.14 shows the decay series of uranium-238, a naturally occurring radionuclide. At each stage, the α or β decay leads to a new nucleus which itself decays, the final product in this case being a stable isotope of lead. At each decay, the rate of growth of the activity of the daughter nuclide depends on the relative values of the decay constants (λ) of the parent and the daughter. Another

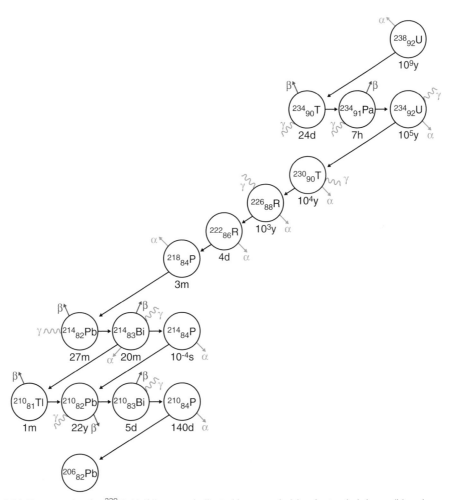

Fig.1.14 Decay series for $^{238}_{92}$U. Half-lives are indicated in seconds (s), minutes (m), hours (h) and years (y).

example, of much more clinical importance, is the decay of molybdenum-99 (see Fig. 1.13) to technetium-99m, which is widely used for imaging.

If we assume that there is no daughter present at time $t = 0$, and that all the disintegrations of the parent lead to the required daughter product, then the activity of the daughter at time t, $A_2(t)$ is given by:

$$A_2(t) = \frac{\lambda_2}{\lambda_2 - \lambda_1} A_1(0) \left(e^{-\lambda_1 t} - e^{-\lambda_2 t} \right) \quad \textbf{(1.18)}$$

where $A_1(0)$ is the initial activity of the parent at time $t = 0$ and are the decay constants of parent and daughter, respectively. Equation 1.18 is of relevance to radionuclide generators as it allows calculation of the optimum time between elutions of the daughter radionuclide.

If the decay of the parent is much slower than that of the daughter, that is, if $\lambda_2 \gg \lambda_1$ then Equation 1.17 reduces to

$$A_2(t) = A_1(0) \left(e^{-\lambda_1 t} - e^{-\lambda_2 t} \right) \quad \textbf{(1.19)}$$

This is the situation for ionisation chamber consistency check devices containing a strontium-90 source. Strontium-90 undergoes beta decay with a half-life of 28.7 years to yttrium-90, which itself decays via beta decay with a half-life of 64 hours. The activity of the long-lived strontium parent determines and maintains the activity of the short-lived yttrium daughter.

Radionuclides of Medical Interest

Table 1.2 lists some common isotopes applied to radiotherapy and nuclear medicine. The choice of isotope for a particular application is based on decay product type (γ, β (+ or −) or α), product energy/ies, half-life, specific activity (activity per unit mass) and availability. The α^- particles (heavy helium nuclei) have a very short range in tissue so will deposit energy close to the site at which a radionuclide is taken up in the body; β^- particles (electrons) have a slightly longer, but still small, range. If the site of disease can be preferentially targeted by these emissions, this leads to significant sparing of surrounding normal tissues in therapeutic applications. If greater penetration is required, of the order of centimetre for brachytherapy, or if imaging of radioactivity uptake through external detection of radiation is required, then photons (γ) or β^+ emissions will be the product of choice.

TABLE 1.2 Characteristics of Some Radionuclides Used in Radiotherapy as Either Unsealed Sources or Sealed Sources

Isotope	Decay Mechanism	Half-Life	Clinical Application
Unsealed Sources			
^{11}C	β^+ (2.0 MeV)	20 m	PET imaging
^{13}N	β^+ (2.2 MeV)	10 m	PET imaging
^{15}O	β^+ (2.8 MeV)	122 s	PET imaging
^{18}F	β^+ (1.7 MeV)	109 m	PET imaging
^{32}P	β^- (695 keV)	14.3 d	Polycythaemia vera
^{89}Sr	β^- (500 keV)	50.5 d	Bone metastases (palliation)
^{99m}Tc	γ (143 keV)	6.0 h	Gamma camera imaging
^{90}Y	β^- (923 keV)	2.7 d	Radiosynovectomy
^{131}I	β^- (264 keV) γ (364 keV)	8.1 d	Thyrotoxicosis and thyroid cancer
^{223}Ra	α (5.7 MeV)	11.4 d	Prostate cancer
Sealed Sources			
^{60}Co	β^-, γ (1.17, 1.33) MeV)	5.26 y	External beam units and gamma knife
^{103}Pd	EC, γ (21 keV)	17 d	Brachytherapy (seeds)
^{125}I	EC, γ (27–36 keV)	60 d	Brachytherapy (seeds)
^{137}Cs	β^-, γ (662 keV)	30 y	Brachytherapy (pellets)
^{192}Ir	β^-, γ (300–400) keV)	74 d	Brachytherapy (wire)

REFERENCES

[1] Interactive Periodic Table Royal Society of Chemistry, http://www.rsc.org/periodic-table/.

[2] Interactive Segre chart. http://people.physics.anu.edu.au/~ecs103/chart/ (Note that this plots Z against N—the opposite of Fig. 1.9. Both versions are commonly used).

FURTHER READING

Dendy PP, Heaton B. Physics for diagnostic radiology. 3rd ed. Baton Rouge: CRC Press; 2012.

Grant IS, Phillips WR. The elements of physics. Oxford: Oxford University Press; 2001.

2

Interactions of Ionising Radiation With Matter

Shakardokht Jafari, Michael Wynne-Jones

CHAPTER OUTLINE

INTRODUCTION

In this chapter we are mostly concerned with the interactions of electrons and photons with matter, as these are the most commonly used particles in radiotherapy (RT).

Charged and Uncharged Particles

The dominating feature of any particle is its charge. Electrons carrying a charge of -1.6×10^{-19} C readily interact via the Coulomb force with other charged particles in the matter they traverse, predominantly with atomic electrons and, to a lesser extent, with protons in atomic nuclei. Photons, by contrast, carrying no charge, interact relatively rarely with matter. The use of clinical proton beams for RT is increasing as new facilities are constructed worldwide. As charged particles, proton beams passing through matter behave in a similar way to electrons, that is, they readily undergo interactions with atomic electrons. The difference between proton and electron interactions lies in the proton having a mass of 1.67×10^{-27} kg, which is roughly 2000 times greater than the electron mass of 9.11×10^{-31} kg. The characteristics of proton energy loss in matter make them highly attractive for RT, offering distinct advantages over photons and electrons, as will be discussed later. Neutron beams are less often selected as the beam of choice for RT at the present time; however, they also offer advantages over photon beams for some tumours because of their biological effect on tissue. Being uncharged, neutrons interact in a similar manner to photons and, in fact, produce very similar depth-dose characteristics.

It should be remembered that RT is not restricted to these particles alone. Ion beams consisting of atomic nuclei stripped of their electrons may also be used. A proton, in fact, can be thought of as a hydrogen atom without its orbital electron. Carbon ions, in particular, have been used to treat a number of cancers in what is, at present, a small number of facilities worldwide, and their characteristics are being actively researched. Negative pions (π^-) were also, at one time, thought to have great potential for RT because of the nature of their interactions and their energy loss at the end of their range. Clinical studies on the use of pions have not demonstrated this advantage to date.

Excitation and Ionisation

Ionising radiation, by definition, has sufficient energy to ionise matter. That is, it has sufficient energy to overcome the binding energy of atomic electrons. Radiation of energy below the binding energy of a particular electron shell may still interact with an electron by raising it to a higher, vacant shell (see Chapter 1). As a result of this interaction, the atom has gained energy and is left in an excited state (Fig. 2.1A). It will eventually lose this excess energy to return to its lowest energy state, or ground state. An electron occupying an outer shell relative to the vacancy may achieve a lower energy state by filling the vacancy (see Fig. 2.1C). The excess energy is released as a characteristic photon (i.e. with an energy equal to the difference in shell binding energies). If this electron is also in an inner shell, it too will leave behind a vacancy, which an outer electron can again occupy (see Fig. 2.1C), again losing energy in the form of a characteristic photon. This process results in a cascade of electrons moving between shells and a corresponding set of characteristic photons, which eventually return the atom to its ground state.

Even if its own kinetic energy exceeds the atomic electron's binding energy, an incoming electron or photon may transfer part of its kinetic energy to an atomic electron to produce excitation. Where the incoming electron or photon transfers more than the binding energy of an atomic electron to the atom, the excited electron is ejected from the

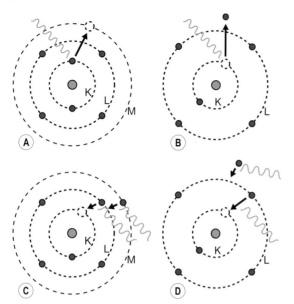

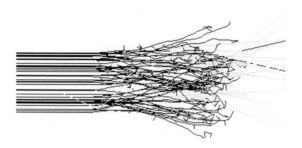

Fig. 2.2 Illustration of the frequent interactions, scattering, and finite range of electrons traversing matter. A beam of 10-MeV electrons (black) strikes a slab of water from the left. Incident electrons readily scatter, losing energy through collisions with electrons in the medium. Occasionally, energy is lost through x-ray production (bremsstrahlung, indicated by light grey lines). Note that (A) no primary electrons escape the slab as it exceeds the finite range of these electrons (x-ray photons and secondary electrons generated by these photons may leave the slab, however), and (B) the total distance travelled by an incident electron (path length) is greater than the maximum depth reached (range).

Fig. 2.1 Excitation and ionisation for a carbon atom. (A) Excitation: an incoming photon raises an inner shell electron to a vacant orbit; the electron has gained energy and, as a result, the atom is left in an excited state. (B) Ionisation: an incoming photon ejects a K-shell electron from the atom; the atom is ionised having an overall positive charge. As no scattered photon was produced, the emitted electron has acquired kinetic energy equal to the energy of the incoming photon minus the electron's binding energy. (C) De-excitation: an L-shell electron drops into the vacancy in the K-shell, emitting a characteristic photon; the L-shell vacancy is filled by the electron involved in the original interaction. (D) De-excitation: an L-shell electron fills the K-shell vacancy and a free electron from the medium is captured to the L-shell.

atom, with kinetic energy equal to the total energy transferred minus the binding energy. As a result of losing an electron, the atom has been ionised (see Fig. 2.1B). The positive ion will seek an electron from its surroundings to return to its uncharged state and so be chemically reactive. In addition, the ejected electron will leave a vacancy behind, which represents an excited state. The cascade process will then follow as described earlier as de-excitation takes place (see Fig. 2.1D).

ELECTRON INTERACTIONS

Collisional and Radiative Energy Loss

The last section was concerned with the dominant interaction that a beam of electrons undergoes when travelling through matter, that of collisions with atomic electrons in the energy range of interest to RT. These interactions lead to excitation and ionisation of the medium traversed, as represented schematically in Fig. 2.2. More rarely, electrons from an incident clinical beam will pass near to and interact with the atomic nucleus, again as a result of the Coulomb force of attraction between negatively charged electron and positively charged nucleus. The path and momentum of the incident electron are changed under the influence of the nucleus, resulting in a loss of electron energy. This loss of energy is the radiative energy loss resulting in a radiated photon, an x-ray. The term, bremsstrahlung (braking radiation), is a helpful descriptive name given to this process, shown schematically in Fig. 2.3. The probability of this interaction occurring is inversely proportional to the square of the incident particle's mass. As a result, bremsstrahlung is only significant for electrons. This important process by which x-ray photons can be produced is described in the following section.

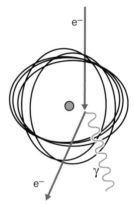

Fig. 2.3 Schematic representation of photon production by electrons (bremsstrahlung). An incident electron deflected by the nuclear Coulomb field loses energy, which appears in the form of an emitted photon.

X-Ray Production

The conversion of electron kinetic energy into photons as a beam of electrons striking a target is decelerated in the nuclear Coulomb field (bremsstrahlung) is the primary method for obtaining clinical photon beams. As suggested earlier, however, for the normal range of energies considered for diagnostic imaging and RT (20 keV to 25 MeV), electrons are far more likely to interact through collisions with atomic electrons. The efficiency of this process is therefore generally low. The likelihood of bremsstrahlung depends on the atomic number of the material traversed, Z (the total charge of the nucleus), and the energy of the incident electron, E, according to:

$$\text{Probability} \sim ZE \qquad \textbf{2.1}$$

The energy of the electron beam is dictated by the maximum photon energy required. The use of high atomic number materials gives the best yield of photons. Table 2.1 presents the proportion of electron beam kinetic energy converted to photons for a tungsten target. The remainder of the incident electron's kinetic energy is lost through collisions with atomic electrons in the target, causing excitation and ionisation.

TABLE 2.1 Percentage of Incident Electron Beam Energy Appearing as Bremsstrahlung for Electrons Incident on a Tungsten Target	
Electron Energy (MeV)	**Photon Yield (%)**
0.05	0.5
0.25	2
1	6
10	30
50	63

Data calculated using the ESTAR program [1].

A large amount of this energy is eventually released in the form of heat, requiring the target to be cooled.

In the bremsstrahlung process, an electron may lose any amount of energy, up to its total kinetic energy. Rather than discrete photon energies, as are observed during de-excitation of atoms, a continuous spectrum of photon energies is produced. An example of the photon spectra produced when electrons are used to generate a 100 kV and 6 MV photon beam is shown in Fig. 2.4.

Photon spectra are commonly designated by kilovoltage (kV) or Megavoltage (MV) to indicate the nominal potential used to accelerate the electrons that created the spectrum. For example, a potential difference of 100 kV between cathode and anode in an x-ray tube will result in electrons with an energy of 100 keV striking the target, producing a 100 kV photon spectrum. Although there is no lower limit on the energy of photons produced, the low-energy components of the spectrum are preferentially removed by photon attenuation within the target and other machine components, so that the peak in the spectrum occurs at approximately one-third of the maximum photon energy.

For electrons striking a thin target, photons are produced in all directions. The intensity (or number) in a particular direction depends on the energy of the incident electrons, and the atomic number of the target. For low electron energies (up to 100 keV), the intensity is almost equal in all directions and as the electron energy increases, the photons produced become more forward directed. This variation in photon intensity with incident electron energy is illustrated in Fig. 2.5, where electrons (indicated by the dashed line) are incident from the left. In this figure, bremsstrahlung production is simulated for a number of incident electrons, with the emitted photon energy and direction sampled from known probabilities (cross sections). Some 2000 photon tracks are represented in each figure, projected from a three-dimensional distribution into a two-dimensional plane. The length and shade of each photon track is representative of the individual photon energy. Note that higher energy photons (lightly shaded, long tracks) appear predominantly in the forward direction. This is one of

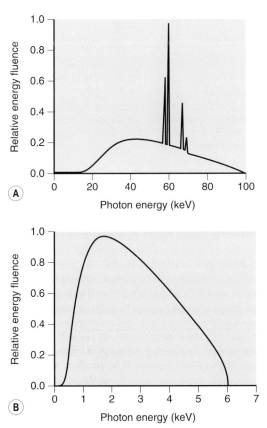

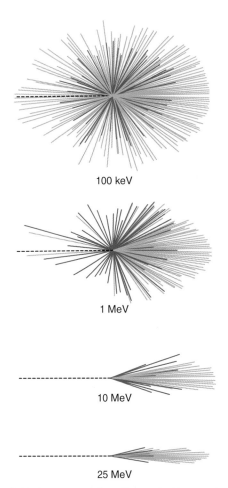

Fig. 2.4 X-ray spectra: (A) 100-kV diagnostic spectrum; bremsstrahlung (continuous) spectrum with superimposed discrete characteristic tungsten x-rays and (B) 6-MV photon spectra from an Elekta SL25 linear accelerator. (A, from IPEM Report 78. Catalogue of diagnostic x-ray spectra and other data. Institute of Physics and Engineering in Medicine; 1997; B, from Baker C, Peck K. Reconstruction of 6 MV photon spectra from measured transmission including maximum energy estimation. Phys Med Biol 1997;42:2041–2051.)

Fig. 2.5 Spatial and energy variation of bremsstrahlung produced by electrons incident on a thin target. Electrons are incident from the left (*dashed line*); bremsstrahlung photons energy is indicated by track length and shade (short/dark = low energy). In each case 2000 bremsstrahlung interactions are simulated from known probabilities.

the reasons for the average photon energy emitted from a linear accelerator target being lower at angles off the beam central axis.

The observed variation in spatial intensity of bremsstrahlung photons affects the design of x-ray targets. At kilovoltage energies, a reflection target is generally used, where photons produced at right angles to the direction of incident electrons are extracted for use. At megavoltage energies, a transmission target is required as photons are mostly travelling approximately parallel to the incident electron beam. This is shown schematically in Fig. 2.6.

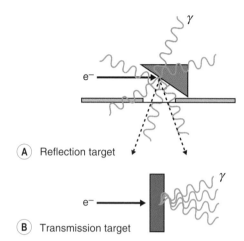

Fig. 2.6 Reflection and transmission targets for the production of x-rays: (A) represents the production of a kilovoltage therapy beam and (B) the production of a megavoltage beam.

Characteristic X-Rays and Auger Electrons

Discrete spectral lines can be seen superimposed on the continuous 100 kV spectrum in Fig. 2.4. These are as a result of characteristic photons being produced during de-excitation of tungsten atoms after inner shell electrons have been excited or ejected through collisions with the incident electron beam. The energies of these characteristic photons correspond to the difference between the binding energies of the inner shell vacancy and the outer shell electron that fills the vacancy. The difference between electron binding energies depends on the atomic number of the target. For tungsten, with a K-shell binding energy of 69 keV and L-shell binding energy of 12 keV, it follows that the minimum energy of a characteristic photon produced by filling an electron vacancy in the K-shell is 57 keV. The same characteristic photons are not observed in the 6-MV spectrum, as they now represent very low energies within this spectrum and are preferentially removed by photon attenuation.

In some instances, the characteristic x-ray does not escape the atom, but excites an outer electron sufficiently for the electron to leave the atom. These electrons are referred to as Auger electrons after the physicist who identified the process.

Stopping Power and Linear Energy Transfer

The rate at which energy from an incident beam of charged particles is lost as it passes through a material is described by the stopping power. If an electron of energy, E, loses a small amount of energy, dE, in a small thickness, dx, of material, the stopping power, $S(E)$, is defined by:

$$S(E) = \mathrm{d}E/\mathrm{d}x \ [\mathrm{MeV\,cm^{-1}}] \qquad \textbf{2.2}$$

If the energy loss is separated into that lost in collisions, S_{coll}, with atomic electrons and that lost through bremsstrahlung (or radiative loss), S_{rad}:

$$S(E) = S_{coll}(E) + S_{rad}(E) \qquad \textbf{2.3}$$

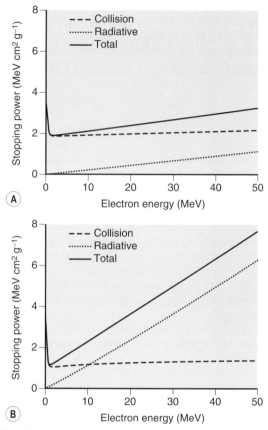

Fig. 2.7 Collisional, radiative, and total stopping power for electrons: (A) in water and (B) in tungsten. Data calculated using the ESTAR program. (From Berger M, Coursey J, Zucker A, Chang J. ESTAR, PSTAR, and ASTAR: Computer programs for calculating stopping-power and range tables for electrons, protons, and helium ions (version 1.2.3), Gaithersburg, MD: National Institute of Standards and Technology; 2005. http://physics.nist.gov/Star.)

If energy is in MeV and distance in centimetres, stopping power has units of MeV cm^{-1}. Alternatively, we may express this in terms of mass stopping power, $S(E)/\rho$, where ρ is the material density (g cm^{-3}). The magnitude of this quantity depends on both the energy of the electron and the material involved. Fig. 2.7 shows the variation of electron mass stopping power with energy in water and lead. Measurement of the energy absorbed in a material is determined using stopping power and the energy absorbed per unit mass is referred to as the absorbed dose. Its units are J/kg, and given the special unit gray, symbol Gy.

Because stopping power reflects the difference in energy absorption between materials, it is used in radiation dosimetry to convert measured radiation dose between materials. For example, using an air-filled ionisation chamber surrounded by water, a direct measurement of energy absorbed, or dose to air, D_{air}, can be made. The dose, D_w, that would be absorbed if the ionisation chamber were replaced by water, which is very close to human soft tissue, would be given by multiplying by the ratio of mass stopping powers between water and air:

$$D_w = D_{air} \times (S_w(E)/\rho_w)/(S_{air}(E)/\rho_{air}) \qquad \textbf{2.4}$$

where ρ_w and ρ_{air} are the densities of water and air, respectively. Strictly, the stopping power used in equation 2.4 must be restricted to energy absorbed within the ionisation chamber volume and must exclude any energy that is lost from the beam but travels beyond the chamber (site of interaction). For example, energy lost in the form of bremsstrahlung, or collisions in which a large amount of the incident electron's energy is transferred to an atomic electron such that it travels beyond the chamber.

Linear energy transfer (LET) also refers to the amount of energy deposited by ionising radiation in matter. Units are also energy per unit length, often expressed in keV μm^{-1}. The LET is commonly used to distinguish between types of ionising radiation. Photons and electrons have a lower LET than protons and alpha particles. The term of low and high LET is often used in radiobiological descriptions. The smaller length units (μm) for LET reflect its application to energy deposition over subcellular dimensions. A schematic comparison between energy deposition for high and low LET beams is illustrated in Fig. 2.8 in relation to radiobiology.

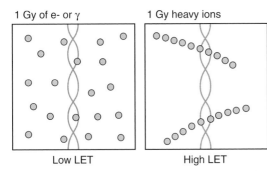

Low LET   High LET

Fig. 2.8 Comparison of dose deposition and biological effect for low and high linear energy transfer (LET) beams. Circles refer to ionising events. The increased track density of ionisation events occurring for the higher LET beam leads to greater biological (DNA) damage. This increase in biological damage in comparison to low LET radiation (e.g. photons) can be expressed as a relative biological effectiveness (RBE), defined as the ratio of radiation doses required to produce the same degree of biological damage. For example, if an RBE of 1.1 is assumed for protons, then a prescribed proton dose of 70 Gy would achieve the same biological effect as a dose of 77 Gy delivered by photons.

Range and Path Length

Electrons have a negative charge and a relatively small mass. As a result, electron transport through matter is characterised by a large number of interactions through which generally a small amount of energy is lost in each interaction and a high degree of scattering occurs (Fig. 2.2). Because of these frequent interactions, it can often be assumed that electrons lose energy continuously as they traverse matter and to a good approximation the energy loss can be assumed to be at a constant rate. It follows that if electrons or any other particles lose energy continuously, then they must have a finite range. This is true of all charged particles. Calculated ranges for charged particles can be obtained using this continuous slowing down approximation (csda), resulting in the csda range. If a beam of monoenergetic electrons is incident on a given material and we assume continuous energy loss, then the total distance travelled, or path length, must be the same for all electrons in the beam. The depth of penetration, or range, will vary because of the different paths traversed by individual electrons as indicated in Fig. 2.2. This range straggling leads to a slope in the measured depth-dose curve, as illustrated in Fig. 2.9A. The steepness of this slope decreases as electron energy is increased, as shown in Fig. 2.9B. Note that the dose does not fall to zero immediately beyond the steep region of dose fall-off, because of bremsstrahlung photons being produced. The intersection between the slope as a result of range straggling and the bremsstrahlung tail gives the practical range of the electron beam, R_p. As a guide, for clinical electron beams produced by linear accelerators (approximately

4–20 MeV), the range of electrons in water (or tissue) can be approximated by:

$$\text{Electron range (cm)} \approx \text{Beam energy (MeV)}/2 \qquad \textbf{2.5}$$

An indication of the accuracy of the aforementioned expression can be made by comparison with electron csda ranges in water, given in Table 2.2.

TABLE 2.2 Electron Continuous Slowing Down Approximation Ranges in Water

Electron Beam Energy (MeV)	Continuous Slowing Down Approximation Range (cm)
0.1	0.01
0.25	0.06
0.5	0.18
1	0.44
5	2.55
10	4.98
25	11.3
50	19.8

Evaluated using the ESTAR program [1].

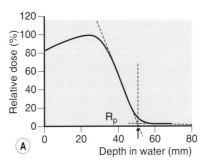

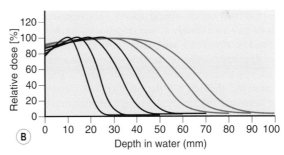

Fig. 2.9 Electron depth-dose distribution in water. (A) 10-MeV electron beam, indicating practical range, R_p. (B) Variation of depth dose with beam energy for (from left to right) 4-, 6-, 8-, 10-, 12-, 15- and 18-MeV beams. (From the Clatterbridge Centre for Oncology NHS Foundation Trust: Douglas Cyclotron. With permission.)

PHOTON INTERACTIONS

In the photon energy range of interest for RT, there are three major interactions that can occur as a beam of photons passes through matter: photoelectric, Compton, and pair production.

The Photoelectric Effect

This interaction, shown schematically in Fig. 2.10, occurs between an incident photon and atomic electron, generally assumed to be an inner

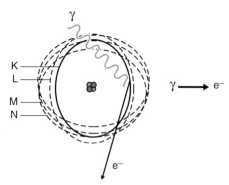

Fig. 2.10 Schematic representation of the photoelectric effect. An incoming photon transfers all its energy to an inner shell electron, ejecting the electron with a kinetic energy equal to the photon energy minus the electron binding energy. Electron shells K to N are indicated.

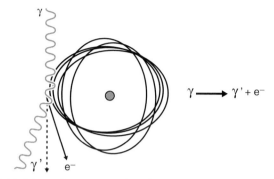

Fig. 2.11 Schematic representation of the Compton effect. An incident photon, γ, transfers part of its energy to an electron and a lower-energy, scattered photon, γ′, is produced.

shell electron. If the photon has sufficient energy to overcome the shell binding energy of the electron, it may disappear by transferring all its energy to the electron. The electron is then emitted from the atom, with kinetic energy, k.e., equal to the energy of the incident photon, E_γ, minus the electron binding energy, b.e.

$$\text{k.e.} = E_\gamma - \text{b.e.} \qquad \textbf{2.6}$$

As a consequence of this interaction, the atom is ionised and in an excited state. De-excitation then occurs, releasing characteristic photons, in the same manner as described above under "Characteristic X-rays and Auger Electrons" after ionisation or excitation by electron interactions. The probability of the photoelectric effect occurring is strongly dependent on the atomic number, Z, of the material traversed and on the energy, E, of the incident photon:

$$\text{Probability} \sim Z_3/E_3 \qquad \textbf{2.7}$$

This strong dependence on the atomic number is put to considerable use in diagnostic imaging because it provides clear differentiation between tissues with different atomic number as well as, or in the absence of, differences in physical density. For example, a 70-kV beam of photons passing through a human pelvis is much more likely to interact and be absorbed when passing through bone, with an atomic number of approximately 13, than it is when passing through adjacent soft tissue, with an approximate atomic number of 7. The photon intensity transmitted through the patient therefore clearly distinguishes between bone and soft tissue, providing a high-contrast x-ray image.

The Compton Effect

The Compton effect dominates in water between 100 keV and 20 MeV and is therefore the dominant interaction in tissue throughout the RT energy range of interest for photons. This interaction involves an incident photon interacting with an atomic electron, overcoming the electron-binding energy, and transferring some of its energy to the electron in the form of kinetic energy and the remainder as a lower energy photon. Unlike the photoelectric effect, no resonance effect is observed, and the interaction is likely to occur with outer shell electrons with binding energies far lower than the energy of the incoming photon. As a result, this interaction is often referred to as occurring with free electrons. The interaction is shown schematically in Fig. 2.11.

The probability of the Compton interaction depends on the density of electrons in a material, which varies as Z/A, ratio of the atomic number Z and mass number A. This ratio is almost constant for elements above hydrogen and, as a result, the Compton effect can be considered to be independent of the atomic number of the material the photons

pass through and is dependent only on the physical density. It is for this reason that medical imaging with megavoltage photons leads to poorer contrast than imaging with kilovoltage photon beams. This represents a benefit for RT to soft-tissue tumours, however, as a significant dependence on atomic number would lead to higher absorbed dose being delivered to bone than soft tissue.

The average proportion of the incident photon's energy transferred to the electron depends on the incident photon energy. For a 100 keV incident photon, on average approximately 10% of its energy, 10 keV, is passed to the electron, whereas the scattered photon retains 90 keV. As the incident photon energy increases, however, a higher proportion of its energy is transferred to the electron; a 10 MeV photon transfers an average of approximately 70%, 7 MeV, to the electron and the scattered photon retains 3 MeV. The variation of average energy transferred to the electron via the Compton effect is illustrated in Fig. 2.12. These characteristics of the Compton effect have implications for RT and radiation dosimetry. For kilovoltage photon beams, electrons set in motion through Compton interactions can be assumed to deposit their energy very close to the site of interaction, whereas for megavoltage photons, these interactions produce high-energy secondary electrons that will travel a significant distance. The latter results in the observed skin-sparing effect of absorbed dose deposition in tissue by megavoltage photon beams, as electrons set in motion near the skin surface deposit their energy over a significant depth. For example, a 3-MeV photon (approximately the average photon energy in a 10-MV photon spectrum) will provide an electron with an average energy of 1.8 MeV (60%), which will deposit energy over a distance of approximately 1 cm

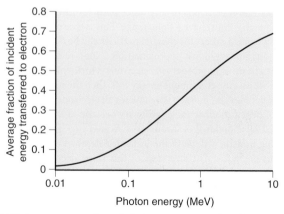

Fig. 2.12 Average proportion of photon energy transferred to secondary electrons during the Compton effect. (From Attix F. Introduction to radiological physics and radiation dosimetry. John Wiley & Sons Inc; 1996.)

in tissue. The angular distribution of electrons set in motion by the Compton effect is also of interest. For kilovoltage photons, the secondary electrons set in motion are emitted over a wide range of angles from the direction of the incident photon. As the incident photon energy is increased, this distribution of electrons becomes more forward directed.

Pair Production

Above a few Mega electron volts (MeV), photons may interact with the nuclear Coulomb field to produce an electron–positron pair, shown schematically in Fig. 2.13. In this interaction, the photon vanishes, and all its energy is transferred to the rest mass and kinetic energy of the electron, k.e.(e^-) and positron, k.e.(e^+). For an incident photon of energy E, conservation of energy demands that:

$$E = 1.022 + \text{k.e.}(e^+) + \text{k.e.}(e^-) \, [\text{MeV}] \qquad \textbf{2.8}$$

Hence the incoming photon must have a minimum energy of 1.022 MeV for the interaction to occur. The probability of a photon being attenuated by pair production is proportional to the atomic number of the material traversed and, for the energy range of interest to RT, increases gradually with the incoming photon's energy.

$$\text{Probability} \sim ZE \, (E > 1.022 \, \text{MeV}) \qquad \textbf{2.9}$$

In water and soft tissue, pair production only becomes significant at photon energies above approximately 10 MeV and so it accounts for very little of the absorbed dose to a patient undergoing RT. With higher atomic number materials, pair production becomes significant at lower energies, for example, at approximately 3 MeV for lead.

The electron and positron produced will lose energy in the medium traversed, mainly through interactions (collisions) with atomic electrons, as discussed earlier. The positron eventually annihilates with a local electron, releasing the remaining positron kinetic energy and rest mass of the positron and electron in the form of photons. This annihilation event becomes more likely as the positron slows down. If it occurs at rest, that is, when the positron has lost all of its kinetic energy, the energy of each photon is equal to 0.511 MeV, the electron (and positron) rest mass. To conserve momentum, these two photons must travel in opposite directions. This feature of positron–electron annihilation is the key to positron emission tomography (PET), as coincident detection of the two photons produced reveals information about the position of the annihilation event, see Chapter 6.

Photons may undergo a similar interaction to the nuclear pair production interaction described earlier in the Coulomb field of an electron. However, the probability of this is very low compared with the interaction in the nuclear Coulomb field.

Exponential Attenuation

An experimental arrangement is shown in Fig. 2.14 for measuring the number of photons that reach a detector as a filter, or attenuator, is placed in the beam path. We are interested in measuring how many photons arrive at the detector without undergoing any interaction in the filter (i.e. how many photons are unattenuated). The purpose of the collimators is to prevent any scattered photons, resulting from an interaction in the filter, from reaching the detector and so causing us to overestimate the number of photons that have not interacted. If scattered photons are excluded, this arrangement is referred to as narrow-beam geometry. The detector records N photons arriving at the detector for a thickness, x, of filter. If the number of photons reaching the detector changes by an amount, dN, when a thin (infinitely thin) filter of thickness, dx, is placed in the beam and we represent the relative change (dN/N) per unit thickness as μ, we have:

$$\mu dx = -dN/N \qquad \textbf{2.10}$$

By integrating this expression, and applying the condition that for zero filter thickness, N_0 photons are recorded at the detector, it is straightforward to show that the number of photons, N, transmitted by the filter and reaching the detector when a filter of thickness x is placed in the beam:

$$N = N_0 e^{-\mu x} \qquad \textbf{2.11}$$

Parameter, μ, is the linear attenuation coefficient (units of per unit distance, e.g. cm^{-1}), and its value is dependent on the filter material and the energy of the photon beam. To compare the effect of varying atomic number on attenuation properties, it is convenient to remove the variation because of material density, ρ. This is achieved by defining the mass attenuation coefficient, μ/ρ. If μ is expressed in units of cm^{-1} and density in $g\,cm^{-3}$, the units of mass attenuation coefficient are $cm^2\,g^{-1}$; the corresponding thickness of filter must then be expressed in terms of mass thickness (linear thickness × density), $g\,cm^{-2}$.

The interactions occurring in a slab of water when irradiated with a beam of 3 MeV photons are illustrated in Fig. 2.15. The mass attenuation coefficient is a macroscopic quantity that, in principle, can be measured relatively simply. It represents the total probability that a photon of a given energy will interact with matter, regardless of the type of interaction. The variation of mass attenuation coefficient with energy for water $(Z = 7)$ and lead $(Z = 82)$ is shown in Fig. 2.16. The reason for the particular shape of the attenuation curves for water and lead is explained by the varying probability with energy of the underlying photon interactions that combine to give the total interaction probability and hence attenuation coefficient. It can be seen that in water the attenuation coefficient is seen to decrease monotonically as photon energy is increased, up to approximately 50 MeV at which point it begins to increase.

In Fig. 2.17 the region of dominance for each interaction type is indicated as photon energy increases from the kilovoltage to

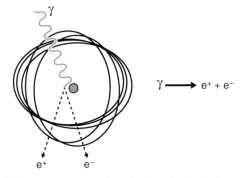

Fig. 2.13 Schematic representation of pair production in the nuclear Coulomb field. *HVL*, Half-value layer.

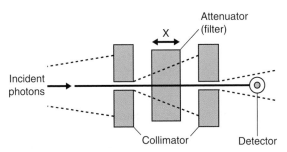

Fig. 2.14 Geometry for photon attenuation measurements. Collimators are present to prevent scattered photons from reaching the detector.

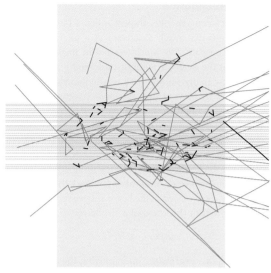

Fig. 2.15 Illustration of photon interactions. A beam of 3-MeV photons *(light grey)* is incident from the left on a 25-cm thick water slab. Photons may escape the slab without interacting, others interact in the water, generating secondary electrons *(black)*, which cause further ionisation and may escape the slab if they are generated close to the exit face. Photons may be backscattered from the face of the slab, along with secondary electrons.

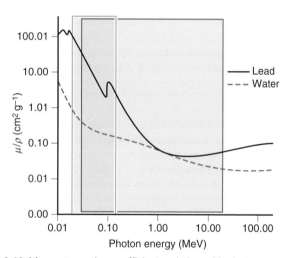

Fig. 2.16 Mass attenuation coefficient variation with photon energy in water and lead. The light and dark shaded *regions* indicate the approximate range of photon energies commonly used for diagnostic imaging and radiotherapy, respectively. (From Hubbell JH, Seltzer SM. Tables of x-ray mass attenuation coefficients and mass energy-absorption coefficients from 1 keV to 20 MeV for elements Z = 1 to 92 and 48 additional substances of dosimetric interest. National Institute of Standards and Technology; 1996. NISTIR 5632; Berger MJ, Hubbell JH, Seltzer SM, et al. XCOM: Photon cross sections database. National Institute of Standards and Technology; 1998. NBSIR 87-3597.)

TABLE 2.3   Energy Regions of Domination for Photoelectric, Compton and Pair Production Interactions

Interaction	Low Z (Water)	High Z (Lead)
Photoelectric	<30 keV	<500 keV
Compton	30 keV to 25 MeV	0.5–5 MeV
Pair production	>25 MeV	>5 MeV

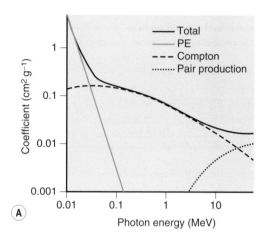

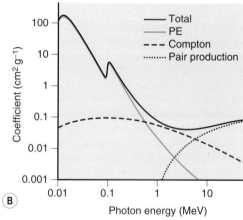

Fig. 2.17 Mass attenuation coefficients, showing the relative contributions from the photoelectric effect *(PE)*, Compton effect, and pair production in (A) water (effective Z = 7) and (B) lead (Z = 82). Note the large region of dominance for the Compton effect in water, because of the lower effective atomic number Z. (From Hubbell JH, Seltzer SM. Tables of x-ray mass attenuation coefficients and mass energy-absorption coefficients from 1 keV to 20 MeV for elements Z = 1 to 92 and 48 additional substances of dosimetric interest. National Institute of Standards and Technology; 1996. NISTIR 5632; Berger MJ, Hubbell JH, Seltzer SM, et al. XCOM: Photon cross sections database. National Institute of Standards and Technology; 1998. NBSIR 87-3597.)

megavoltage range. A summary of the energy ranges in which each interaction dominates is shown in Table 2.3. The photoelectric effect dominates in water, or tissue, for energies up to approximately 30 keV and, in lead, up to approximately 500 keV.

The large discontinuities observed at approximately 15 keV and 88 keV for the mass attenuation coefficient in lead, shown in Fig. 2.17B, are a result of incident photons having sufficient energy to overcome the binding energies of the lead L and K shells, respectively. This large increase in interaction probability around an electron

binding energy suggests that a resonance effect is involved, whereby the probability of interaction is highest when the photon energy is close to that of the electron binding energy. This feature in the mass attenuation coefficient curve is referred to as an absorption edge. The lack of visible absorption edges in water (Fig. 2.17A) is caused by the lower probability of the photoelectric effect occurring in water, relative to the Compton effect and the low binding energies of the K-shell electrons for oxygen and hydrogen.

For lead, the minimum attenuation occurs at a much lower energy of approximately 4 MeV compared with water, after which it begins to rise. It follows that the thickness of lead required to provide a chosen degree of attenuation would be greater for 4-MeV photons than it would be for 20-MeV photons. At higher energies, above approximately 8 MeV, photons may still undergo interactions directly with the atomic nucleus, releasing neutrons and forming radioactive isotopes.

Note that here we are considering monoenergetic photons (MeV), whereas in practice, clinical photon beams contain a spectrum of energies (denoted by MV to indicate this). The effective attenuation coefficients averaged over all energies in the spectra in lead for 6 MV and 15 MV beams are roughly equal. The mass attenuation coefficients of water and lead are approximately equal for 1 MeV photons. At 10 MeV the coefficient for lead is a little over twice that of water, whereas at 100 keV, the coefficient for lead is over 30 times that of water.

The mathematical form of equation 2.12 is identical to that describing radioactive decay. For a chosen material and filter thickness placed in the path of a monoenergetic photon beam, adding additional filters of the same material and thickness will result in the same fraction of beam being transmitted; for example, if 1 cm of a filter results in the beam intensity falling to 70% of its original value, then 2 cm will result in 49% of the original intensity being transmitted. Fig. 2.18A shows a plot of relative transmitted photon intensity ($N/N_0 = e^{-\mu.x}$) for a monoenergetic beam of photons incident on aluminium filters. Taking natural logarithms of this equation yields a linear function, shown in

Fig. 2.18B. The slope of the straight line is equal to $-\mu$. For a filter thickness that reduces the intensity to half the original value, we have:

$$N/N_0 = 0.5 = e^{-\mu\, t_{1/2}} \qquad \textbf{2.12}$$

where $t_{1/2}$ is denoted the half-value layer (HVL) or half-value thickness. Rearranging this expression and taking natural logarithms gives:

$$t_{1/2} = \text{HVL} = \ln(2)/\mu \qquad \textbf{2.13}$$

For a chosen filter material, the HVL of a beam of photons provides a measure of the beam's power of penetration. In the kilovoltage region, HVL is therefore used to represent the quality of a beam of photons. For a monoenergetic beam of photons, it follows that after one HVL, the intensity drops to 50%, after two HVLs 25%, after three HVLs 12.5%, and so on. The presence of inherent filtration for a monoenergetic source of photons would therefore have no effect on the measured beam quality.

Attenuation of Photon Spectra

In practice, photon beams generated by fast-moving electrons striking a high atomic number target will have a spectrum of energies, as described earlier. We may expect the attenuation coefficient to decrease as photon energy is increased (i.e. higher energy photons are more penetrating). As a photon spectrum (i.e. a polyenergetic beam) is filtered, lower energy photons will be preferentially removed from the beam because of their larger attenuation coefficients. This results in the average energy of the beam increasing and the average attenuation coefficient decreasing. As a result of this changing attenuation coefficient, the measured transmission curve will no longer be a true exponential. This is represented in Fig. 2.19, where successive HVLs are no longer constant, but depend on the amount of filtration already present in the beam.

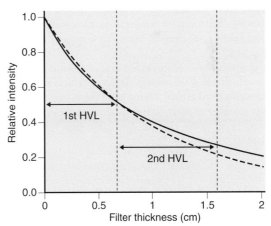

Fig. 2.19 Attenuation comparison between a 100-kV photon spectrum (*solid line*) and a monoenergetic beam (*dashed line*) of the same first half-value layer (HVL). The first and second HVLs (0.7 and 0.9 cm Al, respectively) for the spectrum are indicated. For the monoenergetic beam, the first and second HVLs would be equal, whereas for a spectrum of energies, the subsequent HVLs increase because of beam hardening, as indicated.

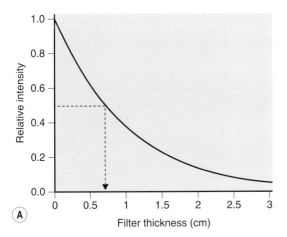

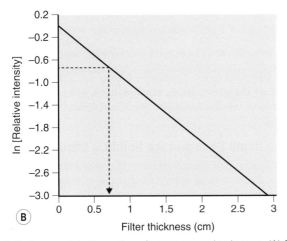

Fig. 2.18 Exponential attenuation of monoenergetic photons. (A) Relative transmission versus filter thickness and (B) in (relative transmission) versus thickness. The half-value layer (HVL) of 0.7 cm Al is indicated on each plot.

Beam Hardening

In addition to the photon attenuation provided by the target and other machine components, referred to as the inherent filtration, additional filters may be placed in the path of the emerging photon beam (Fig. 2.14). This is used particularly in the kV RT beams as well as in the kV photon beams used for diagnostic imaging. The effect of this is to preferentially remove lower energy components from the spectrum, as a result of their higher attenuation. This is a desirable effect as these low-energy photons will reduce the penetration of a RT beam and for x-ray imaging, contribute little to an x-ray image and result in unnecessary radiation dose. Adding filters in the path of the beam reduces the beam intensity (number of photons), but increases the average energy of the beam, referred to as hardening the beam. Comparison of the first and second HVL (HVL_1/HVL_2; Fig. 2.19) gives an indication of the degree of beam hardening occurring and is termed the homogeneity coefficient.

Energy Absorption

As well as being interested in how many photons are transmitted without interacting in a filter (i.e. remain unattenuated), we may also be interested in the amount of energy that is absorbed in the filter, particularly if we replace the filter with biological tissue. This information is given by the energy absorption coefficient, denoted μ_{en}. In a similar approach to that followed for attenuation, we can also define the mass energy absorption coefficient, μ_{en}/ρ. These quantities have the same units as their attenuation counterparts. In terms of the geometry shown in Fig. 2.14, to determine energy absorption, we must detect all unattenuated photons, together with any other energy not absorbed locally. Assuming all charged particles are absorbed (stopped) locally, it is the energy transported away in the form of photons that must be accounted for, that is, all characteristic photons released from excited atoms following photoelectric interactions, scattered photons resulting from the Compton effect, bremsstrahlung photons produced by charged particles (e.g. Compton electrons), and finally, photons arising from positron annihilation following pair production (if the incident photon energy is high enough). The geometry for this situation then represents broad-beam conditions. It follows that the attenuation coefficient for a given monoenergetic photon beam in a given material is larger than the corresponding energy absorption coefficient for the same energy and material as attenuation accounts for both absorption and scatter. Practical measurement geometry will fall between narrow and broad-beam conditions. Fig. 2.20A compares mass attenuation coefficients and mass energy absorption coefficients in water for the range of photon energies of interest to RT.

Energy absorption coefficients are used in radiation dosimetry in a similar way to that in which electron stopping powers are used for electron beams described earlier. Taking again the example of an air-filled ionisation chamber in water, having determined the dose deposited by photons in the air cavity, D_{air}, the dose to the same region when filled with water, D_w, is given by:

$$D_w = D_{air} \times (\mu_{en}/\rho)_w / (\mu_{en}/\rho)_{air} \qquad \textbf{2.14}$$

The variation in the ratio of mass energy absorption coefficients is shown in Fig. 2.20B.

The aforementioned expression assumes that all electrons set in motion by the incident photons deposit their energy within the chamber. This is a reasonable assumption for kV photon beams. For MV photon beams, however, the ranges of secondary electrons become significant and must be considered.

Photo-Nuclear Interactions

At sufficiently high energies, which is above approximately 8 MeV, or a 15 MV spectra, photons may interact directly with the atomic nucleus, releasing neutrons or protons:

$$\gamma + {}^A_Z X \rightarrow {}^{A-1}_Z Y + n \qquad \textbf{2.15}$$
$$\gamma + {}^A_Z X \rightarrow {}^{A-1}_{Z-1} Y + p$$

These interactions do not lead to a significant patient dose, but the production of neutrons can lead to additional shielding requirements

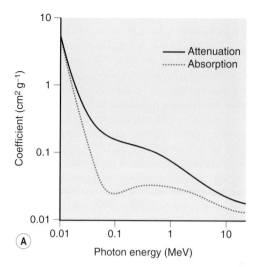

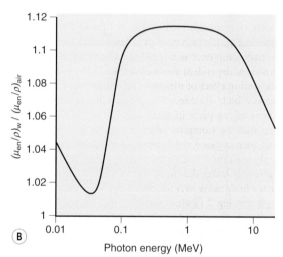

Fig. 2.20 (A) Comparison of photon mass attenuation and mass energy absorption coefficients in water. Note that the difference is largest where the Compton effect dominates because of energy being transported away from the site of interaction by Compton-scattered photons. (B) Ratio of water to air mass energy absorption coefficient. (From Hubbell JH, Seltzer SM. Tables of x-ray mass attenuation coefficients and mass energy-absorption coefficients from 1 keV to 20 MeV for elements Z = 1 to 92 and 48 additional substances of dosimetric interest. National Institute of Standards and Technology; 1996. NISTIR 5632; Berger MJ, Hubbell JH, Seltzer SM, et al. XCOM: Photon cross sections database. National Institute of Standards and Technology; 1998. NBSIR 87-3597.)

for the treatment room. Activation of linear accelerator components, particularly the photon target, can also occur, which must be allowed to decay to acceptable levels before any intervention, such as machine servicing.

Photon Depth Dose and the Build-Up Effect

Fig. 2.18 shows how the transmission of photons decreases exponentially as the amount of matter traversed is increased. The quantity we are generally more interested in, however, is the absorbed dose received at a depth in tissue and how this varies with depth. This quantity is commonly described as percentage depth dose (PDD):

$$\text{PDD} = 100 \times D(d)/D(d_{max}) \qquad \textbf{2.16}$$

where $D(d)$ is the measured dose at depth, d, and d_{max} the depth of maximum dose. Example PDD curves for megavoltage photon beams

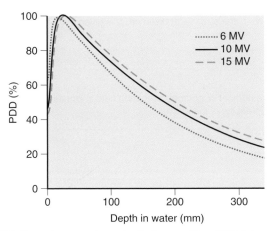

Fig. 2.21 Example percentage depth-dose profiles (*PDDs*) for photon beams in water. (From the Clatterbridge Centre for Oncology NHS Foundation Trust: Douglas Cyclotron. With permission.)

are shown in Fig. 2.21. An important feature of these curves is the fact that the maximum dose is not reached at the surface, but at a depth, d_{max}, which is dependent on the energy of the beam. This provides the skin-sparing effect of megavoltage photon beams.

The dose build-up effect is explained by considering the photon interactions taking place in tissue at the energies involved. Table 2.3 shows us that the Compton effect dominates in low atomic number materials, such as tissue, right across the MeV range of photon energies commonly used for RT. This interaction provides a scattered photon, which generally leaves the site of interaction, and a secondary electron, which has a finite range over which it deposits its energy. For an incident 1 MeV photon, Fig. 2.12 shows us that approximately 0.4 MeV, on average, is passed to the secondary electron, whereas for a 10 MeV incident photon, roughly 6.8 MeV on average would be passed on. This kinetic energy of the secondary electrons is not all deposited at the site of the Compton interaction, but is spread out over the electron's range, which depends on the electron's energy as shown in Table 2.2. Let us now consider the total absorbed dose from secondary electrons as we move between thin layers from the surface to the depth of d_{max}, in steps of some fraction of d_{max}. As illustrated in Fig. 2.22, some energy is deposited in the surface layer by secondary electrons set in motion within this layer and some is transported along with the electrons to underlying layers. Taking a step deeper, we again have a dose from secondary electrons set in motion within this layer, and we have an additional dose contribution from secondary electrons entering from the surface layer (upstream), that is, we now have contributions from two layers. At the next layer, we have three layers contributing, the one we are in and two upstream. At each successive deeper layer, the number of upstream layers contributing electrons increases, so the total absorbed dose rises, or builds up. This process continues until we are at a depth beyond the range of electrons set in motion in the surface layer, at which point we have reached full build up, at d_{max}. The depth of d_{max}, then, corresponds to the average range of secondary electrons set in motion by the incident photon beam, which increases with photon beam energy, as shown in Fig. 2.21 in moving from 6 to 15 MV. In practice, this depth will also be influenced by the field size, by contaminant electrons generated in the head of the accelerator and in any beam-modifying devices in the path of the beam. If we assume that photon attenuation is negligible over a number of layers, then at d_{max} and beyond, the total number of electrons crossing each layer is constant; the number entering a given layer from upstream equals the number moving downstream (see Fig. 2.22). This condition is termed charged-particle equilibrium and is discussed further under Bragg-Gray cavity theory in Chapter 3.

Note that for kilovoltage photon beams, the energies and ranges of secondary electrons will be very much reduced. For example, a 100 keV photon interacting by the Compton effect will produce, on average, a secondary electron of around 15 keV, which has a range of less than 1/100 mm. Secondary electrons generated by kilovoltage photon beams can therefore be assumed to deposit their energy at the site of interaction in tissue and no dose build up or skin-sparing occurs.

For a phantom, or patient, irradiated at a fixed source to surface distance (SSD) with a diverging beam (e.g. that from a small or point source, such as a clinical linear accelerator or x-ray tube), the absorbed dose beyond the depth of d_{max} will decrease with depth because of both increasing attenuation of the incident photons and increasing distance of the point of interest from the source. This latter effect is known as the inverse-square law, as the dose from a point source, in the absence of any attenuating material, will decrease as $1/r^2$, where r is the distance from the source. The derivation of this law is given in Fig. 2.23. We can combine the effect of photon attenuation with the inverse-square reduction in photon intensity, to approximate the PDD beyond d_{max} as:

$$PDD \approx e^{-\mu_{eff}(d-d_{max})} \times (f + d_{max}/f + d)^2 \qquad \textbf{2.17}$$

where μ_{eff} is the effective attenuation coefficient for the beam. The term effective attenuation coefficient is used here, as our geometry does

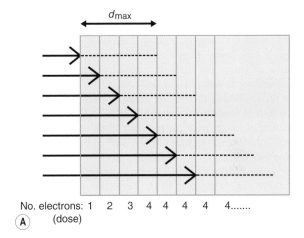

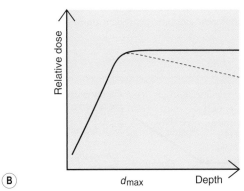

Fig. 2.22 Schematic illustration of dose build-up in MV photon beams. (A) Incident photons (*solid lines*) interact in each layer, liberating secondary electrons (*dashed lines*). These electrons deposit their kinetic energy over their (finite) range, here corresponding to four layers. The total dose in each layer is proportional to the number of electrons crossing it (one to four). (B) The solid line indicates the build-up of dose in the absence of photon attenuation. The dashed line indicates the exponentially decreasing dose beyond d_{max} because of photon attenuation.

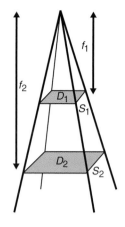

Given a square field of side, s_1 at distance, f_1 the size, s_2, at distance, f_2 is given by:
$s_2 = s_1 \times (f_2 / f_1)$ [1]

Field areas are related by:
$s_2{}^2 = s_1{}^2 \times (f_2 / f_1)^2$ [2]

In the absence of photon interactions, the number of photons over each field is constant (=n, say) and the number per unit area (intensity) is therefore:
$I_1 = n/s_1{}^2$ and $I_2 = n/s_2{}^2$

The ratio of intensities is therefore:
$I_2/I_1 = s_1{}^2/s_2{}^2$ [3]

From [2], we have:
$s_1{}^2/s_2{}^2 = (f_1 / f_2)^2$

So, [3] can be written as: $I_2/I_1 = (f_2 / f_1)^2$ [4]
As dose is proportional to intensity, we can replace Is by Ds in [4] to obtain:
$D_2 = D_1 \times (f_1 / f_2)^2$ or $D_2 \propto 1/f_2{}^2$
This is the inverse-square law; dose, D_2, is *inversely proportional* to the *square* of the distance, f_2.

Fig. 2.23 Illustration of field size scaling and derivation of the inverse-square law.

not exclude scattered radiation and is likely to represent an average over a photon spectrum. μ_{eff} will therefore vary with field size and depth.

KERMA AND ABSORBED DOSE FOR RADIOTHERAPY BEAMS

The various processes by which photons interact with matter produce charged particles, mainly electrons but also positrons which then travel through matter, losing energy by collision processes: ionisation and excitation of atoms and through radiative processes: production of bremsstrahlung, as illustrated in Fig. 2.24.

For photon beams, the transfer of energy from radiation to matter may be seen in two distinct stages:
1. Transfer of energy from the radiation to emitted charged particles
2. Deposition of energy by the emitted charged particles through collision processes

For charged particle beams only the second stage is relevant.

The first stage is governed by the interaction coefficients for photons in matter: photoelectric, Compton, and pair production. The second stage is dependent upon the energies of the charged particles and their subsequent patterns of energy deposition as determined by their stopping powers. The deposition of energy is different from the transfer of energy by different amounts dependent upon the photon energies and materials.

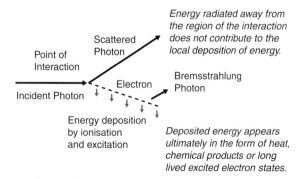

Fig. 2.24 Schematic diagram of energy deposition arising from Compton interaction on matter.

Kerma

The term *kerma,* an acronym for the kinetic energy released per unit mass, is used to quantify the first of the aforementioned stages. It is defined by International Commission on Radiation Units and Measurements (ICRU) [8] as:

$$K = \Delta E_{\text{tr}} / \Delta m \qquad \textbf{2.18}$$

where ΔE_{tr} represents the energy transferred from photons to charged particles and is the sum of initial kinetic energies of all the charged particles liberated by uncharged ionising radiation from an amount of material of mass Δm.

It may be seen from Fig. 2.24 that for the Compton interaction illustrated:
1. The energy of an incident photon is shared between a scattered photon and the ejected electron. The scattered photon carries its energy away from the immediate region of the interaction. The term *terma* represents the total energy removed from the beam per unit mass of matter, including that given to the charged particles and that scattered as photons. Terma is therefore always greater than kerma.
2. The electron travels through matter losing energy continually until its kinetic energy is exhausted.
3. The travelling electron may lose some energy by bremsstrahlung, producing photons, which, like the scattered photon, carry energy away from the immediate vicinity. The term *collision kerma* refers to that proportion of kerma that is deposited via collision processes only. Kerma and collision kerma differ only in accounting for the energy that is re-radiated. In body tissues, the energy re-radiated is small, being less than 1%, so these two quantities are almost equal.

Absorbed Dose

The travelling electrons deposit energy in matter through which they pass, and so the energy deposited by these electrons is displaced in distance from the site of initial transfer of energy from the photon beam. The amount of energy deposited in a small mass of the material is termed the absorbed dose, which is defined by ICRU [1] as:

$$D = \Delta E_{\text{d}} / \Delta m \qquad \textbf{2.19}$$

where ΔE_{d} is the total energy deposited by these charged particles in a volume element of mass Δm.

TABLE 2.4 Proton Range Variation With Energy (CSDA Range Quoted, Calculated Using the PSTAR Program [1])	
Energy (MeV)	Range (cm)
60	3.1
100	7.7
150	15.8
200	26.0
250	37.9

The absorbed dose is similar in value to collision kerma but displaced because of the motion of the secondary charged particles. Absorbed dose equals collision kerma if one of two following conditions are met:

1. The distance travelled by secondary charged particles is sufficiently small for it to be neglected, such that energy may be considered to be absorbed by the matter at the point where it is transferred from photons to the charged particles, a condition known as point deposition of dose. This occurs for low-energy photons, where the emitted electrons can travel only short distances, as detailed earlier.
2. The energy lost from the region of initial transfer by the movement of charged particles away from that region is exactly compensated for by energy brought into the region by other travelling electrons produced elsewhere, a condition known as energy equilibrium, or more generally as charged particle equilibrium.

Units of Kerma and Dose

Both kerma and absorbed dose have units of energy per unit mass, the units for which are joules (J) and kilograms (kg), respectively. The unit gray (Gy) is used for both absorbed dose and kerma and is defined as:

$$1\,Gy = 1\,J/kg \qquad \textbf{2.20}$$

Neither absorbed dose nor kerma are material specific and can therefore be related to any matter: a subscript is generally used to indicate the material. Hence K_a and K_w may be used to refer to air kerma and water kerma, respectively. Likewise for absorbed dose.

HEAVY CHARGED PARTICLE INTERACTIONS

Protons

Carrying the same magnitude, but opposite sign of charge to electrons, protons readily interact with atomic electrons, causing ionisation and excitation as they continuously lose energy passing through matter. The proton mass, being approximately 2000 times larger than that of an electron, results in protons undergoing far less lateral scattering. As bremsstrahlung losses are inversely proportional to the square of the incoming particle mass, such losses are negligible for protons. Rather than the approximately linear relationship between energy and range, as observed for electrons (where range ≈ MeV/2 cm), proton range scales roughly with the square of the proton energy. As protons lose energy far more rapidly than electrons when traversing matter, energies of up to approximately 250 MeV are required to treat deep-seated tumours. Table 2.4 lists proton ranges for a number of beam energies.

A key difference in the characteristics of energy deposition with depth for protons as opposed to electrons is the appearance of a Bragg peak, shown in Fig. 2.25. This results from a reduced amount of lateral scattering and a sharp increase in stopping power (dE/dx) as protons slow down in a material (see Fig. 2.25B). The Bragg peak is ideally suited to RT as the

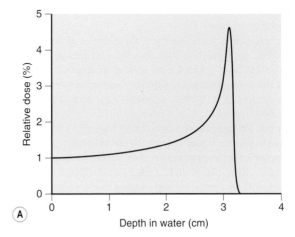

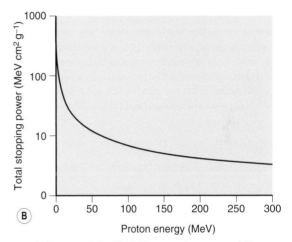

Fig. 2.25 (A) Bragg peak for 60-MeV protons in water, and (B) proton stopping power in water. Note how the shape of the stopping power curve is reflected in the observed depth-dose curve. (From Berger M, Coursey J, Zucker A, Chang J. ESTAR, PSTAR, and ASTAR: Computer programs for calculating stopping-power and range tables for electrons, protons, and helium ions (version 1.2.3), Gaithersburg, MD: National Institute of Standards and Technology; 2005. Available: http://physics.nist.gov/Star.)

high-dose region is concentrated at depth, protecting both overlying and underlying normal tissue. The Bragg peak is also a characteristic of other heavy charged particle beams, such as carbon ions and pions.

Although interactions with atomic electrons is the dominant process by which clinical proton beams (50–250 MeV) lose energy and so deposit dose, an incident proton beam may also interact with the atomic nucleus through elastic or nonelastic scattering. In elastic scattering events, kinetic energy is passed from the incident proton and the internal structure of the nucleus is unchanged. In nonelastic scattering, the nucleus may be fragmented or left in an excited state, in which case kinetic energy is not conserved. Charged particles such as secondary protons, alpha particles produced during these events will deposit their energy close to the site of interaction, whereas neutrons and photons, being uncharged, may carry energy a significant distance away.

To deliver a required dose distribution over a defined target, the Bragg peak is spread out as described in Chapter 9.

Carbon Ions and Pions

In addition to protons, heavier nuclei and other particles may offer potential advantages for RT because of the physical characteristics of their dose deposition in matter and their relative biological effectiveness. Beams of carbon ions and pions, in particular, have been applied clinically for RT.

To reach deep-seated tumours, the energies of heavy ion beams need to be significantly higher than those of protons. For example, although 150 MeV protons have a range of approximately 16 cm in water, the same penetration depth for carbon ions requires a beam energy of close to 3600 MeV, or 300 MeV for each of the 12 nucleons in the ion.

Carbon ion beams have a significantly higher LET in the Bragg peak than in the plateau region. As with the clinical proton beams described in Chapter 9, the Bragg peak of carbon ion beams is spread out across the target, which leads to an increased radiobiological effect across the target region relative to the surrounding low-dose region. Hence, in addition to a lower physical dose, normal tissue is spared further because of a lower biological effect. The increased LET in the Bragg peak is a result of nuclear fragments being produced in collisions, which leads to a dose tail following the Bragg peak, illustrated in Fig. 2.26.

Pion beams have been used clinically to treat over 500 patients at a small number of centres worldwide. Pions are negatively charged particles with a mass approximately 15% of a proton and a half-life of 26 ns (2.6×10^{-8} s). They can be produced by bombarding carbon or beryllium targets with protons. The potential advantage from these particles over alternatives is the star effect, which enhances the dose deposited in their Bragg peak as a result of their capture by atomic nuclei. This capture process causes the nucleus to become unstable and disintegrate into a number of fragments, each of which has a high LET and very short range in tissue.

NEUTRON INTERACTIONS

Clinical beams of fast neutrons, of the order of 60 MV, were the subject of particular interest during the 1970s and 1980s. Being uncharged, they show similar depth-dose characteristics to megavoltage photons (Fig. 2.27). However, they offer potential advantages for some tumours in causing a greater degree of irreparable DNA damage in targets, which have low oxygenation as a result of factors such as poor vascularity. Low-energy neutron beams, referred to as thermal beams, are of interest in their application to boron–neutron capture therapy. This treatment involves first depositing boron (^{10}B) in the tumour, using tumour-targeting compounds, and then applying an external beam of thermal neutrons. These neutrons are captured by boron nuclei within the tumour, creating ^{11}B which subsequently disintegrates releasing helium and lithium nuclei (^{4}He and ^{7}Li, respectively), with kinetic energies of 1.47 and 0.84 MeV, respectively. Being highly charged, these particles deposit their energy within a very short distance of the site of their release.

Aside from their therapeutic applications, fast neutrons are also produced in interactions involving high-energy photons and protons, as mentioned earlier. Fast neutrons lose energy primarily through elastic collisions with atomic nuclei. In the body, this readily produces knock-on protons through collisions with hydrogen, which travel only a short distance in tissue. The proportion of energy that neutrons lose through each collision decreases as the atomic number of the target material increases, with the average energy loss, E, being given by:

$$E/E_0 = 2\,mM/(m+M)^2 \qquad \textbf{2.21}$$

where E_0 is the incident neutron energy, m the neutron mass (1.67×10^{-27} kg), and M the mass of the target nucleus. Materials with a high hydrogen or other low atomic number (e.g. lithium) content are therefore the most effective in slowing down fast neutrons. Wall cladding with a high proportion of low atomic number material may be used in the maze of bunkers housing high-energy photon machines ($\geq$15 MV) to rapidly slow fast neutrons produced by photon interactions (photonuclear interactions) in the photon target.

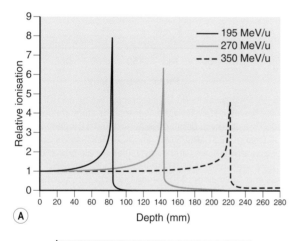

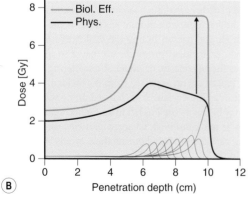

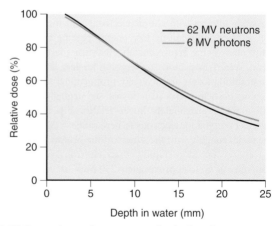

Fig. 2.26 Monoenergetic Bragg peaks for carbon ions incident on water. Note the dose tail beyond the peak because of nuclear fragments. (B) Physical dose and biologically effective dose within a clinical target volume for 170- to 220-MeV carbon ions in water. Note the enhanced biological effect across the target region, resulting in preferential damage to tumour. (From M Krämer, GSI, Darmstadt. With permission.)

Fig. 2.27 Comparison of percentage depth dose in water at 150-cm source to surface distance for 62-MeV neutrons. (From the Clatterbridge Centre for Oncology NHS Foundation Trust: Douglas Cyclotron. With permission.)

Once thermalised, neutrons are captured by a nucleus (nonelastic interactions), for example:

$$n + {}^1H \rightarrow {}^2H + \gamma[2.2\,\text{MeV}]$$

2.22

$$n + {}^{14}N \rightarrow {}^{14}C + p[0.6\,\text{MeV}]$$

In the case of capture by hydrogen (^{1}H), this results in the release of a high-energy photon, which itself presents a potential radiation shielding hazard.

REFERENCES

[1] Berger M, Coursey J, Zucker A, Chang J. ESTAR, PSTAR, and ASTAR: Computer programs for calculating stopping-power and range tables for electrons, protons, and helium ions (version 1.2.3). Gaithersburg, MD: National Institute of Standards and Technology; 2005. Available: http://physics.nist.gov/Star.

[2] Hubbell JH, Seltzer SM. Tables of x-ray mass attenuation coefficients and mass energy-absorption coefficients from 1 keV to 20 MeV for elements Z = 1 to 92 and 48 additional substances of dosimetric interest. NISTIR 5632. National Institute of Standards and Technology; 1996.

[3] Berger MJ, Hubbell JH, Seltzer SM, et al. XCOM: Photon cross sections database. NBSIR 87-3597. National Institute of Standards and Technology; 1998.

[4] Mayles P, Nahum A, Rosenwald J-C, editors. Handbook of radiotherapy physics, theory and practice. London: Taylor and Francis; 2007.

[5] Baker C, Peck K. Reconstruction of 6 MV photon spectra from measured transmission including maximum energy estimation. Phys Med Biol 1997;42:2041–51.

[6] IPEM Report 78. Catalogue of diagnostic x-ray spectra and other data. Institute of Physics and Engineering in Medicine; 1997.

[7] Attix F. Introduction to radiological physics and radiation dosimetry. John Wiley & Sons Inc; 1996.

[8] ICRU. Radiation quantities and units. Report No 33. Washington, DC: International Commission on Radiation Units and Measurements; 1980.

FURTHER READING

[No authors] Central axis depth dose data for use in radiotherapy. A survey of depth doses and related data measured in water or equivalent media. Br J Radiol Suppl 1983;17:1–147.

3

Radiation Detection and Measurement

Andrew Poynter, Andrzej Kacperek, John A. Mills

CHAPTER OUTLINE

INTRODUCTION

The detection of ionising radiation involves using the physical interaction between the radiation and materials in a manner which renders it perceptible through a visual or audible means. Measurement of the radiation requires a depth of knowledge about the physical process which occurs in the physical interaction and being able to quantify this in terms of the energy released in the interaction and how that is deposited in the material as what we refer to as absorbed dose.

In the first section of this chapter, two simple and widely used radiation detectors are described. Their simplicity and ease of use have made them robust and prolific. The modern and universally used means of measuring dose comes from the simplicity and robustness of one of these detectors, the air cavity ionisation chamber. The details and methods of quantifying absorbed dose using air ionisation are described in detail. Although the air-based ionisation chamber forms

the primary technique, the advantages and disadvantages of quantifying absorbed dose with other detectors are described.

Lastly, although accurate measurement of absorbed dose under well-controlled conditions at a single point is essential for effective radiotherapy (RT), it is essential to have in-vivo dosimetry on treatment and patient-specific checks in treatment preparation with the prevalence of dynamically produced RT delivery. Devices for in-vivo dose measurement and the distribution of radiation dose are described.

RADIATION DETECTION

Common types of device that are used in the detection and measurement of radiation and particularly low-intensity radiation use gas amplification and scintillation detectors. The most sensitive devices are event counters, able to detect and record individual photon interactions or the passage of individual charged particles. Each interaction results in an electrical pulse, which is counted either to give a total number of

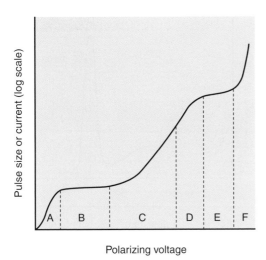

Fig. 3.1 Detector pulse size or current as a function of applied polarising potential. Region A is dominated by recombination of ions. Ionisation chambers operate in region B, proportional counters in region C, and Geiger counters in region E. Region D represents transition between proportional and Geiger regions, and region F illustrates continuous discharge and electrical breakdown.

interactions recorded or the number recorded per unit interval of time to provide a count rate. The decay of a radioactive material may be measured, for example, by monitoring the fall in count rate with time.

Where the radiation intensity is very low, such as in detecting and measuring radiation emitted from a small radioactive source, other more sensitive instruments must be used.

Gas Amplification Devices

In ionisation chambers filled with gas, including air, the ion pairs produced by particles crossing the air cavity are separated, collected, and measured such that the charge collected equates to the number of ion pairs produced. A polarising voltage is placed across the electrodes of the chamber sufficient to separate the ions and direct them to the electrodes of the device. Any kinetic energy gained by ions as they move toward an electrode is continually removed by collision interactions with other air molecules, but the ions do not gain sufficient energy to create additional ionisation. If the polarising voltage is increased, then the charge detected may rise slightly as ion recombination is overcome, but the level will rapidly reach saturation and no further increase in collected charge will occur, as shown in Fig. 3.1.

In gas amplification devices, air in the detector chamber is replaced by a gas, the pressure of which is greatly reduced, thereby allowing any ions produced in it to travel much further before interacting with atoms of the gas. If the electric field across the device is sufficiently high, then ions can gain sufficient energy themselves to cause further ionisation of the gas, producing additional ion pairs. This leads to an increase in the charge collected. As the polarising voltage is increased further, these additional ions may also gain sufficient energy to cause further ionisation, leading to a cascade effect that produces further increase or amplification of the charge, a process that can be repeated many times, as illustrated in Fig. 3.2A. The net result is that the detected pulse of charge is proportional to the amount of ionisation produced by the radiation but is amplified many times. The size of the pulse is determined by both the number of ions initially generated by the radiation and the amount of amplification that takes place. This is in turn dependent upon the applied voltage across the chamber as shown in Fig. 3.1. Gains of many orders of magnitude are possible, and radiation detectors that use this principle are known as *proportional counters*.

If the voltage across the device is further increased, proportionality between initial signal and pulse size starts to break down as the size of the charge avalanche increases. Eventually, the whole chamber volume becomes involved. Ions reaching the electrodes may interact and produce further ions which continue the process. The result is a charge pulse that is determined not by the number of ions initially created, but by the design of the electronics of the detector. Each pulse is of the same height and causes a temporary discharge of the polarising voltage—this temporary reduction in voltage immediately after a pulse allows the counter to recover and any remaining ions in it to be absorbed. Introduction of special materials known as quenching agents into the gas speeds up this residual ion removal. Such detector devices are known as *Geiger counters*.

A typical Geiger counter detector is shown schematically in Fig. 3.2B and consists of a small cylindrical metal tube that forms the negative electrode, with a thin-wire positive electrode running along the axis of the cylinder. The structure is sealed to enclose the low-pressure gas, typically a mixture of argon and ethanol or neon and chlorine. The structure can be designed as either a side-window device (i.e. where radiation enters through the side of the device) for general radiation detection or an end-window device (where radiation enters through the end-cap of the device) for beta-particle detection, the latter having a thin mica window to allow passage of beta particles. The efficiency of a Geiger counter is high for beta particles but is very low for x-rays and gamma rays where the reliance is upon interaction with the wall of the device to generate secondary electrons that pass into the chamber cavity.

Each detected event results in an electric pulse, the size of which is independent of the number of ions initially causing the event, but which lasts for a few microseconds. The chamber then has to recover for a period of a few tens of microseconds, a period known as the dead time during which it will not respond to any further ionisation stimulus. Because the pulse size does not reflect the number of ions initiating the event, the counter cannot distinguish between different types of radiation. Further, the dead time has implications for use in high-intensity or pulsed radiation fields. As the radiation intensity increases, so does the rate of events and the chance of missing pulses because of the extended dead time increases, resulting in under-recording. Similarly, in the pulsed radiation field of a linear accelerator where the pulse lengths are less than the dead time of the detector, the most that a Geiger counter will record will be one count per pulse, regardless of the actual radiation intensity. Hence, Geiger counters cannot be used to

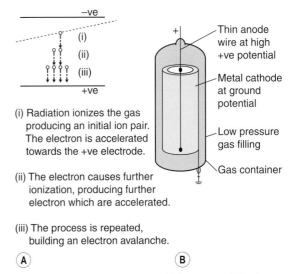

(i) Radiation ionizes the gas producing an initial ion pair. The electron is accelerated towards the +ve electrode.

(ii) The electron causes further ionization, producing further electron which are accelerated.

(iii) The process is repeated, building an electron avalanche.

Fig. 3.2 Schematic diagrams showing (A) the gas amplification process, and (B) a typical Geiger counter.

measure the intensity of a linear accelerator beam and great care must be exercised when using them to monitor radiation levels around a linear accelerator installation.

The pulse height from a Geiger counter varies only slowly with increasing voltage, as shown in Fig. 3.1, making the device relatively insensitive to small changes. At higher voltages, however, the electric field strength can be sufficient in itself to ionise the gas, resulting in continued electrical discharge, or breakdown.

Scintillation Devices

Some materials, such as thallium-doped sodium iodide, are known as *scintillator materials* which are a form of fluorescent material that emit light when irradiated. Scintillator materials are transparent to the light emitted, and so photon interactions cause short flashes of light in the material. The amount of light emitted is proportional to the energy deposited in the crystal. These short flashes of light can be detected by a photomultiplier tube—a device that converts very low levels of light into measurable electrical pulses. Sodium iodide is hygroscopic and is housed within a container that encompasses the material, prevents ingress of water vapour, and reflects light back into the crystal—the inner surface of the container being covered in a reflective coating of titanium dioxide or magnesium oxide. One surface is coupled onto the face of the photomultiplier tube either directly or via a specially constructed light guide. An optical coupling gel is used whenever two material faces are coupled together to reduce scattering caused by any tiny surface irregularities.

The inner surface of the front face of the photomultiplier tube has deposited on it a material (the photocathode) that causes photo electrons to be emitted when subjected to visible light. These electrons are accelerated by electric fields within the device onto a series of dynodes. When an electron hits a dynode, it causes emission of other electrons which in turn are directed onto other dynodes. Eventually, the avalanche of electrons reaches the anode, from where the electrical pulse is extracted. The electrical pulse from the photomultiplier is proportional to the amount of light hitting the photocathode, which in turn is proportional to the energy deposited by the initial radiation interaction in the scintillator crystal. Thus a 300-keV gamma ray will, on average, produce a pulse that is twice as large as that produced by a 150-keV gamma ray provided that in both cases the total energy of the gamma ray is absorbed in the crystal.

A pulse-height analyser is a device that has a number of counters, each representing one channel. Each channel counts the pulses that occur only with a narrow band of pulse heights. Successive channels are set to count increasingly larger pulses. Hence small pulses will appear in the lower channels and large pulses will be counted in the higher channels. When a scintillation detector is connected to a pulse-height analyser, the spectrum of counts produced represents the spectrum of energies deposited in the scintillator crystal. When measuring monoenergetic radiation (e.g. gamma rays from a gamma source), those interaction events that result in all the photon energy being absorbed in the crystal will have similar pulse heights and will be counted together in a narrow series of channels that represent this photon energy level. Interactions that result in less energy being deposited in the crystal (e.g. detection of Compton-scattered photons) will be counted in the wide range of channels below the photopeak channels, as shown in Fig. 3.3. Because the positions of peaks in the spectrum represent specific energy levels, scintillation counters are able to differentiate between different energies of incident photons. By matching measured energy levels and their rates of decay against tabulated energies of emissions and half-lives of known radioactive materials, specific radioactive substances can be identified in any given sample. This process is called *gamma spectroscopy*. This process also underlies the principles of operation of the gamma camera used in nuclear medicine.

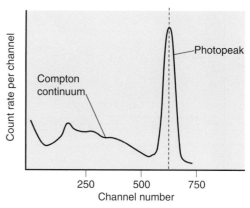

Fig. 3.3 Typical pulse-height spectrum from a gamma source that emits a single-energy gamma ray. The channel number equates to the energy deposited in the detector and the position of the photopeak is dependent on the energy of the emitted gamma ray. The width of the photopeak is dependent on the energy resolution of the detector system.

The pulse from a sodium iodide/photomultiplier detector has a pulse length of a few microseconds. Additional signals that occur within this period combine together and appear as an enlarged signal. These will fall outside the main photopeak channels. The chance of two interactions occurring within the short period will increase as the overall count rate increases (i.e. where the radiation is more intense), resulting in an underestimate of the true radiation intensity. Some plastic scintillators can have much shorter pulse lengths and can be constructed with large surface areas. These can be used to measure higher radiation intensities or to detect and measure radiation distributed over a large area.

Small plastic scintillators connected to distant photomultiplier tubes via long fibre-optic light guides have been used to measure dose distributions in RT [1]. The high sensitivity of the device allows use of tiny detectors that are of particular use in the measurement of rapidly varying intensities, such as in the penumbra of megavoltage beams or in the measurement of distributions from radioactive eye plaques [2]. More recently, tomographic reconstruction techniques have been applied to the optical signals from liquid scintillators to reconstruct full three-dimensional dose distribution maps around brachytherapy sources and eye plaques [3].

Ideal Air Ionisation Chamber

The stable part of the gas amplification response, region B in Fig. 3.1, can be used for the collection of ion pairs. Air, as a readily available medium with its density only affected by pressure and temperature, which can be easily measured, made such a device very attractive and expedient to use for the measurement of dose, thus not only detecting the radiation but also quantifying it. The use of air ionisation is attributed to early work of Pierre Curie [4].

The challenge of using the air ionisation to measure dose is to know the interaction processes, to know the energy related to absorbed dose to the air, and to ensure that all the relevant electrons produced from the ionisation can be measured. The latter represents a physical challenge for the design of the ionisation chamber with which to make the measurement.

The essential aspects of such a physical device is illustrated in Fig. 3.4. In the following sections describing the accurate measurement of absorbed dose all these aspects and how they are addressed are described.

Proton Beam Detection

In principle the same detection systems that are used in x-ray and electron beams can be used for detection of proton fluence, charge, or

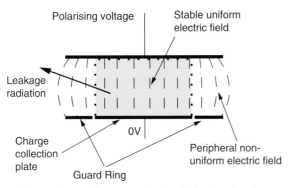

Fig. 3.4 Essential aspects of a free ionisation chamber.

Labels on figure: Polarising voltage; Stable uniform electric field; Leakage radiation; Charge collection plate; Guard Ring; 0V; Peripheral non-uniform electric field

proton dose, albeit with caution and knowledge of their limitations in proton and heavier clinical beams.

Certain instruments such as scintillation counters or silicon- and germanium-based solid-state detectors are single-particle detectors. These are count-rate limited and unable to measure the fluence required at clinical dose rates, which is around 10^9 protons/min. Detection and measurement using ionisation provide a wide dynamic dose range suitable for most clinical conditions.

The energy dependence of dose measurement of protons and other heavy-charged particles is known as Bragg peak quenching or simply low-energy under-response. This is because of the intensely ionising proton tracks at low energy, which saturate detector response. The magnitude of the under-response depends on the mechanism of measurement of a particular detector (e.g. film, thermoluminescent dosimeter (TLD), polymer gels, Fricke gels, or solutions).

Ionisation chambers, usually air filled, are considered the gold standard in particle therapy relative measurements, because they have considerable dose-rate range, insignificant change in response with particle energy, and little degradation with accumulated radiation dose. Some solid-state detectors have been developed which demonstrate minimal under-response.

The proton range, and hence energy, is affected by absorbers, such as detector windows or casings, and these need to be compensated for by calculation or estimation from tables. The use of scintillation detectors for charged particles requires consideration of Birk's law, which describes a nonlinear response with proton energy and an energy threshold.

The use of atmospheric air in ionisation chambers is particularly fortuitous as the stopping power ratio between water and air is relatively constant over a large energy range, and only deviates at very small energies which are not clinically relevant. For dose measurement air ionisation devices require correction for the standard temperature and atmospheric pressure, as well as air humidity. However, some centres have adopted nitrogen filling gas for in-line beam monitors. Nitrogen, unlike air, is not electronegative and free electrons are far less likely to attach to nitrogen molecules and thus will arrive at the chamber anode significantly quicker and more efficiently. This is particularly important when monitoring rapidly changing beam pulses from a synchrotron or synchrocyclotron.

MEASUREMENT AND STANDARDISATION OF DOSE

We have seen that when photons interact in matter, an energy pathway is initiated by which energy is transferred to the matter via emission of charged particles which cause ionisation and excitation of atoms of the matter. The energy eventually manifests as heat or as some form of internal potential energy of electrons and atoms within the matter (e.g. chemical bonds, raised electron energy levels).

Systems detecting radiation use specific parts of this energy pathway. Some systems seek to determine energy deposited in matter by measuring the temperature rise (termed calorimetry). Other detection systems look at chemical changes generated by irradiation of the matter (chemical dosimetry), or utilise long-lived excited electron states (e.g. thermoluminescent dosimetry). Still other systems measure the ionisation produced by the charged particles to calculate the energy transferred to those particles (ionisation chamber dosimetry).

This section describes the systems adopted for the measurement and standardisation of absorbed dose that underpin clinical practice. Later sections consider other methods of radiation detection and measurement, including other systems for measuring absorbed dose.

Dose Standards

It is of particular importance in RT to ensure that a dose of radiation delivered in any one treatment centre is consistent over time and is consistent also with that delivered in other centres, this being a central part of ongoing quality control. It also allows direct comparison of treatment techniques and results between centres and is essential for multicentre clinical trials to be effective. Consistency of measurements on a national or international basis is achieved through a process of central standardisation, with all measurements being traceable to an accepted national or international standard. The National Standards Laboratory (i.e. the National Physical Laboratory (NPL) in the United Kingdom) houses the instruments that are used to determine the national standard for absorbed dose measurement. These instruments are purely laboratory instruments that are impractical for routine use within RT departments.

The U.K. national standard instruments for the standardisation of absorbed dose are of two types:
1. Calorimeters for megavoltage photon and electron beams. Calorimeters are used to provide direct determination of absorbed dose [5].
2. Free-air ionisation chambers for lower-energy photon beams from x-ray generators operating at up to 300 kV [6,7]. These provide a direct determination of air kerma from which the absorbed dose to water can be calculated.

Traceability of Measurement

To ensure consistency of dose measurement between centres, it is necessary for measurements to be traceable back to the appropriate national standard. This is achieved through a hierarchical arrangement shown schematically in Fig. 3.5. Dose measuring instruments within individual hospitals (the field instruments) are used to measure the radiation beams of RT treatment units. These are calibrated periodically (i.e. annually in the United Kingdom) against a secondary standard instrument. The secondary standard instruments are reserved solely for this purpose and are not used to make routine beam measurements. Guidelines on the choice of dosimeter systems for use as secondary standard instruments have been produced by the Institute of Physics and Engineering in Medicine (IPEM) [8]. Each secondary standard instrument is calibrated periodically (i.e. every 3 years in the United Kingdom) by the standards laboratory by comparing the response against national reference level instruments that are in turn compared annually with the national standard instrument. The national standards are themselves compared at intervals with equivalent standard instruments developed by standards laboratories in other countries.

Radiotherapy treatment units, such as linear accelerators and kV therapy units, have in-built dose measuring instruments that monitor and determine the amount of dose delivered—these instruments are known as *monitor chambers*. Field instruments are used to calibrate these monitor chambers so that each monitor unit delivers a known

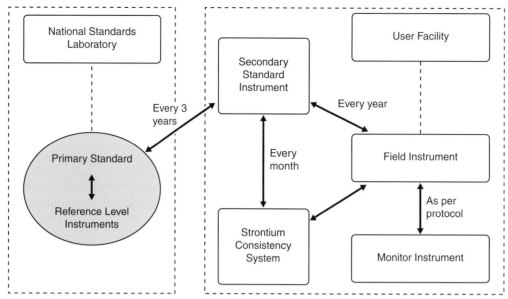

Fig. 3.5 Traceability to the National Standard is assured through a chain of intercomparisons, some of which are carried out at the National Standards Laboratory and others are carried out in local radiation beams. Between intercomparisons, calibration is assured using a consistency system.

amount of radiation. These field instruments may be used to determine not only the amount of radiation delivered, but also the pattern of deposition of energy within matter by measuring dose at different points within the matter. They may be used also to calibrate other dose measuring equipment designed for special purpose measurements, such as in vivo dosimeters.

For the transfer of calibration from instrument to instrument down the chain to be reliable, the method of calibration must be strictly controlled. This is achieved by the adoption of calibration protocols which specify:

- the basis for the standard dose measurement;
- the instrumentation and methods for transfer of dose to field instruments by a series of intercomparisons, including specification of any equipment used and any conditions that must exist for the intercomparison to be reliable;
- instructions for use of the calibrated dosimeter in routine practice.

Each protocol is specific for an energy range and type of radiation: the protocols for calibration of field instruments are covered in a later section.

Standard Calorimeter

In situations where all the absorbed energy is manifest solely as heat (i.e. no energy is lost to form new chemicals or stored in excited electron states), the relationship between radiation dose and change in temperature is given by:

$$\text{Dose (Gy)} = C \times \delta T \qquad \textbf{3.1}$$

where C is the specific heat of the irradiated matter (the amount of energy needed to raise the temperature of unit mass of a substance through 1°C, expressed in units of $J\,kg^{-1}\,{}^{\circ}C^{-1}$) and δT is the change in temperature in degrees Celsius. Equation 3.1 assumes no loss of heat to the surrounding environment or structures. Note that the specific heat may also be expressed in calories rather than joules, in which case an additional numerical multiplier of 4.18 is necessary in the aforementioned equation.

The rise in temperature is extremely small (e.g. a beam of x-rays delivering a dose of 5 gray (Gy) to soft tissue causes a temperature rise of only 10^{-3}°C). Such a small rise in temperature is very difficult to

measure accurately and extreme precautions are necessary to prevent heat loss outside the irradiated vessel.

The national standard calorimeter is based on the irradiation of a known mass of graphite (the core of the NPL high-energy photon calorimeter measures approximately 20-mm diameter by 3-mm thickness) within a graphite phantom. The design of the calorimeter, a photograph and schematic drawing of which are shown in Fig. 3.6, has the core shielded by three jackets, each separated by vacuum to minimise heat loss. Temperature measurements are carried out using thermistors embedded in the graphite core, the resistances of which change with temperature. In practice, because the amount of heat energy lost from the core to surrounding structures is not negligible and may be difficult to determine, the rise in temperature resulting from irradiation is compared with the rise in temperature produced by heating the core using a known amount of electrical energy, allowing absorbed dose to be determined directly instead of using equation 3.1.

Graphite has the advantage of having no chemical defect (i.e. all the absorbed energy appears as heat) and a specific heat that is one-fifth that of soft tissue or water, thereby producing greater changes in temperature per unit dose. The absorbed dose to water may be calculated from the absorbed dose to graphite using the correction factors determined by Nutbrown and colleagues [9].

Measurement by calorimetry is largely independent of whether the radiation is delivered continuously or in pulses and of the pulse intensity. It is therefore ideal for measuring radiation from constant-output sources, such as cobalt units, as well as pulsed output from linear accelerators. The pattern of temperature rise (from irradiation) and fall (from leakage of heat away from the core) may be used to determine both the peak and mean dose rates for pulsed radiation sources.

Because the standard calorimeter cannot be used in a water tank, a number of specially constructed ionisation chambers termed *reference standard instruments* are calibrated annually against the graphite calorimeter in a common graphite phantom. These reference instruments are then used to calibrate in turn the secondary standard instruments using a water phantom. The calibration factor provided for each secondary standard instrument is specific to a stated beam quality and depth of measurement, the latter being important as the spectral content of a radiation beam changes with depth. Table 3.1 shows those

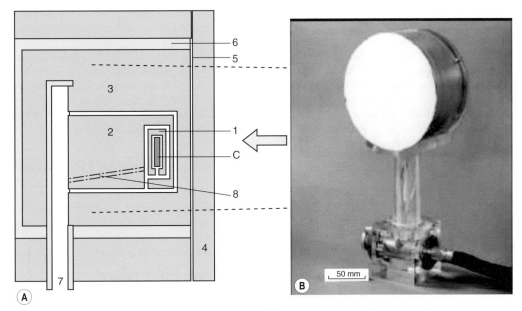

Fig. 3.6 Photograph and simplified schematic drawing of the national standard high-energy photon calorimeter, showing the graphite core (*C*) surrounded by three insulating graphite jackets (*1*, *2*, and *3*). The entire device is housed within a Perspex evacuation vessel (*6*) which has a thin aluminised mylar front window (*5*) and which is evacuated via a port (*7*). A plate (*4*) suitable for the energy to be measured can be added to the front face. Electrical connections to the core pass through the device (*8*). (Modified from DuSautoy AR. The UK primary standard calorimeter for photon beam absorbed dose measurement. Phys Med Biol 1996;41:137–151).

TABLE 3.1 Photon Beam Qualities Used for Therapy-Level Absorbed Dose to Water Calibrations		
Beam Quality (TPR$_{20/10}$)	**Equivalent Beam Energy**	**Reference Depth (cm)**
0.568	60 Co	5
0.621	4 MV	5
0.670	6 MV	5
0.717	8 MV	5
0.746	10 MV	5
0.758	12 MV	7
0.779	16 MV	7
0.790	19 MV	7

The quantity TPR$_{20/10}$ is the ratio of tissue-phantom ratios at depths of 20 cm and 10 cm, respectively, used by standards laboratories as the specifier of beam quality. A number of standards laboratories have developed water calorimeters that directly measure the rise in temperature of a known mass of water. These avoid uncertainties with the national standard instrument in moving from a graphite phantom to a water phantom. Such instruments have been used to confirm doses specified using other systems of dosimetry for photon and charged particle beams and are being increasingly developed as national dosimetry standards [47–51].

photon beam qualities at which calibration factors based on absorbed dose to water, as determined by the standard graphite calorimeter, are provided by the National Physical Laboratory, United Kingdom [10,11]. When used as a basis for calibration in a radiation beam in the user's department, the beam quality for that beam must be determined and the appropriate calibration factor obtained by interpolating from the results provided by the standards laboratory. Calibrations in megavoltage photon beams are carried out at the depths shown in

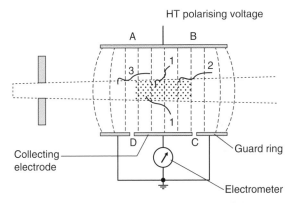

Fig. 3.7 The free air ionisation chamber. Irradiation of the mass of air shown shaded, defined by the cross-sectional area of the radiation beam and the length of the collecting electrode, results in emission of electrons that lose their kinetic energy by ionisation of air. Those ions created within the region ABCD are collected and measured.

Table 3.1 which are beyond the range of contaminating electrons in the radiation beam that have been ejected from the head of the treatment machine [12].

The Free Air Chamber

The free air chamber is the primary standard instrument for kV beams and is shown schematically in Fig. 3.7. The free air chamber effectively determines the energy transferred to secondary electrons as a result of interactions of a photon beam within a defined mass of air (i.e. air kerma [k_a]).

A well-defined beam of radiation, confined by external collimators, is incident upon a volume of air located between metal plates that act as electrodes. The radiation causes ionisation of the air, resulting in electrons being ejected. These electrons in turn cause further excitation and ionisation as they interact with air molecules: the electrons lose kinetic energy with each interaction and will travel an irregular, tortuous path until they come to rest. Each ejected Compton- or photo-electron can produce several hundred ion pairs. An essential requirement of the free air chamber is that the electrons produced by photon interactions lose all their kinetic energy in air and do not reach the metal electrodes. This requirement determines the minimum separation between the metal electrodes, and the overall size of the chamber. For example, measurement of x-rays generated at 200 kV will require a separation of at least 20 cm.

A potential difference, the polarising voltage, is applied between the metal electrodes. This causes positively and negatively charged ions produced in the air to separate, such that positive ions will move towards the negative potential plate while electrons will move towards the other. All ions of one charge sign are collected on one electrode, termed the *collecting electrode*. The charge reaching this electrode is measured and, from this, the number of ions produced may be calculated, because the charge carried by each electron is constant (equal to 1.602×10^{-19} C). The average energy expended by electrons in creating an ion pair, that is allowing for energy lost in exciting atoms as well as energy lost in ionising them, is well determined from experimental work. Hence because the number of ions may be determined using the free air chamber and the average energy necessary to produce each one is known, the total energy transferred to secondary electrons by photon interactions can be calculated.

Fig. 3.7 shows the physical arrangement. The metal plate that forms the electrode which carries the high-tension (HT) polarising voltage runs the full length of the chamber, whereas the other plate has the collector electrode as the central part only, separated and electrically isolated from adjacent metal plates called *guard rings*, which are held at the same electrical potential as the collector electrode. This arrangement ensures that the electric field within the region of the collector electrode is uniform and perpendicular to that electrode. Any ions produced in air within the region ABCD on the diagram will be collected on the collector electrode, whereas any ions produced outside this region will be collected on the guard rings and will not be included in the measurement.

The Proton Beam Dose Standard

There is not a U.K. code of practice for the measurement of absorbed dose with proton beams, but it is in preparation. The primary standard will be a graphite calorimeter with a transfer ion chamber likely to be the Roos chamber which is a parallel-plate design as shown in Figs 3.10 and 3.13B and which has the same dimensions as the calorimeter graphite measurement core. The measurement results will be converted to dose to water using stopping-power ratios and depth displacement factors. In this way the resultant dose uncertainty will approach that achieved in clinical x-ray dosimetry.

Currently the International Atomic Energy Agency (IAEA) TRS 398 Code of Practice [13], which is a Cobalt-60-based dose-to-water, is being used with factors for a particular ion chamber along with the mean proton energy. This code provides correction factors for all commonly available thimble and parallel-plate ion chambers at specified measurement depths in water. In the United Kingdom the Cobalt-60 calibrations are traced back to the U.K. National Physical Laboratory via the local secondary standard.

The code uses the most up-to-date data on proton interactions such as stopping powers, the energy to produce ionisation in air, and perturbation corrections. Some guidance is also offered on ion chamber recombination calculations. This code estimates that the combined uncertainty for proton and carbon beam measurements under reference conditions is 2.3% and 3.4%, respectively. For proton beams, this is approaching the uncertainty of 1.5% achieved with photon beams.

There is no international reference standard for absorbed dose. In the early days of proton beams it was good practice to provide independent checks through dosimetry intercomparisons between new and existing clinical centres. This ensured uniformity of procedure if not absolute dose.

Usually absolute or actual patient dose is measured in the middle of a spread-out Bragg peak (SOBP), see Chapter 9. Although in most clinical cases the SOBP dose curve is quite uniform, there may be a slight ripple effect, and it is important to sample the average beam dose, avoiding the peaks and troughs. This is described in the provisional IPEM Code of Practice for scanned and passive-scattered beams.

PRACTICAL IONISATION CHAMBERS

The aforementioned primary standard instruments are complex, sophisticated, and sensitive and are unsuitable for routine use within a hospital environment where small, relatively robust, simple instrumentation is needed.

One such instrument is the ionisation chamber.

Bragg–Gray Cavity Theory

The absorbed dose within any medium cannot generally be measured directly and so a surrogate has to be used. Ionisation chamber dosimetry is based upon replacing a small volume of the medium by an air cavity within which the ionisation of air by the radiation can be measured and from which the dose to the medium can be determined.

When a medium is irradiated uniformly by electrons, then the fluence of electrons (i.e. the energy carried across unit cross-sectional area) will be the same at all points within the medium. If a small air cavity is introduced of a size such that it does not perturb the electron fluence (i.e. does not introduce changes to the energy spectrum or numbers of electrons), then the fluence of electrons in the air is the same as in the medium and the cavity is termed a Bragg–Gray cavity. Under these conditions, the energy per unit mass (absorbed dose) imparted to the air (D_a) is given by:

$$D_a = J_a W \qquad \textbf{3.2}$$

where J_a is the ionisation produced per unit mass of air, and W is the average energy lost by the electrons per ion pair formed in the air. If the air is now to be replaced by medium, the energy per unit mass imparted to the medium (D_m) would equal the absorbed dose to air multiplied by the electron mass stopping power for the medium divided by that for air $(S/\rho)_a^m$ (averaged over the energy spectrum of the electrons), that is,

$$D_m = J_a W (S/\rho)_a^m \qquad \textbf{3.3}$$

This is the basic equation governing the use of ionisation chambers in the dosimetry of electron beams. For other charged particle beams, the stopping-power ratio for those particles must be used.

Where the medium is irradiated by a photon beam, then photon interactions produce secondary electrons which cause ionisation within the air cavity. Provided that interactions of photons with air molecules are negligible, such that all electrons crossing the air cavity arise as secondary electrons from within the medium and that the aforementioned conditions relating to constancy of electron fluence are met, then the air volume can be regarded as a Bragg–Gray cavity. The aforementioned equation 3.3 still holds.

In practice, when using ionisation chambers, the air volume is enclosed by a wall of material that differs slightly from both air and the medium. The construction of the chamber may introduce perturbations both to the fluence of electrons crossing the air cavity and to the photon beam itself. A wall of infinitesimally small thickness may be considered as having no impact on either, such that the chamber is effectively an air cavity within the medium. As the wall increases in thickness, an increasing percentage of secondary electrons crossing the air volume will be from the wall rather than the medium until, in the extreme, all electrons crossing the air volume originate from within the wall. In this situation, the electron fluence across the air volume is the same as the fluence within the wall, and the dose to the wall (D_w) is given by:

$$D_w = J_a W (S/r)_a^w \qquad 3.4$$

Assuming the photon field is not perturbed by the presence of the chamber, then the dose deposited by photons in the medium is related to that deposited in the chamber wall:

$$D_m = D_w (\mu/\rho)_w^m \qquad 3.5$$

where $(\mu/\rho)_w^m$ is the ratio of mass absorption coefficient for the medium divided by that for the chamber wall.

The conditions for this equation to be strictly valid are not met in practice. For measurement of charged particle beams, the fluence of particles may vary with depth and the introduction of the chamber may cause perturbations to this fluence. In measurement of photon beams, the wall of the chamber may be insufficient to stop electrons from outside it reaching the air volume, and the wall of the chamber differs from the medium in its attenuation and scattering of photons. Energy-dependent correction factors need to be applied to the aforementioned to adjust for these effects.

Dose Determination Based on Calibrated Instruments

The aforementioned correction factors are not necessary when ionisation chambers are used solely as instruments that are calibrated in terms of absorbed dose to water against a suitable primary standard where their effects are taken into account as an intrinsic part of the calibration process. They are required where calibration is in terms of air kerma. Such calibrations are by a series of intercomparisons that are traceable directly to the aforementioned national standard instruments. The absorbed dose is determined using an instrument calibrated in terms of absorbed dose to water (the UK standard for megavoltage photon beams) and is given by:

$$D = R \cdot N_D \qquad 3.6$$

where D is the dose, R is the mean-corrected reading, and N_D is the absorbed dose calibration factor.

For kV-energy photons in the United Kingdom, the chamber calibration (N_k) is in terms of air kerma. The factor $(\mu_{en}/\rho)w_{air}$, which is the ratio of mass energy absorption coefficients for water and air, needs to be included to calculate the dose to water, and a perturbation factor (k) as described earlier needs to be applied. The equation becomes:

$$D = R \cdot N_K \cdot k \cdot [(\mu_{en}/\rho)w_{air}] \qquad 3.7$$

The nature and magnitude of the correction factor k depends on whether calibration is carried out in air (for low-energy x-rays) or in water. Similar expressions may be derived for other modalities of radiation.

Requirements for Practical Ionisation Chambers

Radiation dosimeters based upon ionisation chambers have two basic components: the detector chamber, which produces electrical charge when irradiated, and an associated electrometer, which is an electronic amplifier to which the chamber is connected that is designed specifically for the purpose of measuring charge. The response of the dosimeter represents the response of the chamber to radiation together with the accuracy and consistency of the electrometer in measuring the charge.

Practical instrumentation needs to have a well-determined and predictable, slowly varying response to different energies of radiation, and must be consistent over time.

In addition, other dosimeter requirements are necessary depending upon type of radiation and the nature of the measurement being carried out.

Dosimeter chambers used within standards laboratories are specially constructed or selected. Materials used in their construction are fully investigated to determine chemical content and each chamber is meticulously assessed in terms of its assembly and response to radiation. Electronic equipment used to measure the electrical charge is equally carefully designed, constructed, and calibrated. The prime requirements here are the elimination of sources of inaccuracy in response and the consistency of that response. The overall accuracy of calibration of these instruments depends upon uncertainties in fundamental parameters being measured and to the extent that systematic uncertainties can be avoided. Overall consistency of calibration is between 0.5% and 1%.

Secondary standard instruments are constructed to less stringent standards but are required to operate over a range of beam energies and to remain consistent in response between recalibrations by the standards laboratories (i.e. 3 years). They must be fully transportable so that they can be used to transfer calibrations to other instruments in beams from different treatment machines, or even across different hospital sites. These chambers maintain an accuracy of calibration around 1%. Guidelines covering secondary standards instruments have been published [8].

Field instruments are used in daily measurements within hospitals. Different types of instruments exist, depending upon the nature of those measurements. Thimble chambers, described in detail in the following section, are generally used for calibration of megavoltage photon beams. Chambers based upon the design of the Farmer chamber [14] feature an air cavity of about 0.6 cc, providing a reasonable balance between the response to radiation and smallness of size, and are adequate for measurements in relatively uniform radiation beams with an accuracy of 1% to 2%. Chambers which have much smaller internal dimensions are used to measure variations in dose distributions, which can be very rapid at beam edges. Here, chambers of 0.1 cc or less may be used, with a trade-off between accuracy of response and spatial resolution. Where there is a rapid variation in dose deposited with depth, such as for measurements in the build-up region of photon beams or in the fall-off region of electron beams, parallel-plate chambers are used to ensure good depth resolution for the measurements.

Both thimble ionisation chambers and parallel-plate ionisation chambers are used widely for routine beam calibration and radiation distribution measurements. Other types of detector systems are useful in particular circumstances and may be used as alternatives to ionisation chambers. In particular, in vivo measurements use systems that do not require the application of polarising voltages, thereby reducing electrical risks to the patient. These various forms of radiation detectors are described within the following sections. Some forms, such as TLDs, have no definitive, maintained calibration and are suitable only for comparative measurements of a radiation dose against a known radiation dose, whereas other forms do maintain a definitive calibration and can be used as absolute dosimeters.

THIMBLE IONISATION CHAMBER

Physical Description

The thimble chamber is an ionisation chamber that has a central electrode (the collector electrode) in a volume of air that is contained by a thimble-shaped cap that forms the HT electrode which fits closely onto a metallic stem. The central electrode passes through the inside of the

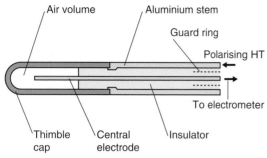

Fig. 3.8 Thimble ionisation chamber. Ionisation produced within the air volume in the thimble cap is collected by the central electrode. The aluminium stem transmits the polarising voltage to the thimble cap. The guard ring minimises charge leakage between the outer (HT) and the inner (signal) elements of the interconnecting cable. A thimble chamber of the Farmer type has the Air volume linked to the atmosphere via a venting aperture (not shown). *HT*, High tension.

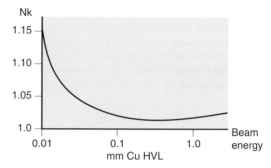

Fig. 3.9 Typical variation in air-kerma calibration versus beam energy for a thimble chamber for photon beam energies within the kV range—expressed in terms of their half value layer (HVL) (see Chapter 2).

stem and is insulated from the metallic stem by a suitable high-quality insulator material such as amber or polythene. This is schematically shown in Fig. 3.8. The cap is generally made of a low atomic number low-density material such as graphite, although various plastic materials have been used where the plastic has been manufactured to be conductive (e.g. Shonka plastic: [15]) or has been coated with graphite to be conductive. The central electrode may be made of aluminium or conductive plastic.

A potential difference (the polarising voltage) applied between the outer cap and the inner electrode drives apart any ion pairs produced in the trapped air and prevents ion recombination, but which is insufficiently large to cause ionisation of the air itself so that in the absence of ionising radiation no current flows. A voltage gradient of a few hundred volts per millimetre is generally sufficient for this purpose. In the presence of ionising radiation, ionisation within the air results in the ion pairs being separated, and with the ions of one sign (depending upon the polarity of the polarising voltage) being collected on the central electrode. The electrometer is generally floating, in that the input to it can be at any voltage level with respect to ground without this affecting the reading. In use, the aluminium stem is held at ground potential and the electrometer is floated to the level of the polarising voltage, so that exposed conductive parts carry no electrical risk to operators. This arrangement allows easy reversal of polarising voltage as required.

When the chamber is introduced into a photon beam, photoelectric and Compton interactions in the walls of the chamber generate electrons that traverse the air cavity, causing ionisation of the air. The wall of the thimble must be sufficiently thick to ensure that all the electrons crossing the air cavity originate in the wall and not in the surrounding material. The wall must therefore be at least as thick as the range of the electrons produced by the photon interactions. However, the wall of the chamber will also attenuate the photon beam and this attenuation will need to be taken into account. If the wall is thick, the attenuation will be large. Practical ionisation chambers such as the Farmer chamber [14] have a wall thickness of about 1 mm. This is sufficient to produce electronic equilibrium for photons generated at kV energies but is insufficient for megavoltage energies when an additional tight-fitting build-up cap is needed to increase the effective wall thickness. This is particularly important when measurements are made in a phantom constructed from a material that differs markedly from the wall material.

The calibration factor of a thimble chamber varies with photon energy. This calibration corrects for wall attenuation, differences in the mass attenuation coefficient between the wall material and water, and perturbations to the photon beam caused when the chamber

(and its associated build-up cap, where applicable) is inserted into a water phantom, thereby displacing water. A typical calibration curve for such an instrument in terms of air kerma for photon beams of kV energies is shown in Fig. 3.9. The calibration factor rises sharply at low photon energies, which limits the lowest energy to which this type of instrument may be used, as small variations in photon energy spectrum for low-energy beams can give rise to considerable uncertainties in calibration factor.

The effective point of measurement for the instrument is taken within U.K. protocols for photon beam calibrations as the chamber centre. The effective point of measurement is forward of the chamber centre for calibration of electron beams. Some international photon calibration protocols are derived for the effective point of measurement being displaced from the chamber centre.

Ionisation of the air volume within the cap of a thimble chamber results in a flow of charge onto the collecting electrode. The rate of flow of charge will depend upon the mass of air within the cavity and on the radiation beam intensity. A balance must be made between the physical size of the chamber and on the ability to measure the charge with sufficient accuracy. Chambers with large air volumes (200–2000 cc) must be used to measure the very low dose rates associated with radiation protection measurements. Chambers with volumes of 10 to 60 cc are available for measurement of diagnostic radiology beams. For measurement of RT beams, chambers of about 0.6 cc are used for calibration measurements, whereas chambers with smaller air volumes may be used for other measurements as described earlier.

Measurement of Dose and Dose Rate

When an ionisation chamber is irradiated, a flow of ions is collected by the collecting electrode. The ions may be accumulated and the total charge determined by the electrometer. Such a measurement would be used to determine the radiation dose delivered over the course of the irradiation. The accumulation of charge is effectively achieved by collecting the charge in a capacitor: the voltage across the capacitor plates increases with the charge stored.

The rate at which dose is delivered may be obtained by dividing the measured dose by the irradiation time. This will produce an average value for the dose rate over the irradiation time, although the actual dose rate may vary during the irradiation period. The actual dose rate at any time point within the irradiation period may be determined by measuring the rate of flow of charge. This is achieved by measuring the potential difference produced as the charge flows through a known high-value resistor.

The charge levels referred to above are extremely small for typical RT doses, typically of the order of nanocoulombs, and dose rate measurements may involve currents of tens of picoamps. The electrometer instrument that measures them must be carefully designed to avoid introducing instrument-induced charges and voltage differences that may interfere with the measurements. Modern instruments are based around purpose-designed high-impedance operational amplifiers with low noise levels, able to measure either dose or dose rate, and which can operate over a range of current and charge levels.

THE PARALLEL-PLATE IONISATION CHAMBER

Although the thimble chamber described earlier is suitable for many dosimetry situations, there are circumstances that require alternative chamber designs:

1. For the measurement of low-energy photons, the wall of a thimble chamber causes too much attenuation such that the calibration factor is large and varies rapidly with energy. This may lead to considerable uncertainties in measurement of dose.
2. The wall of a thimble chamber will also produce too much build up for dose measurements close to the surface for megavoltage radiation.
3. In measurement of electron beams, the cylindrical air volume of a thimble chamber causes significant perturbation of the beam that must be corrected for.

Each of these may be addressed by use of a different design of ionisation chamber. This design has two planar elements: one thin electrode (the HT electrode) forms the entry window for the beam, whereas a second element consists of the collector electrode surrounded by a guard ring. The air between the electrodes is trapped by insulating walls that form the sides of the chamber and which hold the electrodes apart.

The entry window of such a chamber can be made extremely thin—a few micrometres of plastic material on which a conductive surface (e.g. a graphite layer) has been deposited but must be sufficiently rigid so as to maintain chamber geometry. For accurate measurement of low-energy x-rays, it is important that the materials of the chamber have atomic numbers close to those of water to avoid undue perturbation of the beam. The measuring volume of the chamber, shown as the shaded region in Fig. 3.10, is defined by the cross-sectional area of the collecting electrode and the separation between the plates. Interactions with the lateral walls of the chamber generate ions primarily at the edges of the chamber which are collected by the guard ring and not by the collecting electrode.

THE BEAM MONITOR CHAMBER

Linear accelerators and higher-energy kV x-ray units have inbuilt ionisation chambers to monitor and control the amount of radiation being emitted. For these units, the amount of radiation emitted is specified in terms of monitor units, that is, by the quantity of radiation measured by the inbuilt monitor chamber. The sensitivity of these monitor chambers must be adjusted to give the correct amount of radiation dose per monitor unit—a process known as *calibration*.

Monitor chambers are forms of the parallel-plate type that sample the entire radiation beam emitted from the treatment unit. In linear accelerators, each monitor chamber consists of at least two independent ionisation chambers to provide back-up should problems develop with one chamber during patient treatment. One or both chambers may be segmented, having the collector electrode constructed of a number of different and electrically isolated segments, so that assessment of beam uniformity can be made by comparing the current flowing from the various segments. Some monitor chambers are manufactured as sealed units that require no correction for ambient temperature and pressure, but which must be checked to ensure that they remain sealed. Others are manufactured as unsealed chambers that do need correction for temperature and pressure – some modern linear accelerators have inbuilt pressure and temperature transducers and perform this correction automatically, whereas others rely on manual adjustment. All monitor chambers must be calibrated regularly (e.g. daily) as specified in the calibration protocol being followed by the treatment centre or in radiation protection guidance.

In linear accelerators, the monitor chamber is situated below the primary collimator and flattening filter/scattering foil carousel, and before the adjustable collimators, as shown in Fig. 3.11. In this location, although the chamber is protected as far as practicable from backscatter that arises from the adjustable collimator jaws, it will still be subject to some backscatter. The monitor chamber may also be subject to backscatter from any physical wedges placed in the beam. Variations in backscatter contribute to changes in output with field size and to the apparent effect of the wedge. In kV-therapy units, the monitor chamber is located after the exit window of the tube housing and after any added beam filters, so that it samples the final beam. However, the monitor chamber is susceptible to backscatter from the applicator plate and this contributes to differences in output between different treatment applicators.

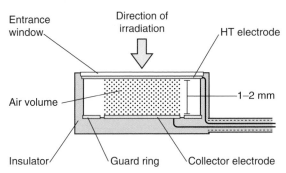

Fig. 3.10 Schematic diagram of a parallel-plate ionisation chamber. Ionisation produced within the shaded volume of air is collected by the collector electrode. The guard rings minimise the effects of the chamber walls. The effective point of measurement is the inside surface of the entrance window.

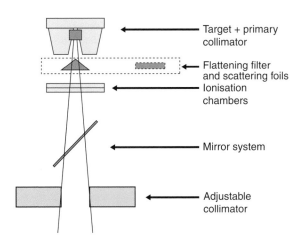

Fig. 3.11 Schematic diagram of a linear accelerator treatment head showing the location of the monitor (ionisation) chambers in relation to other components of the head.

INTERCOMPARISONS WITH SECONDARY STANDARD INSTRUMENTS

Transfer of calibration from the primary standard instrument to the field instrument is achieved via a series of intercomparisons. The response of each field instrument is compared with that of a calibrated secondary standard instrument every 12 months (or following repair to the field instrument) at each beam energy and treatment modality at which it is to be used. Where a specific build-up cap was used in determining the relevant calibration factor of the secondary standard instrument, then the same build-up cap should be fitted during intercomparison measurements, even where those measurements are to be carried out in a Perspex phantom.

Intercomparisons are carried out, wherever possible, by placing the field chamber and the secondary standard chamber side by side in the irradiation field and taking simultaneous readings. Several readings should be taken and averaged for each measurement, and the relative positions of the two chambers should be interchanged to minimise any effects should the radiation beam produce different dose rates at the positions of the two chambers. The relevant conditions (e.g. type of phantom, depth of measurement, field size) under which these intercomparison measurements and subsequent equipment calibration measurements are made are specified in the appropriate dosimetry protocol. In the United Kingdom, separate protocols have been produced by the IPEM or its forerunner organisations covering:

- x-ray beams below 300 kV generating potential [16,17].
- high-energy (megavoltage) x-ray beams [8,18].
- electron beams of energy from 4 to 25 MeV [19].

Because of the very different penetration properties of the beams concerned, the first of these is split into three separate sections covering different energy ranges. For very low energy beams; HVL <1.0 mm Aluminium (Al), measurements are specified for the surface of a phantom. For low-energy beams (HVL 1–8 mm Al), measurements are specified in air, with no phantom present. For medium energy beams; HVL between 0.5 to 1.0 mm Copper (Cu), which are more penetrating, measurements are specified at depth of 2 cm in a phantom.

STRONTIUM CONSISTENCY CHECK DEVICE

Between calibration sessions, the consistency of each instrument has to be checked using an appropriate consistency checking device.

One such device uses a strontium check source [20] and is illustrated in Fig. 3.12. A device of this type for thimble chambers has a ring-shaped source of ^{90}Sr housed within a fully shielded enclosure, into the centre of which the sensitive volume of the ionisation chamber can be accurately placed. ^{90}Sr is a beta emitter and decays at a constant rate with a half-life

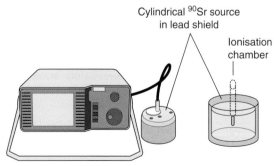

Cylindrical ^{90}Sr source in lead shield

Ionisation chamber

Fig. 3.12 Strontium checking device used to check the consistency of a thimble chamber, together with a schematic of the device showing the source wrapped around the chamber.

of 28.7 years. The chamber response within the device is measured at the time at which intercomparison measurements are made. The response to be expected at any subsequent time can then be calculated simply by accounting for radioactive decay, on the proviso that repositioning of the ionisation chamber can be carried out with sufficient precision. Different source geometries may be used for different types of ionisation chamber, for example, planar ^{90}Sr sources may be used to check the consistency of response of parallel-plate ionisation chambers.

Measurements are carried out periodically (e.g. every month). The chamber response is determined either by measuring the reading achieved for a defined period of measurement or by measuring the time for the chamber to reach a given reading once measurement has been initiated. These measurements ensure the consistency of operation of the measuring device but cannot be used for calibration of the measuring device, because the radiation from ^{90}Sr is not representative of the radiation beams in which the device will be used in clinical practice.

IONISATION CHAMBER CORRECTIONS

Whenever instruments that are based upon collection of ions produced in air are used to determine absorbed dose, a number of factors in addition to the calibration factor have to be taken into account.

Ion Recombination Losses

When the air volume of an ionisation chamber is irradiated, ion pairs are generated as atoms become ionised. To determine the absorbed dose or air kerma accurately, it is necessary to ensure the collection of all the positive or negative ions (depending on polarity) by the collecting electrode. A potential difference is applied across the electrodes to drive the ion pairs apart. If the ion pairs are not driven apart by the applied electric field, they may recombine such that they are lost from collection and the charge is therefore reduced. When ions recombine, the positive and negative ions of an ion pair may recombine with each other (self-recombination), or the negative ion from one ion pair may recombine with the positive ion of a neighbouring ion pair (volume recombination). Both self and volume recombination result in a reduction in the measured charge. The likelihood of recombination is less where the ions are driven apart rapidly, such as when the polarising voltage is high.

Recombination is more likely to occur when ions pairs are created close together, both physically and in time. This occurs when measuring high dose rates, or when measuring in beams in which the radiation is delivered in pulses. The radiation from a ^{60}Co gamma-beam therapy unit is emitted continuously. The radiation from a modern kilovoltage-therapy unit is also virtually continuous, although it does depend somewhat on the type of voltage generator used. For both of these radiation sources, polarising voltages across a thimble chamber of a few hundred volts are generally sufficient that recombination losses are negligible at dose rates commonly used in RT. The radiation from a linear accelerator is strongly pulsed: a linear accelerator delivering a dose rate of 4 Gy/min will deliver the radiation in short pulses, each of a few microseconds duration, with the instantaneous dose rate within each pulse being about 40 Gy/s. Under these circumstances, accurate determination of dose requires knowledge of and correction for recombination losses. The amount of recombination may be determined by carrying out measurements using different levels of polarising voltage across the chamber, applying an empirically derived equation for the equipment being used, or by applying the half-voltage technique [21,22].

Correction for Atmospheric Conditions

It has been previously stated that the rate of flow of ions onto the collector electrode will depend on the amount of air enclosed within the thimble of the chamber, and examples have been given of different instrument sizes for measuring in dose rates at typical protection, radiodiagnostic, and therapy radiation levels. It is, however, the mass of air within the thimble on which the response depends.

For a chamber that is sealed to trap air inside the thimble, variations in atmospheric temperature and pressure will have no impact upon the enclosed mass and will therefore not affect the chamber response. However, the condition of the air within such an instrument may change with time, perhaps because of vapours leaching from the walls of the cap or the surrounding materials. In addition, there is always potential for the seal to fail, allowing some flow of air between the chamber and the environment. If a chamber is unsealed, allowing free passage of air between the inside of the thimble and the general environment, then the mass of air within the thimble will fluctuate with atmospheric temperature and pressure and a correction to any reading will be required to compensate for these changes. As the temperature increases, the air density falls and the mass of air within the thimble will reduce, thereby reducing the chamber sensitivity. As atmospheric pressure rises, the density of air also increases, increasing the mass of gas within the thimble, thereby increasing the chamber sensitivity. If the assumption is made that air affected by temperature and pressure changes in the same way as an ideal gas, then the ideal gas laws can be applied to determine the magnitude of variation in response. If measurements are made at a temperature of T degrees Celsius (°C) and a pressure of P kilopascal (kPa) using an unsealed instrument, the response may be corrected to what it would have been at a standard temperature of 20°C (293 K) and pressure of 101.325 kPa by applying the correction factor:

$$\text{Correction} = (101.325/P) \times [(T+273)/293] \qquad \textbf{3.8}$$

Most practical field instruments are designed and constructed to be unsealed. The design of such an instrument has to ensure that the thimble does not distort with changes in temperature or pressure so that the volume remains constant. Water vapour can affect the chamber response and the aforementioned correction for atmospheric conditions, producing a variation of about 0.7% for change in relative humidity from 10% to 90%. To minimise the impact of relative humidity changes, the secondary standard calibration factor is specified for a humidity value of 50%: variations in chamber response in normal use because of relative humidity changes may generally be ignored.

Chamber Stem Effect

If the stem of the ionisation chamber is within the radiation field, it may perturb the radiation beam and may generate scatter into the air volume of the chamber, thereby affecting the reading (termed the *stem effect*).

During absolute calibration, the chamber is irradiated with a specific field size and a correction is applied for the stem effect with this field size. It is therefore considered whenever the calibration factor is applied. There is, however, potential for the effect to increase or decrease for other field sizes.

With well-designed ionisation chambers, such as the Farmer chamber, the stem effect is small and variations in it can generally be ignored.

Polarity Effect

When an ionisation chamber is used to measure charged particles, some of the charged particles may come to rest on the collecting electrode. These will either add to or subtract from the ionisation charge being collected, depending upon the charge on the particle and on the direction of the polarising voltage (whether the collector electrode is collecting positive ions or electrons). The effect is particularly important when using parallel-plate chambers to measure proton or electron beams and can be overcome by averaging measurements taken with both positive and negative polarising voltages.

A related problem is that, if measurements are carried out in a solid insulating material such as polystyrene, then particles stopped within the material will result in a build-up of charge there, which will perturb the radiation beam being measured. To avoid this, an insulating phantom should be made of thin sheets of material which allows charge built up in this way to leak away.

ALTERNATIVE DOSE MEASUREMENT SYSTEMS

In the aforementioned sections, the primary processes for detection of radiation and measurement of dose centred around calorimetry and ionisation of air. National standard and secondary standard instruments are based on these processes, and field instruments of the thimble or parallel-plate chamber design are recommended for routine measurement of radiation output from therapy machines. There are, however, other techniques that are suitable for measurement of dose or dose rate for different circumstances. These are briefly described in the following section and a selection of such devices is represented schematically in Fig. 3.13.

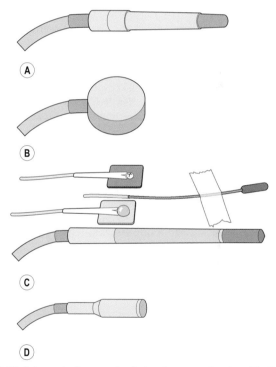

Fig. 3.13 Schematic diagram of radiation detectors showing: (A) a Farmer chamber without an additional build-up cap; (B) a parallel-plate chamber for electron measurements; (C) a selection of diode detectors for phantom and for in vivo measurements, together with a Farmer-type chamber for comparison; (D) a diamond detector.

Film Dosimetry

Film has been used as a system for measuring radiation throughout the whole history of RT. It is particularly useful for measurement of radiation distributions, having applications in phantom measurement of simple and complex radiation beams, in verification of field placements on individual patients, in establishing geometrical accuracy of light beams that delineate radiation beams, and in determination of leakage patterns around the head of a treatment unit.

Standard Photographic Film

Photographic film consists essentially of a transparent polyester material (the base) on which is deposited a layer of silver bromide trapped in a gel (the emulsion). The emulsion may be deposited on one side or on both sides of the base. The emulsion is sensitive to light and so must be used in a light-tight packaging or housing. The silver bromide is in the form of small crystals, each crystal being formed as a lattice of negative bromide and positive silver ions. When irradiated, some lattice bonds are broken and electrons are transferred from the bromine to the silver ions, neutralising those atoms. The presence of neutral silver atoms at key positions of the lattice within a crystal makes the whole crystal developable. In the subsequent development process, the silver ions of developable crystals are converted to atoms of silver. These are fixed in position on the film while the rest of the emulsion, including any nondevelopable crystals, is removed. The deposited silver absorbs light, so these regions of the film appear black while the rest appears transparent.

The degree of blackness depends on the relative concentration of deposited crystals which, in turn, depends upon the intensity of radiation at that location on the film. This is measured by shining light through the developed film and measuring the transmitted intensity. A logarithmic scale is used to define the optical density of the film:

$$OD = \log_{10}(I_0/I) \qquad \textbf{3.9}$$

where I_0 is the incident light intensity and I is the transmitted intensity. The resultant optical density has to be corrected for the intrinsic density of the developed film base. A graph of optical density against absorbed dose is known as the *dose response curve* and can be produced for any film. Accurate dosimetry requires full knowledge of the dose response curve. The response curve may be effectively linear over a restricted range of doses and simple dose comparisons can be made within this range. Used in this way, film has high spatial resolution unmatched by other measuring systems and can provide a full two-dimensional display of dose distribution (such as variation in dose with depth and position across the beam). However, silver bromide has a high atomic number and therefore the response to low-energy photons is greatly increased as a result of increased photoelectric interactions. This makes film unsuitable as an absolute dosimeter and makes accurate comparative measurements difficult in situations where the energy spectrum varies markedly. Although the areas of application of film dosimetry are steadily being reduced as other methods of measurement come to the fore, film dosimetry still has a vital role within RT. It also has a role in radiation protection dosimetry where the film badge has been the historical standard for personal dosimetry, although this is steadily being replaced by other forms of detector.

Radiochromic Film

Standard photographic film as described earlier is sensitive to both ionising radiation and visible light. When used for radiation measurements it has to be kept in a light-free container and processed under controlled light conditions. In contrast to this, radiochromic reactions produce direct coloration of a substance by direct absorption of radiation, without the need for chemical processing.

Radiochromic films have been developed that have little or no sensitivity to visible light, but which demonstrate a change in colour when subjected to ionising radiation.

These may be based upon release of leuco dyes within the material or upon the formation of coloured cross-linked polymers from otherwise colourless monomers. The degree of colour change is dependent upon absorbed dose and may be determined by measuring the attenuation of light of specific frequencies that relate to the colour change. Radiochromic films are commercially available which have good response for doses within the range of 0.5 to 25 Gy and have no high atomic number materials present. Such films therefore have uniform response across a wide range of photon energies. Materials of this type have been used to

determine dose distributions for complex RT treatments and around brachytherapy sources. The most common type is the commercial GAF chromic film [23]. The principle of polymer cross-linkage is similar to that of polymer gels described in a later section.

Semiconductor Detectors

A number of different types of semiconductor-based radiation detectors have been proposed. This text describes the principles of operation of semiconductor diode detectors, metal oxide semiconductor field effect transistors (MOSFETs), and diamond detectors.

The physical process which enables radiation detection and measurement to be achieved with these devices is based upon the way a material can be understood in terms of band structure (see Chapter 1).

These devices use semiconductor material, the most common of which is silicon, to which specific impurities are added at very low concentrations, a process known as *doping*. Two types of doping are used. Doping by an electron donor results in n-type material. For example, arsenic and selenium introduce free electrons into the conduction band of silicon. Doping by an electron receptor produces p-type material. For example, aluminium and gallium effectively introduce additional vacant levels into the valence band of silicon. These unfilled levels are termed holes. If electrons are introduced into a p-type material, they will fill vacant holes and become trapped.

Diode Detector

When adjacent p-type and n-type doping occurs in a single crystal of silicon, a p–n junction is formed. Conduction electrons in the n-type region will diffuse into the p-type region and become trapped, as shown in Fig. 3.14. This results in:
- The region around the interface being devoid of free electrons and unfilled holes. This region is called the depletion layer;
- A transfer of electrons (and hence charge) from the n-type to the p-type side of the interface.

This transfer of charge generates a small potential difference across the depletion layer.

When this depletion layer is irradiated, electrons are released by ionisation, creating electron–hole pairs as shown in Fig. 3.14C. These drift in opposite directions under the influence of the potential

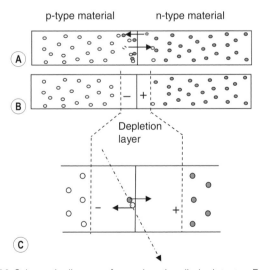

Fig. 3.14 Schematic diagram of a p–n junction diode detector. Electrons from the n-type material and holes from the p-type material diffuse across the junction (A), forming a depletion layer across which an internal potential difference forms (B). Electron–hole pairs formed in the depletion layer are pulled apart by the internal electric field (C).

difference across the depletion layer. Electrons will be drawn towards the n-type material while holes will be drawn towards the p-type, causing charge to flow through the circuit in which the diode is connected. The charge produced is proportional to the dose deposited in the depletion region, and the flow of charge can be measured by an electrometer.

The sensitive region of the diode is very thin, the depletion layer being only a few micrometres in thickness and the cross-sectional area of the silicon crystal being only a few millimetres. However, the sensitivity to radiation is high as the density of the material is over 1000 times that of air in an ionisation chamber and the mean energy to produce an electron–hole pair is about one-tenth of the energy to create an ion pair in air. Diodes can therefore produce measurable signals from extremely small sensitive volumes that make them particularly suitable for measurements that require high spatial resolution. The absence of any applied polarising voltage makes diodes particularly useful for in vivo dosimetry.

Diodes have various inherent problems that must be addressed when they are used as radiation detectors. The size of the depletion layer, and hence the sensitivity of the device, strongly depends on temperature [24]. Diodes therefore need to be calibrated at the temperature at which they are to be used. They are constructed from materials with atomic numbers higher than water, making them over-responsive to low-energy photon radiation. Their response is therefore sensitive to variations in the energy spectrum of any radiation field such as may be caused by changes in depth, radiation field size and position within the field, or energy setting of equipment being measured. In addition, the construction of the device can influence its angular sensitivity [25,26]. A further problem is that diodes may suffer radiation damage after receiving high doses of radiation which causes them to change their sensitivity. It has been shown that diodes formed using predominantly heavy p-type doping are less susceptible to sudden change in sensitivity and have longer working lives than predominantly n-doped diodes [27]. The majority of commercial diodes are of this form.

Diodes are used widely in RT as:

- Individual detectors that are used for measuring dose distributions (e.g. depth doses and profiles, particularly where high spatial resolution is required such as in regions of high dose gradient) of RT beams during initial commissioning and subsequent quality control measurements.
- Individual or groups of detectors for measurement of radiation doses delivered to patients (in vivo dosimetry).
- Arrays of detectors for rapid checking of beam uniformity as part of a quality assurance programme.

Metal Oxide Semiconductor Field Effect Transistor Detector

The structure of a Metal Oxide Semiconductor Field Effect Transistor (MOSFET) is shown schematically in Fig. 3.15 which illustrates a device based upon p-doped silicon substrate material onto which layers of heavily n-doped material and SiO_2 are formed. There are three electrical contacts, which are termed the source, gate, and drain. The source and drain regions may be considered as p–n junctions, which are linked by the SiO_2 channel onto which the gate is deposited.

The device operates essentially like a voltage-controlled switch. If a small voltage is generated between the source and the gate with the drain held at the same potential as the gate, then no current flows initially between the source and drain until the applied voltage exceeds a specific value (called the threshold voltage), whereupon the device switches and a current starts to flow. The application of the applied voltage causes holes to be drawn to the oxide/silicon surface from both the substrate and from the source and drain regions. A conduction channel between source and drain is formed once the concentration of holes becomes sufficient.

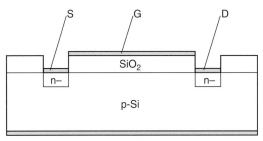

Fig. 3.15 Cross-sectional schematic of a metal oxide semiconductor field effect device. A conducting channel is formed through the oxide layer between the source (S) and the drain (D) when a voltage is applied to the gate (G). The threshold voltage at which this channel is formed is reduced by the effects of radiation.

When the device is irradiated, electron–hole pairs are generated within the SiO_2. The mobility of the electrons allows them readily to migrate away, whereas the holes become trapped at the oxide/silicone surface. These traps, which can survive for a long time, reduce the threshold voltage necessary for the device to switch. The change in threshold voltage is almost linearly related to the radiation dose received by the device.

MOSFET devices are extremely small (<0.1 mm) and are easily fabricated in various shapes and geometries—such that individual detectors can be used for point doses or planar distributions of detectors to measure complex dose profiles. No electrical connections are necessary during irradiation and the electronic equipment needed for readout is relatively simple, making these devices ideally suited to in vivo dosimetry. They do, however, suffer from the same energy response effects as diode detectors.

Diamond Detector

Carbon in the form of diamond is an intrinsic semiconductor with a large energy gap between the conduction and valence bands (5.5 eV). At normal room temperatures, there are very few electrons in the conduction band. If a voltage is placed across a diamond crystal, a tiny current will flow because of these electrons, the magnitude of which is dependent for any given crystal on the applied voltage. The diamond therefore behaves as a resistor.

When irradiated, ion pairs generated within the material increase the number of carriers, and so the resistance falls. The radiation-induced current increases with increasing dose rate. Certain impurities within the diamond can improve the linearity of response between current and dose rate, but the dose rate response has to be considered when using these devices.

A diamond detector consists of a diamond crystal onto which metal contacts have been deposited and to which a voltage of about 100 V is applied. The radiation-induced current is considerably larger than the natural current and so can be measured with precision. Under these conditions, the response is largely independent of temperature. The detector is not readily damaged by radiation, so the device has a long operational life. The diamond crystal may be selected from natural diamonds or grown using chemical vapor deposition processes. They are small detectors and so are useful in measuring in high radiation gradients, with good angular response characteristics. Being composed of carbon, they are low atomic number devices with electron stopping power values similar to those for water [28].

Summary of Direct Reading Radiation Detectors

Various types of radiation detectors have been described in the previous sections. Each type of detector has particular applications for which it is ideally suited. Cylindrical ionisation chambers (Fig. 3.13A) are particularly useful as instruments for calibration of megavoltage photon beams. Parallel-plate ionisation chambers (see Fig. 3.13B) are useful when measuring in regions of high dose gradient, such as in the dose fall-off region of an electron beam. Diodes (see Fig. 3.13C) are useful for in vivo dosimetry. The small size of their detection region makes these devices also useful when measuring in small radiation fields or within beam penumbral regions. Cylindrical forms of these detectors, which include corrections within the design of the device for enhanced low-energy photon response, are readily available. Diamond detectors (see Fig. 3.13D) may be used as an alternative to diode detectors and are especially resistant to radiation damage.

Thermoluminescent Dosimetry

We have seen in the section on the band structure of solids in Chapter 1 that some materials have a normally empty conduction band. When such a material is irradiated, some electrons within the valence band may be given sufficient energy to excite them into the conduction band, leaving a 'hole' in the valence band. These electrons will eventually lose their extra energy and fall back to the valence band to fill the vacant energy level (hole) there. In doing this, the electron has to lose the energy difference between the two energy levels.

The energy lost in this transition may be a few electron volts. In some materials, this energy loss is in the form of emission of electromagnetic radiation, akin to the emission of characteristic x-rays from an x-ray target but at much lower energies. This process appears simple but may actually involve complex energy-level changes for both the electron and the hole that are beyond the scope of this book. The result for some types of material is that it is transparent to the electromagnetic radiation released by these transitions, which is then emitted. The energy of the radiation emitted may be within the visible spectrum in which case the irradiated material emits light. Materials of this type are said to be luminescent in general. When the electrons excited into the conduction band fall back and emit light immediately, the material is said to be fluorescent. Fluorescent screens are used to enhance the response of x-ray film to radiation and are used within some types of portal imaging devices. In luminescent processes, additional energy levels within the forbidden zone, as shown in Fig. 1.3A, formed either from impurities or as a result of discontinuities in the crystal structure, play a part both in trapping the excited electrons and in the emission of light. Energy levels immediately below the conduction band form traps for some of the electrons from that band. Electrons falling into these traps may be held there until they gain sufficient energy to move back into the conduction band, from where they can decay back to the valence band. If the trap level is close to the conduction band, then ongoing energy variations from thermal fluctuations will result in traps being emptied rapidly, producing fluorescence. The further a trap from the conduction band, the longer will be the time for it to empty: traps are therefore characterised by two related features, the distance from the conduction band (the trap depth) and the rate at which it empties (the trap half-life).

In some materials, such as metal-doped lithium fluoride (LiF; i.e. doped with magnesium or manganese), the trap levels are well below the conduction band. At normal room temperatures, these traps would empty exceedingly slowly. If, however, the temperature of the crystal is raised, then the additional heat energy imparted may allow electrons rapidly to escape the traps. The light output from the crystal is dependent upon this supply of heat and these materials are termed thermoluminescent.

When a thermoluminescent material is irradiated, electrons are transported into the conduction band. A small number, about 1%, of these electrons fall into the thermoluminescent traps. When the

material is later heated to a temperature that allows the traps to empty, light is given off. This process is shown in Fig. 3.16. The amount of light is proportional to the number of electrons trapped and hence to the radiation dose delivered to the crystal material. Thermoluminescent dosimetry [29] uses a Thermoluminescent Dosimeter (TLD) reader that both heats the detector and simultaneously measures the amount of light emitted, as indicated in Fig. 3.17.

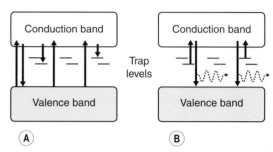

Fig. 3.16 Illustration of thermoluminescent dosimeter processes. Irradiation of the material raises electrons into the conduction band. Some of these fall back to the valence band while others become trapped in intervening energy levels, as shown in (A). When heat is applied, the electrons in the traps are raised back into the conduction band and subsequently fall back to the valence band, releasing visible photons as shown in (B).

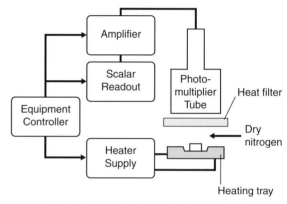

Fig. 3.17 Schematic diagram of a thermoluminescent dosimeter readout system. The heat filter protects the photomultiplier tube and reduces thermal counts. The dry nitrogen atmosphere prevents oxidation of the detector surface.

A material such as LiF, which is the most common TLD material in clinical use, will have a number of traps at differing depths. The light output from LiF as a function of temperature of the crystal is known as a glow curve and a typical glow curve is illustrated in Fig. 3.18. The traps closest to the conduction band empty first, producing the glow peaks labelled I to III. These traps have relatively short half-lives at room temperatures such that the signal falls too rapidly for reliable dose estimates, so the output from these bands is usually ignored. The signal from the higher temperature peaks IV and V is from traps with half-lives measured in years, so that timing between irradiation and readout is not generally relevant—the light from these traps is measured to estimate the dose. After use, the material is thermally annealed, a process which resets the electron energy levels and traps occupancies to their initial values, after which the material may be reused.

The light output from a specific dosimeter will depend upon a number of factors:

- The amount of intrinsic thermoluminescent material.
- The nature and extent of the doping.

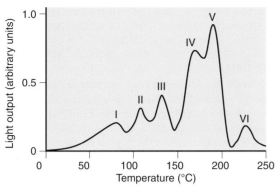

Fig. 3.18 Schematic illustration of the glow curve from LiF:Mg,Ti showing the six peaks representing different trap depths.

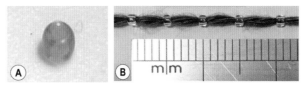

Fig. 3.19 (A) A magnified view of a microsilica bead thermoluminescent dosimeter (hollow, with 0.5-mm internal diameter). The bead is coloured for illustration only. (B) microsilica beads arranged on a piece of cotton with 5-mm spacing distance.

- The previous thermal history in general and the postanneal cooling in particular.
- The radiation history of the material—radiation-induced damage may alter the energy band structure of the material.
- The surface condition of the crystalline material—marks and scratches attenuate and scatter the light.
- The detailed nature of the readout cycle.

Some of the aforementioned cause differences in response between different dosimeters, whereas others cause differences in response of a single dosimeter from use to use. In addition, the response is not strictly linear with dose but increases with increased dose, a feature known as *supralinearity*. TLD is not used as an absolute dosimeter (i.e. where the calibration is stable and constant). To address these issues, TLD dosimeters are used in batches, where the dosimeters in each batch have the same handling and general history and where some are selected as measuring dosimeters whereas others are irradiated to known doses to calibrate the batch response in a traceable manner.

LiF is the most commonly used TLD material and is available in various forms that include powder; single-crystal chips (size 4 mm × 4 mm × 1 mm approximately), and rods (size 6-mm long × 1-mm diameter); sintered chips, disks, and rods; and Teflon-embedded disks and rods. The effective atomic number is slightly greater than that of water, leading to over-response of between 1.3 and 1.7 for photon energies of less than 100 keV, but the response is virtually uniform for megavoltage radiation. The detector response does not vary with dose rate up to dose rates of greater than 10^6 Gy/min. Other materials are available, including lithium borate which has a more uniform energy response at low energies, and calcium sulphate which has a high sensitivity to low-energy photons.

TLD materials are currently used as in vivo dosimeters for both surface dose and interstitial measurements. For measurements on the patient surface to estimate the dose at the depth of dose maximum, care must be taken to ensure that appropriate build-up is used, both for the patient measurement and for calibration irradiation. Despite the variations in response described earlier, TLD is used to provide a traceable postal calibration service both to centres without access to a primary or secondary standards laboratory and to check on the accuracy of calibration across various centres as part of clinical trial quality control procedures.

Microsilica bead TLDs have recently been introduced as a high spatial resolution detector for use in complex high-gradient dose distribution measurements such as advanced radiation therapy techniques [30,31]. They are spherical doughnut shaped with a hole in the middle with approximate size of 1.5-mm outer diameter and 1.0-mm thickness (Fig. 3.19A). This physical shape allows for two-dimensional and three-dimensional arrangements (e.g. Fig. 3.19B, where bead TLDs are arranged on a cotton thread for a line profile of dose measurement). This along with robustness and inert nature makes them an ideal passive in-vivo dosimetry system when it is difficult to control the environmental factors such as humidity and temperature inside the patient's body.

Although they can be read out using a conventional TLD reader, one might use a large number of bead TLDs for high-resolution measurements in complex two-dimensional and three-dimensional arrangements which require significant labour resources for readout and data analysis. In such occasions use of a fully automated TLD reader and data processor that is introduced specifically for the readout process of bead TLDs seems to be a more practical approach.

The detector response does not vary with beam angle and dose rate. The effective atomic number of silica bead TLDs is almost two times greater than that of water, leading to a significant energy dependency, similar to that of bone, for beam energies of kV range where photoelectric effect is the main radiation interaction process. Being bone equivalent makes them a suitable detector if one wants to measure dose to the bone. However, when dose measurement to water or soft tissue is intended, a careful calibration using the same beam energy is required. Moreover, silica bead TLDs together with a soft tissue equivalent detector can be used as a means of beam energy discrimination.

Chemical and Biochemical Detectors

Energy deposited in matter may be manifest ultimately in various forms, one being altered chemistry. RT relies upon this to a large extent in the process of damaging and destroying tissue cells. In some cells, direct interaction of the radiation with DNA causes irreparable damage leading to death of those cells. In others, radiation-induced chemical changes within the cells produce active free radicals that cause similar damage to DNA.

In some materials, the altered chemical make-up remains and can be detected. Where the effect is stable and proportional to dose, this may be used in chemical and biochemical dosimetry. If the chemical yield is known (number of chemical molecules formed per unit of energy absorbed), then chemical dosimetry could be used as a primary standard. Fricke dosimetry was used for a short period in the past in this way to provide a definitive calibration of electron beams for which the yield was well established.

Fricke Dosimetry

Fricke dosimetry is based upon conversion of ferrous sulphate ions (Fe^{2+}) to ferric ions in a weak sulphuric acid solution [32]. The concentration of ferric sulphate is determined by measuring the attenuation of light passing through the solution. Light of a particular wavelength (304 nm) is used as this is attenuated differentially by ferrous and ferric ions. The instrument used for accurate measurement of attenuation at a particular frequency of light is a spectrophotometer. The ferrous sulphate solution has to be carefully prepared and handled to avoid chemical contaminants that can affect the result.

The dose is given by:

$$D = k\Delta A / [\varepsilon \delta \rho\, G(Fe^{3+})] \qquad \textbf{3.10}$$

where k is a constant, ΔA is the change in absorption (optical density), δ is the optical path length, ρ is the Fricke density, ε the difference in molar extinction coefficient, and $G(Fe^{3+})$ is the chemical yield.

This system is not very sensitive such that doses of greater than 10 Gy are required to produce sufficient concentration of ferric ions, but accuracies of better than 2% are readily achievable. The process is effectively insensitive to dose rate and can be used to determine doses up to 400 Gy. The detector is 96% water and is therefore essentially water equivalent. It can be used over a wide range of energies and modalities. Fricke dosimetry has been used in the past by standards laboratories to confirm measurements of absorbed dose using other dosimetric techniques.

Ceric Dosimetry

Similar to Fricke dosimetry, ceric dosimetry relies on the reduction by radiation of ceric ions (Ce^{4+}) to cerous ions (Ce^{3+}) in a mixture of ceric and cerous ions in 0.4 M sulphuric acid. The concentration of cerous ions is determined by spectrophotometry using light with a wavelength of 320 nm.

Gel Dosimetry

The techniques described previously are suitable for producing single-point measurements of dose (e.g. ionisation chambers) or measurements of two-dimensional distributions (e.g. film). In contrast to these, gel dosimeters allow measurement of three-dimensional distributions. These are ideally suited to determination of distributions arising from complex treatments such as intensity-modulated RT. In addition, gel dosimetry is proving useful in situations where other forms of measurement are difficult, such as in dosimetry of very small radiation fields (e.g. stereotactic RT and proton beams) and measurements around brachytherapy sources where the radiation dose varies rapidly with position relative to the source. Phantoms to hold the gel material can be made to reflect anatomical shapes.

There are currently two forms of gel detectors in use: Fricke gel and polymer gel. For each, various ways of reading out the signal have been developed, the most common of which are magnetic resonance (MR) and optical computed tomography (CT). Gel detectors in general are insensitive to dose rates, are effectively water equivalent, and the signal is relatively linear with dose. Overall accuracy is limited (typically around 5%), although spatial resolution is excellent.

Fricke Gels and FXG Gels

In 1984, Gore and colleagues proposed the use of MR techniques on Fricke solutions [33] and Fricke-infused gels in which ferrous ions are held within the gel matrix. When reduced by radiation to ferric ions, the spin–spin (T2) relaxation times of linked protein atoms change. This change in relaxation times in each small volume of the material can be measured using an MR scanner. Each measurement is accompanied by a test irradiation that is used to determine the sensitivity of each detector batch to different dose levels.

Although able to produce accurate dose distributions, the process has two main drawbacks. First, measurement is time-consuming and requires ready access to an MR scanner. Second, the ferric ions migrate through the gel matrix with time, so that measurements have to be undertaken shortly after irradiation [34].

A development of this technique led to the introduction of xylenol orange into the gel mix [35]. This material is photochromic and has the property of changing colour from orange to purple when the mix is irradiated. This change in colour can be determined by measuring optical attenuation of filtered light. A set of two-dimensional slice readouts can be obtained using an optical CT device.

Polymer Gels

Polymer gels are based upon the polymerisation of monomers embedded in the gel matrix which produces long polymer chains and cross-linkage of polymers [36]. These reduce the T2 relaxation time which can be determined using an MR scanner. A common polymer gel in current use is the commercial BANG® gel of Maryanski and colleagues [37], which is based upon polymerisation of the monomer acrylamide. This may be produced in forms that allow optical readout using an optical CT device, as radiation induces white opacity in an otherwise transparent material. Because cross-linkage of monomers stabilises the material, there is no migration away from irradiated areas, such that these devices are stable over time.

BANG gels have to be produced and sealed while under a nitrogen atmosphere to avoid oxygen-induced polymerisation affecting the results. This necessity has been removed in newer gel formulations in which oxygen in the gel is bound into a chemical matrix which prevents it from causing polymerisation, making the production of gels for dosimetry far more simple [38].

Alanine-Electron Paramagnetic Resonance Dosimetry

Alanine is a polycrystalline amino acid which has the chemical formula $CH_3CH(NH_2)COOH$. When irradiated, stable free radicals are formed within the material. These radicals can exist unchanged for long periods, allowing separation of irradiation from the readout process [39]. Some of these free radicals have a single unpaired electron attached to one of the atoms of the radical. The single unpaired electron exists in one of two energy states. When subjected to a magnetic field, these energy states equate to what is referred to as parallel and antiparallel spin states, the difference in energy between them being proportional to the strength of the magnetic field.

The electron normally occupies the lower state but may be excited into the higher state by absorbing a specific resonant wavelength of electromagnetic radiation of photon energy ($h\upsilon$) equal to the energy separation between the two states, for magnetic field strengths of 300 mT and frequency of about 9 MHz, which is within the microwave part of the electromagnetic spectrum. The concentration of free radicals can be assessed by measuring the degree of absorption of this resonant radiation, a process known as electron paramagnetic resonance (or traditionally electron spin resonance) [40]. A number of free radicals are involved, the most important one involving the loss of the NH_2 group.

Dosimeters are formed by mixing known quantities of alanine with one or more binding agents to produce a compact, solid detector, which has both density and atomic number values that differ only slightly from water and which is suitably sensitive to radiation. The dose response is almost linear from 10 to 10^4 Gy and is largely independent of dose rate. Lower doses down to below 1 Gy can be measured provided that the device is calibrated to account for nonlinearity of response at these dose levels. Accuracies of better than 2% are achievable under controlled conditions. The combination of accuracy and stability has led to them being used by a number of standards laboratories as a basis for a remote calibration service which rivals the use of thermoluminescent dosimetry. Alanine dosimetry systems are also available commercially. A number of research groups are currently investigating the development of two-dimensional and three-dimensional measurement systems based upon spatially distributed alanine. Other groups are investigating chemical variations of alanine (e.g. 2-methylalanine) to develop dosimeters more suited to lower dose ranges for in vivo dosimetry [41].

Biological Dosimetry

The response of biological systems has been used as an indicator of the dose delivered since the very first applications of radiation to the treatment of human disease. Early dosimetry standards were based upon skin erythema levels, with the absorbed dose determined by the degree of reddening of the skin and on the resultant type of erythema produced. This system was very inaccurate and was abandoned in favour of other physical forms of radiation dosimetry long before the introduction of skin-sparing megavoltage treatments. There are, however, circumstances, such as accidental exposures, where other forms of dosimetry are not applicable and where doses have to be estimated on the basis of the biological responses. There are various possible biological indicators of absorbed dose based upon the response of different biological systems. These include effects on biological molecules and genetic structures, but also effects on cells and structures.

Biological Molecules

The process described earlier in relation to alanine dosimetry in which the concentration of long-lived free radicals can be determined by using electron spin resonance may also be applicable to estimate doses to specific tissues. This process is relatively insensitive but has been used to estimate doses received around sites of nuclear explosions and accidents [42,43].

An alternative method to assess absorbed dose is based upon quantifying changes in the chemical composition of body fluids. The concentration of thymidine in blood serum has been shown to be a sensitive indicator of absorbed dose in mice [44] but is unfortunately less applicable to primates.

Genetic Structures

The most advanced and established method of biological dosimetry is based upon determining the concentration of chromosome aberrations by counting the number of dicentrics in human peripheral blood lymphocytes [45]. This form of dosimetry is able to estimate doses down to about 0.1 Gy and is used in cases of accidental overexposure.

An alternative method is based upon determining the concentration of micronuclei formed as a result of the radiation exposure. This method may possibly be developed to compete with dicentric concentration analysis [46].

Cells and Biological Structures

The dose responses for various biological systems are well documented in the literature. Radiation inhibits the production of blood cells, inhibits the production of sperm in males and leads to the death of hair follicles—all of which may be used to estimate the absorbed dose shortly after exposure. For high doses of radiation, breakdown of other organs may be used where the absorbed dose exceeds tissue tolerance levels for those organs.

COMPOSITE DETECTORS AND ARRAYS

Measurement of radiation dose distributions has been important in RT, primarily to assess the uniformity of radiation beams and determine the size of the radiation beam. Radiographic film (see the 'Film Dosimetry' section above) densitometry was extensively used for this and it provided a high-resolution detector with uniform response. Film provided a simple, practical, and easily assessed hard copy of the results with almost no data processing.

The alternative method used a single scanning ionisation chamber, or solid-state photon or electron detector which traversed the beam. Single-detector scanning and film techniques were time-consuming to undertake and to process. However, while treatment techniques

remained simple, there was little impetus for greater measurement complexity. In addition, in the past the consistency of detector production and performance was variable and multiple detector arrays were problematic because of nonuniform performance.

This situation has changed dramatically with dynamic and intensity-modulated beam delivery. It is worth mentioning at this point that there have been two approaches to performing quality control measurements on volumetric modulated dose distribution such as those delivered by volumetric modulated arc therapy (VMAT). The first technique measures the two-dimensional distribution of fluence from a beam and compares it with the intended delivery. The second technique measures a distribution delivered to a regular phantom with the modulated beams intended for treatment. Both techniques are used; the first requires an area detector array, whereas the second needs a volumetric detector array.

Linear Detector Arrays

As mentioned earlier, single-detector scanners (Fig. 3.20) could provide measurement of the radiation distribution within the beam and the use of a single detector ensured that the measurements were entirely consistent with each other and there were no inherent artefacts because of detector response variation. The first complication with the use of single-detector scanner arose with the introduction of dynamic wedges (see Chapter 9).

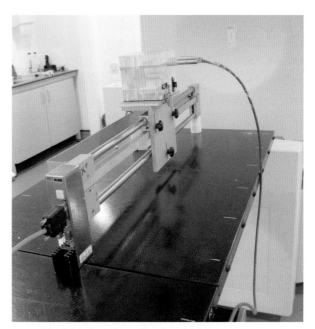

Fig. 3.20 One-dimensional single-detector scanner.

The variability in detector response was overcome in a linear array by checking and correcting the response of each detector on an individual basis before its practical use. Fig. 3.21 shows such a system, known as a Schuster array. An initial calibration of the array before its use would step through all 88 detectors in the array, placing each on the central axis of the radiation beam and determining calibration factors for each detector to provide a uniform response across the entire array. Following this calibration, the equipment users could confidently interpret the beam profiles and make adjustments to the RT beams as required.

Area Arrays

One of the earliest two-dimensional measurement devices used a radiofluorescent screen and imaging system which captured a digital image using a camera (Fig. 3.22). This enabled the beam fluence to be captured

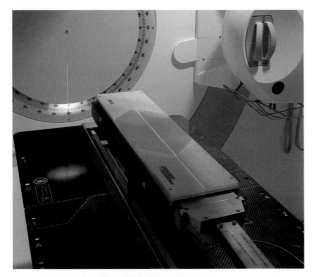

Fig. 3.21 Schuster array.

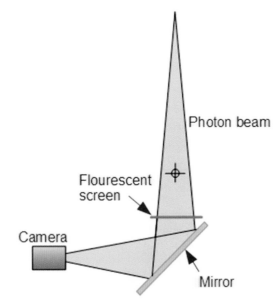

Fig. 3.22 The main components of a beam imaging system to measure fluence in two dimension.

for analysis. The system was a logical extension of film to a measurement system which would effectively process the image data to assess the fluence distribution, the beam size, and the field edges. The system was large, cumbersome, and did not lend itself to easy use.

With improved consistency of detector production and electronic processing performance, detector arrays which could be used with confidence of insignificant inherent detector variation became practically feasible. Modern, two-dimensional arrays are light-weight devices (Fig. 13.4), which can be used on couch tops or mounted to the radiation head of the machine. Detectors can be solid-state diodes or ion chambers depending upon the manufacturer. They provide real-time monitoring of beam profiles along major axes and diagonal axes of the radiation beam. They also enable intensity-modulated beam fluences to be readily measured and assessed as part of patient-specific quality control (PSQC)—see Chapter 13.

Digital two-dimensional fluence measurements whether from densitometered film or two-dimensional arrays require analysis software to fully use the information acquired. Commercial software packages were

developed for this and could be applied to any digital two-dimensional measurement.

Volume Detectors Arrays

The introduction of intensity-modulated treatment delivery has meant that there is a need for patient-specific checks to be undertaken, often on an individual patient basis. With the widespread adoption of volumetric intensity-modulated treatment delivery, the need to rapidly assess a treatment delivery in three dimensions as part of the patient pretreatment verification has made volumetric arrays essential. Although gel systems as described in the Gel Dosimetry, Fricke Gels and FXG Gels and Polymer Gels sections can provide high-resolution three-dimensional measurements, the processes they use are time consuming and lend themselves to research work and quality audit. For routine PSQC work the consistent performance of modern radiation detectors have enabled reliable three-dimensional arrays to be developed (see Fig. 13.5).

ELECTRONIC PORTAL DOSIMETRY

From the start of developing megavoltage electronic portal imaging devices (EPIDs) it was envisaged that such an imaging system could be used to measure the dose distribution within the patient by combining CT images of the patient with the beam fluence detected by the EPID. Initially, the CT data set was considered to be the planning data set. However, with cone beam CT routinely used to verify treatment setup, the CT data set acquired at treatment could now be used to improve accuracy. As has been seen in this chapter, physical radiation detectors need to be considered carefully and their performance understood to obtain accurate measurements. In addition, the beam model needs to be able to accurately model the dose distribution from the measured fluences. The value of portal dosimetry depends upon the measurement accuracy. Currently this accuracy is to within ±5% at best depending upon the physical situation with regard to the patient and beam delivery. This method of treatment verification is used clinically, often still on a trial and evaluation basis.

ALTERNATIVE SYSTEMS FOR PROTON BEAMS DOSE MEASUREMENT

There are three types of measurement to be considered in proton and carbon therapy clinical measurements:
- Relative dose measurements
- Reference dose measurements
- Absolute dose measurements

Relative measurements of proton beams refer to measurements proportional to dose but expressed in either units of percent or simple ratios. Because cyclotron beam intensity can vary, any measurements are referenced to the incoming primary beam. Relative measurements encompass lateral two-dimensional scans, and importantly depth-dose scans of the pristine Bragg peak and of the prescribed depth-dose or SOBP (see Chapter 9).

Many devices used in RT physics quality analysis are unsuitable for proton therapy purposes. X-ray film, Fricke and polymer gel, and TLD detectors are categorised as one-hit detectors and exhibit significant under-response in the low-energy Bragg peak region, where the proton tracks are highly ionising and therefore of high linear energy transfer. These devices may be used where only measurements at a single energy or depth is being monitored. Radiochromic films, based on density change by radiation-induced polymerisation, show a much reduced quenching effect, which has led to their wider adoption in proton therapy quality control of field area homogeneity and aperture verification checks.

Measurement of the pristine Bragg peak at particular energies, and also the prescribed SOBP, is performed by central axis depth-dose scans as in photon and electron radiotherapy beams. The gold standard for proton and carbon beam depth-dose measurement is considered to be the use of a waterproof parallel-plate ion chamber in a water tank. The ion chamber, if used at an appropriate bias potential, does not exhibit Bragg peak quenching and there is no evidence of significant ion recombination effect changes with energy.

For the convenience of rapid measurement, flat silicon photo-diodes have been used with rotating polymethacrylate (PMMA) wheels, offering a variable depth. The latter has to be converted to water-equivalent depth by correcting with PMMA/water stopping-power ratios. It should be noted that in certain cases, semiconductor diodes can exhibit slight over-response at the Bragg peak, and a gradually reduced sensitivity induced by radiation damage. It should be noted that recent work with microdiamond detectors, which are essentially a carbon detector and close to being water equivalent, has demonstrated excellent spatial resolution and both negligible quenching at the proton Bragg peak and negligible response fading with accumulated dose. Although water tank measurements are well suited for horizontal beam orientations, these measurements are more problematic for rotating gantry treatment beams. In these cases, a solid multilayer Faraday cup device which consists of conducting foils sandwiched between insulating absorbers is employed. This yields charge-with-depth information, and in particular the distal fall-off depth, from which beam energy can be obtained. There are commercial devices which provide multilayer ion chambers, sandwiched between solid water-equivalent plastic absorbers.

Raster or spot-scanned beams also require measurements of the reproducibility of individual spots at a particular energy or depth layers. For this purpose, two-dimensional diode or ion chamber arrays are available which automatically analyse and store results. Miniature ion chamber arrays are becoming the preferred choice to avoid any dose degradation and energy dependence issues.

Three-dimensional dose distributions are particularly problematic for small proton fields and when measuring in the vicinity of high dose gradients. This is because of the limited choice of detectors, whether semiconductor diodes or miniature ion chambers. More recently, pin-point thimble ion chambers with volumes less than 0.03 cm^3 have become available (PTW N31015), offering excellent spatial resolution for higher energy proton beams. The use of PRESSAGE® radiochromic gels has also shown promise in showing small three-dimensional dose distributions, but have a quenching under response which requires correction.

REFERENCES

[1] Beddar AS, Mackie TR, Attix FH. Water-equivalent plastic scintillation detectors for high-energy beam dosimetry: 1. Physical characteristics and theoretical considerations. Phys Med Biol 1992;37:1883–900.

[2] Fluhs D, Heintz M, Indenkampen F, Wieczorek C, Kolanoski H, Quast U. Direct reading measurement of absorbed dose with plastic scintillators—the general concept and applications to ophthalmic plaque dosimetry. Med Phys 1996;23:427–34.

[3] Kirov AS, Piao JZ, Mathur NK, et al. The three-dimensional scintillation dosimetry method: test for a ^{106}Ru eye plaque applicator. Phys Med Biol 50:3063–3081.

[4] Marie and Pierre Curie, "Quartz piezo electrometer," *The College of Physicians of Philadelphia Digital Library*, https://www.cppdigitallibrary.org/items/show/2593.

[5] DuSautoy AR. The UK primary standard calorimeter for photon beam absorbed dose measurement. Phys Med Biol 1996;41:137–51.

[6] Marsh ARS, Williams TT. 50 kV Primary standard of exposure: design of free-air chamber. NPL Report RS(Ext) 54, 182. Teddington: National Physical Laboratory; 1982.

[7] Palmer JA, Duane S, Shipley R, Moretti CJ. The design and construction of a new primary standard free air chamber for medium energy x-rays. Med Biol Eng Comput 1997;35:1086.

[8] Morgan AA, Aird EGA, Aukett RJ, et al. IPEM guidelines on dosimeter systems for use as transfer instruments between UK primary dosimetry standards laboratory (NPL) and radiotherapy centres. Phys Med Biol 2000;45:2445–57.

[9] Nutbrown RF, Duane S, Shipley DR, Thomas RAS. Evaluation of factors to convert absorbed dose calibrations from graphite to water for the NPL high-energy photon calibration service. Phys Med Biol 2002;47:441–54.

[10] Rosser KE, Owen B, DuSautoy AR, Pritchard DH, Stoker I, Brend CJ. The NPL absorbed dose to water calibration service for high-energy photons. In: Proceedings of symposium on measurement assurance in dosimetry. IAEA-SM-330/35. Vienna: IAEA; 1994. p. 73–81.

[11] NPL. Practical course in reference dosimetry. National Physical Laboratory; 2006.

[12] Lillicrap SC, Owen B, Williams JR, Williams PC. Code of practice for high-energy photon therapy dosimetry based on the NPL absorbed dose calibration service. Phys Med Biol 1990;35:1355–60.

[13] IAEA. Absorbed dose determination in external beam radiotherapy. An international code of practice for dosimetry based on standards of absorbed dose to water. IAEA TRS-398. Vienna: IAEA; 2000.

[14] Farmer FT. A substandard x-ray dose-meter. Br J Radiol 1955;28:304.

[15] Shonka RF, Rose JE, Failla G. Conducting plastic equivalent to tissue, air and polystyrene. In: 2nd United Nations conference on peaceful uses of atomic energy. New York: UN; 1958. p. 160.

[16] IPEM. The IPEMB code of practice for the determination of absorbed dose for x-rays below 300 kV generating potential (0.035 mm Al–4 mm Cu HVL; 10–300 kV generating potential). Phys Med Biol 1996;41:2605–25.

[17] IPEM. Addendum to the IPEMB code of practice for the determination of absorbed dose for x-rays below 300 kV generating potential (0.035 mm Al–4 mm Cu HVL; 10–300 kV generating potential). Phys Med Biol 2005;50:2739–48.

[18] IPSM. Code of practice for high-energy photon therapy dosimetry based on the NPL absorbed dose calibration service. Phys Med Biol 1990;35:1355–60.

[19] IPEM. The IPEM code of practice for electron dosimetry for radiotherapy beams of initial energy from 4 to 25 MeV based on an absorbed dose to water calibration. Phys Med Biol 2003;48:2929–70.

[20] Barish RJ, Lerch IA. Long-term use of an isotope check source for verification of ion chamber calibration. Med Phys 1992;17:203–6.

[21] Burns JE, Rosser KE. Saturation corrections for the NPL 2560/1 dosemeter in photon dosimetry. Phys Med Biol 1991;35:687–93.

[22] Havercroft JM, Klevenhagen SC. Ion chamber corrections for parallel-plate and thimble chambers in electron and photon radiation. Phys Med Biol 1993;38:25–38.

[23] Lewis DF. A processless electronic recording medium. In: Electronic imaging proceedings of SPSE's symposium. Arlington, springfield, VA: Society for imaging science and Technology; 1986. p. 76–9.

[24] Grusell E, Rikner G. Evaluation of temperature effects in p-type silicon detectors. Phys Med Biol 1986;31:527–34.

[25] Rikner G. Silicon diodes as detectors in radiation dosimetry of photon, electron and proton radiation fields. Thesis, Sweden: Uppsala; 1983.

[26] Shi J, Simon WE, Ding L, Saini D. Important issues regarding diode performance in radiation therapy applications. In: Proceedings of the 22nd annual Engineering in Medicine and Biology Society (EMBC), annual international conference, Chicago; 2000.

[27] Rikner G, Grusell E. Effects of radiation damage on p-type silicon diodes. Phys Med Biol 1983;28:1261–7.

[28] Khrunov VS, Martynov SS, Vatnitsky SM, et al. Diamond detectors in relative dosimetry of photon, electron and proton radiation fields. Radiat Prot Dosimetry 1990;33:155–7.

[29] Kron T. Thermoluminescence dosimetry and its applications in medicine: Part 1. Physics, materials and equipment. Australas Phys Eng Sci Med 1994;17:175–99.

[30] Jafari SM, Bradley DA, Goldstone CA, Sharpe PHG, Alalawi AI, Jordan TJ, Clark CH, Nisbet A, Spyrou NM. Low cost commercial glass beads as dosimeters in radiotherapy. Radiat Phys Chem 2014;97:95–101.

[31] Jafari SM, Jordan TJ, Hussein M, Bradley DA, Clark CH, Nisbet A, Spyrou NM. Energy response of glass bead TLDs irradiated with radiation therapy beams. Phys Med Biol 2014;59:6875–89.

[32] Fricke H, Morse S. The chemical action of roentgen rays on dilute ferrous sulphate solutions as a measure of radiation dose. Am J Roentgenol Radium Ther Nucl Med 1927;18:430–2.

[33] Gore JC, Kang YS, Schulz RJ. Measurement of radiation dose distributions by nuclear magnetic resonance (NMR) imaging. Phys Med Biol 1984;29:1189–97.

[34] Baldock C, Harris PJ, Piercy AR, Healy B. Experimental determination of the diffusion coefficient in two dimensions in ferrous sulphate gels using the finite element method. Australas Phys Eng Sci Med 2001;24:19–30.

[35] Appleby A, Leghrouz A. Imaging of radiation dose by visible colour development in ferrous-agarose-xylenol orange gels. Med Phys 1991;18:309–12.

[36] Maryanski MJ, Gore JC, Kennan RP, Schulz RJ. NMR relaxation enhancement in gels polymerized and cross-linked by ionizing radiations: a new approach to 3D dosimetry by MRI. Magn Reson Imaging 1993;11:253–8.

[37] Maryanski MJ, Schuklz RJ, Ibbott GS, et al. Magnetic resonance imaging of radiation dose distributions using polymer gel dosimeter. Phys Med Biol 1994;39:1437–55.

[38] Fong PM, Keil DC, Does MD, Gore JC. Polymer gels for magnetic resonance imaging of radiation dose distributions at normal room atmosphere. Phys Med Biol 2001;46:3105–13.

[39] Bradshaw WW, Cadena DG, Crawford GW, Spelzler HAW. The use of alanine as solid dosimeter. Radiat Res 1962;17:11.

[40] Regulla DF, Deffner U. Dosimetry by ESR spectroscopy of alanine. Appl Radiat Isot 1982;33:1101.

[41] Olsson S, Sagstuen E, Bonora M, Lund A. EPR Dosimetric properties of 2-methylalanine: EPR, ENDOR and FT-EPR investigations. Radiat Res 2002;V157:113–121.

[42] Mascarenhas S, Hasegawa A, Takeshita K. EPR dosimetry of bones from the Hiroshima A-bomb site. Bull Am Phys Soc 1973;18:579.

[43] Guskova AK, Barabanova AV, Baranov AY. Acute radiation effects in victims of the Chernobyl nuclear power plant accident. In: UNSCEAR report on sources and effects of ionizing radiation, Appendix 613–631. New York: United Nations; 1988.

[44] Feinendegen LE, Muhlensiepen H, Porchen W, Booz J. Acute non-stochastic effect of very low dose whole body exposure, a thymidine equivalent serum factor. Int J Radiat Biol 1982;41:139–50.

[45] Bender MA, Awa AA, Brooks AL, et al. Current status of cytogenetic procedures to detect and quantify previous exposures to radiation. Mutat Res 1988;196:103–59.

[46] Prosser JS, Lloyd DC, Edwards AA. A comparison of chromosomal and micronuclear methods for radiation accident dosimetry. In: Goldfinch EP, editor. Radiation protection: theory and practice. New York: Institute of Physics; 1989. p. 133–6.

[47] Damen P. Design of a water calorimeter for medium energy x-rays: a status report. CCRI(I)/05-38, NMi Van Swinden Laboratorium, Netherlands; 2005.

[48] Krauss A. The PTB water calorimeter for the absolute determination of absorbed dose to water in 60Co radiation. Metrologia 2006;43(3):259–272.

[49] Palmans H and Seuntjens JP Construction, correction factors and relative heat defect of a high purity 4° Calorimeter for absorbed dose determinations in high-energy photon beams. NPL Calorimeter Workshop, 1214; 1994.

[50] Ross CK, Seuntjens JP, Klassen NV, Shortt KR. The NRC sealed water calorimeter: correction factors and performance. Proc NPL Workshop on Recent Advances in Calorimetric Absorbed Dose Standards – ed. Williams AJ & Rosser KE, 90–102, NPL Teddington; 2000.

[51] Willaims AJ, Rosser KE, Thomson NJ, DuSautoy AR. Recent advances in water calorimetry at NPL. Proc 22nd Annual EMBS International Conference, Chicago; 2000.

Radiation Protection

Mike Dunn

INTRODUCTION

The biological effects of ionising radiation are described in detail in Chapter 17 of this book, and are summarised in the following section. Because there are known risks of radiation exposure, levels of acceptable risk have been specified by international expert groups, principally the International Commission on Radiological Protection (ICRP). Based upon these acceptable risks, dose limits have been recommended and in most cases adopted into national legislative requirements.

To understand these dose limits and the associated risks, it is necessary to have an understanding of the dose units that they are measured in and this chapter will explain these dose values. In addition, as there are known risks of radiation, most countries have regulatory requirements that have to be met to limit the risk to radiation workers, patients and members of the public arising from the use of radiation. The legislative requirements within the United Kingdom will be described and some of the methodology used to comply with these, including personal radiation monitoring, equipment testing, appropriate construction of radiation areas and the administrative arrangements surrounding the application of radiation.

BIOLOGICAL EFFECTS OF RADIATION

The block diagram (Fig. 4.1) details the various biological effects that radiation may cause resulting from the absorption of energy associated with the radiation. As will be seen later, different areas of the body have different degrees of radiation sensitivity, which is mirrored in the fact that there are different dose limits for specific areas of the human body.

Almost since the discovery of ionising radiation, its potential for causing deleterious effects has been known. These effects are caused by the absorption by the human body of the energy associated with the radiation. Such energy absorption can cause ionisation (charged particles) and excitation in the body and or subsequent chemical changes by the formation of such things as free radicals. The end result, however, is a potential for some form of biological change or damage to occur. A measure of this absorbed energy is a fundamental value used for radiotherapy treatment and has been given the units of gray (Gy) (see Chapter 2).

These changes can cause three types of effects, which are summarised subsequently. The first two effects have no known threshold dose below which the effects will not occur and are the origin of the concept of there being no safe dose of radiation.

Stochastic Hereditary Effects

These effects are expressed not in the exposed individual but in the exposed individual's subsequent offspring or future generations. Effects such as one eye a different colour from the other or, more grossly, one limb shorter or missing, are examples. Genetic defects appear in the population as a result of many causes, radiation being just one of them, with about 1 in 200 live births having a genetic defect expressed. As such, the possibility of radiation being the cause of any defect can only be shown statistically, the probability being dose dependent, rising with dose. The current risk estimated by ICRP 103 [1] of severe hereditary effects from radiation is one in 500,000 for a radiation dose of 1 mSv (see later), that is, about 2500 mSv would double the natural occurrence of genetic defects (1 in 200 to 2 in 200). This is significantly less than the previous risk estimation in the previous ICRP 60 [2].

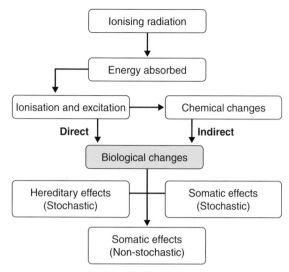

Fig. 4.1 Effects of radiation.

The ICRP notes that there remains no direct evidence from human epidemiologic studies of heritable effects of radiation exposure and justifies the inclusion of a component of heritable risk in detriment estimates based on observed mutational effects in experimental animals.

Stochastic Somatic Effects

These effects are expressed in the exposed individual in the form of cancer induction. Again, cancer has a number of causes, radiation being only one. About 4 in 10 of the population is likely to have a cancer in their lifetime. The probability of this being caused by radiation increases with dose. The current risk estimated by ICRP 103 [1] of a cancer from radiation is 1 in 18,000 for a radiation dose of 1 mSv (see later). The extra cancer risk from very low doses is extremely small and, in practice, undetectable in the population. However, the extra cancer risk at higher doses may be detectable using statistical methods. Even after high-dose exposure, it is rarely possible to be certain that radiation was directly responsible for a cancer arising in an individual. There are a number of scientific uncertainties in making these estimates of cancer risk at low doses. In 2000, the highly respected United Nations Scientific Committee on the Effects of Atomic Radiation [3] suggested that uncertainties in cancer risk estimates may be about twofold higher or lower for acute doses where cancer risk can be directly assessed and a further factor of two (higher or lower) for the projection of these risks to very low doses and low dose rates.

Nonstochastic Somatic Effects

These effects, sometimes known as *deterministic*, are expressed in the exposed individual in the form of acute effects of radiation, such as radiation burns, hair loss, sterility, vomiting and diarrhoea. These effects will only occur once the level of dose received exceeds the threshold dose for that effect, with the severity of the effect increasing with dose beyond the threshold. Dependent on the area irradiated and the level of dose received, such effects will be displayed by patients undergoing radiotherapy exposures. A picture showing some of these effects is given in Fig. 4.2. Details of dose thresholds that need to be exceeded for different effects are given in Table 4.1. These thresholds should be considered as minimum dose thresholds and may vary upwards due to variance in the physiology of the target organ. e.g. skin vascularity and period of time over which the radiation dose is received.

The risk factors quoted previously have been assessed from data arising from five main sources of information. These are the effects

noted shortly after the discovery of radiation, evidence from radiation accidents, effects of the atomic bombs exploded in Hiroshima and Nagasaki during World War II, evidence from radiotherapy treatments and results from animal experiments. These information sources have given data relating to the effects of relatively high doses of radiation, and an assumption is made currently that there is a linear no threshold (LNT) relationship between dose and risk from these high-dose data points by extrapolation to the lower dose levels encountered as part of occupational exposure to staff working with radiation, with an assumption that no dose threshold exists below which no stochastic effect will occur. This assumption has not been proven and the relationship may not be linear, which would mean that we could be either over- or underestimating the stochastic risks of cancer by using the LNT response model.

DOSE DESCRIPTORS

Two different dose quantities have been quoted in the aforementioned text. These are sieverts (Sv) and Gy.

Gy is a measure of absorbed dose or energy in joules per kilogram as described in Chapter 2. Two other quantities are relevant when discussing radiation protection matters, these are *equivalent dose* and *effective dose* which have the units of Sieverts to indicate a change in dose descriptor.

Equivalent Dose

The same absorbed dose delivered by different types of radiation may result in different degrees of biological damage to body tissues. The total energy deposited is not the only factor which determines the extent of the damage. The equivalent dose was introduced to take into account the dependence of the harmful biological effects on the type of radiation being absorbed. The equivalent dose is therefore a measure of the risk associated with an exposure to ionising radiation. Risks caused by exposures to different radiation types can be directly compared when expressed in terms of equivalent dose.

The unit of equivalent dose is Sv and is defined for a given type of radiation by the relationship:

$$\text{Equivalent dose (Sv) } H = \text{Absorbed dose (Gy)} \times \text{Radiation weighting factor } W_R$$

4.1

The radiation weighting factor is a dimensionless number which depends on the way in which the energy of the radiation is distributed along its path through the tissue.

The rate of deposition of energy along the track is known as the *linear energy transfer* (LET) of the radiation and has units of keV μm^{-1} measured in water which is considered equivalent to tissue.

Radiation with a high LET (such as protons and alpha particles) is more likely than radiation with a low LET (such as x-rays or beta particles) to damage the small structures in tissue such as deoxyribonucleic acid molecules. This is because the energy from high LET radiation is absorbed in a small volume surrounding the trail of dense ionisation produced by this radiation. The radiation weighting factor is directly related to the LET of the radiation. The radiation weighting factors given in ICRP 103 [3] are used to correct for differences in the biological damage to tissue caused by chronic exposure to different radiations (Table 4.2).

Effective Dose

Equivalent dose accounts for the varying biological effects of different types of radiation on a particular tissue type or organ,. However, it

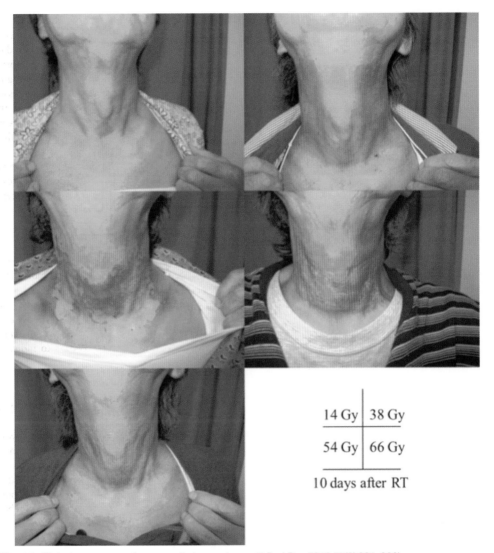

14 Gy | 38 Gy

54 Gy | 66 Gy

10 days after RT

Fig. 4.2 Clinical symptoms of acute radiation erythema (J Rad Res 2016;57(3):301–306).

TABLE 4.1 Dose Thresholds for Biological Effects		
Threshold Dose (Gy)	**Area Irradiated**	**Effect**
>0.15	Testes	Temporary sterility
>0.5	Eye	Cataracts
>2.0	Skin	Burns
>2.5	Gonads	Permanent sterility
>20	Central nervous system	Death in hours

From ICRP 60. Ann ICRP 1991;21(1–3). ICRP Publication 60. 1990 Recommendations of the International Commission on Radiological Protection. Pergamon Press.

TABLE 4.2 Weighting Factors for Different Types of Radiation	
Radiation Type and Energy Range	**Radiation Weighting Factor (W_R)**
Photons—all energies	1
Electrons—all energies	1
Protons	2
Alpha particles	20

From ICRP103:2007:37 (2-4). ICRP Publication 103. The 2007 Recommendations of the International Commission on Radiological Protection. Elsevier.

should come as no surprise to find out that the same radiation exposure to different parts of the body can have very different results. If the entire body were irradiated with a uniform beam of a single type of radiation, some parts of the body would react more dramatically than others. To take this effect into account, the ICRP have developed a list of tissue weighting factors, denoted W_T, for a number of organs and tissues that most significantly contribute to an overall effective biological damage

to the body. It should be noted that areas of the body with a high cell turnover are more radiosensitive than areas with a slower cell turnover and thus have a larger weighting factor. Table 4.3 presents values of the tissue-weighting factor W_T based upon standard man which is a 70-kg male. Figures would be different for females, for instance, as they have more radiosensitive breast tissue. As such, the effective dose for a

TABLE 4.3 W_T Values

Tissue Weighting Factors According to ICRP103 (ICRP 2007)

Tissue	Tissue Weighting Factor W_T	$\sum W_T$
Bone marrow (red), colon, lung, stomach, breast, remaining tissue[a]	0.12	0.72
Gonads	0.08	0.08
Bladder, liver, oesophagus, thyroid	0.04	0.16
Bone surface, brain, salivary glands, skin	0.01	0.04
Total		**1.00**

[a]Remaining tissues—adrenals, extra thoracic region, gall bladder, heart, kidneys, lymphatic nodes, muscle, oral mucosa, pancreas, prostate (♂), small intestine, spleen, thymus, uterus/cervix (♀).
From ICRP103:2007:37 (2-4). ICRP Publication 103. The 2007 Recommendations of the International Commission on Radiological Protection. Elsevier.

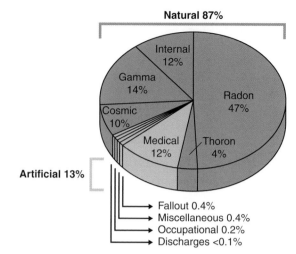

Fig. 4.3 The average background radiation levels in the UK is 2.7 mSv per year from the sources detailed in this pie chart. (Courtesy of the National Radiation Protection Board now the Health Protection Agency.)

particular examination should not be viewed as a precise figure, but merely a figure giving an indication of relative risk.

To arrive at an effective dose for a particular examination, it is necessary to determine the equivalent dose to the different listed tissues or body parts, multiply these doses by the relevant tissue weighting factor and then sum the constituent parts. The units of effective dose are the Sievert and a worked example is given in Table 4.4.

BACKGROUND RADIATION

We are all exposed to radiation, regardless of our occupation, from natural radiation sources in the environment and from man-made sources. We have no control over the level of exposure to these sources of natural radiation other than by choosing a particular lifestyle. For example, cosmic rays from outer space are attenuated by the Earth's atmosphere and the more atmosphere there is, the more the attenuation. This means that people who live at high altitudes or travel in high flying aircraft will get a greater radiation dose from cosmic rays. Other sources of natural radiation and the proportions that they contribute to the overall dose are shown in Fig. 4.3.

The major sources of natural radiation are the radioactive gases radon and thoron. Together they contribute over 50% of the average background radiation dose in the United Kingdom. These gases are generated in granite rock and, as a consequence, the intensity of the radon exposure varies considerably around the world, being higher in areas where there is more granite rock. In addition, if the rock is cracked, the gas can escape into the environment more easily leading to higher levels in the environment. Such a situation exists in Cornwall where the level of radon gas is up to 3 times the national average. This has consequences in terms of the gas entering the homes of people living in these areas. Because the trend is to insulate homes more rigorously, this can have the effect of trapping the gas in the homes, leading to elevated doses to the inhabitants. Constructing well-ventilated houses and incorporating a special membrane into the foundation of new houses can alleviate this. Installing extraction fans and increasing under-floor ventilation may improve older properties. These natural sources contribute an average dose of about 2.3 mSv per annum to a member of the UK population.

Another 0.4 mSv per annum is contributed to by artificial or man-made sources, such as discharges from nuclear power stations, making the average total dose 2.7 mSv. However, the biggest contribution is from the diagnostic uses of radiation where, although the individual doses are small, a large number of x-rays are performed with, on average, every member of the UK population undergoing at least one x-ray examination per year. Because this is a controllable exposure to some

TABLE 4.4   Effective Dose From a Chest X-Ray With a Skin Entrance Dose of 500 μGy

Organ	% Entrance Dose	Dose (μGy)	Equivalent Dose (μSv)	Weighting Factor	Tissue Weighted Dose (μSv)
Gonads	0.2	1	1	0.08	0.08
Breast	2	10	10	0.12	1.2
Bone marrow (red)	1	5	5	0.12	0.6
Lung	30	150	150	0.12	18
Thyroid	1	5	5	0.04	0.20
Bone	1	5	5	0.01	0.05
Heart	10	50	50	0.01	1.25
Stomach	5	25	25	0.12	3
Liver	10	50	50	0.04	2.0
			Effective dose (μSv) =		26.38

Based on the above ICRP figure of 1 in 18,000 cancer incidences per mSv, this implies an additional risk of 1 in 682,335.

extent, a great deal of effort has been put into reducing both the individual dose per patient and the number of examinations carried out. This has been brought about by both legislative requirements (see later) and good practice guidelines.

LEGISLATIVE REQUIREMENTS

Until 1985, there were no legislative requirements specifically relating to the use of radiation in place within the United Kingdom. The use of radiation in medicine was relatively well self-regulated by compliance with good practice guidelines developed by the professionals involved. The United Kingdom's membership of the European Community required the Government to enact a number of legislative requirements, which are common across the Community. The withdrawal of the UK from the European Community will not affect this, and the regulations have recently been revised. These will now be discussed in some detail.

The Ionising Radiations Regulations 2017

The Ionising Radiations Regulations 2017 [4] revised the Ionising Radiations Regulations 1999 and deal with the protection of workers and members of the public from ionising radiation from any source. The Approved Code of Practice—*Work with ionising radiation* [5]—supports these. These documents are legally enforceable, and breaches of their requirements could lead to prosecution by the regulators, normally the Health and Safety Executive. Good practice guidance is given in the Medical and Dental Guidance Notes [6]. The Ionising Radiations Regulations require three basic requirements to be met; these are:

1. That no practice involving radiation be adopted unless there is a positive net benefit, either to the exposed individuals or to society, that is, it can be justified.
2. All exposures must be as low as reasonably achievable or practicable. This is often referred to as the ALARA or ALARP principle. The principle requires that any particular source, the number of people being exposed, and the likelihood of incurring exposures where these are not certain to be received, be optimised to a minimum, taking account of social and economic factors. In practice, there may be a number of options where an assessment would show that costs are not grossly disproportionate. The option, or combination of options, which achieves the lowest level of residual risk, should be implemented, provided grossly disproportionate costs are not incurred. In general, the greater the risk, the more that should be spent in reducing it, and the greater the bias on the side of safety. The judgment as to whether measures are grossly disproportionate should reflect societal risk, that is to say, large numbers of people (employees or the public) being killed at one go. This is because society has a greater aversion to an accident killing 10 people than to 10 accidents killing one person each.
3. Dose equivalents to individuals do not exceed certain dose limits. The exposure of individuals resulting from the combination of all relevant practices should be subject to dose limits, or to some control of risk in the case of potential exposures. These are aimed at ensuring that no individual is exposed to radiation risks that are judged to be unacceptable from these practices in any normal circumstances.

The original regulations were enacted in 1985 and were revised in 1999 and again in 2017.

The revision of the 1985 regulations was brought about largely because of a reassessment of the risks of radiation. The new assessment indicated that the risks had previously been underestimated by a factor of about 3 times. This has meant a reduction in the whole-body dose limit by a factor of about three. The reassessment was based on the fact that many of the biological data were based upon the effects observed in the victims of the Hiroshima and Nagasaki bombs. The effects observed were equated to dosimetry data gathered from atomic bombs dropped in the Nevada desert. Unfortunately, the atmospheric conditions in the Nevada desert are very dry in comparison to the humid conditions in Hiroshima and Nagasaki. These humid conditions attenuated the radiation to a greater degree than the atmospheric conditions in the Nevada desert by a difference of about three. Consequently the biological effects observed in Hiroshima and Nagasaki were occurring at levels of dose some 3 times lower than originally thought. This led to a requirement to reduce the previous dose limits by a factor of about three. The revision of the 1999 regulations has occurred in part because of a reassessment of the risk of radiation to the lens of the eye. This led to a requirement to reduce the previous dose limit from 150 to 20 mSv per year. Another change introduced by the 2017 regulations was a three-tier system of informing the Health and Safety Executive of uses of ionising radiation. This is known as the *graded approach* because what needs to be applied for depends on the size and likelihood of exposure. The risk increasing as you go down the list with an increasing fee payable. Depending on the level of risk of the ionising radiation work that is undertaken, an application will need to be made to either:

- notify
- register
- or get consent

Applications are made electronically at: https://services.hse.gov.uk/Account/Login/Register?returnUrl=/en-US/Account/Manage/ConfirmEmailRequest

Risk Assessments

Before any work being undertaken with ionising radiation, the employer is responsible for carrying out a risk assessment. This is in common with the requirement under the Management of Health and Safety at Work Regulations [7] to carry out risk assessments for other work involving hazards. The purpose of this risk assessment is to identify the measures needed to restrict the exposure of employees and other persons to ionising radiation. The assessment must be suitable and sufficient enough to demonstrate that all hazards, with the potential to cause a radiation accident, have been identified and the nature and magnitude of the risks arising from those hazards have been evaluated. Where the risk assessment identifies a radiation risk, the employer must take all reasonable steps to prevent any such accident, limit the consequences of any accident that does occur and provide employees with the information, instruction and training to restrict their exposure. These risk assessments should normally be recorded and reviewed regularly to ensure their continued relevance. The factors that should be considered in performing a radiation risk assessment are given in the Approved Code of Practice [5] and include such things as the nature of the sources and the estimated radiation dose rates to which anyone can be exposed.

Dose Limits

The annual dose limit has remained largely unchanged for the past 40 years and, despite the new dosimetric evidence, the absolute whole-body dose limit per year remains at 50 mSv. However, such a level of dose is only allowable in special circumstances as the dose averaged over a 5-year period must not exceed 20 mSv per year for those occupationally exposed and aged over 18 years. For those employees under 18 years old, the whole-body dose limit is 6 mSv per year. The current dose limits are summarised in Table 4.5. It should be noted that there are currently no dose limits for patients undergoing examination or treatment with radiation, only that their doses must be as low as reasonably practicable and that any dose given must be justified in terms of

TABLE 4.5	**Current Dose Limits**		
	Classified Workers and Trainees Under 18 Years	Unclassified Workers	Members of the Public
Whole body	20	6	1
Individual organ	500	150	50
Lens of eye	20	15	15
Fetus of pregnant worker	1	1	

Dose limits per year in mSv.

the risk to the patient from not carrying out the exposure (see The Ionising Radiation (Medical Exposure) Regulations (IRMER) [8] later).

There are two things to note in Table 4.5. First, there are different dose limits for different areas of the body because different organs within the body have different radiosensitivities and radiation exposures are very often nonuniform. Areas of the body where cell division is quicker are more radiosensitive. An area of the body with the quickest cell division and therefore the most radiosensitive is the fetus. This, in regulatory terms, is considered to be a member of the public from the point of the dose limit to be applied. A dose limit of 1 mSv to the fetus equates to a dose to the abdomen of the mother of about 2 mSv for diagnostic x-ray energy radiation, and is the limit that the employer has to apply for the declared term of the pregnancy. As such, the period of time for the dose limit to be exceeded starts when the worker declares herself to be pregnant to her employer. Secondly, there are three groups of people with different dose limits, classified workers, unclassified workers and members of the public. Classified workers are those workers who, by virtue of the work they undertake, are likely to exceed the dose limits for unclassified workers. Before a worker can be classified, they are required to be declared fit to do so by a relevant doctor or employment medical adviser. This is a registered medical practitioner who has been appointed in writing to undertake the role of a relevant doctor. Once a worker has been classified, the employer is legally obliged to issue the worker with an individual radiation dosimeter and keep a cumulative dose record until the person to whom the record relates has or would have attained the age of 75 years but in any event for at least 30 years from when the record was made. This must be undertaken by a Health and Safety Executive (HSE) approved dosimetry and record keeping service. An annual report is sent to a body known as the *Central Index for Dose Information* of the doses received by all classified persons, with the intention of being able to undertake epidemiologic studies in subsequent years and to provide a central record of doses received by a classified worker which, if the worker changes employers, is passed onto their new employer. Reports of any investigation into a real or suspected overexposure of a member of staff patients or visitors must be kept until the person to whom the record relates has or would have attained the age of 75 years but in any event for at least 30 years from the date of the relevant accident. The HSE has defined an exposure significantly more than intended as being the reporting criteria to be used in determining if a patient has been overexposed because of equipment failure. This information is given in Appendix 2 of the Guidance Note PM77 [9]—*Equipment used in connection with medical exposure.* This specifies that notification to the HSE should be made if the dose given to a patient from beam therapy or brachytherapy arising from equipment failure exceeds 1.1 times the intended dose for a whole course or 1.2 times the intended dose for any fraction. For unsealed radionuclide therapy, the guideline multiple is 1.2 for any administration where the overdose occurred because of equipment failure.

Although a large number of hospital staff are individually monitored with a radiation dosimeter, very few are classified radiation workers. Possible exceptions are staff, such as radiopharmacists, interventional radiologists and radiotherapists, handling sealed brachytherapy sources although with the advent of high-dose rate after-loading brachytherapy devices, this is becoming less and less common. Radiation monitoring has shown that the vast majority of hospital staff receives less than 0.1 mSv per year from the work they undertake. Nevertheless, employers are obliged to demonstrate that staff working with radiation do not require to become classified and the best way of doing this is to provide them with a radiation monitor. The regulations can be interpreted as requiring that any dose monitoring records of nonclassified staff are kept for a minimum of 2 years.

The whole-body effective dose limit for all other persons including anyone below the age of 16 years is 1 mSv per year with equivalent dose limits for specific areas in the body as detailed in Table 4.5.

Carers and Comforters

A special case is made in the regulations for members of the public who are carers and comforters of patients undergoing or who may have undergone a medical exposure, for example, a parent who holds a child while being x-rayed or a member of the family of a patient treated with radioactive material who is discharged from hospital with relatively large amounts of radioactive material still in their bodies. To fall into this category, the carer has to knowingly and willingly accept the risks in providing comfort and support to the patient. This means that the carer must be provided with information about the risks by the hospital treating the patient. In this case, there are no specific dose limits for the carer, however, information should be given to them regarding steps to be taken to control, as far as reasonably practicable, the dose they receive. Public Health England, a body set up by the Government to provide impartial advice on radiation protection matters amongst other things, has recommended that, in this context, the exposure received by persons acting as carers and comforters should not in general exceed 5 mSv from their involvement in one series or course of treatment. Normally, it should be possible to design procedures that will keep doses received by carers below this level.

There will also be occasions when members of the public who are not carers and comforters and therefore cannot knowingly or willingly be exposed to radiation, come into contact with patients who have undergone a therapeutic administration of a radiopharmaceutic, for example, sharing public transport or accommodation. In such cases, an effective dose limit of 5 mSv in any period of 5 consecutive years is used. In practice, sufficient action is normally taken by hospitals following accepted practice on release of such patients from hospital for this not to be a problem.

Controlled and Supervised Radiation Areas

If the dose limits are to be adhered to, it is necessary to impose strict controls on how and where radiation generating equipment and radioactive materials are used. Such equipment and material should be housed in areas where sufficient protection is afforded by the surrounding structures so that people in adjacent areas will not get a significant exposure. Where persons are required to enter radiation areas or adjacent locales, then engineering controls and design considerations must be used to protect them. For example, concrete walls and door interlocks to terminate an exposure if entry to the treatment room is made, are preferable to mobile lead screens, which may be placed incorrectly or written instruction prohibiting entry, which may not be obeyed.

Radiation areas are defined under UK legislation as being either a controlled or a supervised radiation area. These should have been identified as part of the risk assessment (see previously).

A controlled area is any area where persons entering are required to follow special procedures to limit the risk of a significant exposure contained within local safety rules, (see later) or where they are likely to receive an effective dose of more than 6 mSv per year or an equivalent dose greater than three-tenths of any other applicable dose limit. A controlled area must, wherever possible, be defined with reference to physical boundaries; for example, the whole of an x-ray room must be defined as a controlled area, even though the dose definition of a controlled area would mean that the controlled area perhaps does not extend more than 2 metres from the x-ray tube and patient. Once a controlled area has been defined, access into it must be controlled, wherever practicable radiation warning signs and notices are required to be placed on entrances to the area, explaining the nature of the radiation, for example, x-rays, gamma rays and so on, and the control measures to help avoid the risk, for examples signs saying, 'Do not enter when red light is on'. An example of such signing is given in Fig. 4.4.

Where a source of radiation is mobile, for example, a mobile x-ray unit used on several wards, then such signing would be impracticable and is therefore not used. However, a controlled area is still defined and controlled by the radiographer, for example, 2 metres around the x-ray set and patient and anywhere in the main beam until it is sufficiently attenuated by a solid object or distance.

In a medical situation, access to a controlled area is limited to four groups of people; these are:

1. The patient undergoing the exposure, for whom there are stringent controls both on the equipment that is used and the process. These are governed by the Ionising Radiation (Medical Exposure) Regulations 2017 (see later).
2. Classified workers who are subjected to individual monitoring. Where a classified worker of another employer enters someone else's controlled area, then the owner of the controlled area must make an entry into a passbook carried by the classified worker. This gives an estimate of the dose received by the classified worker while working in the controlled area [10].

3. Unclassified radiation workers and others who have been issued with written schemes of work which, if followed, ensure that they do not receive a dose greater than any applicable dose limit. Where an unclassified worker enters a controlled or supervised area of another employer for the purpose of work, for example, an x-ray service engineer, then cooperation between the person's employer and the employer in control of the supervised/controlled area should exchange information about the risks so adequate arrangements can be made for worker protection.
4. Regulatory inspectors, who enter to inspect the area for checking compliance with requirements.

A supervised area is any area where a person is likely to receive an effective dose of greater than 1 mSv per year (publics dose limit) or an equivalent dose greater than one-tenth of any relevant dose limit. If a supervised area has been defined, it is necessary to keep the conditions of the area under review to determine if the area needs to be designated a controlled area. Supervised areas should be suitably signed to indicate the nature of the radiation source and warning that a supervised area exists and the risks arising therein.

Local Rules, Radiation Protection Advisers and Supervisors

Once a controlled or supervised area has been defined, then it is necessary to have written local safety rules, referred to as local rules. These should be drawn up taking into account the findings of the prior risk assessment. These rules must be drawn to the attention of any worker who needs to enter a controlled or supervised area. Among other things, they should contain written schemes of work for safe entry into the controlled areas and contingency plans for any foreseeable accident, for example, radioactive source spillage. They should also contain the name of the Radiation Protection Adviser (RPA), who needs to be appointed by any employer who has set up a controlled area. Their duty is to advise the employer on compliance with the regulatory requirements, assistance in undertaking a prior risk assessment of areas where ionising radiation is to be used, the correct identification of controlled and supervised areas and the prior examination of plans for radiation

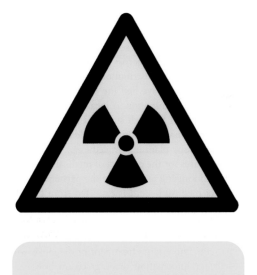

Fig. 4.4 Radiation warning signs.

installations and the acceptance into service of new or modified sources of ionising radiation. In the Health Service, an RPA is normally an experienced radiation physicist. An RPA is required to have a certificate of competence to act as an RPA, which is issued by an HSE-approved certification body every 5 years to candidates who can provide evidence of their suitability to act as an RPA.

In addition, the name of the Radiation Protection Supervisors (RPSs) for the area should be included in the local rules. Their responsibility is to supervise that the work with radiation that is being undertaken on a day-to-day basis is in compliance with the local rules. They should also be involved in the preparation of the local rules for the area that they supervise to ensure that they are both practical and not prohibitive. To act as an RPS, the person must have received training in a core of knowledge that has been specified by the HSE. In addition, they should be someone in a position of authority and familiar with the work of the area they are supervising. The HSE has also indicated that there should be approximately one RPS for every 20 members of staff working in the radiation areas for adequate supervision to be undertaken.

Local rules must contain the following as a minimum:
- Identification and description of controlled and supervised areas
- Names of RPSs
- Arrangements for restricting access to radiation areas
- Dose investigation levels. These are levels of dose which, if received, will trigger an investigation into the circumstances. They are lower than any applicable dose limit.
- Summary of work instructions, including written arrangements for nonclassified persons (schemes of work)
- Contingency arrangements for any foreseeable accident or incident

Radiation Safety Committee

Ultimate legal responsibility for compliance with the regulations, as with all Health and Safety legislation, lies with the employer. Although not a legal requirement, it is seen as good practice for large establishments, such as hospitals, to set up a radiation safety committee to assist the employer in complying with the regulations and to discuss matters relating to radiation safety including considering reports on any incidents that may have happened. This committee normally has representatives from each area where radiation is used and for each staff group who encounters radiation, together with the RPA and employers' representative. The outcome of the radiation protection committee meetings is very often reported to more general health and safety committees, to ensure as wide as publication of radiation protection matters as possible and to keep employees informed.

The Ionising Radiation (Medical Exposure) Regulations 2017

The Ionising Radiation (Medical Exposure) Regulations 2017 [8], often abbreviated to IRMER, are designed to protect a patient undergoing treatment or diagnosis with ionising radiation; they also cover persons exposed to radiation as part of research and medico-legal procedures, such as preimmigration chest x-rays. These regulations are policed by the Care Quality Commission. A set of amendment regulations were published shortly after the publication of the 2017 regulations in relation to safety measures regarding radioactive substances and the emission of ionising radiation.

They define four groups of people with legal responsibility under the regulations.

The Employer

The employer is responsible for ensuring there are a number of written procedures in place and that the staff involved adhere to these procedures. This will help protect staff members from individual criminal liability.

The procedures required are as follows:
- Procedures to identify correctly the person and the area to be exposed. The majority of errors that occur in procedures involving radiation to patients are caused by patient misidentification.
- Procedures to identify correctly who is entitled to act as referrers, practitioners and operators. It is the responsibility of the employer to decide whom they are willing to let fulfill these roles and to ensure that those undertaking the roles are adequately and appropriately trained. This training has to be role specific and cover those areas relevant to the role being undertaken that are outlined in schedule 3 of the Regulations. There is also a requirement for staff acting in these roles to demonstrate continuing education in radiation protection of the patient.
- Procedures to be observed in the case of medico-legal exposures.
- Procedures to make enquiries of females of childbearing age to establish whether they may be pregnant or breastfeeding. As we have seen, irradiation of the fetus can be detrimental. In addition, radioactive material administered to the mother may be expressed in the breast milk, which would then give a potentially large radiation dose to a breastfed baby.
- Procedures to ensure that quality assurance programmes are carried out. These relate to ensuring that these procedures are adhered to and are still relevant and quality assurance programmes performed on radiation equipment as required by the Ionising Radiations Regulations 2017 [4].
- Procedures for the assessment of patient dose and administered activities.
- Procedures for the use of diagnostic reference levels. These are levels of patient dose which are not expected to be exceeded when good and normal practice regarding diagnostic and technical performance is applied. Levels should be set in terms of easily checked dose parameters, such as fluoroscopic screening time or dose area product (DAP) readings. A DAP reading is obtained by the use of a flatbed ion chamber placed upon the collimator of the x-ray unit and it provides a measurement of the dose multiplied by the area of the applied radiation field. As such, the measurement units of a DAP reading are $Gy.cm^2$. The levels should be set locally with due regard to any national or international data that are available. Such levels have been set by the Public Heath England, based upon surveys performed across the country and set at the 75th percentile value of the dose distribution found. Over a period, this and changes in technology have had the effect of reducing the doses given for particular examination. A local series of diagnostic reference levels should be set for each standard radiologic examination, including interventional procedures, nuclear medicine investigations and radiotherapy planning procedures.
- Procedures for the conduct of medical research involving the exposure to ionising radiation of the participating individuals where no direct medical benefit is expected from the exposure. This should include the use and setting of dose constraints that are levels of dose associated with the research, which are not allowed to be exceeded.
- Procedures for giving written information and instruction to patients undergoing treatment or diagnosis with radioactive materials for information to be given on how the exposure from the patient can be restricted so as to protect persons in contact with the patient following discharge from the hospital (see carers and comforters previously).
- Procedures for the carrying out and recording of an evaluation of each medical exposure including factors relating to patient dose. That is a procedure to ensure that no exposure is undertaken

without a net benefit to the patient, for example, if x-ray images were not examined by a radiologist, no benefit would ensue from the exposure. This is usually fairly straight forward and apparent in exposures undertaken in radiotherapy.

- Procedures to ensure that the probability and magnitude of accidental or unintended doses are reduced as far as reasonably practicable. This should include things such as routine servicing and postservicing quality assurance checks on the equipment.

The employer is also legally obliged to keep training records of those identified as undertaking practitioner or operator roles. They must also draw up and keep up to date an inventory of the radiation equipment at each radiologic installation they control. They are also responsible for establishing referral criteria for medical exposures and for making these available to the referrers.

The Referrer

The referrer must be a registered medical or dental practitioner or other registered health professional entitled to act as a referrer under the employer's procedures (see earlier). Such a requirement therefore does not allow referrals from staff groups, such as Associate Practitioners, as they are not currently registered.

The legal responsibility is to provide sufficient detail on the referral request to allow for the correct identification of the patient and, where relevant, their menstrual status. They are also required to provide sufficient details of the clinical problem to allow justification and authorisation of the radiation exposure.

The Practitioner

The IRMER practitioner is a registered medical or dental practitioner or other registered health professional who is entitled by the employer's procedures to undertake this role. Their legal duty is to justify a medical exposure on the basis of the information provided to them by the referrer, taking into account the specific objectives of the exposure, the total potential benefits and risks to the individual undergoing the exposure and the possibility of using alternative techniques which do not use ionising radiation but which would attain the same objective.

In radiotherapy applications, there will normally be only one IRMER practitioner, for both the treatment exposures and any concomitant exposures as part of the planning process, for example, simulation, computed tomography (CT) scans and verification images. The number of concomitant exposures has increased as the developing technical capabilities for conformal, image-guided radiotherapy make target and critical organ definition an increasingly important aspect of radiotherapy. Estimation of doses and risks to critical organs in the body from all sources is thus necessary to provide the basis for adequate justification of the exposures as required by IRMER. Although negligible in comparison with the target dose, realistic numbers of concomitant exposures give a small but significant contribution to the total dose to most organs and tissues outside the target volume. In general, this is in the range of 5% to 10% of the total organ dose but can be as high as 20% for bone surfaces [12].

The Operator

The operator is any person recognised by the employer's procedures who carries out any practical application of the medical exposure. This covers a range of functions, each of which will have a direct influence on the medical exposure. Some of these will be undertaken in the presence of the patient, for example, making the exposure, identifying the patient. Other aspects are performed without the patient being present, for example, machine calibration and radiotherapy planning. Anyone who evaluates a medical image and records the result of this evaluation is also considered to be an operator.

A requirement of the legislation is that practitioners and operators are adequately and appropriately trained and that they undertake continuing education in radiation protection of the patient. Medical and dental practitioners who act as referrers do not require any additional training, although other health professionals performing this role should be trained in the clinical aspects of a patient's presentation that would warrant an exposure.

Medical Physics Expert

A medical physics expert (MPE) is defined as a state registered clinical scientist with corporate membership of the Institute of Physics and Engineering in Medicine or equivalent and at least 6 years of experience in the clinical specialty. A certification process is being introduced to allow formal recognition and validation of a person's competency to act in this role. An MPE is a legal requirement for radiotherapy practices. They must be full-time contracted to the radiation employer and available at all times for radiotherapy practices. Their roles in radiotherapy are, among other things, to provide consultation on the suitability of treatment techniques, with responsibility for the dosimetry and accuracy of treatment, optimisation of treatments by ensuring that equipment meets adequate standards of accuracy and the definitive calibration of radiotherapy equipment and dosimeters.

Legal Liability

IRMER requires that any cases of exposures significantly more than intended be reported to the Care Quality Commission for them to carry out an investigation. The employer should of course also perform such investigations. In so doing, it should be possible to determine if the IRMER procedures are correct or if they were not adhered to. By failing to adhere to the employers' procedures, individuals take on the legal liability which, in certain circumstances, may lead to a criminal prosecution of that individual.

Administration of Radioactive Substances Advisory Committee

Regulation 2 of the Medicines (Administration of Radioactive Substances) Regulations 1978 [14] (MARS Regulations 1978) and as amended in 1995 [15], requires that any doctor or dentist who wishes to administer radioactive medicinal products to humans should hold a certificate issued by Health Ministers. The Regulations also established a committee to advise Ministers on applications. This is known as the Administration of Radioactive Substances Advisory Committee (ARSAC) and issues certificates to medical staff (normally of consultant status) who wish to administer radioactive materials to patients. To become certificated, a practitioner is required to demonstrate that they have received IRMER training and an apprenticeship with an ARSAC certificate holder. To make the process more streamlined, individual IRMER practitioners who wish to authorise the use of radioactive materials will be issued with a certificate allowing them to prescribe, authorise and administer radionuclide and treatment type specific radioactive materials. Hospitals and other establishments that wish to administer radioactive materials for treatment, diagnosis or research must also be in possession of an ARSAC certificate covering all the radionuclides and uses that they wish to undertake. An ARSAC radiation practitioner can then work at any establishment where the allowed practices on both their individual certificates and the establishments certificate are consistent. Further details can be found in Notes for Guidance on the Clinical Administration of Radiopharmaceuticals and Use of Sealed Radioactive Sources (https://assets.publishing. service.gov.uk/government/uploads/system/uploads/attachment_data/ file/694951/ARSAC_notes_for_guidance.pdf).

Environmental Permitting (England and Wales) Regulations 2016

To keep, use and dispose of radioactive materials in the quantities used in a hospital that performs radiotherapy and diagnostic applications of radionuclides, The Environmental Permitting (England and Wales) Regulations 2016 [13] require that the premises are in possession of permits to keep the material and authorised to dispose of any waste arising from its use. The Department of the Environment pollutions inspectorate regulates this. Permits will detail the maximum activity and number of sources that may be held on the premises of individually named radionuclides. Authorisation for keeping and disposal of radioactive waste will be given providing the radiation user has performed an environmental impact assessment, which shows that, in the worst case scenario, doses to members of the public and others who come into contact with the radioactive waste are acceptable and that the disposals follow the best practical means for the environment. Authorisations will indicate the maximum activity of individual radionuclides that may be kept and subsequently disposed of over noted time periods by various routes.

Allowed routes of disposal are:

- in general, domestic refuse provided that it is to be disposed of by land filling or incineration and that it is below certain very low activity limits and concentrations;
- by incineration via a similarly authorised incinerator for higher activity waste;
- disposal of liquid waste in the sewage system, this is by far the most common route in terms of the activity disposed because of the majority of material being excreted by patients; and
- gaseous disposal of radioactive gases normally from a discharge point on the top of a building.

High Activity Sealed Radioactive Sources and Orphan Sources Regulations 2005

These regulations were introduced to reduce the loss of such sources either through a terrorist act or incorrect disposal. These regulations were incorporated into Environmental Permitting (England and Wales) Regulations 2016 but remain in force in Scotland and Northern Ireland. A special permit issued by the Department of Environment is required for sources which are designated as High Activity Sealed Sources (HASS). This designation is dependent on the radionuclide involved and its activity and form. If a source falls into a HASS category, additional security arrangements are required to be put in place and the source owner must demonstrate that they have adequate financial provisions in place for its subsequent future disposal. Without this, a permit will not be granted.

PROTECTIVE MEASURES

There are a number of protective measures that may be used, either singularly or, more commonly, in combination to reduce or limit the amount of radiation personnel are exposed to. By minimising the radiation dose people receive, you will minimise the risk of stochastic effects occurring and eliminate the risk of deterministic effects.

Time

The dose someone receives when exposed to radiation depends on the dose rate of the source and the time spent exposed to it, because high-dose rates will give a higher dose in a shorter time. Therefore anything that can be done to minimise the time exposed to a radiation source will minimise the exposure. For complex procedures, staff should carry out practice runs with dummy sources until they become proficient in the procedure; for fluoroscopic screening procedures, such as simulation, the use of a last image hold device will minimise the exposure time.

Distance

Radiation arising from a point source reduces in intensity in proportion to the square of the distance from the source. That means doubling your distance would quarter your exposure, quadrupling your distance would reduce the exposure to one-sixteenth. As such, this is a relatively easy way of reducing exposure and, importantly from the employer's point of view, does not usually cost anything. The use of long-handled forceps when dealing with radioactive sources will significantly reduce exposure, particularly to the hands. However, in radiotherapy installations, for example, linear accelerators, because the original source intensity is usually high, the distance required to move to reduce the intensity to an acceptable level makes this method of protection unusable by itself, because the distance required would be in the order of kilometres. Distance is very often employed as a protective measure in linear accelerator installations by the installation of a maze type entrance into the treatment area which requires scattered radiation generated within the treatment area to undergo a number of scattering interactions along the maze corridor before reaching the maze entrance or door, thus increasing the distance the radiation travels and reducing the dose rate. A correctly designed maze can mean no requirement for a radiation protective door to be used at the entrance.

Barriers

By placing an appropriate protective barrier between the radiation source and the area you are trying to protect, the level of the radiation reaching that area will be attenuated and reduced. However, care must be taken in choosing the correct material for the radiation type you are shielding against. If dense materials are used as the initial attenuator for beta particles (electrons), then x-rays will be generated from the attenuating material because of bremsstrahlung or braking radiation. Consequently, beta particles should be initially shielded by low-density material, such as Perspex, followed by a denser outer shield, such as lead. The thickness of shielding required is dependent upon the initial dose rate, the dose rate that is required after passing through the attenuator and the energy of the radiation, thickness increasing with any of these. Therefore lead aprons, with a thickness of approximately 0.25 mm of lead that are successfully used for shielding personnel using diagnostic x-rays, with a typical energy of 30 to 60 keV, would be completely inadequate to provide protection from the radiation from a cesium-137 radiation source (energy 662 keV) and the much higher energies employed in radiotherapy treatment rooms.

Because lead is the most common radiation shielding material, it is normal to quote the amount of protection afforded by different materials in terms of the lead equivalence of that material. The lead equivalence thus forms the basis of comparing one absorber to another at a given radiation energy. At diagnostic x-ray energies, the photoelectric absorption in lead is significant, because attenuation caused by photoelectric absorption is proportional to the atomic number of the material cubed and the density. For higher energy radiation where Compton scatter starts to predominate as the attenuation process, the reduction in radiation is proportional to the density of the material. As a consequence, as the energy of the radiation increases, the advantage of lead over other absorbing material diminishes because of the strong interdependence of photoelectric absorption on energy. With radiation above about 1 MeV in energy, where the Compton process predominates, there is no real advantage in using lead because all materials show very similar attenuation properties depending solely on their density.

For high-energy linear accelerator installations (generally taken as a minimum 10 MV) the possibility of neutron generation and activation must be considered and appropriate protective material employed.

Contamination

Where unsealed radioactive materials are used, either in the gaseous or liquid state, the possibility of contamination of the surfaces and the environment in which the material is being used needs to be considered. Such contamination may be subsequently internalised within the body either through inhalation, ingestion or absorption through the skin or wounds in the skin. Such absorptions will then counter the protective measures noted earlier as it will not minimise the exposure time; it will minimise the distance from the source to the tissues and no barriers could be put in place. As a consequence, other controls are essential when unsealed sources are used. These are source confinement, using trays, fume cupboards, glove boxes, etc., ensuring that the environment in which the sources are being used is well ventilated and easily decontaminated and good basic hygiene standards, such as wearing gloves and protective clothing and washing hands after dealing with such sources. These simple precautions will help to reduce the risk of internal exposure rather than eliminate it altogether. Adequate contamination monitoring with a radiation detector, such as a Geiger counter, should also be undertaken.

Building Materials

The correct choice of building material is essential for adequate protection of surrounding areas at the least possible cost. Various factors need to be taken into account when specifying the level of protection required and the material with which to protect. The radiation beam itself can consist of three components, primary beam radiation, that is radiation that is in the main beam of the radiation source, this will be the most intense and energetic. With the advent of flattening filter-free linear accelerators, the radiation dose rate has increased by 3 to 6 times, which can require additional protection to be installed. Scattered radiation originating from objects, such as the patient that the primary beam has struck, is less intense than the primary beam radiation but is taken to be of the same energy and, finally, for x-ray tubes, linear accelerators and sealed source units, leakage radiation originating from the radiation source housing. This is limited to certain maximum levels by regulatory requirements and typical leakage levels are less than 10% of the maximum allowed. Those factors that need to be taken into account in determining the levels of barrier thickness required are such things as:

- the attenuation properties of the material at the energies of radiation to be used
- the area you are trying to protect (i.e. is it going to contain radiation sensitive material, such as radiographic imaging plates?)
- the occupancy of the area to be protected
- the energy of the radiation that is to be used; the higher the energy the greater the penetration
- the possibility of neutron production (see later)
- the beam use factors (i.e. is the area to be subjected to the primary radiation beam at any time and if so for how long, or is it only exposed to scattered and leakage radiation?)
- the amount of radiation that is going to be used in a week, more commonly called *the workload* (e.g. beam on time)
- what is above, below and surrounding the area where radiation is being generated
- what is the acceptable exposure level to the areas you are protecting; such areas should be designed to conform to the As Low As Reasonably Practical requirement but, for public areas, should not exceed 1 mSv per year and in general are designed to be less than 0.3 mSv per year.

Having taken the aforementioned factors into consideration, calculations are made to determine the lead equivalence that is needed to protect the areas to the required degree. For diagnostic x-ray and radionuclide uses, the level of protection required varies from about 0.5 mm to 2 mm of lead, dependent on whether the barrier is subjected to the primary beam. This is usually achieved either by using sheet lead or concrete. Other material may be used but care must be taken because the design and density of alternative building materials vary. For example, clay bricks come in various densities ranging from 1600 to 2000 kg m^{-3}. In addition, they may be designed to reduce their weight by introducing cavities into the brick. In practice, because of these variables, it is advisable to perform transmission measurements on the intended material before construction with it is undertaken, to verify the lead equivalence provided by it. Many lightweight building blocks are available with densities of less than 1000 kg m^{-3} but, by themselves, they are unsuitable for use in a radiation area and need to be used in conjunction with other protective material, such as barium (barytes) plaster or lead lining. Conventional plaster is made with calcium sulfate. Replacing the calcium sulfate with barium sulfate to plaster x-ray room walls significantly increases the attenuation of the wall owing to the relatively high atomic number of barium (56) compared with calcium (20); indeed this is the reason why barium is used in barium meals and enemas. Care needs to be taken with wall and door furniture, such as handles and coat hooks, to ensure that the protection of the barrier is not compromised. Occasionally, breaches in the protection are essential to supply room services, such as air conditioning and electrical supply. In such circumstances, thought needs to be given as to how this is achieved. Such breaches should never occur in primary barriers and the use of mazes and careful angulations of the ducting passing through the wall will retain the protective ability. Whenever possible, it is better to take the services through a wall below the level of a solid floor. This is normally tested during room commissioning with the use of a radioactive source and radiation detectors. With increasing energy and the photoelectric effect becoming less predominant, lead becomes less favourable as the attenuating medium because of the large amounts that would be required and its tendency to creep or pool under its own weight. Therefore, for radiotherapy applications, concrete is the usual attenuating medium with occasionally barium or baryte concrete being used in areas subjected to the primary beam, particularly where space is at a premium. This type of concrete is relatively expensive and because of its higher density, much heavier than normal concrete. The typical wall thickness (primary barrier) for a 10 MeV linear accelerator is of the order of 1.2-metre dense concrete. Lapped steel plate can also be used in conjunction with concrete for an installation where space needs to be conserved, but it is best avoided where neutron production is likely. Such activation is brought about when linear accelerators are operated above 10 to 15 MV, by photonuclear reactions of the high-energy photons or electrons in the various materials of the target, flattening filter collimator and other shielding materials [19]. Neutron contamination increases rapidly as the energy of the beam increases from 10 to 20 MV and then remains approximately constant above this. Measurements have shown that, in the 16 to 25 MV x-ray therapy range, the neutron dose equivalent along the central access is about 0.5% of the applied x-ray dose and falls off to about 0.1% outside the field. If concrete has been used to shield from the photons, then sufficient protection from the neutrons will be provided by these structures. However, great care needs to be taken if iron or lead is used for part of the shielding as not only is the neutron attenuation poorer but neutron interactions in such material produce gamma radiation. Indeed, gamma production can arise in dense concrete which has metal bearing aggregate and care must be taken to avoid this type of aggregate. In such cases, it is necessary to use a combination of shielding materials with a sandwich construction of lead, steel, and polyethylene or concrete. Polyethylene is used as an efficient attenuator of neutrons and the steel or lead is then used as a photon attenuator.

If designing an area where unsealed (e.g. liquid) radionuclides are to be used, then thought needs to be given to ensuring that the floors and walls are constructed and finished in such a way as to make them easy to decontaminate. Decontamination is usually achieved by a washing process, occasionally using caustic solutions. Consequently, providing the surfaces are easily washable without degradation and are impermeable to the cleaning solutions, then they will be suitable for use. Care should be taken in ensuring that joints between benches and so on are sealed. Thought also is required in the correct selection of the material used for drains as some radionuclides are absorbed preferentially by plastics.

In conclusion, a number of factors need to be taken into account in designing a radiation room; its walls and barriers must be such that the levels of radiation received by staff, waiting patients and members of the public are kept to a minimum. This can be achieved by the correct use of shielding material. A certified and appropriately experienced RPA should always be consulted in any design process involving radiation.

MONITORING OF RADIATION LEVELS

Monitoring of radiation levels can be performed in a number of ways. The Ionising Radiations Regulations only require employers to provide personal radiation dosimeters to their classified radiation workers and to demonstrate that nonclassified workers do not need to become classified. One way of avoiding issuing personal radiation monitors to nonclassified staff is to perform environmental monitoring and then making a judgment as to the probability of workers requiring to become classified. Environmental monitoring must also be carried out on all new or modified protective structures to ensure that they meet with the radiation protection required by the design specification worked out, considering those matters described in the aforementioned section. A number of different instruments can be used to perform this monitoring, each with their own advantages and drawbacks; some of these are now described (see also Chapter 3).

Ion chambers can be used for such measurements; they have the advantage that they have a relatively uniform response over a wide range of energies and can be used to make both dose and dose rate measurements. The lower the level of dose that is to be measured, the larger the ionisation chamber needs to be for there to be sufficient ionisation current to make a measurement. Doubling the volume of an ion chamber will double its sensitivity, all other things being equal. Ion chambers with volumes in excess of 1 litre are available to measure transmission through protective walls. Smaller volume ion chambers are used to measure radiation output in the primary beam of an x-ray unit ranging in volume from about 0.5 to 6 mL. One disadvantage of such devices is that they have a relatively long time constant, which means they do not respond quickly to changes in the incident radiation intensity. In addition, the pulsed nature of the radiation emitted from linear accelerators can lead to accuracies in radiation dose measurements because of recombination effects in ion chambers.

Instruments involving Geiger counters or scintillation detectors are more sensitive than ionisation chambers, respond more quickly and use detectors of smaller size. This is because the signals that are initially generated are further amplified. Such instruments are more often used in detecting surface contamination in radionuclide laboratories; their chief disadvantage is that they are energy dependent, their response varying with the energy of radiation being measured. As such, unless the monitor has been calibrated with the energy of radiation being measured, the reading will not be correct. Such instruments can be used in diagnostic x-ray installations, together with a radioactive source, such as Americium 241, to check the integrity of barriers, at positions, such as handles and light switches.

Mains operated radiation detectors are often placed at exits and other strategic places in radiation areas where either the level of radiation may fluctuate or the radiation sources are mobile and a warning is required if the source leaves the area. Detectors with either an audible or visual indication of a high reading are often placed on exit doors of the rooms of patients being treated with radioactive materials such that, if they try to leave the area, an alarm will alert the ward staff. Similar alarms are required in radiotherapy departments, to provide independent confirmation that the source(s) on gamma beam generators or remote after loading units have returned to the safe position.

Personal Radiation Dosimeters

There are a number of different types of personal radiation dosimeters, which can be used to assess the dose individual staff members receive as part of their work activity; these are detailed subsequently, together with their relative advantages and disadvantages. These must be worn when at work and not be exposed to radiation when the person is not at work, as these monitors are used to determine the exposure a person receives as part of their work. This includes those cases where the person undergoes a medical exposure to radiation as part of their care pathway. The dosimeters are usually worn at waist level and changed on a regular basis, normally monthly. If a protective apron is being worn, the dosimeter should be worn underneath, because the whole-body radiation exposure to the trunk is the quantity to be measured. Occasionally, dose is assessed to other areas of the body and providing the dosimeter is small enough, can be placed on the fingers, wrists, legs or forehead. These are used to demonstrate that the doses these areas receive are within the dose limits for the individual organs noted in Table 4.5. To carry out definitive measurements of dose, which will be accepted by the regulators, the dosimeters used must be of an HSE approved type. To meet this type of approval, the dosimeters have to meet certain minimum performance and measurement specification.

Direct Readout Dosimeters

These have a radiation detector associated with an electronic display, so that a direct readout of the dose received can be made at any time. More sophisticated devices allow interrogation of the dose time profile via connection to a computer, to help establish when peaks of dose have occurred, and also recording of the dose received. A picture of such a device is shown in Fig. 4.5.

The advantage of such dosimeters is that there is no delay in knowing what dose has been received as the equipment provides a direct readout; the disadvantages are that they are relatively expensive (£200–£400), susceptible to damage and some are energy dependent so different readings will be obtained on them for the same received

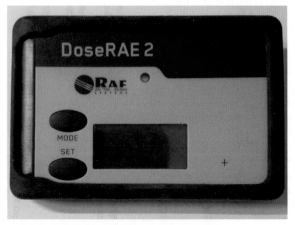

Fig. 4.5 Personal radiation dosimeter.

dose. Less expensive versions also have the disadvantage that there is no permanent record of the dose received unless logged by the user.

Thermoluminescent Dosimeters

The thermoluminescent dosimeter (TLD) consists of a crystal or powder (e.g. calcium sulfate or lithium boride), which can record the dose of radiation it is exposed to and store this information. When heated (thermo), the material gives off light (luminescent); the amount of light being given off is proportional to the radiation dose to the material. The material is usually placed in a holder which enables the dosimeter to distinguish between penetrating and nonpenetrating radiations; this is done by placing a portion of material underneath a dome of plastic and another portion merely under a thin protective envelope.

The advantages of TLD's include:

- Can be used as personal and environmental dosimeter
- Use thermoluminescent (TL) materials
- Electrons are raised/trapped at higher energy levels
- The energy is released as light when heated
- Light emitted is converted into an electrical signal
- Light emitted is proportional to incident radiation
- Lithium (LiF:Mn) based TLDs for personal dosimetry: because they are tissue-equivalent
- Calcium (CaF_2:Dy, $CaSO_4$:Dy) based TLDs for environmental monitoring: caused by their high sensitivity
- Lithium borate ($Li_2B_4O_7$:Mn) TLDs for high-dose range dosimetry
- TL materials are available in many different forms: for example, powder, hot pressed chips, pellets, impregnated Teflon disks
- Read-out instruments (reader) are required
- Method to heat the TLD material: electrical, hot gas or a radio-frequency heater, heated in an inert gas during read-out
- Device to convert the light output to an electrical pulse
- Light signal is amplified using a photomultiplier
- Small size (only milligram quantities of TL material is needed)
- TLDs can be reused
- Doses down to 0.1 mSv accurately readable

The disadvantages of TLDs are:

- only one reading during heating, cannot be repeated
- subject to fading (because of temperature or light effects)
- requires careful handling to avoid dirt on the dosimeters interfering with light emission.

Optically Stimulated Luminescent Dosimeter

These measure radiation through a thin layer of aluminium oxide. During analysis, the aluminium oxide is stimulated with selected frequencies of laser light causing it to become luminescent in proportion to the amount of radiation exposure. This is very similar in principle to the computed radiography imaging plates that have film in diagnostic radiology. The dosimeters give accurate readings down to 0.01 mSv, representing another revolution in dosimetry. This new degree of sensitivity is ideal for employees working in low-radiation environments and for pregnant employees. Another advantage is that they can go through a washing machine cycle without being affected. The increased sensitivity does have a potentially disadvantage in that does that would have been previously unreported will now appear of dose records. This sudden reporting of a dose may raise concern in monitored staff but good education should alleviate this.

Radiation Records

In addition to the personal dose monitoring records mentioned earlier, a number of other records are also required by the regulators to be kept. These are detailed subsequently.

Contamination Checks

In areas using unsealed radioactive materials, regular checks are required to be made on both the personnel working in the area and on the work surfaces of the area to ensure that radioactive contamination is not building up or being spread. Records of these measurements need to be made and are subjected to inspection by both HSE and Department of the Environment inspectors.

Leak Tests, Disposal and Movement Logs

All sealed radioactive sources must undergo an annual leak test to verify the integrity of the source housing; in addition, whenever sources are moved from their storage area, a note of where they have gone to needs to be made. Reports of any loss or damage to radioactive sources also need to be kept. The Environmental Permitting Regulations 2016 requires that records be kept of receipt and disposal of radioactive materials together with the quantities and types of radionuclide (see Environmental Permitting Regulations earlier).

Equipment Checks and Calibration

On an annual basis, contamination monitors, dosimeters and dose rate meters require to be calibrated and the results of this calibration logged. The calibration of such equipment needs to be traceable back to a national calibration standard so that it can be assured that what is measured at one centre will be the same as measured at another. This is often arranged by sending one instrument away for calibration by a national calibration service, such as the National Physical Laboratory, and then cross-calibrating other equipment held with the one that was sent away.

Having calibrated the measurement equipment, these can then be used with a degree of confidence for carrying out dose measurements on radiotherapy treatments machines, diagnostic x-ray equipment and for contamination and dose rate measurements. Such measurements in radiotherapy form part of a comprehensive quality assurance programme that is required to be in place in every radiotherapy department to help ensure that the risk of incorrect or inaccurate treatments being given is minimised.

Other Requirements

A number of other matters, some of which do not directly relate to radiation, will now be discussed, all of them are however safety related and are therefore worthy of note.

Transport of Radioactive Materials

Prior to a change in legislation in 1996 it was permissible for professional users of radioactive materials, for example, a radiotherapist, to transport radioactive materials on the road without any requirements placed upon them for their safe carriage. This professional user's exemption was removed with the introduction of the Radioactive Material Road Transport Regulations. These required that anyone carrying more than certain limited quantities of radioactive material on the road have received adequate and appropriate training, that the material is contained in approved packaging and that the packages and vehicles are labelled and placarded to indicate the risk of ionising radiation. Further requirements were established by The Carriage of Dangerous Goods and Use of Transportable Pressure Equipment (Amendment) Regulations 2011 [20]. Anyone involved in the transportation of radioactive materials is also required to appoint a Dangerous Goods Safety Adviser, who needs to be certificated to undertake such a role in the type of dangerous goods they are providing advice on. The advisers' role is to provide guidance to ensure compliance with the regulatory requirements.

Critical Examinations, Commissioning and Quality Control

Before new equipment is used clinically, the installer has a legal responsibility to carry out a critical examination of the installation, to ensure that all safety critical parts of the equipment are operating correctly. A report of the examination should be made to the customer who should keep it for reference throughout the life of the equipment. The critical examination should be repeated after any major upgrade or repair to the equipment, which may affect the radiation output or other safety critical factors, for example, source or x-ray tube change.

Once the installer has performed a critical examination, the user should carry out an adequate number of tests and measurements to establish a quality control baseline and ensure that the equipment is working within the purchasing specification. All safety related features of the equipment should be checked including those associated with the room containing the equipment.

A Medical Physics Expert should be responsible for acceptance testing of the equipment. For radiotherapy equipment, compliance with the Guidance Notes [6], Guidance Note PM77 [9]—Equipment used in connection with medical exposure, and the appropriate sections of British Standard BS EN 60601 [16], relevant to equipment safety should be checked. Further guidance on the acceptance testing and commissioning of radiotherapy equipment can be found in the (Institute of Physics and Engineering in Medicines) IPEM 94 [17] Commissioning and Quality Assurance of Linear Accelerators and IPEM 81 [18] Physics Aspects of Quality Control in Radiotherapy.

Personal Protective Equipment

A range of personal protective equipment (PPE) (lead aprons, gloves, thyroid shields and eye protectors) should be provided in all diagnostic x-ray rooms and for use with mobile x-ray equipment. When not in use, these should be stored appropriately so as to avoid damaging their protective properties. Lead aprons for instance should never be folded but should be hung on dedicated hangers or rails of sufficiently large diameter to prevent creasing.

All PPE should be visually examined at frequent intervals and any defective items removed from use. Protective clothing must be examined at least annually to ensure that no cracks in the protective material have developed. This has to be done by radiographic or fluoroscopic examination if the protective material is not directly visible. The results of the inspection should be recorded and the protective devices themselves should be individually identifiable, for example, by a serial number. It should be noted that PPE is of insufficient lead equivalence to protect personnel from the much higher energy radiotherapy treatment radiations, but will provide adequate protection from radiation emitted from CT scanners, diagnostic units and On Board Imaging devices used as the part of the treatment planning and set up process.

Mechanical, Electrical and Fire Hazards

In addition to the hazard from the radiation being generated from radiotherapy and diagnostic x-ray equipment, hazards also arise from the mechanical structure of the equipment in the form of the weight associated with the equipment. Radiotherapy equipment, in particular, normally has a large amount of high-density material (lead or depleted uranium) surrounding the radiation source to ensure that radiation is only directed to the area intended and leakage radiation from the x-ray tube or around the radiation source is minimised. The overall weight of the equipment is also increased by the need for counterbalancing weights in supporting structures. Where megavoltage equipment is concerned, merely rotating the gantry from one position to another involves the acceleration and retardation of several tonnes. Care should be taken in moving such equipment, ensuring that there is nothing in the intended path of travel as a lot of damage can be caused quite easily if such weights crash into something, for example, a trolley left beside the treatment couch.

Even low-voltage electrical equipment has the potential to kill. The voltages that radiotherapy and x-ray equipment work at ranges from a few volts to hundreds of thousands of volts; as a consequence, such equipment should never be operated with wet hands or in wet conditions. All major components of any installation should be visibly connected to 'earth' using either a continuous copper tape or a single core wire covered with a green or green and yellow sheath. These connections should all be brought together at a common earth reference terminal (often labelled as *ERT*), which is normally a large copper bar placed close to the control console or x-ray generator. All areas of the equipment that are potentially electrically hazardous will be housed in cabinets either behind fixed panels or locked doors. These must always be kept secure and only opened by authorised personnel after they have isolated the electricity supply. In addition, large capacitors may be present and are likely to hold their charge even after the mains supply has been switched off and special precautions need to be taken to discharge them safely before maintenance work is undertaken.

Because of the high voltages employed in radiotherapy and x-ray equipment, there is an increased risk of fire. As a result of the requirement for radiotherapy installations to have a minimum number of entrances/exits, such rooms normally only have the one. As such, it is important that any fires starting in such rooms are detected as early as possible and fire detection devices, such as smoke alarms, are essential. In some situations, patients undergoing treatment will be immobilised on the treatment table by securing them to it with treatment moulds. This makes the release of these patients time consuming in an emergency situation, such as fire. Rehearsals of removing patients from treatment rooms should be undertaken regularly so staff are aware of problems that they may face. Fire extinguishers should be of a type suitable for tackling electrical fires, the use of water being avoided, as this would present a potential electrocution hazard. Procedures should be in place to provide advice to the fire brigade if a fire occurs in radiation areas and a list of the location of radioactive material should be provided to the fire service on an annual basis. In a fire situation, if the fire brigade sees a radiation warning sign they will err on the safe side until the nature of the hazard has been established.

By complying with all the regulatory requirements and guidance, it is possible to remove the risk of acute radiation effects and limit the probability of stochastic effects occurring. As such, anyone working routinely with radiation should be made aware of what is expected of them in terms of protecting both themselves and others from the use of radiation.

REFERENCES

[1] ICRP103:2007:37 (2-4). ICRP Publication 103. The 2007 Recommendations of the International Commission on Radiological Protection. Elsevier.

[2] ICRP 60. Ann ICRP 1991;21(1–3). ICRP Publication 60. Recommendations of the International Commission on Radiological Protection. Pergamon Press; 1990.

[3] United Nations. Sources and effects of ionising radiation, vols. 1–2. UNSCEAR 2000 Report to the General Assembly with scientific annexes. United Nations sales publications E.00.IX.3 and E.00.IX.4. New York: United Nations; 2000.

[4] The Ionising Radiations Regulations 2017—Statutory Instrument 2017 No. 1075. HMSO. http://www.legislation.gov.uk/uksi/2017/1075/pdfs/uksi_20171075_en.pdf.

[5] Work with ionising radiation. Approved Code of Practice and Guidance. L121 HSE; 2017. 2nd ed. March 2018;

[6] Saunderson JR, Mayles WPM, Mairs W, Rowley L, Worrall M. Medical and Dental Guidance Notes. A good practice guide on all aspects of ionising radiation protection in the clinical environment. 2nd ed. Bristol: IoP Publishing Limited; 2018.

[7] The Management of Health and Safety at Work Regulations 1999—Statutory Instrument 1999 No. 3242. HMSO. http://www.legislation.gov.uk/uksi/1999/3242/pdfs/uksi_19993242_en.pdf

[8] Ionising Radiation (Medical Exposure) Regulations 2017. Statutory Instrument 2017 No. 1322. HMSO. Available: http://www.legislation.gov.uk/uksi/2017/1322/pdfs/uksi_20171322_en.pdf.

[9] PM 77 Guidance Note. Equipment used in connection with medical exposure. 3rd ed. Health and Safety Executive; 2006. http://www.hse.gov.uk/pubns/guidance/pm77.pdf.

[10] HSE. Protection of outside workers against ionising radiation. HSE information sheet Ionising Radiation Protection Series 4. 2000 and http://www.hse.gov.uk/radiation/ionising/doses/index.htm.

[11] Radiation The Ionising. (Medical Exposure) (Amendment) Regulations. No. 121 HMSO. Available: http://www.legislation.gov.uk/uksi/2018/121/contents/made; 2018.

[12] Harrison RM, Wilkinson M, Shemilt A, Rawlings DJ, Moore M, Lecomber AR. Organ doses from prostate radiotherapy and associated concomitant exposures. Br J Radiol 2006;79:487–96.

[13] Environmental Permitting (England and Wales) Regulations, 2016. Available: https://www.legislation.gov.uk/uksi/2016/1154/pdfs/uksi_20161154_en.pdf.

[14] The Medicines (Administration of Radioactive Substances) Regulations 1978–Statutory Instrument 1978 No. 1004. HMSO.

[15] The Medicines (Administration of Radioactive Substances) Amendment Regulations 1995–Statutory Instrument 1995 No. 2147. HMSO.

[16] BS EN 60601. Medical electrical equipment British Standard. From British Standards online at http://bsonline.techindex.co.uk. 2000.

[17] IPEM 94. Commissioning and quality assurance of linear accelerators. IPEM Report No. 94. IPEM; 2007.

[18] IPEM 81. Physics aspects of quality control in radiotherapy. IPEM Report No. 81. 2nd ed. IPEM; 2018.

[19] Axton E, Bardell A. Neutron production from electron accelerators used for medical purposes. Phys Med Biol 1972;17:293.

[20] The Carriage of Dangerous Goods and Use of Transportable Pressure Equipment (Amendment) Regulations 2011 SI 2011 No. 1885. Available: http://www.legislation.gov.uk/uksi/2011/1885/pdfs/uksi_20111885_en.pdf.

Imaging With X-Ray, Magnetic Resonance Imaging and Ultrasound

Andy Rogers, Carl Tiivas, Sarah Wayte

CHAPTER OUTLINE

INTRODUCTION

X-Ray, magnetic resonance imaging (MRI) and ultrasonic images play a key role in the diagnosis, staging, planning and delivery of treatment and follow-up of patients with cancer.

In everyday language, an image is a picture and, more generally, it is a representation of the distribution of some property of an object. It is formed by transferring information from the object to an image domain. In practice, this requires the ordered transfer of energy from some source via the object of interest to a detector system. The detected signal may be processed in some way before being displayed and stored by suitable devices.

Medical imaging modalities covered in this chapter are classified according to the type of energy used to carry information: x-rays, radiofrequency (RF) waves and high-frequency sound waves.

X-Ray imaging enables tumours to be localised with respect to normal anatomic structures and to external markers. Because x-rays travel in straight lines until they are absorbed or scattered, they can produce images which faithfully represent spatial relationships within the body. It is principally for this reason that x-ray images of various kinds are essential to the planning and delivery of radiotherapy. A further reason is that interactions of ionising radiation with matter are an essential feature of both imaging and therapy, so that information on properties of tissues relevant to treatment planning, such as electron density, may be obtained from suitable images.

MRI is an excellent technique for imaging soft tissue and is often used to diagnose and stage cancer in the head, neck and body. It can also be used to monitor the response to treatment. The extent of the cancer can be seen on anatomic images. Other specialised MRI techniques, such as diffusion weighted imaging and dynamic imaging with a contrast agent, can also be used to refine the diagnosis and cancer staging. Magnetic resonance spectroscopy (MRS) provides information regarding the metabolism of the tumours and can also be used to monitor treatment response.

Diagnostic ultrasound imaging has several advantages over other imaging modalities [1]. It is relatively cheap, safe, gives real-time images and has good soft tissue contrast. As well as anatomic detail, ultrasound can exploit the Doppler effect to give information about blood flow and the vascularity in tissues. The distortion of tissue under pressure in ultrasound images can give images related to the elasticity of tissues.

Radionuclide imaging, including positron emission tomography-computed tomography (CT), which is primarily concerned with the function of organs and tissues, is dealt with in Chapter 6.

X-RAY IMAGING

Overview of X-Ray Imaging Process

The energy source in medical x-ray imaging is usually an x-ray tube and electrical generator though, in the case of radiotherapy portal imaging, it may be the linear accelerator. As the x-ray beam passes through the patient, some radiation is absorbed or scattered. The intensity of the emerging primary beam varies with position and carries information about the interactions that have occurred in the body. The emerging beam can be detected by a variety of devices, for example, film/screen cassette, image intensifier, solid state electronic detector. These are typically large area devices and the image is a two-dimensional shadowgraph of the intervening anatomy. Radiographic film is unique in combining all three roles of image detection, recording and display. Image intensifiers are usually joined to a charge-coupled device (CCD) camera and display monitors: static images or dynamic (i.e. moving) series may be stored on analogue video media or, more likely these days, digitised for storage on hard disks or other removable storage media, such as digital video device (DVD). Digital fluoroscopy and radiography systems use digital computers and their storage and display devices as integral components of the imaging system, as does CT. In CT, the x-ray beam is collimated in the longitudinal direction to a narrow slit and this is aligned with an arc of solid state detectors. The tube and detectors are mounted on a gantry that rotates about the patient. While the x-ray tube/detector assembly is rotating, the patient is fed through the aperture on a moving couch creating a helix of irradiation on the patient and detector. These projections are processed in a digital computer to form images of transverse slices through the patient.

Production of X-Rays for Imaging

The general topic of x-ray production is covered in Chapter 2. This section highlights some aspects of specific relevance to imaging.

X-Rays are generated by causing electrons, which have been accelerated to high energies in a vacuum tube, to collide with a metal target. The electrical supply is normally from a generator, which takes power from the mains three phase alternating current (AC) supply and converts it, using a transformer and associated circuits, to an approximately constant kilovoltage (kV) direct current (DC) output. Older models used rectification and smoothing circuits which resulted in appreciable ripple on the kV waveform, that is, the output voltage varied by several percent over a mains cycle. For this reason, the kilovoltage is specified as the peak value, denoted by the abbreviation kV_p. Modern generators use converters, operating at a frequency of several kHz, which produce voltage waveforms with very little ripple. Diagnostic imaging work mostly uses accelerating potentials in the range 50 to 150 kV_p, though lower values are used in mammography.

At megavoltage energies, as in linear accelerators used for radiotherapy, the x-rays are produced mainly in the forward direction of the electron beam and hence a transmission target is used. At kilovoltage energies, as used in diagnostic x-ray equipment, radiotherapy simulators and CT scanners, x-rays are produced more isotropically and a reflection target is used. This allows the tube to be constructed with a rotating anode (Fig. 5.1), which permits the heat generated to be dissipated over a much larger area than with a stationary anode. This is important because, at kilovoltage energies, more than 99% of the electron beam energy is converted to heat in the anode and less than 1% appears as x-rays. Moreover, to produce images with good spatial resolution, the focal spot must be as small as possible and short exposure times are used to reduce blurring caused by patient movement. With a stationary anode, a large quantity of heat would be deposited in a short time over a very small area, resulting in serious damage to the target. In fact, most x-ray tubes offer two sizes of focal spot, the larger being used for higher exposure rates (higher filament current) that impose higher heat loading demands on the filament.

The x-rays produced have a spread of energies, that is, a spectrum as shown in Fig. 5.2, and there are two main components. One is the bremsstrahlung produced when electrons experience large accelerations as they pass close to atomic nuclei. This produces the major part of the spectrum, the smooth curve. Superimposed on this, is the second component, the line spectrum caused by characteristic radiation emitted when orbital electrons move to lower energy levels to fill vacancies which have been caused by ionisation because of the accelerated electrons from the filament interacting with the anode material. The area under the spectrum represents the total quantity of radiation produced.

The shape of the spectrum determines the quality of the radiation, that is, its penetrating properties. Increasing the tube current (mA) or the exposure time (s) both increase the quantity of radiation produced but do not affect its quality. Increasing the applied voltage (kV_p)

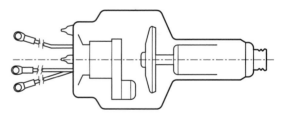

Fig. 5.1 X-ray construction and rotating anode tube. (Courtesy Elekta Ltd.)

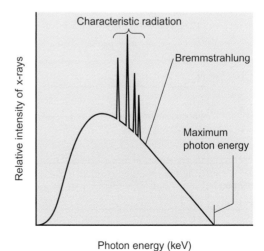

Fig. 5.2 X-ray spectrum produced from a tube.

increases both the quality and quantity of radiation produced and the output is approximately proportional to the square of the applied voltage $(kV_p)^2$. Other factors, such as anode material and filtration of the beam, further affect the quality and quantity of radiation produced. For imaging, the lower energy components are usually selectively reduced by suitable filtration, as they only contribute to patient radiation dose and not image quality.

Information From Absorption and Scattering

When x-rays, generated from a suitable source, are incident upon an object, such as the human body, some pass straight through while others interact with the material in the object by processes of absorption and scattering. In biological tissues at kilovoltage energies, the interactions of importance are photoelectric absorption and Compton scattering. The photoelectric effect depends strongly on atomic number Z and the energy E of the x-rays. Calcium, found in bone, has a relatively high atomic number and hence bone strongly absorbs kV x-rays. At megavoltage energies, it is the Compton effect that predominates and this depends primarily on electron density ρ_e.

The beam emerging from the object contains primary radiation together with scattered radiation. It is the varying intensity of the transmitted primary beam that carries useful information to produce an image.

Differential Attenuation in the Primary Beam

Consider the simple situation in Fig. 5.3, which shows a slab of some homogeneous material A of thickness X_A and linear attenuation coefficient μ_A, which contains a region of some other material B of thickness X_B and linear attenuation coefficient μ_B. Suppose a parallel x-ray beam of intensity I_O is incident on this slab. Then the intensity of the primary beam transmitted through A is:

$$I_A = I_O \exp(-\mu_A x_A) \qquad \textbf{5.1}$$

and that transmitted through both A and B is:

$$
\begin{aligned}
I_{AB} &= I_O \exp(-\mu_A(x_A - x_B))\exp(-\mu_B x_B) \\
&= I_O \exp(-\mu_A x_A)\exp((\mu_A - \mu_B)x_B) \qquad \textbf{5.2} \\
&= I_A \exp((\mu_A - \mu_B)x_B)
\end{aligned}
$$

Hence the ratio of the transmitted intensities is:

$$I_{AB}/I_A = \exp((\mu_A - \mu_B)x_B) \qquad \textbf{5.3}$$

By taking the (natural) logarithm of both sides, this may also be expressed as:

$$
\begin{aligned}
\ln(I_{AB}/I_A) &= \ln(I_{AB}) - \ln(I_A) \\
&= (\mu_A - \mu_B)x_B
\end{aligned} \qquad \textbf{5.4}
$$

This ratio, which determines the contrast visible in the image, increases with the thickness of B (X_B) and with the difference between the linear attenuation coefficients of A and B ($\mu_A - \mu_B$).

The linear attenuation coefficients for air and bone are very different from those of soft tissue at kV energies, so even quite thin structures containing these materials can be visualised on the x-ray image. The differences between the linear attenuation coefficients for different soft tissues are, however, much smaller and special techniques such as CT are needed to reveal them.

Contrast Media

Some structures may be made visible by deliberately introducing contrast agents, such as air or liquids containing iodine or barium, which have a very different value of μ from the surrounding tissues.

Scatter as Unwanted Background

Scattered radiation generally contributes a more or less uniform background signal to the image, which does not convey useful information but which reduces contrast. The amount of scattered radiation emerging from the patient can be several times greater than the transmitted primary beam, increasing with the energy of the x-ray beam, the size of the area irradiated and the thickness of the body part being imaged. It is possible to reduce the amount of scatter reaching the detector by using antiscatter grids or by using an air gap technique. The latter relies on an appreciable separation between the patient and the image detector, which is often the case when using a radiotherapy simulator. The principle is illustrated in Fig. 5.4, which shows that the amount of scatter reaching the detector falls off much more rapidly than the intensity of the primary beam as this distance is increased.

Antiscatter Grid

The antiscatter grid consists of an array of long, thin lead strips, separated by some relatively radiolucent spacer material (Fig. 5.5). Only radiation travelling perpendicular to the grid can pass through to the detector. Most of the scattered radiation is travelling at other angles and is intercepted and absorbed by the lead strips. Some primary radiation is absorbed too, but the net effect is greatly to increase the ratio of primary to scattered radiation reaching the detector, thus improving image contrast. To ensure that the detector receives the requisite number of photons to ensure adequate image quality, the use of antiscatter grids results in an increased dose to the patient. If the angle between the primary beam and the perpendicular to the grid becomes too great, for

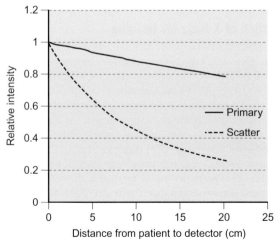

Fig. 5.4 Diagram showing the fall off in scatter reaching detector with distance.

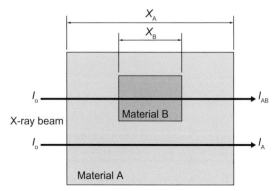

Fig. 5.3 Simple inhomogeneous situation to illustrate contrast.

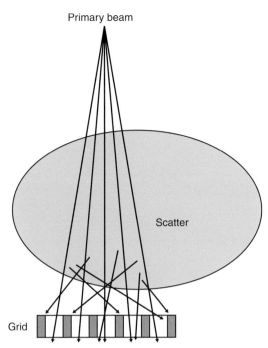

Fig. 5.5 Antiscatter grid principles.

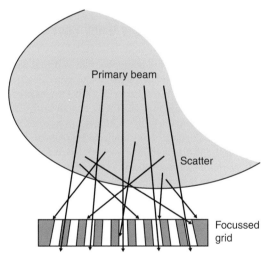

Fig. 5.6 Focussed antiscatter grid.

example, towards the edge of large fields, then a significant fraction of primary radiation will be absorbed. This can be overcome by using a focused grid, as shown in Fig. 5.6. To avoid shadows from the lead strips producing distracting lines on the image, it is possible to move the grid to and fro laterally during the exposure and thus to blur out those lines.

PLANAR IMAGING

Film and Screen Detection

For many years, radiographic film has been used as a combined detector, storage and display device for x-ray images. It is usually used in conjunction with intensifying screens, which have a higher absorption efficiency than film for x-rays and which emit many visible light photons for each x-ray photon absorbed (Fig. 5.7).

Radiographic film consists of a transparent polyester base, approximately 0.2 mm thick, usually coated on both sides with an emulsion containing crystals of silver bromide and this, in turn, is coated with

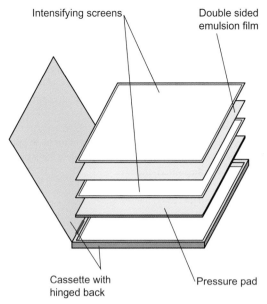

Fig. 5.7 Radiographic film cassette.

a protective layer. When the emulsion is exposed to light or x-rays, some electrons are transferred from bromide ions to silver ions, which are reduced to silver atoms. These form a latent image which is not visible until it is chemically developed, a process in which the remaining silver ions in the affected crystals are also reduced to silver atoms, which cause blackening of the film. The more silver atoms present per unit area in the developed image, the darker the film appears.

Exposed films are normally processed automatically, in several stages:

1. Development of the latent image using an organic reducing agent;
2. Fixing the developed image by dissolving away undeveloped silver bromide from the emulsion;
3. Hardening the emulsion to protect it from damage; and
4. Washing the film and drying it.

Films may be manually loaded into the processor in a darkroom or automatically from suitable cassettes using a so-called daylight processor.

The intensifying screen (Fig. 5.8) uses a fluorescent material that emits visible light when irradiated with x-rays and it is this visible light that is then detected by the film. (The same principle is used in image intensifier systems and in some digital imaging devices: see later). A

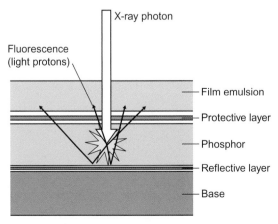

Fig. 5.8 Intensifier screen principles.

cassette is used that contains a separate screen for each side of the film and is constructed so as to ensure close contact between screen and film over their whole area. This reduces blurring. Many visible photons are produced for each x-ray photon absorbed and so the exposure required to produce a given degree of blackening on the film is greatly reduced compared with direct exposure of the film to x-rays. With modern rare earth screens, this reduction may be by a factor of about 100.

Characteristic Curve

The degree of blackness of the film is measured in terms of optical density (D). If a beam of light of intensity I_o is incident on a piece of film and intensity I_t is transmitted, then:

$$D = \log_{10}(I_o/I_t) \qquad \textbf{5.5}$$

Hence, a region of film that transmits one-tenth of the incident light intensity has optical density 1.0, whereas a region which transmits one hundredth of the incident light intensity has optical density 2.0. A perfectly transparent region would have $D = 0$.

A graphic plot of D against log (exposure) is called the *characteristic curve*. A typical example is shown in Fig. 5.9. If an unexposed film is developed, its optical density is a little greater than zero because the film base is not perfectly transparent and also because some of the silver bromide crystals are reduced to metallic silver (film fog). Over a range of exposures, the characteristic curve is approximately linear, and the gradient (slope) in this region is known as *gamma for that film/screen combination*. At very high exposures, all the silver bromide crystals are reduced on development and no increase in D occurs for higher exposures: the film/screen response is said to be saturated.

Contrast is the difference in D between different parts of an image. Under favourable conditions, the human eye can detect density differences as small as 0.02. If the slope of the characteristic curve is steep (i.e. has a high value of gamma), this means that the density increases rapidly over a relatively narrow range of exposure values, so the image has high contrast. On the other hand, only a narrow range of exposures can be represented before the image saturates, that is, the latitude is low, and careful radiographic technique is needed to ensure that all features of interest are properly imaged. A lower gamma film/screen combination produces lower contrast but can encompass a wider range of exposure levels, that is, it has greater latitude.

If only a relatively small exposure is required to produce a given density, as in curve A on Fig. 5.10, the film/screen combination is said to be fast. Conversely, a slow combination requires a greater exposure to

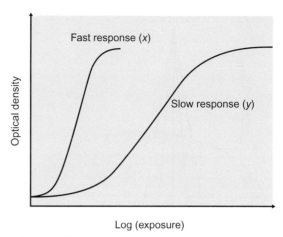
Fig. 5.10 Fast and slow film/screen response curves.

produce the same density (curve B). It might be thought that fast systems would always be desirable, to minimise the patient dose required to produce the image, but this is not necessarily so for two reasons:

1. The image has a more grainy appearance because faster films have larger silver bromide crystals which produce larger individual spots of silver in the developed image.
2. Fewer x-ray photons (quanta) are used to produce the image and this increases quantum mottle, or noise (see later).

Digital Computed Radiography Using Photostimulable Phosphors

An alternative to imaging on radiographic film is digital radiography using photostimulable phosphor plates as the x-ray detector. These are similar to intensifying screens used with film but, instead of emitting visible light immediately on absorbing x-rays, they store a fraction of the absorbed energy as a latent image by exciting electrons to occupy energy level traps where they remain until stimulated by a suitable light source. The spatial density and distribution of trapped electrons forms the latent image. This latent image is subsequently read out by scanning the plate with a laser beam, in a light-tight enclosure, and this causes light of a different wavelength from that of the laser to be emitted as the trapped electrons return to a lower energy level in the phosphor. The emitted light is detected by a sensitive photomultiplier tube that produces an electrical signal proportional to the intensity of the light. The electrical signal is digitised and stored in a computer as an image matrix, which might typically contain 2000×2000 pixels (picture elements).

The term *computed radiography* is sometimes used for these systems to distinguish them from digital radiography using electronic solid state detectors (see later).

Fluoroscopic Imaging With Image Intensifier Chain

It is possible to view a time-varying (dynamic) image by using a fluoroscopic system, in which the x-rays are absorbed by a fluorescent material that emits visible light, as in the intensifying screens used with film. Because the brightness of this image is low, an image intensifier is used to increase the brightness and this secondary image is viewed by a CCD camera (Fig. 5.11). The CCD camera signal is recorded in digital format.

The image intensifier tube is an evacuated glass envelope with an input phosphor, which is typically in the form of a layer of caesium iodide (CsI) crystals. In contact with this is a photocathode, which absorbs the visible light from the phosphor and emits photoelectrons. These are accelerated through a large potential difference (≈ 25 kV) and focused onto a much smaller output phosphor, which again produces visible light

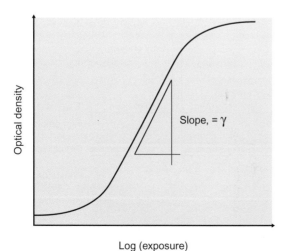
Fig. 5.9 Graphic plot of optical density against exposure.

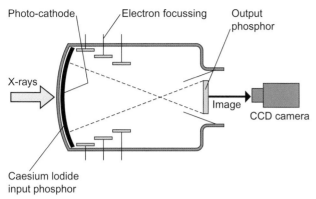

Fig. 5.11 Charge-coupled device (CCD) camera viewing of the intensifier, the II chain.

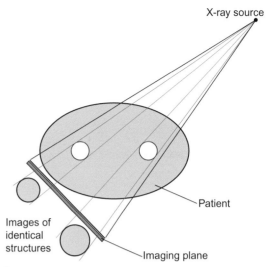

Fig. 5.12 Magnification of objects lying in different planes.

when it absorbs these electrons. As a consequence of the energy gained by the electrons and the fact that they are concentrated onto a smaller area, the brightness of the image at the output phosphor is much higher than at the input. This image is then viewed by a CCD camera, usually via close coupled optics to minimise any distortions and scatter.

At each stage in this process there is some loss of fidelity in the image and this can be serious if the electron optics are poorly adjusted or if there is significant interference from external magnetic fields. Even the Earth's magnetic field can affect the output image.

Digital Fluoroscopy and Radiography Using Solid State Detectors

Large area solid state detectors based on amorphous silicon (a-Si) technology are now available as an alternative to the image intensifier, CR systems and film screen systems. These comprise an array of semiconductor elements, each of which acts as a capacitor storing electric charge. Overlying this a-Si matrix of pixels is normally a phosphor layer, such as Cs-I. This turns the incident x-rays into light photons that are captured by the a-Si photodiodes that turn the incident light photons into electric charge. The charge pattern is read out electronically by control electronics that open transistor 'gates' in each pixel to allow the charge trapped to flow, thus creating a voltage across readout resistors. This voltage is then turned into a digital signal via an analogue-digital converter. This all happens quickly enough to allow up to approximately 4 million pixel signals to be read out virtually in real time (unlike computed radiography systems, which require the image plate to be transferred to a reader) and the digital signal stored as a digital image matrix in a computer. Hence, dynamic imaging can be performed with these systems and pulse mode acquisition is also possible to produce higher quality fluoroscopic and radiographic images.

ASSESSMENT OF IMAGE QUALITY

Magnification Distortion

Because x-rays diverge from a small focal spot and travel in straight lines through the patient before reaching the image detector, the image is magnified as shown in Fig. 5.12. Object features which lie in a given plane, parallel to the image detector, are magnified by the same factor. Planes closer to the x-ray source have a higher magnification factor; planes nearer to the image detector have a lower magnification factor. It is often said that a particular image is taken at a certain magnification: strictly this only applies to one specific plane, usually that passing through the isocentre. Any anatomic feature which does not lie in a single plane parallel to the detector will appear distorted in

the image, since different parts of it will be magnified to different degrees.

Resolution, Geometric Unsharpness and Movement

The resolution of an imaging system is a measure of its ability to represent separate features in the object as separate features in the image. Because no imaging system is perfect, the image of a point in the object is to some degree blurred and sharp edges are rendered unsharp. The image of a point is called *the point source response function* for the system.

There are several sources which contribute to the unsharpness of an x-ray image: the finite size of the x-ray focal spot, patient movement and resolution of the detector system.

X-ray Focal Point Size

Diagnostic x-ray tubes usually offer a choice of two focal spot sizes: fine (typical diameter 0.4–0.8 mm) or broad (typical diameter 0.8–1.5 mm). Fig. 5.13 shows how such a source gives rise to a penumbra when imaging a sharp edge. The penumbra is wider for a larger focal spot. Because of the bevelled angle of the rotating anode, the apparent size of the focal spot, and hence the degree of blurring, varies across the image in the direction of the axis of rotation of the anode. The blurring is also increased for detail lying in planes with greater magnification. This is especially important for the image of field defining wires in a physical simulator as these are located relatively close to the x-ray source and are thus greatly magnified (Fig. 5.14). Sometimes, especially if the broad focus is used, a double image may be produced: this results from the

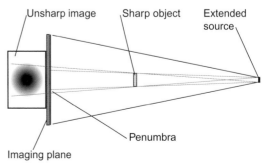

Fig. 5.13 How a source gives rise to a penumbra.

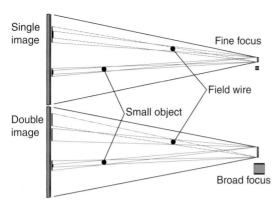

Fig. 5.14 Magnification of the field wires in the simulator.

fact that the focal spot in fact often consists of two relatively intense linear sources of x-rays, separated by a region of lower intensity.

Patient Movement

If the patient moves during the exposure, then features will be blurred in the image. This can be minimised by using short exposure times, by asking the patient to keep still and to hold his/her breath and, if necessary, by using patient immobilisation devices.

Resolution of the Detector

The detector resolution is inherently related to the number of distinct and independent samples which are detected within the image. This can be thought of as the spatial sampling rate of the detector. For film, the sampling rate is directly related to the grain size, so for example, if a grain size was 1.0 μm by 1.0 μm, a 1 mm^2 area of film would contain 1,000,000 samples. Hence the sampling rate can be expressed as 1,000,000 samples per mm^2. With digital systems, the sampling rate is dependent upon the density of sensitive electronic devices that can be manufactured per square mm. This depends upon the pixel size that is effectively the size of the a-Si sensitive element. The resolution required is determined by clinical need and detector design has had to evolve to meet various clinical requirements.

Image Signal and Noise

An ideal x-ray image would represent the distribution of attenuation coefficient in an object with perfect fidelity. In practice, even the image of a homogeneous object of uniform thickness is not perfectly uniform. The signal exhibits variations about its mean level and these are called *noise*. Noise can make it difficult to distinguish signal levels which only differ by a small amount, that is, areas of low contrast in the image.

There are various sources of noise but one that is always present to some degree is quantum noise, or mottle. This results from the fact that any image is made using a finite number of x-ray photons (quanta) and the processes of interaction in the patient and of absorption in the detector are random. This means that there is a statistical variation in the number of photons detected even over an area of uniform attenuation. If the average number of photons per unit area is N, then the statistical uncertainty in the number detected in any particular unit area is $\sqrt{N}$. Expressed as a percentage of the average number this is $100 \times \sqrt{N}/N\%$ or $100/\sqrt{N}\%$. So, relative to the detected signal, the noise decreases as the number of x-ray photons increases, but it is never quite equal to zero.

Other sources of image noise can be the finite size of the fluorescent crystals in intensifying screens, the finite size of silver grains in radiographic film and electrical noise in various components of an imaging chain or digital detector system.

Dose

All x-ray imaging procedures, including those discussed later, give some radiation dose to the patient. This is believed to entail a (usually small) risk of harmful effects, such as future cancer induction. It is normally a requirement of national regulations (e.g. in the United Kingdom the Ionising Radiation [Medical Exposure] Regulations [2]) that the doses from medical imaging exposures should be kept as low as reasonably practicable consistent with the intended purpose. Doses from different procedures can be measured or calculated in various ways. For a given patient, it is often convenient to combine these into an estimate of the total effective dose received, which may be regarded as an index of the total radiation risk from the combined imaging procedures. However, it should be noted that dose limits for patient exposure do not exist and each and every medical radiation procedure should be justified on its own merits as contributing to the medical management of the patient (e.g. [2]).

TOMOGRAPHIC IMAGING

Planar x-ray imaging is limited in its ability to show low-contrast features, especially in soft tissues, and to allow accurate localisation of features in all three spatial dimensions. This results from the fact that it projects a three-dimensional object onto a two-dimensional image domain, coupled with limited ability to reject scattered radiation. Tomographic imaging addresses these limitations by imaging selected planes of the patient separately, that is, two-dimensional sections of the patient as two-dimensional images.

Historically, so-called *conventional* tomography used linked movements of the x-ray tube with planar detectors to image selected longitudinal planes of the patient in focus, with more distant planes increasingly blurred out into a more or less uniform background. Ingenious methods were devised to optimise the use of these systems and there is continuing interest in digital processing of the component images, for example, in the technique called *tomosynthesis*. Although these techniques can improve localisation and contrast, they do not reduce the effect of scattered radiation.

Computed Tomographic Reconstruction From Projections

CT uses the principle of mathematically reconstructing the internal structure of an object from a set of images of the object taken from different projections. To acquire data from which to reconstruct a single slice, the x-ray beam is collimated and aligned with an arc of narrow solid state detectors. The tube and detectors are mounted on a gantry that rotates about the patient (Fig. 5.16). With this set up, it is possible to reject a large proportion of the scatter, while detecting the transmitted primary beam with high efficiency. Essentially, one-dimensional projection images are acquired from many angles and the data are processed in a computer to form images of transverse slices through the patient. There are several mathematical techniques which can be used to do this, including filtered back-projection (see Fig. 5.15), and iterative methods, but most commercial systems use some variant of interactive reconstruction.

Practical Configurations

Almost all modern CT scanners are of the so-called third-generation design shown in Fig. 5.16. Electrical connections with the rotating gantry are made using slip-rings and sliding contactors operating at low voltage, the high-voltage generator being mounted on the rotating gantry itself. This allows the gantry to rotate continuously in the same direction, which is necessary for helical, often known as *spiral acquisitions* in which the patient on the table top is slowly advanced through

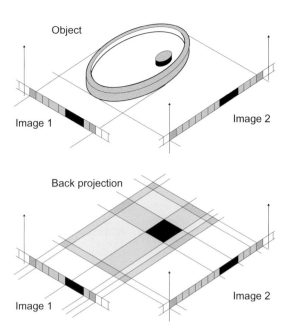

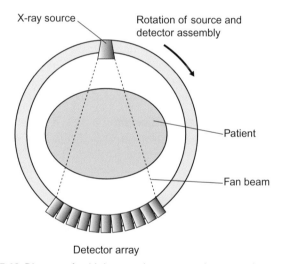

Fig. 5.15 The principle of filtered back projection.

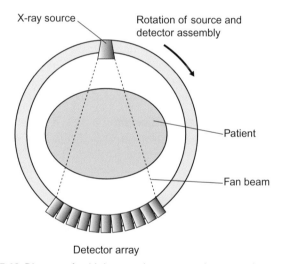

Fig. 5.16 Diagram of a third-generation computed tomography scanner.

the gantry aperture and data are acquired continuously during several rotations.

Multislice Computed Tomography

Since the early 1990s multislice CT scanners have become available, in which several arcs of detectors are stacked together longitudinally and the divergence of the x-ray beam can be adjusted so as to irradiate them simultaneously. This permits more rapid collection of projection data from a given length of the patient and makes for efficient use of the x-rays generated by the tube, thus easing the heat loading requirements.

Cone Beam Computed Tomography

It is possible to acquire projection data using devices other than a dedicated CT scanner. Using a solid-state detector and rotating this about the patient during data acquisition, a set of cone beam projections is obtained from which a set of transverse slices can be reconstructed.

Dynamic Imaging

Many structures in the body move. Some motion is more or less regularly repetitive or periodic, as in the beating heart or respiratory movement. Some may be quasiregular, for example, peristalsis, and others, motion intermittent, for example, swallowing or coughing. A single image will only represent the situation within the time-frame over which it is acquired: if that is short compared with the time over which the movement occurs, then it will be a 'snapshot' of a particular phase of the movement; otherwise it will be a blurred image, averaged over some range of movement.

By taking a time sequence of images, a so-called dynamic series can be acquired, which represents the anatomy of interest at its various positions. This can be useful for diagnosis and staging, for example, a barium swallow to demonstrate oesophageal or gastric abnormalities, or for planning treatment, for example, a fluoroscopic study of the chest to demonstrate movement of a lung tumour.

Gated Imaging

Where periodic motion is present, gated imaging may be a useful option. This represents data over a typical cycle of the motion as a series of images at different times or phases of the cycle. The image acquisition is linked to some suitable physiologic gating signal, for example, from an electrocardiograph or respiratory monitoring device.

DEDICATED RADIOTHERAPY SYSTEMS

The basic principles of x-ray imaging have been described earlier. However there are some x-ray devices which are exclusive to radiotherapy with either x-ray imaging embedded into the device or by using image data obtained with x-rays.

Simulator

The radiotherapy simulator is a machine which replicates the movements and geometry of a treatment machine (linac) but uses a diagnostic x-ray tube to produce kV images. It includes beam limiting diaphragms and field-defining wires to allow accurate simulation of the treatment beam and patient geometry. The gantry and couch of the simulator should reproduce all the movements of the treatment machine and to the same accuracy or better (see Chapter 10).

Computed Tomography Virtual Simulator

By acquiring a series of CT slices over a suitable longitudinal range, it is possible to generate a digital representation of the body in all three spatial dimensions. This can be used as the basis of virtual simulation, in which digitally reconstructed radiographs can be generated to provide beam's eye views of the patient from arbitrary directions for various shapes and sizes of field (see Chapter 10).

Treatment Verification Systems

A check on the accuracy of positioning of treatment fields can be made by acquiring portal images, that is, images of the transmitted treatment beam emerging from the patient. These may be acquired directly onto film or by an electronic portal imaging device. Because photoelectric absorption is relatively unimportant with megavoltage x-rays, contrast between bone and soft tissue is much poorer than with kV images so identification of anatomic features depends more on contrast with air.

Manufacturers now offer a range of kilovoltage imaging devices integrated with linear accelerators for image guided radiotherapy. These include kV tubes and amorphous silicon imagers mounted on the same gantry at 90 degrees to the megavoltage beam. Such systems can acquire data during a rotation about the patient to produce cone-beam CT images.

Another system uses two fixed x-ray tubes mounted in the floor of the treatment room, used in conjunction with ceiling mounted detectors to acquire oblique views of the patient. The images can be analysed by computer software to compare with reference images to indicate required set-up corrections. It can, however, be difficult for operators to interpret images taken from these angles.

At one time, a linac manufacturer offered a CT scanner in the treatment room so that, by rotating the treatment couch by 90 degrees from the usual treatment position, a CT scan can be obtained with the patient set up.

MAGNETIC RESONANCE IMAGING

Overview of the Magnetic Resonance Imaging Process

MRI uses a strong magnetic field (typically 0.3–3.0 T) and RF pulses to produce images of the hydrogen distribution within the body. By altering the interval between the RF pulses and the time at which the signals are detected, images with different tissue contrast are produced. Nuclei with odd numbers of protons and neutrons act like tiny magnets and in the presence of a strong magnetic field, they have a net alignment with the field. After a pulse of RF energy is applied, some of the nuclei will flip and align themselves against the field. Following the pulse, the nuclei will return to the original alignment producing an RF signal at the same frequency as the one applied. Images are generated that reflect the distribution of these nuclei within the tissue.

Producing a Signal

Magnetic resonance occurs when a magnetic field is applied to systems that possess both a magnetic moment and angular momentum. The nuclei of hydrogen atoms are a single proton which has both a magnetic moment and angular momentum. When the hydrogen nuclei or protons in the human body are placed in a strong magnetic field (B_o), they will precess around the direction of the magnetic field at a frequency (f_o) given by the Larmor equation:

$$f_o = \frac{\gamma}{2\pi} B_o \qquad \textbf{5.6}$$

where γ is a constant called the *gyromagnetic ratio*. $\gamma/2\pi$ is approximately 42.6 MHz T^{-1}.

The protons also have a quantum mechanical property called *spin*. When a magnetic field is applied, the protons can either precess parallel or antiparallel to the magnetic field, as shown in Fig. 5.17. The parallel energy state requires less energy. At a field strength of 1.5 Tesla, at body temperature (37°C), the excess of parallel protons is around 4 per million. The excess of parallel protons (or 'spins') in the lower energy state produces a net magnetisation vector (M_o) parallel to the magnetic field (B_o). By convention, the direction of the applied magnetic field is the z-axis.

M_o is of the order of microtesla. Therefore in all MRI sequences, a RF pulse is applied to move it away from the magnetic field (B_o), so it can be detected. The applied RF pulse needs to be at the Larmor frequency, or it will have no effect. The RF pulse brings all the spins into phase, so the net magnetisation vector rotates about the z-axis at the Larmor frequency, as shown in Fig. 5.18A. As the RF pulse continues to be applied, the motion of the net magnetisation vector during the RF pulse in the rotating frame and the laboratory frame is shown in Fig. 5.18B and C. The angle through which M_o is rotated depends

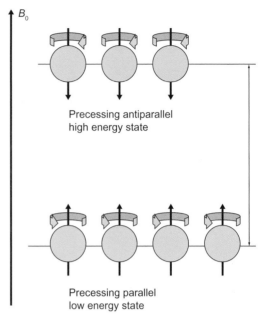

Fig. 5.17 Protons precessing parallel or antiparallel to the applied magnetic field.

on the amplitude and duration of the RF pulse. A 90-degree pulse will rotate M_o into the x-y or transverse plane.

The rotating magnetisation vector induces a voltage in a receiver coil. The detected signal oscillates at Larmor frequency, and decays exponentially, as the individual spin components of M_o rapidly dephase.

Returning to Thermal Equilibrium

Once the RF pulse is switched off, the net magnetisation vector M_o will return to its thermal equilibrium state parallel to the magnetic field. Felix Bloch described this process, called *relaxation*, using two different time constants, T_1 and T_2.

T_1 relaxation is also called *longitudinal relaxation*, as it governs the rate at which the z-component of M_o recovers. The recovery process occurs when spins, which have been excited by the RF pulse, give up their energy to their surroundings (or lattice in early experiments). Following a 90-degree RF pulse, the Bloch equation simplifies to:

$$M_z(t) = M_o\left[1 - e^{\left(-t/T_1\right)}\right] \qquad \textbf{5.7}$$

T_2 relaxation occurs because each proton experiences a very slightly different magnetic field strength, as the surrounding protons and molecules move around it on a microscopic scale. As a result, each proton experiences slightly different magnetic fields over time, causing them to rotate at different frequencies (equation 5.6), leading to a de-phasing of the signal in the transverse plane. This de-phasing, viewed in the rotating frame, is shown in Fig. 5.19. Following a 90-degree RF pulse, the Bloch equation simplifies to:

$$M_{xy}(t) = M_{xy}(t=0)e^{\left(-t/T_2\right)} \qquad \textbf{5.8}$$

As well as the random movement of protons and molecules causing the de-phasing of the protons, de-phasing is also caused by magnetic field inhomogeneities and because of the change in magnetic field at some tissue boundaries. The combined relaxation caused by both random spin–spin interactions, and the magnetic field inhomogeneity and changes at some tissue boundaries is called T_2* *relaxation*.

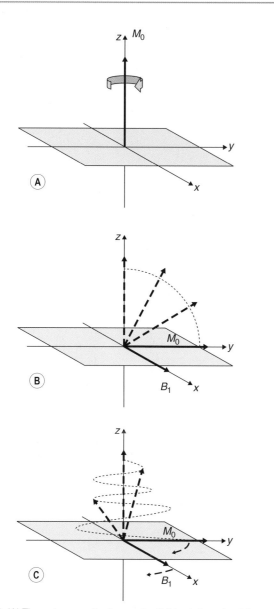

Fig. 5.18 (A) The net magnetisation vector (M_o) rotating about the z-axis at the Larmor frequency. (B) Motion of M_o in the rotating frame during the application of a 90-RF pulse (B_1). (C) Motion of M_o in the laboratory frame during the application of a 90-RF pulse (B_1).

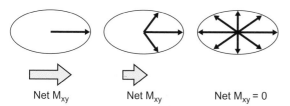

Net M_{xy} Net M_{xy} Net M_{xy} = 0

Fig. 5.19 De-phasing of transverse magnetisation over time shown in the rotating frame.

Imaging Sequences

An MRI sequence provides spatial information, and also controls the contrast within the image. We will discuss image contrast first using the Bloch equations, and then two-dimensional spatial encoding.

How Contrast Is Altered in a Magnetic Resonance Image

To produce an MRI image, a series of RF pulses must be applied. The reason for this will become clear when spatial encoding of the signal is discussed. The time between the 90-degree RF pulses is called the *repetition time* (*TR*). The echo time (TE) is the time between the 90-degree RF pulse and the central point of signal detection.

If no transverse magnetisation remains when each 90-degree RF pulse is applied, the signal (S) produced at time TE is:

$$S(TE) \propto M_0 \left[1 - e^{\left(-TR/T_1\right)}\right] e^{\left(-TE/T_2\right)} \qquad \textbf{5.9}$$

An image with the contrast dependent on the T_1 times of the tissues is called a T_1 *weighted image*. From equation 5.8, to remove any T_2 weighting requires $e(-TE/T_2) \approx 1$ which is achieved by keeping TE$\ll T_2$. To make the signal dependent on T_1 requires TR around the minimum T_1 time. Typically, brain imaging at 1.5 T would use a TR of approximately 500 ms and TE of 20 ms. Table 5.1 shows the T_1 and T_2 times of white matter, grey matter, cerebral spinal fluid (CSF) and fat. equation 5.9, with TR around the minimum T_1 time and TE$\ll T_2$, also indicates that tissues with shorter T_1 will produce a higher signal than tissues with a long T_1. So, on a T_1 weighted image, white matter is brighter than grey matter, and CSF is dark. (Fat will also be bright because of its short T_1 time and long T_2 time.)

To produce a T_2 weighted image, with contrast dependent upon T_2 times requires T_1 weighting to be eliminated. Again, looking at equation 5.8, this is achieved when $e(-TR/T_1) \approx 0$ which occurs when TR ≈ 3 to 5 times T_1. To make the signal dependent on T_2 requires a TE around the T_2 time of tissue. For brain imaging at 1.5 T, the TR is at least 3000 ms and echo times of 80 to 120 ms would be typical. equation 5.9, with TR 3000 ms or higher and TE equaling 80 to 120 ms, shows that tissues with long T_2 will produce more signal than those with a short T_2. So, from Table 5.1 in a T_2 weighted image, CSF is very bright, and grey matter is brighter than white matter.

A third type of image, called a *proton density image*, aims to produce weighting dependent only on the density of protons within a given region and is independent of the T_1 and T_2 relaxation times. So, again looking at equation 5.9, T_1 weighting is eliminated by using a TR of 3 to 5 times the T_1. T_2 weighting is removed by keeping TE$\ll T_2$. The parameters for a brain image at 1.5 T would typically be TR of at least 3000 ms, and TE around 20 ms.

The three image contrasts, using different parameters, are shown in Fig. 5.20.

How Positional Information Is Encoded in the Signal

Next, how the signal is spatially encoded to produce an image will be considered. The two-dimensional spin warp [3] imaging method will be described. Other imaging methods are used in MRI, but this method is the most common.

Fundamental to the imaging process are gradients which produce a linear spatial variation of the magnetic field in either the *x, y,* or *z* direction. The hardware that produces these gradients will be explained later. When switched on, the gradients produce a linear spatial

TABLE 5.1	T_1 and T_2 Relaxation Times of Common Tissues at 1.5 T	
Tissue	T_1 (ms)	T_2 (ms)
White matter	560	82
Grey matter	1100	92
Cerebrospinal fluid	2060	1000–2000
Fat	200	$\approx$110

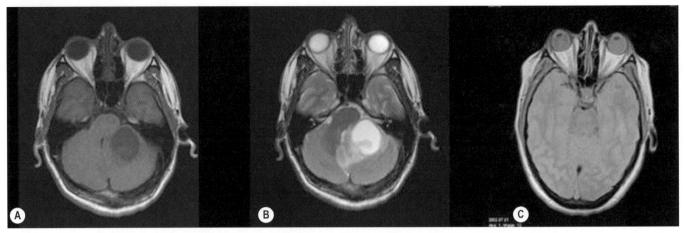

Fig. 5.20 T_1 weighted image (repetition time [TR] = 554 ms, echo time [TE] = 13 ms), T_2 weighted image (TR = 5070 ms, TE = 98 ms) and proton density (TR = 370 ms, TE = 15 ms).

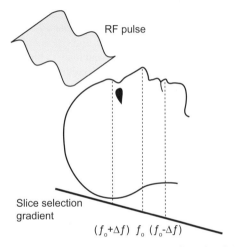

Fig. 5.21 Slice selection gradient applied head to foot. A radiofrequency pulse at the Larmor frequency (fo) will tip all the spins in an axial slice through the nose.

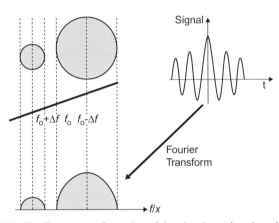

Fig. 5.22 The Fourier transformation of the signal as a function of time, produces the amount of signal present at each frequency or spatial position along the x-axis.

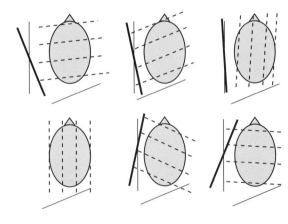

- - - - Lines at the same frequency

Fig. 5.23 The phase encoding gradient is shown as a *thick black line*. As the strength of the phase encoding gradient is varied, the angles of lines of equal frequency change (shown as *dotted black lines*).

variation of the magnetic field along their length. This will also produce a linear variation in the rotation frequency of the spins along the gradient (see the Larmor equation 5.6).

The first step of the two-dimensional spin warp imaging process is to select a slice. This is achieved by applying simultaneously an RF pulse and a gradient perpendicular to the slice direction. Fig. 5.21 shows a gradient applied along the z-axis (or head–foot direction). At the same time as the gradient is applied, an RF pulse is applied. If the RF pulse is at the Larmor frequency, it will flip the spins which are precessing at the Larmor frequency (in line with the nose on Fig. 5.21), but at no other spatial location. Spins at different slice positions are selected by varying the frequency of the RF pulse; for example, in Fig. 5.21, an RF pulse at $(f_o + \Delta f_o)$ will flip the spins at eye level. In each case, an axial or transverse slice will be selected. To produce sagittal images, a gradient is applied from left to right across the patient, and for coronal slices from anterior to posterior. Angled slices are produced by applying two gradients at the same time.

Once a slice of spins has been excited, the positions of the spins within that slice need to be determined. Along one dimension/direction of the slice, this is achieved using a frequency encoding gradient. In Fig. 5.22, the frequency encoding gradient is shown applied horizontally to two different sized test tubes. The signal is collected during the application of the frequency encoding gradient, and Fourier transformed. The Fourier transform of a signal as a function of time is a

signal as a function of frequency. However, by applying the frequency encoding gradient, we have made frequency directly proportional to spatial position. So, the Fourier transform of the time signal is a summation of the signal at each position along the gradient. This is shown in Fig. 5.23, where the Fourier transform of the signal gives the amount of signal in each column.

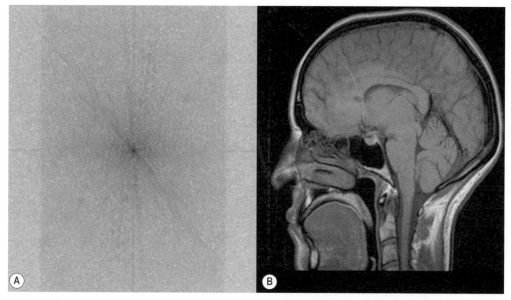

Fig. 5.24 (A) K-space data. (B) The two-dimensional Fourier transform of the k-space data.

How the spatial position in the final dimension of the image is determined is conceptually the most difficult part of the imaging process to understand. For readers who want a much more comprehensive understanding than will be attempted here, I would suggest referring to a good MRI text book, such as *MRI: from picture to proton* [4] or an online resource such as mriquestions.com [5]. A gradient, called the *phase encoding gradient*, is applied along the slice, perpendicular to the frequency encoding gradient. For a 256×256 matrix image, the phase encoding gradient is applied with 256 different amplitudes. In Fig 5.23, some different amplitudes of phase encoding gradient are shown, and it can be seen that these different amplitudes rotate the angle of the lines of equal frequency in the image. The different amplitudes of phase encoding gradient can be thought of as analogous to the different back projections obtained at different tube angles in CT. An RF pulse and slice selection gradient, followed by one of the 256 amplitudes of phase encoding gradient and the frequency encoding gradient, are applied for each signal collected. The signals produced are digitised and stored in turn in a computer. This complete data set (called the *k-space data*) undergoes a two-dimensional Fourier transform to produce the final MRI of the slice. Fig 5.24 shows the k-space data and corresponding MRI.

MAGNETIC RESONANCE IMAGING SCANNERS

The main components of an MRI scanner are the main magnetic, *x*, *y* and *z* gradient coils, a RF transmitter coil and a receiver coil. A computer controls the timings of the RF pulses and currents through the gradient coils. Image reconstruction may be performed by the main computer or an additional specialised computer.

The majority of clinical MRI scanners use superconducting magnets. These currently have field strengths between 0.5 and 3.0 T, but there are 7 and 8 T research systems. (The signal to noise ratio increases with field strength, but so does the potential for RF burns and scanner cost.) The superconductivity (no electrical resistance) is achieved by cooling the wire coils which produce the magnetic field to around −269°C using liquid helium. These magnets have a cylindrical design, with the patients lying inside the bore (or tunnel), and the magnetic field direction aligned with the bore. Fig 5.25 shows a commercial MRI scanner with a superconducting magnet.

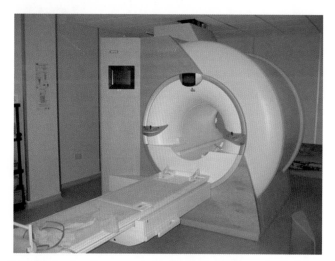

Fig. 5.25 A magnetic resonance imaging system with a cylindrical superconducting magnet.

Other types of magnet are available in commercial MRI systems. For example, Fig. 5.26 shows an open 0.35-T permanent magnet. Although the magnet is heavy (around 10 tonnes), running costs are low.

The remainder of this section will concentrate on the cylindrical superconducting magnet system because it is by far the most common. The field produced by the magnet is not completely uniform, therefore it must be shimmed. A fixed shim is achieved either passively using small pieces of steel positioned around the magnet, and/or actively using computer determined current magnitudes inside special superconducting coils called *shim coils*. As the patient affects the magnetic field homogeneity, additional shimming is also performed each time a patient is imaged. This dynamic shimming uses the gradient coils and sometimes extra (resistive) shim coils. The RF pulses are transmitted through a 'body' coil which is inside the bore of the magnet, and the signal is normally picked up by a dedicated receiver coil. At its simplest, this receiver coil is a loop of wire, orientated perpendicular to the main magnetic field. An MRI scanner would typically have five or more different coils dedicated to imaging different body parts, for example head, knee, spine, body, heart and breast coils, and a few general purpose coils for imaging the remaining parts of the body. The RF coils can be used both to transmit the RF pulses and to detect the voltage signal produced. The most common design of coil which both transmits and receives RF pulses is a birdcage coil (Fig. 5.27). This coil design

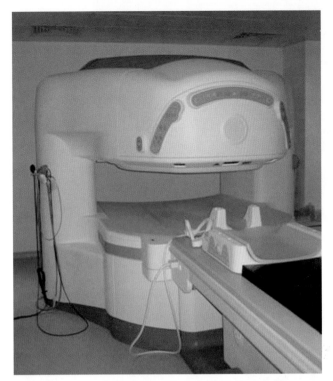

Fig. 5.26 An open magnetic resonance imaging system with a permanent magnet.

produces a uniform RF field with good penetration and is often still used in knee coils and head coils of older systems.

SPECTROSCOPY

Single voxel MRS is a technique which produces a spectrum of the metabolites present in a voxel. Most MRS is performed on hydrogen nuclei as they are the most abundant nuclei and MRI systems and coils are already tuned to hydrogen's resonant frequency. MRS can also be performed on ^{23}Na and ^{31}P. In the limited space available here, only hydrogen MRS will be discussed.

The voxel which produces the MRS spectrum is normally selected using RF pulses and gradient. For single voxel spectroscopy, two techniques called *point-resolved spectroscopy* (PRESS) [6] and *stimulated echo acquisition mode* (STEAM) [6] are commonly used. A Fourier transform of the signal detected from the voxel gives the spectrum (Fig. 5.28). A spectrum is produced because each metabolite has a slightly different

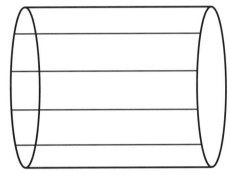

Fig. 5.27 Schematic diagram of a birdcage coil.

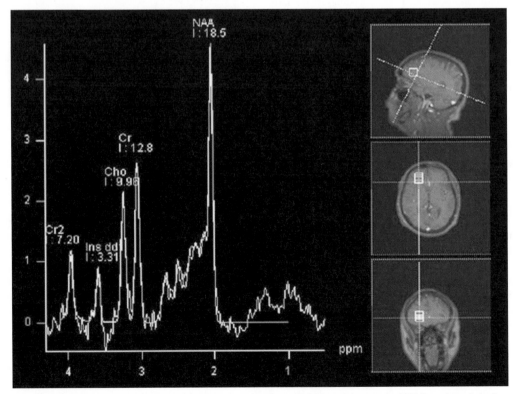

Fig. 5.28 Spectrum from a voxel normal brain tissue showing a high N-acetyl aspartate (*NAA*) peak, and choline (*Cho*) levels below those of creatine (*Cr*). Obtained using a stimulated echo acquisition mode sequence TE = 30 ms.

local magnetic field strength, because of its chemical environment. Therefore each metabolite resonates at a slightly different frequency. The area under each peak is proportional to the amount of metabolite present. The water peak has to be suppressed or this would dominate the spectrum.

Chemical shift imaging is another spectroscopic technique which produces a matrix of spectra from a matrix of voxels encoded with a phase encoding gradient.

CLINICAL APPLICATIONS OF MAGNETIC RESONANCE IMAGING IN ONCOLOGY

Anatomic MRI is often used in the head, neck, abdomen and pelvis for the detection of cancer, and staging the disease. Contrast agents, which are gadolinium based, and injected intravenously, shorten the T_1 of tissue. Areas of tumour with high vasculature are therefore highlighted on T_1 weighted images obtained after the administration of contrast agent.

Complete textbooks have been written on the use of MRI in cancer diagnosis, staging, treatment planning and for treatment monitoring. In this section, the application of MRI in brain tumour imaging is briefly outlined. MRI can be used to diagnose and stage cancer in most organs of the body including bladder, pancreas, bowel, and breasts, cervix and ovaries in women, and prostate in men. The use of MRI in bowel cancer will be concentrated on as an example of this vast area.

Brain Tumours

MRI scanning is unsurpassed as the ideal imaging medium for the diagnosis of brain tumours. Brain tumours make up around 9% of all adult cancers. Approximately one-half are primary tumours and half are secondary. Gliomas are the most common type (45%–50%) of primary brain tumour. Fig. 5.29 of a patient with a large left occipital lobe glioma shows the extent of the tumour which appears as an area of hyperintense signal on the T_2 weighted image. Pathologic processes, such as a tumour or infarction, increase the amount of extracellular water, which can lead to cerebral oedema. T_2 weighted images (see Fig. 5.30A) are best at showing an increase in the amount of extracellular water, which also appear as hyperintense areas (white). On T_1 weighted images, oedema appear as a hypointense (black) area.

Discrimination between the tumour and surrounding oedema can be helped by the use of gadolinium contrast, which can enhance the tumour in the image. Gadolinium is a rare earth metal with seven unpaired electrons. These unpaired electrons enable nearby protons to align more quickly with the magnetic field and therefore shortens the T_1 and T_2 relaxation times. Usually, low-grade gliomas do not enhance on T_1 weighted images with gadolinium; however, high-grade gliomas enhance avidly, often with a heterogeneous appearance because of haemorrhage or necrosis. Fig. 5.29B and C shows areas of strong contrast enhancement where the glioma has broken down the blood–brain barrier. However, isolated tumours cells can penetrate beyond the tumour margins visualised using MRI. This is significant with regard to the margins used in planning (see Chapter 10).

The type of brain tumour can usually be determined by its location and appearance. However, the tumour shown in Fig. 5.30 from its visual appearance and location could have been a glioma or metastasis.

The single voxel spectrum from the lesion is shown in Fig. 5.31. For comparison, a spectrum obtained from normal brain tissue was shown in Fig. 5.28. The very high level of lactate, and only slightly increased choline level, show that this lesion is likely to be a metastasis.

Body Tumours

The role of MRI in body cancer diagnosis and staging is vast. As a purely illustrative example, we will look at the role of MRI in staging rectal cancer and the difference that it makes to treatment.

The very close proximity of the rectum to other organs makes the very exact staging of rectal cancer critical. Fig. 5.32A and B shows an early stage of rectal cancer, with the cancer confined within the rectum muscle wall. This patient was managed by surgical resection. Fig. 5.32C–E shows a patient with the later stage of rectal cancer; the cancer has extended outside the rectal muscle wall along the veins into the surrounding fatty tissue (extra mural venous invasion). This patient required combined radiotherapy and chemotherapy, followed by surgery. MRI was used again at the end of the combined radiotherapy and chemotherapy to monitor the response of the tumour. The patient then had surgery. All patients with rectal cancer will have continued monitoring with CT at 6 to 12 month intervals, to check for liver and other metastases.

MRIs of tumours in the abdomen and pelvis can be fused with CT images for use during treatment planning. The nonrigid nature of the anatomy makes fusion more difficult than in the brain.

ULTRASOUND IMAGING

In this chapter, the emphasis is on the use of ultrasound in imaging. However, at higher power levels than those used for diagnosis, it can be used in various ways in the treatment of cancer and other conditions. These include lithotripsy to smash kidney stones, hyperthermia to enhance radiotherapy and high intensity focused ultrasound (HIFU) to ablate soft tissue.

Overview of Ultrasound Imaging Process

Ultrasound is defined as a vibration with a frequency above the upper limit of human hearing at 20 kilohertz (20 kHz). One hertz (1 Hz) equals 1 vibration cycle per second. In fact, medical ultrasound most often uses much higher frequencies, usually between 1 and 20 MHz, and higher frequencies than these can be used for acoustic microscopy. The passage and interactions of the ultrasound wave as it penetrates through tissue, interacts with it and is scattered, reflected and attenuated enables information about tissue to be derived from the wave [1].

Physical Characteristics of Ultrasound Waves

Ultrasound usually travels as a longitudinal pressure wave moving through the soft tissue producing areas of compression and rarefraction. Considering a small area of tissue—this will vibrate to and fro along the direction of travel of the ultrasound wave as the pressure wave passes.

The amplitude of the ultrasound wave can be defined in various ways, such as the peak pressure, the peak distance displaced or peak velocity of a small area of tissue. A way of characterising the energy carried in an ultrasound wave is to measure the intensity, which equals the power transmitted per cross-sectional area of the beam in Watts per square centimetre.

$$C = f \times w \qquad \textbf{5.10}$$

where C = speed of sound (m/s), f = frequency (Hz) and w = wavelength (m).

For soft tissues, the average speed of sound is 1540 m/s. So, for medical ultrasound, the wavelength is from about 0.075 to 1.5 mm. The resolution of ultrasound images is related to the wavelength, so higher frequency ultrasound, which has a smaller wavelength, gives better resolution.

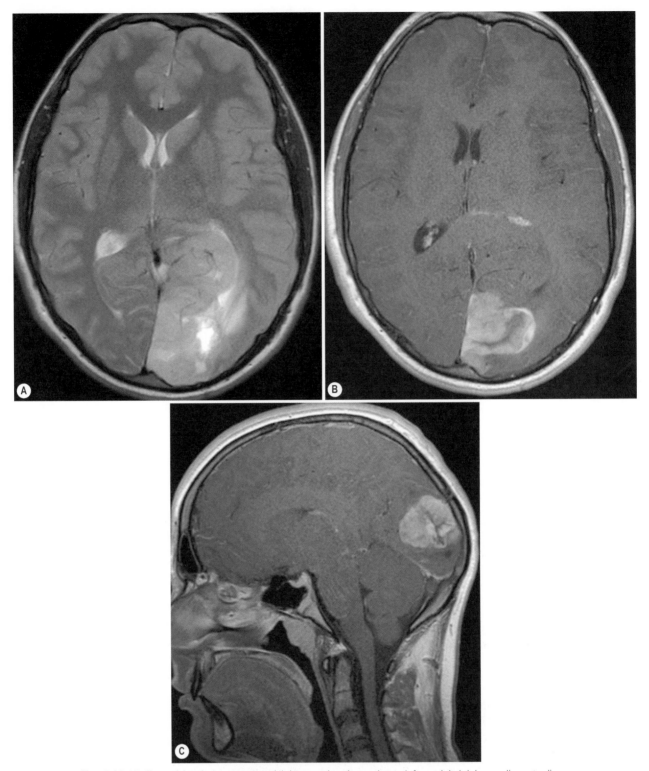

Fig. 5.29 (A) T_2 weighted precontrast axial image showing a large left occipital lobe malignant glioma. (B) Postcontrast T_1 weighted axial image. (The same slice position is shown as previous image.) (C) Postcontrast axial T_1 weighted image. The contrast agent clearly defines the area of the glioma where blood/brain barrier has broken down.

The speed of ultrasound in tissue is related to the bulk modulus and the density of the tissue through which the ultrasound travels. The bulk modulus is defined as the change in pressure divided by the fractional change in volume for a material. So, for harder materials, where a given change in pressure will result in a small change in volume, the bulk modulus is large. Higher density results in a lower velocity.

$$C = \sqrt{(B/D)} \qquad \textbf{5.11}$$

where C = speed of sound (m/s), B = bulk modulus (N/m^2) and D = density (kg/m^3).

$$B = dP/(dV/V) = V \times dP/dV \qquad \textbf{5.12}$$

where P = pressure (N/m^2) and V = volume (m^3).

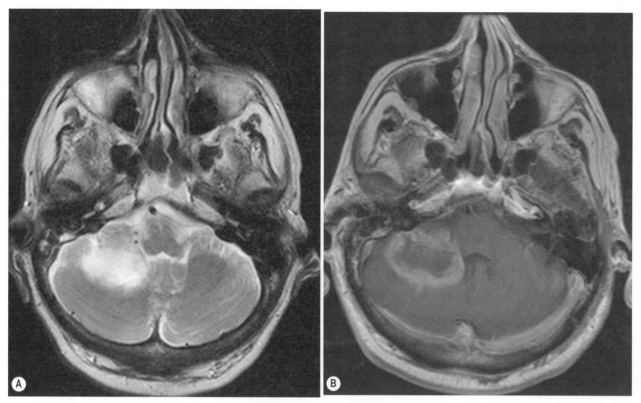

Fig. 5.30 Axial T_2 weighted image of a glioma or brain metastases. (B) Axial T_1 weighted image post contrast.

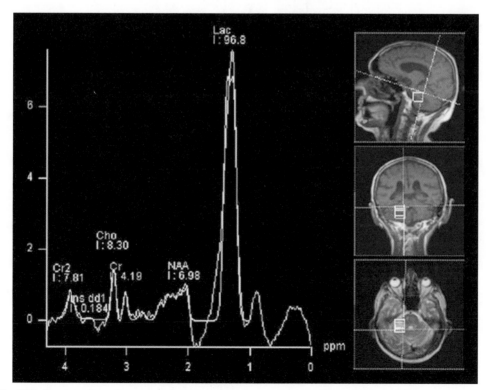

Fig. 5.31 Spectrum from the metastasis showing an extremely elevated lactate peak, and slightly elevated choline levels. The spectrum was obtained using stimulated echo acquisition mode with echo time = 30 ms.

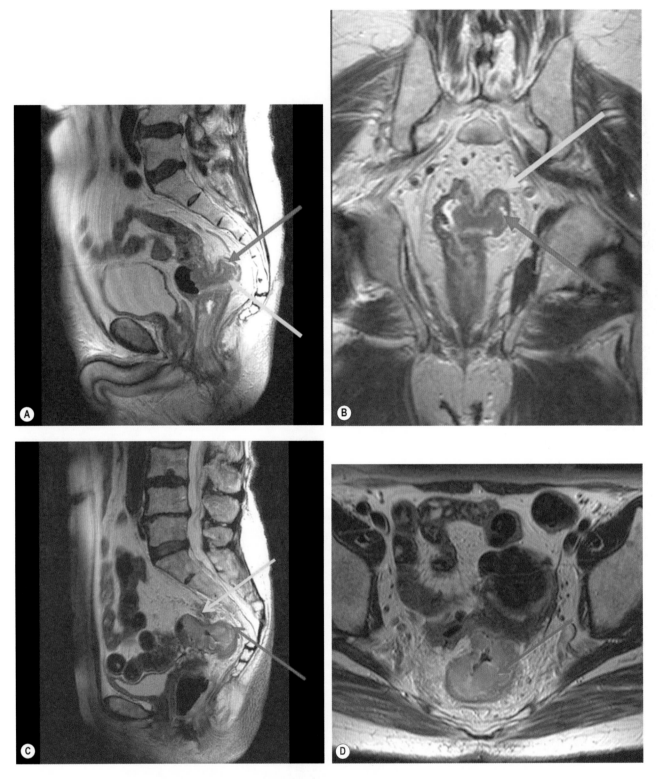

Fig. 5.32 (A) Sagittal image of early stage rectal carcinoma (*red arrow*) still contained within the rectal muscle wall (*yellow arrow*). (B) Coronal image of early stage rectal carcinoma (*red arrow*) still contained within rectal muscle wall (*yellow arrow*). (C–E) Sagittal, axial and coronal images of a stage 3 rectal cancer, which has extramural venous invasion. The *red arrows* point to the tumour and the *yellow arrows* to areas of extramural venous invasion.

Continued

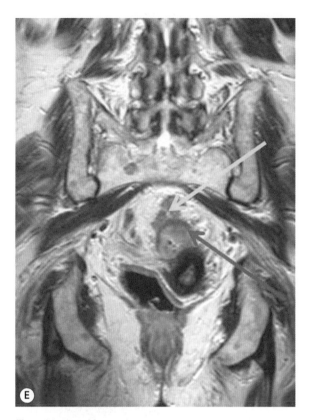

Fig. 5.32—cont'd

The speed of ultrasound in different soft tissues is generally within about ±6% of 1540 m/s. The speed of ultrasound in harder tissues, such as bone, is much higher at about 3200 m/s. Air, which has a low bulk modulus and low density, has a much lower speed of sound at 330 m/s.

For diagnostic purposes, ultrasound gives us information related to the mechanical properties of tissue. Ultrasound is reflected from interfaces between tissues with different mechanical properties. The amount of ultrasound reflected depends on the acoustic impedance of the material.

Considering a small area of tissue, the acoustic impedance is defined as the ratio of the pressure amplitude divided by the velocity amplitude of this small area of tissue as the ultrasound wave passes through it. The acoustic impedance can also be defined relative to the speed of sound and tissue density.

$$Z = \rho \times C \qquad \textbf{5.13}$$

where Z = acoustic impedance, ρ = density and C = speed of sound in tissue.

The fraction of ultrasound reflected from an interface between tissues of different acoustic impedances can be calculated as subsequently.

$$R = (Z_1 - Z_2)^2 / (Z_1 - Z_2)^2 \qquad \textbf{5.14}$$

where R = fractional intensity of ultrasound reflected.

Interactions at Interfaces

For interfaces between different soft tissues, the amount reflected is usually between 0.01% and 1%. For a soft tissue to air interface, 99.9% of the ultrasound is reflected. The practical consequence of this is that ultrasound cannot image beyond gas, so that lung tissue cannot be imaged. Bowel gas can be a problem in the abdomen. Also, the air gap between the ultrasound transducer and the skin must be eliminated using ultrasound gel when scanning. Imaging into and beyond bone is usually impractical, as bone both reflects a lot of the ultrasound and highly attenuates the ultrasound beam.

For smooth interfaces between different tissues, reflection will be mirror like, so that the angle of reflection equals the angle of incidence. Also the transmitted part of the wave may be bent slightly (refracted) because of the difference in sound velocity between the materials. Usually, for soft tissues, the angle of refraction is small and is neglected.

For rough interfaces, the ultrasound will be reflected at a variety of different angles. For small scatterers, which are much smaller than the wavelength, the ultrasound is scattered in all directions. This is called *Rayleigh scattering* and occurs for instance with red blood cells.

As it travels through tissue, energy will be lost from the ultrasound beam by scattering of ultrasound away from the beam direction and by energy absorption in the tissue. Energy absorption occurs when the coherent vibration of the ultrasound wave is degraded into random motion of the tissue, that is it heats the tissue.

Attenuation and Interference

Attenuation of the ultrasound beam is usually proportional to the frequency of the ultrasound, so higher frequency ultrasound is more highly attenuated. This results in a compromise between attenuation and image resolution. For superficial structures, a higher frequency is usually used to give better resolution. For deeper structures, a lower frequency with poorer resolution may be needed to allow sufficient ultrasound to penetrate the tissues.

In addition to the aforementioned interactions, because ultrasound is a wave phenomena, we must consider interference effects. If two waves arrive at a point and the peaks of the waves are aligned, the peaks add up, resulting in constructive interference. If however, the peak of one wave arrives at the same time as a trough from the other wave, then the waves will cancel each other out, resulting in destructive interference.

When considering the intensity of the echo from a small area of tissue, this is the sum of the echoes from a group of microscopic scatterers within this area. The overall intensity of the echo will be a weighted sum of all the echoes from all the microscopic scatterers in this area, which will depend randomly on the degree of constructive or destructive interference. These random interference effects produce variations in echo intensity called *speckle*, which is considered a type of structured noise in the image. When looking at the texture of echoes in an image of an organ, these will be partly related to the physical variations in underlying mechanical properties of the tissue and partly related to random interference. Luckily, in diagnostic images, speckle is a minor problem and it is possible to reduce its effects.

ULTRASOUND SCANNERS

Production of Ultrasound for Imaging

Ultrasound machines use piezoelectric materials to generate and detect ultrasound.

The piezoelectric effect was discovered by Pierre and Jacque Curie in 1880 and occurs in some materials where there is a polarised crystal structure. When a piezoelectric material is compressed, it generates a voltage across the crystal structure. An opposite voltage is generated if the crystal is subjected to rarefraction (low pressure). Thus a piezoelectric crystal will generate an alternating voltage across it as ultrasound passes through and thus it can be used as a detector. Conversely, if an alternating voltage is applied across a piezoelectric crystal, it will vibrate and hence can be used to generate ultrasound.

The most commonly used piezoelectric material is a ceramic material, lead zirconate titanate.

Originally, a focused beam of ultrasound was produced by using a flat disk piezoelectric element with an acoustic lens attached to the front. Modern ultrasound transducers use an array of many small piezoelectric elements, often in a row called a linear array but also in a two-dimensional array. The depth of focus and steering of the beam can be controlled electronically by altering the relative timing delay between the pulses applied to each element.

Derivation of an Ultrasound Image

To produce an ultrasound image, the sound navigation and ranging principle, Sonar is used. This was originally used to detect submarines. A short pulse was directed along a narrow beam and the depth from which the echoes were generated within the tissue was calculated from the time delay between the transmitted pulse and the echoes return, knowing the speed of ultrasound in the tissue. For each pulse transmitted, the intensity of the echoes can be used to modulate the brightness of the image on a screen along a line in the image.

By moving the line along which the beam is directed for subsequent pulses, a two-dimensional image of the amplitude of echoes from the tissue can be built up. This is called a *brightness mode image*, usually referred to as a *B mode image* (Fig. 5.33). In modern scanners, the line of the beam is moved by electronically switching which piezoelectric elements along the array are energised for each pulse.

As ultrasound travels very quickly in soft tissue (1540 m/s), each ultrasound image can be acquired very quickly and frame rates of between 5 and 40 images per second can be achieved, allowing real time imaging. This makes it possible to follow movements of the heart, guide biopsy needles to sample tissue from lesions in real time and facilitate live image guidance during various invasive ablation techniques.

Brightness Mode Ultrasound Imaging

When B mode ultrasound images are produced, simplifying assumptions are made about how the ultrasound beam travels and interacts. The main assumptions are that the ultrasound travels along a straight narrow path at constant velocity, with similar attenuation across the image. Also it is assumed that the pulse only bounces once on its path before travelling back to the transducer. Deviations from these assumptions result in various

artefacts in the images. For example, in reality, the beam is not quite straight because of refraction and the velocity of ultrasound changes slightly when passing through different tissues. This results in slight horizontal and vertical distortions in the images. Ultrasound operators become skilled in recognising these artefacts and minimising their effects. Some artefacts can be useful. For instance, the image beyond a highly attenuating structure will be darker as less ultrasound penetrates beyond the object. Thus a gallstone usually shows a characteristic shadow beyond it. Conversely a low attenuation structure, such as a clear fluid filled simple cyst, will show a bright enhancement streak beyond it, as more ultrasound penetrates to the tissue below. This can be used as a diagnostic feature suggesting a simple cyst.

Linear Array Ultrasound Imaging

Linear transducer arrays, consisting of a single row of piezoelectric crystals usually produce a two-dimensional image. The depth of focus can be controlled electronically by altering the relative amount of delay between the voltage pulses applied to each of the elements. Likewise, a continuously incremented electronic delay across the elements can be used to steer the ultrasound beam. The focussing and steering delays are combined to control the overall beam from the array. The image is built up with brightness proportional to the intensity of the echoes along directional lines exactly the same as the B mode imaging described in the Derivation of an ultrasound image section.

It is possible by moving the transducer perpendicular to this two-dimensional image plane to produce a three-dimensional stack of images. The spatial orientation of these images can be determined using a detector that clips to the ultrasound probe to detect the spatial position of the probe and hence the image plane in space. Alternatively, specialised two-dimensional arrays of piezoelectric elements can be used to produce three-dimensional images by electronically steering the beams across a three-dimensional block of tissue.

Intracavitary and Endoscopic Probes

Sometimes image quality is limited when imaging from outside the body. Small endoscopic ultrasound probes can improve local image quality.

Intracavity probes can be introduced into the body to allow the ultrasound transducer to be as close as possible to the tissue of interest. This allows higher resolution, clearer images to be produced. Transrectal and transvaginal ultrasound probes can be used in imaging of the prostate, ovary or uterus for instance.

Harmonic Imaging

Most of the time in ultrasound imaging, the echoes detected are at the same frequency as the transmitted pulse. However, gas bubbles and soft tissue produce harmonic echoes at multiples of the transmitted frequency. Most commonly, harmonic echoes are detected at twice the transmitted frequency. This technique was originally used in conjunction with ultrasound contrast agents, which consisted of suspensions of encapsulated microscopic gas bubbles that are injected into the circulation. The gas bubbles produce strong harmonic echoes, so it is possible to produce images that largely reflect the distribution of the contrast agent.

Later, it was discovered that soft tissue generates enough harmonic echoes to produce images. These harmonic images of soft tissue tend to have better contrast and fewer artefacts at depth than conventional images.

Dynamic Imaging

The movement of blood and tissues can be measured using the Doppler effect. The Doppler effect occurs when a wave is reflected from a moving structure. If the structure is moving towards the sound source, the

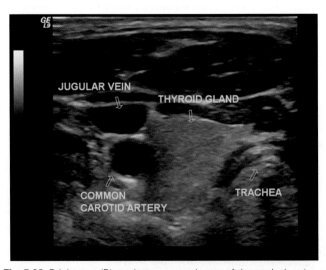

Fig. 5.33 Brightness (B) mode transverse image of the neck showing a map of the brightness of reflection of ultrasound from different tissues. Blood vessels are dark on B mode images as blood reflects relatively little ultrasound.

wavefronts are compressed and this increases the frequency of the ultrasound. Likewise, the frequency is decreased when the structure is moving away from us. The most familiar everyday example of this is a car horn, which sounds higher pitched when the car approaches and lower as the car passes and moves away from us.

Pulsed mode Doppler ultrasound uses repeated sampling of the ultrasound from a sample volume in a blood vessel and gives a detailed real time blood flow velocity spectrum, allowing the changes in flow during the heart cycle to be studied and the blood velocity to be calculated. Fig. 5.34 shows a pulsed Doppler mode blood velocity spectrum in the lower half of the image.

It shows the blood flow velocity spectrum (vertical axis) in a small sample volume as it changes with time (horizontal axis). Each peak represents high systolic flow at the start of each heart cycle. The small upper image shows where the sample volume was located.

Colour Doppler ultrasound measures the shift in frequency from moving blood and overlays this on the B mode grey scale image. The colour on the image is coded according to the direction of the flow relative to the beam and the size of the frequency shift, which is related to the blood flow velocity. Colour Doppler images can give an idea of the vascularity of tissue. Fig. 5.35 shows a colour flow Doppler image of blood flow in the common carotid artery.

Contrast and Tissue Characteristic Imaging

Encapsulated microbubbles can be injected into the blood stream as a contrast agent to increase the reflections from blood vessels and vascular tissue [7].

A newer technique, called *elastography*, can give images related to how hard various tissues are [8]. It achieves this by measuring the distortion of the tissues on ultrasound images with and without applying pressure to the tissue. Other techniques involve generating transverse (shear) waves in tissue. Sometimes, elastography can demonstrate changes in the hardness of tissue surrounding a mass demonstrated

on the B mode image. This suggests that infiltration into the surrounding tissue has occurred and that the B mode image alone may underestimate the extent of the tumour local involvement in some cases.

Ultrasound has some heating effects and other biological effects related to the activity of gas bubbles in the acoustic field (cavitation) are possible. However, if used prudently at diagnostic power levels, it is considered safe.

CLINICAL APPLICATIONS OF ULTRASOUND IMAGING

General Imaging

Probably the best known application of ultrasound is its use in obstetrics to image the fetus. The age of the pregnancy, fetal growth and fetal abnormalities can be monitored and detected. It can also be used to guide the sampling of amniotic fluid (amniocentesis) to analyse the genetic makeup of the fetus.

Ultrasound is used widely in cardiology to analyse the size and shape of heart chambers, the pumping action of the heart and analyse flow through stenosed or faulty heart valves.

In the venous system, ultrasound can be used to detect deep vein thrombosis and analyse the function of venous valves. In the arterial system, ultrasound can detect stenosis, occlusion or aneurysmal disease in the main arteries.

Advantages and Disadvantages

Ultrasound gives good soft tissue contrast and can identify abnormal structure, size or texture of many different organs in the body. It is one of the cheapest imaging modalities, and small portable ultrasound machines can be used in clinics, in accident and emergency, by paramedics in the field or in operating theatres.

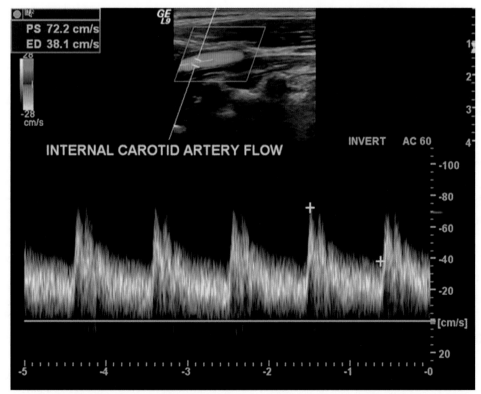

Fig. 5.34 Pulsed mode Doppler sonogram of flow in the internal carotid artery.

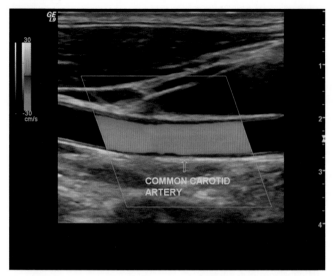

Fig. 5.35 A colour Doppler image of flow in the common carotid artery. The background brightness mode information shows the echoes of stationary tissue. Within the colour box, flowing blood is colour coded according to the direction of flow and size of the frequency shift, which is related to the blood flow velocity and the angle of the flow relative to the beam direction.

However, as previously mentioned, the dependence of ultrasound imaging on the transmission and reflection at tissue interfaces and the poor transmission through an air-tissue interface limits the clinical applications of ultrasound imaging. It is of no value in examining the lungs. Bowel gas can limit the quality of images in the abdomen. Ultrasound cannot usually be used to image beyond bone, although some useful Doppler flow information can be obtained transcranially, using low-frequency ultrasound directed through the thinnest parts of the skull. Calcified tissue can also cause imaging problems notably in renal patients and diabetics.

Also the ultrasound appearance of a solid mass may not be specific enough to diagnose whether a lesion is cancerous and a biopsy is still required to establish its histology.

Imaging for Cancer

Ultrasound imaging is used widely in the diagnosis of cancer, assessment of its local extent and staging. Masses can be identified and characterised, helping to differentiate solid masses from benign fluid-filled cysts [7].

Good images are produced if there is a tissue-fluid interface and, therefore ultrasound is particularly effective at showing whether lumps are cystic or solid. For this reason, ultrasound is frequently used to examine the breast. Ultrasound can distinguish between solid (often malignant) and cystic (often benign) lumps within the breast.

Small endoscopic ultrasound probes can be used to assess the invasion of a tumour into the bowel wall and surrounding tissue for instance.

Colour Doppler can detect the distribution of small vessels within a mass and can help to characterise how vascular it is. Vascular lesions are more likely to be malignant.

Ultrasound is a sensitive technique for detecting metastases within the liver, as metastases often reflect the sound wave poorly and produce hypoechogenic areas. The use of gas bubbles as an ultrasound contrast agent can help to characterise the blood supply in liver tumours. Liver tumours often derive their blood supply from the hepatic artery, which makes them enhance early on contrast studies. Liver tissue that has a blood supply from the portal vein will enhance later.

Ultrasound contrast agents are usually eventually incorporated into the liver parenchyma by phagocytosis. Harmonic images, taken a few minutes after injection, can be used to selectively image the distribution of gas bubbles in the liver tissue. Areas where no bubbles are shown, often correspond to liver metastases, which sometimes cannot be detected on the conventional ultrasound images.

Transvaginal ultrasound can be used to measure the thickness of the lining of the uterus, the endometrium and is a sensitive measure for screening for endometrial cancer in patients with postmenopausal bleeding. It also produces good images of ovarian cysts and solid areas within these cysts can be demonstrated which helps decide whether the lesion is likely to be benign or malignant.

When the ultrasound appearance of a solid mass is not specific enough to diagnose whether a lesion is cancerous, and a needle biopsy is required, this can be done under ultrasound guidance.

Ultrasound imaging can be used to guide various invasive therapies. Ablation devices can be inserted percutaneously or endoscopically into tumours under ultrasound guidance and the local tumour tissue can be ablated using heat, cold or chemical means.

CLINICAL THERAPEUTIC ULTRASOUND

It is worth considering the use of ultrasound in direct cancer therapy. HIFU can be used to ablate areas of soft tissue. A large focussed ultrasound transducer can produce a high temperature increase in the focal area and spare surrounding tissue. HIFU machines often combine MRI and ultrasound. MRI is used to image the area to be ablated and temperature sensitive MRI sequences can be used to optimise and measure the treatment. This technique has been used in various soft tissue and bony lesions. It can be used in areas of previous radiotherapy and can be repeated but tends to be slow to treat a large tumour area.

REFERENCES

[1] Hoskins P, Martin K, Thrush A. Diagnostic ultrasound: physics and equipment. Cambridge University Press; 2010.

[2] Statutory Instrument 2017 No. 1322. The Ionising Radiation (Medical Exposures) Regulations 2017.

[3] Edelstein WA, Hutchison JMS, Johnson G, Redpath TW. Spin warp NMR imaging and application to the human whole-body imaging. Phys Med Biol 1980;25:751–6.

[4] McRobbie DW, Moore EA, Graves MJ, Prince MR. MRI: from picture to proton. Cambridge University Press; 2003.

[5] Questions and Answers in MRI. Elster AD, ELSTER LLC 2018, https://www.mriquestions.com/index.html.

[6] Keevil SF. Spatial localisation in nuclear magnetic resonance spectroscopy. Phys Med Biol 2006;51:R579–636.

[7] Rumack CM, Levine D. Diagnostic ultrasound. 5th ed. Philadelphia: Elsevier; 2018.

[8] Ophir J, Alam SK, Garra B, et al. Elastography: ultrasonic estimation and imaging of the elastic properties of tissues. Proc Inst Mech Eng 1999;213:203–33.

Imaging With Radionuclides

Paul Hinton

INTRODUCTION

Radionuclide imaging plays a key role at all stages in the management of cancer patients. This includes diagnosis, staging, planning the delivery of treatment for both radionuclide and external beam radiotherapy (RT), monitoring of treatment response and follow-up.

An ever-increasing range of radiotracers are available, and the challenge is to localise their distribution as accurately as possible within the patient by the external detection of radiation emitted from the patient involving gamma rays, annihilation photons or bremsstrahlung radiation.

The main advantage of radionuclide imaging is its incredible sensitivity to detect very small amounts of tracer and to demonstrate the function of cells, tissues and organs. Other modalities such as x-ray, magnetic resonance imaging (MRI) and ultrasound primarily provide structural or anatomical information, although the distinction between structural and functional imaging is not absolute.

As new radiotracers become more specific to particular cancer cells, multimodality combinations of imaging systems (hybrid imaging), as in positron emission tomography (PET) and x-ray computed tomography (CT) or PET and MRI, can provide powerful tools for discriminating between normal and malignant tissues [1,2].

A radiotracer is produced when a suitable radionuclide is combined with a pharmaceutical compound or a molecule that targets a particular biological function or process. The behaviour of this radiolabelled compound is monitored by radiation detectors external to the body, allowing the noninvasive measurement of in vivo biochemical function, aspects of tissue function, and dynamic biological processes.

As novel targeting molecules are discovered, a new branch of nuclear medicine is becoming more prevalent, where the same targeting molecule can be used with different radionuclides either designed for accuracy of localisation (diagnostics) or to deliver a treatment dose of radiation with a therapeutic radionuclide, which is known as theranostics. Radionuclide imaging is increasingly becoming essential for cancer diagnosis and RT treatment.

OVERVIEW OF THE RADIONUCLIDE IMAGING PROCESS

A full-ranging nuclear medicine service includes diagnostic imaging, nonimaging and radionuclide RT treatments. This chapter will only cover radionuclide imaging; radionuclide therapeutic applications is covered in Chapter 7. A radionuclide is an unstable isotope of an element that will spontaneously 'decay' by the emission of particles and/or electromagnetic radiation. The three most common emissions from radionuclides are alpha and beta particles and gamma rays. There are two types of beta particle: beta minus ($\beta-$) and beta plus ($\beta+$). Both have the mass of an electron with negative and positive charges, respectively, and a beta plus ($\beta+$) particle is referred to as a positron, the antiparticle of the electron. Of the different types of radioactivity, gamma rays are the only one with sufficiently penetrating characteristics to enable them to be detected externally to the patient.

Radionuclide imaging has two branches. One uses a relatively limited number of radionuclides that emit gamma rays and is referred to as single-photon imaging. The other uses radionuclides that decay by emitting positrons, which are referred to as PET. As mentioned previously, a positron is not penetrating but does interact locally with an electron, with both annihilating to form two photons travelling in opposite directions. These photons are penetrating and can be detected as they leave the body.

A radiopharmaceutical is formed by attaching a radionuclide to a molecule, a process also known as radiolabelling. These are introduced into the body by some means, usually by intravenous injection, but can also be administered by oral ingestion, intradermally, intraarterially or by inhalation. Each radiotracer has a known biodistribution within the body, which is related to the physiology or function of an organ, tissue or tissue type. This is in contrast to x-ray, magnetic resonance, or ultrasound imaging which, to a large extent, image anatomical structure.

Gamma rays are imaged by a device known as a gamma camera and the device used to detect annihilation photons resulting from the decay of positron emitting radionuclides is referred to as a PET camera. Gamma cameras are large-area-detection devices capable of forming an image of the distribution of a radiopharmaceutical within the body. The majority of devices have two detector heads, although it is possible to purchase single or triple head equipment. Imaging with a gamma camera can take place with the detector heads and patient in a stationary position (called *planar mode*), or with the detector heads stationary and the patient moving through the heads on the couch (termed *whole body mode*), or with the detector heads rotating around the body through, typically, 180 or 360 degrees. This mode of acquisition is known as single photon emission computerised tomography (SPECT). PET cameras work on the basis of a series of rings of stationary detectors, identifying the location of a nucleus decaying via positron emission, by coincident detection of both annihilation photons within a predefined time window (of picosecond to nanosecond length). This is sometimes referred to as coincidence imaging.

Most gamma and PET cameras being installed currently are hybrid systems with an x-ray CT scanner incorporated into the gantry. In both cases, the primary purpose is to allow hybrid three-dimensional imaging that is intrinsically coregistered. The use of the structural (transmission) CT image has an additional benefit in that it can improve the quality of the radionuclide images by allowing them to be corrected for attenuation, with the CT scan being converted into an attenuation map [3,4]. This map is used to correct the nuclear medicine functional, emission images for variations in body tissue thickness and density. Having the CT imaging incorporated into the cameras allows the emission and transmission images to be acquired sequentially in the same patient imaging session. Assuming there is no patient movement, the data derived from the transmission image can be accurately applied to the emission images. This process is applicable to SPECT images acquired on gamma cameras and all images acquired on PET cameras. Consequently, imaging techniques associated with these devices are known as SPECT/CT and PET/CT. Initially, the CT units were not of a standard comparable to the most up-to-date helical multislice devices, and the structural images obtained were not of a diagnostic quality. However, gamma cameras and PET scanners are now purchased with high-specification CT units attached and the registration or fusion of high spatial resolution structural images with the sensitive but poor resolution functional images results in an imaging device that is extremely effective at identifying and localising pathology.

GAMMA CAMERAS

Gamma cameras (Fig. 6.1) are imaging devices used to detect and record the distribution of a radiopharmaceutical within the body. Historically these have involved the use of scintillation crystal detectors to convert the gamma rays into flashes of light, but commercial, large field of view, solid-state gamma cameras are now available.

Scintillation Gamma Cameras

Gamma rays are detected by using large area crystals, typically 50 cm × 40 cm with a thickness of about 1 cm, of sodium iodide doped with trace quantities of thallium [NaI(Tl)]. The crystal structure has the property of absorbing gamma radiation and reemitting photons of visible light and is referred to as a scintillator. Smaller detector systems are available for specialised purposes, such as cardiac or brain imaging. A schematic of a scintillation gamma camera detector head is shown in Fig. 6.2. The crystal, collimator and photomultiplier array are mounted inside a lead shield. Further information about the design of gamma cameras may be found in Wolbarst et al. and/or Cherry et al [4,5].

The process of recording a single gamma ray event by the camera is as follows:

- A γ-ray emitted from the body and travelling towards the detector, in a direction approximately parallel to collimator holes (parallel hole collimator), will be able to pass through and interact with the NaI(Tl) scintillator crystal.

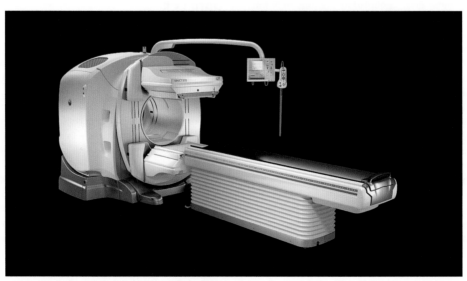

Fig. 6.1 Gamma camera.

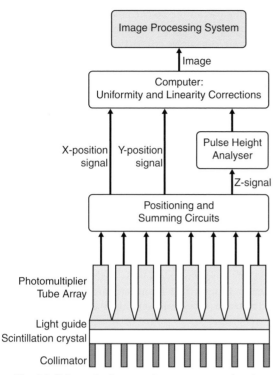

Fig. 6.2 Schematic diagram of gamma camera head.

- The γ-ray will be absorbed by the crystal and the energy will be reemitted as a plume of photons with a wavelength associated with visible light.
- The light photons travel through a light guide to the front face of the photomultiplier tube (PMT) array where they are converted into photo-electrons.
- The photo-electrons are multiplied between the increasing voltage dynodes of the PMT, amplifying the signal.
- Comparison circuitry between the signal produced by the PMTs localises the position of the detected event.

- The total output from the PMT array also gives information about the energy of the detected event. Energy discriminators (windows) allow photons of a specific energy, usually only unscattered photons, to contribute to the image.

Solid-State Gamma Cameras

The scintillation gamma camera has remained of the same basic design since its development in the late 1950s. Many attempts have been made to replace various performance-limiting components, such as the photomultipliers, with solid-state devices to improve the gamma camera's capabilities, but only now are fully solid-state gamma camera systems becoming commercially available for use in routine nuclear medicine imaging. The cameras generally use cadmium zinc telluride (CZT) modules sitting behind a collimator. One of the first clinical systems was the Spectrum Dynamics D-SPECT cardiac camera [6] and now GE Healthcare are producing large field of view CZT systems capable of a full range of nuclear medicine imaging studies [7]. The gamma rays are directly converted to electron–hole pairs in the CZT crystal (Fig. 6.3). With the dedicated counting electronics attached to the CZT, several gains in performance are achieved in terms of sensitivity, spatial resolution, and energy discrimination.

Image Construction

Images of the distribution of radiopharmaceuticals within the body are made up of hundreds of thousands to millions of detected events with each event individually detected. Most gamma cameras have two detector heads and the orientation of these heads is variable. The structure of the collimator affects directly two important performance characteristics of the gamma camera: spatial resolution and sensitivity.

The function of a gamma camera collimator is to permit gamma rays travelling in a predefined direction to reach the detector. This is achieved by absorbing all other gamma rays in the septa between the holes of the collimator. A number of different types of collimators are available, but by far the most widely used are parallel-hole collimators.

Parallel-hole collimators consist of a thick lead plate with several thousand small parallel holes perpendicular to the plane of the plate. For this type of collimator, there is a 1:1 relationship between the size

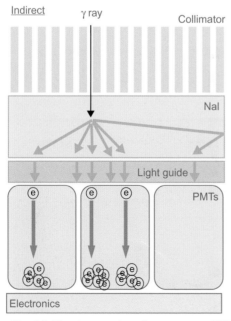
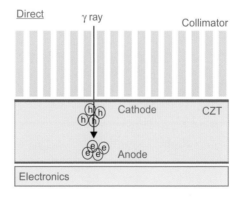

Fig. 6.3 Direct conversion of gamma rays. *CZT*, cadmium zinc telluride; *PMTs*, photomultiplier tubes.

of the distribution of imaged activity and its projection on to the detector. Thus the size of the image is independent of the distance from the subject to the detector face. The characteristics of a parallel-hole collimator depend on the hole diameter, hole length, and septal thickness (amount of lead between the holes). Sensitivity and spatial resolution are inversely related; the higher the sensitivity the poorer the spatial resolution and vice versa. Parallel-hole collimators are purposely designed to image gamma rays of a specific energy ranges, usually denoted as low, medium and high energy. Imaging technetium-99m (Tc-99m) requires a low-energy collimator. The size of hole, length of septa, and number of holes influence the characteristic of a collimator designed for a specific energy. Low-energy collimators are available with descriptions such as high sensitivity, general purpose, high resolution, and very high resolution. The exact characteristics of each collimator can vary immensely between manufacturers.

Imaging Techniques
Planar Imaging

Reference has been made to planar and tomographic imaging. Planar imaging can take a number of forms. The simplest is with the camera directed at the part of the body containing the organ or organs of interest and acquiring a predefined number of events or period of time. These are sometimes referred to as spot views. Keeping two camera heads in a fixed position in front of and behind the patient and moving the patient slowly between the detectors is commonly referred to as whole body imaging. The bone scans (Figs 6.4 and 6.5) shown use this form of imaging. A dynamic acquisition is when a series of images, often sequential and of the same duration, is obtained. With these data, temporal changes in distribution guide the diagnostic results. An example of dynamic imaging is shown in the 'Kidney imaging' section. A final form of planar imaging is when the acquisition is synchronised to a physiological signal obtained from the patient, known as gating. A gated blood pool study shown in the 'Cardiac imaging' section is the most widely used form of this mode of imaging used to estimate the left ventricular ejection fraction (LVEF). The cardiac cycle is divided into a fixed number of frames (the example shown in Fig. 6.10 includes 24 frames each of 41 ms). The dynamic acquisition is triggered by the R-wave on the patient's electrocardiogram (ECG). Images from multiple heart beats are obtained and corresponding frames (first, second etc.) are summed together to produce a dynamic series representing a composite beat. Without

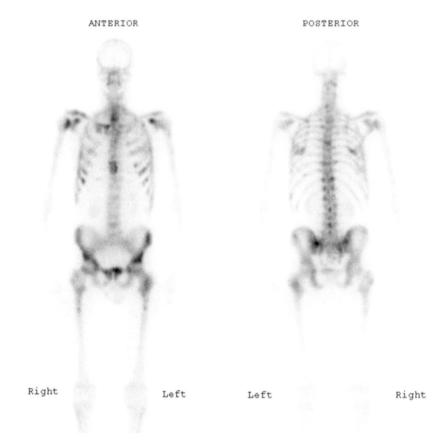

ANTERIOR   POSTERIOR

Right   Left   Left   Right

Fig. 6.4 Normal bone scan.

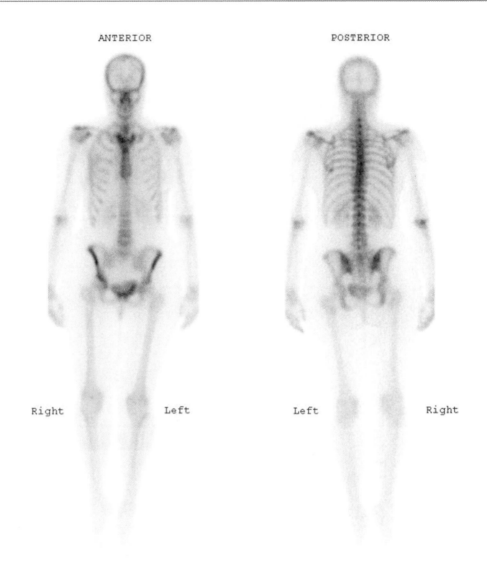

ANTERIOR   POSTERIOR

Right   Left   Left   Right

Fig. 6.5 Bone scan with secondary deposits.

this technique, the quantity of data in each frame would be insufficient to achieve the accuracy of the ejection fraction calculation required.

Tomographic Imaging

Tomographic imaging is performed with a gamma camera, by rotating the detector system around the patient while acquiring images. The image data may be obtained with the camera heads stationary at a number of fixed positions around the body known as *step-and-shoot* mode, or acquired continuously as the camera rotates. Two-dimensional cross-sectional images are reconstructed using mathematical algorithms, in a similar way to x-ray CT. The two-dimensional cross-sectional images can be stacked to form a volume of data that gives the appearance of having acquired a three-dimensional data set.

Knowledge of the three-dimensional distribution of the radiopharmaceutical within the body allows correction for the attenuation of the emitting gamma radiation if the size and density of surrounding structures can be determined. This is achieved with the aid of a CT attenuation map. A CT acquisition represents the variation of x-ray absorption throughout the image volume and a direct relationship

can be made between this and the attenuation of the emitted gamma radiation. An example of nuclear medicine images that have been attenuation corrected and fused with the CT structural images is shown in Fig. 6.6.

Note that the CT device in this example is a low-dose unit, not in the diagnostic category.

Gamma Camera Performance Characteristics

It is essential that gamma camera performance is maintained to achieve the highest possible sensitivity and specificity of each investigation undertaken on it. The performance of gamma camera detectors is characterised by a number of parameters:
- spatial resolution
- sensitivity
- uniformity
- linearity and energy response
- energy resolution
- multiple window registration

Detailed descriptions of the precise definitions of these parameters, factors influencing their stability, measurement methodologies, and how they may be specified during equipment procurement are covered

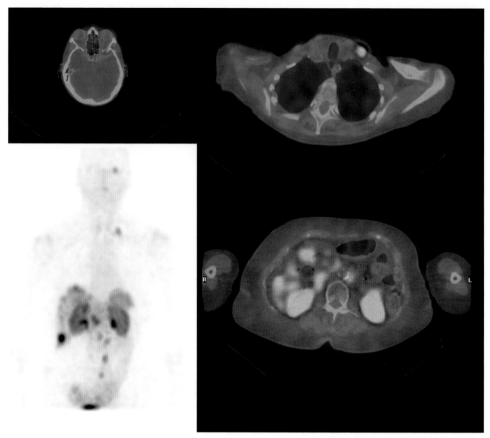

Fig. 6.6 Tc-99m Tektrotyd single-photon emission computerised tomography/computed tomography image of a patient with multiple neuroendocrine tumour metastases.

in two publications: Institute of Physics and Engineering in Medicine (IPEM) Report 111 2003 [8] and National Electrical Manufacturers Association (NEMA) 2012 [9]. Brief outlines are given here.

Spatial resolution. This is the ability to distinguish an object from its surroundings and is a measure of the sharpness of the image. It is defined by a full-width half-maximum distance and this is about 3 mm for the intrinsic (no collimator) resolution of a current gamma camera.

Sensitivity. This term relates to the number of gamma events per megabequerel (MBq) detected by the gamma camera.

Uniformity. This refers to the variations in count rate across the field of view when the detector is exposed to a uniform source of a gamma ray emitting radionuclide.

Linearity and energy response. These refer to the gamma camera's ability to determine the true location and energy of a gamma ray detected anywhere in the field of view. These are the fundamental parameters that influence detector uniformity.

Energy resolution. Statistical variations in the detection of gamma rays by the crystal and photomultiplier assembly result in a characteristic broadening of the total absorption peak of the energy spectrum. Energy resolution is defined by an energy full-width half-maximum.

Multiple window registration. This refers to the ability of the gamma camera to determine the location of a detected gamma event as a function of its energy.

Corrections can be made during data acquisition to overcome some of the nonrandom defects in camera performance. These include corrections for nonuniformity of sensitivity, nonuniformity of energy resolution and nonlinearity.

There are additional performance characteristics to take into account when performing SPECT imaging and still further with SPECT/CT. SPECT imaging requires the centre of rotation of the rotating camera heads to be within predefined limits. Failure to do so will result in artefacts on the reconstructed SPECT images. It is also important that the parameters defining the detector heads' performance remain stable at every angle of rotation. SPECT/CT relies on the accurate registration of the SPECT and CT images and phantoms should be routinely used to assess the gamma camera SPECT capability and SPECT/CT alignment. The performance of the CT is assessed as for all CT equipment, as covered by IPEM Report 91 [10].

POSITRON EMISSION TOMOGRAPHY SCANNERS

PET imaging systems (Fig. 6.7) are designed specifically for radionuclides that decay by positron emission. Scintillator crystals with high stopping power are used, such as lutetium oxyorthosilicate or lutetium–yttrium oxyorthosilicate. These are positioned in rings around a gantry. As coinciding annihilation events need to be detected for PET imaging, electronic timing circuitry registers if two crystals detect a photon within a defined time window, ranging from picoseconds to nanoseconds, allowing 'true' events to be detected. Many single events and random coincidences will also be detected (Fig. 6.8A). The size of the crystal elements depends on the make and model, but is generally 3 mm to 6 mm. The elements are arranged in 360 degree rings, with typically 15 to 30 rings consisting of the order of 10,000 individual crystal elements. The crystal size is one of the main factors in limiting the

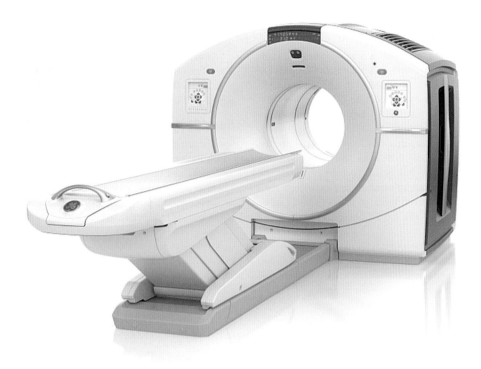

Fig. 6.7 Positron emission tomography camera.

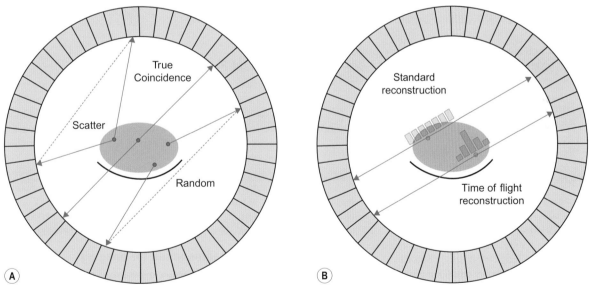

Fig. 6.8 (A) Positron emission tomography (PET)-detected events. (B) PET time-of-flight rebinning.

spatial resolution, commonly 4 mm (full-width half-maximum) [11,12] although systems designed for special purposes, such as brain scanning, can achieve 2 mm.

The computer system is able to reconstruct the line connecting two detected events in opposite crystals as a line of response (LOR). Millions of LORs are acquired over a period of time and reconstructed to form cross-sectional images using appropriate image reconstruction software.

Attenuation of the annihilation photons within the body degrades the image quality in the similar manner as it does for SPECT imaging. Ironically, although the 511-keV photon energy is much higher and

therefore much more penetrating than the Tc-99m 140-keV emission most widely used in single-photon imaging, attenuation effects are more pronounced on the reconstructed PET images. This is because each pair of detected photons will have had to pass through the equivalent of the total body thickness, the exception being activity located close to the body surface. Correction for the qualitative and quantitative impairment of PET images because of attenuation is achieved by the acquisition of CT attenuation correction maps. CT was introduced for this purpose in the early 2000s and PET equipment now routinely has diagnostic quality CT units attached for its correction function, but the quality of the CT greatly enhances the diagnostic capability of the modality as functional and structural information is fused on a single set of images.

As with gamma camera systems there is a move towards solid-state electronics and although PET still uses scintillator crystals for the initial detection, these can now be connected to silicon photomultipliers. This advance allows time-of-flight (TOF) PET to deliver significantly improved image performance. By being able to measure very small differences in the detection time of the coincident photons the information can be used to more precisely locate the origin of the annihilation (see Fig. 6.8B). In non-TOF image reconstruction, the origin of the annihilation event has equal probability along the LOR within the patient outline, but by using exceptionally fast electronics the slight difference in arrival times at the detectors can be used to weight the rebinning of the events more accurately along the LOR.

Other reconstruction improvements such as resolution modelling have also helped improve the quality of PET images. Resolution modelling uses known performance characteristics of the imaging system and compensates for this in the reconstruction of the images.

RADIOPHARMACEUTICALS

A wide range of radiopharmaceuticals are available [13,14]. Most of these are administered intravenously, but radiopharmaceuticals can be administered by many routes, including orally, by inhalation, intraarterially and subcutaneously. When deciding upon the efficacy of a given radiopharmaceutical, the physical and chemical properties of the radionuclide, together with biochemical, physiological and pharmacological properties of the pharmaceutical, must be considered.

The Radionuclide

The best possible radionuclide to use for any given procedure will depend upon its properties, which include:

- type of radiation emitted, its energy and abundance
- half-life
- specific activity
- radionuclidic purity
- chemical properties of the element
  Each of these properties is considered in the following sections.

Type of Radiation

Diagnostic imaging involves external detection of the radiation. Therefore the required physical characteristics include the emission of gamma or x-radiation.

The photon energy should be high enough to avoid serious attenuation in tissue, but low enough to allow the photon to be stopped by and interact with the detector. The design characteristics of a gamma camera favour photons with energies between 75 and 300 keV. Selecting radionuclides that have a monoenergetic emission is an advantage as a single-energy window will minimise the quantity of scattered radiation incorporated into (and degrading) the final image. Absorbed radiation dose to the patient will be kept as low as reasonably practicable if the radionuclide has no particulate emissions and decays with a high abundance of gamma photons. Tc-99m does not emit any particles and provides 89 photons of 140 keV for every 100 disintegrations.

Physical Half-Life

The half-life of the radionuclide must be sufficiently long to allow for radiolabelling, administration, localisation and imaging of the radiopharmaceutical within the organ of interest. At the same time, it should be remembered that the radiation dose to the patient is proportional to the half-life of the radionuclide and therefore the half-life should be as short as possible.

As a rule of thumb, radionuclides used for imaging ideally have half-lives of similar duration to that of the study. However, there are exceptions and some of these are described and explained with regard to biological half-life (see Chapter 7).

Specific Activity

Specific activity should not be confused with radioactive concentration, which has units of activity per volume. Specific activity is activity per unit mass and therefore it has units of Becquerel per gram or mole. There is a maximum specific activity for each radionuclide, which depends upon its physical half-life. Specific activity gives an indication of the ratio of radioactive to nonradioactive atoms of the element in the sample.

Generally, for radiopharmaceutical production, it is best to use radionuclides with as high a specific activity as possible as this allows very small quantities to be used, which will help to ensure that the radiolabel does not significantly alter the chemical or biological properties of the pharmaceutical to which it is attached. However, carrier-free samples can be difficult to work with because there is so little mass of the element present; for example, 500 MBq of carrier-free Tc-99m has a mass of 2 ng.

Radionuclide Purity

Radionuclide purity is the fraction of the total radioactivity in the sample that is in the form of the desired radionuclide. It is important to have the highest radionuclide purity possible as any contaminants of other radionuclides will increase the radiation dose to the patient and may degrade the image. Impurities can arise from the manufacturing process, from daughter radionuclides or from parent radionuclides.

Chemical Properties

Even if a radionuclide has ideal physical properties, it is of little value if it has no useful chemical properties that can be used for localisation or if it cannot be efficiently and securely attached to a suitable pharmaceutical. The success of Tc-99m as the radionuclide of choice in diagnostic imaging is due in no small part to the way in which its chemistry has been exploited.

Chemical toxicity is normally not a matter of concern as radiopharmaceuticals are administered in such extremely small quantities, of the order of nanograms. This amount is so small that it is uncommon for the administration of radiopharmaceuticals to a patient to cause any interference at all with the physiological effects being investigated.

The Ideal Radionuclide for Imaging

Tc-99m comes close to meeting the requirements of a near ideal radionuclide for imaging. It has a monoenergetic gamma emission of 140 keV, high abundance, no accompanying particulate emissions, a half-life of 6 hours and decays to an effectively stable daughter product. It is readily available from a molybdenum-99 generator in a chemical form that can be simply attached to a range of pharmaceuticals.

Mechanisms of Localisation

Radiopharmaceuticals can be divided into two major categories depending upon whether or not their localisation within the body involves their participation in a specific chemical reaction. Many traditional radiopharmaceuticals, such as Tc-99m macroaggregated albumin (MAA) for lung perfusion imaging, are not incorporated into specific biochemical pathways but rely for their utility on the correct molecular size and route of administration. The most exciting developments in recent years have involved radiopharmaceuticals whose precise chemical nature has allowed specific biochemical pathways to be investigated; for example, Tc-99m octreotide (Tektrotyd), a somatostatin analogue used to localise neuroendocrine tumours that overexpress somatostatin receptors [15].

A more detailed breakdown of mechanisms that determine the localisation and behaviour of radiopharmaceuticals is given later.

Diffusion and Dilution

Tracers may be used that distribute themselves throughout the space in the body into which they were introduced. Imaging of their distribution can identify the extent of these areas or demonstrate where their natural boundaries have broken down. For example, ventilation imaging, which depends upon the inhalation of a suitable tracer, such as krypton-81m gas, into the lungs where it diffuses throughout the functioning air spaces, allowing them to be visualised.

Radiotracer dilution is a quantitative (generally nonimaging) method which depends on complete mixing of a radiopharmaceutical throughout a body space. Knowledge of the administered activity and the radioactive concentration of a sample of the fluid within the space once mixing is complete will allow the volume of the space to be calculated. An example is the determination of red cell mass.

Capillary Blockade and Cell Sequestration

If radioactive particles in the size range 20 to 50 μm are injected into the vascular system, they will partially occlude the first capillary bed they encounter (the size of capillaries is 8–10 μm). An intravenous injection of 200,000 Tc-99m-labelled particles of MAA will block around 0.02% of the capillaries of a normal lung, thus permitting the visualisation of the vascular bed of the lungs. A protein such as albumin is chosen for production of the particles, as it will be broken down naturally and removed from the lungs.

Phagocytosis

The reticuloendothelial cells in the body have the capacity to ingest bacteria and small particles in the range 0.01 to 10 μm. This is known as phagocytosis. If a radiolabelled colloid is injected intravenously, the phagocytic action of the reticuloendothelial cells, in particular the Kupffer cells in the liver, will remove the colloid from the circulation, enabling the organ to be visualised. Areas of nonfunctioning liver tissue will not remove the colloid material.

Metabolic Pathway

The metabolic pathway of a huge number of substances can be investigated using radioactive techniques. They may be designed specifically to investigate a particular body function, such as Tc-99m-labelled mercaptoacetyltriglycine (MAG3) for the investigation of kidney function.

Iodine is incorporated into the hormones produced by the thyroid gland, and a study of the metabolic behaviour of iodine in the body gives valuable diagnostic information on thyroid function. Radioactive iodine introduced into the body therefore enables iodine metabolism to be studied easily. iodine-131 and iodine-123 are two radionuclides commonly used for imaging thyroid tissue (see discussion later).

Metabolic Trapping

Some radiopharmaceuticals become trapped within the tissue into which they have been transported by metabolic processes. Certain radiopharmaceuticals have been developed specifically to exploit this behaviour. For example, Tc-99m tetrofosmin and methoxyisobutylisonitrile (MIBI) were developed to mimic the distribution of uptake of thallium-201 used in myocardial perfusion. Thallium-201 washes out of the tissues quickly, but the Tc-99m-labelled analogues are trapped,

allowing more time for the tracer distribution to be imaged and generating better quality images.

Fluorine-18 fluorodeoxyglucose (F-18 FDG) is the most widely used radiopharmaceutical in PET imaging. It is commonly described as a metabolic marker. Its chemistry is modified by the label so that it becomes trapped within the cells and its method of localisation comes under the heading of metabolic trapping rather than metabolic pathway (see discussion later).

Antibodies and Antibody Fragments

Antibodies are large Y-shaped molecules consisting of proteins. They form part of the body's immune response and the body manufactures them as needed to neutralise a threat posed to the body by foreign or harmful material. The material that triggers the antibody response is called the antigen. Antibodies are produced in the body at the site of need and are not designed to be carried in the blood seeking out suitable receptors but splitting them into fragments can retain their functionality and remove some of the drawbacks of using the whole antibody.

Antibodies can also be raised against substances that are not foreign to the body. For example, there are antileukocyte antibodies and fragments of these can be radiolabelled and used to investigate the distribution of circulating leukocytes and their sites of accumulation in the body (see later).

Radiolabelling of antibodies has been seen as very promising in nuclear medicine but nonspecific uptake, particularly in the liver, has meant that few radiolabelled antibodies are in routine use for radionuclide imaging.

Receptor Binding

However, the experience gained in attempting to label antibodies did pay dividends in the area of receptor labelling. Receptors are found in all areas of the body and their specificity has been exploited in various commercially available products. One example is somatostatin receptors, which can be used to investigate and treat neuroendocrine and other tumours (see later). Other receptor targets that are looking promising are prostate-specific membrane antigen for prostate cancer and human epidermal growth factor (HER) for breast cancer.

Production and Quality Control of Radiopharmaceuticals

For the vast majority of studies, radiopharmaceuticals are bought from a supplier; either as the labelled compound ready for administration or as a sterile kit containing the chemicals to label the desired radionuclide on site. The chemicals are supplied freeze dried in a vial ready to be reconstituted when needed. The most common type is the Tc-99m cold kit. There are many examples of these. They all contain the pharmaceutical itself, some form of reducing agent to pull the technetium away from its pertechnetate environment, and additional material required to bulk out the contents so that they freeze-dry successfully. There may be additional chemicals to buffer the solution to ensure that it maintains the correct pH and other substances required to ensure optimum chemical binding between the radionuclide and the pharmaceutical. The pertechnetate itself is produced by a molybdenum-99 generator, obtained from a manufacturer once or twice a week, and eluted once or twice a day.

The bulk of the quality control of a radiopharmaceutical or its components is the responsibility of the manufacturer. However, each nuclear medicine department is required to ensure the quality of the radiopharmaceuticals it uses. For the majority of diagnostic tests, intravenous injection is necessary, so great care must be taken to produce a sterile radiopharmaceutical in a solution of the correct pH value and free from foreign proteins arising from previous bacteriological activity (pyrogens). To ensure this, they are obtained from an onsite or off-site radiopharmacy, which is either licensed by the Medicines and Healthcare Products Regulatory Agency or can claim an exemption under the Medicines Act 1968 [16].

Specialised cabinets are used to provide an environment that caters for the conflicting requirements of the radiation safety of the operator and the need for aseptic production. For radiation safety, it is customary to provide an environment at a lower pressure than its surroundings to contain any airborne contaminants. However, the preparation area must be bathed in sterile air at a pressure higher than that of the surroundings so as to avoid inward leakage of nonsterile air and microorganisms. Labelling of a patient's own cells is classed as a medical procedure and is undertaken in specialised facilities with more stringent requirements for protection of the operator and the product.

Before administration, the information on the label on the vial, syringe or capsule, if oral administration, is checked against that prescribed for the procedure. The activity given to the patient is checked independently in a radionuclide calibrator, which measures the amount of radioactivity (generally in MBq) for the radionuclide specified. The constancy of the radionuclide calibrator is checked daily and its calibration should be traceable to national standards. The amount of activity administered is noted in the patient record. These checks are required under the Ionising Radiation (Medical Exposures) Regulations 2017 [17].

If the binding of the radionuclide to the pharmaceutical is poor, the distribution of radioactivity in the body may appear unusual or abnormal. Poor binding can be as a result of problems with the radiopharmaceutical or one of its components or it may be as a result of a fault in reconstitution. Radiopharmacies measure the radiochemical purity, usually by chromatography, to check the binding. Unusual distributions in images should be reported to the radiopharmacy for investigation, although other situations can arise that will modify the distribution. For example, a woman who is breastfeeding may exhibit increased uptake of radioactivity because of uptake into milk. In addition, prescribed and over-the-counter drugs taken by the patient may affect the biodistribution of a radiopharmaceutical.

CLINICAL APPLICATIONS

Imaging of the distribution of a radiopharmaceutical within tissues and, in some cases, how it changes with time, enables deductions to be made about the function of the tissue. An abnormal distribution may appear as an increase in radioactive concentration above the surroundings or the expected margins, revealing lesions as hot spots; or as reduced activity in the visualised pattern. The appearance of hot spots does not necessarily mean that a lesion is larger than the minimum resolvable power of the gamma camera; if the amount of activity accumulated in the lesion is large enough compared with its surroundings, the lesion will be detected in the image. Cold spots are sometimes referred to as photopenic areas; they are more difficult to detect than hot spots because the margins are blurred with respect to the surroundings.

The purpose of imaging is to investigate tissue function rather than anatomical definition. The following provides a brief description of some of the more important clinical applications of radionuclide imaging, directly or closely applicable to imaging cancer.

Table 6.1 is a list of commonly used radiopharmaceuticals with notes on their more important uses, details of the diagnostic reference level, the absorbed dose to the critical organ and the effective dose to the whole body from International Commission on Radiological Protection (ICRP) 53 and subsequent addenda [18].

Bone Imaging

Bone imaging is the most widely used investigation in nuclear medicine and the majority of referrals relate to patients with known primary tumours (breast or prostate cancer) and suspected metastatic spread of the disease to the bones. Bone is made up of collagen and minerals, mainly calcium, phosphates and hydroxides. The minerals form a crystalline lattice known as hydroxyapatite. Following intravenous injection, a bone-seeking agent will be transported to the bone and become adsorbed on to the newly forming hydroxyapatite crystals, thus reflecting the bone-forming (or osteoblastic) activity at a given skeletal site. Hence areas where there is an abnormally high increase in bone turnover will show increased uptake and will appear as hot spots on the image. Because localisation in bone depends on transportation in blood, avascular areas will appear cold. Conversely, areas of locally increased blood flow may appear as areas of increased uptake on the scan.

All current commercially available bone-seeking radiopharmaceuticals are based on phosphate-containing compounds, which can be labelled with Tc-99m. A variety of analogues are available, but the most widely used is methylene diphosphonate (MDP). Typically, 400 to 600 MBq of Tc-99m MDP is administered intravenously and, after a period of 3 to 4 hours (to enable circulating activity to clear), approximately 40% of the injected activity will be localised in the bone, with the majority of the remainder being excreted via the kidneys. Multiple static views or a combination of a whole body imaging and selected static views is acquired. Tomography may also be helpful where a higher dose of 800 MBq can be given. A normal bone scan is shown in Fig. 6.4 and a bone scan showing secondary deposits is shown in Fig. 6.5.

The bone scan is a very sensitive technique for demonstrating bone lesions and shows changes earlier than conventional x-ray. For musculoskeletal problems SPECT/CT scans are particularly useful.

Tumour Imaging

Nuclear medicine can employ many agents to aid in tumour localisation and to follow the progress of the disease and treatment. This section describes nonspecific tumour agents, such as gallium, thallium, and MIBI, as well as several specific tumour agents and studies.

Gallium

Gallium-67 citrate has a long history of use in radionuclide imaging. It was the first agent used for the investigation of infection and has also been used in many different tumour types and in suspected osteomyelitis. Its use has gradually decreased over the years as more specific agents have been developed, but it still has a place in the investigation of sarcoidosis of the lung and, in oncology, for the investigation of inflammation or neoplastic disorders, where other modalities have been unhelpful, and in fever of unknown origin.

It is injected intravenously and binds immediately to transferrin which localises in normal spleen, liver, gastrointestinal tract, kidneys and, to a certain extent, in bone. It also localises in inflammation, infection and many tumour types. Uptake is therefore widespread and diffuse.

Thallium

Thallium-201 as thallous chloride is handled by the body in a similar way to potassium, which is why it has been employed to investigate the parathyroid and myocardial perfusion. Incidental findings on such studies indicated that it could also be taken up by some tumours. The mechanism is uncertain, but it has found a role in some centres in the localisation of viable tissue, particularly in brain tumours and osteosarcoma.

MIBI

Tc-99m MIBI was developed to replace thallium-201, and was also noted to localise in tumours while it was under clinical evaluation as

TABLE 6.1   Examples of Some Radiopharmaceuticals in Common Diagnostic Use With Critical Organ, Effective Dose, and Diagnostic Reference Activity

Radionuclide	Chemical Form	Clinical Use	DRL Activity (MBq)	Physical Half-Life	Route	Critical Organ	Dose to CO (mSv)	Effective Dose (mSv)
Fluorine-18	Fluorodeoxyglucose	Tumour imaging	400	110 minutes	IV	Bladder	64	8
Gallium-68	Prostate-specific membrane antigen	Prostate cancer imaging	150	68 minutes	IV	Kidneys	30	3
Gallium-68	Dotatate	Somatostatin Receptor Imaging	250	68 minutes	IV	Spleen	70	6.4
Gallium-67	Gallium citrate	Tumour and inflammation imaging	150	78.3 hours	IV	Gonads	10	15
Krypton-81m	Gas	Lung ventilation imaging	6000	13 seconds	Inhalation	Lungs	1	0.2
Indium-111	Indium oxide–labelled leukocytes	Infection and abscess imaging	20	2.8 days	Leukocyte labelling and IV	Spleen	110	7
Iodine-123	Sodium iodide	Thyroid imaging	20	13.2 hours	Oral or IV	Thyroid	90	4 for 35% uptake
Iodine-131	Sodium iodide	Thyroid metastases imaging	400	8.1 days	Oral or IV	Bladder	244	24 for 0% uptake
Technetium-99m	Sodium pertechnetate	Thyroid imaging	80	6 hours	IV	Colon	3	1
Technetium-99m	Sodium pertechnetate	Meckel diverticulum imaging	400	6 hours	IV	Colon	17	5
Technetium-99m	Macroaggregated albumin	Lung perfusion imaging	100	6 hours	IV	Lungs	7	1
Technetium-99m	Exametazime HMPAO	Regional cerebral blood flow imaging	500	6 hours	IV	Kidney	17	5
Technetium-99m	HMPAO attached to leukocytes	Infection imaging	200	6 hours	Leukocyte labelling and IV	Spleen	30	2
Technetium-99m	Pentetate (DTPA) as aerosol	Lung ventilation imaging	80	6 hours	Inhalation	Lungs	1	0.5
Technetium-99m	MAG3	Renal imaging	100	6 hours	IV	Bladder	11	0.7
Technetium-99m	Phosphonate (MDP, HDP)	Bone imaging	600	6 hours	IV	Bladder	29	3
Technetium-99m	Succimer (DMSA)	Kidney imaging	80	6 hours	IV	Kidneys	14	0.7
Technetium-99m	MIBI or tetrofosmin	Myocardial perfusion at rest or exercise	400	6 hours	IV	Colon	7–10	3–4
Technetium-99m	Octreotide	Somatostatin Receptor Imaging	740	6 hours	IV	Kidneys	15	3.7
Thallium-201	Thallous chloride	Myocardial perfusion imaging	80	73.1 hours	IV	Gonads	47	18

CO, Critical organ; *DMSA*, dimercaptosuccinic acid; *DTPA*, diethylenetriamine pentaacetic acid; *HDP*, hydroxymethyl diphosphonate; *HMPAO*, hexamethylpropyleneamine oxime; *IV*, intravenous; *MAG3*, mercaptoacetyltriglycine; *MDP*, methylene diphosphonate; *MIBI*, methoxyisobutylisonitrile.

a myocardial perfusion agent. It has found an application in the localisation of breast tumours.

mIBG

Metaiodobenzylguanidine (mIBG) is an analogue of norepinephrine (noradrenaline) and guanethidine. It is available radiolabelled with iodine-123 for diagnostic imaging and with iodine-131 for pretreatment dosimetry and therapy. Normal adrenal medulla tissue will concentrate the agent as will neuroendocrine tumours or tumours of neural crest origin, such as pheochromocytoma, neuroblastoma, carcinoid tumours and medullary carcinoma of the thyroid. Uptake into tumour can be inhibited by many drugs, including tricyclic antidepressants; therefore care must be taken to withdraw any potentially interfering medication well in advance.

Somatostatin Receptor Imaging

Somatostatin is a peptide found in the brain, where it acts as a neurotransmitter, in the gastrointestinal tract, and the pancreas, where it is manufactured. It inhibits the release of neuroendocrine hormones, such as growth hormone and insulin.

Somatostatin receptors are found in normal pituitary, pancreas and upper gastrointestinal tract from the stomach to jejunum. They are also expressed by a variety of endocrine tumours, such as carcinoid, small cell lung cancer, in tumours of the ovary, cervix, endometrium, breast, kidney, larynx, paranasal sinus, salivary gland, and some skin tumours and tumours arising from glial cells in the central nervous system. It can be surmised that somatostatin receptor imaging could therefore be clinically useful in a variety of tumours. However, somatostatin has a half-life of only 2 to 3 minutes in the body so such imaging was not feasible until the availability somatostatin analogues with much longer clearance times.

Initially in single-photon imaging, an indium-111-labelled somatostatin (^{111}In-pentetreotide) was used, but now a technetium-labelled somatostatin analogue is available: ^{99m}Tc-HYNIC-Tyr3-Octreotide (Tektrotyd). Somatostatin receptors can also be labelled with gallium-68, a positron emitter with a half-life of 68 minutes for PET imaging.

Sufficient uptake for visualisation can occur with many carcinoid tumours, pituitary tumours, gastrointestinal tract endocrine tumours (although disappointing in insulinoma), small cell lung cancer, medullary carcinoma of thyroid, neuroblastoma, pheochromocytoma, meningioma plus Hodgkin and non-Hodgkin lymphoma. Many of these tumours may be better visualised with CT and MRI, but somatostatin receptor imaging may be used to demonstrate small symptomatic tumours and metastatic spread, although hepatic metastases are difficult to visualise because of uptake in normal liver. Evidence of somatostatin receptor uptake is an essential step when considering radionuclide therapy for these tumours. Fig. 6.8 shows a Tc-99m SPECT/CT image of a patient with multiple neuroendocrine tumour metastases in the liver.

Imaging Thyroid Cancer

Nuclear medicine imaging of the thyroid plays a minor role in the initial diagnosis of thyroid cancer. Ultrasound and fine-needle aspiration are first-line imaging techniques [19].

The normal function of the thyroid gland includes the concentration of iodine from the circulation, and the synthesis and storage of thyroid hormones. Iodine may also be trapped in the salivary glands and the gastric mucosa. Iodine-131 was once the radionuclide of choice for all thyroid imaging. However, because it delivers a relatively high radiation dose to the patient and has poorer imaging properties, it has been almost completely superseded by iodine-123 and Tc-99m pertechnetate

for routine diagnostic thyroid imaging. Iodine-131 continues to be used for therapy (see Chapter 7) and, in some centres, for whole body imaging in patients who have previously undergone treatment for thyroid cancer and where further disease is suspected.

Fig. 6.9 shows a whole body iodine-131 scan on a patient previously treated for thyroid cancer but with widespread metastases. Sometimes suspected thyroid metastases do not appear 'hot' on the iodine-131 scan. In such circumstances, they may be designated to be not iodine avid and an F-18 FDG study may be considered for further evaluation.

Cardiac Imaging

The commonest cardiac investigation performed in the nuclear medicine department on oncology patients is gated blood pool imaging. It is correctly called equilibrium radionuclide ventriculography, but more often termed a MUGA (multiple gated acquisition) scan. It is used to evaluate cardiac function, in terms of LVEF, before and in response to the administration of potentially cardiotoxic chemotherapeutic drugs.

The heart is a muscular organ divided internally by a septum into right and left sides, each side having two chambers. The right and left atria receive blood returning from the pulmonary and systemic circulations. The right and left ventricles are pumping chambers and are more muscular, particularly the left ventricle, which pumps the blood to the systemic circulation.

LVEF is one of the major indicators of cardiac function. It can be investigated by means of a MUGA scan, which is performed generally following a two-stage injection procedure. A nonradioactive or 'cold' injection of pyrophosphate is followed 20 minutes later by administration of 400 to 800 MBq of Tc-99m pertechnetate, both administered intravenously. The 'cold' preinjection allows labelling of the patient's red cells to take place in vivo. By using the R-wave of the patient's ECG to gate (i.e. control) image acquisition, a series of 16 to 24 images is recorded during each cardiac cycle and stored in time order on the computer. Data collection continues for 10 to 15 minutes. Images of adequate spatial resolution for the purpose are obtained by summing images of identical time segments from several hundred cardiac cycles. The MUGA images can be processed to produce amplitude and phase images that aid the delineation of the left ventricle and the demonstration of paradoxical motion. Amplitude refers to the magnitude of the change of the LV image intensity, whereas phase refers to the timing of the intensity change within the cycle. The LVEF is derived from the maximum counts (C_{max}) and minimum counts (C_{min}) in the left

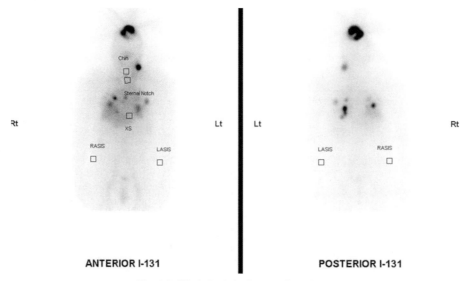

ANTERIOR I-131   **POSTERIOR I-131**

Fig. 6.9 Whole body iodine-131 (I-131) scan.

ventricle over the cardiac cycle (Equation 6.1), and is usually expressed as a percentage. All counts are corrected for background.

$$LVEF = (C_{max} - C_{min})/C_{max} \qquad \textbf{6.1}$$

The technique is recognised as the gold standard [20,21] for LVEF estimation among competing modalities as it does not rely on geometrical approximations to the shape of the heart chamber, but instead derives its values from the entire ventricle, including any effect caused by paradoxical motion. It is also less operator dependent than other assessments. Fig. 6.10 shows images from a patient with a normal LVEF.

MUGA scans image radioactive-labelled blood within the heart. Blood flow to the heart muscle itself (myocardial perfusion) can be imaged using Tc-99m MIBI or tetrofosmin. Thallium-201 was once the most common agent but, because of its higher radiation dose, more limited availability, and less favourable imaging characteristics, has been superseded by the Tc-99m agents. This group of radiopharmaceuticals distribute themselves within the heart muscle according to blood flow through the coronary arteries. Tomographic images are taken under stress and at rest and the results are used in the differential diagnosis of normal myocardial perfusion, ischemia and infarction. These studies have an important role in diagnosis of heart disease in patients with low to medium probability and in prognosis. The LVEF can be derived from gated myocardial perfusion tomography, but the results are not as reliable as those from a MUGA scan, particularly where the position of a substantial part of the myocardial wall must be inferred because there is no blood flow within it. MUGA scanning is used extensively in patients being treated for breast cancer, particularly those receiving Herceptin and the anthracycline group of cytotoxic agents that can be cardiotoxic.

Kidney Imaging

The kidney produces urine and disposes of metabolic waste products. It is divided into an outer cortical and an inner medullary region. Urine drains from the medullary region via the renal pelvis into the ureter and into the bladder. Several radiopharmaceuticals are available for imaging the kidney and investigating renal function.

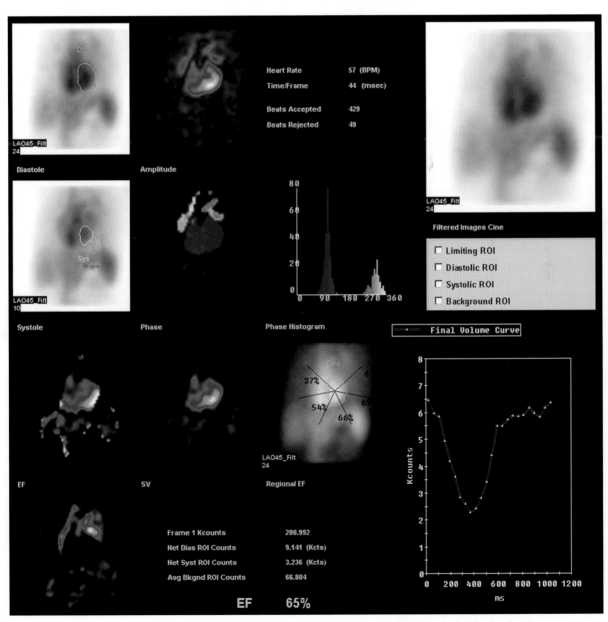

Fig. 6.10 Multiple gated acquisition images from a patient with a normal left ventricular ejection fraction.

The choice of pharmaceutical depends on the specific renal function measurements required and the clinical condition being studied. The commonest reason for renal investigation in oncology patients within nuclear medicine is to investigate suspected obstruction to urine drainage through the ureters caused by primary tumours, such as gynaecological pelvic malignancy or bladder and prostate carcinomas, or by secondary metastatic disease spread to lymph nodes in the para-aortic or iliac chains, which lie adjacent to the ureters. The nonimaging test, glomerular filtration rate, is also common in oncology patients, as part of the workup for the prescription of nephrotoxic drugs (e.g. carboplatin).

The most widely used radiopharmaceuticals for kidney function imaging are Tc-99m tiatide (MAG3) and pentetate (diethylenetriamine pentaacetic acid). They are suitable for the assessment of individual kidney function, and investigation of drainage. With the kidneys and bladder in the field of view of the gamma camera, up to 80 MBq of Tc-99m

MAG3 is injected intravenously. For the following 20 minutes a series of images (generally 20-second frames) is acquired. Regions of interest are defined around the kidneys and bladder and, after suitable background correction, activity–time curves can be generated for each region. This set of curves is termed a renogram. Often, this term is also used to denote the entire investigation.

Fig. 6.11 shows the renogram results from a patient with one normally functioning kidney and one obstructed kidney.

Other renal agents include Tc-99m dimercaptosuccinic acid (DMSA) which is fixed in the kidneys and not excreted and is used primarily in the investigation of renal scarring, often in children.

Infection Imaging

A patient's own leukocytes (white cells) will accumulate at the site of an infection, so one method of localising infection is to label autologous white cells with a suitable radionuclide. Two are available: indium-111

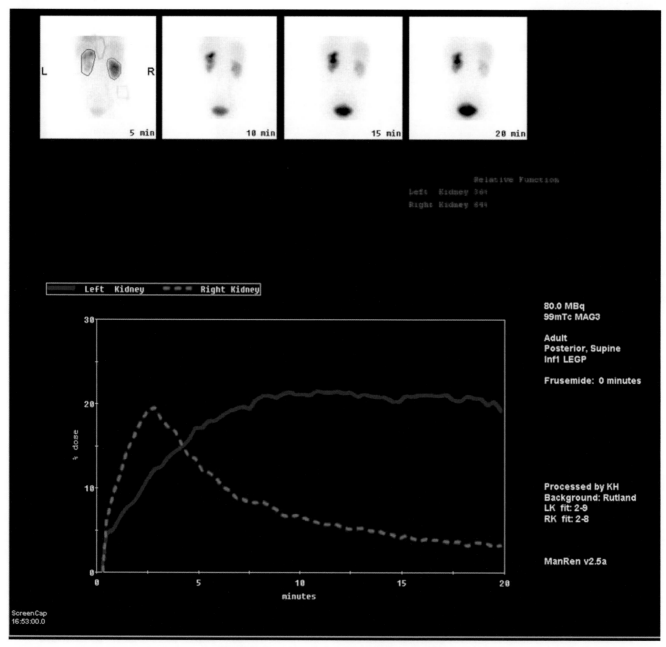

Fig. 6.11 Renogram images and clearance traces.

and Tc-99m. Both labelling processes involve taking up to 200 mL blood from the patient and leaving it to settle under gravity for about an hour. This enables reasonable separation of white cells from the rest of the blood. The cells are incubated with either indium-111 as oxine or tropolonate or Tc-99m as hexamethylpropyleneamine oxime (HMPAO) marketed as Ceretec, which was originally developed for cerebral perfusion studies. The labelling technique is not available in many centres as it is labour-intensive, requiring skilled experienced staff and specialised aseptic facilities. The use of gallium-67 citrate in the localisation of infection is discussed under its general entry in a previous section.

Sentinel Node Mapping

Lymphatic vessels receive cellular waste and discharge it from the body. The waste is filtered through nodes within the vessels. Metastatic spread from some tumours is carried by the lymphatics, and sites of disease are found within the lymph nodes.

Breast cancer is known to spread in this way and almost all of the associated lymph nodes are located in the axilla. Historically, the usual approach by breast surgeons was to perform a full axillary clearance of lymph nodes along with surgical removal of the breast in patients with breast carcinoma. Should histology have subsequently failed to find any evidence of metastatic spread in the nodes, this signalled a good prognosis for the patient. Unfortunately, some of these patients went on to suffer serious morbidity associated with the removal of the lymph nodes, including severe oedema of the arm.

A technique has been developed, initially for breast cancer patients [22], to locate the node(s) nearest to the tumour site, which is referred to as the sentinel node(s). Tc-99m-labelled nanocolloid is injected subdermally or intradermally in the peripheral region of the breast containing the tumour. Gamma camera imaging postinjection will identify the location of the sentinel nodes to help guide the surgeon. Fig. 6.12 shows the sentinel lymph node images of a patient immediately before surgery. Injection and imaging may take place either on the morning of the surgery or on the previous day. Patients will have the still radioactive sentinel nodes located in theatre with the aid of an intraoperative probe system (Fig. 6.13). Histological evaluation of the sentinel nodes will influence the patients' subsequent treatment pathway. The technique is now being used for many other tumours and tumour sites including melanoma, vulval, penile, and head and neck tumours.

POSITRON EMISSION TOMOGRAPHIC IMAGING

Compared with normal cells, tumour cells are highly metabolically active and tend to have higher glucose metabolism. This makes the positron emitting tracer F-18 FDG particularly useful in oncology to identify hypermetabolic tissues that may be malignant. Detailed descriptions of clinical PET/CT can be found in Barrington et al. and Lin et al. [23,24] as well as in the Royal College of Radiologist guidance [25]. Glucose is actively transported into cells via a group of glucose transport proteins (GLUT) on the cell membrane and once inside

Anterior

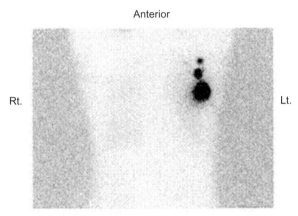

Rt.   Lt.

Images at 2 h 15 min post injection

Left Lateral

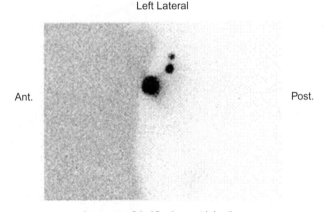

Ant.   Post.

Images at 2 h 15 min post injection

Fig. 6.12 Sentinel lymph node images of a patient immediately before surgery.

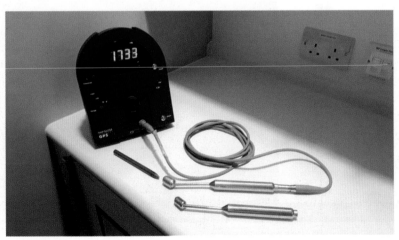

Fig. 6.13 Intraoperative lymph node probe system.

the cell, the glucose is phosphorylated by a hexokinase enzyme as part of the glycolysis pathway. FDG enters the cells, in the same way as glucose via GLUT, particularly GLUT1 and GLUT3. FDG is phosphorylated similar to normal glucose, but then is trapped inside the cell as it cannot enter further into the glycolysis pathway. The increased metabolism of glucose in malignant cells is because of upregulation of the enzyme hexokinase and increased levels of the membrane transport proteins GLUT1 and GLUT3. Overexpression of GLUT1 and GLUT3 is primarily seen in the rim of hypoxic tumour tissue. The production of adenosine triphosphate is maintained by upregulation of glucose transport and glycolysis even in the presence of hypoxia. Indeed, tumour cells favour the more inefficient anaerobic pathway thereby increasing

glucose demands further. The metabolism of glucose is partly regulated by the transcription factor hypoxia-inducible factor 1 (HIF-1). HIF-1 stimulates the expression of more than 40 genes, including vascular endothelial growth factor, insulin-like growth factor 2, GLUT1 and 3, and several glycolytic enzymes such as hexokinase 1 and 3. It has been demonstrated that the activity of tumour cell hexokinase, which can be indirectly measured by FDG-PET, is correlated with the growth rate of tumours.

Therefore determination by PET of FDG uptake during and after antineoplastic treatment may be used as an early indicator of response to treatment. The reaction to RT or chemotherapy treatment may be an initial rise in FDG uptake, followed by a decrease, the magnitude of

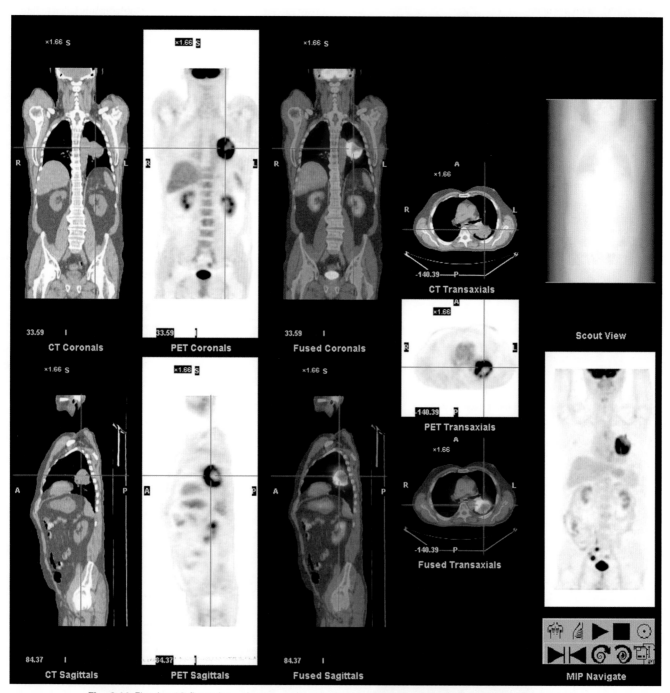

Fig. 6.14 Fluorine-18 fluorodeoxyglucose positron emission tomography/computed tomography image of a patient with a lung tumour.

which can serve as a marker of treatment response. However, FDG is also taken up in inflammatory lesions giving rise to nonspecificity. This presents interpretational limitations and requires caution in the reporting of PET/CT scans. The optimal timing of posttreatment evaluation by PET/CT is not established and is the subject of current research and will be dependent on tumour type and treatment modality.

A growing body of literature has now led to FDG-PET being used routinely in the clinic for the detection and staging of malignant tumours, determining the extent of spread of disease (including assessment of the suitability of patients for radical surgery), differentiation of benign from malignant mass lesions, measuring response to therapy, and long-term follow-up for detection of recurrent disease.

A great number of other compounds have also been labelled with fluorine-18, such as fluorocholine, fluorofatty acids, fluoroamino acids, spiperone derivatives, fluoromisonidazole and fluoroaltanserin with fluorocholine finding the most use clinically.

Several other medium half-life, inorganic positron emitting radionuclides are becoming available. Their half-lives of several hours offer considerable advantages for supply from regional distribution centres. Iodine-124 ($t_{1/2} = 100$ hours) or iodine-120 ($t_{1/2} = 1.4$ hours) may be used to label tracers and ligands that have previously been labelled with iodine-123 or iodine-131. 5-Iododeoxyuridine offers potential as a radiotracer for functional imaging of cell proliferation. Bromine-76 ($t_{1/2} = 16$ hours) has also been used as a PET label for a variety of compounds, including deoxyuridine derivatives as proliferation markers and antibodies. Macromolecules, such as peptides (e.g. octreotide) and proteins (e.g. monoclonal antibodies), are also amenable to radiolabelling with such radionuclides. Perfusion and permeability clinical studies have been demonstrated using copper-64 ($t_{1/2} = 12.7$ hours) as a label for the perfusion/flow marker copper-64 PTSM (Cu(II)-pyruvaldehyde-bis(N4-methylthiosemicarbazone)).

Further opportunities are possible using positron emitter generator systems, where the parent radionuclide has a much longer half-life than the daughter. Commercial, fully licensed germanium-68/gallium-68 generators are now available with parent/daughter having half-lives of 268 days and 68 minutes, respectively and licensed cold kits are also becoming available for ease of preparing these radiopharmaceuticals. These Ga-68 radiopharmaceuticals show fast target blood clearance and localisation. ^{68}Ga-DOTATOC, ^{68}Ga-DOTATATE, and ^{68}Ga-DOTANOC are radiolabelled somatostatin analogues used for imaging and differentiating lesions of various somatostatin receptor subtypes, which are overexpressed in many neuroendocrine tumours. The use of radiometals for labelling peptide targeting agents also provides an additional value following a positive scan where the use of beta or even alpha emitting radionuclides can be labelled to the same peptides to allow radionuclide treatment. For localising other tumours there have been promising results in the use of ^{68}Ga-DOTA-rhenium-cyclised alpha-melanocyte-stimulating hormone and ^{68}Ga-DOTA-NAPamide in melanoma, ^{68}Ga-DOTA-PEG(4)-BN(7-14) (PESIN) for the imaging of bombesin receptor-positive tumours, and ^{68}Ga-ethylene dicysteine-metronidazole for imaging tumour hypoxia. Aside from tumours, inflammation can also be imaged using ^{68}Ga-DOTA peptide inhibitor of vascular peptide protein 1 (VAP-P1). This has potential clinical utility in systemic inflammatory disease diagnosis and monitoring.

Fig. 6.14 shows an F-18 FDG PET/CT image of a patient with a lung tumour.

CONCLUSIONS

Radionuclide imaging is continually developing and plays an invaluable role in the diagnosis, staging and assessment of treatment response in cancer patients.

REFERENCES

[1] Lonsdale MN, Beyer T. Dual-modality PET/CT instrumentation–today and tomorrow. Eur J Radiol 2010;73:452–60.

[2] Musafargani S, Ghosh KK, Mishra S, et al. PET/MRI: a frontier in era of complementary hybrid imaging. Eur J Hybrid Imag 2018;2:12.

[3] Dendy PP, Heaton B. Physics for diagnostic radiology. 3rd ed. CRC Press; 2011.

[4] Wolbarst AB, Capasso P, Wyant AR. Medical imaging: essentials for physicians. John Wiley & Sons; 2013.

[5] Cherry SR, Sorenson JA, Phelps ME. Physics in nuclear medicine. 4th ed. Saunders; 2012.

[6] Patton J, Sandler M, et al. D-SPECT: a new solid state camera for high speed molecular imaging. J Nucl Med 2006;47(suppl 1):189.

[7] Keidar Z, Raysberg I, et al. Novel cadmium zinc telluride-based detector general purpose gamma camera: initial evaluation and comparison with a standard camera. J Nucl Med 2016;57(suppl 2):259.

[8] Institute of Physics and Engineering in Medicine (IPEM). Quality control of gamma camera systems. IPEM Report 111. IPEM; 2003.

[9] National Electrical Manufacturers Association (NEMA). Performance measurements of gamma cameras. NEMA NU-1; 2012.

[10] Institute of Physics and Engineering in Medicine (IPEM). Recommended standards for the routine performance resting of diagnostic x-ray imaging systems. IPEM Report 91. IPEM; 2005.

[11] Bailey DL, Townsend DW, Valk PE, Maisey MN, editors. Positron emission tomography. Springer-Verlag; 2005.

[12] Bushberg JT, Seibert JA, Leidholdt EM, Boone JM. The essential physics of medical imaging. 3rd ed. Philadelphia: Lippincott Williams & Wilkins; 2012.

[13] Welch MJ, Redvanly CS, editors. Handbook of radiopharmaceuticals, radiochemistry and applications. Wiley; 2003.

[14] Kowalsky RJ, Falen. Radiopharmaceuticals in nuclear pharmacy and nuclear medicine. 3rd ed. Washington, DC: American Pharmaceutical Association; 2011.

[15] Decristoforo C, Mather SJ, et al. 99mTc-EDDA/HYNIC-TOC: a new 99mTc-labelled radiopharmaceutical for imaging somatostatin receptor-positive tumours: first clinical results and intrapatient comparison with 111In-labelled octreotide derivatives. Eur J Nucl Med 2000;27:1318–25.

[16] Her Majesty's Stationary Office. The human medicines regulations. statutory instrument 2012/1916. London: HMSO; 2012.

[17] Her Majesty's Stationary Office. The ionising radiations regulations 2017. London: HMSO; 2017.

[18] ICRP Publication 53 and subsequent addenda. Radiation dose to patients from radiopharmaceuticals. Ann ICRP 1988;18(1–4).

[19] Schoedel KE, Tubin ME, et al. Ultrasound-guided biopsy of the thyroid, a comparison of technique with respect to diagnostic accuracy. Diagn Cytopathol 2008;36:787–9.

[20] Bartlett ML, Srinivasan G, Barker WC, et al. Left ventricular ejection of results from planar and SPECT gated blood-pool studies. J Nucl Med 1996;37:1795–9.

[21] Harel F, Finnerty V, Ngo Q, et al. SPECT versus planar gated blood pool imaging for left ventricular evaluation. J Nucl Cardiol 2007;14:1795–9.

[22] Mansel RE, Fallowfield L, et al. Randomized multicenter trial of sentinel node biopsy versus standard axillary treatment in operable breast cancer: The ALMANAC Trial. J Nat Canc Inste 2006;98(9):599–609.

[23] Barrington SF, Maisey MN, Wahl RL, et al. Atlas of clinical positron emission tomography. 2nd ed. Hodder Arnold; 2006.

[24] Lin EC, Alavi A. PET and PET/CT. Thieme.

[25] The Royal College of Radiologists. Evidence-based indications for the use of PET-CT in the UK. Ref BRCR (16)3 2016. London: RCR.

7

Therapy With Unsealed Radionuclides

Matthew Aldridge, Sofia Michopoulou

CHAPTER OUTLINE

INTRODUCTION

Radionuclide therapy, molecular radiotherapy and internal radiation therapy are some of the terms used for treatments involving administration of unsealed or dispersible radioactive sources to patients.

Radionuclide therapy is used for both benign and malignant conditions. Cell targeting can be as a result of chemical or physical properties of the radiopharmaceutical, such as the mechanical entrapment of microspheres in liver capillaries, or by means of carrier molecules that attach to receptors guiding the radionuclide to the target tissue.

The aim of radionuclide therapy is to deliver sufficient radiation dose maximising the cytotoxic effect to the target tissue, while sparing normal tissues and thus limiting toxicities to normal organs at risk. This can be achieved by selecting pharmaceuticals that maximise the ratio between the amount deposited in the target tissue and the amount deposited in nontarget tissue. Furthermore, the radionuclide properties are chosen so as to deposit energy locally to the target tissue. Most radionuclide therapies use beta-emitting radionuclides with a soft tissue range of a few millimetres. Recently, alpha-emitting radionuclides were also introduced in clinical practice. Alpha emitters have a range of just a few micrometres in tissue and very high linear energy transfer, resulting in local energy deposition and a highly targeted cytotoxic effect. Some alpha- and beta-emitting radionuclides additionally emit gamma photons which enable imaging the distribution of the radiopharmaceutical in the body using a gamma camera as described in Chapter 6 and can provide data for dosimetry calculations. The physical properties of radionuclides commonly used in therapeutic applications are outlined in Table 7.1.

Dosimetry for radionuclide therapy is performed using the medical internal radiation dosimetry (MIRD) scheme [1]. The radiation dose, D, delivered from a source organ, s, to a target organ, t, is given by the accumulated activity, Ã, in the source organ and the S-factor, S $(t \leftarrow s)$, as outlined in Equation 7.1. Representative absorbed doses for commonly used radiopharmaceuticals are outlined in Table 7.2. The accumulated activity in the source organ is calculated by integrating the radioactivity in this organ over time as shown in Fig. 7.1C. The radioactivity in the source organ clears with an effective half-life (T_{eff}), which depends on the physical half-life of the radionuclide (T_{phys}) and the biological clearance of the pharmaceutical (T_{biol}) as outlined in Equation 7.2. The S-factor depends on the physical properties of the radiation, that is, the type of radiation and the energy, as well as the size and shape of the target organ and its distance from the source organ. S-factor values are calculated using Monte Carlo simulations based on anthropomorphic models of the body. Tables of these factors are available in the literature for a variety of radionuclides and source-target organ combinations [1,2]:

$$D = \tilde{A} \cdot S \qquad \text{7.1}$$

$$\frac{1}{T_{eff}} = \frac{1}{T_{phys}} + \frac{1}{T_{biol}} \qquad \text{7.2}$$

Radionuclide therapy has been in use since the 1940s, but has since 2010 seen a rapid growth with new therapies being introduced into clinical practice [3], such as radium-223 (^{223}Ra) dichloride for bone palliation, lutetium-177 (^{177}Lu) DOTATATE for the treatment of neuroendocrine tumours and selective internal radiation treatment (SIRT) for liver metastasis, as shown in Fig. 7.2.

Many of these new therapies are performed in a theranostic context. The principle of theranostics is the use of a diagnostic and therapeutic pair of radionuclides, generally using the same pharmaceutical as a carrier, with pretreatment imaging used to stratify patients for molecular radiotherapy. A good example of a theranostic pair is ^{68}Ga/^{177}Lu, which when labelled with a somatostatin analogue such as DOTATATE, can identify appropriate patients using positron emission tomography (PET)/computed tomography (CT) imaging, as outlined in Fig. 7.1A, B. Furthermore, the diagnostic component of theranostics allows for personalised evaluation of biokinetics and dosimetry, providing a useful tool in predicting which patients will respond optimally to therapy.

In clinical practice, the radionuclide therapy service is delivered by a multidisciplinary team of health care professionals. Typically, treatment

TABLE 7.1 Properties of the Radionuclides Used in Therapy

Radionuclide	Physical Half-Life (Days)	Therapeutic Radiation	BETA EMISSION Mean Energy (MeV)	BETA EMISSION Mean Range in Soft Tissue (mm)	GAMMA EMISSION Energy (MeV)	GAMMA EMISSION % Abundance
^{131}I	8.02	Beta	0.182	0.6	0.364	81.7
^{223}Ra	11.4	Alpha	5.78	<0.1	0.154	6.04
					0.269	13.6
^{177}Lu	6.7	Beta	0.13	0.6	0.208	11
					0.117	6.4
^{90}Y	2.7	Beta	0.935	3.6	—	—
^{32}P	14.3	Beta	0.70	3.0	—	—
^{89}Sr	50.5	Beta	0.58	2.4	0.909	0.01
^{153}Sm	1.9	Beta	0.22	0.6	0.103	28
^{169}Er	9.4	Beta	0.099	0.3	—	—
^{186}Re	3.8	Beta	0.33	1.1	0.137	9

TABLE 7.2 Radiation Absorbed Dose for Some Radiopharmaceuticals

Radiopharmaceutical	Effective Dose (mSv/MBq)	Typical Administered Activity A (MBq)	Effective Dose From A (mSv)
^{131}I sodium iodide: carcinoma	0.061	3500	214
^{131}I sodium iodide: thyrotoxicosis	24	400	9600
^{223}Ra dichloride	30	3.850	116
^{131}I MIBG	0.2	1100	220
^{177}Lu-DOTATATE	0.174	7400	1288
^{90}Y microspheres	1.88	2100	3948
^{32}P sodium phosphate	2.4	200	480
^{89}Sr strontium chloride	3.1	150	465

selection is jointly performed by oncologists and nuclear medicine physicians, based on clinical examination, prior imaging and blood indices. Dosimetry calculations are performed by medical physicists. The therapy administration is supported by nuclear medicine physicians, technologists and physicists working together, although this may vary from centre to centre.

IODINE-131 IN THE TREATMENT OF THYROID DISEASE

Iodine-131 (^{131}I) is the radionuclide most widely used therapeutically and has been used in the treatment of thyroid conditions since the 1940s. Iodine accumulates in the thyroid gland and the use of Iodine-131, with the emission of beta particles with a maximum range of 3 mm in tissue allows a high radiation dose to be delivered to the thyroid and a low dose to the rest of the body. It is most commonly used in the form of sodium iodide [^{131}I] for treatment of the benign thyroid diseases, thyrotoxicosis and nontoxic goitre and in thyroid carcinoma.

The characteristics of ^{131}I are shown in Table 7.1. As specified by the Society of Nuclear Medicine (SNM) [4] and the European Association of Nuclear Medicine (EANM) [5], it is essential that, before any treatment, all thyroid hormones, iodine-containing preparations and supplements and any other medications that could suppress thyroid uptake are discontinued for a sufficient length of time. Almost all thyroid treatments are given orally, as a capsule or a liquid.

Thyroid Cancer

Within differentiated thyroid cancer (DTC), the carcinoma retains characteristics of healthy thyroid tissue including the expression of the sodium iodide symporter, enabling the uptake of radioiodine. The treatment is associated with a 10-year overall cause-specific survival of 85%.

Radioiodine therapy may be subdivided into ablation, a postsurgical procedure used to eliminate thyroid remnants, or as a component of primary curative treatment in the setting of nonresectable or incompletely resectable lesions.

Following total thyroidectomy, the aim of remnant ablation is to destroy any remaining normal thyroid tissue and any microscopic deposits of thyroid carcinoma [6]. The usual activity administered for ablation is 3.7 GBq, although in the low to intermediate risk group, lower activity of 1.1 GBq is being used instead [7]. By destroying any remaining thyroid tissue, the theory is that the only remaining source of thyroglobulin production is any remaining malignant cells, thus making the measurements of thyroglobulin level a sensitive test of any local recurrence or metastatic disease.

Metastatic lesions have a lower avidity for iodine than normal thyroid tissue and it is customary to administer higher activities of 3.7 to 5.5 GBq [7]. Treatments for thyroid cancer require an in-patient stay in a dedicated treatment room with appropriate facilities including radiation shielding, due to the high external dose rates from these patients contributing to significant dose to the public, their family and to any comforter and carer. As such, the patients are monitored during the

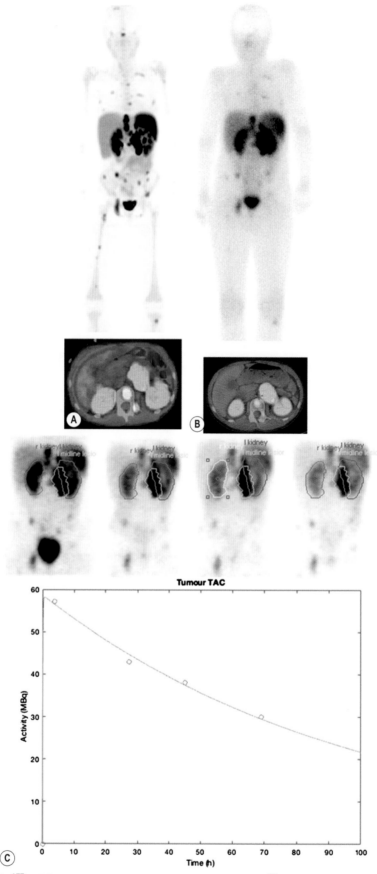

Fig. 7.1 ^{68}Ga/^{177}Lu-DOTATATE theranostic example. (A) Diagnostic ^{68}Ga-DOTATATE positron emission tomography/computed tomography (PETCT) imaging scan showed multiple DOTATATE avid lesions confirming patient eligibility for treatment,normal uptake is visualized in kidneys, liver, spleen and bladder (B) ^{177}Lu-DOTATATE posttherapy single-photon emission computed tomography/(SPECT/CT) verified distribution of therapeutic activity and facilitated dosimetry, (C) kidney dosimetry based on (SPECT) ^{177}Lu-DOTATATE therapy scintigraphy: the accumulated activity in the kidney was calculated from the kidney counts obtained at 2, 24, 48 and 70 hours postadministration.

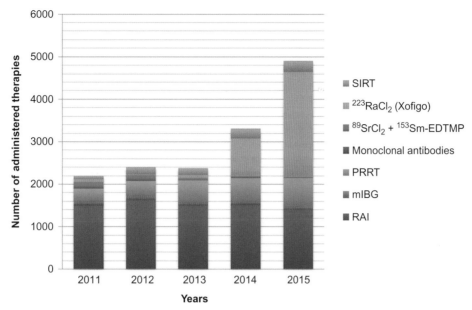

Fig. 7.2 Number of administrations for common types of radionuclide therapy in U.K. centres participating in the Internal Dosimetry Users Group Survey between 2011 and 2015. (Courtesy of Bruno Rojas).

stay until the level of radioactivity has fallen sufficiently for safe discharge as outlined in the Medical and Dental Guidance Notes (MDGN) [8].

To improve the effectiveness of treatment, the remaining thyroid tissue may be stimulated by elevating the level of thyroid-stimulating hormone (TSH), with the effect of aiding the absorption of radioiodine [7]. One method is to withhold thyroid hormone medication for 2 to 4 weeks and allow TSH to increase. However, this is associated with hypothyroid symptoms in most patients. The alternative is to administer Thyrogen, a protein designed to be identical to TSH, as a prescription medication given in two injections before treatment or diagnostic testing.

Gamma camera images, using 364 keV photons of ^{131}I may be obtained after treatment to confirm uptake in residual thyroid, recurrence or metastases [7]. Scanning protocols may also be used after surgery and before ablation. It may also be used for instance, to determine the completeness of ablation as part of a patient's treatment. [123]Iodine may provide a suitable alternative for follow-up. Hybrid single-photon emission computed tomography (SPECT/CT) imaging described in Chapter 6 enables precise anatomical localisation of any residual disease and metastatic spread.

Benign Thyroid Disease

The over-production of thyroid hormones manifests in patients as hyperthyroidism, arising from benign conditions such as Graves' disease, toxic or nontoxic goitre and solitary hyperfunctioning thyroid nodule. As iodine is a component of thyroid hormones LT4 (tetraiodothyronine, T4) and T3 (L-triiodothyronine), it is readily extracted from the blood and trapped and organified in the thyroid gland when administered as radioiodine. Approaches to radionuclide therapy have included giving enough radioiodine to render the patient hypothyroid and giving low activities of ^{131}I in combination with antithyroid drug [9]. However, the RCP recommend that the aim of treatment should be to render the patient euthyroid, while accepting that there will be a moderate rate of hypothyroidism [10].

Assessment of thyroid function and eligibility for treatment may be performed using ^{123}I-labelled sodium iodide or ^{99m}Tc-pertechnetate. Pertechnetate ions are trapped through the active transport mechanism

in the same manner as ^{123}I or ^{131}I-labelled sodium iodide and thyroid function may be evaluated by measuring the percentage uptake of administered activity.

According to national regulations, the treatment may be given on an out-patient basis, assuming that an appropriate risk assessment has been undertaken, principally with regard to contact patterns with other members of the public [8]. The range of activities currently prescribed varies between 200 and 800 MBq [9]. If therapy is performed on an in-patient basis, particularly in the case of paediatric patients, then this should take place in the appropriate environment with the necessary resources required by national legislation.

PALLIATION OF BONE PAIN

Radionuclide therapy gives an additional possibility for the palliation of bone pain arising from osteoblastic metastases, which are seen in some cancers with a high prevalence, such as prostate and breast carcinoma. This systemic approach may be used for patients with multifocal osteoblastic metastases as an alternative to external beam radiotherapy, or for those whose pain is refractory to conventional analgesia or antitumour therapy [11]. Before administration of the treatment, it is essential to verify that there is evidence of focal increased uptake on bone scintigraphy (Chapter 6). Such increased uptake is due to an osseous reaction to the development of metastases and, if it is not present on a gamma camera bone scan using a ^{99m}Tc imaging agent (e.g. MDP or HDP, see Chapter 6), there will be no selective uptake of the therapeutic radionuclide and, therefore, no benefit.

A variety of bone seeking radionuclides are available for bone palliation, including beta emitters such as ^{89}Sr and [153]Sm and more recently, [223]Ra, an alpha emitter. [223]Radium-dichloride (Xofigo®) has rapidly become the most widely used radiopharmaceutical and has been shown to not only provide pain relief but also improve overall survival in patients with castration-resistant prostate cancer (CRPC) [12]. It is currently undergoing clinical trials to assess its efficacy for breast carcinoma [13]. [223]Radium dichloride selectively accumulates in areas of high bone turnover by forming complexes with hydroxyapatite, the inorganic component of the bone. [223]Ra has a half-life of 11.4 days and a mean alpha energy of 5.78 MeV. The alpha particles have a high linear energy transfer and can thus deposit their energy over a short range (<100 μm) resulting in double-strand DNA breaks and highly localised cytotoxic effects. Additionally, this short range of ^{223}Ra minimises myelosuppression, a known risk of beta emitters such as ^{89}Sr with a range of 2.4 mm [12]. ^{223}Ra also emits low abundance (<2%) gamma photons with energies of 82, 154 and 270 keV. These can be imaged with a gamma camera to confirm uptake on bone metastasis.

A standard treatment course of ^{223}Ra comprises six administrations at 4-week intervals, and the activity delivered is typically adjusted by patient weight, with 55 kBq/kg^{-1} given to patients with prostate cancer [14]. Posttherapy imaging offers the additional opportunity to perform personalised dosimetry and customise the injected activity of subsequent administration to the individual patient [15].

^{223}Ra is routinely given as an outpatient treatment and is generally well tolerated with the most common side effects being diarrhoea or vomiting as the radiopharmaceutical is mostly eliminated through the fecal route. Being an alpha emitter, the posttherapy radiation protection restrictions required are minimal and focus on good hygiene to reduce the risk of radioactive contamination [14].

MOLECULAR RADIOTHERAPY TREATMENT OF NEUROENDOCRINE TUMOURS

Neuroendocrine tumours are a complex group of tumours derived from the primitive neural crest, which develops to form the sympathetic nervous system (SNS): malignant neuroendocrine tumours include phaeochromocytoma, neuroblastoma, carcinoid tumours—including gastro-entero-pancreatic tract (GEP NETs), paraganglioma and medullary thyroid cancer.

Neuroendocrine tumours demonstrate targets for molecular radiotherapy in that they frequently express somatostatin receptors (SSTRs) on their cell surface, enabling them to be imaged with somatostatin analogues such as ^{111}In-Pentreotide (commercially available as Octreoscan) or ^{99m}Tc-HYNIC-TOC (commercially available as Tektrotyd) on a gamma camera. More recently, somatostatin imaging has been achieved using PET radiopharmaceuticals such as ^{68}Ga-DOTATATE and using the advantages conferred by PET imaging over planar imaging: improved spatial resolution, contrast and the ability to perform whole-body scanning in a short time [16].

Peptide-receptor-radionuclide-therapy (PRRT) uses similar somatostatin analogues as in diagnostic imaging, but instead labelled with therapeutic radionuclides, with the most commonly used being yttrium-90 (^{90}Y) and lutetium-177 (^{177}Lu) [17]. Both are beta emitters, ^{90}Y having a maximum energy of 2.3 MeV and tissue penetration of 12 mm, whereas ^{177}Lu emits lower energy particles of 0.5 MeV and tissue penetration of 2 mm. Both ^{90}Y and ^{177}Lu peptides demonstrate rapid blood and urinary clearance, with the main dose-limiting organ being the kidneys. For this reason, it is common to co-administer amino acids L-lysine and L-arginine, to block the renal tubules and hence afford protection [17].

^{177}Lu emits gamma radiation of low abundance, making it suitable for gamma camera imaging, and the half-life of 6.7 days enables dosimetric evaluation. Typical administered activities are between 3.5 and 7.4 GBq, although this may be modulated, taking into account renal toxicity and individualised dosimetry. A fractionated approach is optimal with at least four administrations each separated by 8 to 12 weeks. Patients may require admission to a dedicated radionuclide therapy room for a period of time determined by national regulations [17]. A Phase 3 Neuroendocrine Tumors Therapy Trial (NETTER-1) found that ^{177}Lu-DOTATATE therapy increases progression-free survival in patients with advanced midgut neuroendocrine tumours [18].

These tumour types offer another target for MRT in the form of noradrenaline transporter expression, which can be a predictor of tumoural uptake of metaiodobenzylguanidine (mIBG). A noradrenaline analogue, mIBG can be labelled with iodine-131 (^{131}I).

Before treatment, any drugs known to interfere with the uptake and/or retention of ^{131}I-mIBG must be withdrawn in accordance with the European guidelines [19]. A thyroid blocking agent such as potassium iodide must be prescribed, starting before and continuing for an extended period after treatment, to protect the gland from taking up any free ^{131}I with the subsequent risk of developing hypothyroidism. The dose-limiting toxicity is haematological and monitoring of blood counts is essential after treatment.

Eligibility for treatment can be assessed by ^{123}I-mIBG imaging on a gamma camera or ^{124}I-mIBG on a PET/CT camera to confirm uptake in tumour sites. Uptake can also be confirmed with a low activity of ^{131}I-mIBG, and all radionuclides exhibit gamma emissions such that dosimetry can be assessed.

In routine practice, the majority of centres administer fixed ^{131}I mIBG activities of 3.7 to 11.1 GBq at 3- to 6-monthly intervals. Because several therapeutic doses may be required to achieve objective response, these activities are often repeated at varied intervals [16].

Neuroblastoma is a predominantly childhood cancer that peaks in incidence in young children. Over 50% of patients present with high-risk disease, and ^{131}I-mIBG may also be used in relapsed or refractory neuroblastoma, with 90% of neuroblastoma mIBG avid. Treatment of very young children poses challenges resulting from radiation safety requirements associated with the administration of ^{131}I-mIBG therapy.

Myelosuppression is the main dose-limiting toxicity, necessitating stem cell reinfusion at higher administered activities [20].

These treatments are well tolerated by patients with very few side effects reported.

SELECTIVE INTERNAL RADIATION THERAPY

SIRT or radioembolisation is a safe and effective treatment for unresectable primary and secondary liver cancer.

SIRT uses yttrium-90 (^{90}Y) microspheres, which are injected through a catheter into the liver vasculature. The microspheres are mechanically trapped inside the tumour, delivering high radiation dose to the tumour with relatively low dose to the normal liver parenchyma [21].

^{90}Y is a high-energy beta-emitting radionuclide. Its physical properties are provided in Table 7.1; ^{90}Y has an average range of 4 mm in tissue and can travel over 10 metres in air but can be easily shielded by 10 mm of acrylic. ^{90}Y does not have any gamma emissions but is accompanied by the emission of secondary bremsstrahlung X photons, which can be exploited for imaging.

As of 2018, two commercial microsphere products are available worldwide:

1. Glass spheres (Theraspheres) with a diameter of 20 to 30 μm. These are injected in limited numbers (1 to 4 million particles at 2500 Bq per particle), producing lower embolic effects (blockage of the vessels), which makes them suitable for patients with compromised portal venous flow [21].
2. Resin spheres (SIRTEX) of 20 to 60 μm diameter, which use a large number of spheres for the same desired activity (20 to 60 million particles at 50 Bq per particle) resulting in more uniform distribution of radiation dose and also larger embolic effect than Theraspheres [21].

The SIRT patient pathway is complex and requires combined expertise from oncology, interventional radiology and nuclear medicine departments.

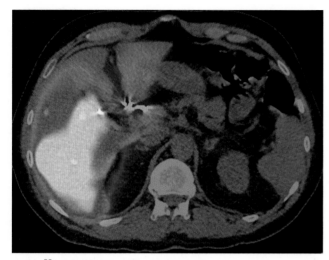

Fig. 7.3 ^{90}Y-Selective internal radiation therapy. Posttherapy bremsstrahlung single-photon emission computed tomography/computed tomography scan of the liver acquired for treatment verification indicated uptake in targeted segments of the left and right liver lobes.

In the 2 weeks before treatment a planning angiography is performed to identify the tumour-perfusing vessels and to assess portal vein patency. Once the optimal catheter position has been identified, ^{99m}Tc-labelled albumin macroaggregate (MAA) is administered acting as a surrogate for the microspheres.

Planar scintigraphy and/or SPECT/CT imaging of the ^{99m}Tc-MAA distribution is used to evaluate the tumour perfusion, to quantify shunting to the lung, which could result in radiation pneumonitis and finally, to exclude any reflux to the gastrointestinal tract [21]. Chapter 6 outlines the imaging principles of planar scintigraphy and/or SPECT/CT.

The required therapeutic activity is then determined by dosimetry evaluation of the ^{99m}Tc-MAA images using the MIRD methodology, or by using empirical calculations such as the body surface area method, or by Monte Carlo simulation techniques [22].

Treatment is performed in the angiography suite, with the catheter placed at the same position as for the ^{99m}Tc-MAA injection. Following the therapeutic injection, patients are hospitalised for clinical reasons. Radiation protection precautions following therapy relate to external dose rate from bremsstrahlung radiation and a small amount of urinary excretion [23].

Posttherapy verification of the ^{90}Y distribution can be performed through bremsstrahlung imaging using planar or SPECT scintigraphy as shown in Fig. 7.3. Alternatively, posttherapy PET imaging exploiting the low abundance of pair production, which occurs in the ^{90}Y decay, may be used.

PHOSPHORUS-32 IN THE TREATMENT OF REFRACTORY MYELOPROLIFERATIVE DISEASE

Phosphorus-32 (^{32}P)-phosphate is used in the treatment of polycythaemia rubra vera (PRV) and essential thrombocythaemia. Although its use is in decline it has a role in patients over 70, who are resistant to other treatments such as venesection and conventional chemotherapy [24].

The ^{32}P radionuclide is a pure beta-emitting radionuclide, with a mean particle range in tissue of 3 mm and a maximum of 8 mm. It is typically administered by intravenous injection with an activity

of between 150 and 250 MBq and there is no requirement for an in-patient stay [25].

INTRAARTICULAR AND INTRACAVITARY TREATMENTS

Radiation synovectomy/radiosynoviorthesis (RS) is a molecular radiotherapy modality used for treatment of chronic inflammatory joints. It involves the intraarticular injection of radiopharmaceuticals either on an in-patient or out-patient basis, dependent on local regulations.

Beta emitting radiopharmaceuticals ^{90}Y, ^{186}Re and ^{169}Er (see Table 7.1) can be used to penetrate and ablate the synovial tissue. It is injected as a colloid with an ideal particle size of 10 nm, which results in a homogeneous distribution within the joint cavity and minimal lymphatic clearance. The affected joint should be immobilised for 48 hours postinjection, Eligibility for treatment can be assessed with ^{99m}Tc-MDP/HDP/HEDP, used to detect synovial inflammation.

As a general rule, yttrium-90 (^{90}Y) silicate/citrate is used for large joints like the knee, rhenium-186 (^{186}Re) sulphide is used for medium-sized joints such as the hip, shoulder or ankle, and erbium-169 (^{169}Er) citrate is used for small joints as in the fingers [26]. This is because of the differences in soft-tissue range with the greater range of ^{90}Y used for larger joints.

Appropriate radiation protection considerations are required to protect both the patient and the medical staff performing the procedure. It is essential to use Perspex syringe shields to reduce radiation exposure to the fingers.

RADIOIMMUNOTHERAPY

Radioimmunotherapy (RIT) uses engineered monoclonal antibodies paired with radionuclides. When injected into the bloodstream, they bind to cancer cells and deliver a high radiation directly to the tumour. In contrast to most treatments already discussed that are well established, RIT is a relatively new and growing field.

In non-Hodgkin's lymphoma (NHL), ^{90}Y-ibritumomab tiuxetan (Zevalin®) is an approved treatment targeting the CD20 antibody for the treatment of relapsed follicular NHL, which is refractory to chemotherapy. It is prescribed as 15 MBq/kg, with a maximum of 1.2 GBq and the dose-limiting toxicity is haematological [27].

^{177}Lu-prostate-specific membrane antigen (PSMA) was recently introduced for the treatment of metastatic prostate cancer. PSMA receptors can be found in high abundance at the surface of these cancerous cells and have an internalisation process that allows endocytosis of the PSMA-labelled radionuclides, which are then concentrated within the cell. The ^{177}Lu-PSMA treatment can be provided by using the monoclonal antibody J591, or by using peptide-labelled radiopharmaceuticals such as PSMA–Division of Radiopharmaceutical Chemistry (DKFZ)-617. The treatment is delivered in up to six fractions at a minimum of 6-week intervals and the administered activity varies between the different studies with a range of 3 and 8 GBq per fraction. Excretion is mainly renal, and the organs most at risk are the kidneys, salivary and lacrimal glands.

Patient selection for ^{177}Lu-PSMA treatment follows a theranostic pathway. The diagnostic arm uses either ^{68}Ga PSMA PET/CT or ^{99m}Tc-PSMA SPECT/CT to localise metastatic disease pre- and posttherapy. ^{177}LuPSMA SPECT imaging is then used for treatment verification and dosimetry. So far, trial results have indicated positive response to ^{177}Lu-PSMA treatment, but it is still early days and prospective randomised trials are needed to confirm any potential benefits [28].

RADIATION PROTECTION, WASTE AND REGULATIONS

Radiation protection is an important component of molecular radiotherapy for the patient, comforter and carers, and staff involved in both the administration and care of the patient. The type of therapy agent used will affect the protection requirements. Treatments with predominantly beta emitters and low abundance gamma rays, such as [90]yttrium present a lower external dose rate to others, whilst radionuclides such as [131]iodine with a long half-life of 8 days, and the high abundance of high energy, 364 keV gamma rays, present a more complex problem.

Requirements and guidance are drawn from several sources. In the United Kingdom, the Ionising Radiation Medical Exposure Regulations (IRMER17) [29] and the Ionising Radiation Regulations (IRR17) [30] apply for radionuclide therapies, whereas the Medical and Dental Guidance Notes (MDGN) provides guidance on the implementation of legislation [8]. In particular, an individualised risk assessment is used for each patient to estimate likely contact patterns with other people, their home circumstances and the risk of contamination and ingestion and inhalation of radionuclides. Specific requirements can include restricting any contact with young children and pregnant women.

Hospital Requirements

- Appointed Trust Radiation Protection Advisor (RPA)
- Appointed Trust Radiation Protection Supervisor (RPS)
- Medical Physics Expert (MPE) with expertise in radionuclide therapy
- Appropriate certification for radiopharmaceutical administration from the Administration of Radioactive Substances Advisory Committee
- Procedures for compliance with Ionising Radiation Regulations (IRR2017) such as designation of controlled areas, dose limits, contamination monitoring and risk assessments
- Registration and authorisation for holding and disposing of relevant radioactive materials, referred to as the Environmental Permitting Regulations (EPR2010) license [31]
- Method of checking activity before administration
- Facilities for oral and intravenous administration of radiopharmaceuticals

Facilities

Dependent on national and local regulations, there may be a requirement for the patient to be admitted and cared for in a specialised and dedicated radionuclide therapy facility as follows:

- A room with sufficient lead lining, which is designated as a controlled area
- Exclusive use of a toilet and shower facility with appropriate disposal route
- Method for monitoring for room and equipment contamination. Facilities for wash and decontamination of bed linen, towels and clothing. Appropriate facilities for storage of contaminated items. These facilities should be adequately shielded, labelled and designed with appropriate security measures to prevent risk of escape or theft of material

- Staff and comforters and carers must wear appropriate personal protective equipment such as gloves, gowns and overshoes. They should also have access to appropriate decontamination facilities, including wash basin and decontamination shower
- Appropriately trained nursing and care staff who are also trained in radiation protection

Comforters and Carers

Patients undergoing molecular therapy may require additional support by a family member or friend. For paediatric patients, their parents would typically act as comforters and carers for the duration of their treatment. Comforters and carers are defined in IRMER17 as those individuals who are 'knowingly and willingly helping (other than as part of their occupation) in the support and comfort of patients undergoing medical diagnosis or treatment'. They are not subject to the public dose limit, but their radiation exposure should be justified by the IRMER practitioner. The dose to comforters and carers should be kept as low as reasonably achievable (ALARA) and for this reason radiation protection measures are put in place and advice is provided to help individuals minimise their personal radiation exposure [29].

Outpatient Therapies

The MDGN contains a table of restrictions which are suitable when discharging patients who have undergone radioiodine therapy for thyrotoxicosis. This includes restrictions on contact with children and any restrictions on the mode of transport used [8]. Self-discharge must be firmly discouraged on the grounds of the hazards to others.

Where risk assessment has shown it necessary, all patients should be given written instructions on leaving hospital about precautions to be taken to minimise the dose to others. This may take the form of a card. Even many weeks after precautions have elapsed, patients may retain enough radioactivity in their bodies to set off radiation alarms at airports. Travel plans and arrangements should be discussed with patients before discharge.

Following discharge of the patient from in-patient accommodation, the room may not be re-used until it has been monitored and declared free from contamination.

In the case of the death of a patient following the administration of a therapeutic dose of radioactivity, due regard must be given to the safety of the relatives, pathologists and undertakers etc. The MDGN [8] contains a section giving advice on this, but a local policy should be written for each treatment offered in that centre.

Waste Disposal

The disposal of radioactive waste from a hospital must be organised, carefully controlled and documented in compliance with the U.K. regulations to avoid hazard to staff, patients and the general public. The Environment Agency will authorise limits of activity for gaseous, aqueous and solid waste discharge for each site [31]. Solid waste refers to items contaminated with radioactivity, such as syringes, swabs and paper tissues. Aqueous waste refers to waste discharged to the sewage systems and can include radioactive solutions from radionuclide administration and body fluids from patients. The site must show that it disposes of all waste by the best practicable means before authorisation is granted. Detailed records must be kept of all disposals of radioactive materials, irrespective of which route has been used. These records should include the type of radionuclide, its activity at disposal, the route of disposal and the date of disposal.

REFERENCES

[1] Loevinger R, Budinger TF, Watson EE. MIRD primer for absorbed dose calculations. Society of Nuclear Medicine; 1988.

[2] Stabin MGMIRDOSE. personal computer software for internal dose assessment in nuclear medicine. J Nucl Med 1996;37(3):538–46.

[3] Rojas B, Hooker C, McGowan DR, Guy MJ, Tipping J, Rojas B, Hooker C, McGowan DR, Guy MJ. Eight years of growth and change in UK molecular radiotherapy with implications for the future: Internal Dosimetry Users Group survey results from 2007 to 2015. Nucl Med Comms 2017;38(3):201–4.

[4] Silberstein EB, Alavi A, Balon HR, Clarke SE, Divgi C, Gelfand MJ, Goldsmith SJ, Jadvar H, Marcus CS, Martin WH, Parker JA. The SNMMI practice guideline for therapy of thyroid disease with [131]I 3.0. J Nucl Med 2012;53(10):1633–51.

[5] Luster M, Clarke SE, Dietlein M, Lassmann M, Lind P, Oyen WJ, Tennvall J, Bombardieri E. Guidelines for radioiodine therapy of differentiated thyroid cancer. Eur J Nucl Med Mol Imag 2008;35(10):1941–59.

[6] Robbins RJ, Schlumberger MJ. The evolving role of ^{131}I for the treatment of differentiated thyroid carcinoma. J Nucl Med 2005;46(1):28S–37S.

[7] Perros P, Boelaert K, Colley S, Evans C, Evans RM, Gerrard BA, Gilbert J, Harrison B, Johnson SJ, Giles TE, Moss L. Guidelines for the management of thyroid cancer. Clin Endocrinol 2014;81(s1):1–22.

[8] Medical and Dental Guidance Notes. A good practice guide on all aspects of ionising radiation protection in the clinical environment. Institute of Physics and Engineering in Medicine; 2002.

[9] Stokkel MP, Junak DH, Lassmann M, Dietlein M, Luster M. EANM procedure guidelines for therapy of benign thyroid disease. Eur J Nucl Med Mol Imag 2010;37(11):2218–28.

[10] Dottorini ME, Mansi L. Radioiodine in the management of benign thyroid disease: clinical guidelines. Report of a Working Party, 2007. Royal College of Physicians (RCP). Eur J Nucl Med Mol Imag 2007;34(12):2148–9.

[11] Lewington VJ. Bone-seeking radionuclides for therapy. J Nucl Med 2005;46(1 suppl):38S–47S.

[12] Parker C, Nilsson S, Heinrich D, Helle SI, O'Sullivan JM, Fosså SD, Chodacki A, Wiechno P, Logue J, Seke M, Widmark A. Alpha emitter radium-223 and survival in metastatic prostate cancer. N Engl J Med 2013;369(3):213–23.

[13] Coleman R, Aksnes AK, Naume B, Garcia C, Jerusalem G, Piccart M, Vobecky N, Thuresson M, Flamen P. A phase IIa, nonrandomized study of radium-223 dichloride in advanced breast cancer patients with bone-dominant disease. Breast Canc Res Treat 2014;145(2):411–8.

[14] Poeppel TD, Handkiewicz-Junak D, Andreeff M, Becherer A, Bockisch A, Fricke E, Geworski L, Heinzel A, Krause BJ, Krause T, Mitterhauser M. EANM guideline for radionuclide therapy with radium-223 of metastatic castration-resistant prostate cancer. Eur J Nucl Med Mol Imag 2018;45(5):824–45.

[15] Flux GD. Imaging and dosimetry for radium-223: the potential for personalized treatment. Br J Radiol. 2017;90(0):20160748.

[16] Gains JE, Bomanji JB, Fersht NL, Sullivan T, D'Souza D, Sullivan KP, Aldridge M, Waddington W, Gaze MN. ^{177}Lu-DOTATATE molecular radiotherapy for childhood neuroblastoma. J Nucl Med 2011;52(7):1041–7.

[17] Zaknun JJ, Bodei L, Mueller-Brand J, Pavel ME, Baum RP, Hörsch D, O'Dorisio MS, O'Dorisiol TM, Howe JR, Cremonesi M, Kwekkeboom DJ. The joint IAEA, EANM, and SNMMI practical guidance on peptide receptor radionuclide therapy (PRRNT) in neuroendocrine tumours. Eur J Nucl Med Mol Imag 2013;40(5):800–16.

[18] Strosberg J, El-Haddad G, Wolin E, Hendifar A, Yao J, Chasen B, Mittra E, Kunz PL, Kulke MH, Jacene H, Bushnell D. Phase 3 trial of ^{177}Lu-Dotatate for midgut neuroendocrine tumors. N Engl J Med 2017;376(2):125–35.

[19] Giammarile F, Chiti A, Lassmann M, Brans B, Flux G. EANM procedure guidelines for ^{131}I-meta-iodobenzylguanidine (^{131}I-mIBG) therapy. Eur J Nucl Med Mol Imag 2008;35(5):1039–47.

[20] Gaze MN, Chang YC, Flux GD, Mairs RJ, Saran FH, Meller ST. Feasibility of dosimetry-based high-dose ^{131}I-meta-iodobenzylguanidine with topotecan as a radiosensitizer in children with metastatic neuroblastoma. Canc Biother Rad 2005;20(2):195–9.

[21] Giammarile F, Bodei L, Chiesa C, Flux G, Forrer F, Kraeber-Bodere F, Brans B, Lambert B, Konijnenberg M, Borson-Chazot F, Tennvall J. EANM procedure guideline for the treatment of liver cancer and liver metastases with intra-arterial radioactive compounds. Eur J Nucl Med Mol Imag 2011;38(7):1393.

[22] Garin E, Rolland Y, Laffont S, Edeline J. Clinical impact of ^{99m}Tc-MAA SPECT/CT-based dosimetry in the radioembolization of liver malignancies with ^{90}Y-loaded microspheres. Eur J Nucl Med Mol Imag 2016;43(3):559–75.

[23] Kennedy A, Nag S, Salem R, Murthy R, McEwan AJ, Nutting C, Benson A, Espat J, Bilbao JI, Sharma RA, Thomas JP. Recommendations for radioembolization of hepatic malignancies using yttrium-90 microsphere brachytherapy: a consensus panel report from the radioembolization brachytherapy oncology consortium. Int J Radiat Oncol Biol. Phys 2007;68(1):13–23.

[24] Parmentier C. Use and risks of phosphorus-32 in the treatment of polycythaemia vera. Eur J Nucl Med Mol Imag 2003;30(10):1413–7.

[25] Tennvall J, Brans B. EANM procedure guideline for ^{32}P phosphate treatment of myeloproliferative diseases. Eur J Nucl Med Mol Imag 2007;34(8):1324–7.

[26] Clunie G, Fischer M. EANM procedure guidelines for radiosynovectomy. Eur J Nucl Med Mol Imag 2003;30(3):BP12.

[27] Wiseman GA, White CA, Stabin M, Dunn WL, Erwin W, Dahlbom M, Raubitschek A, Karvelis K, Schultheiss T, Witzig TE, Belanger R. Phase I/II ^{90}Y-Zevalin (yttrium-90 ibritumomab tiuxetan, IDEC-Y2B8) radioimmunotherapy dosimetry results in relapsed or refractory non-Hodgkin's lymphoma. Eur J Nucl Med 2000;27(7):766–77.

[28] Emmett L, Willowson K, Violet J, Shin J, Blanksby A, Lee J. Lutetium 177 PSMA radionuclide therapy for men with prostate cancer: a review of the current literature and discussion of practical aspects of therapy. J Med Radiat Sci 2017;64(1):52–60.

[29] The Ionising Radiation (Medical Exposure) Regulations 2017. Statutory Instrument No. 1322; 2017. Regulated by the Care Quality Commission.

[30] The Ionising Radiation Regulations 2017. Statutory Instrument No. 675, 2017. Regulated by the Health and Safety Executive.

[31] Permitting the Environmental. (England and Wales) Regulations, Environmental Protection. In: England and Wales; 2010.

8

Radiotherapy Devices With Kilovoltage X-Rays and Radioisotopes

Claire Fletcher, John A. Mills

CHAPTER OUTLINE

INTRODUCTION

There are a variety of radiotherapy (RT) machines based on radioactive sources and x-rays. Radioactive sources have provided gamma rays and beta rays for many years. X-rays range from accelerating voltages as low as 10 kV to megavoltage beams with equivalent accelerating potentials of up to 25 MV and electron and particle beams are also used. Clinical practice has developed to use these devices where applications have been found. Over time, this has established niches for different machines where clinical expertise has become well understood and the therapeutic benefit of particular techniques has been demonstrated. In this chapter the range of RT machines and devices that use kilovoltage x-rays and radioisotopes are described.

KILOVOLTAGE X-RAY PRODUCTION

X-Rays From Electrons

X-rays are produced by using the process described in Chapter 2 (see the X-Ray Production section) and normally referred to as bremsstrahlung. In the process accelerated electrons are slowed down and lose energy to x-rays produced in the interaction with a material. In x-ray machines, the interaction takes place in a target, referred to as the x-ray target. An energetic beam of electrons is produced by the machine using high-voltage acceleration and this electron beam is directed onto the x-ray target.

High-Voltage Circuits

It is essential to have a high voltage to accelerate an electron beam for x-ray production. On early machines, step-up transformers were used to provide high voltages to excite the x-ray tube. The transformers operated at mains frequency and were very bulky because of the large iron core required.

Modern units employ switched-mode power supply techniques, to improve voltage stability and make savings in size and efficiency. The power supply comprises an input rectifier to convert mains alternating current (AC) to a direct current (DC) voltage. A switching inverter converts the DC to a high-frequency (25 kHz) pulsed waveform that is stepped up to 10 kV via a high-frequency transformer. Finally, the waveform is rectified and passed through a number of cascaded multiplying stages (Cockcroft–Walton) to produce a DC voltage in the 100- to 300 kV range.

The extra High Tension (HT) voltage is monitored and a control signal fed back to alter the pulse width of the waveform leaving the inverter stage. In this way, a stable voltage is maintained across the x-ray tube.

The intensity of the x-ray beam produced at a particular kilovoltage depends on the number of electrons emitted from the filament. This tube current is a function of the filament temperature and hence of the filament current. The filament drive voltage is controlled electronically to respond to changes in the AC supply and stabilise the beam current. A schematic is shown in Fig. 8.1. Typically, for voltages in excess of 200 kV, two high-voltage power supplies are used in series.

The HT generator is controlled externally so that safe operating parameters can be set for the particular tube in use. The generator status can also be fed to the operating system to indicate faults, to link into the interlock system to ensure safe treatment, and to assist in fault diagnosis.

The high-voltage and filament power supply is connected to the x-ray tube by means of a high-voltage cable. To prevent voltage

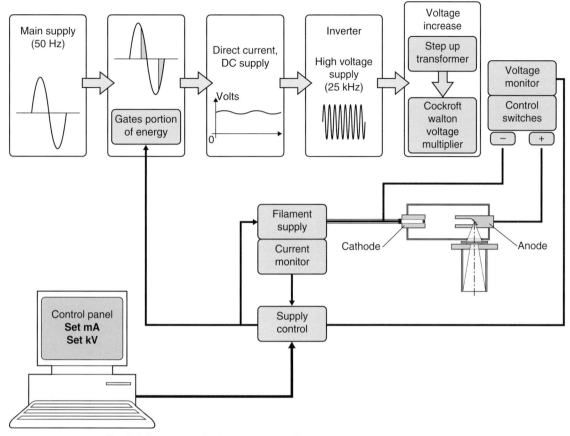

Fig. 8.1 Schematic of HT generator with feedback and connection to controller.

flashover in the connectors, care must be taken to keep all parts clean and use high-voltage insulating grease during assembly and reassembly following maintenance inspection.

KILOVOLTAGE X-RAY CHARACTERISTICS

The x-ray beam from any bremsstrahlung target consists of a range of energies up to the maximum accelerating potential produced by the machine. Hence, for a 120-kV machine, 120 keV will be the accelerated electron energy and, in turn, the maximum x-ray photon energy will be 120 keV. This spectrum of energies is modified using a filter to remove lower-energy x-rays and so reduce the dose to the skin. The beam that emerges from the tube through the x-ray window has undergone what is called inherent filtration. However, additional filtration is chosen to provide a beam with the desired depth-dose (DD) penetration. The energy characteristics of the beam are often referred to as its quality and are dependent upon both the accelerating potential and filtration. The beam quality is normally measured using the thickness of aluminium or copper and specified in terms of the half-value layer (HVL), which is the thickness of the layer of metal required to reduce the intensity of the beam by half. Typically, when this is measured it is done in a narrow beam, obtained by additional collimation to a broad clinical beam. The measuring ionisation chamber is also placed at sufficient distance from the machine, floor, and walls to ensure there is no additional scattered radiation. In practical terms, the penetration of the beam is also as a result of the source to surface distance (SSD) and the field size. DD data indicating the penetration of different HVL beams can be compared [1].

SUPERFICIAL AND DEEP KILOVOLTAGE MACHINES

Deep x-ray (DXR) and superficial x-ray (SXR) units provide x-ray beams in the keV energy range. The term orthovoltage is also used and this term reflects the arrangement whereby the x-rays are produced in a direction at right angles to that of the accelerating voltage. The units typically take the form of a tube assembly which can be manually manipulated to direct the beam onto the patient. The SSD is typically in the range of 20 to 50 cm and the field is defined at the surface by a mechanical applicator. An example of such a machine is shown in Fig. 8.2.

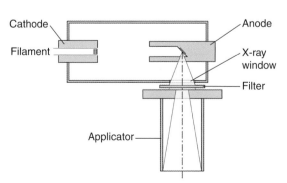

Fig. 8.2 Example of an orthovoltage machine.

Tube Stand

The tube is mounted on a mechanism commonly referred to as the tube stand (Fig. 8.3). The design of the tube stand enables manipulation of the beam direction by the machine operator to direct it at the patient's lesion. There are both floor-mounted and ceiling-mounted stands. The design allows translational and rotational movement of the beam and there may be scales of distance and angle which enable the setup position or changes to it to be recorded and monitored. Electrical or mechanical brakes are fitted to the rotational axes and translational runners in order that the position can be reliably fixed in position before treatment and monitored during treatment.

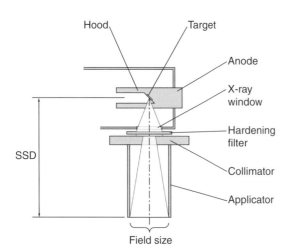

Fig. 8.3 Orthovoltage machine on a stand.

Collimation

The anode construction provides the initial collimation of the beam as the x-rays come off the target almost omnidirectionally (Fig. 8.4). This is referred to as a hooded anode and the aperture defines the maximum size of conical x-ray beam that could be provided. The collimation is completed by use of an applicator that is fixed directly below the tube aperture and provides the following:
- The base of the applicator consists of a collimator which defines the shape and size of the radiation field at the end of the applicator.
- The end of the applicator is the shape and size of the radiation beam.
- The end of the applicator determines a fixed distance from the source.

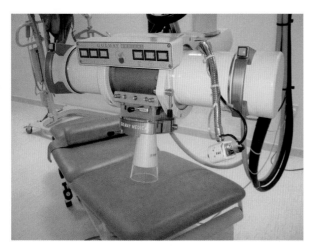

Fig. 8.4 Anode construction, hood, and omnidirectional emission with applicator to collimate beam and set source to surface distance and define field size.

- The axis of the applicator is mechanically aligned to the axis of the radiation beam.

Skin and Eye Shielding

Beam collimation is provided on orthovoltage machines with a range of applicators, which have regular field sizes. These applicators are usually chosen by the user when the unit is purchased. The choice is made to provide a nominal range of sizes for coverage of typical lesions. Often, it is necessary to treat lesions of nonstandard size and irregular shape. It is common practice to manufacture a lead cut-out to define the treatment field exactly to the area specified by the radiotherapist. The cut-out is used in conjunction with one of the regular sized applicators to irradiate the treatment area and shield the surrounding normal skin from the rest of the beam. For lesions on the face and in close proximity to the eyes, a lead mask is manufactured based upon a plaster cast of the patient. As well as defining the treatment field and shielding the normal skin and the eyes, the lead mask can also be used to provide direction and localisation of the beam (Fig. 8.5).

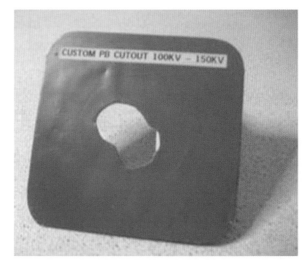

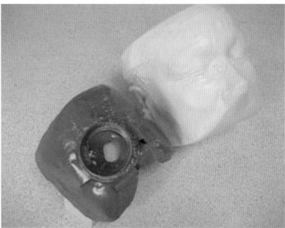

Fig. 8.5 Irregular lead cut-out and mask.

To provide effective shielding, the thickness of lead for the cut-out has to be chosen taking into account the energy of the beam. This can be done from tabulated data of attenuation in lead against field size and beam energy as expressed by HVL. It is always prudent, however, for the RT physicists to undertake measurements and verify the shielding that is being obtained with the chosen thickness of lead.

When the treatment area impinges onto the eye, it is possible to insert eye shields to provide some protection to the lens. There are commercial lead and tungsten shields available. The problem encountered with eye shields is the contribution from scatter which reaches into the region under the shield from the surrounding field.

Control of Output

The stability of the output from the unit is directly related to the electrical stability of the tube voltage and current. Stabilised electrical supplies as described earlier ensure that this is achieved consistently. Typically, a timer is used to control the amount of dose that is delivered. The timer is normally a countdown device and starts to operate when the treatment is initiated and the voltage and current are supplied to the tube. After the set time has elapsed, the voltage and current are switched off and treatment terminates. A timed exposure requires that the output dose rate is stable and that is dependent upon the aforementioned electrical control stability. There is always an inherent increase in the dose rate as the voltage and the current ramp-up to their operating value and this effect is normally taken into account using a transit time to accommodate the underdose which this would otherwise lead to. The transit time is added to the calculated time based upon a nominal dose rate to produce a total set time.

Most modern DXR and SXR units use a full-field ionisation monitor chamber through which the beam passes. By measuring the charge released against the absolute dose under particular set-up conditions, it is possible to control the output from the machine by a system which terminates the beam when the accumulated charge equals the required dose. The units of charge from the ionisation chamber are referred to as monitor units and the specific dose delivered to any individual patient is achieved by calculating the required number of monitor units to be set.

Calibration of Dose Output

As described earlier, there are two types of exposure control used on orthovoltage equipment. For a great many years, it has been done using a timer. However, in more recent years, exposure is controlled by a full-field ionisation monitor chamber mounted in the radiation beam.

For timer control, the machine operator requires to know the dose rate of the machine and, for ionisation chamber control, the response of the chamber must be directly related to an absolute dose. The ionisation chamber response is normally quantified in monitor units and calibrated to be dose per monitor unit. Hence, for both systems of control, it is necessary to measure the absolute dose delivered by the beam under a very specific set up, often referred to as the calibration conditions. The time to be set or the monitor units to be set are then determined using relative factors from the calibration setup. For example, the specific dose rate may be measured for a 5-cm diameter applicator at 30-cm SSD. To calculate a time to set, relative factors for other applicators, difference in SSD, and changes in the irradiated area are used.

The absolute dose is measured in accordance with a protocol or code of practice. This ensures uniformity of practice between institutions. It will use the absolute dose calibration of the ionisation chamber being used for the measurement and this will be traceable to a standards laboratory. The calibration can be done in air with the use of mass absorption coefficient ratios to determine the dose to water or tissue. Alternatively, the measurement can be done directly at depth in water. For superficial kV units with HVL values up to 8-mm Al, it is typical to determine the surface dose rate as this is where the dose is to be applied. However, for DXR units with HVL values higher than 8-mm Al, it can be preferable to quote the dose deeper than the surface and closer to the target. In the latter case, it is preferable to calibrate at depth in water.

CONTACT KILOVOLTAGE MACHINE

Contact RT began in the 1940s with very short SSD x-ray treatments. The characteristics of these beams are a rapid fall in DD from the

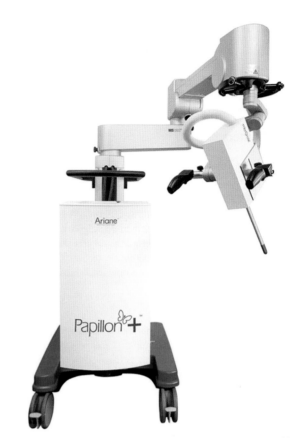

Fig. 8.6 A contact radiotherapy machine. (Courtesy Ariane Medical Systems.)

surface as a result of the short SSD. Therefore in contrast to moving from SXR to DXR to gain penetration, these beams can provide a very high dose to 1 mm to 2 mm of the incident tissue while considerably limiting the dose given deeper. This does mean that the DD variation and the incident dose are very sensitive to displacement. For example, a 1-mm stand-off at 20-cm SSD changes the incident dose by 1%, whereas at 4-cm SSD it changes by 5%. Similarly, the change in DD at 1-cm depth is 2% at 4-cm SSD, compared with 0.1% at 20-cm SSD.

The HT generator is of a standard design as already described in section above on High-Voltage Circuits and typically 50 kV accelerating potential is used with filtration occurring intrinsically in the construction materials as well as in the x-ray target which may well be a transmission design. The design of the target and its cooling system as well as monitoring the output is challenging. A contact beam will have an HVL of about 0.35 mm Al [1]. These machines have a gantry stand to enable direct treatment onto a surface lesion, which may be inside the rectum or intraoperatively aligned to an applicator inserted into the surgical cavity. Such a machine is shown in Fig. 8.6.

GRENZ KILOVOLTAGE MACHINE

Very-low kV x-ray generation was explored from the 1920s and the term *Grenz*, which is border in German, was used for beams with HVL less than 0.04 mmAl, because their biological effect was observed to lie between x-rays and UV for skin conditions. In some designs, the x-ray target was the window of the tube. However, in all designs the hardening effect of the tube limited the softness of the x-rays produced. There are typical beam characteristics [1]. HT generation, cooling, and gantry systems remain the same as for SXR and DXR machines.

RADIONUCLIDE CHARACTERISTICS

Radionuclides provide a range of materials to make a variety of ionising radiation beams available as RT devices. These devices range from teletherapy beams of gamma rays to physical encapsulations of material which enable direct RT with electrons. By far, the majority of devices used is collectively described as brachytherapy.

Gamma Emitters

Radium

Radium-226 was the first radioisotope used in brachytherapy. It has a half-life of 1600 years and a mean photon energy of approximately 800 keV. The major source of gamma rays is the gaseous daughter product radon. For medical applications radium was encapsulated in a tube which had to be gas tight and frequently checked for leaks. The gamma rays used are highly penetrating and very thick lead shields are required to provide adequate radiation protection. Other radioisotopes with more suitable properties are now available and as a result this material is no longer in use.

Caesium

Caesium-137 is a fission product derived from spent uranium fuel rods used in nuclear reactors. Caesium-137 has no gaseous daughter products and largely replaced radium as the nuclide of choice in the 1960s. It has a half-life of 30 years and a mean photon energy of 662 keV.

Iridium

Iridium-192 has a mean gamma energy of 380 keV and half-life of 73.83 days. It has been in use since the late 1950s and has a high specific activity. Its physical form for RT is of a flexible wire and this has many advantages over traditional radium and caesium needles for interstitial implants.

Iodine

Iodine-125 has a half-life of 60 days and has been used clinically since the early 1960s. It is the daughter product of xenon-125 which is produced by a neutron-gamma reaction and the average photon energy of iodine-125 is only 28 keV.

Cobalt

Cobalt-60 has a half-life of 5.3 years and an average photon energy of 1.253 MeV. This high photon energy makes it a highly penetrating RT beam and it is used for teletherapy.

Beta Emitters

Strontium

Strontium-90 has a half-life of 28.8 years. It is only useful when in radioactive equilibrium with its daughter product (yttrium-90) and that equilibrium is achieved with silver encapsulation. Strontium-90 emits electrons of 546 keV and the daughter product, yttrium-90, emits an electron with a maximum energy of 2.27 MeV.

Ruthenium

Ruthenium-106 has a half-life of 369 days. It is a fission product of uranium and decays with a low-energy beta emission to rhodium-106 which has a maximum high-energy beta emission of 3.54 MeV.

BRACHYTHERAPY AND AFTERLOADING MACHINES

Brachytherapy is a mode of treatment in which the radioactive sources are placed in close or direct contact with the tissue to be treated. It has the advantage of delivering a highly localised radiation dose to a small tumour volume. There is a sharp fall-off of radiation dose in the surrounding normal tissue and therefore the risks of complication are reduced.

There are three main delivery techniques:

1. Intracavitary—Radioactive sources are inserted into a natural body cavity such as the vagina, uterus, bronchus, oesophagus, or rectum to directly treat a tumour.
2. Interstitial—Radioactive sources are inserted directly into the tissue at the tumour site, via needles or implants.
3. Surface applicators—Radioactive sources are applied to the external surface of a patient, directly onto the tumour.

Most radionuclides used in brachytherapy are photons emitters; however, beta- and even neutron-emitting sources are used for some applications.

Caesium-137 was incorporated into zirconium phosphate for needles and tubes used for manual interstitial and intracavitary brachytherapy. Sources were doubly encapsulated and had a recommended working life of 10 years, during which their activity falls by approximately 20%. Caesium-137 tubes were favoured for gynaecological insertions and extensively used in low dose rate (LDR) and medium dose rate (MDR) treatments. An extensive guide to the use of initially radium tubes and needles and then caesium tubes and needles is The Manchester System [2]. Manually inserted LDR caesium produced excellent tumour control rates in gynaecological tumours and the serious complication rate was also low, at 5% or less. Such results remain the gold standard against which modern techniques must be judged. The most widely used technique was the Manchester System in which preloaded sources were placed in the uterus and against the cervix (Fig. 8.7). The dose rate at point A was approximately 0.5 Gy/h, which proved to be biologically very advantageous. A typical regimen used to treat an early stage 1b carcinoma of the cervix was two insertions of approximately 72 hours given 1 week apart to achieve a total dose of 75 Gy to point A. From about the year 2000, imaging using computed tomography (CT) and magnetic resonance imaging (MRI) became much more common for brachytherapy, leading to departures from the Manchester system in favour of conformal planning and using

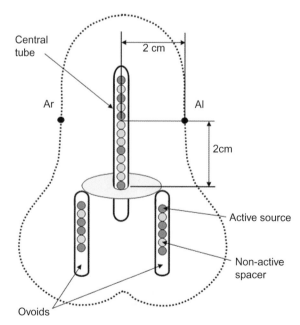

Fig. 8.7 Medium dose rate source positions and the Manchester A points.

the three-dimensional dose-volume parameters recommended by GEC-ESTRO in 2005 and 2006 [3,4].

Iridium-192 wire has also been extensively used for all forms of brachytherapy. The Paris System [5] was a guide to the use of this wire. Coils of thin wire (0.3 mm diameter) can be cut to convenient lengths and inserted into flexible nylon tubes or rigid hollow afterloading needles similar to hypodermic needles, which have been previously implanted into tumours. Thicker wires, 0.6 mm in diameter, in the form of hairpins (Fig. 8.8) can also be inserted directly into tumours through suitable guides. Lead shields of only 2-cm thickness provide very good protection from the gamma rays given off by iridium-192. The only major disadvantage of iridium is its relatively short half-life and the need for fresh material for each implant, at LDR.

Iodine-125 is used for permanent implants of the prostate. It has been used clinically since the early 1960s and because the average photon energy of iodine-125 is only 28 keV, the thickness of lead required for protection is only 0.02 mm. In tissue, the HVL is in the region of 1.7 cm and very little radiation is emitted from the patient. Therefore permanent implants in the form of seeds which remain after the radiation has decayed completely can be performed using this relatively short half-life isotope.

The major use of plaques emitting beta radiation is in the treatment of eye tumours.

Strontium-90 compound is incorporated in a rolled silver foil bonded into a silver applicator and formed so that it presents an active concave surface of 15-mm radius to the cornea, with a surface filtration of 0.1-mm silver. Strontium-90 is only useful when in radioactive equilibrium with its daughter product, yttrium-90. The silver filter is designed to absorb low-energy beta particles from the strontium decay (0.546 MeV max) while transmitting the higher-energy beta particles from the yttrium-90 (2.27 MeV max). The back of the applicator is finished with a much thicker (0.9 mm) layer of silver to reduce the transmitted dose rate to a relatively safe level. The plaques are designed to give a useful dose rate of approximately 1 Gy/min at the surface, which is reduced to 50% at approximately 2 mm depth.

The ruthenium-106 applicator is made of silver with a window thickness of 0.1 mm of silver and a thicker protective layer of 0.9 mm of silver on the back. The applicator is designed for suturing to the sclera for 7 to 10 days. The useful dose rate is typically 0.1 Gy/min at the surface, reducing to 50% at approximately 2.7 mm depth. A 15-mm acrylic visor is recommended to protect the eyes of the operator when using the ruthenium applicators.

Treatment of retinoblastoma has been effected using cobalt-60 ophthalmic applicators of similar construction to the ruthenium applicator.

The longer half-life was an advantage, but the high-energy gamma radiation gave high doses to other vital structures (e.g. the lens, macula, and optic nerve) than with the ruthenium-106 beta-particle radiations.

From when brachytherapy was first introduced up until the mid-1970s, brachytherapy sources were loaded into rubber applicators and positioned by hand. Sources remained in place during the treatment and then were manually retrieved except for the permanent iodine-125 prostate implants which were not removed after delivery of the prescribed treatment dose. Consequently, staff involved in the process from the beginning to end were exposed to ionising radiation. For the latter reason, manual insertion of radiation sources should be avoided if possible.

Afterloading is when radioactive material is loaded into hollow needles, catheters, or applicators that have been previously inserted into the tumour area. Manipulation of these applicators carries no radiation hazard for medical and nursing staff so that time can safely be taken to ensure optimal source geometry.

In the late 1970s, sources with a high specific activity were readily available, for example, caesium-137. In addition, developments in computer-controlled delivery and new flexible carriers made it possible to produce devices that could automatically deliver and retrieve treatment sources.

When used with LDR afterloading systems, caesium-137 was most commonly used in the form of spherical pellets. This was achieved by mixing the caesium with glass to form beads that could be encapsulated by spherical stainless steel shells. These pellets could then be used in the form of a source train. Caesium-137 continued to be favoured for gynaecological insertions and was extensively used in LDR and MDR afterloading systems from the late 1970s. This has now been mainly replaced by high dose rate (HDR) afterloading systems using iridium-192.

Iridium-192 became the radioisotope of choice for both HDR afterloader units and interstitial implants, taking advantage of its high specific activity and the properties of a flexible wire. HDR sources are normally renewed every 3 months. Cobalt-60 can be used as an alternative source in HDR units, but higher thickness of lead is required for radiation protection than with the lower-energy iridium-192.

HDR and also pulsed dose rate (PDR) afterloading systems have become the main systems of choice worldwide. The PDR, as its name suggests, delivers in pulses and was developed on the basis of theoretical radiobiological work which predicted better radiobiological equivalence with LDR treatment. PDR involves short pulses of radiation, typically once an hour, to simulate the overall dose rate and radiobiological effectiveness of LDR treatment. The source strength

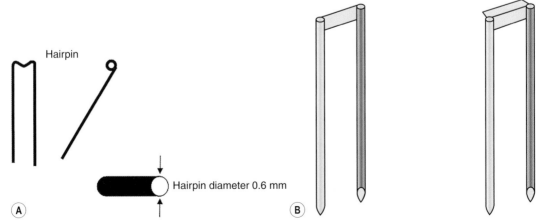

Fig. 8.8 Iridium-192 wire implants. (A) 0.6-mm diameter hairpins and (B) guides for insertion.

of a PDR machine is approximately one-tenth of that of an HDR source. With HDR, treatment is completed in a matter of minutes, whereas PDR lasts a few days.

HDR has the advantage in that treatment can be carried out in about 20 minutes. Theoretically, HDR is more likely to cause normal tissue damage than LDR. However, this has not been seen in practice and is thought to be largely caused by the effects of fractionation. HDR brachytherapy treatment is usually divided into two to four fractions, given over weekly intervals.

THE HIGH DOSE RATE AFTERLOADING MACHINE

HDR machines essentially consist of a high-activity iridium-192 source at the tip of a transfer wire which can be positioned within applicators or catheters already inserted into the patient and attached to the afterloader by a transfer tube. The source activity is typically 400 GBq to 500 GBq and provides an air kerma rate (AKR) of about 50 mGy/h at 1 m when initially installed. The source is an iridium pellet, whose diameter is about 0.6 mm and length 3.5 mm. It is encapsulated in stainless steel, whose diameter is about 0.9 mm and length 4.5 mm, and welded onto the transfer wire (Fig. 8.9). The source resides in a shielded safe when not irradiating a target volume (Fig. 8.10).

The HDR is connected to a treatment control system (TCS) and treatment planning system (TPS). Treatment plans are transferred to the TCS for treatments to be carried out.

For treatment, the machine is programmed to drive the transfer wire out of the machine along the transfer tube, taking the source out of the safe into a number of predetermined treating positions for set dwell times. These treating positions lie within an applicator or catheter, located adjacent to or inside the target that has been previously inserted into the patient. The source can be fed into different types of applicators and catheters for different types of treatment. In this way the high-activity source can be positioned as required by the TPS to deliver the chosen isodose distribution. During the treatment planning, the dose distribution is manipulated by changing source dwell time and position before the final, approved plan is transferred to the TCS.

There are other distinct features of HDR machines and these are illustrated in Fig. 8.10.

A nonradioactive check wire is driven along the transfer tube and into the treatment catheter or applicator immediately before irradiation to ensure that the passage is clear and without problem. Both wires are driven by identical, accurate motor-drive mechanisms. Limit detectors monitor the end of or absence of the wire and a radiation monitor verifies the presence of the source in the safe. Interlocks are also required to ensure there is no possibility of inadvertent or inappropriate irradiation of patient and staff.

IMPLANTED KILOVOLTAGE MACHINE

The miniaturisation of x-ray sources has led to the opportunity of implanting a non-radioactive source to deliver treatment to a target volume. This is also referred to as electronic brachytherapy. Essentially these miniature devices generate electrons with 50 keV energy in a very short distance and bombard a transmission target such as tungsten or gold to produce an almost omnidirectional point source distribution of x-rays. As with contact therapy (see the Contact Kilovoltage Machine section), the source is in direct contact with tissue and has a rapid fall off in DD.

The aspects of such a device are shown in Fig. 8.11.

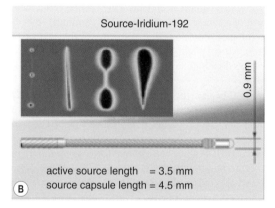

Source-Iridium-192

0.9 mm

active source length   = 3.5 mm
source capsule length = 4.5 mm

B

Fig. 8.9 Iridium-192 high dose rate source and dose distributions.

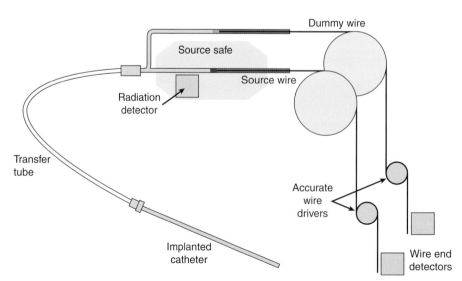

Dummy wire

Source safe

Source wire

Radiation detector

Transfer tube

Accurate wire drivers

Implanted catheter

Wire end detectors

Fig. 8.10 Schematic of the essential features of a high dose rate afterloading machine.

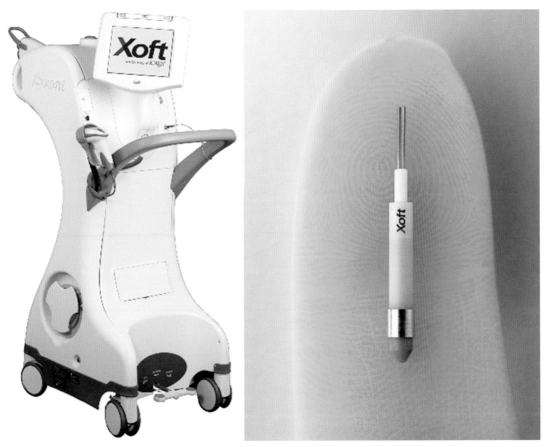

Fig. 8.11 Miniaturised 50-kV x-ray source system for x-ray brachytherapy. (Courtesy Xoft.)

BETA-RAY MACHINE

As mentioned earlier with regard to brachytherapy, beta-particle emitters have found applications in superficial treatment using the superficial penetration of the beta particles and delivery of a dose to a small thickness of tissue.

A beta-ray device has also been developed to deliver a RT dose from a small strontium-90 source directly to the central area of the retina using an intraocular probe during eye surgery.

Most early teletherapy machines that were developed for both medical and industrial applications used gamma-emitting radionuclides such as caesium-137, iridium-192, and cobalt-60. However, one notable attempt was made to deliver a teletherapy beam of electrons for total skin irradiation with strontium-90. It used a 900 MBq source, which was 53cm long by 2cm wide. The machine traversed along the patient for 40 cm to deliver a skin dose. The treatment times were in excess of 15 minutes to deliver a therapeutic 2 Gy dose fraction, and the penetration of the dose was limited to about 2 mm by the maximum energy of the daughter yttrium-90 emission of 2.27 MeV. The limited penetration and dose rate illustrate why there was no widespread use of such a teletherapy machine and megavoltage accelerators went on to provide much more effective electron beams for total skin electron treatment.

GAMMA-RAY MACHINE

The penetrative limitations and high skin dose of even 300-kV x-rays drove the desire for higher-energy x-rays. The radioisotope cobalt-60 (^{60}Co) was discovered at the University of California by Seaborg and Livingwood [9] in the 1930s and, in Canada in 1951, it was used for teletherapy. The isotope is produced by neutron bombardment through the following process:

$$^{59}\text{Co} + n \rightarrow {}^{60}\text{Co} + \gamma \qquad \textbf{8.1}$$

Nuclear reactors provided an ideal production platform for the substance. The attraction of cobalt-60 was the high-energy gamma emission produced in the radioactive decay process (Fig. 8.12) and also the relatively long half-life of the isotope of just over 5 years. The energy of the gamma rays are almost four times that of the highest DXR unit.

The DD characteristics of a nominal 10cm × 10cm field size cobalt-60 beam at 80 SSD are compared in Fig. 8.13 with those for a 10cm diameter, 0.4Cu HVL kilovoltage beam. The latter would typically be produced from acceleration with about 300 kV and appropriate filtration. The DD characteristics for a 10cm × 10cm field size 6 MV

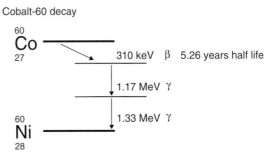

Fig. 8.12 Cobalt gamma-ray decay process.

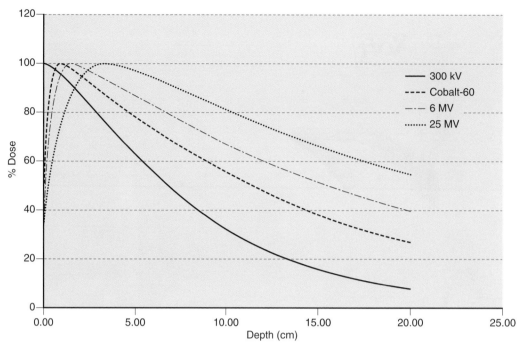

Fig. 8.13 300-kV, cobalt, 6- and 25-MV depth-dose curves.

and 25 MV beams at 100 SSD from a linear accelerator are also shown for comparison.

The advantages are immediately obvious. First, the dose at depth, say 7 cm, is increased by almost a factor of 1.5. Second, however, the forward scattering of the electrons produced from the photon interactions produces the skin-sparing effect with a maximum dose at 0.5-cm depth rather than at the surface. Cobalt units provided the clinician with an enormous technical advantage for teletherapy.

The cobalt unit represents an extremely simple method to generate a megavoltage treatment beam. There is no requirement for the highly skilled maintenance and costs associated with linear accelerators and this enables teletherapy to be provided at low cost in situations where technical support is not readily available. This is the enormous potential for these machines: simplicity and economy.

Radioisotope Source

The radioactive cobalt-60 source consists of a small container that encapsulates pellets or disks of cobalt with an activity of typically 200 TBq. The typical dimension of such a source is a 2-cm diameter by 2-cm long cylinder. Herein lies one of the deficiencies of the cobalt treatment unit as this large source in turn produces a large penumbra in its radiation fields. The source is housed within a large shielded safe, which has a shutter mechanism to transport the source into an exposed position. Typical mechanisms are spring-loaded wheels, jaws, and sliding mechanism and there were electrical, mechanical, hydraulic, and pneumatically driven systems developed. Periodic testing is required to ensure that there is no leakage of radioactive material from the source encapsulation. Swabs are taken from the aperture to the safe to detect contamination. Emergency personnel procedures are also required to be in place to ensure that, in the event of a failure of the transport mechanism, the patient can be safely removed from the room and the source returned to the safe by manual means. One noticeable feature of a cobalt head is that it is continually warm. This arises from the radioactive decay and absorption in the shielded housing and, in particular, all the β-decay indicated in Fig. 8.12. It is testament to the reality of the energy release from the cobalt source.

Beam Collimation

The collimation of the beam is achieved using a system of primary collimator, secondary collimator, and penumbra trimmers as shown in Fig. 8.14. The primary collimator is adjacent to the source and can form part of the drum assembly within which the source is stored. It forms the initial beam which will set the maximum size possible for the final treatment field. The penumbra of a radiation field is dependent upon three aspects: the size of the source, the distance of the secondary

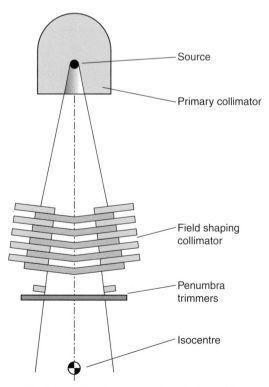

Fig. 8.14 Collimation system for cobalt machine.

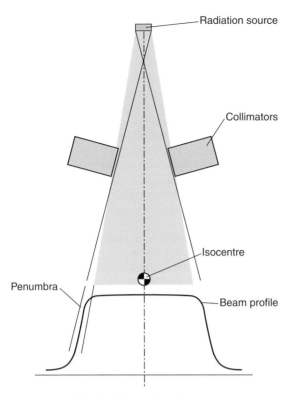

Fig. 8.15 Penumbra diagram.

collimator jaw from the source, and electron scatter at the edge of the beam (Fig. 8.15). Scatter really only becomes a problem at very high energies above 15 MV photon beams. However, the radiation source at 2 cm is very large. If then the secondary collimator jaws were placed one above the other, the penumbra across the inner jaws would be larger than across the outer jaws. Therefore to provide a more equitable size in both directions, the jaws are interlaced as shown in Fig. 8.14. The distance from the source is extended even further by the use of penumbra trimmers, which can be fitted to the ends of the main secondary collimators. Although this technique is effective, it is not always practical because of patient positioning.

Design of Gamma-Ray Teletherapy Machines

Initially, there were fixed-head cobalt treatment machines followed by rotating gantry-mounted machines (Fig. 8.16). The rotating gantry machines were arranged in such a way that the axes of the radiation head rotation and the gantry rotation intersected. This enabled isocentric treatment of the patient with multiple beams intersecting within the target and enhancing the dose there simply by rotation of the gantry. Because of the massive shielding for the radioactive source, the radiation head presented a considerably heavy load for the gantry assembly to accommodate. This led to relatively large displacements between beams at the isocentre and could well be of the order of 10 mm with gantry rotation.

One additional set of movements that was available on several machines was pitch and roll (Fig. 8.16). The advantage of these two movements was that, for some poorly non-ambulant patients, the beam could be directed for treatment with them upright in a chair or even remaining in their bed. Such treatments would be single field and often single-shot treatments for palliation. Nevertheless, it provided a valuable treatment technique for the clinician and operator.

In compact rooms, the radiation head was balanced on the gantry by a shield to reduce the radiation protection requirements in the room. Wedges were also available for these machines and consisted of metal filters placed on trays directly below the secondary collimators. No dosimetry monitoring was installed to control the radiation delivery. The delivery was controlled by a timer which controlled the period during which the source was exposed to the patient from its safe. Because there was a finite time during which the source would be transported to the fully exposed position, this was accommodated by modifying the exposure time with a transit time. The dose rate of the source was checked periodically by absolute measurement under reference calibration conditions. This would typically be monthly, and, in addition, a comparison would be made against the known physical decay prediction to ensure the purity of the isotope.

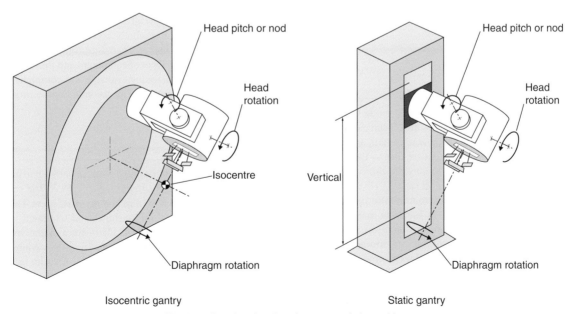

Isocentric gantry   Static gantry

Fig. 8.16 Rotational and static gantry cobalt machines.

RADIOSURGERY

The Gamma Knife or Leksell Gamma Knife is a trademark for a specific commercial device. It is a dedicated cranial radiosurgical machine which uses a large number of collimated cobalt-60 sources to provide an ablative dose to a small treatment volume. The target volume may be in the order of 5- to 40-mm diameter and multiple spherical volumes can be used in combination. This machine was pioneered by Lars Leksell in Sweden in the 1960s to 1980s. The device now has widespread use and the main principle behind the design of the source collimation is shown in Fig. 8.17. There were up to 200 cobalt sources in the early machines and all the beams intersect at a point, giving a high dose volume within the patient who was positioned so that the intersection volume is located at the target. In the early machines there were several helmet collimators with different collimator diameters. Using tungsten plugs, the source, and therefore beam array, was configured for the particular treatment by helmet selection and arrangement of plugs. In the modern machines there is a single moveable helmet with multiple collimator holes of between 4- and 16-mm diameter and the combination of beams is automated.

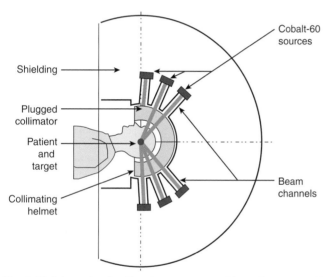

Fig. 8.17 Schematic of collimation system used in radiosurgery with cobalt sources.

RADIATION SAFETY

Radiation safety, a statutory requirement well set out in Chapter 4, is an intrinsic design feature of RT devices and facilities. Protection needs to be afforded to the patient, the operating staff, and members of the public. Devices are designed to ensure that to the maximum extent possible, the patient is exposed to only the clinically required radiation field and dose. The former aspect relates to the beam shaping and the shielding built into the device to minimise any peripheral radiation present outside the useful beam. Ensuring that an accurate dose is delivered for the patient is dependent upon the operation of machine control systems, such as dose monitors, timers, and safety interlocks, and working practices to ensure, for example, the presence of the correct applicator, the correct energy of a beam, and the mechanical operation of shutters and drive mechanisms. The design of the machine and the room also includes radiation shielding and design features to provide protection during clinical treatment, and

equipment testing and maintenance to operational, scientific, and technical staff. Lastly protection of the public is ensured by adequate interlocks and room shielding design.

The types of radiation, range of energies, activity of sources, and treatment dose rates make for a varied range of design of the treatment room. For example, in the case of iodine-125 radioactive sources, the self-shielding of the body reduces the hazard substantially. By contrast, a HDR afterloader poses a substantial requirement on the room design with regard to wall thickness and entrance, possibly requiring a maze. Consideration should also be given to the direction of therapy beams and where in the room or adjacent rooms or corridors a hazard could occur and can be reduced by design. Room design for Co-60 teletherapy machines is comparable with that for high-energy linear accelerators as described in Chapter 9. Design guidance and principles [6] are readily available.

One final and recent issue with regard to radiation safety has been the possibility of radioactive materials being used for terrorist purposes. Although the threat of terrorism has led to heightened security throughout many facets of life, it has also impacted on the security provision for radioactive sources, their storage, and transport.

COMMISSIONING AND QUALITY CONTROL

The role of commissioning and quality control to ensure the protection of individuals against the dangers of ionising radiation in relation to medical exposure is set out in Article 8 of the European Commission (EC) Directive 93/47/Euratom [7]. Chapter 13 deals in detail with the principles of quality control. However, it is worth emphasising that it applies to all RT devices, although Chapter 13 deals primarily with examples for megavoltage equipment.

The Directive specifies the following three aspects with regard to maintaining safe and effective equipment to protect individuals:
1. Commission the equipment by conducting measurements to ensure it operates within a required specification for clinical use.
2. Undertake routine quality control checks to ensure its ongoing performance.
3. Undertake quality control checks following repair and modification to ensure its ongoing performance.

These three principles should be applied to all RT devices, including those discussed in this chapter. There is considerable guidance available for quality control of all types of equipment and these are referenced in Chapter 13. However, a readily available and comprehensive guide is published by the Institute of Physics and Engineering in Medicine (IPEM) [8].

CONCLUSION

The diversity of RT machines and devices can be seen to have developed as the needs for clinical treatment were explored and scientific, engineering, and technical knowledge and expertise grew. This exploration has led to many devices and machines and treatment techniques. In recent years many devices, particularly intra-operative devices with kV beams, have rekindled the availability of this equipment. At the same time, concerns for radiation safety and security have diminished others which use radioactive sources. Overall, however, the absence of alternative treatments, along with the continued efficacy of RT as a treatment method, has maintained and revived the use of many devices and machines.

REFERENCES

[1] Central axis depth dose data for use in radiotherapy. A survey of depth doses and related data measured in water or equivalent media. BJR 1996;(Suppl. 25), British Institute of Radiology. BJR25.

[2] Council Directive 93/47/Euratom. Official J Eur Communities 1997; L180:22–7.

[3] IPEM (Institute of Physics and Engineering in Medicine). Physics aspects of quality control in radiotherapy. IPEM report 81. 2nd ed. York, UK: IPEM; 2018.

[4] Meredith WJ. Radium dosage—the Manchester system. 2nd ed. Baltimore: Williams and Wilkins; 1967.

[5] Perquin B, Dutriex A, Paine CH, Chassagne D, Marinello G, Ash D. The Paris system in interstitial radiation therapy. Acta Radiologica:oncology, radiation, physics, biology 1978;17(1):22–48.

[6] Radiation protection in the design of radiotherapy facilities. IAEA SafetyReport Series No 47. Vienna, Austria: IAEA; 2006.

[7] Potter R, Haie-Meder C, Van Limbergen E, et al. Recommendations from gynaecological (GYN) GEC ESTRO working group (II): concepts and terms in 3D image-based treatment planning in cervix cancer brachytherapy—3D dose volume parameters and aspects of 3D image-based anatomy, radiation physics, radiobiology. Radiother Oncol 2006;78:67–77.

[8] Haie-Meder C, Potter R, Van Limbergen E, et al. Recommendations from Gynaecological (GYN) GEC-ESTRO Working Group (I): concepts and terms in 3D image based 3D treatment planning in cervix cancer brachytherapy with emphasis on MRI assessment of GTV and CTV. Radiother Oncol 2005;74:235–45.

[9] Livingwood JJ, Seaborg GT. Radioactive Isotopes of Cobalt. Phys Rev 1941; 60:913–918.

Beam Production: Megavoltage Accelerators

Andrzej Kacperek, John A. Mills

INTRODUCTION

Radiotherapy (RT) treatment is dominated by the use of megavoltage x-ray beams between 4 and 25 MV. These beams are generated by medical linear accelerators (linacs) which can also deliver electron beams. The advantages of proton beams have been recognised and have led to their wider use with an increasing availability of proton therapy throughout the developed world. Neutron beams are no longer widely used, but advantages of light ion beams are still being explored clinically. There are also development programs to improve the understanding of the absolute dose and the radiobiological effect of both proton and light ion beams.

This chapter deals with megavoltage machines producing x-ray, electron beams, and proton beams. Clinical applications have affected the design, characteristics, and use of these machines.

Particle physics required the development of accelerators to provide high-energy particle beams. This development in part provided the accelerator technology for radiotherapeutic beams and often a beam line was used for radiobiological research work and even clinical treatment. For example, at the large research accelerator facility called TRIUMPH in Vancouver, treatment with pions was used to first explore radiobiological effects on cells and animals followed by clinical treatment for selected patients. This type of arrangement was often the case and there are many examples. However, orientation of the beam to the site of treatment could often be problematic and there was a need for development of dedicated megavoltage accelerators which would enable maximum exploitation of the therapeutic benefits by directing and shaping the RT beams effectively to the target in the patient.

THE MEDICAL LINEAR ACCELERATOR

The workhorse of modern RT is the linac [1,2] which owes its development to the pioneers who worked to produce higher-energy beams than kilovoltage beams upon which teletherapy started. The modern medical linac was born out of the development of megavoltage treatment machines in the 1950s. At this time, betatrons, autotransformers, and Van de Graaff generator designs were used to accelerate electron beams to high energy. However, the elegance of acceleration based upon radiofrequency (RF) electromagnetic waves became universally adopted to provide high-dose-rate megavoltage treatment beams.

The fundamental components remain unchanged, although the performance, construction, and control systems have been developed considerably to take advantage of modern engineering, technology, electronics, and computers. Today, such medical linacs are prolific and provide the vast majority of RT treatments.

LINEAR ACCELERATOR LAYOUT AND COMPONENTS

The major core sections of a linac serve the purpose of producing a high-energy electron beam. These components consist of an electron source, a source of RF electromagnetic waves, and an accelerating waveguide. These core sections can now be found in some custom machines, such as the tomotherapy units, and the principles of operation are identical. In this section, however, the description will be with regard to the isocentric gantry-mounted machines which are now in widespread use throughout the world.

Besides the major core components, a modern medical linac consists of a gantry assembly to direct the beam into the patient and a radiation head which enables beam shaping. For x-ray beams, the target, which is bombarded by the electron beam to produce the x-rays, is contained in the radiation head. Steering and stability of the electron beam require focussing, bending, and steering. This is achieved using magnetic fields generated electrically with inductive coils. High-voltage and high current sources are also needed along with vacuum pumping systems and cooling systems to create a stable machine environment for production of the beam.

Fig. 9.1A illustrates the typical layout of the major components of a linac.

The gun filament assembly produces electrons by raising tungsten to a sufficiently high temperature through electrical heating. There are two types of waveguide: standing waves (see Fig. 9.1C) and travelling waves (see Fig. 9.1B). Although this affects the waveguide structure, both types use electromagnetic waves at an RF of approximately 3 GHz. In the travelling type, the electrons are carried along on an accelerating wave, whereas the standing type uses the electric component of the wave to exert an accelerating force on the electrons.

The source of the radiowaves is either a klystron or a magnetron. The klystron uses a low-power RF signal from a small cavity oscillator. This is applied to a high-power electron stream in the klystron and results in a high-power RF wave. By contrast, the magnetron is a multiple cavity device which produces a high-power RF wave directly. Waveguide sections transport the RF from the magnetron or klystron to the accelerating waveguide section.

Because electrons are charged particles, there is a tendency for an electron beam to disperse as it travels along the accelerating waveguide. Fortunately, this can be countered by using the interactive force which is applied to any charged particle as it passes through a magnetic field. The magnetic fields that are used to counter this dispersion are produced by focussing coils. These coils are wound around the accelerating waveguide and produce a magnetic field flux parallel to the direction of the electron beam.

This interactive force between a magnetic field and the travelling electrons is further used with magnetic fields at right angles to the direction of the electron beam. One of these fields is generated by

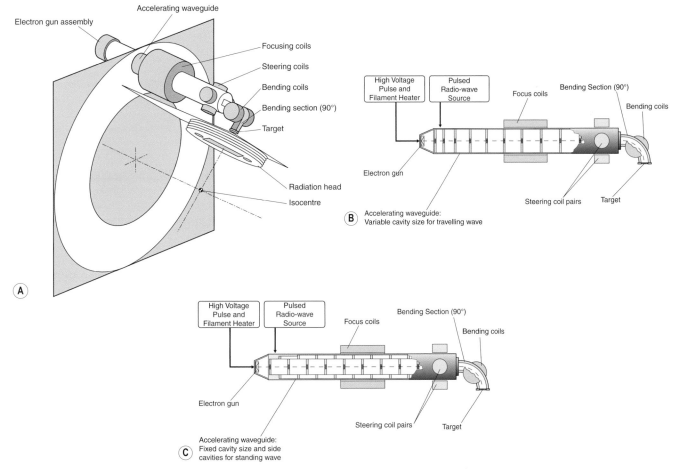

Fig. 9.1 Typical layout of the major components of a medical linear accelerator. (A) General. (B) Travelling waveguide. (C) Standing waveguide.

the bending magnet which bends the electron beam round into a trajectory appropriate for the radiation head. This magnet also plays a crucial role in the selection of beam energy. By altering the strength of the magnetic field, which can be controlled by the electrical current flowing in the bending magnet coil, the appropriate energy selection can be made.

The other use of magnetic fields at right angles to the electron trajectory is to steer the beam into and out of the accelerating waveguide. It is important to maximise the number of electrons that are accelerated and therefore ensuring the most efficient trajectory of the beam along the guide minimises the losses experienced. These magnetic fields are produced by the steering coils and control of the electric current within them can be used to adjust the trajectory for efficiency and correct beam alignment through the radiation head.

Beam production is not an energy-efficient process and there is a lot of energy dissipated within the machine as heat. The stability of beam production relies on the stability of component dimensions, such as, for example, the RF cavities in the waveguide. These can be subject to expansion and contraction with heating. Hence there is a need for a great deal of water cooling on the machine; the target, all the magnetic coils, the accelerating waveguide, the RF source, and large electrical devices such as transformers. Adequate and stable cooling is essential for effective beam production.

The other essential ancillary aspect of the linac is the need for the accelerating waveguide to be under high vacuum. For some machine designs, the waveguide is factory sealed, whereas for others vacuum pumps work continuously to maintain the high vacuum required.

The gantry construction of the standard medical linac is referred to as being isocentric. In effect, this means that all the main axes of rotation concerning the gantry, the radiation head, and the patient couch intersect approximately through the same point in space referred to as the isocentre. This is illustrated in Fig. 9.2. The benefit of this isocentric system is that placement of the patient such that the tumour is centred on the machine isocentre simplifies treatment with the superposition of multiple beams.

X-RAY BEAM

The x-ray beam is produced through bremsstrahlung or braking radiation by bombardment of a tungsten transmission target by the electron beam. The tungsten target is placed directly in the path of the accelerated electron beam, immediately after it exits from the accelerating waveguide and the bending coil section. As shown in Fig. 9.3, this raw x-ray beam is collimated into the useful beam by the primary collimator. The raw beam has a peak intensity in the forward direction (Fig. 9.4). Conventionally, the aim in RT has been to deliver as uniform a dose as possible to the tumour. To achieve this simply from a direct beam, the raw beam is made uniform or flattened using a flattening filter made from steel. The profile of the flattening filter provides the maximum attenuation in the centre and the detailed shape of the filter is specific to the profile of the raw beam which is energy dependent.

Following flattening of the beam, the x-rays pass through an ionisation chamber before going on to field shaping with secondary collimators. The ionisation chamber consists of three sections, with each section covering the full area of the useful beam. The first two sections are the dosimetry channels one and two (Ch1 and Ch2). Ch1 is the primary channel, which provides a signal to terminate the beam after a required dose has been delivered. Ch2 is identical to Ch1 and acts as a safety back-up to guard against excessive overexposure should a fault occur with Ch1. The third section is a segmented chamber, which is used to monitor characteristics of the beam such as uniformity and symmetry. The uniformity refers to the variation of dose across the beam and will be characteristic of the beam energy. The symmetry refers to a tilt in the beam between positions equidistant from the central axis of the beam and is dependent upon the alignment of the electron beam onto the target (Fig. 9.5). These signals can be used to control the operation of the machine. For example, the uniformity signal can be used to control the gun filament electron emission and the symmetry signal can be used to control the steering coil currents.

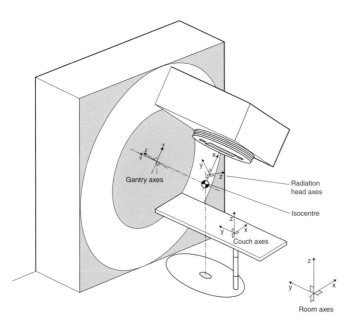

Fig. 9.2 Linear accelerator axes, and gantry, collimator, and couch—per International Electrotechnical Commission (IEC) 1217 convention.

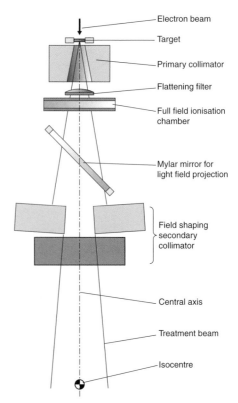

Fig. 9.3 Linear accelerator radiation head.

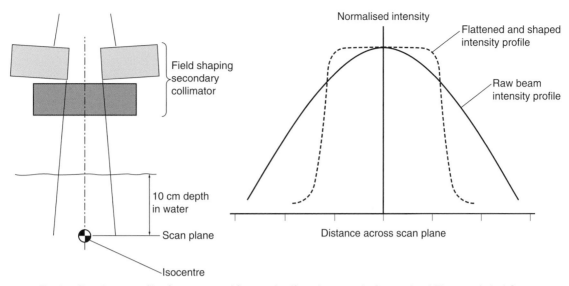

Fig. 9.4 Raw beam profile after target and flattened uniform beam under International Electrotechnical Commission (IEC) conditions.

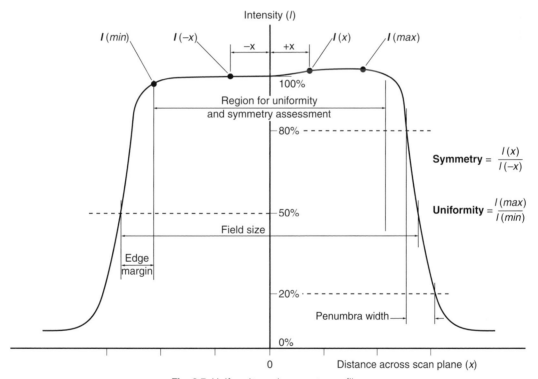

Fig. 9.5 Uniformity and symmetry profiles.

Final beam shaping is done using the substantial secondary collimation system. In early machines these consisted of two sets of jaws which could set rectangular field shapes by movement in orthogonal directions. In modern machines these jaws have been replaced entirely or replaced in part or supplemented by multileaf collimation (MLC) with leaf widths at the isocentre ranging from 4 mm to 10 mm. This has provided the opportunity for simplified conformal shaping of the beam to the target volume as well as the varying of the beam intensity by rapidly changing the beam shape within the overall field and, in some cases, by dynamic control of the MLC while the machine is radiating.

A standard conventional method of varying the intensity of the beam has been the use of metal wedges placed across the beam to modify the uniformity of the beam profile in a controlled manner. This modification of the beam intensity has been found to be extremely useful in obtaining uniform dose distribution within the target. Fig. 9.6 shows the effect which a typical metallic wedge has on the uniform profile. Although in the past these wedges were fitted manually by the operator, they can now be provided in two ways. First, by having a metallic wedge mounted on a motorised platform in the radiation head which can be automatically moved into and out of the radiation beam. The other way is to have one of the secondary collimator jaws move across

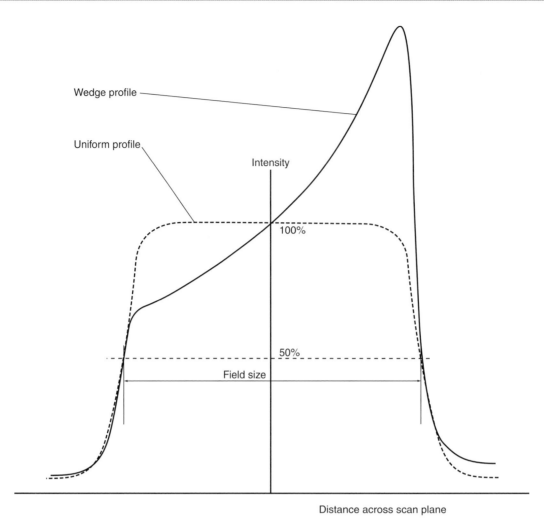

Fig. 9.6 A uniform and wedge beam profile.

the field during radiation. For example, at the start of the radiation, the jaws would be entirely closed with both jaws on the same side of the central axis. As radiation continues, one jaw would open and traverse across to the opposite side of the central axis. The three methods are referred to as fixed wedges, motorised wedges, and dynamic wedges.

ELECTRON BEAM

As well as the x-ray mode of operation, high-energy linacs are also used to deliver electron treatment beams. In this mode of operation, the transmission target is automatically moved out of the beam so x-rays are no longer deliberately produced. As mentioned earlier, x-ray production is not efficient and with the target removed, an electron beam dose rate comparable to that of an x-ray beam can be obtained with approximately 5% to 10% of the electron beam required from the accelerating waveguide for x-ray production. With this significant reduction in beam current the problem of leakage radiation from the accelerating waveguide is significantly reduced. The accelerating waveguide can be set to produce a spectrum of energies with the magnetic field produced by the bending section being used to select the required energy. The bending section thus acts as a spectrometer allowing passage of only the electrons with the required energy into the primary collimator for production of the treatment beam.

The electron beam as it emerges from the window after acceleration and bending has a very narrow width compared with the required treatment field size, and scanning and scattering systems have been developed to provide adequate field coverage. Scanning systems employ electromagnets to steer the electron beam across the treatment field. However, by far the most predominant technique employs a dual scattering system along with an applicator attachment to the radiation head (Fig. 9.7). In a dual scattering system, a primary scatterer is introduced to the electron beam before the primary collimator. A secondary scatterer is substituted for the flattening filter and this may be profiled for the specific electron beam energy which has been selected. These scatterers and the flattening filters are mounted on a carousel which moves them automatically into the beam with the energy selection. Typically, a treatment machine would have two photon beams and five or six electron beams, each with a different energy. Both primary and secondary scatterers are specific to the energy selected. The secondary collimators used for shaping the photon fields are used to set an initial field size for the electron beam as it leaves the radiation head. The electrons are scattered in air and so an applicator is used to produce a sharp edge to the treatment field at the patient. The applicators have open sides and consist of a set of field trimmers which reduce the field down to the required size. The treatment is either with the applicator in contact with the patient or with a small stand-off of typically 5 cm. The practice at any centre depends upon local preference. The electron beam passes through the same ionisation chamber with multiple sections and segments as the x-ray beam. The signals from these are used to monitor and control the performance of the beam and ensure delivery of the correct dose.

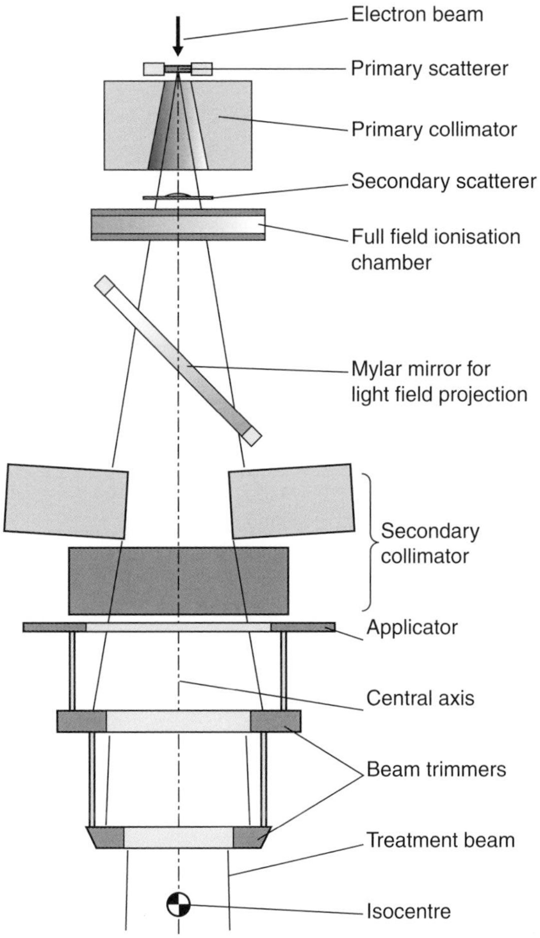
Electron beam
Primary scatterer
Primary collimator
Secondary scatterer
Full field ionisation chamber
Mylar mirror for light field projection
Secondary collimator
Applicator
Central axis
Beam trimmers
Treatment beam
Isocentre

Fig. 9.7 Double scattering foil system with applicator for electron beam production.

LINEAR ACCELERATOR CONTROL SYSTEMS

Effective and safe performance of a linac depends upon two types of control system. The first concerns the operation of the systems within the accelerator, for example, the control and tuning of the magnetron. The second relates to the stability controls on voltage and current supplies. The importance of this second type of control is apparent in considering the use of the bending magnet for energy selection. The current supply system is controlled to ensure a stable current is supplied to the magnet coils and maintain a stable energy. Although this second control system is essential, it is not directly controlled by changes in the radiation beam. One example of a system that is directly controlled by the radiation beam concerns detection of field symmetry using the ionisation chamber in the radiation head. Using the symmetry information, the electron beam is steered using the steering coils to maintain a symmetric field (Fig. 9.8). In this example, an asymmetry in the field is detected by the segments of the ionisation chamber in the radiation head. These signals are electronically or computationally processed to alter the current supplied to the steering magnet coils and restore the symmetry of the field.

Satisfactory beam delivery by a linac relies on the dynamic operation of several such systems. All operate automatically and result in an interplay between the electron emission from the gun, the tuning of the RF source, the steering of the beam, and the stability of all the currents and voltages which ensure the correct focussing and bending of the accelerating electron beam.

NONSTANDARD LINEAR ACCELERATORS

Although the basic waveguide system for the acceleration of electrons has remained the same, this system has been incorporated into different delivery systems and specialised beam delivery systems have been provided to enhance the RT treatment.

Intensity-Modulated Radiotherapy

With the development of MLC beam shaping, the possibility to produce a radiation field made up from multiple shaped fields rapidly was brought about. This enabled intensity-modulated beams to be delivered which could be tailored to the individual requirements of a patient's target and anatomy. The resolution of MLCs have been improved and it is recognised that for standard RT a 3-mm leaf width is ideal. However, modern machines have a minimum width of 5 mm at the isocentre. Intensity-modulated RT (IMRT) has thus become a treatment mode which has found many applications and is likely to eventually become the standard routine method of delivery for all treatments.

CyberKnife

Robotic technological development in industry has led to robots with a very wide ranging directional and positioning ability. Whereas with a standard treatment machine the beams were almost always delivered in the same plane, the dexterity of a robotic arm meant that the beam could be directed in any direction in space with high accuracy and precision. The CyberKnife is a commercial system which exploits this. The linac is mounted at the end of a robotic arm. Small-diameter x-ray beams are produced and the beams are directed into the target, shaping the dose distribution around the target in a conformal manner by combining a multiple of beams. This treatment machine has found applications in the treatment of targets close to critical tissue, such as the spine.

Tomotherapy

The pioneering development of IMRT led to the development of Tomotherapy, a commercial device now widely used. A standard waveguide producing a 6-MV beam was mounted on a computed tomography (CT) scanner gantry so that an IMRT beam could be delivered around and along the patient. The radiation field consisted of a narrow strip across the axis of the machine gantry rotation. A fast MLC device modulated the beam.

Volumetric-Modulated Arc Therapy

The delivery of IMRT was initially based upon multiple static beams and typically for a prostate this would consist of five fields. The success of tomotherapy and the development of the standard linac MLC and the machines control system led to the development of volumetric-modulated arc therapy (VMAT). In this mode, the treatment delivery is executed by modulation of the beam through MLC shaping adjustment as the machine rotates around the patient. The rotation can be a single arc or multiple arcs depending upon the site. The most significant impact of VMAT has been on the treatment delivery time, which was reduced significantly compared with the initial static field technique. The ease of overall treatment delivery with VMAT has led to its use being widely adopted.

Stereotactic Ablative Radiotherapy

Another adaptation of the linac has been stereotactic RT and radiosurgery. It is also referred to as stereotactic ablative radiotherapy (SABR) and stereotactic body RT (SBRT). Although dedicated small field collimators were initially used, micro-MLC and even the higher resolution of standard MLCs are used for the small fields involved. These small

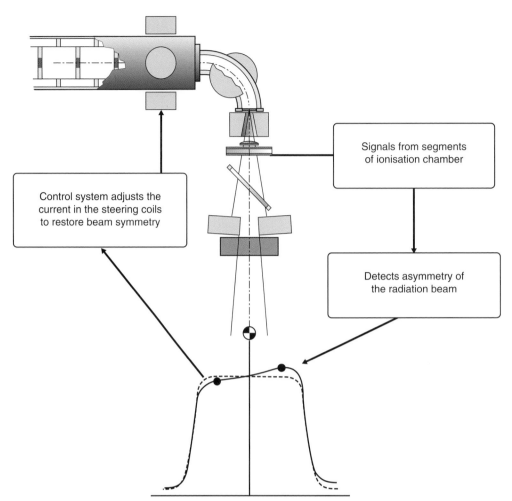

Fig. 9.8 Control system to maintain a symmetric field.

fields are delivered statically or, in arc treatment techniques, with very accurate patient positioning. Stereotactic techniques are used for liver, lung, and cranial tumours and also cranially for arterio-venous malformation.

Flattening Filter-Free Dose Delivery

With the advent and widespread use of IMRT there came a realisation that for the IMRT mode of treatment there was no need to make a treatment field have a uniform dose distribution (see the X-ray beam section above). There were two significant aspects that arose from a flattening filter free (FFF) beam. One was that the dose rate increased considerably, sometimes by a factor of 3. Second, the beam modelling for dose prediction was simpler. Many treatment sites have had FFF-type treatment evaluated and the most useful has been for the SABR method mentioned earlier. In this type of treatment there are advantages in having a high dose rate and delivering the dose quickly to avoid missing or compromising the dose to the target.

PATIENT ALIGNMENT FOR X-RAY AND ELECTRON THERAPY

In both the x-ray and the electron mode of operation, the radiation beams are aligned with the mechanical rotation of the radiation head (Fig. 9.9). The system for patient to beam alignment can be considered to consist of three parts. The first is indicators which are aligned with the axes of the radiation head rotation and hence the radiation beam.

The second is indicators which locate the isocentre of the machine in space. The third has become established now as the final verification of alignment based upon cone beam CT or portal imaging and the registration of patient anatomy with reference images. In combination, the beam alignment to the patient can be achieved and verified. Only the first two systems will be described here and Chapter 10 describes image verification.

There are three main indicators of the radiation beam axis: treatment front pointer, treatment back pointer, and light field cross wires. These are illustrated in Fig. 9.10 and the pointers are attached to the radiation head during the patient setup. The light field cross wires projection is achieved through an optical system in the radiation head. Essentially, this system generates a light source which, by using mirrors, is effectively positioned at the x-ray target. Cross wires are introduced into the light field using a thin transparent sheet and with the light source and the cross wire centre exactly on the radiation head axis of rotation, an optical projection of the axis is produced.

The isocentre is indicated by three optical and mechanical systems. The first uses the treatment front pointer and the tip of the pointer is set to the isocentre (Fig. 9.11). A second indicator is referred to as a distance meter and, effectively, this uses the coincidence between the cross-wire projection and the distance meter projection to determine distances from the x-ray source to the surface of the patient (Fig. 9.12). In the third indicator, the alignment lasers are independent of the machine and consists of room-mounted lasers that through cylindrical lenses project sheets of light through the isocentre,

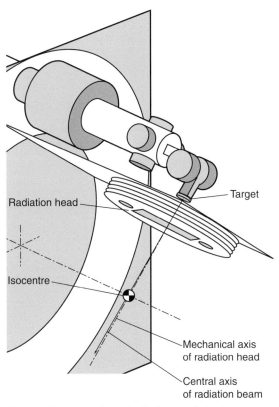

Fig. 9.9 Alignment of mechanical and radiation beam axes.

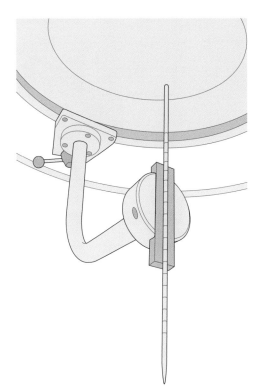

Fig. 9.11 Treatment front pointer for isocentre indication.

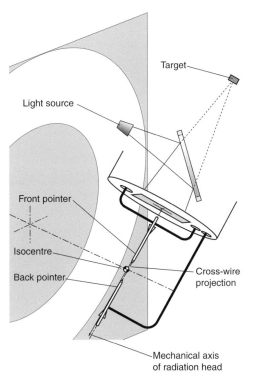

Fig. 9.10 Cross wires and treatment pointers; front and back.

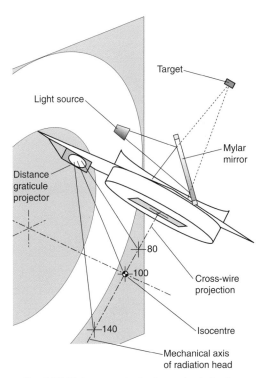

Fig. 9.12 Distance meter for isocentre indication.

providing a set of cartesian coordinate planes with the isocentre at the origin (Fig. 9.13). With the use of surface marks from the planning stages of the patient's treatment preparation, the laser sheets enable the patient to be set up with the isocentre at the appropriate place within the patient.

The mechanical treatment back pointer has now been replaced by a laser system. A laser is mounted on the treatment machine which projects a sheet from the base of the gantry through the isocentre and the axis of gantry rotation. Intersection of the machine-mounted sheet and the wall sheets produces a line coincident with the axis of rotation (Fig. 9.14).

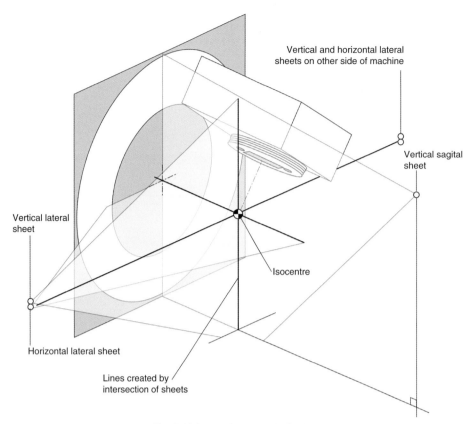

Fig. 9.13 Lasers isocentre indication.

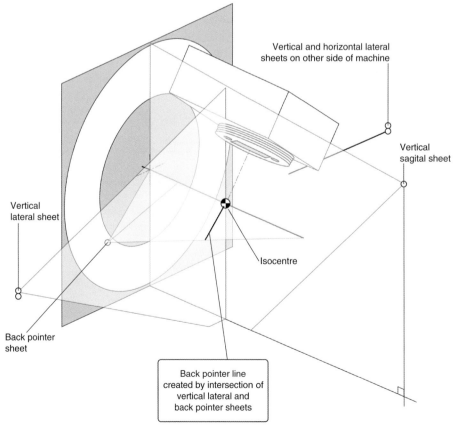

Fig. 9.14 Laser back pointer.

RADIATION SAFETY

Radiation safety is of paramount importance with regard to treatment machines and relates to several aspects of the machine construction and its operation. The legislative requirements and practical means to achieve effective radiation protection are described in Chapter 4. Another significant aspect with regard to radiation protection is the room design described below.

However, besides these aspects, there is a need for protection of the staff and patients by the provision of machine interlocks and shielding. The radiation head itself is constructed with shielding to minimise the radiation leakage outside of the treatment beam. For electron treatment this is also addressed within the applicator design and the diaphragm settings.

Room door and maze barrier interlocks are installed to try and ensure that no accidental irradiation of staff can occur. Besides these, the treatment machines have many interlocked circuits. These interlocks are of two types. The first type is to ensure that the beam is operating within chosen performance limits. An example of such would be the monitor on a linac which ensures that the beam is uniform and symmetric about the central axis. Another would be the monitor of the bending current which ensures that the energy of the beam remains stable and would detect any fault in the electrical circuit that could affect it and hence the energy of the beam. The second type ensures that fitments on the machine are correctly set. An example of this would be the flattening filter for photons and the scattering foil for electrons. Another would be the position or presence of an x-ray target for photons and whether the electron applicator was correctly fitted and agreed with that in the treatment prescription.

One well-established safety system on linacs is the provision of two monitoring ionisation chambers which are completely independent and monitor the entire field. The primary chamber, often referred to as Channel1 (Ch1), is calibrated to deliver a known dose to a reference point from which doses can be calculated and predicted. The other chamber, referred to as Channel2 (Ch2), is a back-up chamber and set so that in the event of a Ch1 failure the difference between the two channels will be detected and the irradiation terminated. Should the difference detection and Ch1 fail completely, Ch2 is set so that it will terminate the treatment having delivered a very small additional dose than that intended by the clinician. There is also a tertiary termination system provided by a timer which should be set so that it would terminate the treatment in the event of both Ch1 and Ch2 termination system failures with only a small additional dose being given to the patient.

ACCEPTANCE, COMMISSIONING AND QUALITY CONTROL

Following supply of a treatment machine, two conditions have to be established. The first is that the equipment supplied meets the specification required by the customer. This involves a formal acceptance of the machine by the customer based upon a demonstration by the supplier that the machine meets the performance and safety specification upon which purchase of the machine was agreed.

It is then essential that the characteristics of the machines beams and the performance of the machine are established by measurement. This commissioning period sets out to provide the data upon which all calculations and dose predictions will be made for a patients treatment. In addition, it provides the baseline set of performance data against which subsequent check or quality control measurements will be made. Besides measuring standard data, such as output factors, depth dose, and tissue phantom ratios, specific data for beam-dose algorithms in the computer treatment planning systems along with verification data for the dose predictions are gathered and used for validation. In the case of imaging and any other ancillary equipment relevant commissioning measurements should also be devised.

Quality control (see Chapter 13) of the equipment is required to ensure subsequent satisfactory operation. It is required routinely and on a periodic basis to demonstrate the continued satisfactory operation of the machine. It is required following machine breakdown and repairs to ensure that the operation has been returned to a satisfactory level and, lastly, it is required following adjustments to the running of the machine to ensure again that the satisfactory operation of the machine has been maintained.

Formal acceptance, the period of commissioning and quality control had become an established practice, and is now recognised in statutory legislation: Euratom 97 and IRMER 2000 [3,4].

TREATMENT ROOM DESIGN FOR X-RAY AND ELECTRON PROTECTION

The details of the treatment room design are very dependent upon the treatment machine and there are two main aspects to consider. The first concerns radiation safety and the protection of personnel[5], whereas the second concerns the ergonomics of the room. The layout of the room is important to ensure efficient treatment, patient access, as well as machine maintenance.

For radiation protection, many of the features employed and the materials used can also be related to the actual location of the room, either its adjacencies to public areas or whether it is a new room or a re-used and modified room. Although there can be many aspects to detailed room design, there are general features that all room designs use to exploit very fundamental characteristics of radiation.

The purpose of shielding is to protect members of the public and workers associated with the treatment centre, particularly those who will spend a considerable portion of their working day in the vicinity of the room and are involved with patient treatment.

These general features concern first, the direction of the primary beam and providing sufficient shielding to attenuate the direct beam. Also with regard to beam direction, the position of room access and the access of penetrations into the room for services such as water and electrical supply, cabling, and ventilation should be placed to avoid the primary beam irradiation. Away from the primary shielding, the room walls should be adequate for scattered radiation.

The next feature concerns room access which may be direct or using maze. Here there are considerations such as staff access and patient's apprehension of being left alone in a room. Direct access requires a substantial shielding door to be fitted which will be motorised, extend the time for entry, and require contingency for access in the event of motor failure. For a maze entrance, three aspects are of significance: cross-sectional area, distance along the maze, and bends in the maze. The area concerns the cross section at the maze entrance in the room, in effect the amount of scattered radiation in the room which enters into the maze. The smaller this can be made consistent with patient access including a bed, the less radiation will enter the maze. Reduction of the cross-sectional area of the maze at the room by use of a lintel can make a substantial contribution to protection. Second, the length of the maze will increase the distance between entrance and exit and provide a dose reduction in line with the inverse square relationship. Lastly and significantly, the scatter from a right-angled bend within a maze can make a very significant contribution to reducing the dose which can be measured at the end of the maze outside the room.

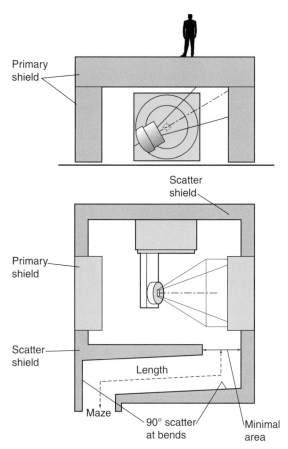

Fig. 9.15 Major features of radiation protection for a linear accelerator treatment room.

neutron flux. Second, care should be taken to avoid metal content in the construction materials including the concrete aggregate, as gamma activation can occur trading a neutron problem for a photon problem. This is also the case for wood lining which was considered appropriate in the past. Lastly, specialised lining, including commercial lining substances for the maze and other penetrations, can be used to reduce significantly the problem to well below radiation protections limits.

For more details on protection requirements, legislation, and the choice of materials, see Chapter 4.

Besides safety, the layout within a room for equipment and storage should be given consideration. Adequate storage will ensure that the treatment machine accessories such as applicators and specific patient devices such as immobilisation shells can be stored properly. This will help to avoid damage which may compromise treatment because of the incorrect operation of the equipment, for example, electron applicators or treatment pointers. It also avoids treatment delays by having equipment readily available and avoiding repair of damaged devices. Also worth considering at the room design stage are the layout of the room, the access to the room and the treatment control terminals, visibility of information screens, and the location of lasers. Furthermore, hand controls for manoeuvring the machine should be accessible and readily available to avoid damage and enhance the ease of treatment. The distance and access from the treatment control area into the room is important to maximise throughput and ease workload. In addition to patient and treatment staff considerations, it is important to facilitate speedy access to the machine for repairs. This will reduce downtime by enabling effective equipment, such as hoists to be used easily, and ensuring adequate clearance is available for the removal and fitting of components. Lastly, adequate lighting and dimming controls will ease patient setup and again assist with increasing patient throughput and easing workload. Similarly, clear and controllable CCTV (closed-circuit television) is essential.

SPECIAL TECHNIQUES WITH LINEAR ACCELERATORS

Although linacs have been designed to deliver beams which will superimpose on each other within the patient in an effective manner, they have also been adapted to fulfil some other treatment requirements.

One of the major adaptations has been to provide total-body irradiation (TBI) treatment with x-rays and total skin electron (TSE) treatment. For both these types of treatment the limitation of the accelerator is its field size. However, by treating patients at greatly extended distance of up to 4 m, full body coverage has been achieved for megavoltage TBI (Fig. 9.16).

In Fig. 9.15, a typical megavoltage medical linac room layout is shown with the aforementioned features indicated for clarity.

For high-energy photon beams, neutron production because of a photon–neutron interaction in the nucleus needs to be considered. This interaction occurs at megavoltage photon energies but is nominally considered a problem at 10 MV and above. It occurs in, for example, the collimation system on the machine. The aspects described earlier are not readily applicable and expert advice needs to be sought. Nevertheless, despite the problems which neutrons bring, there are readily available solutions which enable safe room design with direct and maze access, even up to 25 MV. Several aspects concerning neutrons are worthwhile mentioning. First, sharp corners in the rooms aid in reduction of the

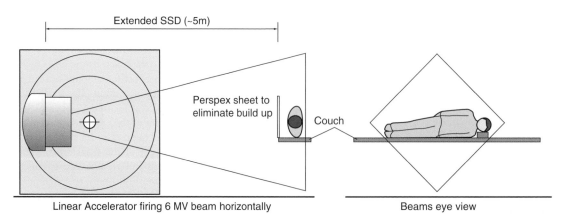

Fig. 9.16 Linear accelerator for total-body irradiation.

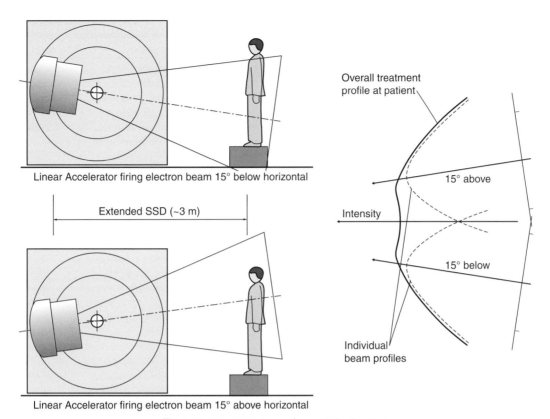

Linear Accelerator firing electron beam 15° below horizontal

Extended SSD (~3 m)

Linear Accelerator firing electron beam 15° above horizontal

Fig. 9.17 Linear accelerator for total sin electrons.

Likewise, techniques to provide electron fields large enough to cover the entire patient have been devised for TSE. Fig. 9.17 shows the well-acknowledged Stanford technique; however, there are other techniques involving gantry rotation and patient movement. For these extended source-to-patient TSE treatment distances, high dose rates can be specially generated by the linac to reduce treatment time.

THE DEVELOPMENT OF CLINICAL PROTON AND HEAVIER CHARGED PARTICLE ACCELERATORS

Treatments using heavier charged particle beams, particularly protons, have now moved from decades of development in research centres to being accepted as a formidable tool in mainstream RT. Despite the considerable improvements in x-ray treatments in precision, conformal quality, and speed, proton therapy beams and carbon particle therapy are addressing lesions that are both radiation resistant and positioned adjacent to critical organs. The much reduced level of secondary integral dose makes this form of therapy of particular interest in paediatric treatments. Commercial and technical developments have helped in producing accelerators of high reliability, compact size, and more economic price. The quality of treatments has been further improved by the advantages of the latest developments in image verification and patient positioning. However, the heavier mass and energy of therapy protons require the use of large, heavy gantries to support powerful bending and focussing magnets, and beam delivery head. Equally demanding is a gantry rigidity that must offer mechanical isocentre reproducibility no different from that found on x-ray linac machines.

It is estimated that the number of patients who could benefit from proton therapy varies from 2% (United Kingdom) to 12% (Sweden) of those currently receiving x-ray RT. This would represent a substantial

patient throughput and stimulates the present-day expansion for this radiation modality.

The first patient proton beam treatment (PBT) facilities were necessarily based in research centres, particularly in the United States (Berkeley 1954; Harvard 1961) and Sweden (Uppsala 1957). This was followed by their establishment in other countries, for example, in Russia (JINR 1967; ITEP 1969) and Japan (the National Institute of Radiological Sciences 1979; Tsukuba 1983) [6–8].

The first hospital-based PBT centre commenced treatment in 1989 at Clatterbridge in the United Kingdom, albeit only with an energy suitable for treating ocular tumours. The first purpose-built high-energy proton centre started treating patients in 1990, at the Medical Centre at Loma Linda in California. This pioneering project used a synchrotron to provide proton beams, with selected energies, being directed to three large gantries, as well as a fixed horizontal beam [9].

The majority of PBT centres are now based in clinical environments rather than research centres, and are now considered a part of mainstream RT. There are over 75 PBT centres in operation worldwide in 2018, with 29 in North America alone. Eleven other centres provide carbon beam therapy alone or with PBT. The increase in patient treatments is shown in Table 9.1.

TABLE 9.1	**Annual patients treated with PBT world-wide**	
Year	All treatments	Ocular treatments
2015	14,300	1650
2016	17,500	1800
2017	20,350	1820

(Particle Therapy Co-operative Group (PTOG), M Jermann PSI, CH, https://www.ptcog.ch)

In fact, 170,250 patients were treated with PBT by the end of 2017, of which 26,000 received ocular treatments. In addition, another 28,600 patients were treated with carbon beams. Ocular treatments with a low-energy proton beam commenced in 1975 [10] and although the basic technique has changed very little in over four decades, it has improved by adoption of digital imaging for diagnosis and verification. This remains the most successful PBT treatment in terms of local tumour control, with 22 centres performing this treatment modality. Most treatments are of four or five high-dose fractions [10,11] with lower-energy cyclotrons providing particularly sharp beam penumbra and distal fall-off.

PARTICLE ACCELERATOR LAYOUT AND COMPONENTS

The majority of PBT beams are produced with circular particle accelerators. The development of the cyclotron was prompted by the need to produce higher proton energies as a tool in nuclear physics experiments. It was necessary to overcome the limitations of the drift-tube linac of Wideröe, the Van de Graaf generator, and the Cockcroft–Walton accelerator tube. Ernest Lawrence extended the Wideröe concept of accelerating particles by small incremental energy steps, but in a circular path maintained by a strong magnetic field, whereby the particles would gain energy across the same electrical potential. In 1931, after earlier attempts, the group of Ernest Lawrence built an 11-in. (approximately 280-mm) diameter circular accelerator which produced protons of over 1 MeV albeit at very low currents. Within seven years, a larger 60-in. (1525-mm) version was being used to produce medical radioisotopes and supply deuterons for neutron therapy. The cyclotron concept of accelerating charged particle beams, guided in circular orbits by a magnetic field, with incremental increases in energy across electrodes was established.

Basic Components of a Cyclotron

The main components of a cyclotron are listed in Table 9.2.

Basic Theory of Classic Cyclotron Operation

Positive ions, in this case protons, are accelerated by incremental amounts across an alternating potential, as shown in Fig. 9.18. The protons take a circular path in a plane that lies at right angles to a uniform magnetic field which causes the proton to travel in a circular path. The circular path can be described by considering the balance between the rotational centripetal force and the magnetic Lorentz force which acts normal to the magnetic field and the direction of motion (inset in Fig. 9.19). It can be shown that the radius of the ion orbit will increase with the increasing momentum of the ion (Fig. 9.20). However, the period of the ion orbit is independent of ion momentum and of the orbital radius. Thus although the ion energy and path length increase for each orbit, the ion will arrive at the accelerating gap at the correct time to receive further increment of energy from the alternating potential. This is called *cyclotron resonance*. The beam will have a finite energy spread, so faster charged particles will arrive earlier at the gap and will experience reduced acceleration or *phase slip*; and slower particles which arrive later at the gap will experience smaller or no acceleration and may be lost to the beam; this is termed *phase stability*. This type of circular accelerator is termed as *isochronous* because the ions and the RF accelerating potential remain in phase. Thus the repeated traversing of the dee gap by the circulating proton beam incrementally increases the beam energy by the RF potential (V_{dee}) on the dee which is typically 30 kV to 100 kV. This enables high energies to be achieved on

Component	Function	Details
Ion source	To provide a source of charged particles by ionising a neutral gas (usually hydrogen).	Types: PIG, ECR, duoplasmatron, or microwave
RF power source	To provide an alternating potential to the dee electrodes.	30–50kV; 20–50 MHz
Main magnet	To provide a high magnetic field.	Resistive or super-conducting
Vacuum tank	This volume includes the dee electrodes and the accelerating beam, and deflector assembly.	Main accelerating chamber
Dee electrodes	Provide an acceleration gap between the two electrodes.	The hollow dee-shaped conductors provide a field-free cavity between accelerations.
Electrostatic deflector	A channel, at negative potential, to provide an exit from the cyclotron tank into a beam pipe.	Other types of deflector are used in synchrotrons.
Vacuum pumps	high vacuum required (10^{-5}–10^{-7} mbar) to avoid beam losses.	Oil diffusion pumps or ion getter pumps; turbo-molecular pumps are not used due to vulnerability of stray magnetic fields.
Cooling system	Water-cooling to dissipate heating of magnets, RF, all magnet power supplies.	Ensure that water is of correct pH to avoid corrosion in copper coils.

ECR, Electron cyclotron resonance; *mbar*, megabar; *PIG*, Penning ionisation gauge; *RF*, radio frequency.

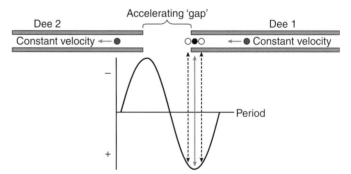

Fig. 9.18 Phase stability of ions in a cyclotron. The dees are viewed edge-on.

exiting the cyclotron after multiple passes across the dees. For example, if the dee potential was sufficient to increase the proton energy by 200 keV per orbit, a final beam energy of 240 MeV would be achieved in 1200 proton orbits. An overview of the construction and path of the accelerating proton is shown in Fig. 9.19.

The RF potential across the dees acts as a focussing electrostatic lens [12] which helps maintain the proton beam in the central plane. However, this effect is less with increased proton energies, and the main focussing is provided by the main magnetic field. Clearly, the design of

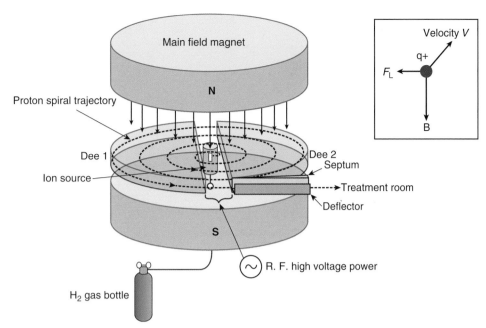

Fig. 9.19 Proton path in a constant magnetic field.

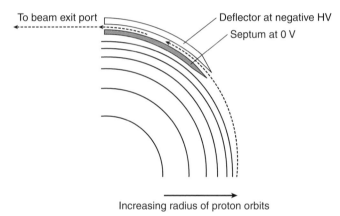

Fig. 9.20 Simplified quarter plan view of proton orbits and conventional electrostatic deflector.

cyclotrons requires stable RF frequency and power, and precise and constant magnetic fields for optimal performance.

The ability of a magnet to bend a charged particle beam is expressed as magnetic rigidity and can be expressed numerically in terms of the magnetic field intensity B, the bending radius, the ion beam momentum, and the charge on the ion. This parameter is useful when considering the bending required for ions of different mass, charge, and energy in switching magnets, scanning beam magnets, and accelerators.

The limitations of the classic design of the Lawrence cyclotron became apparent when progressing to higher particle energies and beam currents. Relativistic effects begin to become significant when increasing the proton energies beyond the 30-MeV range because of an increase in proton mass. The mass will increase by 6% at 60 MeV and by 27% at 250 MeV. The increase in ion mass will reduce proton velocity and orbit period, thereby causing the particles to become gradually out of step with the RF accelerating potential and thus loose isochronicity. The classic cyclotron uses a uniform magnetic main field across the tank, but the weakening of the field at the edge of the magnetic poles creates a vertical focussing component which maintains the beam in the central plane and improves beam output. This is called *weak focusing*. However, the increase in proton energy with the use of wider pole diameters to encompass the increasing orbit radius causes difficulty in the radial and axial focussing which is required to maintain the ion beam in a medial plane, leading to significant loss of beam current. The classic cyclotron design is now limited mainly to low-energy (<30 MeV) proton or other ion beams with high currents for production of radioisotopes for medical applications.

Ion Source Operation

Protons or other light ion charged particles are produced in an ion source, where for example for protons, hydrogen gas is ionised, by various means, to create a localised plasma of protons and electrons. This is illustrated by a simplified image in the case of a cold-cathode Penning ionisation gauge (PIG) ion source (Fig. 9.21). Electrons are emitted from the two opposing cathode surfaces by a strong electric field, and as they oscillate between the cathodes, they ionise the hydrogen gas. The ionisation is intensified by the main magnetic field of the cyclotron, and with the heating of the electrodes, produces a self-sustaining plasma. The protons are then introduced into the cyclotron tank by diffusion through a chimney slit and by attraction from a puller electrode, which is at the same potential as the dee RF power. At this point the protons come under the influence of the RF accelerating potential of dees and of the main cyclotron magnetic field. The earliest ion source functioned by the ionisation of hydrogen gas by energetic electrons from a hot tungsten filament. Because of the high availability requirements in modern clinical ion therapy facilities, ion sources are required to provide more intense currents, reliability, and ease of maintenance. Types of ion sources which create ion plasmas, such as PIG, duo-plasmatron, electron cyclotron resonance (ECR), and microwave plasma, are described in detail elsewhere [13,14]. Ion sources are required to contain intense plasma produced with high power input [alternating current (AC), direct current (DC), RF, or microwave] usually with a strong magnetic field. The gas flow must be sufficient to maintain the plasma but not overload the main tank

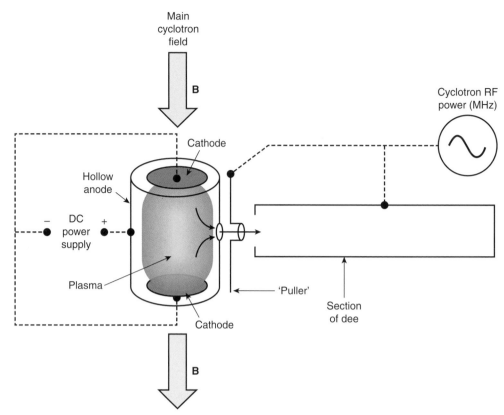

Fig. 9.21 Simplified operation of a Penning ionisation gauge ion source.

vacuum system. The ECR and microwave-driven ion sources are considered to deliver reliably high currents with considerably lower maintenance. However, experimental clinical centres delivering different particle beams may require separate ion sources because of quite different operating conditions.

Characteristics and Limitations for Therapy

Clinical therapy requires an accelerator to produce a maximum particle energy to achieve a range of prescribed proton dose penetration depths. A sufficient beam current should be available to deliver clinical dose fractions in minutes. This requirement refers to accelerators with continuous beams; it is noted that many modern clinical machines are configured to produce narrow pencil beams for spot-scanning or raster beams. These necessitate the production of necessarily short but high dose-rate pulses; thus mean current and maximum currents have to be specified. The maximum beam current must take into account beam losses along long beam tubes and gantry systems, as well as energy selection systems (ESSs) which function by energy absorption.

Synchrocyclotrons

This type of circular accelerator was developed to increase the beam energy of the proton beams, and additionally to reduce the size of the diameter of the main magnet. The limitations of the classic cyclotron design were loss of accelerating phase with increasing proton energy because of a weakening magnetic field with orbit radius and reduction in proton velocity because of relativistic increase in proton mass.

The synchrocyclotron incorporated a reducing RF to match the reduction in the orbit period. Thus the increasingly energetic protons would remain in-phase until extraction at the edge of the main field. In earlier designs this was performed by a rotating-vane condenser which functions at a duty cycle of the order of several hundred cycles. The

frequency variation of the RF power from f_{intial} to f_{final} is approximately 30%. An additional feature which reduces beam losses is where the accelerating phase occurs at a voltage which is offset from the maximum voltage. Thus later arriving protons will receive an additional boost in acceleration whilst those more energetic protons arriving at the gap earlier will receive reduced accelerating potential. This type of synchronisation can be seen as a self-correcting feedback loop and is more tolerant of RF and magnetic field variations. Although beam losses are reduced during orbits, the varying phase synchronisation means that bunches of protons are produced which match the varying RF frequency, as protons which are out-of-phase will be lost to the beam. Overall, synchrocyclotrons will produce a significantly reduced beam current of less than 1% compared with the continuous beam current from a classical cyclotron. This type of circular accelerator has been used in passive-scattered beam mode, but it also lends itself for spot scanning. The pulse frequency, with suitable pulse duration, of the order of 1 Hz, can be programmed to complete the required dose spots of individual energy layers, accompanied by fast mechanical energy degraders to decrease the depth of the beam scan as shown in Fig. 9.22. Several commercial PBT synchrocyclotrons such as the Proteus S2C2 and Mevion Hyperscan 250i are used in single-room treatment configurations (Table 9.3). These machines benefit from the use of powerful superconducting main field magnets to reduce size and weight; the latter can be related approximately to the magnetic field by $1/B^3$ [15]. Thus relatively small increases in magnetic field can improve the compactness of cyclotron accelerators.

Azimuthal Vertical Focussing or Isochronous Cyclotrons

This was an early concept proposed by Thomas in 1938. The classical cyclotron accelerator used weak vertical focussing as a result of the reduction of the main field with orbit radius to maintain the beam stability.

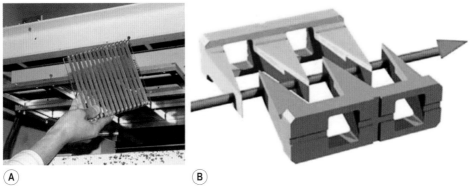

Fig. 9.22 (A) Static ridge energy modulator (National Institute of Radiological Sciences, Japan). (B) Fast-moving carbon multiwedge degrader as part of energy selection system (ESS) used at Paul Scherrer Institute (PSI). *Red arrow* indicates beam direction. (Courtesy PSI, Villigen.)

TABLE 9.3 Comparison of compact accelerators with single-room systems

Vendor	Model	Machine Type	Proton energy (max.)	Weight/ size	Magnetic field (Tesla)	Dose-rate	Field (cm × cm)	Beam delivery options
MEVION	S250 (mounted on gantry) (Room footprint)	Synchro-cyclotron (500 Hz)	250 MeV	22 T; 1.8 m (gantry 80T)	8-10 T; superconducting (Nb_3Sn)	2–0.4 Gy.min^{-1}	20 × 20	Passive beam; scanning (Hyperscan© option)
IBA	S2C2 ProteusOne (centre footprint = 395m^2)	Synchro-cyclotron (1 kHz; 1 μS pulse)	230 MeV	50T; 2.5 m	5.7–5.0 T; superconducting (NbTi);	2 Gy	24 × 20	Pencil beam scanning
VARIAN	ProBeam Compact© (Superconducting); Centre footprint 260m^2	Cyclotron	230 MeV (4 cm–30 cm)	90T	1.4 T (max.); NbTi	>2 Gy.L^{-1}. min^{-1}	30 × 40	ProScan (IMPT)
HITACHI (Hokkaido)	Compact synchrotron (machine footprint (27 m^2)	Synchrotron (slow extraction)	70–220 MeV	N/A; (mean 5.1 m diameter)	N/A			Spot-scanning and passive-scattered.

To design an increase in the final proton energy, or design a smaller cyclotron pole diameter, it is necessary to increase the magnetic field with radius to compensate for the relativistic mass increase of the protons and maintain synchronicity with the dee gap RF. However, this results in vertical defocussing with increasing orbit radius, and thus loss of beam intensity. The solution was to apply strong vertical focussing by means of a stepped variation of the main magnetic field intensity along the proton orbit or azimuthal direction. This is produced by alternate stronger and weak fields by wedge-shaped sectors machined within the pole face as shown in Fig. 9.23. These are known as hills and valleys, respectively, because of the stepped changes of the pole gap. The sharp change of field at the hill and valley interface causes a deviation in orbit radius from a circular path, depending on whether a hill or valley sector is being traversed. The proton path is no longer perpendicular to the field change—this fact causes vertical focussing and defocussing. The overall effect is strong vertical focussing. Thus isochronicity is maintained with the increasing main field, B, with proton orbit and with much reduced beam losses. At higher energies, greater than 30 MeV, the wedge-shaped sectors are modified to produce swirl-shaped sectors which greatly enhance the strong vertical focussing. Most modern therapy cyclotrons are of this design which is known as azimuthal vertical focussing (AVF). The Varian ProBeam and IBA Proteus C230 are of this type and Fig. 9.24 shows the curved dees and pole gap swirls of a high-energy AVF cyclotron.

Synchrotrons

This type of circular accelerator was developed at the same time as the synchrocyclotron in the late 1940s, to increase the final energy of the accelerated protons and heavier ions. The concept lies in maintaining an ion beam path circumference of fixed radius, where individual dipole magnets guide the beam in a circular path. Particles are preaccelerated to low energies of say 5 MeV to 8 MeV by means of a radiofrequency quadrupole (RFQ) and linac, before injection into the synchrotron ring. Particle energy increase is provided by an RF accelerator cavity as shown in Fig. 9.25, with an RF deflector or kicker to extract the required amount of beam and at the requested energy. Thus low-energy protons or ions have their energy increased by simultaneously ramping both the frequency of the RF cavity gap and the magnetic field of the individual dipole magnets. The configuration can be considered figuratively as dividing the single pole face of a cyclotron main magnet into individual magnets, as equal slices of a cake. Clearly, if more magnets are employed, then each dipole magnet would have a lesser beam bending or magnetic strength requirement. Thus the final design circumference is dependent on the magnet strength of the bending dipoles, required final energy, and particle types.

As in the case of synchrocyclotrons, the beam is bunched rather than continuous. As the low-energy ions are introduced into the synchrotron ring, an increase in dipole magnet field strength is

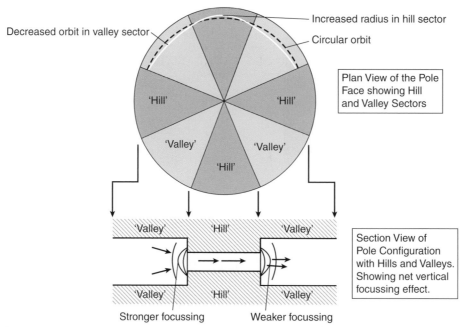

Fig. 9.23 Focussing effect of dees acting as electrostatic lens, to maintain beam on central plane.

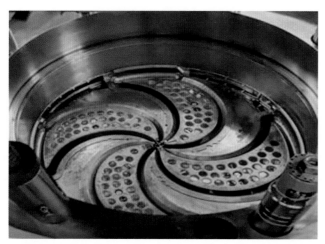

Fig. 9.24 Example of swirl-shaped wedged sectors (Courtesy NYPC, Varian ProBeam).

synchronised with the increasing RF accelerating field. After the required particle energy is attained, the steering and accelerating field strengths are maintained constant for durations of seconds during which time the beam is extracted by an electrostatic kicker [16,17]. This beam is of sufficient intensity and duration to complete a layer of spot scanning at a particular proton energy corresponding to the required depth. The beam is then decelerated by decrease in the accelerating and steering fields. If all the spots in the required depth slice have been completed, the following proton bunch may be of a reduced energy, E_2, to spot-scan the next shallower depth. The average beam intensity is much reduced compared with that from a cyclotron, but the extraction process is highly efficient (typically >90%). In addition, modern clinical synchrotrons are designed with quite fine energy selection which can move penetration by 1-mm steps. This avoids the significant beam losses of fixed energy accelerators which use energy degradation to affect depth changes. For both passive-scattered and pencil scanning beam modalities these can be in excess of 95%. The requirement of fast changing magnetic fields for energetic ions necessitates these magnets to be resistive with iron cores. The footprint of synchrotrons is necessarily large to accommodate the dipole bending magnets if smaller superconducting magnets cannot be used. The greater the number of magnets, the smaller the magnetic strength required of each dipole. In addition, synchrotrons can accommodate the acceleration of heavier ions of higher magnetic rigidity like carbon and oxygen as well as protons.

For a clinical carbon and proton facility the footprint is larger than other circular accelerators depending on whether heavier ion therapy was intended and if superconducting dipole magnets were used. The bending magnet requirements of a carbon therapy gantry are challenging, as the magnetic rigidity is approximately three times that required with a proton beam for a similar penetration of 30 cm. The HIT (Heidelberg Ion Therapy Centre) carbon therapy gantry is 22 m in length and 13 m in height. The weight is approximately 600 t, which is approximately four times the weight of proton beam gantries. Rotating X-ray linacs may weigh between 1 to 2 t. A rotational deviation of the isocentre of less than 1 mm is achieved despite this mass and size. The increasing use of superconducting magnets with more compact designs will reduce significantly the footprint of the gantries and accelerator rings.

PASSIVE-SCATTERED BEAMS AND PENCIL BEAM SCANNING BEAMS

The advantage of proton therapy lies in the possibility of delivering a three-dimensional dose distribution which is both uniform over the treatment volume and highly conformal to the outlined tumour shape. This exploits the sharp proton beam penumbrae, particularly at shallower depths, and the rapid distal fall-off because of the Bragg peak phenomenon. The incident beam area can be shaped to the tumour outline at a particular depth, and the beam penetration can be conformed to the posterior edge of the treatment volume and uniformly spread across the target—see the spread-out Bragg peak (SOBP; Fig. 9.26). The delivery techniques with proton beams to the patient can be grouped in a simplified manner into two types:

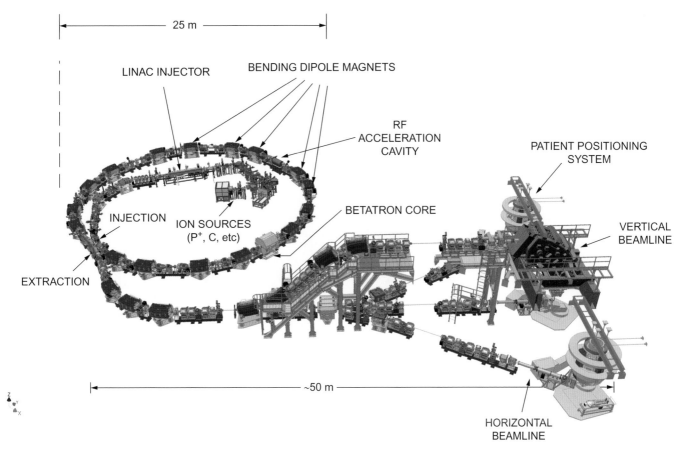

Fig. 9.25 Schematic plan view of clinical synchrotron based loosely on Hitachi and Siemens configurations (not to scale). The beam transport to treatment rooms is a notional disposition, but similar to the HIT, CNAO, and MedAustron facilities.

- passive-scattered beams, with energy modulation and collimation
- pencil beam scanning with narrow monoenergetic beamlets

The optimisation of both delivery methods requires consideration of the type of accelerator producing the proton beam and in particular its pulse structure. Early developments in proton therapy used the passive-scattering technique to produce large and uniform treatment fields, particularly with synchrocyclotrons. Several possible configurations of passive scattering are available. These are analogous to those found in linear accelerators producing x-ray and electron beams, and may consist of one or two high-Z metal foils, with central stoppers, placed upstream of the patient nozzle and normal to the beam. These serve to scatter the raw beam to form an approximate Gaussian distribution which broadens along the beam direction, as shown in Fig. 9.27. This creates a clinically satisfactory homogeneous central region, which is then collimated at various stages along the beam line by antiscatter diaphragms and the treatment nozzle. The selected scatter-foil configuration depends on the maximum field size required, the amount of beam energy and beam current losses that can be accepted, the uniformity of dose and beam energy over the beam aperture, consideration of the activation of beamline components and production of secondary neutrons, and the appropriate shielding and radioprotection issues. Single or double-scattering, with or without central stopper, or contoured double-scattering is selected according to the aforementioned criteria, and has been used in all types of circular accelerators, and on fixed horizontal beam lines and rotating gantries [6,17,18]. Generally, the thinner double-scattering foil combinations have much greater beam and energy efficiency than single thicker foils.

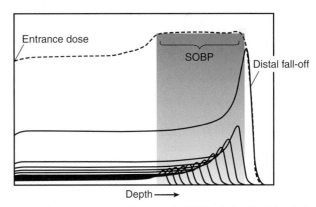

Fig. 9.26 Typical spread-out Bragg peak (SOBP; *dashed line*) depth dose for a high-energy proton beam, showing the component Bragg peaks (*solid lines*). The SOBP region covers the target volume and margins.

Passive-scattered beams require proton beam energy selection for maximum prescribed treatment range, and a method of modulating, or scanning, the pristine Bragg peak in depth, to produce a uniform dose over the target volume with the SOBP. The component Bragg peaks are produced by a variable energy absorber shown in Fig. 9.27. This is essentially a rotating wheel with precisely stepped thicknesses of plastic or metal, which intercepts the proton beam upstream. Various examples are shown in Fig. 9.28.

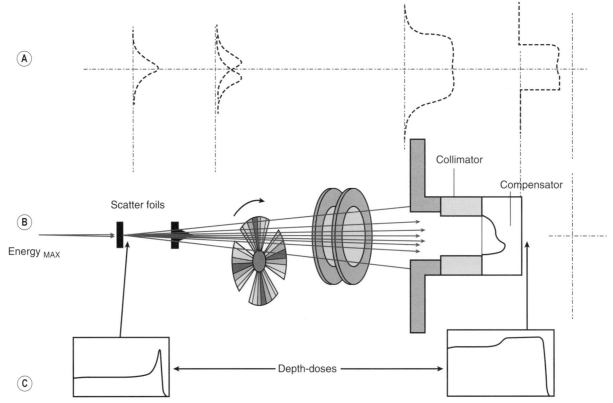

Fig. 9.27 Schematic of proton beam modulation and shaping.

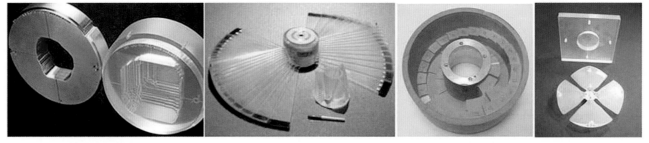

Fig. 9.28 Examples of proton beam modulators and beam shaping (Courtesy ACC, HCL, IBA, CCC).

The time structure of the accelerator beam needs to be considered when employing rotating modulators. The short pulses and kilohertz range of duty cycle of synchrocyclotrons require the rotation speed to be either much faster or slower than the beam pulse frequency to ensure even sampling of beam energies. This poses little problem with the essentially DC beam current from cyclotrons because of the high megahertz range of RF on the dees and the slow-extraction synchrotron pulses, which are of the order of the order of seconds. This problem is avoided at the National Institute of Radiological Sciences for example, by use of a static modulator called a ridge filter (fig. 9.22), due its triangular wedge-shaped absorber strips. The wedge angle and maximum thickness define the extent of the SOBP.

Dose conformity of the lateral field is achieved by patient-specific collimators, which are machined to the required shape by CNC milling machines from treatment planning data (see Fig. 9.28). Collimators for proton therapy were usually manufactured with brass 350. However, the low melting point metal compound Cerrobend has been used, which could be moulded to the required aperture shape and thickness,

allowing reusability and economic use of the material. Multileaf collimators in passive-scattered beam lines were not developed because of the required weight, control complexity, and the coarseness of the leaf thicknesses which would not match the precision of a machined brass aperture. However, multileaf collimators are being employed in pencil beam scanning systems to improve lateral penumbrae, particularly at lower energies.

Patient-specific compensators, used in conjunction with brass apertures for proton therapy treatments, are constructed to contour the proton field to the posterior edge of the target volume. These are machined from either PMMA or blue wax. Like the apertures, the process requires the use of precision milling machines. Several sets of aperture and compensator would be required for each treatment field. A disadvantage is that the compensators cause full dose proximal to the tumour edges [6,18].

Cyclotrons and synchrocyclotrons produce a single maximum energy at extraction. The prescribed treatment energy is thus obtained by reducing the primary energy using an ESS, which is simply an energy absorber with either fixed or adjustable thickness. This can be situated after beam extraction in multigantry facilities, or on individual gantries. This is usually coupled with beam analysis devices which are basically slits, to reduce downstream beam scatter and energy spread. However, the ESS and analyser are a source of scattering of the proton beam, leading to significant instantaneous neutron and gamma-ray dose rates and high induced radioactivity in beam line components. This requires design of appropriate neutron and gamma-ray shielding compatible with radiation protection limits.

Rapid developments in beam control technology have enabled pencil beam scanning with proton or ion beams to offer the most dose conformity to a three-dimensional tumour volume, with significantly reduced integral dose, especially when used with multiple fields. This is achieved by scanning monoenergetic pencil beamlets, at programmed intervals, in the transverse direction, also referred to as an energy slice. This is repeated in the longitudinal, depth direction by stepped energy changes. The distribution of beamlets, or spots, in a depth slice is dependent on spot size and the planned transverse area. Whereas beamlets describe the pristine Bragg peak depth doses, the spots refer to the proton dose because of the Bragg peak and the intensity of the spot delivered takes into account the dose from the Bragg peak tails from higher-energy beamlets. Equally, the beam energy changes, corresponding to changes of transverse slice depth, are dependent on the resolution of the Bragg peak beamlets and energy change interval of a facility. These will lead to ripple effects that need to be minimised and the planned spot distributions are calculated to deliver dose homogeneity of less than 2.5% in the transverse and depth directions. Pencil beam scanning offers the possibility of intensity-modulated proton therapy, which is the application of multiple heterogeneous fields to create a resulting uniformly irradiated volume. As with x-ray IMRT, this reduces risk to organs at risk, improves sparing of healthy tissue, and potentially offers better target dose conformity to complex tumour volumes with much reduced integral dose.

The pencil beam scanning technique requires fast-acting scanning magnets, rapid changes in beam energy, responsive power supplies with range sufficient for required beam rigidities, and on-line in-beam dose and position monitoring for precise beam spot control. A simplified diagram of the main features of spot-scanning beams is shown in Figure 9.29. The beamlet must be of sufficiently narrow divergence to fulfil the spatial resolution required for a conformal treatment, but of sufficient width and spacing to produce the required field uniformity of less than 2.5%. The interval of energy change, hence of scanned depth, is dependent on the ESS and the inherent depth–width of the monoenergetic Bragg peak. Many commercial vendors now provide a finely spaced selection of available beam energies (70–250 MeV) in approximately 50 to 70 steps, which correspond to range differences of only a few millimetres. The lower limit of 70 MeV is mainly as a result of severely reduced beam intensity and difficulties in beam scattering and focussing below that point. It is noted that the continuous beam from cyclotrons, and slow-extraction synchrotrons, requires only relatively small beam current of the order of nanoamperes (nA) n for pencil beam scanning, whereas the short pulses with longer duty cycle machines require higher instantaneous current availability to complete volume scans in clinically acceptable times. The parameters required for pencil beam scanning are summarised in Table 9.4.

At present, there are basically two techniques of moving and delivering pencil beam dose to the required spatial position [8,16,17,19]. These can be described as (1) dose-dependent and (2) time-dependent scanned dose delivery to a particular volume element (voxel). The dose-dependent delivery requires the beamlet to remain at a fixed voxel coordinate until the planned dose is delivered, and then move to the

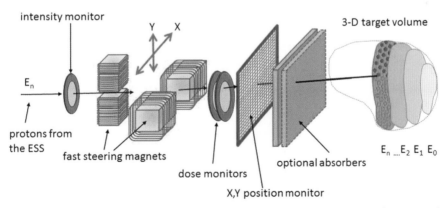

Fig. 9.29 Schematic of proton beam scanning control and Bragg Peak depth control using energy change.

TABLE 9.4 Basic parameters required for pencil beam scanning

Basic Requirements	Lateral: scan speed (cm.mS^{-1})	Speed of energy change	Range of field size (mm × mm)	Spot diameter (mm)	Dose delivery (Gy.Litre^{-1}.min^{-1}.)	Gantry switching time (s)
Small beam divergence; spot; spot interval.	1–0.2	100 mSec per 5 mm depth	200 × 200–400 × 400	<5 mm @ full width at half maximum	1–2, with dose uniformity of <2.5%	<30

next adjacent voxel. In the time-dependent delivery the beamlet or spot will remain in the voxel position for a fixed time interval and then move to the adjoining voxel. This presupposes that the machine beam current is relatively stable; otherwise, returning to the voxel would be necessary. In both cases, the beam monitoring and intensity control must be rapid to minimise errors in the finite beam switch-off time. A slower beam current would reduce this uncertainty at the expense of longer treatment times.

The beam movement options may be briefly summarised as:

- Spot scanning, where the beam is switched-off between voxels, thus creating a dead-time between spots.
- Raster scanning, where the beam is on between spots albeit reduced in intensity. Beam-off only for longer spatial intervals. This is a generally used option.
- Line scanning of continuous modulated dose in one-dimensional lines. This is in development at Paul Scherrer Institute (PSI), where Gantry 2 potentially offers fast and flexible scanning, with fast dose redelivery as required [19,20]. The scanned beam, in one-dimensional direction, is delivered at a constant high velocity, and the planned spot dose is modulated along a horizontal axis.

Although pencil beam scanning is capable of almost ideal target conformity and dose homogeneity, there are several inherent issues. In particular, patient or organ movement could cause significant dose heterogeneity with hot and cold spots. Development of very much faster scanning speeds with advanced beam measurement and feedback control offers the possibility of multiple dose redelivery during a single field. Gating of the scanned beams with organ motion or body respiration and inadvertent movements may increase treatment time but permit tighter conformal margins. Likewise, the fast scanning speeds would permit consideration of breath-

hold gating which has been practised with cyclotron beams and slow-extraction synchrotrons.

Adaptive pencil scanning is being investigated to address interfraction and intrafraction anatomical changes. It is made easier because imaging and replanning are performed rapidly and patient-specific beam modifiers are not required. The structure of a working pencil beam scanning system is shown in Fig. 9.30. In some configurations, the long traversal in air causes subsequent beam dispersion which is countered by use of helium- or vacuum-filled chambers. The second scanning magnet is necessarily larger than the first as the spread of the beam in space and velocity is increased by the first magnet. Note that some superficial fields may need penetration depths lower than those provided by the low-energy limit of approximately 70 MeV. In these cases, calibrated range absorbers are applied at the nozzle to minimise proton scattering and maintain adequate field penumbrae. The sharpness of the penumbrae is dependent on the Gaussian width of the beamlets, particularly at the field edge. Several approaches at improving edge penumbrae include the use multileaf collimators, and programming heavier weighting factor to the edge beamlets [21].

GANTRIES

The use of fully rotational gantries permits the planning and delivery of optimal treatments in conventional x-ray linac therapy. To fully exploit the advantage of proton and carbon therapy, most commercial systems provide rotational gantries (Fig. 9.31). However, these gantries require considerable mechanical and beam transport design. The weight of the focussing quadrupoles and bending dipoles, and shielding and beam monitoring devices lead to total weight of more than 100 to 200 t for 250-MeV proton beams. The beam rigidity required of high-energy carbon

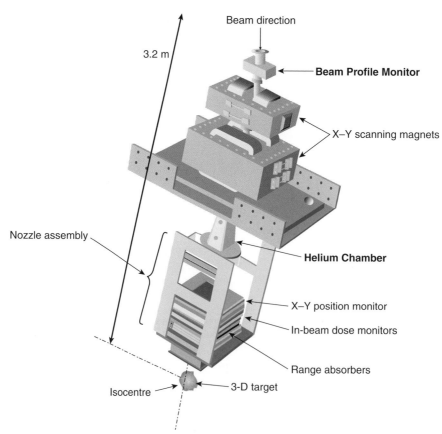

Fig. 9.30 The structure of a pencil beam scanning system (Courtesy MDA/Hitachi).

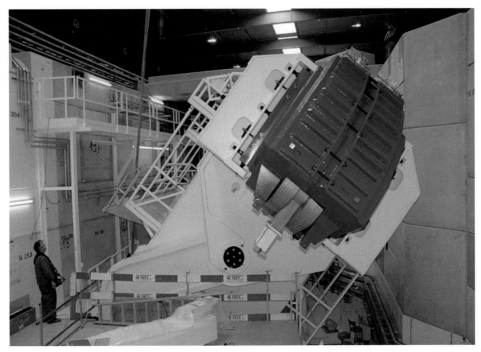

Fig. 9.31 Paul Scherrer Institute (PSI; Gantry 2) compact isocentric design at commissioning, showing main bending dipole (*blue*) weighing approximately 40 t. The diameter of rotation 7.5 m and total weight 220 t. The maximum treatment field at isocentre is approximately 12 × 20 cm. (Courtesy David Meer, PSI, Villigen, Switzerland.)

therapy beams is three times that of clinical proton beams. For example, the total weight of the HIT carbon gantry components is more than 600 t.

Where compact PBT facilities are planned on existing hospital sites, the floor footprint is an important consideration for both the accelerator and the gantry system. Many vendor systems offer reduced gantry rotation such as 270 degrees to 180 degrees. The rotational axis is necessarily large to obtain as near a parallel beam as possible. Fig. 9.32 illustrates the PSI-designed (+180 degrees to −30 degrees) gantry, but the scanning X–Y magnets are situated upstream of the main bending dipole which necessarily has to have a large acceptance aperture. This has been motivated by near-parallel beams presenting much reduced surface dose than finite source beams which have their focal point downstream of the beaning dipole.

TYPES OF PROTON AND ION ACCELERATORS

Table 9.5 briefly summarises the main features of circular accelerators used clinically and available commercially. This does not include beam transport and the treatment rooms. A proton linac is included for comparison. It is noted that the footprint is related to magnet size and field strength. Energy change and thus depth of the beam for cyclotron and synchrocyclotrons are by hardware absorbers, whilst for the synchrotron and proton linac this is by RF and magnet control.

CLINICAL PROTON THERAPY CENTRES

Table 9.6 lists the proton therapy systems that are being built by commercial vendors. Usually the beams from an accelerator will be directed, via beam lines, to a treatment room, or will be switched between several treatment rooms, which may have either gantries or fixed beamlines. An accelerator, feeding beams into multiple treatment rooms, with either gantries or fixed beamlines, or combination of both. The beam control systems are required to switch rapidly from one room to another as soon as patient setup has been achieved. The larger purpose-built proton therapy centres are designed for higher patient throughput and specialist treatments (e.g. paediatric tumours) using multiple treatment rooms with gantries or fixed beams. Although the proton gantries are up to three stories in diameter, the patient treatment room appears quite small. The matching of treatment beam characteristics between rooms is required to achieve optimum treatment flexibility. In addition, the majority of new treatment rooms now offer the spot or raster scanning for optimal three-dimensional radiation conformity. Fast, in-room CT scan verification and precise positioning by robotic couches further underpin accurate beam volume delivery, with treatment setup and irradiation times similar to those in conventional x-ray therapy.

With the expansion and acceptance of PBT, and allied with technical developments particularly in smaller, superconducting magnets, suppliers offer more compact accelerators or single-room solutions as shown in Table 9.3. As can be inferred, these compact single-room systems have footprints considerably larger than linac rooms with areas of approximately 25 m^2. However, these are considered sufficiently small to be installed in, or adjacent to, existing cancer hospitals, to complement conventional x-ray RT.

Table 9.1 shows that there is a continued requirement for proton energies in the 60- to 70-MeV range to treat rare intraocular tumours, with their numbers increasing from 1650 in 2015 to 1820 in 2017. Ocular treatments constitute 10% of the total proton referrals. The first ocular proton therapy was performed in 1975 at the Harvard Cyclotron Laboratory (HCL), Cambridge, USA, followed by European centres. The beam quality, produced with accelerators with little or no energy degradation, exhibits highly conformal fall-off and penumbrae characteristics [11]. They are well adapted to such small field treatments,

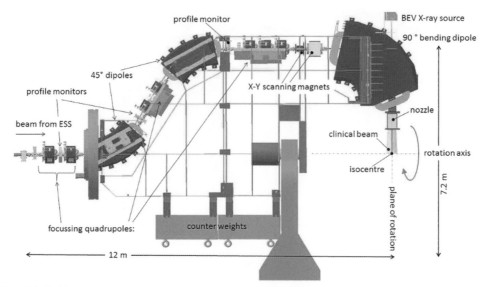

Fig. 9.32 Profile schematic view of the Paul Scherrer Institute (PSI) Gantry 2 with raster scanning capability. Nozzle can be extended to reduce air gap from exit window to patient. Parallel scanning in X and Y axes, with fast energy degrader. (Courtesy E. Pedroni, PSI, Villigen Switzerland.)

TABLE 9.5   Main features of circular accelerators used clinically and available commercially

| Feature | TYPE OF ACCELERATOR | | | |
	Cyclotron	Synchrocyclotron	Synchrotron	Proton linac
Radio frequency	Fixed	Variable	Variable	Variable
Magnetic field	Fixed	Fixed	Variable	–
Proton radius	Fixed	Variable	Fixed	–
Particle energy	Fixed	Fixed	Variable	Variable
Energy change	Manual	Manual	Electronic	Electronic
Particle current	High	Low	Low	Low
Beam waveform	Continuous	Pulsed	Pulsed	Pulsed
Footprint	Compact	Compact	Large	Compact

TABLE 9.6   Comparison of commercial proton beam treatment centres with multiroom and gantry systems

Vendor	Machine	Type	Weight	Max energy range	Dose-rate or maximum current	Room switching time (s)	Field size (cm × cm)	Beam delivery options
IBA	Proteus PLUS, C230	Isochronous cyclotron	220T; 4.3 m	230 MeV	2 Gy/min	20	30 × 40	Pencil-beam, scattered
VARIAN	ProBeam	Super-Conducting (NbTi); isochronous cyclotron	90T; 3.1 m	250 MeV	800 nA	<30	30 × 40	Pencil-beam
HITACHI	ProBeat-V (footprint 42.5m²)	Synchrotron (slow extraction)	25 m diameter	70–230 MeV	Approx. 1.5 Gy/L/min	<0.45	30 × 30	Spot-scanning
PROTOM INTERNATIONAL	Radiance 330	Synchrotron	16T; 4.8 m diameter	330 MeV imaging; Therapy (70–250MeV)	2GyL/min	<1.2	30 × 40	Pencil scanning only

TABLE 9.7 Comparison of carbon-ion centres

Centre	Country	Type of accelerator, (diameter)	Max carbon beam energy (proton energy)	Particle types	Field-size cm², scanning mode	Treatment rooms	Year of clinical start
HIT, Heidelberg	Germany	Synchrotron (20 m)	88–430/u (221 MeV)	C (p, He, O)	20 × 20, raster scanning	1 gantry; 2 H beams	2009
CNAO, Pavia	Italy	Synchrotron (25 m)	120–400/u (60–220 MeV)	C (p, He)	20 × 20; spot scanning	1 H+V; 2 H beams	2011
MIT, Marburg	Germany	Synchrotron (21 m)	430/u (221 MeV)	C (p)	20 × 20, raster scanning	4 fixed beams (3 × H; 1X 45)	2015 (recommissioned)
MedAustron	Austria	Synchrotron (25m)	400 MeV/u (60–250MeV)	C (p)	Quasi-discrete spot scanning-raster	2 fixed beam (1V + 1H); 1 gantry (p)	2017
HIMAC (NIRS), Chiba	Japan	Synchrotron (2 rings) (41 m)	100–800 MeV/u	C (He)	22 × 22; 3D scanning (in 2012); broad beam	1 × h; 1 × V; 1 × V+H beams. Gantry in 2016.	1994
HIBMC, Hyogo	Japan	Synchrotron (30 m)	70–320/u (190 MeV)	C (p, He)	15 × 15; Wobbler + filter	3 + H; 1 × V and 45 degrees; 2 p gantries.	2001
GHMC, Guma	Japan	Synchrotron, (22 m)	400 MeV/u	C	15 × 15; wobbler + filter	3 rooms (H, H + V, V)	2010

3D, Three-dimensional.

which require submillimetre precision. There are now 22 centres reporting ocular treatments and the majority of treatment centres use chair patient positioning with a gaze angle optimised for a particular treatment. Several eye treatment centres have been developed from high-energy neutron therapy such as Clatterbridge and Nice, or from research machines (Berlin, Catania, San Francisco, Krakow).

CLINICAL CARBON ION THERAPY CENTRES

Synchrotrons which are designed specifically for proton beams have diameters of 6 to 8 m, whereas synchrotrons for carbon beam therapy extend to 22 to 25 m in diameter. This was necessary to achieve what is referred to as high magnetic rigidity of the carbon beams used clinically. Table 9.7 provides the basic information on clinical carbon therapy facilities. At present, the size and cost render them to be clinical research facilities rather than routine RT centres. They are suitable for clinical trials, studying the effects of highly conformal isodose and elevated relative biological effectiveness (RBE) on radiation-resistant tumours. Included in Table 9.7 are three of the earlier Japanese facilities which represent the worlds largest clinical experience, having treated over 11,000 patients by 2017.

Note that recent developments in superconducting magnets, to counter the high magnetic rigidity of carbon beams, have enabled the adoption of compact gantries for carbon beams offering stronger bending fields at three of the Europe centres. All European centres have adopted either raster-beam or spot scanning to optimise three-dimensional dose conformity and minimise extraneous secondary radiation from the treatment nozzles. It is noted that the Heavy Ion Medical Accelerator Centre in Japan has added both three-dimensional spot scanning and a compact gantry to its facility. The latter weighs 200 t compared with the 600 t of the HIT gantry. The design of the HIT facility emerged from a collaboration of the GSI-Darmstadt and Siemens Medical, whilst the National Centre of Oncological Hadrontherapy in Italy and MedAustron designs were based on Proton-Ion Medical Machine Study initiated at European Council for Nuclear Research

(CERN) [22]. This offered the advantage of a smaller surface area with the ion injectors and drift-tube linac situated inside the synchrotron circumference [23]. Although present facilities are solely based on synchrotron acceleration, an isochronous superconducting cyclotron-based C-400 design is proposed by IBA and is capable of accelerating protons to 250 MeV and carbon ions to 400 MeV/u. Although heavy at 700 t, it has a diameter of only 6.6 m and height of 3.4 m. The design incorporates ion injectors beneath the cyclotron.

NONCIRCULAR ACCELERATORS

A linac for image-guided hadron therapy (LIGHT) for producing therapeutic-range protons has been proposed by Ronsivalle et al [24] using high-gradient (15–20 MV m^{-1}) 3-GHz linac technology. Much development has been performed by a spin-off company from the CERN. This consists of a low-energy proton source which passes protons into an RFQ device. This is a radial arrangement of four long vane electrodes which provide alternating RF electrostatic fields. The transverse fields provide focussing and the longitudinal fields acceleration. It bunches and accelerates the beam up to 5 MeV and further acceleration with linear acceleration increases the energy to 38 MeV. Finally, acceleration to the therapeutic 180–230 MeV range is obtained by addition of a cell-coupled linac with each cell providing 13 MeV. A maximum energy of 230 MeV would require a length of approximately 25 m. The 200-Hz pulse repetition rate is similar to existing RT x-ray linacs and is very suitable for clinical spot scanning. A degree of energy selection is possible by altering the accelerating gradient of the cells. Further developments suggest variable control of beam intensity and proton energy between repetition pulses. The low beam spread characteristics promise minimal beam losses, with shielding mainly required for the treatment rooms. Although testing is still taking place, the Advanced Oncotherapy Consortium have planned and are developing a clinical therapy installation in an existing U.K. clinic and the reductions in size, weight, and footprint may offer further advantages over circular accelerators, beamline, and gantry configurations.

NEUTRON AND OTHER BEAMS

Fast Neutron Beam Therapy

In the 1970s and 1980s there was great interest in using neutron beams for treating radiation-resistant solid tumours. Owing to the high linear energy transfer (LET) of neutrons, and decreased dependence on the oxygen enhancement ratio, these beams were able to deliver highly effective clinical doses with an RBE (Relative Biological Effectiveness) of approximately 3.0. Neutron beams were shown to be highly penetrating in tissue, deposit dose by means of collision with tissue oxygen and carbon, and produce highly ionising knock-on low-energy protons. Most clinical neutron beams were produced by proton or deuteron bombardment of beryllium or sometimes lithium targets. These machines could produce the large proton currents of 30 to 50 µA required for delivering clinical doses of 2 Gy/min. Most acceleration was achieved with cyclotrons, although at the Fermilab in Chicago, Illinois, United States, a 66-MeV proton linac was used. It should be noted that neutron beams required significant development in collimation which usually consisted of steel, tungsten, and high-density polythene and weighed up to 1 t. Earlier machines, as well as D-T generators, had limited neutron penetration in tissue. Later versions were designed with higher acceleration energies to produce fast neutron doses with penetration characteristics similar to 6- and 8-MV x-ray linacs. In addition, facilities with isocentric gantries, improved collimation, wedges, blocks, and couch rotations enabled comparative studies and randomised trials between neutrons and x-rays to be performed. However, the initial promise was not fulfilled mainly because of increased normal tissue toxicity. This was related to uncertainties in RBE, difficulties in neutron collimation, and dilution of the RBE by significant gamma-ray beam component. Results from parotid and air sinus lesions showed some benefit; however, this benefit may now have been eclipsed by highly conformal x-ray therapies. There are now few active centres offering fast neutron therapy; however, it should be noted that the first gantry-mounted and superconducting cyclotron was developed by H. Blosser for the Wayne State University Medical Center (Detroit, USA) and opened in 1991. This produced neutrons by the d,n reaction on Be; it weighed only 25 t, with a 360° gantry, and offered multirod collimation as well as blocks for improved dose conformity. The experience gained with this compact superconducting cyclotron, on a gantry mounting, eventually led to the development of the Mevion proton therapy system, and the single-room proton therapy facility.

Boron Neutron Capture Therapy

Boron neutron capture therapy (BNCT) involves the labelling of a tumour seeking compound with a target nuclei and neutron irradiation. It is a twofold form of RT based firstly on the administration of a boron-10 (^{10}B)-labelled compound which concentrates on or in tumour cells. This tumour volume is then irradiated with a low-energy neutron beam. The nuclear reaction which occurs for thermal energy neutrons (typically 0.0025 eV) has a high probability of 94% and excites ^{10}B to ^{11}B. The excited atom then disintegrates into lithium-7 (^{7}Li), an alpha particle (^{4}He), and a 478-keV gamma ray. As seen in Fig. 9.33 the particles have a high LET compared with the gamma ray, so are highly ionising short-range tracks of 5 µm to 9 µm, respectively, and would wholly or partially traverse the width of a tumour cell.

Fig. 9.34 shows a schematic view of a clinical irradiation using epithermal neutron beams from a nuclear reactor. The efficacy of BNCT is still being tested by research centres. Because of the decrease in availability of reactor neutron beams, development of BNCT is directed towards low-energy proton cyclotrons producing mA current

$$n(\text{thermal}) \quad + \quad {}^{10}\text{B}$$
$$\rightarrow \quad {}^{4}\text{He} \quad + \quad {}^{7}\text{Li} \quad + \quad \gamma\text{-ray}$$

	Energy	LET	Range
^{7}Li	840keV;	175 keV/µm	5 µm
^{4}He	1470 keV	150 keV/µm	9 um
γ-ray	478 keV	~1 keV/µm	-----

Fig. 9.33 Nuclear reaction and physical data for boron neutron capture therapy.

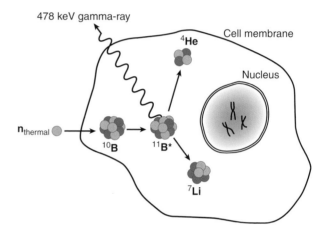

Fig. 9.34 Schematic of boron neutron capture therapy.

proton beams [25]. These beams then bombard Be or Li targets to produce an epi-thermal neutron beam. The thermal neutron uniformity is further improved by reflecting materials of Al or Bi.

Proton Boron Capture Therapy

Recent work has suggested that boron capture of low-energy protons [26] may amplify the dose released at the Bragg peak and form a dose enhancement. This process is also described as a proton–boron fusion reaction as it resembles a nuclear fusion reaction with the proton being absorbed. However, as in BNCT the therapeutic effect is dependent on the boron compound uptake in tumour cells.

The phenomenon is described by the following reaction:

$$\text{Proton} + {}^{11}\text{B} \,(80\%\ \text{abundance}) \rightarrow {}^{12}\text{C} \rightarrow 3\ \text{alphas}\,({}^{4}\text{He})\,(\sim 4\,\text{MeV})$$

$$\textbf{(9.1)}$$

The dose enhancement is achieved, at the Bragg peak, by the release of three short-range, highly ionising alpha particles, and by the greater (80%) abundance of the ^{11}B isotope. The ranges of the 2- to 3-MeV alphas are about 30 µm and encompass a cell diameter with high probability of traversing the cell nucleus [26]. This proposal would combine the physical advantages of low-LET proton therapy with the biological enhancement of localised high-LET particles. Like BNCT, the decay of the immediate carbon nucleus produces a 719-keV gamma ray, which offers the potential of real-time monitoring and range verification with gamma camera imaging. Unlike BNCT, this technique would be a dose enhancement to conventional proton therapy, without the requirement of a source of thermal neutrons.

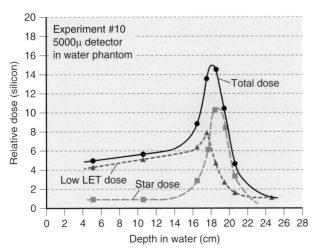

Fig. 9.35 The star burst phenomenon, enhancing the low-linear energy transfer (LET) dose with that from the short-range high-LET particles. (Courtesy M Kligerman (LAMPF)).

Pion Therapy

This accelerator-based therapy involves creating negative pi-meson (pion) beams by bombarding proton beams onto low-Z target nucleons. This produces pions, with mass 278 times that of an electron. These charged particles produce increasing ionisation along their path length, culminating in a broad Bragg peak at the end of their range. At the end of the range the pion is captured by an oxygen or carbon nucleus, causing disintegration of the nucleus into short-range high-LET particles, such as protons, alphas, deuterons, as well as neutrons and electrons. This is the star burst phenomenon which enhances the dose delivered by the pions alone. The combined total dose from a pion beam is shown in Fig. 9.35. Pion treatment was considered of interest in treating radiation-resistant tumours. Clinically useful pion beams require the bombardment of beryllium (Be) or carbon targets with high currents (0.1 mA to 1 mA) of high-energy protons in the 500–800-MeV range. This produces pion beams with penetration from 22 cm to 31 cm. The short lifetime of pions (2.5×10^{-8} s) necessitates short beamlines of the order of 10 m, with collimation and focussing magnets. Generally, clinical pion beams used computer controlled movement of patient couches, to enable the fixed beam to cover the required treatment area. The PIOTRON at PSI used the channelling of 60 radial pion beams into a cross-sectional slice, with axial patient couch movement to irradiate a three-dimensional treatment volume.

There have been three clinical pion programmes as shown in Table 9.8. The majority of treated indications were in the brain, mainly glioblastomas, and also in prostate cancers. Although the high-LET

component in the star burst was attractive clinically, spreading this depth dose over larger volumes diluted the biological effectiveness of the star burst peak. Much of this was as a result of dispersion of neutron energy from the star burst peak. In addition, the pion beams had significant contamination with muons and electrons. The effective RBE was considered to be 1.1 to 1.5. Although much was learnt from biological and physical dose treatment planning, normal tissue response, and precise beam delivery, clinical results were considered to show no significant benefit compared with x-ray therapy. The power and the size requirements of pion-producing accelerators would have prohibited their development in a hospital environment. For example, the TRIUMF cyclotron requires 18 kA for magnet currents with a weight of 4000 t.

Antiproton Therapy Beams

The potential use of antiprotons has been studied at the CERN [27]. Antiprotons are known to have slightly greater range than protons with a much greater dose at the Bragg peak. This is caused by the annihilation of the slowing antiproton with a target nucleon. The rest mass energy of 1.8 GeV is released by pions and about 20% of these are absorbed by a nucleus. This leads to fragmentation and release of low-energy highly ionising particles. This is reflected in an increased measured biological effect. However, as with pion therapy, the biological effectiveness may be diluted by modulation of the antiproton energy, and by the accompanying whole-body dose as a result of neutrons and pions. The penumbra has been shown to be poorer than protons at depth and the requirement of a very-high-energy accelerator, as well as sufficient antiproton fluence, is very unlikely to be fulfilled outside a few international research laboratories. However, the emission of energetic pions during therapy would offer real-time monitoring of the annihilation peak and hence of the treatment range.

Laser-Induced Proton and Particle Beams

The use of very-high-intensity laser light to produce particle fluence has important attractions, and recent progress [28,29] has demonstrated therapy-level doses in conventional treatment times. The protons are produced by extremely short, intense pulses of laser light incident on a small area of thin metallic foil. This impact creates a localised plasma where the faster accelerated electrons will almost instantaneously create extremely high electric fields of the order 10^{12} V m^{-1} when leaving the back of the target material. Protons and other positive ions emerging from the foil will be accelerated by this electric field, normal to the surface of the foil, to energies of tens of MeV. This process is illustrated in Fig. 9.36. Intensities of at least 10^{19} W cm^{-2} are required in the laser pulse. So far, measured results have produced up to 60 MeV, albeit with a multienergetic proton spectrum describing a quasi-exponential distribution, to a maximum cut-off energy. This is caused by the

TABLE 9.8	Pion treatment centres				
Institute (country)	Accelerator type	Years of operation	Proton beam energy MeV and beam current	Clinical pion beam arrangement	No. of patients treated
LAMPF (USA)	Linear accelerator	1974–1981	800 (1 mA)	vertical beam	230
PSI/SIN (Switzerland)	Isochronous ring synchrotron	1980–1993	590 (100 μA)	horizontal with 3D scanning (Piotron)	503
TRIUMF (Canada)	Large-pole (50') diameter cyclotron, negative ion	1979–1994	500 (100 μA)	horizontal beam, scanning couch	367

3D, Three-dimensional.

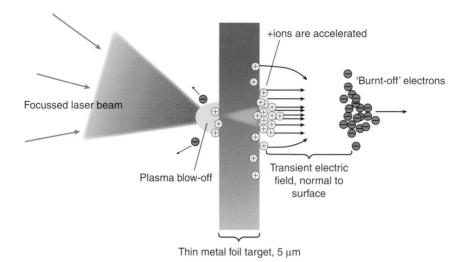

Fig. 9.36 The process to produce particle fluence using very short pulse, high-intensity laser light (after K Ledingham).

inhomogeneous transverse field resulting in a distribution of proton energies. Thus the maximum proton energy is dependent on the initial laser beam intensity. Furthermore, significant quantities of other contaminant particles are produced. Reduction of the target area, application of small hydrogen-rich inclusions, and use of gaseous hydrogen targets have been shown to improve beam intensity and narrow the energy spectrum of the protons.

The interest for proton therapy lies in the possibility of compact layout and footprint. A single power laser would be used to distribute light beams by optics to treatment gantries, where the proton beam intensity and energy would be produced. This would eliminate the beam transport, steering magnets, beam monitoring, and vacuum systems, as well as reducing stray neutron production and shielding. This will be dependent on reducing the costs and size of lasers as well as increasing both the laser pulse rate and power intensity. The improvements in the latter, coupled with improvements in energy selection and narrow beams, make laser-induced proton beams well suited for the spot-scanning technique. At present, the Sultan Centre at Selçuk University in Konya, Turkey, is being established to demonstrate such a laser-driven therapy system.

SHIELDING OF PROTON THERAPY ACCELERATORS AND TREATMENT ROOMS

Many of the design criteria for reducing scattered radiation in high-energy linacs are also applicable to proton therapy accelerators and their treatment rooms. More detailed considerations are given in reference handbooks [3,30]. One significant difference is that, with the exception of the Mevion single-room facility (Table 9.3), all proton therapy centres have separate bunkers for the accelerator with long beam lines and associated diagnostic equipment transporting the beam into different treatment rooms as required. The principal radiological concern is secondary neutron dose rates produced by the scattering of the proton beam in the accelerator, beam line diagnostics, and treatment head. Higher-energy neutrons are rapidly reduced in energy by high-Z elements such as iron, then further moderated by low-Z elements such as the water content in concrete, and then finally absorbed by doping elements such as B or Li, if required.

As in other radiation treatment facilities, the building shielding design is dominated by the staff or public usage of adjacent areas. Space

limitations will determine the nature and economic cost of the planned shielding. For example, earth-fill would be considerably more economical than doped concrete, whilst Pb-backed boron-doped polythene composite material would represent significant space saving but at substantial cost.

Activation of air by primary proton beam and secondary neutron fluences produces short-lived positron-emitting isotopes such as ^{11}C, ^{13}N, and ^{15}O. Their half-lives are 20.3 minutes, 10 minutes, and 2 minutes, respectively, and the amount produced will depend largely on field size and whether scanning or passive-scattered mode is employed. However, the short-lived nature of these isotopes and adequate ventilation in the treatment room should minimise any radiological concern. However, the ^{41}Ar (beta/gamma-ray) produced by thermal neutron reactions on the natural argon in air, requires consideration due to its longer half-life (1.83 hours).

Activation of the concrete shielding by secondary neutrons will be more of a consideration around the accelerator and beam lines as a result of longer running times and proton beam losses. Most radioisotopes produced in normal high-density concrete will be relatively short-lived. However, other additive or trace elements may need to be considered, such as Co, Ba (barytes concrete), and Eu, which will produce longer-lived daughter radioisotopes.

NANOPARTICLE-ENHANCED THERAPY

The use of high-Z nanoparticles (NPs) as radiosensitisers has been shown to enhance the dose effect in both in vitro and in vivo studies with x-ray therapy. The effectiveness with x-ray beams is because of interaction with the high-Z atom and the subsequent creation of low-energy secondary electrons. In comparative studies using different ionising radiations, the enhancement effect is highest for x-ray photons. The modelling of gold NPs in proton beam therapy [31] has been shown to offer some degree of radio enhancement in clinical SOBP proton beams, depending on NP size and quantity of NP absorbed internally through the cell wall. Although the radiosensitisation mechanism of high-Z NPs are not fully understood, it has been shown that the secondary electron spectrum from protons is of considerably lower energy than that induced by x-rays, meaning that for protons, high-Z NPs need to have penetrated the cell wall to achieve dose enhancement.

FUTURE DESIGN

It has been shown that much expertise from nuclear physics and engineering has been directed to the commercial provision of particle accelerators particularly for proton beams. In addition, clinical proton accelerators are necessitated to have reliability requirements or uptime at least equal to that of modern x-ray linacs. This is due in part to (1) the extended treatment hours necessitated by the capital outlay and expected patient throughput, and (2) that as accelerators are unique at a clinical facility, and thus represent a single point of failure as patients cannot be transferred to another proton facility. Any gantry or nozzle downtime at multigantry facilities can be assuaged by redirecting patients to the other gantries. Single-room proton facilities are either planned to operate with adjoining x-ray linacs, or in some cases may be configured to operate as a suite of single-room treatment rooms as suggested by Mevion. This emphasises the importance of siting of proton beam treatments in larger RT centres which have the capacity to transfer treatment to x-ray linacs if required.

The ability of ion accelerators to deliver prescribed dose and conformal fields reliably and in conventional treatment times has been described. Future developments in proton or heavier charged particle accelerators, and their advance into tertiary RT centres will be dependent on:

1. The accumulation of patient follow-up data confirming the expected benefits of particle therapy.
2. The increase of clinical indications expected to show clinical advantage compared with x-ray treatments.

Improved determination of the precision of beam delivery, particularly with the positioning of the distal Bragg peak, or proton end of range. Developments are following two main directions: the in vivo monitoring of proton end of range by measurement in two-dimensional or three-dimensional gamma rays induced by protons, either high-energy inelastic scattered photons or positron emissions; and improving the accuracy of proton treatment planning by better determination of proton stopping power when converting x-ray CT data, or from direct patient-specific CT obtained from proton tomography using high energy.

RECORD AND VERIFY SYSTEMS

The task for the machine operators who deliver the treatment has always involved setting up the patient and the machine for the treatment. Part of this task has involved the treatment setup being checked as independently as possible before treatment being delivered. The increasing complexity of machines and treatments and the introduction of quality systems which require the process to be traceable have made automatic verification of the treatment setup essential. With the availability of fast computing systems, record and verify (R + V) systems have been developed to fulfil this automatic role. Essentially, the R + V system consists of three distinct components: storage, check, and record. The patient prescription is stored, a check is made that the machine parameters at treatment match the prescription, and a record is built-up of the treatment delivered. The structure of a system is illustrated in Fig. 9.37.

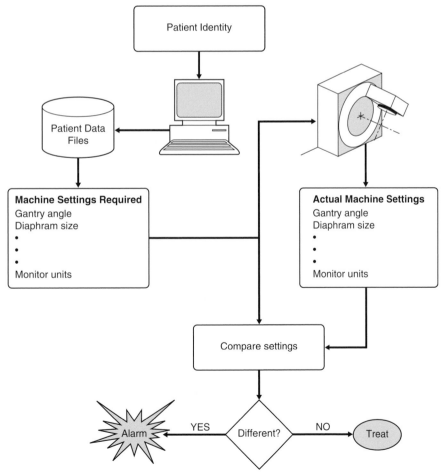

Fig. 9.37 Structure of record and verify (R + V) system.

For each patient, a treatment parameters file is held and the parameters are downloaded from the R+V system to the treatment machine at each occasion of treatment. The machine is then set up for treatment of the patient by the operators and the R+V system compares the settings on the machine with the values stored in the system file. Any differences must be resolved by the operators before treatment can commence. This will normally be done by adjustment of the patient and machine setup to bring it in line with the treatment parameters. However, in exceptional circumstances, parameters can be over-ridden subject to appropriate checking and supervision. The patient's file is also used to record the dose delivered to the patient on each treatment to maintain an accumulated record of the treatment dose to the patient.

Although these systems provide an invaluable aid to treatment delivery, it should be borne in mind that such systems can fail. As with any computerised data transfer process, acceptance checks and routine checks are required to verify that systems assign the data correctly to a patients treatment.

CONCLUSION

The x-ray and electron beam medical linac has become very well established and reached a very consistent level of performance. Although 20 years ago individual machines could vary, they now have identical beam characteristics and are interchangeable as machines. The availability of these machines is high and widespread, with satellite treatment centres made easier because of the high reliability of the equipment. Beam shaping with high-resolution MLC, VMAT, FFF beams, and SABR have taken the megavoltage x-ray machine treatment delivery to a very sophisticated level. The inclusion of on-board imaging with kV cone beam and MV treatment beam imaging has meant that the treatment accuracy and reproducibility have been enhanced. These MV imaging systems have also enabled the development of on-board MLC calibration systems, routine quality control systems, and transit dosimetry. This has improved the efficacy of machine maintenance and monitoring of machine performance. Transit dosimetry has provided the means for rapid treatment verification of dose delivered.

The worldwide advent of heavy charged particle therapy in hospital or clinical research facilities, in the last two decades, has confirmed its place within mainstream RT for certain clinical indications. The commercially available facilities have:

- automated and stable operation
- high availability of at least 98%
- low-maintenance designs, with long-term service contracts
- lower power requirements
- smaller-sized accelerators with smaller footprint facilities commercially available

Modern proton beam therapy facilities are now expected to have the same reliability as modern RT x-ray linacs. This is a necessity to service the expected large patient throughputs for PBT. The latter will be driven by the experience of the growing number of proton and carbon therapy centres. The larger PBT centres in particular will rapidly increase clinical evidence from clinical trials and follow-up data. The commercially available smaller one-room PBT facilities are to be considered as an addition to existing large RT departments. By contrast, developments on circular accelerator-based machines are directed at smaller weight, size, and reliability, particularly with the adoption of superconducting main coils. The main developments in alternative accelerator technology are linac-based proton beams and laser-driven proton sources. Progress in further PBT machine developments remains predicated on increasing patient throughput and proven clinical indications.

REFERENCES

[1] Thwaites DI, Tuohy JB. Back to the future: the history and development of the clinical linear accelerator. Phys Med Biol 2006;51:R343–62.

[2] Karzmark CJ, Morton RJ. A primer on theory and operation of linear accelerators in radiation therapy. 2nd ed. Medical Physics Publishing; 1997.

[3] Council Directive 93/47/Euratom. Official J Eur Communities 1997; L180:22–7.

[4] The Ionising Radiations Regulations 2017 – Statutory Instrument 1999 No. 3232. HMSO.

[5] Stedeford B, Morgan HM, Mayles WPM. The design of radiotherapy treatment room facilities. IPEM; 1997.

[6] Paganetti H. Proton therapy physics (series in medical physics and biomedical engineering). 1st edition. ISSN 978-1-4398-3644-3646. Boca Raton, USA: CRC Press; 2011.

[7] Smith A. Proton therapy, Phys Med Biol 2006;51:R491–504.

[8] Flanz J, Smith A. Technology for proton therapy. Cancer J 2009;15 (4):292–7.

[9] Coutrakon G. Accelerators for heavy-charged-particle radiation therapy. Technol Cancer Res Treat 2007;6(4 Supp):49–54.

[10] Gragoudas ES. Proton beam irradiation of uveal melanomas: the first 30 years. The Weisenfeld Lecture. Invest Ophthalmol Vis Sci 2006;47 (11):4666–73.

[11] Kacperek A. Ocular proton therapy centers. In: Linz U, editor. Ion beam therapy. Biological and medical physics, biomedical engineering, vol. 320. Heidelberg: Springer, Berlin; 2012. https://doi.org/10.1007/978-3-642-21414-1_10.

[12] Baird D, Faust T. Scientific instruments, scientific progress and the cyclotron. Br J Philos Sci 1990;41(2):147–75.

[13] Muramatsu M, Kitagawa A. A review of ion sources for medical accelerators (invited). Rev Sci Instrum 2012;83(2):02B909.

[14] Kleeven W. Injection and extraction for cyclotrons, In: CERN Accelerator School (CAS) – Small Accelerators, Zeegse, The Netherlands, 24 May-2 June, 2005. Proceedings CERN-2006-012; 26 October 2006. p. 271–96.

[15] Owen H, Lomax A, Jolly S. Current and future accelerator technologies for charged particle therapy. Nuclear Instruments and Methods in Physics Research Section A: Accelerators, Spectrometers, Detectors and Associated Equipment 2016;809:96–104.

[16] Owen H, Holder D, Alonso J, MacKay R. Technologies for delivery of proton and ion beams for radiotherapy. Int J Modern Physics 2014. A 29, 1441002.

[17] Schippers M. In: CERN-2017-004-SP. Proceedings of the CERN Accelerator School "Accelerators for Medical Applications"; 2015. p. 165–76. https://doi.org/arXiv:1804.08551.

[18] Goitein M, Radiation Oncology M. A physicists-eye view. New York, NY: Springer; 2008. https://doi.org/10.1007/978-0-387-72645-8.

[19] Giordanengo S, Donetti M. In: Dose delivery concept and instrumentation in Proceedings, CAS-CERN Accelerator School: Accelerators for Medical Applications. Presented at CAS- CERN Accelerator School on Accelerators for Medical Application, Vösendorf, Austria, 26 May - 5 June; 2015. p. 13–47. 10.23730/CYRSP-2017-001.13.

[20] Pedroni E, Scheib S, Böhringer T, Coray A, Grossmann M, Lin S, Lomax A. Experimental characterization and physical modelling of the dose distribution of scanned proton pencil beams. Phys Med & Biol 2005;50 (3):541–61.

[21] Safai S, Bortfeld T, Engelsman M. Comparison between the lateral penumbra of a collimated double-scattered beam and uncollimated scanning beam in proton radiotherapy. Phys Med Biol 2008;53:1729–50.

[22] Degiovanni A, Amaldi U. History of hadron therapy accelerators. Physica Medica 2015;31(4):322–32.

[23] Amaldi U, Bonomi R, Braccini S, Crescenti, M.; Degiovanni, A.; Garlasché, M. et al. Accelerators for hadrontherapy: from Lawrence cyclotrons to linacs. Nuclear Instruments and Methods in Physics Research Section A. 620; 2-3: 563-577.

[24] Ronsivalle C, Picardi L, Ampollini A, et al. First acceleration of a proton beam in a side coupled drift tube linac. In: Europhysics Letters. 111. 1:29 July 2015. 14002.

[25] Forton E, Stichelbaut F, Cambriani A, Kleeven W, Ahlback J, Jongen Y. Overview of the IBA accelerator-based BNCT system. Appl Radiat Isot 2009;67(7–8):S262–5.

[26] Cirrone GAP, Manti L, Margarone D, et al. First experimental proof of Proton Boron Capture Therapy (PBCT) to enhance protontherapy effectiveness; 2018. Nature, Scientific Reports 8; no. 1141. https://doi.org/10.1038/s41598-018-19258-5.

[27] Bassler N, Holzscheiter MH, Jäkel O, Knudsen HV, Kovacevic S. The antiproton depth–dose curve in water. Phys Med Biol 2008;53 (3):793–805.

[28] Schwoerer H, Pfotenhauer S, Jäckel O, Amthor K, Liesfeld B, Esirkepov T, et al. Laser–plasma acceleration of quasi-monoenergetic protons from microstructured targets. Nature 2006;439(7075):445–8.

[29] Ledingham K, Bolton P, Shikazono N, Ma C. Towards laser driven hadron cancer radiotherapy; a review of progress. Appl Sci 2014;4(3):402–43.

[30] Radiation protection in the design of radiotherapy facilities. IAEA SafetyReport Series No 47. Vienna, Austria: IAEA; 2006.

[31] Lin Y, McMahon SJ, Paganetti H, Schuemann J. Biological modeling of gold nanoparticle enhanced radiotherapy for proton therapy. Phys Med Biol 2015;60(10):4149–68.

10

Radiation Treatment Planning: Immobilisation, Localisation and Verification Techniques

Andrew Penny, Phil Sharpe

CHAPTER OUTLINE

INTRODUCTION

The treatment planning process consists of a series of patient-related work tasks that eventually result in a custom plan of the external beam treatment and will enable the radiation dose prescription to be applied. The radiation treatment planning (RTP) system provides a three-dimensional dose distribution of the beams arranged around the body using a mathematical model of the megavoltage x-ray field. The composite dose map is displayed in relation to the target volume and the critical anatomical structures within the body.

Integral to the planning process are devices that ensure the treatment is reproducible on a daily basis; the most important of these is a method of reducing movement of the patient during treatment, and this is called *immobilisation*. The specification of such a device is dependent on the area of the body for which it is required. For treatments of the head and neck, some form of immobilisation device is essential to ensure reproducible set-up and to avoid displacement of the plan isocentre from its intended position. The relatively small field sizes used in the head and neck, compared with pelvic or thorax plans, require a high degree of beam positional accuracy, because of the proximity to critical organs (e.g. eye, spinal cord), which depends on effective immobilisation of the head. Other devices that facilitate reducing movement of the patient are site specific. For example, external beam radiation treatment of the breast uses a board that supports the patient at an inclined angle and provides hand grips that raise their arms above their head to meet the requirements for glancing beams arranged to the breast. Other devices stop the patient from moving their legs to reduce lower body movement or can make the treatment more sustainable over the few minutes of the beam exposure time.

Complete eradication of patient movement is impossible to achieve, although reducing this to within acceptable tolerance (e.g. 3 mm for head and neck, 3 to 5 mm for stereotactic ablative body radiation therapy [SABR] and 5 mm for thorax and pelvis) is commonly achieved. Another technique to improve beam positional accuracy is to track the movement of the patient or movement of anatomical landmarks using an external device that is integral with the treatment accelerator. This method is called image-guided radiotherapy (IGRT). IGRT requires monitoring of the patient using a real-time imaging device (e.g. video, ultrasound, x-ray, cone beam computed tomography [CT]) and the information is compared with the patient plan to correct for any positional inaccuracy. This technique enables a precise level of beam positioning control that can allow for any inadequacies in immobilisation or effects of organ movement (e.g. lung displacement during respiration).

With more advanced IGRT techniques such as four-dimensional CT and even a linear accelerator combined with a magnetic resonance imaging (MRI) scanner, internal anatomy can be imaged in real time during treatment, movement can be seen and the radiation beam only turned on while the target is in the correct place; this is known as gated radiotherapy.

Anatomical information of the patient in the treatment position is required to undertake three-dimensional treatment planning. The process of localisation includes the acquisition of radiological images from a CT scanner. The localisation process provides external contour information and anatomical data that enable definition of planning target volume (PTV) contours and organs at risk (OAR); methods of providing this information range from x-ray CT, MRI through to positron emission tomography (PET). However, the basic requirement, to define the external contour and internal structures for treatment planning, is provided by a CT data set of the patient that can be transferred to the treatment planning system (TPS) where attenuation data are converted to electron density values for heterogeneity correction of the megavoltage beam data. Non-x-ray CT imaging modalities cannot provide this attenuation correction, however with the ability of MRI to visualise soft tissue far greater than that of CT, some companies have developed an MRI planning tool that assigns bulk densities to different structures such as dense bone, spongy bone, muscle, fat and air to produce a synthetic CT to plan with.

The production of an optimised treatment plan for external beam megavoltage treatment is highly dependent on the following:
- The size and shape of the PTVs
- The limiting (tolerance) dose to the critical structures (OAR)
- The positional reproducibility of the linear accelerator and couch support system
- Limitation dictated by the patient's position within the immobilisation device
- Selection of optimum beam parameters (e.g. field size, collimator rotation).
- Limitation of other medical procedures (replacement hips, pacemaker)

A customised treatment plan for the patient must be checked before first treatment to ensure the accuracy and validity of the plan; this process is called *verification*.

Verification of the plan was previously undertaken on a simulator where radiographic images of each beam portal ensured the accuracy of the isocentre position and verified the beam size and shape against the treatment plan. Most modern radiotherapy centres now use a process called *virtual simulation* which allows the use of the original CT information to produce a digitally reconstructed radiograph (DRR) of the beam portal that provides a virtual film that is comparable to the simulator image.

With the implementation of more complex treatments such as intensity modulated radiotherapy (IMRT) and arc therapy, beam portals are used as orthogonal isocentre verification images rather than treatment fields. Also, this is done less frequently now with the introduction of cone beam CT on the treatment machine that can be matched to the original CT scan for verification.

PATIENT IMMOBILISATION

Thermoplastic Shells

The majority of patients receiving radiotherapy to the head and neck region are immobilised using commercial systems that use a combination of head and/or neck rests to get the patient in the correct treatment position. A perforated thermoplastic material is softened in a hot water bath or warm oven and shaped directly onto the patient (Fig. 10.1A). This system uses a U-frame (for head only) or S-frame (head and shoulders) in which the thermoplastic will attach when heated and softened and stretches from the tip of the nose to the baseplate, where the U- or S-frame is indexed and locked down. Although this system is very easy to use and provides a snug fit for excellent fixation, it also can, in some cases, exhibit shrinkage; to compensate for this, it is usually prepared with spacers added at the initial stage with thickness dependent on the amount of shrinkage observed by the user. Removing these spacers, during treatment, when tightness and shrinkage become apparent makes things more comfortable for the patient and reduces the need for a new shell, which would, in turn, need a new plan.

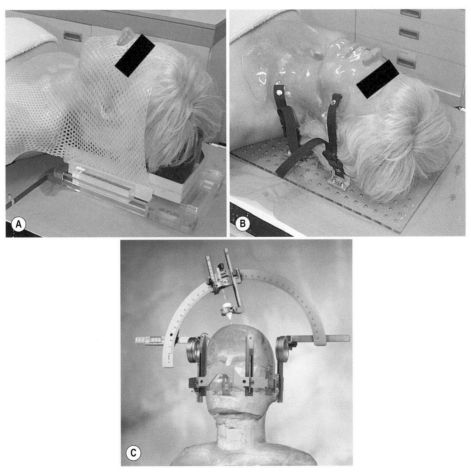

Fig. 10.1 (A) Thermoplastic shell (Orfit). (B) Vacuum-formed Perspex shell. (C) Stereotactic frame (Leksell). (With kind permission from Elekta, Stockholm.)

A reinforced thermoplastic is also available that improves rigidity, comfort, and immobilisation. Solid thermoplastic reinforcement strips, melted into the perforated sheet, provide rigid fixation and rotational stability necessary for treatments requiring more precise immobilisation, such as IMRT and conformal radiotherapy treatments.

These thermoplastic shells are a particularly attractive alternative to the vacuum-formed shells to those centres that do not have extensive pretreatment preparation facilities. The material is easily moulded, generally transparent and the perforations allow visual assessment of the final fit.

Patient Head Shells

Previously, the majority of patients receiving radiotherapy to the head and neck region were immobilised using a custom-made shell that accurately fits to provide effective and reproducible positioning of the head at all stages of planning and treatment. However, in most cases, thermoplastic shells have taken over because of improvement in speed of production and reproducibility. The custom-made plastic shell is still used by some centres for electron treatments where wax build up is to be moulded to the shell.

Typically, the process used to fabricate a clear plastic shell (see Fig. 10.1B) requires a plaster cast of the patient's head to first be produced. The transparency of the plastic enables the accuracy of fit to be checked with minor adjustments being made to ensure the shell is a good fit to achieve the optimal position for treatment, while maintaining patient comfort.

Typically, the following steps are required to produce a full head shell:

1. The patient should assume the position to be adopted in the treatment room; this usually involves a headrest that supports the neck and inclines the head at the required angle for treatment. Separate impressions are taken of the front and back halves of the head.
2. An impression of the back half of the patient's head is made, using for example, a plaster of Paris bandage or dental alginate, which covers an area up to a coronal plane at the level of the ears.
3. Before taking a similar impression of the front half of the head, a few precautions are necessary to ensure patient comfort. The patient should breathe normally through the nose and separating cream should be used on the skin to enable easy removal of the plaster cast. In some circumstances, a tissue-equivalent mouth insert will be required to depress and fix the tongue.
4. The plaster bandage should be shaped carefully around the bony protuberances of the head to facilitate good fitting of the shell and to provide effective immobilisation. The two plaster impressions, front and back, must fit uniquely together once they are removed from the patient. Further, layers of plaster bandage are applied to the two halves to provide rigidity and, once hardened, are removed from the patient.
5. The two halves are fixed together with further plaster bandage over the joints and the impression is filled with a thin mix of plaster and allowed to set overnight.
6. The final solid cast is trimmed and sawed in half along a suitable coronal plane. The cast is now ready for vacuum forming.
7. The flat surface of each half cast is placed on the vacuum forming machine. A large plastic sheet is heated and stretched into a bubble before the casts are raised and the vacuum applied to form a tight skin around the surface of the moulds.
8. The excess plastic is trimmed from each shell to provide a flange that enables the two halves to be held together with plastic press-studs. Side supports are moulded and attached to the shell to enable it to be fixed to the treatment head support.

Three Dimensional Printing

With the advent of three-dimensional printing, some departments have started to use the technology to help with patient immobilisation devices. An electron mask can be created by scanning the patient's face with a three-dimensional hand scanner. The three-dimensional hand scanner can obtain a three-dimensional surface image of a patient in approximately 5 minutes and is much less stressful to the patient compared with an impression using traditional methods. This information is then used to create a surface file that can be edited to include an end-frame localisation point or a mouth-bite localisation and printed using acrylic or other plastic materials.

Information can also be obtained and printed from CT scans using the TPS. Structures that have been outlined in a TPS can be exported and used to print immobilisation devices or bolus as defined on the TPS.

Nonshell Fixation Systems

These systems of head restraint are based on a custom impression of the patient's maxillary teeth and hard palate fixed to a plastic dental bite block (tray). Some designs incorporate a vacuum applied through the bite block that secures it to the maxillary structures; a vacuum pump is placed on the treatment couch and attaches to the mouth tray via a suction tube. Any decrease in pressure indicated by the vacuum gauge is indicative of a misplacement of the bite block. The mouthpiece is attached to two hollow carbon-fibre composite columns mounted on a baseplate by a patient-specific fixation set consisting of a transverse plate and an angle plate. Moving the plates against each other gives enough degrees of freedom to provide exact positioning. Once adjusted, the fixation set stays assembled throughout the entire treatment ensuring precise repositioning for the next fraction. A laser localiser box, consisting of side Perspex plates and top plate, are attached to the baseplate for daily set-up. Etched lines on the plate aid in visualising the laser lines projected on the plates. This localiser box is removed before treatment.

This type of nonshell fixation can be as accurate as head shell methods provided that no displacement of the mouth bite occurs that could compromise the rigidity of the system. Patients that may be unsuitable for shell-type immobilisation, such as children and phobic patients, will often prefer this technique; however, because of limitations imposed by the system design, it is unsuitable for use with tumours of the lower oral cavity and neck.

Stereotactic Frames

Stereotactic frames were originally designed for stereotactic intracranial surgery, biopsy and electrode placement, but have since been extensively adopted for radiosurgery head immobilisation, (see Fig. 10.1C). The high level of precision required for radiosurgery, such as Gamma Knife® and X-knife® systems, necessitates a means of relating three-dimensional patient image coordinates to three-dimensional locations in frame coordinates to submillimetre accuracy. The most common system in use is the Leksell Stereotactic System® Frame, which is rigidly attached to the patient's head using four small screws placed with local anaesthetic. The frame is shown in Fig. 10.1C. The frame provides the basis for target coordinate determination and is used to immobilise and position the patient's head within the radiosurgery collimator helmet. The centre coordinates of the target volume are positioned at the intersection of the beams (from 200 cobalt sources for the Gamma Knife) so that target-centering is always achieved within this geometrically rigid system. Relocatable versions of the stereotactic frame are also available that are closer in design to the head-arc fixation method.

Body Immobilisation

Numerous techniques are available for immobilisation of areas other than the head and neck. The major devices used are best discussed in relation to their site-specific needs:

Breast. Treatment of the breast commonly requires the use of three fields: two coplanar glancing beams to the breast and a supraclavicular field. All fields will often make use of the asymmetric collimators to bring one edge of each field to the beam central axis, thereby removing the effect of beam divergence from that one edge. This does not remove the penumbra, and the alignment of the superior edges of the breast fields with the inferior edges of the supraclavicular fields is critical. To achieve accuracy in this set-up requires careful positioning of the patient so that all fields can be treated without moving the patient. The use of a specially designed breast board is preferred. The device may consist of a support which inclines the patient's upper body and provides an elbow support and/or a hand-grip for the patient to grasp while holding the arm/s above the head; all these positions can be varied to meet the individual requirements of the patient's treatment and locked into position. Linear and angular measurement scales allow the set-up to be recorded and reproduced at each fraction.

There is significant evidence that cardiac doses received by patients undergoing left breast radiotherapy lead to increased risk of long-term cardiovascular side effects [1].

Modern techniques such as deep inspiration breath hold (DIBH) is when the patient inhales a comfortable 70% of their maximum inhale and holds their breath during gated treatment where the beam is only on during breath hold. This technique utilises the patient's own anatomy to reduce dose to the heart and lung [2]. An inflated lung pushes the breast tissue up and away from the body isolating it more, while simultaneously pushing the heart inferiorly and posteriorly away from the treatment field.

For patients with large pendulous breasts, there are several immobilisation devices available, such as the Vac-Fix™ bag, a wireless bra or breast cups.

Pelvic region. This is one of the most difficult areas of the body to provide effective immobilisation. Some systems use a single sheet of thermoplastic over the entire abdomen or pelvis that fixes to a baseplate; this is a larger version of that described for the head. An alternative to this is to use a large sealed plastic bag loosely filled with small expanded polystyrene spheres, the Vac-Fix™. The bag is manually formed round the patient while the air pressure in the bag is gradually reduced using a vacuum pump. At approximately half atmospheric pressure, the bag becomes rigid and fits firmly around the patient, preventing any significant movement. The rigidity can be maintained throughout a course of treatment and until the vacuum is released, when the bag and contents may be re-used for another patient. A variety of shapes and sizes of bag are available to immobilise any part of the anatomy or the whole of the patient, for total body irradiation (TBI), for example. The attenuation in the polystyrene is minimal, but being opaque, consideration must be given to the beam entry ports during the initial evacuation. Radiation damage to the plastic will eventually cause vacuum failure and necessitate the replacement of the bag. Other devices, such as ankle stocks and foot rests, can minimise movement by impeding body rotation or slippage on the treatment couch. The use of a belly-board for prone patients, providing a cut-out in the patient support, which allows the abdomen to fall anteriorly, ensures that much of the radiosensitive small intestine falls out of the high dose region.

Thorax. For modern radiotherapy, the problems imposed by respiratory movement can be considerable. Normal breathing causes movement of the chest wall and introduces uncertainties with regard to target volume position during treatment. These uncertainties are usually allowed for by introducing appropriate margins to the volume definition at the planning phase. However, these increased margins may have a significant effect on normal tissue doses and therefore have a limiting effect on the target dose. Effective compensation for these movements may involve either tracking of markers on the skin surface or identification of internal lung movement. Tracking the movement of the chest can be achieved using markers that can be followed using video cameras and calculating coordinate shifts that trigger a treatment pause if tolerances are exceeded. The tracking of internal organ movement is called IGRT; these systems use either ultrasound or x-ray tomographic imaging methods to monitor and compare organ positions with the original CT planning images. This topic will be discussed further later in this chapter.

STEREOTACTIC ABLATIVE BODY RADIATION THERAPY

SABR uses large doses of radiation to ablate the tumour which results in a long treatment time for the patient. With the additional length of each treatment fraction, the focus moves further to patient comfort, positional stability and reproducibility of treatment position. It is suggested that patients are positioned supine in a comfortable and reproducible position with their arms above their heads, although alternative positions may be required for individual patients.

Devices such as vacuum bags and thermoplastic moulds can be used to achieve patient comfort and stability. Custom devices may also be used for immobilisation and to facilitate abdominal compression. The immobilisation device should allow for patient and tumour imaging as necessary using any required imaging techniques and not interfere with dose calculation or treatment delivery. The most popular immobilisation solution in the U.K. is the use of a wing board with knee support, with or without vacuum immobilisation.

SURFACE-GUIDED RADIOTHERAPY

Surface guided radiotherapy (SGRT) is a rapidly growing technique that uses sets of stereoscopic cameras and projectors to track a patient's surface in three-dimensional for both set up and image guidance during treatment. It can be used for most areas and works by the system having two or more sets of stereoscopic cameras and a projector. Each projector emits its own unique dot matrix image over the patient. The cameras can individually see the pattern projected and use the information to extrapolate the three-dimensional contour of the patient in real time. This information can then be matched to the expected contour of the patient from the planning CT scan. The addition of this equipment can help with set-up as it will show set-up errors as the patient is being positioned. It can also be used as part of IGRT to track the patient to make sure they do not move during treatment, or combined with gated radiotherapy, to allow implantation of breath-hold techniques and automatically switch the beam off when the patient is out of position.

VOLUME DEFINITIONS

Accurate treatment depends on voluming. The parameters used in defining treatment volumes are described in detail in two documents published by the International Commission on Radiation Units and Measurements (ICRU), Reports 50 and 62, 'Prescribing, Recording and Reporting Photon Beam Therapy' [3,4].

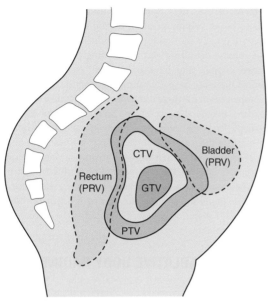

Fig. 10.2 Prostate showing clinical target volume (*CTV*, gross tumour volume (*GTV*, planning organs at risk volume (*PRV*), planning target volume (*PTV*), bladder and rectum.

The following are a transcript of the definitions:

- *Gross tumour volume (GTV)* is the gross palpable or visible/demonstrable extent and location of the malignant growth.
- *Clinical target volume (CTV)* is a tissue volume that contains a GTV and/or subclinical microscopic malignant disease, which has to be eliminated. This volume thus has to be treated adequately to achieve the aim of therapy: cure or palliation.
- *Planning target volume (PTV)* is a geometrical concept, and it is defined to select appropriate beam size and beam arrangement, taking into consideration the net effect of all the possible geometrical variations and inaccuracies to ensure that the prescribed dose is actually absorbed in the CTV.
- *Treatment volume* is the volume enclosed by an isodose surface, selected and specified by the radiation oncologist as being appropriate to achieve the purpose of treatment.
- *OAR* are normal tissues whose radiation sensitivity may significantly influence treatment planning and/or prescribed dose.

ICRU 62 is the supplementary report to ICRU 50 and discusses in more detail the complex factors that account for delineation of the PTV. An internal margin (IM) is defined to accommodate for the variations in size, shape and position of the CTV as a result of anatomical variations caused by organ movement. An additional set-up margin (SM) must be then added to allow for the uncertainties of patient-beam position. Whereas the IM is required to allow for a physiological process, the SM is required to allow for the technical factors that cause uncertainties. The SM may be reduced by improved immobilisation of the patient and improved set-up accuracy. The IM can only be reduced through techniques such as respiratory gating or IGRT The OAR volumes will also exhibit the same uncertainties in position and these will also require a margin to be added; the concept of planning organs at risk volume (PRV) is analogous to the PTV (Fig. 10.2).

NONCOMPUTED TOMOGRAPHY CONTOURING DEVICES

Contours are all important in producing dose distributions. The value of radiation treatment planning depends on the reproducibility of the shape of the patient on a day-to-day basis throughout the course of treatment. The couch where the patient contour will be taken, therefore should be identical in every respect to the couch on which that patient will be treated. It is imperative that the patient is correctly positioned before the contour is taken for planning purposes. Since the advent of radiotherapy treatment planning, a variety of physical devices have been available for taking patient contours. The simplest of these consists of a material (lead strip, flex curve) that can be bent around the patient and retains the shape, while being transferred to paper to trace the contour.

Adjustable templates have been used that allow for more complex shapes to be transposed. A large number of adjustable pins or rods (3-mm diameter) held in a frame can accurately reproduce the surface shape in an axial plane. The frame is transferred to a drawing board and the contour traced onto paper.

Another simple method of obtaining a contour(s) from an immobilisation shell is by fixing the shell within a frame so that a movable pin that can rotate around the plane to be contoured provides radial distance measurements; this system relies on radial coordinate measurements to transpose the contour shape of the required plane to paper. Many of these physical devices involving the use of contact techniques have been superseded by noncontact devices such as laser imaging/optical devices or through the use of computerised axial tomography; the latter will be described in detail in the following sections.

The use of optical systems, which have the benefit of no direct patient contact, have been used to provide both single and multiple contours of the patient in the treatment position. These systems are commonly installed within the simulator room and use the in-room alignment lasers (two laterals and one sagittal) that project both an axial and a vertical line onto the patient's skin. Multiple views of these laser projections can be imaged by using four Charge-coupled device cameras, mounted at ceiling height in each corner of the room, focused on the laser lines. Software manipulation of these four images enables a reconstruction of an axial contour and a sagittal contour. Multiple contours of the patient can be acquired by moving the couch either longitudinally (axials) or laterally (sagittals) and capturing images at each position.

This remote method of contour acquisition has many advantages over the physical methods described above; the key benefits are its inherent noncontact with the patient and the technique requires no manual handling of a device. Optical systems provide digital images of the patient's external contour that can quickly and easily be transferred to the TPS and are generally compatible with the planning software. The ability of these systems to provide three-dimensional skin contours are generally obsolete in all but the very rarest of cases (e.g. bariatric patients). See Fig. 10.3.

PHYSICAL SIMULATION

The treatment simulator is essentially a diagnostic x-ray unit that emulates the geometrical movement of an isocentric linear accelerator. The simulator had been an aid to radiotherapy for nearly half a century, and enabled highly accurate localisation of the target volume, the verification of the proposed treatment plan and, in some cases, even precise visualisation of the organs at risk.

The unit allowed real-time imaging of the beam portal and a facility to produce x-ray films of each treatment field.

These machines have now been superseded with the advancements of virtual simulation (CT simulation) as a result of the power of modern computers and advancements in CT scanning technology.

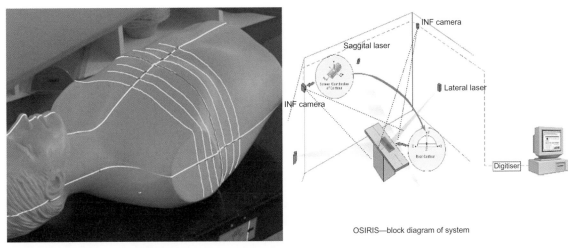

Fig. 10.3 OSIRIS system. (With kind permission from Qados Ltd., Sandhurst.)

COMPUTED TOMOGRAPHY SIMULATION

The term *CT virtual simulation* was first introduced in a publication by George Sherouse in 1987 [5] who recognised that a suitable software package in conjunction with a diagnostic CT scanner could be developed that would emulate a conventional radiotherapy simulator. In the early 1980s, the use of CT scanners in treatment planning amounted to providing axial images that could be transferred to the TPS. The process of plan optimisation and verifying the set-up before treatment was purely a role for the TPS and the physical simulator with no significant manipulation of the three-dimensional CT data to augment this process. At this time, the use of the beam's eye view (BEV) allowed the visualisation of a beam shape relative to the target contour, bony anatomy and other contoured organs. The BEV gave the planner the ability to optimise beam positions, shapes and orientation in the same manner as could be achieved radiographically on the simulator.

In 1983, Goitein and Abrams [6] introduced the use of the digitally reconstructed radiograph (DRR), a virtual radiograph or film of the patient. The calculation of DRRs is computationally intensive consisting of ray-line projection, interpolation, line integration and grey-scale mapping of the CT data. For many years, the inability of computers to provide fast array processing slowed the introduction of virtual simulation into the treatment planning process.

The automatic registration of the BEV and DRR has provided powerful tools to enable the planner to achieve on the TPS what was available on the simulator but with the added benefits of CT visualisation (Fig. 10.4A). With the increased computing power of the modern age, the speed of DRR calculation is subsecond, which has led to the extinction of the simulator in most departments.

In the early 1990s, specialised graphics workstations were introduced that allowed fast three-dimensional array processing for ray-tracing, volume rendering and image reconstruction. Commercial systems became available at this time and, with the rapid improvement in PC processor speeds in recent years, have resulted in CT virtual simulation becoming more available and widely used in radiotherapy (see Fig. 10.4B).

CT virtual simulation is a combination of the physical process of using a CT scanner as an alternative to the physical simulator described above and the virtual process of simulator emulation using software programs.

CT localisation requires the patient to be supported and immobilised in the same position as for radiotherapy treatment. This can be more difficult compared with the conventional simulator, which is designed specifically to mimic the linear accelerator patient support systems. The CT scanner must have a flat-top couch that can accept all these patient support accessories.

The process of marking the patient is facilitated by a laser system consisting of two fixed lateral lasers, the plane of these lasers being offset from the CT aperture plane by typically 500 mm, and a sagittal laser that can be moved laterally to overcome the fixed nature of the CT couch. The laser system can define the origin of a coordinate system that relates to the treatment machine coordinate system by shift distances or, in some cases, define the precise plan isocentre coordinates.

CT scanners used for simulation are invariably diagnostic scanners that have been adapted with flat table-top and external (to the gantry) laser systems. However, the advent of large bore scanners specifically for radiotherapy planning has enabled these systems to be not only complementary but adopted as an alternative to the physical simulator. These scanners have apertures of 80 to 85 cm compared with the conventional 70 cm and have scan field of view (SFOV) that is 10 to 15 cm larger than the diagnostic SFOV. For breast treatments, where the ipsilateral arm is raised above the head and subtends an angle close to 90 degrees, then the large aperture scanners provide increased functionality (Fig. 10.5).

The CT simulation process requires a scout (pilot) view to be taken to identify the required scan volume and suitable scan parameters. Axial image acquisition can be performed in either axial or spiral mode; the latter enables a continuous movement of the tube/couch rather than stepped movement in the axial mode. The patient CT study is passed to the virtual simulation workstation.

VIRTUAL SIMULATION

The physical simulator used a real-time image using either a fluoroscopic screen with image intensifier or an amorphous silicon panel; this may have been followed by exposure of a radiographic film to provide localisation of the treatment volume, visualisation of the treatment field and verification of the plan design.

The CT simulator equivalence to the physical simulator includes software capabilities to contour target volumes and critical structures, placement of treatment isocentre, beam design and generation of DRRs. Many of the software control features are incorporated into three-dimensional planning systems and are often merged into one

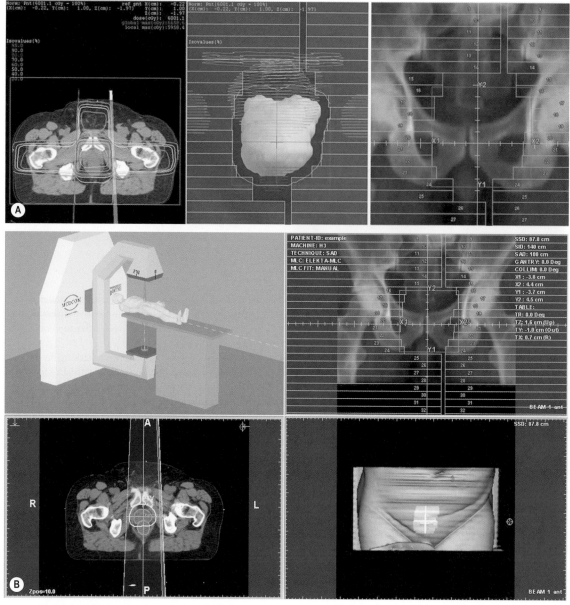

Fig. 10.4 (A) Beams eye view on a treatment planning system with digitally reconstructed radiograph on virtual simulator. (B) Screen shot of virtual simulator with surface rendering and transverse slice.

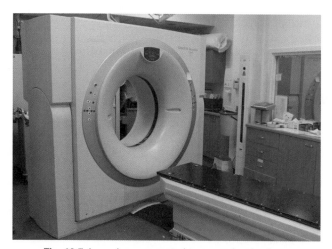

Fig. 10.5 Large bore computed tomography simulator.

software suite. The ability to bring in and fuse other images to the dataset (MRI, PET-CT) and view simultaneously with a press of a button has major advantages.

The treatment planning portion of the CT simulation process starts with the definition of a treatment reference point that can either coincide exactly with the position of the isocentre or alternatively, can be an estimate of its position. The former method will require the definition of the target volume to precisely define the treatment isocentre and will require the oncologist to be present; whereas the latter method does not require the target volume to be defined and the final isocentre position can be found using shift coordinates. These shift distances (Fig. 10.6) are relative to the reference point and can be applied at the first treatment to align precisely the isocentre to the target. The shift coordinate method is commonly used in a busy department where there is limited time to wait until targets are contoured or where the oncologist is not available during the scanning session.

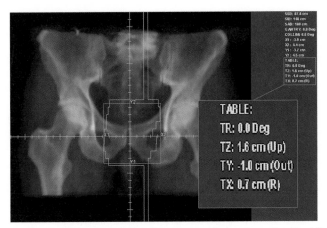

Fig. 10.6 Beam's eye view/digitally reconstructed radiograph with shift information.

A TYPICAL HEAD AND NECK COMPUTED TOMOGRAPHY SIMULATION PROCEDURE

Localisation requires the thermoplastic shell to be attached to the flat indexed CT couch to emulate exactly the patient positioning on the treatment machine.

The scanning parameters are usually a trade-off between maximising DRR resolution and keeping the number of slices to a manageable size (typically a 3-mm slice thickness and a 1.5-spiral pitch). The scanning extent is determined from the pilot (scout) view and the external contours are often produced at a remote virtual simulation workstation while previewing the scanned slices.

A reference slice plane is selected and the patient reference origin coordinates created and transferred to the CT couch and/or lasers. The CT longitudinal couch, vertical couch and sagittal laser positions are set to define the patient reference origin and the patient's thermoplastic shell is marked. The patient session is now finished. An alternative approach is to mark the patient before scanning and to set this position as the patient reference origin.

Virtual simulation requires marking of the GTV, CTV, PTV and OARs; the isocentre and field parameters can then be defined using the TPS. The plan is sent for calculation and optimisation to the TPS and exported back to the virtual simulator workstation for verification. The DRRs for all beams are printed (laser imager) and approved by the oncologist.

Shift coordinates are printed from the relationship between the isocentre to patient reference origin coordinates. These are transferred to the treatment machine with the plan details. Worksheets and DRRs are then printed (see Fig. 10.6). Note that most radiotherapy centres are moving toward a 'paperless' environment where plans and images are transferred and approved electronically.

The advantages of CT virtual simulation can be summarised as follows:

- Full three-dimensional simulation allowing unique verification of beam coverage and avoidance in three dimensions
- Beams can be simulated and verified that are not possible with conventional simulation, for example, vertex fields
- The verification image, the DRR, can contain more information than conventional simulation and can be manipulated to enhance tumour visualisation
- There is a much closer connection to diagnostic information with CT simulation allowing integration of multimodality images

During the early use of CT simulation, it was evident that the inability to image organ movement (e.g. lung) was a significant disadvantage over the fluoroscopy of physical simulation. However, the improvement in image acquisition and reconstruction speeds has provided the ability to follow respiratory movement. The technique is often called respiratory gated acquisition and four-dimensional viewing. This method enables images to be acquired at a rate of more than 16 frames per second that enables the full movement of the patient's diaphragm to be visualised within a movie loop. The definition of lung tumour margins can now be assessed in three dimensions.

MULTIMODALITY IMAGES FOR PLANNING

CT imaging plays a crucial role in radiotherapy planning as it provides the electron density information that is required to correct the absorbed dose for the different tissues through which the beams will pass.

CT imaging also provides excellent definition between tissues having marked differences in x-ray attenuation values (e.g. air/bone/soft tissue); however, the contrast of these images is poor for structures with similar electron densities (e.g. tumour/soft tissue).

MRI is based on the measurement of radiofrequency radiation resulting from transitions induced between nuclear spin states of hydrogen atoms (protons) in the presence of strong external magnetic fields. Unlike CT, where the signal intensity is dependent on x-ray attenuation and its contrast on the electron density of tissues, MRI depends on the intrinsic tissue properties associated with proton densities and spin relaxation times. Therefore MRI has the ability to differentiate between tissue of similar density, thus providing better delineation, not only of tumour extent, but also of the adjacent critical soft tissue organs.

MRI also provides unrestricted multiplanar, volumetric, vascular and functional information.

Some of the problems associated with using MRI for treatment planning are:

1. inherent image distortion, particularly at the periphery of the image (typically 3 mm for heads and up to 15 mm for pelvic images).
2. pixel intensities are not related to electron density values and therefore cannot be used for heterogeneity correction (i.e. density/dose) when calculating treatment plan dose distributions.
3. the physical restrictions of the MRI scanner mean that a patient cannot be easily positioned in the treatment position. A quantitative method called *image registration* is used that provides fusion of CT and MRI image studies.

MRI data are transferred to a TPS where the therapy CT images and the MRI images are registered. Manual and automatic methods of registration are now available as part of sophisticated software systems provided with CT simulators. The manual methods involve matching fiducials that are visualised on both CT and MRI; these fiducials are opaque markers or bony structures so that image translation in the three coordinates directions achieve a match between the two studies. The accuracy of image registration can be assessed by the accuracy to which the fiducial markers match.

Once the two image data sets are matched, then volume contouring on the MRI images is automatically translated to the CT study. This technique provides the advantages of the MRI images for tumour delineation while maintaining the CT study for accurate calculation of the treatment dose distribution.

Automatic registration methods, such as mutual information, use rigid and nonrigid matrix transformations that are able to compensate for rotational as well as translational differences between the two image sets.

Imaging modalities that provide functional or tumour kinetic information for radiotherapy treatment planning have become widely available. PET and single photon emission CT (SPECT) produce nuclear medicine images that enable improved staging of malignant disease and improved treatment planning by ensuring that gross tumour volumes are more accurately defined. Information from these functional imaging modalities can be used to design more conformal radiation dose distributions and to prescribe additional dose to specific tumour micro-regions.

The specific activity of the radiopharmaceutical, fluoro-2-deoxyglucose (^{18}F-FDG), produces uptake in malignant tissue that enables highly accurate determination of the extent of solid tumour spread. FDG is taken up by glucose transporters and its concentration can be measured (images) by the retained activity within various tissues. FDG uptake correlates strongly with the presence of cancer.

The introduction of combined PET/CT scanners has improved the availability of this new modality. The PET images are superimposed upon the CT images, both of which are simultaneously acquired during a single scan session. Planning can be performed either in treatment position, requiring modifications to the scanning protocols, or in diagnostic position with image registration being used to accommodate the change in patient position between functional image and treatment planning patient position.

Specialised software can register the PET/CT study with the therapy planning CT study to enable contours on the PET images to be transposed to the planning images.

There is increasing evidence that, in many clinical situations, radiotherapy treatment may be planned more accurately if supplementary functional images of the patient are available. In practice though, the lack of access to PET and the problem of image registration have restricted the use of combined anatomical and functional information.

- PET is prohibitively expensive, which has limited its routine clinical use to only larger oncology facilities.
- Multimodality image registration is a difficult problem, which is further complicated by the significant anatomical changes that may occur between the different imaging sessions because of surgery, chemotherapy, patient weight change or fluid collection.

PORTAL VERIFICATION AND IMAGE-GUIDED TREATMENTS

Portal Imaging

Confirmation of the accuracy of the delivered beam is an essential part of quality assurance. This is achieved primarily by imaging the beam portal using the linear accelerator before, during or after a treatment exposure.

This can be achieved using a choice of film. Therapy verification film, a slow film housed in a light-proof packet, can be left in place for the full treatment exposure. Alternatively, a faster film housed in a cassette with stainless steel intensifying screens requiring a smaller incident dose can be used; the advantage of this method is that it is possible (although perhaps not practical) to develop the image and analyse the outcome before delivering the full treatment dose.

The disadvantages of film are the need for on-site processing facilities, the time delay in processing, inability to manipulate the image quality without re-exposure and the resultant long-term storage considerations.

Hardcopy films are now superseded by electronic or digital forms of imaging. Solid state devices or electronic portal imaging devices (EPID) are now integral components of the linear accelerator. These devices may consist of an amorphous silicon detector panel housed on a retractable arm, which is an integral component of the linear accelerator gantry. In this way, the panel is always perpendicular to the beam central axis, thus avoiding image distortion. Detector panels have a physical size of 30 × 40 cm and this allows practical imaging of fields, typically 20 × 25 cm. Image quality from amorphous silicon devices is considerably superior to that which can be achieved with film or optical camera-based systems.

Protocols for the frequency of imaging are determined locally, although typically, these consist of imaging the fields for the first three to five fractions to establish accuracy and reproducibility, and then periodically throughout the rest of the course to ensure consistency.

Analysis of the images produced may be qualitative; that is, an eyeball assessment in conjunction with the software measuring tools or, increasingly, may use the assistance of an automatic image registration tool to provide quantitative displacements. The image registration or matching process requires user-defined anatomy to be outlined on a reference image (typically the DRR or the conventional simulation image). The same anatomical features are then outlined on the portal image and the software will overlay these contours, thus providing a field-edge displacement value for the lateral, longitudinal and rotational positions. As a result, it is possible to determine whether the isocentre position is within predetermined tolerances or whether adjustment is required.

There are many advantages to digital imaging systems; physical storage problems are removed, although consideration must be given to the need for future data retrieval. Software tools can be used to manipulate the image to aid viewing and analysis; multiple users can view the image and remote access facilities can be implemented. From a treatment delivery aspect, however, the biggest advantage is the ability for on-line assessment of images and immediate adjustment of patient position to achieve greater accuracy.

Image-Guided Radiotherapy

Conformal radiotherapy depends on geometrical and dose shaping to optimise the dose distribution to the known planning target volume. Techniques to achieve this involve the use of multileaf collimation to shape each field to a beam's eye projection of the PTV (geometric conformality) and intensity modulation of the beam (IMRT) to achieve dose shaping of the beam (dose conformality). These methods do not take into account the fourth dimension to radiotherapy, time, which can extend from seconds to days.

A number of time-related factors introduce significant uncertainties in radiotherapy.

1. The movement of target and critical tissues during treatment (seconds to minutes).
2. The movement of organs between treatment fractions (days).
3. The dynamic movement of the beam delivery method (seconds to minutes).

The interplay between the dynamic beam delivery motion and tissue motion during treatment can result in both over- and under-dosage of the target volume.

Two questions that have involved considerable debate are: What are the effects of organ motion on treatment planning images? And, How can we acquire information on organ motion? The advent of ultra-fast CT acquisition from multislice scanners has enabled time-dependent organ position data to be captured. This large quantity of data can be used during the treatment planning process, but the contouring of the hundreds of image slices is not possible using conventional manual methods. Automatic organ tools have been developed that enable tracking of organ movement (four-dimensional imaging).

During treatment, these organ movements must also be monitored to correlate with planning (verification) data.

Several methods of image-guided techniques are available:
- Radiopaque markers that can be tracked using video cameras.
- Ultrasound systems that determine organ positions before treatment.
- Diagnostic x-ray systems mounted on the linear accelerator that can provide orthogonal images or CT (cone beam reconstructed) images including four-dimensional cone beam images.

- Treatment room CT scanners that are adjacent to the linear accelerator and can provide pretreatment or posttreatment CT images.
- MRI-Linac, whereby a patient can have an MRI scan during treatment.

The advantages of real time daily imaging allow for the assessment of organ motion, patient weight loss or tumour shrinkage, and action can be taken to improve treatment accuracy by adapting treatment [7].

REFERENCES

[1] Taylor C. Radiation-related heart disease following treatment of breast cancer (abstract). Radiother Oncol 2011;99:S76.

[2] Latty D, Stuart KE, Wang W, Ahern V. Review of deep inspiration breath-hold techniques for the treatment of breast cancer. J Med Radiat Sci 2015 Mar;62(1):74–81.

[3] ICRU Report 50. Prescribing, recording and reporting photon beam therapy. International Commission on Radiation Units and Measurements; 1993.

[4] ICRU Report 62. Prescribing, recording and reporting photon beam therapy (supplement to ICRU Report 50). International Commission on Radiation Units and Measurements; 1999.

[5] Sherouse GW, Mosher CE, Rosenman J, Chaney EL. Virtual Simulation: Concept and Implementation. In: Bruinvis, et al. editors. The Use of Computers in Radiation Therapy. North-Holland: Elsevier; 1987.

[6] Goitein M, Abrams M. Multi-dimensional treatment planning: beam's eye view, back projection, and projection through CT sections. Int J Radiat Oncol Biol Phys 1983;9:789–97.

[7] Kataria T, Gupta D, Goyal S, Bisht SS, Basu T, Abhishek A, et al. Clinical outcomes of adaptive radiotherapy in head and neck cancers. Br J Radiol 2016;89:0085–6.

11

Radiation Treatment Planning: Beam Models, Principles and Practice

Maria Mania Aspradakis

CHAPTER OUTLINE

INTRODUCTION

Radiation therapy is being administered using either externally applied radiation beams of low (kilovolt) or high (megavolt) energy photons, electrons, protons, or heavy ions or internally or superficially applied radiation sources (brachytherapy). Whatever the type of radiation used, treatment planning (TP) is the necessary step in the treatment chain that enables the treatment of a patient with radiation. It encompasses all work involved in the preparation of a clinically acceptable and deliverable treatment. The goal is to determine a dose distribution within the patient that will destroy the tumour while sparing healthy tissue as much as possible. In palliative radiotherapy (RT) the goal is to provide relief from pain usually from metastatic disease. In curative or radical RT the aim is to kill cancer cells while taking into account the radiosensitivity and proximity of healthy organs—organs at risk (ORs). Table 11.1 contains examples of typical dose tolerances for normal tissues.

Appropriate imaging techniques are needed to identify tumour volumes. Treatment volumes for TP, referred to as the planning target volume (PTV), usually contain those outlined from imaging, as it is important to account for uncertainties in volume definition and motion

during treatment. The methodology followed in the prescription of radiation therapy in terms of volume definition as well as production of a treatment plan is provided in a series of International Commission on Radiation Units and Measurements (ICRU) reports [1–6]. The radiosensitivity of healthy tissues must be taken into consideration during TP and this is possible through the knowledge of tolerance doses for the OR. The most recent compilation of tolerances doses can be found in a series of publications by Quantitative Analyses of Normal Tissue Effects in the Clinic (QUANTEC) [7]. Serial organs are those that loose functionality when they receive a dose above a certain threshold; for example, the spinal cord. Organs classified as parallel continue to provide functionality even if part of them is completely damaged by radiation (e.g. lung), and there are organs that respond as both serial and parallel, such as the heart. In this case it is important to minimise the volume of the organ that receives more than a threshold dose. For example, in the case of lung the aim is to minimise the volume of lung receiving more than 20 Gray (Gy), because it is known that doses above this threshold lead to radiation pneumonitis.

The first step in TP is volume definition (referred often as contouring) and dose prescription. Target volumes and OR together with the

TABLE 11.1	Typical Normal Tissue Tolerance Doses for Generally Accepted Risks		
Organ	**Typical dose limits**		**Comments**
Spinal cord	45 Gy		Although a serial organ, the length of the cord receiving the dose may be taken into account
Lung	V20 (e.g. <32%) mean lung dose <18 Gy		Normally consider total volume of both lungs (if the GTV or PTV lies within the lung then its volume should be subtracted from the total lung volume and higher V20 volumes may need to be accepted)
Heart	<40 Gy to entire heart		Normally the heart volume outlined will include blood
	No more than 1/3 of heart volume to receive 60 Gy		
Kidney	Whole kidney 12 Gy		Essential to ensure unirradiated kidney is functioning or a non-functioning kidney is preferentially sacrificed
	1/3 kidney 16 Gy		
Liver	Whole liver <21 Gy		
	1/3 liver 30 Gy		
Lens	6 Gy		If cataract formation is the concern then consider the consequence of any treatment compromise against future cataract removal
Rectum	% of 2 Gy/fraction dose for 74 Gy prescribed dose	(%) Max. vol.	
	68	60	An example of a DVH based dose constraint rather than a single volume or dose threshold
	81	50	
	88	30	
	95	15	
	100	3	

Note that these values may vary for individual situations because of clinical condition and other therapies increasing radiosensitivity and that correction must be made for different fractionation.

dose prescription are specified by clinicians. A prerequisite for this step is the information on the anatomy of the patient. Modern radiation therapy in most cases uses three-dimensional patient information from computed tomography (CT) or magnetic resonance imaging (MRI). The patient is ideally imaged in the treatment position and planning volumes are either identified exclusively on these images or with the aid of additional imaging modalities (such as positron emission tomography) providing further information on the location and extent of the tumour.

The second step in TP involves the generation of a treatment plan. A treatment plan contains all information needed to realise the dose prescription. Prerequisite for this is an adequate description of the radiation device used for the treatment, the anatomical information of the patient, and a method to calculate the dose in the patient. This task is carried out by staff groups (medical physicists, planning radiographers, dose planners, or dosimetrists) specifically trained in the generation of treatment plans, nowadays almost exclusively using computerised systems. Modern treatment planning systems (TPSs) are software suites comprising different tools for the visualisation of the patient anatomy, the definition of volumes, and the simulation of the treatment unit and of radiation transport and energy deposition in different media, as well as tools for the calculation of dose statistics and the evaluation of metrics on plan quality.

The final step in the TP chain is quality assurance (QA) and verification of the planned treatment. This is typically referred to as plan or patient-specific verification, where the treatment plan is checked and its parameters are verified through an independent dose calculation method and/or measurement, depending on the complexity of the plan.

In what follows, the key aspects regarding TP are discussed in detail: patient data, beam modelling, dose calculation and treatment plan evaluation. Following this the most common TP techniques currently implemented in external beam RT are presented. Basic concepts on QA in TP are discussed in the final section of this chapter.

REPRESENTATION OF THE PATIENT FOR TREATMENT PLANNING

The Planning CT

Approximate representation of the patient anatomy for the purpose of TP is a practice of the past. Nowadays the planning CT is the minimum requirement of input on information about the anatomy of the patient needed to generate a treatment plan. A CT study comprises a series of sequential two-dimensional images of the patient. These provide a three-dimensional reconstruction on the patient anatomy required for volume definition. Sophisticated software tools on TPSs allow clinicians and planners to specify the extent of volumes of interest and design any additional volumes that could aid the production of an optimal treatment plan.

CT images, by definition, are reconstructed from the attenuation of kilovolt x-rays through the imaged body and thus they also reflect the attenuation properties of the different materials present in the body in the particular kilovolt energy used for imaging. Through a calibration procedure of materials of known properties (primarily electron or mass density) scanned under CT, a relationship between the type of material and the signal registered by the CT is derived. The CT calibration curve as implemented in any TPS defines the relationship between relative mass or electron density of media and CT numbers in terms of Hounsfield units (HU). Thus, CT images also provide information in three dimensions on the properties of tissues. This is used to calculate how radiation is attenuated and how particle energy is deposited in the patient. One of the first tasks in setting up a TPS for clinical use is to provide the correct mapping between CT numbers and relative material density and/or material properties. Whether the calibration of CT numbers is in terms of relative electron density or relative mass density and perhaps also on additional material properties depends on the input requirements of the dose calculation method.

In three dimensions, and for the purpose of dose calculation, the matrix of CT numbers is divided in voxels. The size of these becomes important when dose is to be calculated in volumes of organs of size comparable with the resolution in the original CT image study. Typical CT image separation and voxel size used for calculations in standard TP calculations is 2.5 mm. The resolution of the CT image data set can affect both how faithfully volumes are represented in a treatment plan and subsequently how accurately dose can be calculated for these volumes.

To improve visualisation of certain organs (e.g. nodes in head and neck images) on CT images contrast materials may be injected in the patient before the acquisition of the CT scan. This aids volume definition, but depending on the contrast agent used, the material composition in the patient, as present in the CT scan, may differ from that during treatment where there is no contrast material present. In most cases it has been shown that these differences are negligible, but this is something that requires verification for the contrast materials used in a clinic.

Another consideration when using CT images for TP is the presence of high-density materials in the patient, such as dental fillings and metal prosthesis. Such materials create artefacts on the images where regions of the anatomy around the metal appear distorted and with incorrect CT numbers assigned to these regions. The use of CT scanners operating in an extended CT range (up to about 30,000 HU) together with the appropriate CT calibration derived for that range can ensure that the correct material density is assigned to very large CT numbers. In addition, some CT scanners provide artefact reduction algorithms to process images and improve image quality. In the absence of both techniques to address the presence of artefacts, and as an approximation for dose calculation, it is common practice to manually identify regions with artefacts and override the CT numbers in these with those of the neighbouring structures as appropriate. Detailed guidance on the dosimetric considerations with implanted hip prostheses can be found in the report of AAPM (American Association of Physicists in Medicine) task group 63 [8].

Implanted devices in the patient, such as cardiac pacemakers, also produce artefacts, but with these the primary concern is the influence of radiation and electromagnetic interference from a linear accelerator (linac) on the operation of the device. Before TP it is advisable to obtain information from the manufacturer of the implanted device and in any case limit the dose received from scattered radiation to below 2 Gy [9,10].

Patient Immobilisation for Treatment Planning

Planning CTs are typically acquired using a flat couch top, similar to that used for treatment. However, modern patient immobilisation devices available on treatment machines use couch tops that differ in design and composition than those used during CT. In this case it is important that the couch top as well as any immobilisation device used to reproducibly position the patient for treatment is taken into consideration during TP, especially when the irradiation beam traverses through the device. A comprehensive report by the AAPM task group 176 summarised the dosimetric implications when different couch tops and immobilisation devices are involved in the treatment plan [11]. Careful dosimetry is needed to evaluate skin doses as a result of build-up effects from such devices. It is important that these devices are modelled in TP calculations either by including these as part of the patient anatomy (provided they have been present during CT scanning as in the case of body immobilisation bags or thermoplastic masks/shells), or by adding these from a library of support models representing each particular device. This is a common approach in planning systems for commercial couch tops available from different manufacturers.

Motion Management in Treatment Planning

Respiratory motion of thoracic and abdominal regions not only causes artefacts during image acquisition but also has implications on the delineation of tumour volumes. Following the nomenclature from ICRU reports (and in particular ICRU report number 62) margins are added to the gross tumour volume (GTV) to account for suspected microscopic spread, intrafraction and interfraction motion and patient setup errors. An additional margin to account for tumour motion could lead to either an overestimation or an underestimation of the dose delivered to the moving tumour [12]. From the methods to account for respiratory motion reviewed in the report of AAPM Task Group 76, the most commonly used are motion encompassing methods and in particular deep inhalation breath hold (DIBH), four-dimensional CT approaches, and respiratory gating methods. In all cases, initially the patient's free breathing pattern is recorded. In DIBH the planning CT is taken during deep inhalation and the treatment plan is prepared based on this, with treatment being delivered while in DIBH. In four-dimensional CT approaches, CT scanning is correlated with the breathing pattern with multiple CT scans taken during at least 10 different breathing phases. From all these data typically two single-CT data sets are reconstructed and registered. In the maximum intensity projection scan each voxel in the image is assigned the maximum CT number from all phases. In the average scan, each voxel is assigned the average CT number from all phases. The former is used for the delineation of the volume encompassing the tumour in its full range of motion, whereas the latter is used for dose calculation.

Magnetic Resonance–Based Planning

MRI offers superior soft tissue contrast in comparison to CT and for this reason it is common practice to register MR images with CT so that tissue delineation is carried out on the MR image with contours transferred to the CT for planning and dose calculation. Recent developments in technology lead to specific commercial solutions for certain anatomical sites, such as the prostate, where planning is based only on MRI and the information on electron density required for dose calculation is derived using mDIXON imaging and models that classify the different tissues based on that imaging [13]. This is clearly an approximation that can work for areas of the body with small tissue differentiation.

BEAM MODELLING AND DOSE CALCULATIONS FOR EXTERNAL MV PHOTON BEAM TREATMENT PLANNING

Dose calculation algorithms used for RT TP must be general to model all particle transport and energy deposition in arbitrary irradiation geometries, flexible in their implementation, and accurate (better than 3%) and fast enough to be practically useful in the clinical environment. Designing models that fulfil these requirements has been challenging and the introduction of computer technology and its availability in hospitals from the early 1990s have led to the development of the sophisticated methods currently available on most commercial TPSs. Fig. 11.1 shows the physical processes that need to be accounted for in megavolt photon beams.

Modelling the dose in the patient is a two-step process: in the first step the energy fluence from the treatment head reaching the patient surface is calculated (energy fluence modelling), and in the second this energy fluence is transported and energy is deposited in the patient (dose modelling). Mathematically this is described as the multiplication

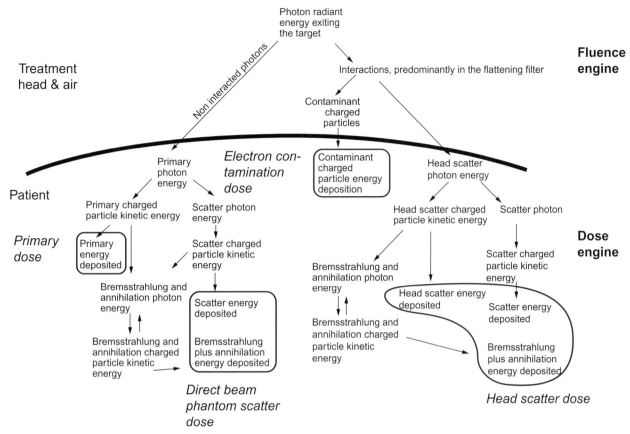

Fig. 11.1 The physical processes to be modelled in MV photon beams. From these the different components of dose are classified: primary dose, phantom scatter dose, head scatter dose and dose from contaminant electrons. The physical processes taking place in the treatment head are modelled by the fluence engine, whereas the physical processes in the patient are modelled by the dose engine (see main text). (From Ahnesjö A, Aspradakis MM. Dose calculations for external photon beams in radiotherapy. Phys Med Biiol 1999; 44(11): R99–R155.)

of two factors, both derived by modelling, and this is described in the following equation [14]:

$$\frac{D(x, d; A)}{M(A)} = \frac{D(x, d; A)}{\Psi(x; A)} \cdot \frac{\Psi(x; A)}{M(A)} \qquad \textbf{11.1}$$

where D is the dose, x is an arbitrary calculation point, d the treatment depth, A the collimator setting, M the monitor signal, and Ψ the energy fluence (Fig. 11.2). The first factor in equation 11.1 is the dose per energy fluence from direct photons at the plane of the isocentre in air and this is the outcome of dose modelling. The second factor in the equation is the calibration of the dose engine, expressed as the relationship between direct energy fluence and monitor units (MUs) under reference conditions. What follows provides some insight into fluence and dose engines as well as the calculation of MUs as implemented in modern TPS.

Modelling of the Source of Radiation

The radiation reaching the patient surface originates directly from the primary source (on linacs operating in photon mode this source is the target) and from components of the treatment head as a result of primary particles interacting with these. Extrafocal radiation, also referred to as head-scattered photon radiation, is the radiation that is scattered from the flattening filter, primary collimator, secondary jaws, physical wedges and multileaf collimators (MLCs). This can amount up to 10%

of the total radiation reaching the isocentre and at large collimator settings up to 12% of this can originate from the flattening filter.

An energy fluence engine needs to model the finite size of the radiation source, geometrical penumbra, all sources of head-scattered radiation, the backscatter into the monitor ionisation chamber, leakage radiation from collimating devices, transmission between MLC leaves and through the rounded MLC ends and changes in beam spectrum and electron contamination in megavolt (MV) photon beams. The design of such an engine needs to be flexible and tailored to different designs of treatment heads and easily configurable using a small number of measured data.

Energy fluence engines provide the number, energy, and location of particles that reach the patient. With Monte Carlo (MC) methods the total photon energy fluence and contaminant electron fluence (in photon beams) exiting the head of the accelerator can be modelled explicitly. In practice it has proved efficient and sufficient to implement what are known as multisource beam models instead. In these models different parts of the treatment head are handled as different sources of origin of scattered photons, which can be modelled separately. The algorithms modelling each of these sources implement semianalytical functions to describe the separate physical processes that take place when primary particles interact with different components in the treatment head. The parameters of these functions are typically derived through processes that minimise the differences between measured and calculated data under predefined radiation conditions. The main source of head-scattered photon radiation is the flattening filter.

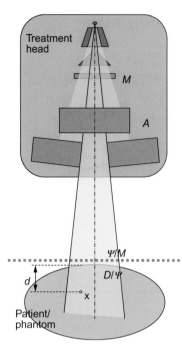

Fig. 11.2 Illustration of the separation of energy fluence modelling and dose modelling. (From Karlsson M, Ahnesjö A, Georg D, et al. Physics booklet Nr 10: independent dose calculations concepts and models. ESTRO physics booklets. Brussels: European Society for Therapeutic Radiology and Oncology; 2010. With permission.)

Charged-particle contamination in high-energy photon beams is usually modelled as a separate effect. Modelling the finite size of the direct radiation beam exiting the target, for example, becomes important at narrow collimated fields, where the field size becomes comparable to the size of the source and this influences both beam output and the shape of the penumbra of the dose profile [15,16]. Multisource beam models and the consideration of effects such as transmission from the ends and edges of MLC leaves differ among TPSs, and there are only a few scientific publications or TPS manuals that describe these in detail [6,14,17].

Modelling of Dose in the Irradiated Medium

Dose engines refer to the mathematical models that characterise and model particle transport and energy deposition in the irradiated medium. Dose engines are classified in two categories, see Table 11.2. It is the methods in the second category that are of interest nowadays and are discussed in more detail in this chapter.

Explicit Dose Modelling

In explicit dose modelling, the paths, interactions, and location of energy deposition from particles traversing the irradiated medium are simulated in detail. These are calculations from first principles and with few approximations to radiation transport physics.

The radiation transport problem is described by the radiation transport equation, also known as the Boltzmann transport equation (BTE). The equation is mathematically established by considering energy conservation when particles traverse a small volume and it separately addresses the number of particles entering and leaving this volume and being attenuated or generated in the volume. The equation provides a deterministic solution for the calculation of total differential particle fluence in the irradiated medium (the number of particles at a given energy and direction of transport). For the radiation transport problem in photon dose modelling it is assumed that positrons can be treated as electrons, bremsstrahlung radiation is neglected, and photons transported in the medium are treated either as primary or scattered photons.

Once the primary energy fluence reaching the patient is computed by the multisource fluence engine, the primary photon fluence is calculated by ray-tracing in the irradiated medium. The medium is divided in a grid matrix of calculation points, and particle transport equations are solved for this grid so that electron fluence is calculated. The multiplication of electron fluence with appropriate stopping powers gives the dose deposition at each point on the grid. At the time of writing, only one of the commercial TPSs offers this approach as an option for external beam and brachytherapy planning [18–20].

Alternative to solving the BTE is the stochastic approach based on the MC method [21–23]. This is a numerical method where pseudorandom numbers are used to sample from probability functions that describe physical phenomena. The input for probability functions is radiation attenuation data. Radiation interaction data (interaction cross sections) are needed to describe particle interactions in the media.

TABLE 11.2	Classification of Dose Engines		
Category	**Method**	**Modelling Approach**	**Characteristics/Remarks**
Factor-based	**Empirical**	Based on broad beam measured data stored as fan-line matrices divergent from a point source	Implemented together with sector integration methods to model scatter dose in irregular fields together with 1D, 2D or 3D heterogeneity corrections
Model-based	**Explicit modelling** of secondary particle transport and interaction	Deterministic solvers to the Boltzmann transport equation (BTE)	Accurate approaches; distributions tend to be influenced from discretisation effects. Only one type of this method is available on a commercial TPS (Eclipse Acuros),
		Stochastic approaches based on the Monte Carlo method	Accurate approaches; distributions tend to be noisy.
	Implicit modelling kernel-based approaches	Pencil beam kernel convolution methods	Not accurate in heterogeneous media. Ideally suited for optimisation calculations and second checks.
		Point kernel methods (superposition/ collapsed cone approaches)	Accurate in heterogeneous media, with limitations at media interfaces and high-density media. These are the current workhorses in treatment planning calculations.
		Hybrid approaches: FSPB with lateral scattering	Performance analogous to that of point kernel methods. Only one type of this approach is implemented on a commercial TPS (Eclipse AAA).

Additional input to simulations with MC is a detailed description of the irradiation geometry. Probability distributions describe how particles are transported and sampling from interaction cross-section data determines the type of interaction that each particle will undergo. With the MC method, modelling the transport of photons is more straightforward as these tend to undergo fewer interactions as they traverse media, whereas for electrons, which undergo a lot more interactions (of the order of 10^4 interaction events for an electron with energy of 1 MeV), modelling their transport involves the use of special modelling techniques. These tend to consider many electron transport steps or interactions in groups of fewer events. This is necessary for realistic computation times. Variance reduction techniques are needed to practically implement techniques based on the MC method for radiation dosimetry and TP applications. These are the methods to reduce the uncertainty in the results, with the aim to increase efficiency in the simulation, while faithfully addressing all involved physical processes. The implementation of appropriate electron transport physics and of variance reduction techniques differs among different dose engines based on the MC method.

Keeping track of the location of each particle in relation to the irradiation geometry and its energy in comparison to the energy thresholds defined for the simulation is essential for the calculation of a dose distribution. During the simulation the following properties are assigned to each particle: its type, energy, location, and direction of travel. A further assigned property is its weight, which relates to the contribution and importance of the particle in the simulation as a result of the different variance reduction techniques employed. The array of data containing all information for all particles constitutes the beam's phase space. In an MC simulation, random numbers are drawn to transport a particle and determine the position where this will experience its next interaction. The type of interaction is subsequently sampled and for each particle originating from this event, its properties (energy, position, direction and weight) are stored. Particles are placed on a priority list (the stack) and the simulation continues for each particle on the stack until the particle either leaves the medium or until the energy of the secondary electrons produced is less than a specific threshold; at that position, further transport of this particle stops and its energy is deposited locally (their energy is being scored).

Implicit Dose Modelling: Kernel-Based Approaches

Implicit solutions to the radiation transport problem are known as *kernel-based* methods. These use precomputed data, the energy deposition kernels (EDKs), which describe the spatial distribution of the expectation value for the energy deposition caused by an elemental beam in water. EDKs are classified into different types with the most common being the point kernels and the pencil kernels. Point kernels describe the energy distribution from photons forced to interact at a given location (usually at the centre of homogeneous water medium), whereas pencil kernels describe the distribution of energy in a semiinfinite homogeneous medium from a point monodirectional (infinitesimally narrow and monoenergetic) photon beam (Fig. 11.3).

Point kernels are calculated from simulations using the MC method [24]. They can be separated into different components depending on the interaction history of different particles, where the primary dose component results from energy deposited by the first-scattered charged particles and the scattered photon component originate from first-scattered photons and so on. There are several ways to compute pencil kernels. One way is through simulations using the MC method or from an integration of point kernels along the direction of the pencil beam. Other methods use radial differentiation of measured scatter functions, or deconvolution of measured dose profiles, or curve fitting (parameterisations) of kernels originally generated with the MC method. The

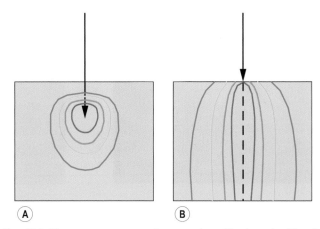

Fig. 11.3 Most common types of energy deposition kernels: (A) point kernel; (B) pencil kernel. (Reproduced from Ahnesjö A, Aspradakis MM. Dose calculations for external photon beams in radiotherapy. Phys Med Biol 1999;44(11):R99–155. With permission.)

latter approach has been recently extended so that the fitting parameters can be obtained as a function of a single beam parameter, the beam quality index, $TPR_{20,10}$ [25].

It is perhaps of interest here to clarify the difference of common terms that appear similar but have different meaning. Pencil beams result in dose distributions from a monodirectional beam (namely a beam of zero area) and this is not the same as a beamlet, which is a finite-size pencil beam (FSPB) that is very small in cross section. By small photon field one typically refers to beams with an area greater than that of a beamlet and less than 3 cm × 3 cm.

Pencil Beam Models

In pencil beam methods dose is calculated from the integration (convolution) of the two-dimensional energy fluence with the pencil beam kernel over the area of the beam aperture (Fig. 11.4).

This integration is straightforward for uniform circular beams. In the case of irregular field apertures, the field can be divided into sectors of constant energy fluence over the sector area. Pencil beam convolution can be executed using fast convolution algorithms, such as fast Fourier transform (FFT) [26]. Such an implementation is only appropriate in a homogenous medium and when the pencil kernel is assumed to be laterally invariant, that is, when changes of the energy spectrum off-axis (off-axis softening) are ignored and the medium is homogeneous. To account for heterogeneities pencil beam models incorporate scaling of the pencil kernel with changes in the medium density, usually in two dimensions, along the kernel axis and off-axis position at the depth of the calculation point. A correction for off-axis spectral variations is in principle possible, but differs among implementation of this model. If ignored, it can lead to errors in dose calculations up to 5% at large off-axis distances [14].

Point Kernel Models

Point kernel models, also known as convolution/superposition models, calculate dose from the integration of point kernels with the total energy released per unit mass, or terma (T), in the irradiated medium [27–29]. Terma is the total energy released by primary photon interactions per unit mass and includes the energy imparted to both charged particles and scattered photons; in other words, it is the energy lost or removed from the primary beam per unit mass. Before performing this integration, these models first calculate terma. Terma is calculated by tracing and attenuating the incident photon energy fluence along rays of transport in the three-dimensional calculation volume (phantom or patient).

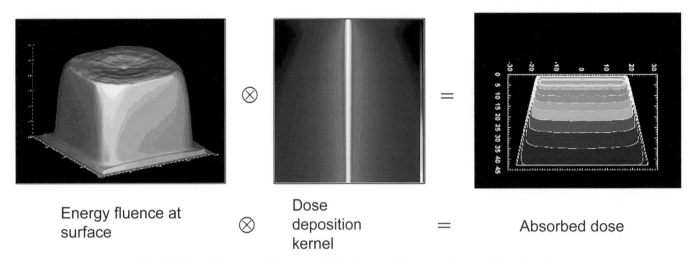

Energy fluence at surface ⊗ Dose deposition kernel = Absorbed dose

Fig. 11.4 Pencil beam model: the convolution of energy fluence with a pencil beam kernel.

Once terma at each voxel is known, point kernels are weighted by their value and the dose distribution is then calculated from an integration over the entire three-dimensional matrix (Fig. 11.5).

The advantage of these approaches is that they enable a complete three-dimensional modelling of the energy deposition process. Important modelling considerations introducing approximations (and these differ among implementations in commercial TPSs) include beam divergence, beam hardening, off-axis softening and electron contamination. To model beam divergence accurately point kernels need to be tilted to be aligned with the divergent path of primary photons as they are transported in the medium. The polyenergetic nature of the megavoltage photon beam is taken into account from the knowledge of the beam spectrum and from an additional integration over this. Some TPSs use published (generic) beam spectra as an approximation of the clinical beam, but most derive an estimate of the clinical spectrum through an optimisation procedure, which minimises the difference between measured and calculated depth-dose data for a range of field sizes. The spectrum is used for the calculation of a polyenergetic terma and kernels. As with pencil beam models, spectral changes laterally can be modelled by taking into consideration the variation off-axis of the mass attenuation coefficient.

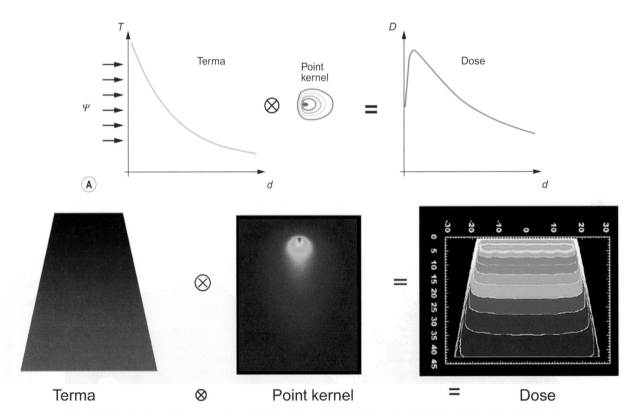

Fig. 11.5 Illustration of the convolution of terma and a point kernel in one and two dimensions: (A) along the depth; (B) on a plane. (From Karlsson M, Ahnesjö A, Georg D, et al. Physics booklet Nr 10: independent dose calculations concepts and models. ESTRO physics booklets. Brussels: European Society for Therapeutic Radiology and Oncology; 2010. With permission.)

For contributions to dose in the build-up region from contaminant-charged particles (in MV photon beams these are primarily electrons originating from the flattening filter, monitor chamber jaws and air) kernel-based approaches incorporate a separate model. Contaminant electrons can be dealt with as an additional source in the multisource model or can be modelled from a separate dose engine using pencil kernels that describe the change of dose from contaminant electrons laterally and with increasing depth. The heterogeneous and finite nature of the patient is more accurately accounted for in point kernel models than in pencil beam models because scaling of terma with changes in medium density is possible along the path of transport of primary photons, and rectilinear scaling of point kernels with variations of density between points of interaction and energy deposition can be performed in three dimensions, thus taking full advantage of the available three-dimensional information from CT data sets.

A challenge in the implementation of superposition models in the clinical environment has been the reduction in computation time to perform all numerical operations for the direct summation of the energy deposited in each voxel by each other voxel in three-dimensions. Superposition may offer high accuracy in the calculation of dose, but it is time consuming. FFT techniques can be employed, but these require that point kernels remain spatially invariant (cannot be scaled with density variations). This is not sufficiently accurate for modelling dose in heterogeneous media. As a compromise between accuracy and speed of calculation, approaches have been developed in which the resolution of the dose matrix is varied depending on the gradients present in the terma matrix. The most common approach, however, has been the collapsed cone approximation [30]. With this, the space around a point kernel (the point where energy is released in the medium) is discretised into cones, and energy is transported and deposited only along the axis of these cones. To calculate the dose deposited in the medium one integrates energy contributions along transport directions that are aligned with the axes of several cones. With the collapsed cone approach the numerical operations are proportional to the total number of voxels in the dose calculation matrix multiplied by number of transport directions chosen for the calculations (Fig. 11.6).

Finite-size Pencil Beam Models

In FSPB models the beam aperture is divided into small beams of identical, finite cross section over which energy fluence is considered

constant [31]. FSPBs are precomputed (usually from pencil kernels calculated using the MC method). FSPB-based models sum up contributions from individual FSPBs weighted by the incident energy fluence. The best-known implementation of this approach is the analytic anisotropic algorithm (AAA) available in a widely used commercial TPS. In Eclipse/AAA the FSPB kernels are represented by an analytical fit to a weighted sum of four Gaussians [32,33]. This implementation saves computation time. Beam divergence, depth hardening, off-axis softening, and electron contamination are taken into consideration similar to point kernel models. Because FSPB kernels are scaled with density variations along the axis of the FSPB as well as laterally the performance in terms of dose accuracy of the AAA in heterogeneous media is better than pencil beam models and comparable to that of superposition/collapsed cone approaches.

Factor-Based Approaches

Traditionally dose calculations for high-energy photon beams were entirely based on the use of large sets of stored measured data (percentage depth doses, profiles, tissue-air ratios, tissue-phantom ratios etc.). Dose was calculated from the multiplication of a series of factors, each of which described a change in the dose with a change of a parameter in the irradiation geometry, such as depth or field size, from that under reference conditions [34–37]. These methods are classified as factor-based or broad beam data-based models where some factors were derived directly by interpolation from the stored data or from simple modelling, if possible. Additional algorithms were needed to provide an estimate of the dose in heterogeneous media. Typically the stored data correspond to collimator settings down to 4 cm × 4 cm. Factor-based approaches have been used extensively in TP for conformal RT where the aim is to encompass the planning target by a homogeneous dose, and where the penumbra is not contributing to the dose in the target. They have limited application when it comes to the accurate prediction of dose from complex irradiations, which differ substantially from those during the experimental determination of the input data. In complex irradiation geometries such as in intensity-modulated RT, beam portals comprise of many narrow collimated beams. In these cases it is often desirable to plan an inhomogeneous dose distribution to the target. To accurately compute the dose in such cases it becomes important to model the beam penumbra, the influence of collimating devices, such as MLCs, and/or the occlusion of the direct beam source.

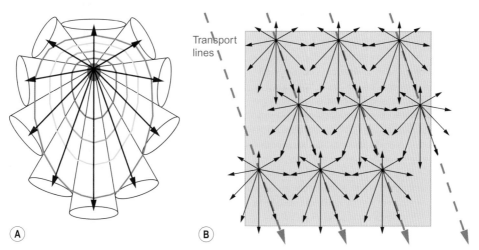

Fig. 11.6 Illustration of the collapsed cone approximation: (A) the point kernel is divided into cones; (B) superposition is performed along transport lines aligned with the axis of each cone. (From Karlsson M, Ahnesjö A, Georg D, et al. Physics booklet Nr 10: independent dose calculations concepts and models. ESTRO physics booklets. Brussels: European Society for Therapeutic Radiology and Oncology;2010. With permission.)

Factor-based approaches are ideally suited to the calculation of dose at a point on the central axis from irradiation geometries that do not differ substantially from those of the input data. These methods may still play a role as an approximate secondary independent method for the verification of dose at a point, but are no longer implemented in modern TPSs.

Conclusion on Model-Based Approaches

The accuracy in the calculation of dose in homogeneous and heterogeneous media has been the subject of many investigations and comparisons. One can conclude that the most accurate approaches are those based on the MC method and the deterministic solution of the BTE. However, the workhorses in TP calculations are point kernel models (superposition/collapsed cone approaches) and the AAA based on an FSPB approach. These are less accurate in computing dose in the build-up region, media interfaces, and high-density media in comparison to the solutions based on the MC method and the deterministic solutions, but more accurate than pencil beam models in computing dose in heterogeneous media. They are computationally more intensive than pencil beam models but fast enough to be used in the clinical routine.

Nevertheless, pencil beam models have an important role in RT planning. They are used in plan optimisation engines during inverse planning and for independent dose calculations as part of plan-specific quality assurance (PSQA). In addition, they are being implemented in software tools together with complex detector systems designed specifically for the verification of intensity-modulated radiation therapy (IMRT)/volumetric modulated arc therapy (VMAT) treatment plans as part of pre-treatment QA.

DOSE PER MONITOR UNIT FORMALISM: CALCULATION OF MONITOR UNITS

The outcome of any explicit or implicit dose calculation model is essentially dose per amount of incident radiation (Fig. 11.2). Linacs are calibrated to a given dose per MU under reference conditions. This traditionally corresponds to 1 cGy/MU at the depth of maximum build-up, at source-to-surface distance (SSD) of 100 cm and collimator setting of 10 cm × 10 cm. Thus for model-based doses engines to calculate MUs, it is necessary to establish a relationship between incident radiation and MUs under reference conditions. This defines the calibration of the dose engine and is derived from a measurement of dose per MU under reference conditions and from a calculation of dose per incident radiation under the same reference conditions [3].

The formalism used to calibrate dose engines varies among TPSs. Strictly an additional model is needed to account for the effects of backscattered radiation into the monitor chamber at different collimator settings [3,17,21]. Depending on the design of the linac head and its monitor chamber, the signal from the chamber can be affected from particles which have backscattered from the upper part of the jaws into the chamber. At collimations narrower than 10 cm × 10 cm (reference collimator setting) the amount of backscattered radiation into the monitor chamber increases, influencing the signal of the monitor chamber, so that the chamber would reach its preset value faster (leading to a decrease in relative output); at collimations greater than 10 cm × 10 cm the amount of backscattered radiation is less that than at 10 cm × 10 cm (leading to an increase in relative output). In factor-based approaches this effect is inherently accounted for in the measured data (measured total output factor and in air output factors). Most commercial TPSs with model-based dose engines do not explicitly consider this effect (which can reach the order of 2% at a 40 cm × 40 cm field), but account for this through a correction factor derived from measured output factors.

TREATMENT PLAN EVALUATION TOOLS

The ideal RT treatment plan produces a uniform coverage of the target volume without giving significant dose to surrounding normal tissue. three-dimensional planning is a realistic option for many cases, because of the increased availability of RT CT scans, virtual simulation, MR, fast computer hardware, and improved algorithms. Treatment plans are therefore more difficult to compare and evaluate, hence the need for plan evaluation tools. Several such tools are in use as discussed.

Isodose Distributions

Isodose information is presented as lines or surfaces of equal dose. They show either relative or normalised dose, if the dose is expressed as a percentage of a reference dose or they give absolute dose (in units of gray or centigray), and if the dose prescription has been included in the treatment plan. It is a matter of local protocol as to which method is used, although prescriptions specifying different doses to different volumes within the same plan are best displayed in terms of units of absolute dose.

To calculate dose to a surface or volume, a matrix of reference points spread over the volume of interest is required. The number of points and their spatial resolution are always a trade-off between speed and accuracy. The finer the grid of calculation points, the greater the calculation accuracy in regions of steep dose gradients, for example, close to the beam edges. The disadvantages of a fine grid are the increased computation time and the creation of large data files. In general, two criteria are specified:

- the desired dose accuracy
- the maximum acceptable distance between the estimated and actual isodose contours

For example, 2% dose accuracy or 2-mm isodose positional accuracy will be achieved with a grid spacing of 5 mm.

Typically, the x and y coordinates of these points are in the transverse plane and the z coordinate is in the superior–inferior plane. The z coordinate is frequently interpolated as the slice thickness of the planning CT scan can vary. The isodose contours are produced by linear interpolation between points, therefore the separation of these points needs to be small enough to allow sufficient dose detail at organ and PTV boundaries.

Conventionally isodose curves were normalised to give 100% to a reference point, in accordance with the recommendation in reports [1,4] on dose-at-a-point prescription and reporting. In complex, three-dimensional conformal radiation therapy the normalisation of isodose distributions follows the recommendations in ICRU reports [3,6] on dose–volume prescription and reporting. Typically in complex three-dimensional conformal RT isodoses are being normalised so that 100% of the prescribed dose is delivered to the mean of the target. The aim is usually to cover the PTV with the 95% isodose curve while ensuring the maximum dose within the volume does not exceed 107% [1,4].

The dose distribution can be displayed on multiple views of reconstructed sections (e.g. transverse, sagittal, and coronal sections on a single screen), and also on a three-dimensional reconstruction of anatomy with isodose surfaces displayed.

Useful features include the following:

- opaque and translucent colour wash displays give a good overall impression of the dose distribution, but can obscure target volumes, so should be interchangeable with conventional isodose lines (Fig. 11.7);
- zoom and pan facilities;
- isodose surfaces displayed as wire frames superimposed on rendered surfaces, with real-time manipulation;
- a volume of regret is a dose reduction technique applied to the dose distribution. A window of acceptability of dose level is chosen and

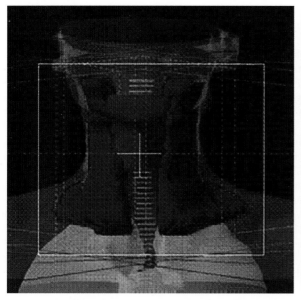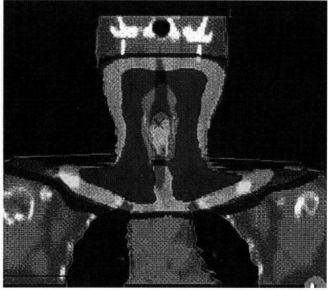

Fig. 11.7 Tumour and nodal volume in the left image with the right image showing an intensity-modulated radiation therapy plan delivering different doses to the tumour and nodal volumes.

portions of organs outside this window can be highlighted. For critical organs, this is a one-sided test, in which regions where the dose is above the acceptable level are displayed. For target volumes, regions of either too high or too low dose can be shown. This display feature is particularly useful when checking the coverage of arcing beams (e.g. for stereotactic RT).

Beams Eye View

A useful three-dimensional tool for field placement is the beams eye view (BEV), which shows the patients anatomy from the source position of the therapy machine, looking out along the axis of the radiation beam. The BEV approach is useful for identifying the optimal beam angles at which to irradiate the target and avoid irradiating adjacent normal structures, by interactively moving the patient and the treatment beam. Using BEVs, it is possible to set up noncoplanar radiation beams.

- Because there can be a great deal of information displayed via the BEV, it is important to show different structures in colour and be able to highlight, include, exclude, and shade them interactively while adjusting beam parameters.
- A visual and quantitative representation of machine and treatment couch parameters is also necessary, together with customisable limits and restrictions of beam, collimator, and couch angles for specific treatment machines.
- The limitation of BEVs is that it is a one-field presentation, so that field overlap is not immediately observed until the dose calculation is done.
- Another view available on some planning systems is the physicians eye view or observers eye view which enables the viewer to look at the patient from all angles to obtain an overview while multiple fields are being displayed.

An extension of the concept of a BEV is to use a digitally reconstructed radiograph (DRR). The DRR is reconstructed by various methods from the CT scan data set, which has been used for patient volume definition and planning. This has the advantage of being the same data set, so that any possible transfer errors which may occur between simulator and CT scanner are eliminated. The accuracy of the reconstruction of the DRR depends on the slice thickness of CT data and the computing tools available to reconstruct the radiographs. CT

information can be enhanced to extract more bony structure from the CT data and suppress the soft tissue to obtain an image with well-differentiated bony landmarks. Using such tools, one can also produce an image that is closer in appearance to either a megavoltage portal image or a diagnostic image.

Dose Volume Histograms

Volume calculations on a three-dimensional TPS provide a large amount of data that can be difficult to interpret and evaluate when displayed as isodose curves on several transverse, sagittal and coronal planes. It is much easier to condense the three-dimensional dose distribution data to a graph which displays the radiation distribution within a specifically defined volume of interest, so that summarising and analysing the data are possible. Such a graphical representation is called a dose volume histogram (DVH). The DVH can be expressed as the summed volume of elements receiving dose in a specified dose interval against a set of equally spaced dose intervals. This is a differential DVH and shows the absolute or relative volume in each dose interval (bin) directly. An example is shown in Fig. 11.8 of the evaluation of a breast dose distribution using selected dose bins as the measure of homogeneity over the treatment volume for two differently compensated plans. The standard plan gives a wider spread of dose over the volume of

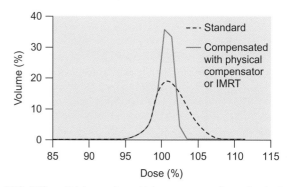

Fig. 11.8 Differential dose volume histogram comparing a standard and a compensated breast plan.

interest compared with the compensated plan, which shows a large volume receiving much less variation in dose.

More often used are cumulative dose volume frequency distributions, which are plots of the volume receiving a dose greater than, or equal to, a given dose. The volume accumulates starting at the highest dose bin continuing towards zero dose, eventually reaching 100% of the total volume. In most cases, the volume is specified as the percentage of the total volume of a particular structure receiving dose within each interval; however, it may be expressed as absolute volume in some cases.

DVHs can be used during the planning process to check whether the dose is adequate and uniform throughout the target volume. They show that hot and cold spots exist, but do not indicate where they occur, nor whether there are several of them. However, because they do not display spatial information, they should not be the only method of plan evaluation used.

The main use of DVHs is as a plan evaluation tool. They can be used as a graphical way of comparing different treatment plans on a single graph, for specifically identified OARs and PTVs. DVH PTV comparisons should show a uniformly high dose throughout the volume—the shape approximates to a step function and a steep slope shows that a large percentage of the volume has a similar dose (Fig. 11.9).

For OARs, the DVH should have a concave appearance (Fig. 11.9B) but, for different critical organs, it may be acceptable to deliver either a relatively high dose to a small volume or a small dose to a large volume.

An example of plan comparison for three different dose distributions is shown in Fig. 11.10A and B.

DVHs for OARs have a concave appearance. Fig. 11.10B shows comparative DVHs for a rectal volume where 50% of the volume is receiving 60, 63 or 66.5 Gy depending on the different treatment plan. It is also useful to display both absolute dose and absolute volume, together with normalised values, on the same graph.

Dose Volume Histogram Calculation Requirement and Methods

The three-dimensional image is made up of a sequence of CT scans. This can be represented as a three-dimensional grid with cubic volume elements, equally spaced in the x and y directions, but not necessarily in the z direction. The volume of the voxel can then be defined by the product of the x and y grid spacing and the slice thickness. A reasonable

resolution for sampling the volume of typical anatomical structures is about 2 to 3 mm.

Structures with irregular boundaries can give calculation errors when calculating with a regular rectangular grid. In addition, structures that are long and thin require a finer resolution in one direction than the other. The ideal solution is to be able to adjust the voxel size dynamically to the dimensions of the structure in x, y and z independently.

The dose for each voxel can be determined at the same time for the outlined volume of interest, by linearly interpolating the dose to the centre of the voxel from the dose matrix. All contributing voxels are collected into the appropriate dose bins of the histogram for each structure. The user can specify the number and dose interval of the bins to customise the resolution of the DVH plots. These bin values can then be expressed in graphical form. It is important that the dose and volume calculation windows are large enough to totally include all the voxels in any specific structure.

The range of expected dose values is divided into equal intervals when constructing a histogram. For each interval, the volumes of the voxels receiving dose within that interval are accumulated in the appropriated element of an array, or bin. Cumulative DVHs are obtained by adding volumes accumulated in each bin with the volumes in all bins corresponding to higher dose intervals. For cumulative DVHs, the appropriate dose interval for the bins depends on the dose–response curve for the structure of interest. A dose of 0.5 Gy has been shown to be reasonable, whereas 2 Gy is too wide an interval. Differential DVHs treat the volume in each bin as a separate quantity, and a bin interval between Gy 2 and 5 Gy is reasonable.

Clinical Use and Limitations of Dose Volume Histograms

It is not strictly correct to compare plans with different doe computational parameters because different dose calculation algorithms may not handle heterogeneities, or penumbra etc., in the same way. The dose matrix resolution can affect the results of the DVH, especially in regions of steep dose gradient.

Interpretation of the DVH plot is fairly subjective and implications of small differences between DVHs are not well understood. This indicates the usefulness of an objective numeric score such as tumour control probability (TCP) or normal tissue complication probability (NTCP) to provide a ranking when comparing plans. (Small changes

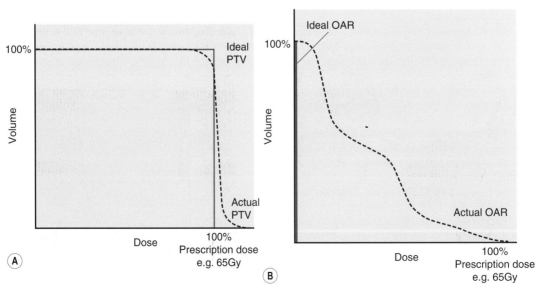

Fig. 11.9 Ideal and typical dose volume histograms: (A) for planning target volume *(PTV)*, (B) for organ at risk *(OAR)*.

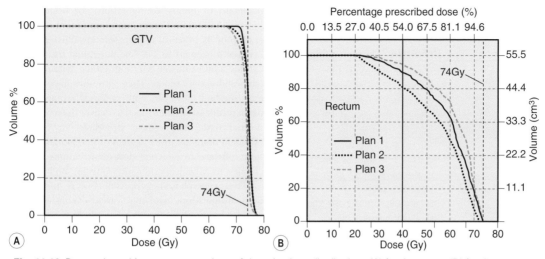

Fig. 11.10 Dose volume histogram comparison of three isodose distributions (A) for the target; (B) for the rectum.

in DVH often result in significant differences in the computed TCP and NTCP values.)

DVHs do not indicate the complexity of the field arrangements and will not show any use of illegal couch, collimator angles and so on.

In summary, the DVH is a very useful tool for three-dimensional plan comparisons and as an input parameter for TCP and NTCP calculations. TCP and NTCP are quantitative methods of predicting the likelihood of local control. DVHs and the predicted behaviour of the cell population in question are used as input data. There is, however, large uncertainty in the clinical data, so absolute probabilities are not attainable, but relative probabilities can be used to assess different treatment plans. DVHs should, however, be used in conjunction with other plan evaluation tools, especially those which will give spatial information. They can also be used to compare different treatment modalities such as protons and photons when performing TP studies, before doing clinical trials.

Dose Surface Histograms and Dose Wall Histograms

There are some clinical organs where it could be more relevant to consider the wall of the organ rather than the whole volume, such as the rectum. Dose to rectal wall is more likely to represent patterns of

morbidity than dose to volume and rectal dose maps can be extracted from dose surface histograms to give an estimate of areas of high dose that may relate to patterns of morbidity. An example of such a map is shown in Fig. 11.11.

Dose Statistics

Dose statistics as outlined in Table 11.3 give a simplified view of the dose in a specified structure for evaluation purposes.

Other Tools

A publication by Willoughby et al. [38] describes a system of evaluating and scoring RT treatment plans using an artificial neural network. Treatment plans were assigned a figure of merit by a radiation oncologist using a 5-point rating scale. DVH data extracted from a large training set were correlated with the physician-generated figure of merit using an artificial neural network, and the net was tested on another set of plans. The accuracy of the neural net in scoring plans compared well with the reproducibility of the clinical scoring, and the system is promising for the reliable generation of a clinically relevant figure of merit.

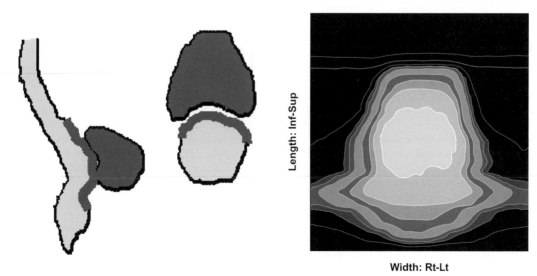

Fig. 11.11 Dose surface map.

TABLE 11.3   Definitions of the Dose Statistics

Statistic	Definition
Total volume	The sum of all dose volume histogram (DVH) voxels found within a set of boundary contours
International Commission on Radiation Units and Measurements (ICRU)-50 dose	The specification dose as defined in the ICRU report 50 [1]
Mean dose	The sum of the doses assigned to each voxel divided by the total number of voxels
Min dose	The minimum dose in the volume
Max dose	The maximum dose in the volume
Volume greater than or equal to the prescribed dose	The sum of all voxels within DVH bins corresponding to a dose greater than or equal to the prescription dose
Volume greater than or equal to the reference dose	The total volume within DVH bins corresponding to a dose greater than or equal to the user-supplied reference dose

Also useful are:

- side-by-side transverse/sagittal/coronal plans
- video loop stepping through two plans displayed side by side, particularly with colour wash displaying isodoses
- zoom facility over the relevant area to be compared can be useful
- dose at a point interactively integrated and displayed simultaneously on both plans
- dose difference displays
- surface dose display (e.g. on the surface of the spinal cord)

The other aspect of plan evaluation which has not been addressed is the accuracy of the actual dose delivery, which is dependent on complexity of plan, size of margins, reproducibility of set up and so on. Some sort of uncertainty analysis should be developed to include these other aspects of treatment plan evaluation.

TREATMENT PLANNING TECHNIQUES IN EXTERNAL MV PHOTON BEAM RADIOTHERAPY

This section concerns TP with megavoltage photon beams.

Forward and Inverse Planning

The terminology of forward and inverse planning applies to the planning process of any type of beam arrangement: photon, electron or proton. Forward planning has been the tradition for many years and is what RT clinical experience has been built upon. Basically, from a knowledge of the beam characteristics in terms of field size, depth dose, and even intensity modulation with wedges and compensators, the dose planner manually would iteratively devise a treatment beam arrangement that can deliver the prescribed dose.

In essence, in inverse planning one starts with the required dose distribution and finds the beam delivery method to achieve it. Inverse planning was introduced together with the concept of intensity modulated radiation therapy (IMRT), where optimisation algorithms were used to predict the optimal radiation pattern [39,40]. Since the introduction of inverse planning in the early 1980s on a racetrack microtron and of MLCs for beam shaping [41–43], an enormous technical effort led to the development of software and hardware using the MLC (standard or binary configuration) for beam intensity modulation [44,45]. IMRT with photons was a significant development and consideration of its practical implementation illustrates the complexity and benefits it brought to TP. The individual treatment beams for IMRT can be delivered using MLCs in either dynamic or multiple-segment (step-and-shoot) mode. There are advantages and disadvantages of each method; however, both methods require the intensity of each beam profile to be determined to deliver the intended dose to the target, normal tissue and critical structures. In volumetric arc therapy (VMAT) there are more degrees of freedom available to the optimisation software to generate dose distributions, through simultaneous changes in MLC leaf and gantry position and beam dose rate.

The inverse planning process not only requires sophisticated computational algorithms involving a variety of control theory–type processes, but also requires that the operators obtain an understanding on how to steer these processes to provide the effective use of them for various clinical sites and individual clinical situations. The solution space for the delivery is in theory infinite and although there are some limiting aspects dictated by hardware design (e.g. the width of the MLC leaf and minimum separation between leaves), which can be taken into account in the computation, the operator brings an overview which is essential to control the inverse planning process and obtain a robust solution.

Forward Planning With Standard Beam Arrangements

An enormous amount of clinical practice, knowledge, and treatment grew from the many years of forward planning. This clinical experience is still relevant today with regard to the management of patients and practical delivery of treatment. It also provides simple solutions where that may be appropriate.

This section does not attempt to provide a comprehensive atlas of treatment plans or an in-depth planning guidance for each site but uses a few clinical examples to demonstrate planning techniques.

The first step in preparing a plan is to decide on the position of the isocentre. Although the centre of the PTV might appear to be the best location, in practice, it may be preferable to set the isocentre to predefined skin marks which have been set at the time of CT scanning. The skin marks will have been chosen to lie on a stable skin location, perhaps at a standard anatomical point or height above the couch and avoiding steep body contour gradients. This results in a simpler and safer set up and the fields will then be aligned to the PTV by asymmetric collimator settings.

Another strategy is to select the isocentre position based on the internal anatomy of either the PTV or adjacent critical structures. This can minimise the dose to critical structures by eliminating beam divergence without complicating the field arrangement. Examples are breast treatments without the beams diverging into the lung or abutting nodal fields, or brain treatments avoiding beam edges diverging into critical structures, such as the lens. Another aspect regarding choice of internal anatomy relates to the dose computation algorithm and placement of the isocentre in solid material and not in an air cavity to improve the dose prediction accuracy at that point for checking.

The beam energy is chosen by considering the depth of maximum build-up d_{max} and the penetration properties of the beam (Table 11.4 shows typical values for commonly used energies). Low-energy beams (e.g. 4–6 MV) are suited to more superficial volumes (e.g. head and neck PTVs), whereas deep pelvic PTVs will require 10 to 20 MV. Beam energies above 15 MV do not give a great benefit to the planner, but their frequent use on a linac can introduce radiation protection problems because of neutron production.

The build-up region is a significant feature of the MV beam in that it gives skin sparing, allowing doses that would severely damage the skin to be delivered deep into the patient. However, a PTV which extends

TABLE 11.4 Typical Depth-Dose Characteristics for 10 × 10-cm² Radiotherapy Beams

X-Ray Energy	Source-to-Surface Distance (cm)	D_{max} Depth (cm)	$D_{80\%}$ (cm)	Dose at 10 cm (% of D_{max})
60 kV	30	0	0.5	2
100 kV	30	0	1.0	10
220 kV	50	0	2.5	29
4 MV	100	1.0	5.9	63.0
6 MV	100	1.5	6.7	67.5
10 MV	100	2.3	8.0	73.0
15 MV	100	2.9	9.1	77.0
25 MV	100	3.8	10.9	83.0
Electron Energy (MeV)				
4	95	0.9	1.4	1
6	95	1.3	1.9	1
10	95	2.2	3.2	1
15	95	2.6	4.9	3
20	95	2.6	6.7	10

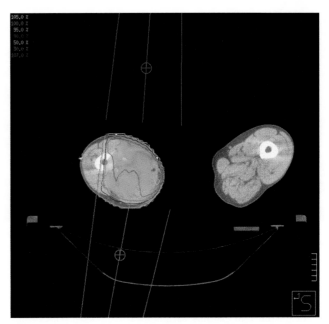

Fig. 11.13 Sarcoma with parallel-opposed field; isocentres outside target.

from near the surface to a depth requiring MV photons may require bolus to be added to the skin. By placing this tissue-equivalent material on the skin, the build-up region is shifted into the bolus and the maximum dose of the beam is delivered on or near the skin. Unless the PTV is superficial, the planner should consider the impact of patient immobilisation devices acting as build-up and increasing the surface dose.

Standard field arrangements may be modified for specific patient situations such as metal hip implants. Here, it is preferable to avoid beams entering through the implant so a three-field arrangement must be modified such as shown in Fig. 11.12.

Single Fields

Most plans are based on the intersecting of multiple field paths to create a high-dose region, but single fields may sometimes be the ideal choice especially for superficial PTVs. The spine can be treated with a single posterior field, although this will usually be done as part of a multifield arrangement to treat the whole central nervous system. To cover a PTV length of greater than 40 cm, the field may need to be treated at

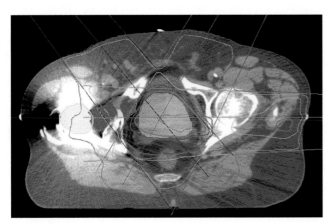

Fig. 11.12 Modified three-field beam arrangement to avoid prosthesis.

extended SSD (i.e. the isocentre will be positioned off the skin surface; Fig. 11.13). To produce a uniform dose to the cord lying at varying depths, a compensator may be employed, but the most efficient technique is to use top-up fields all centred on a single isocentre, delivering a few MUs to otherwise underdosed sections of the PTV.

Turned Wedges

Wedges are usually most beneficial with the wedge in the plane of the plan (usually the transverse patient plane). However, if the patient contour varies out of this plane, a turned or longitudinal wedge may be required to produce an even dose in the superior–inferior direction. This may be accomplished by overlying two fields with identical dimensions, but with the collimator rotated 90°. For multibeam plans, it may be possible to achieve uniform dose with a single turned wedge on one field only.

Parallel-Opposed Fields

The typical isodose distribution arising from a parallel-opposed field is shown in Fig. 11.14. If the separation is not too great for the available beam energy, then a dose range of +7% to −5% is perhaps just achievable. The high-dose regions may present a problem at wide separations and also the hourglass-shaped contour at about the 90% to 95% level may result in unacceptably low doses at the midplane of the volume. Wedges may be employed where the contour slopes or internal heterogeneities are present, and the use of shielding can produce irregular dose distributions conforming to complex PTV shapes. Clinical applications include large pelvis volumes and whole-brain treatments.

Beams Weighted in 2:1 Ratio

The standard parallel-opposed distribution can be modified to deliver a higher dose to one side of the PTV without resorting to a more complex plan. It must be clear what the plan request means by 2:1 weighting. For simple manually calculated plans, it would usually mean that the ratio of MU set is 2:1. However, with computerised plans, a dose reference point may be positioned somewhere other than at the midplane depth, so it must be clear to which point the 2:1 ratio applies. The presence of heterogeneities further complicates the issue as the TPS may adjust the

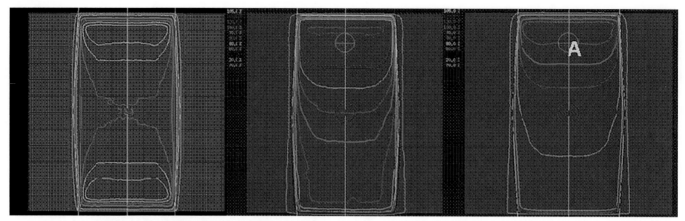

Fig. 11.14 Isodose distributions produced by parallel-opposed beams. Left-image beams are equally weighted, central image weighting is 2:1 at midplane, and right-image weighting is 2:1 at point A.

set MUs to deliver equal dose from each field to a point by compensating for the different densities each beam has traversed. This demonstrates the potential hazards arising from changing from basic manual calculations to CT-based dosimetry where a seemingly simple request for 2:1 weightings can take on several different interpretations (see Fig. 11.14).

Breast Treatments

The breast can be treated with a parallel-opposed pair, but the technique is generally refined to minimise lung dose by creating a non-diverging edge, either by fully asymmetric fields with the central axis along the field edge or by slightly angling the fields so that the central axes are not parallel to one another but the back edges are (Fig. 11.15).

Wedges will usually be required to produce a uniform PTV dose by compensating for the missing tissue and the presence of lung. Because of time constraints, the PTV is not outlined if treating the entire breast and the PTV is normally defined during simulation or virtual simulation and will not be specifically contoured and the gantry angles determined by the accepted amount of lung in the field. For postmastectomy chest wall treatments, the contour shape combined with the significant presence of lung may result in open fields or even a wedge orientated with the thin end at the apex of the breast.

A beam of typically 5 MV is adequate for most breast treatments but, as the separation between the medial and lateral field edges increases beyond about 22 cm, a higher-energy beam is required. The increased energy results in reduced breast tissue coverage superficially because of the increased build-up depth so should be avoided unless essential.

Segmented fields can produce a more uniform dose especially in larger or irregular outlines (see Fig. 11.15A–C). Usually, a single segment on one field is sufficient to bring the dose range within ICRU-50 [1] and ICRU-62 [4] requirements. For left-sided breast treatments it may be necessary to shield the heart.

Limb Sarcomas

These are usually treated with two opposed fields slightly angled to produce a sharper dose gradient to maximise the drainage channel along the limb. The PTV is often greater than 40 cm long and, for a standard linac, extended SSD fields are necessary. These require carefully described set up instructions (Fig. 11.13).

Wedged Pairs

For superficial PTVs that extend quite deeply, the wedged pair can produce the optimum dose distribution (Fig. 11.16). Highly wedged beams are required to maintain a uniform dose across the depth of the PTV. A greater hinge angle tends to produce a more uniform dose gradient and may be necessary for deeper PTVs, but is likely to increase normal tissue dose adjacent to the PTV. The exit doses from a two-field plan can be significant for critical structures, such as the mouth or cord in parotid treatments, and sometimes a lightly weighted third field can be beneficial if the relative weighting of the two fields cannot be adjusted.

Multiple Field Plans

For PTVs lying deeper in the patient, three or more fields with paths intersecting at the PTV usually offer the best dose distribution for the PTV while avoiding excessive dose to normal tissue. The clinically useful dose will normally only be delivered where all the beam paths overlap, unless complex inverse planning is employed or an intentional dose gradient is required inside the PTV. The field arrangement is designed to ensure that the treated volume conforms as closely as possible to the PTV while complying with critical structure constraints and minimising the volume of normal tissue irradiated, the irradiated volume as defined in ICRU-50 [1].

Pelvis Plans

Three fields will often be sufficient to deliver the required dose to the PTV while maintaining acceptably low normal tissue doses. Unless the PTV extends close to the surface (e.g. some rectum PTVs), a high energy (10 MV or more) is desirable. A posterior plus two lateral fields (as shown in Fig. 11.17) represent a good starting point for a plan. The wedges on the lateral fields compensate for the fall off in dose from the posterior field and also the missing tissue because of the patient contour. The weightings are adjusted to obtain an acceptable PTV dose while also considering the normal tissue doses in the beam entry path and, in this case, the beam exit path from the posterior field. The lateral maximum doses for typical pelvis patients may be around 80% of the PTV dose, or more for patients with a wide separation. The maximum dose that the posterior field contributes to normal tissue will usually be lower—typically 60% of the prescribed dose because of the presence of more radiosensitive structures

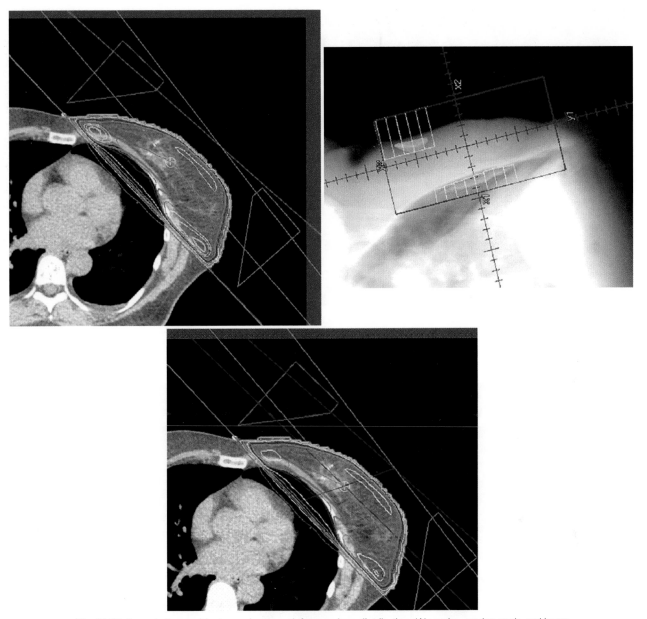

Fig. 11.15 Aspects to consider to produce a satisfactory dose distribution: (A) varying wedge angle and beam weights alone, which may not be satisfactory; (B) adding a segmented field with the high-dose regions shielded and the lower-dose regions thus boosted; (C) introduction of a segmented field to enhance (A).

within its entry and exit paths. Four fields may be required, especially for large volumes in large patients, a four-field box arrangement being the standard technique.

The lateral fields in the three-field plan may be angled by either a few degrees or perhaps 20° or more. Angling a few degrees posteriorly in a supine patient will produce a sharper dose gradient on the posterior PTV edge, which can reduce the dose to the adjacent critical structure, the rectum, in the case of a prostate PTV for example. Angling the fields more posteriorly will reduce the normal tissue doses as the exit dose from one lateral will not contribute so much to the contralateral entrance dose. For some PTV shapes, a better conformality may be achieved with oblique angles but, in many cases, the rectum dose will be increased by the use of posterior oblique fields.

Thorax Plans

The optimum field arrangement will significantly depend on the location of the PTV in the chest. Three fields are usually required (but see combined two-phase example in the next section) although occasionally, a parallel-opposed pair is the best arrangement. Examples of bronchus PTV field arrangements are shown in Fig. 11.18. The cord dose tolerance must not be exceeded and the heart dose minimised where relevant. The total left and right lung volume must be outlined so that the total volume is displayed in the DVH. A field arrangement that minimises the lung volume irradiated should then be found usually by analysing the V20 from the DVH.

The choice of beam energy needs careful consideration as at high energy, the increased path length of the electrons released can be detrimental to the target coverage if the target is adjacent to low-density

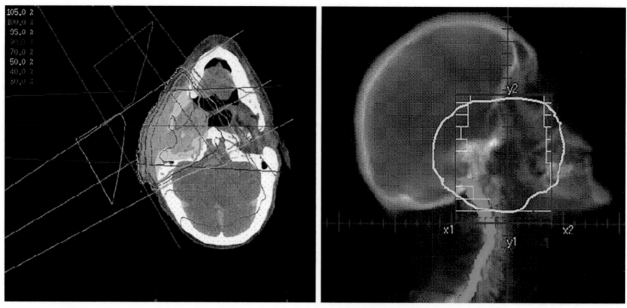

Fig. 11.16 Left image shows transverse view of wedged pair with low-weighted segment field used to boost the dose to part of the planning target volume (shown in *blue*). On the right, the beam's eye view of the boost field showing partial shielding of the cord.

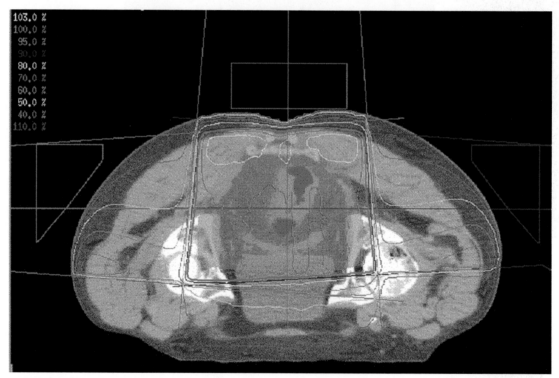

Fig. 11.17 Three-field rectum treatment.

tissue and air. Dose algorithms do not provide accurate dose predictions for these situations and generally the choice of a low-energy beam is considered preferable.

Phased Treatments

For many sites, the treatment plan will comprise two or occasionally more stages. For example, phase one will deliver dose to a known primary lesion and to surrounding nodal involvement or other disease spread. Phase two will then be a reduced PTV covering the primary lesion only.

Another reason for phased treatment would be to spread the dose to critical structures by employing a different field arrangement in phase two but still targeting the same PTV.

Another form of phased treatments is the use of feathered junctions when treating large PTVs to minimise the risk of overdose or underdose occurring at matched field edges and, typically, three phases are

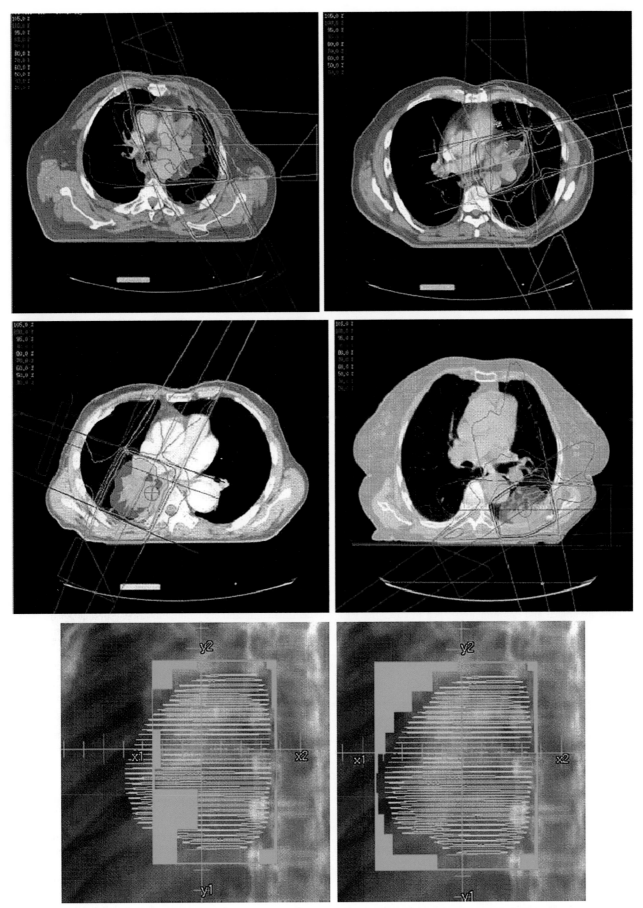

Fig. 11.18 (A–D) Bronchus treatment with (E) segments used in the left anterior oblique instead of (C) a wedge.

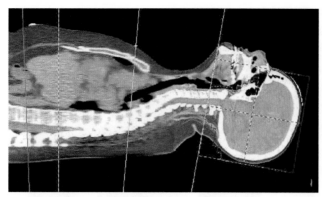

Fig. 11.19 Central nervous system junction.

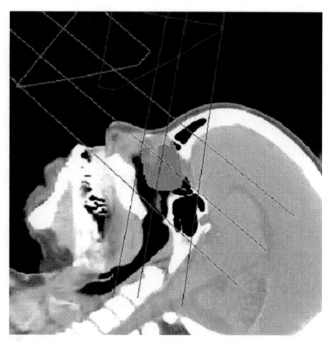

Fig. 11.20 Planning in the sagittal plane to avoid adjacent critical structures, in this case the contralateral eye.

employed in this technique. An example is the treatment of the entire central nervous system with a spine field matched to brain fields with collimators angled to follow the divergence of the spine field (Fig. 11.19).

There may be radiobiological and/or practical advantages in delivering the phases concurrently in each daily fraction rather than consecutively, when a new plan must be produced and checked for each phase.

Oesophagus

Traditionally, the oesophagus has been treated with two phases with the intention of minimising the cord and lung critical structure doses. Phase one is an anterior–posterior parallel-opposed pair, which also irradiates the cord usually to a dose slightly higher than the dose the PTV receives during this phase. As cord tolerance is approached, a phase two plan is introduced, usually an anterior and two posterior oblique fields. The oblique fields avoid the cord completely, but it continues to receive an exit dose from the anterior field. Therefore, it is essential to plan the phase two before much of the phase one treatment has been delivered as if the phase two is not started in time, the total cord dose may exceed the tolerance over both phases. This arrangement is intended to minimise lung dose by using the anterior–posterior beam arrangement up to cord tolerance. More recently, cardiac toxicity has become a concern, especially where chemotherapy is also administered, and the heart is outlined as a critical structure. The treatment is delivered using a single four-field plan and the lateral fields are angled and conformally shaped to cover the PTV while shielding the heart from as much high dose as possible. Thus the cord maximum dose and the lung and heart volume doses are all optimised in a single plan.

Noncoplanar Planning

The majority of plans have the central axes of all the fields in one plane—usually the axial patient plane, although a sagittal, coronal, or oblique plane may be preferable in some circumstances (e.g. a wedged pair to treat the orbit; Fig. 11.20).

Coplanar planning simplifies the planning process as if all beams project the same out-of-plane dimension, then they will each cover the out-of-plane PTV dimension equally. Beam path lengths through normal tissue are minimised and collimator rotations on opposing fields can be easily matched. For most of the body, coplanar fields are preferable with a few exceptions when small angulations from the treatment plane are used. Examples of such angulations are some breast treatments where floor and collimator rotations are introduced to establish a vertical junction between the breast and nodal fields (Fig. 11.21) and avoiding the shoulders in lateral neck beams.

One disadvantage of coplanar fields is that the exit path of one field will often overlap the entrance path of another with potentially significant cumulative doses. Noncoplanar plans can be most beneficial in the skull where the beam paths can avoid each other except at the PTV, without increased path lengths because of the approximately spherical body contour. However, greater care is needed to avoid critical structures in three-dimensional as beams can deliver significant dose well beyond the PTV area. For example, the thyroid irradiated by beams in the sagittal plane treating a brain (Fig. 11.22).

Field Matching

Matching two fields may be essential to treat large volumes as described in the previous section, with feathering used to spread the uncertainty of the set up, especially when a single isocentre technique cannot be utilised. Fig. 11.23A and B show how asymmetric fields can simplify field matching and are commonly used, especially in head and neck treatments to match two distinct but abutting PTV shapes into a single treatment.

However, matching may also be necessary when a previous treatment is adjacent to a PTV currently being treated. Matching diverging fields can be complex, and a compromise is usually a pragmatic approach, especially in palliative, low-dose treatments. If the planner has confidence in the location of the previous set up, then an attempt to match the beam divergence may be practical. Alternatively the match may be made at a critical structure, such as the spinal cord, and the overdose and underdose regions adjacent to the cord are accepted (Fig. 11.24).

Forward-Planned Intensity-Modulated Radiotherapy

The field-in-field technique is particularly useful in forward planning, where just additional segments are used to produce improvements in homogeneity, delivery of integrated boosts, and/or improved sparing of OARs.

A simple example is a forward-planned breast technique, which retains the preferred tangential beam arrangement, but allows shaping

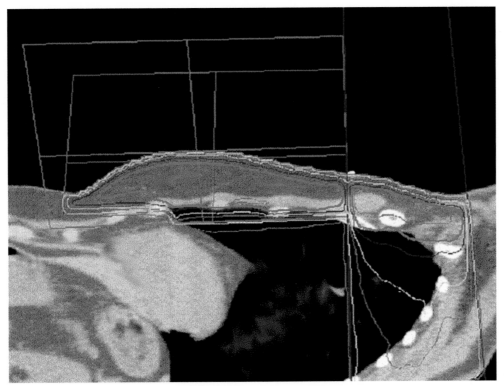

Fig. 11.21 Breast junction.

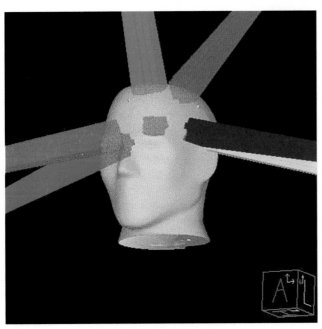

Fig. 11.22 Noncoplanar skull.

of dose to areas within the breast that would be underdosed or over-dosed without such customised compensation. This is illustrated in Fig. 11.25B, where the dose uniformity has been improved compared with that in Fig. 11.25A by the addition of four segments within the standard field.

Patients with prostate cancer can also be treated using a forward-planned technique. This is done where the aim is simultaneously to boost the dose to the prostate, while delivering a lower dose to prostate and seminal vesicles PTV, within the same treatment fraction. This can be achieved using a three-field technique, with two to three segments per beam. Segment shapes can be determined according to rules based on the patient anatomy and the weights adjusted to give the required dose distribution.

Forward planning can also be used to generate more complex plans, such as the generation of concave dose distributions in the pelvis [46] or head and neck. Although the dose distribution of such plans may not be quite as conformal as those produced by inverse planning, they may be an improvement on a standard treatment plan.

Inverse Planning
Intensity-Modulated Radiotherapy With Fixed Beam Configurations

Inverse-planned IMRT involves devising a set of dose constraints which are entered into an optimisation routine to generate a solution deliverable with usually a limited number of beam configurations using intensity-modulated fields. Essential to this is a fully outlined set of three-dimensional volumes of interest and defined values as to the acceptable dose levels to be delivered to or avoided by those volumes.

Typical dose constraints for all IMRT plans on the PTV are 99% of the volume needs to receive at least 90% of the prescribed dose, and 95% of the volume should receive at least 95% of the prescribed dose. Simultaneously, there is a constraint that only 5% of the volume receives no more than 105% of the prescribed dose, and 2% of the volume receives no more than 107% of prescribed dose. In addition, there are dose constraints on the OARs similar to the dose constraints that would be used for conformal RT. There may also be the need for constraints to avoid high-dose regions throughout the irradiated volume by adding false structures with appropriate dose constraints to force the calculation.

There is a lot of published work on finding class solutions for IMRT plans, to define numbers, angles, and energies of beams. A number of

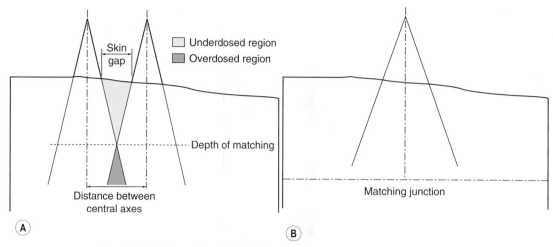

Fig. 11.23 Field matching with (A) divergent beams and (B) asymmetric fields.

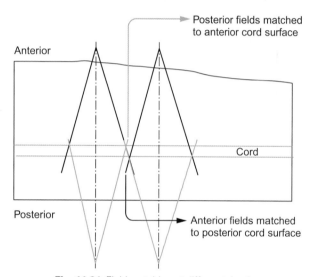

Fig. 11.24 Field matching at different depths.

authors have found that, for some sites, a small number of appropriately selected beam orientations can provide dose distributions as satisfactory as those produced by a large number of unselected equispaced orientations [48]. The general increase in numbers of incident gantry angles means that lower energies are suitable for deep-seated tumours [49] although some groups [50] have preferred to continue using higher energies.

During the inverse planning process, the optimisation algorithm will only attempt to cover or spare those volumes that have been completely outlined. It may therefore be necessary to outline volumes where strict dose sparing is not required; however, the planner would prefer to avoid hot spots and ideally reduce the dose within these volumes. A volume that does not strictly relate to anatomy may be drawn to apply a dose constraint with a relative low priority that will help to avoid dose overspill in this area. Expanded volumes (i.e. extra margins) can be used to ensure coverage of targets. Depending on the leaf widths and motions, this may require differing margins in different directions.

Optimal fluences converted to deliverable leaf motion sequences must take into account the MLC limitations of the machine. This should be considered when choosing beam orientations and selecting gantry and collimator angles to ensure, for example, that the width of the target volumes in BEV is not larger than the maximum beam width that can be delivered at one time. Deliverable fluences can be

realised using either multiple static-field segments, and this is known as segmental MLC delivery or step-and-shoot IMRT, or by having pairs of leaves dynamically move across the beam portal at varying speeds during beam-on, which is known as dynamic MLC or sliding window IMRT delivery.

Each planning system has its own characteristics, therefore, practice with the system when developing class solutions to achieve local planning techniques is important.

The calculation process is in two stages. First, the TPS calculates the optimum energy fluence for each beam. Second, this is converted to a deliverable set of field segments that the treatment unit can deliver. There may be significant differences between the ideal and achievable fluences, so the planning process will be more efficient with access to the final distribution being available during the planning stage. The planner must still ensure that the calculated plan is reasonable and deliverable and that skilled manual intervention to an inverse plan is usually required, for example, removing very small segments, or those with a low number of MUs. The planner must also be aware of the limitations of the TPS algorithm as there may be significant errors in calculations of small or elongated fields, or fields with small MLC apertures compared with the secondary collimator settings.

Intensity-Modulated Radiotherapy With Rotating Arcs

Tomotherapy. The first implementation of a rotating arc approach was based on the serial or sequential tomotherapy concept [45]. This concept used a narrow beam collimated with two sets of binary MLC (the position of the jaws was either open or closed) mounted as an add-on on a gantry of a conventional linac. During a gantry rotation and stationary couch position two slices were irradiated at once and following this the couch was translated for the irradiation of the next two slices. This was the Peacock system with the pneumatically driven MIMiC binary collimator, where the couch motion was controlled by the Crane system and the patient was immobilised with an invasive head immobilisation device (Talon). Treatments were inversely planned using the Corvus optimisation engine. The Peacock was the first commercial solution (by Nomos Corporation) for the treatment of patients with IMRT. This technology was primarily available in the United States for IMRT treatments, but has been nowadays superseded by helical tomotherapy and other rotational therapy solutions.

The concept of helical tomotherapy uses a single bank of binary MLC with the compact linac rotating and the treatment couch translating in a continuous manner, thereby delivering a fan beam similar to a CT scanner [44,51]. The photon beam is a flattening filter-free

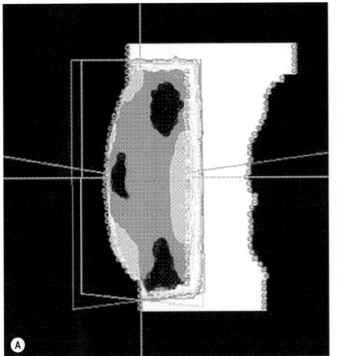 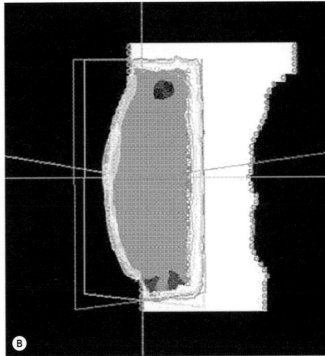

Fig. 11.25 The use of additional segmented fields within the two wedged fields which alone produced the dose distribution on the left improves the dose uniformity to that shown in the right image.

beam. Each leaf delivers a rotating pencil beam and the pencil beam modulation is carried out by changing the fraction of the time the leaf is open during gantry rotation so that the desired energy fluence can be delivered from each gantry angle. There is a backup collimator that is used to adjust the field width and there is the possibility to use multiple field widths. An integrated planning system is used for optimisation and dose calculation. The original helical tomotherapy system, Hi-Art by TomoTherapy Inc., has been further developed into the Tomotherapy and Radixact systems (Accuray).

Volumetric arc therapy. VMAT is a rotational IMRT delivery technique nowadays widely available on conventional-type linac using a standard MLC. VMAT is possible through continuous gantry rotation, with the MLC leaf, the gantry rotation speed, and the dose rate varying throughout the 360° arc [52]. VMAT is a volumetric delivery, with the patient on a static couch and with the patient volume treated simultaneously during gantry rotation. Optimisation calculations for VMAT delivery are performed in a series of stages starting initially with an arc that is subdivided into a small number of gantry positions at which the MLC leaf positions are determined. Subsequently the optimisation continues using an increasingly larger number of gantry positions where beam segment apertures are being interpolated from gantry positions from the previous optimisation stage. VMAT technology (optimisation and delivery software) is available nowadays on all modern TPS and linacs and has become the most commonly used approach for IMRT.

Specialised Techniques With MV Photons

Over the years, highly specialist treatment techniques have been developed often with dedicated treatment machines. Although often some form of the treatment can be delivered on a standard linac with specialised accessories or modification, there are also examples of highly specialised treatment facilities being developed to exploit and explore the potential of the special treatment techniques.

Total-Body Irradiation

Total-body irradiation (TBI) is employed in the treatment of leukaemia to kill leukaemic cells and to suppress the immune system before a bone marrow transplant. The target site is therefore all malignant stem cells, immunocytes (cells of the immune system), and bone marrow stem cells, whereas the most important critical structure is the lung, as radiation-induced pneumonitis is a common side effect and can limit the total dose administered. TBI is administered in conjunction with chemotherapy before bone marrow transplant so a reliable treatment delivery is essential as once the chemotherapy commences, the bone marrow transplant cannot be delayed.

The only practical RT technique is to give a uniform dose to the entire body (including the skin). There are wide variations in the delivery technique, the dose administered, the dose specification point, and the dose rate [53]. However, most techniques employ a standard linac beam with the patient at an extended SSD of approximately 4 to 5 m treated with lateral fields. A Perspex sheet is placed in the beam to reduce the depth of the build-up region and bolus may be placed close to the patient to even out the body contour and provide a more uniform dose. The low density of lung means that the thorax will receive a higher dose than the rest of the trunk, so it is important to provide some form of lung compensator, which can range from positioning the patients arms over the chest to MLC compensation.

The beam characteristics will differ considerably from those at the standard treatment distance so extensive measurements are required to establish a TBI technique. The effect of scatter from the wall behind the patient, the floor, and the air all create a unique beam condition, and these affect not only the patient dosimetry, but also the measuring devices such as thermoluminescent dosimeter (TLD) and diodes, which must also be calibrated in these conditions.

TP may be based on CT data if the TP computer can accurately account for extended SSD fields. However, all techniques rely on in-vivo dosimetry to confirm or establish the MU required. These surface dose measurements must be carefully related to the dose at depth – usually the midplane dose at the abdomen, or dose to the lung, and may be significantly influenced by electron contamination and the unpredictable scattered radiation doses in this set up.

Stereotactic Radiotherapy and Radiosurgery

The term stereotactic means the three-dimensional localisation of a point in space by a unique set of coordinates that relate to a fixed external reference frame (Fig. 11.26). The first radiotherapeutic use of stereotactic radiotherapy (SRT) was in the treatment of brain tumours, following the principles that had evolved with its neurosurgical use. Although mainly used in the brain, stereotactic principles can be used to treat any tumour site in the body (known as stereotactic body radiotherapy (SBRT)), provided that a good, reproducible fixation system is used, whether the treatment is given in single or multiple fractions. Stereotactic radiosurgery (SRS) is the technique by which narrow, well-defined beams of radiation are focused precisely onto a small target. It is particularly used in brain RT because of its highly focused nature and the importance of reducing dose to sensitive structures, such as brain stem and optic nerves. As the patient fixation, target localisation, treatment delivery, and verification are so precise, the PTV margins around the GTV are generally smaller than for conventional treatment.

SRT/SRS/SBRT treatments can be realised on gantry-mounted linacs as well as on other types of treatment delivery systems.

Stereotaxy on gantry-mounted delivery systems. Modern gantry-mounted linacs provide the capability to treat using narrow radiation fields collimated with MLCs or special add-on collimators or cones. Imperative on such systems is maintaining the alignment of mechanical, radiation, and imaging isocentres to better that 0.5 mm. Flattening filter-free beams allow deliveries at high dose rates. MLCs with leaf widths between 2 and 5 mm are preferable for use in stereotaxic applications. Linac-mounted and external imaging systems are in most cases available for image guidance prior and/or during treatment (image-guided radiotherapy (IGRT)).

Stereotaxy on specialised delivery systems. In addition to gantry-mounted linacs, there are a range of other technologies available for stereotaxy. Multisource SRS systems use a large number of Co-60 sources, which are focused on the volume to be treated. Most commonly used systems on this category are Elektas Gamma Knife model C and Perfexion systems.

Alternatively, there is the robot-mounted linac CyberKnife system by Accuray. This is a compact linac with a single-energy flattening filter-free beam at a dose rate of 1000 MU/min collimated with either cones of different diameters or an adjustable collimator made of two hexagonal banks of tungsten or an MLC with leaf width of 2.5 mm. The robot has six movable joints and typically treatments are planned and delivered using predefined irradiation geometry (treatment templates or paths) dictated by the body site to be treated.

Image-assisted stereotaxy. More recently radiation therapy systems are being developed by research groups or are commercially available that combine MRI together with radiation delivery from either multisource or linac-based systems. These systems offer superior imaging capabilities for volume definition, IGRT, and adaptive RT. The challenges still under investigation are the interference of radiation delivery and MR systems, the limited MR field of view, image distortion issues and artefacts, correct assignment of electron and material properties to voxels for dose calculation purposes, and accounting for the deviation of the paths of charged particles in magnetic fields for dosimetry and TP calculations [13].

Stereotactic treatment planning. The determination of dosimetric parameters needed for factor-based dose calculations often used in TPSs dedicated for cranial stereotactic TP is challenging because of the perturbations introduced by the size detectors used for the measurements in very narrow collimated fields [16,54,55]. It is recommended to follow a careful experimental methodology and use more than one detector with appropriate corrections for the determination of dose. Comprehensive guidance on small MV photon field dosimetry is provided in the dosimetry code of practice of International Atomic Energy Agency (IAEA)/AAPM [54].

The accuracy in dose calculations for stereotactic planning using model-based approaches relies primarily on the design of fluence engine. A prerequisite for this is that the finite source size is modelled (source occlusion effects) as well as the influence of the rounded MLC leaf ends on shaping the overlapping beam penumbras.

TP requires the facility to plan multiple noncoplanar arcs focused to one or more isocentre, or to use multiple, fixed, noncoplanar conformal beams (conformed either with narrow add-on collimators or MLCs). Planning systems will generally allow planning with dynamic

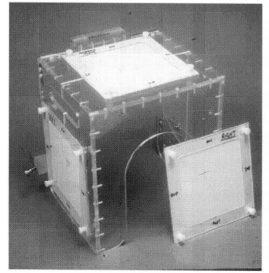
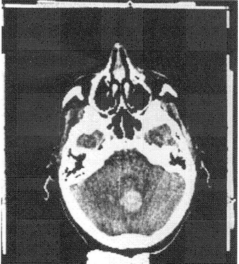

Fig. 11.26 Early approach using a localization frame for setting up the patient for cranial stereotaxy. This technique is now obsolete and image guidance is used instead.

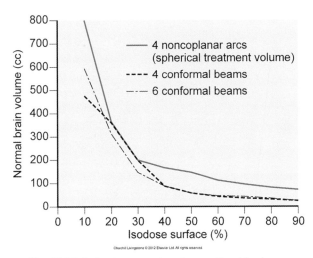

Fig. 11.27 A simple comparison for an ellipsoid volume.

noncoplanar conformal arcs linked to a microleaf delivery system. This directly replaces the original multiple arcs of pencil beams produced with tertiary collimators. VMAT technology with appropriate narrow MLC leaf width is also available.

DVH analysis of brain treatment plans has shown that three to five arcs provide sufficient normal tissue sparing (while giving good dose uniformity to the PTV). However, if stereotactic treatment is being used for young patients or for benign conditions, it is relevant to consider increasing the number of arcs to reduce the exit dose to the whole body from any sagittally orientated arcs. For larger, irregular target volumes (35–70 cc), four to six fixed, noncoplanar fields are probably a better technique, with either conformal blocking or MLC-defined shielding based on the BEV of each portal. Fig. 11.27 shows DVHs comparing three different beam configurations used in a stereotactically planned, elliptically shaped brain lesion. The sparing effect of conformal beam shaping for four and six fixed fields compared with a spherical treatment volume produced by single-isocentre, multiple arcing with a circular collimation is clearly shown.

Although MLCs make it very efficient to produce conformality, conventional 1-cm leaf systems are often unacceptably coarse for SRT and SRS. Typically MLCs with leaf widths of 0.5 cm and 0.25 cm are being used.

ELECTRON THERAPY

Electron beams provide an ideal treatment for superficial PTVs extending from the skin surface to typically down to a depth of 5 cm. The major advantage over photon beams is the sharp fall-off in the dose at depth. The radiobiological effect (RBE) is the same as that for x-rays. Besides the standard fields of circles, squares and rectangles defined by the end frames at the patient end of the applicator, custom cut-outs may be constructed for individual patient PTV shapes.

Electron beams interact with patient contours in unexpected ways and these interactions vary significantly over the clinical range of electron energies (typically 4–20 MeV) so computer planning, or experimental verification can be essential in some treatments. Because the computer dose predictions have the greatest uncertainty in these non-uniform conditions, they should be used with care and with dose measurements (experimental determination of output factors) when appropriate.

Dose Calculations for Electron Beams

Conventionally electron treatments are not computer planned as the set-up is fairly straightforward and the patient can be considered as a uniform water medium. In these cases, standard depth doses and output factor charts may be employed to select beam energy and calculate the MU required. Manual calculations are usually based on the central axis depth dose of the standard applicators, but it is important to understand the limitations of applying these standard data to real clinical conditions.

Dose calculation models for electron beams implemented on planning systems have been either based on pencil beam methods or the MC method. The first commercial pencil beam method was that developed by Hogstrom et al [56,57]. Pencil beam models assume Gaussian characteristics of the incident beam. Hence deviations from these characteristics as a result of collimator scattering, for example, yield errors in the calculation of profiles, leading to an inaccurate prediction of the beam output. To model accurately the penumbra there are corrections needed to the incident pencil beam and these tend to give inaccurate results in the presence of heterogeneities. The width of the incident electron pencil beam is narrow at shallow depths and widens as the depth increases. Dose deposition in voxels at shallow depths tends to be modelled well in the presence of heterogeneities because the size of the voxel is larger than the width of the pencil beam. Dose calculations at voxels located at greater depths at the end of the electron range, where the pencil beam widens, do not account for influence of heterogeneities localised at those depths. Methods to correct for such effects are usually computationally intensive. In most cases pencil beam models tend to be used for the display of a dose distribution, whereas a factor-based formalism is used for the calculation of the MUs.

There is increasing use of dose calculation models based on the MC method. One implementation is based on the macro Monte Carlo (MMC) method developed by Neuenschwander et al [58]. Key concept to this approach is use of precomputed energy deposition data stored in macroscopic spheres of various radii and for a variety of media. Using these data electrons are transported in macroscopic steps through the absorber. The method proves efficient for implementation in a clinical setting. An alternative dose calculation model based on the MC method is the voxel-based Monte Carlo (VMC) approach by Kawrakow et al [59]. Unlike the MMC method, the VMC approach does not use precomputed data but introduces approximations and simplifications in the elementary electron processes without significant losses in accuracy for TP applications and with substantial savings in computation time.

Energy and Depth-Dose Characteristics

Fig. 11.28 shows how an electron beam energy is selected for a specific PTV depth. At low energies, the surface dose may be less than 95% of the prescribed PTV dose and bolus may be needed to shift the isodoses deeper within the patient. Bolus may also be used to modify the treatment depth if a limited range of electron energies is available. The bolus may be applied to the patient skin (in the form of wax or other flexible tissue-equivalent material), or it may be more convenient and comfortable for the patient if the bolus is attached to the end of the applicator, when a solid material such as Perspex may be used. In the latter situation, standoff of up to about 5 cm between the bolus and the patient surface will produce the same penetration of the beam in the patient as if the bolus had been applied directly to the skin surface.

If the 90% isodose is selected to cover the PTV and the dose prescribed to this isodose, then this will result in a 111% maximum dose at the depth of d_{max}. However, this will always be within the PTV. The 90% or 95% isodose is selected as they provide a useful range to cover the PTV, whereas the 100% peak would, at most beam energies, be of

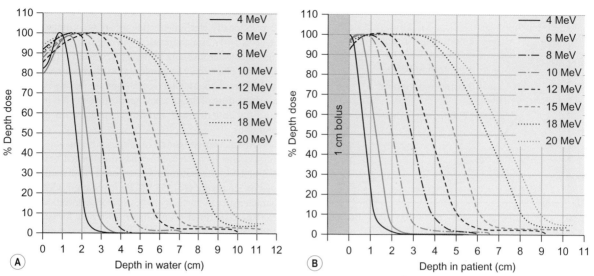

Fig. 11.28 Typical central axis percentage depth doses in water for 10 × 10-cm² electron fields. On the left, no build-up and on the right, with 1-cm build-up.

insufficient range to deliver the prescribed dose to more than a few millimetres in depth.

Penumbra

The penumbral region of any treatment beam determines the field margin that must be applied around the PTV. Because this is complex in electron beams, varying with depth and energy, the clinician must appreciate the dose profile and whether adequate coverage at the field edges will be achieved. If coverage of the 95% isodose at d_{max} is the only point of interest, then the margin can be taken as A in Fig. 11.29A. However, for small fields in particular, the rounded profile of the 95% contour becomes significant and the field could be described as being entirely formed of penumbra as shown in Fig. 11.29B.

Standoff and Stand in

It may be impossible to position the applicator at the standard treatment position. For example, neck treatments may be obstructed by the shoulders, or the patient surface may present a variable SSD across the field area. The inverse-square law cannot usually be applied in the

same way as for photon beams produced by the same treatment machine as each electron energy has a virtual source distance because of the multiple sources of electrons ranging from the scattering foils through to the photon collimators and the electron applicator. Therefore either standard standoff correction tables should be used, or an inverse-square calculation made, based on the virtual source distance. Where the patient contour varies within the field, it is a matter for clinical judgment as to where the prescribed dose is delivered and where an overdose or underdose is acceptable.

Patient Contour Effects

If an electron beam is incident on a steep gradient in the patient contour, then the uniform scattering that produces the standard isodose and depth-dose characteristics no longer exists, and the light field projected onto the skin gives a misleading indication of good coverage. Electrons are cascaded along the edge of the gradient to greater depths before depositing their dose. For shallow gradients, this effect may only result in a small modification to the depth dose; for steep gradients, the cascaded electrons deposit a significant dose, often beyond the targeted volume. All these effects are highly energy dependent and therefore require a reliable planning algorithm or careful experiment to confirm the actual dose distribution. Whenever practicable, this situation should be avoided. The beam angle of incidence should be carefully set up by gantry, collimator, and couch rotations to minimise nonorthogonal incidence. If the electron beam is incident on a cavity such as the ear, then the ear should be filled with a wax plug or wet gauze. Bolus should always extend beyond the field edge so as to avoid a sharp gradient and variations in bolus thickness should be gradual. It may be necessary to employ bolus to block up some target volumes (e.g. around the ear pinna or nose) to provide lateral scatter into the PTV and to generate the uniform dose distribution predicted by the standard isodose distributions. Note that field defining collimation will not produce a significant scatter contribution because of self-absorption. However, shielding within the field must be coated with wax or similar materials to prevent backscattered electrons from enhancing the dose to adjacent tissue. Examples of internal shielding are nasal and mouth shields to prevent the beam from penetrating beyond the PTV.

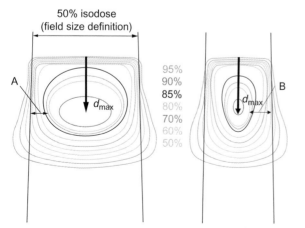

Fig. 11.29 Electron isodose distributions for (A) 8 × 8-cm² and (B) 3 × 3-cm² fields.

Heterogeneities

Bone will attenuate an electron beam because of its higher density and this can be advantageous where the PTV lies above bone as this reduces the dose to underlying tissue. The lung and other air cavities can be a significant hazard in electron beams as their transmission is minimal compared with water and the electron beam entering the lung will not be significantly attenuated until it reaches the lung tissue interface. Therefore, great care should be taken when using higher-energy beams (greater than 12 MeV) to ensure that the dose limits of critical structures underlying the air cavity are not exceeded. The most common example of this is in electron breast boosts where the heart may receive a significant dose.

The use of CT planning can demonstrate the effects of heterogeneities, but unless the calculation algorithm has been verified under all conditions, the isodose distributions should be considered for indication only. CT planning can be useful for identifying the depth of critical structures (e.g. the spinal cord in neck node treatments) even if the TPS dose calculation is not used.

Field Matching

A perfect match between electron–electron or electron–photon fields is not possible, and a compromise is always needed—either to underdose at the junction and risk recurrence or overdose and accept potential tissue damage. The underdose or overdose regions are not in the same location and are dependent on the electron beam energy. Typically, a gap at the skin surface between the 50% isodose edges of an electron and photon beam of 2 mm will give an acceptable compromise. No gap will produce doses of typically 120% or more, whereas a 5-mm gap will result in a significant low-dose region of 70%. Angling the photon beam a few degrees away from the electron beam will give a very small reduction in the overdose region. The use of spoilers, for example, Perspex build-up, in the electron beam can broaden its penumbra and make the set up less critical [60].

Matching two electron beams is similarly very difficult and will often be complicated by the fact that the beams are not parallel to one another as the reason for matching is to cover a large or highly curved contour (e.g. the skull). The match border on a curved surface may be created by a lead strip which shields the surface from one field and is then positioned on the other side of the junction to shield the surface from the abutting field. Even with careful immobilisation, such junctions are prone to significant overdosing or underdosing, especially with oblique fields and where the lead cannot be perfectly positioned in direct skin contact. Therefore, junctions should generally be feathered by moving the junction two or three times during the treatment course to reduce severe overdosing and underdosing. However, many electron treatments are boost fields so a high-dose region of 120% of the boost dose may only be present for say 25% of the overall treatment and thus represents a total dose of 105%.

Verification measurements should be performed with thermoluminescent dosimetry or film to estimate the dose distribution in unusual electron treatment setups.

Specialised Techniques With Electrons

The majority of electron treatments are undertaken with direct single fields using the standard beams on the linac. However, there are two established special techniques, which, although not used widely, are worthy of description.

Total Skin Electron Therapy

The treatment of mycosis fungoides and similar malignancies requires irradiation of the entire skin surface and, given the rarity of the disease, this complex treatment delivery is performed at only a few specialised centres. An even dose distribution is required to a depth of only typically 6 mm for the 90% isodose level, but often encompassing the entire skin surface of the body. It is extremely difficult to come close to achieving 95% to 107% uniformity however complex the treatment technique may be.

A wide variety of techniques have been developed to attempt to achieve this dose coverage. A small single field at an SSD of 1 to 2 m which scans, or arcs, over the patient is one option, but the commonest technique is to use an extended SSD of between 3 m and 7 m so that the patient is covered in one or two beams. The dose rate of a standard linac is increased to reduce treatment times and the dose delivered in daily fractions over several weeks, for example, 36 Gy in 1-Gy daily fractions, as not all treatment positions are delivered in each fraction. The x-ray component of the electron beam is in the range of 1% to 4% of the maximum electron dose for these techniques, so the whole-body dose is not normally of concern.

Beam energies of between 4 and 10 MeV are usually employed, although the energy at the patient is reduced by scattering in air, and energy degraders and scattering screens are placed in the beam to improve dose uniformity and appropriate beam penetration.

The standard depth doses will not be applicable under these conditions and extensive commissioning work is required to determine depth dose and dose rates under these unique treatment conditions. The patient is usually standing and will adopt a different pose at each fraction to be treated effectively at different beam angles to deliver an even dose and to minimise self-shielding. Additional static fields may be required to boost regions that have not received sufficient dose because of self-shielding or extreme obliquity of the incident beam (e.g. the soles of the feet and top of the head).

Evaluation of the dose delivered is difficult as the dose from different beams with a wide range of angle of incidence must be measured at very shallow depths. Thermoluminescent dosimetry is ideal in this area. There is limited scope for precise TP for individual patients before treatment delivery and in-vivo dosimetry is important in verifying the delivered dose to the individual patient and potentially leading to small adjustments in treatment position in subsequent fractions.

Arcing Electron Treatment

Initially, many treatment sites appear good candidates for arcing electron therapy, where multiple fixed fields are replaced by a single beam arcing over the patient and thus eliminating problems of matching junctions. However, in practice, arcing therapy is of no practical value in all but a small number of cases. Fig. 11.30 shows the cross-sectional view of an arc with a narrow slit beam (typically 2–5-cm wide), centred

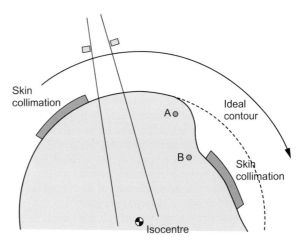

Fig. 11.30 Electron arc treatment.

on a deep isocentre, sweeping over the patient. The arc commences and terminates with the slit irradiating shielding so that each part of the patient receives the same exposure to the slit beam.

Fig. 11.30 shows why this treatment is rarely applicable to widespread surface lesions. The dose to each point depends on the dose rate of the treatment machine, the slit width, and the time that each point of the patient is in the beam. This in turn depends on the arcing speed but, more crucially, it also depends on the distance from the isocentre. If points A and B in the diagram are at the same depth and the SSD at point B is 3 cm greater than that at point A, then the dose at point B will be approximately 6% less than that at point A because of the inverse-square law. However, point B is closer to the isocentre so the sweeping beam will spend much longer irradiating this point than point A resulting in a much higher dose at this point. Therefore contours with any significant variation in curvature will introduce large dose ranges across the arc. There are few sites where this can be achieved for more than 30° of arc and the back is probably the best location for this treatment. The head is unlikely to be a site where arcing therapy offers any advantage over fixed fields even when the matching of abutting fixed fields is the alternative.

In principle, varying the slit width during the arcing could adjust the output, but this requires specialised technology to perform and is not available as a standard treatment option. A specialised TP computer is also required to design this complex treatment as the contour will vary along the slit as well as around the arc. As arcing beams have entirely different characteristics to fixed fields of the same energy, and the inevitable variation of contour through the arc, many hours of pretreatment phantom measurements and in-vivo verification during the treatment are required to design the treatment.

KILOVOLTAGE PHOTON THERAPY

Although opposed fields may be suitable if the separation is small, kilovoltage beams are generally used as a single field to treat very superficial lesions. The field size may be defined by the applicator, but often a lead cut-out will be placed on the skin surface to define the field (see Chapter 8, Fig. 8.5). This needs to be only 2-mm thick for beam energies up to 160 kV. The sharp penumbra of the kV beam means that the high dose part of the field can be matched to the PTV edge. At depth, however, there is some bowing out of the low-value isodose contours.

Although there is some variation of depth dose with field size, this tends to be pronounced beyond the clinically useful depths so will usually only be relevant if considering the dose to underlying structures.

If a lead cut-out on the skin is used, the calculation of treatment time or MU must be based on the cut-out size as well as the applicator output. To calculate the dose in a cut-out, the applicator output must be corrected by the ratio of the backscatter factors for the applicator and cut-out dimensions. This ratio is greater than unity, so that the MUs required for the applicator are increased if a cut-out is used.

The equivalent square or diameter of the cut-out needs to be calculated if the outputs of square or circular fields and backscatter factors are tabulated. The equivalent diameter may be more appropriate as these areas tend to be more circular than rectangular. For irregular cut-outs, and cut-outs on irregular contours, this area measurement is difficult, and realistically the output may not be calculated to better than ±2% to 3%, and probably less accurate for the smallest fields. It may vary by more than this across the area of the cut-out because of the field shape, beam profile, and varying standoff.

The limited applicator size means that fields may have to be abutted to treat long PTVs or for high curvature surfaces. The sharp penumbra means that fields can be abutted and give a uniform dose. The most practical method of achieving this is to use lead on the skin to define the junction rather than an applicator. Care should be taken to ensure the beams are as parallel to each other as possible to minimise overdosing at depth.

DIFFERENCES BETWEEN KILOVOLTAGE AND ELECTRON THERAPY

Although both modalities are suited for superficial treatments, the mechanism of dose deposition is different, resulting in clinically significant differences in the features of the dose distribution.

Depth-dose characteristics will usually favour electron beams because of the sharp fall-off in dose beyond the PTV, although if the prescribed dose is to be delivered to the patient, surface bolus material may be required for lower-energy (typically <10 MeV) electron beams. This is because of the build-up effect present in electron beams, but which is negligible in kV x-ray beams where the maximum dose is at the surface.

The predominant interaction of a low-energy kV photon beam is photoelectric absorption with a probability of interaction in tissue approximately depending on Z^4 (Z being the atomic number). Therefore there is an enhanced dose absorption in bone, which can be significant if high doses are prescribed to superficial regions with underlying bone, such as the scalp. At 100 kV (3-mm Al half-value layer (HVL)), the dose absorption in bone will be 4.5 times greater than in water. By 300 kV (3-mm Cu HVL), this is reduced to 1.05 times the dose in water as Compton interactions predominate and the atomic number of the absorbing material is no longer significant.

The relatively high energy of electrons in an electron beam compared with those generated in a kV beam results in a large range and they can therefore penetrate into tissue well beyond the field edge. The consequence of this is a much broader penumbral region than is present in a kV x-ray beam, and this penumbra varies with depth. Therefore the use of electron beams to treat PTVs very close to critical structures, such as the lens, should be avoided if possible. The sharp penumbra of a kV beam makes it the ideal modality where critical structures are adjacent.

The SSD of a kV machine will typically be far shorter than a linac, usually ranging from 25 cm to 50 cm. Therefore, the inverse-square law dependence of dose will be far more significant in kilovoltage than electron treatments (e.g. a 2-cm air gap results in a dose reduction of approximately 12% at an SSD of 30 cm compared with a reduction of approximately 4% for an electron beam at a standard linac SSD).

There is usually less demand on a kV treatment machine than on a linac, so where the physical differences in the beam are of no clinical significance, then the use of kV may reduce departmental waiting times and facilitate a treatment starting sooner than on a linac. For a few patients, the increased treatment time arising from the lower dose rates of a kilovoltage unit compared with those from a linac may be a disadvantage.

PROTON AND HEAVY-ION THERAPY

The general formula for proton pencil beam algorithm for both passive-scattered and scanned beams is similar to that of photons. The dose distribution within the pencil beam, $D(x, y, z)$ may be described with a single- or double-Gaussian spread across the transverse beam dimensions in x and y axes and the dose distribution along the z axis for a particular proton range depth. These characteristics alter with different incident proton beam energies.

The principal benefit of clinical proton beam therapy is the adjustable range with its sharp distal fall-off. This, however, is also the cause of its inherent uncertainty in target coverage as there is no exit dose to be monitored on treatment. There are several important considerations when planning with proton and ion beams which differ from conventional x-ray and electron planning, mainly relating to uncertainties in calculating proton or ion beam range:

1. The conversion of Hounsfield CT data to proton stopping power, or range.
2. The proton beam modality employed. That is whether it is a scanning pencil beam or a passive-scattered beam with collimation and compensators.
3. The use of planning robustness where uncertainty of complete target volume coverage particularly at the distal fall-off, or avoidance of adjacent OAR, necessitates planning of beam directions, which rely preferentially on beam penumbrae rather than on proton range to achieve complete target coverage.
4. Compensation for biological effectiveness for high-linear energy transfer (LET) ion beams, as well as the high-LET portions of proton beams.

The Hounsfield CT number to proton stopping power conversion has been the subject of much research and development where there was particular concern in regions of bone and air gap interfaces, as well as the proximity of high-Z metal implants.

Robust planning has particular importance in pencil beam scanning where nonideal setups, and inadvertent intrafraction movement or respiratory motion would cause significant errors in delivered dose volume. These issues are less problematical with passive-scattered beams, which are planned with static beams and appropriate range and lateral margins.

Pure Bragg peak beam data at each preferred energy for either passive-scattered or pencil beams would be tabulated in the TPS. In addition, pencil beam scanning requires precise knowledge of the pencil beam dimensions with energy. These may be described by the full-width half-maximum or a Gaussian distribution profile factor, sigma, as well as the position of the delivered beam spots. Recent developments in proton TPS have included the option of correcting for the increasing biological effects with increasing proton LET or RBE at the distal fall-off. Although these effects are not generally considered significant, they are subject to much discussion. The proton range uncertainty when considering all aspects of the planning and measurement processes has been estimated by Paganetti from between 2.7% and 4.6% +1.2 mm of the computed range [61].

Ion beam therapy, for example, with carbon ion beams, is known to produce beams of high RBE, although these are not uniformly distributed. The physical dose distribution of the ion depth-dose distribution has to be modified to produce a uniform biologically effective depth dose (see Chapter 2, Fig. 2.26). The increasing LET of the ion tracks, with decreasing beam energy towards the Bragg peak, causes the ions to become increasingly ionising. Thus biological survival data, which would be dependent on tumour type to be treated, fractionation, and total dose, are folded into the pencil dose algorithm. An additional complexity arises from the effect of carbon beam fragmentation into short-range high-LET particles such as helium and lithium. This dose correction can be shown to amount to 30% to 40% at the carbon beam distal fall-off. Sophisticated TPS is required for proton beam therapy, which requires biological survival data and modelling of LET or RBE data compensation with beam energy, dependence of proton stopping power, and biological survival data.

In general, single Bragg peak data are tabulated for each energy, and then used to form a prescribed spread-out Bragg peak (SOBP) to cover the target. Typically only two to three different fields are employed in modern proton beam therapy plans, whether pencil beam scanning or passive-scattered beams.

The need for an inverse-square correction for variation in SSD depends on the beamline setup and the apparent origin of the proton source. In passive-scattered systems, the scatter foils and/or modulators may be only several metres upstream of the isocentre and thus need an inverse-square correction. The same would apply to a pencil beam setup where the scanning magnets would act as the virtual source. Some gantries, for example, the Gantry 2 at Paul Scherrer Institute, have been designed to produce a parallel beam as they arrive at the patient. In effect the beam has infinite source to axis distance and this reduces surface dose and simplifies the use of matched fields when large target areas are needed to be treated.

The need for custom modulation wheels depends on whether the conformity produced by a scanned pencil beam is needed, or whether treatment using a passive-scattered beam would suffice. The latter would apply to centres with beam lines that offer both proton beam modalities: scanned and passive. Passive-scattered techniques require a large set of modulator wheels whether for a gantry or fixed horizontal beam line and also require some set ups to use these in conjunction with beam timing to produce the required modulation and uniformity. However, most commercial systems offer pencil beam scanning with a finely spaced range of energies (as explained in Chapter 9). This enables millimetre resolution in depth.

For passive-scattered beams the coverage is according to the prescribed SOBP and range, thus the modulator is custom-made. The modulation depends upon energy resolution and affects the quality of the SOBP, that is, the ripple effects.

The aperture is always tailored to the target. Usually, brass apertures, and polymethyl methacrylate (PMMA) compensators, are used in passive-scattered beams; these are created from planning data of the target shape and volume. The manufacture of patient-specific beam modifying equipment is normally not required for pencil beam scanning as the intensity and positioning of the beamlets, or spots, deliver the prescribed three-dimensional dose volume. However, certain improvements have evolved to improve the field edge penumbrae by using collimators. Plastic energy absorbers, which are applied at the beam nozzle and close to the patient, are used to achieve very superficial penetration depths, but in these cases the increased lateral spread of the beamlets would be incorporated at the planning stage.

With passive-scattered beams there are beam output factors to account for the beam aperture area, metal collimators, distance, and energy. This does not apply to pencil beam scanning where the intensity of each beam spot or beamlet is calculated to deliver the prescribed field, whether in a uniform field mode or in an intensity-modulated mode.

QUALITY ASSURANCE IN TREATMENT PLANNING

The TPS is an essential component in the RT process as it is used to define treatment volumes and design and evaluate treatment plans. The role of the TPS is illustrated in Fig. 11.31. It is a software suite comprising a range of different software tools, of which the most unique and complex are the fluence and dose calculation engines. QA in TP can be examined in two parts. The first part incorporates all quality control checks on different aspects of functionality of the TPS. The second part is specific to the individual patient's treatment and referred to as patient- or plan-specific quality assurance (PSQA). The next two paragraphs address these two aspects.

Treatment Planning System Commissioning and Performance Testing

The general performance of a TPS is at first level checked by its vendor. The vendor and the user subsequently are responsible for the generic

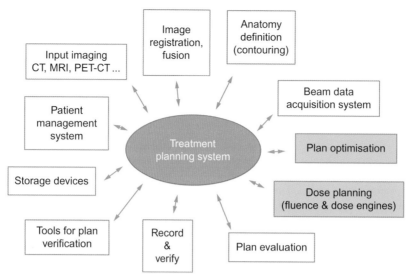

Fig. 11.31 The treatment planning system as the hub of radiotherapy.

performance of the system in the clinical setting (the user's environment). As with other medical equipment this second step refers to the acceptance testing of the TPS on-site just after installation. Following this, it is the user's responsibility to check the performance of the TPS under the specific conditions in which it is to be used clinically. The medical physicist is solely responsible for this task. This involves both commissioning the TPS, verifying this before clinical use, and designing an appropriate QA program for periodically checking its performance.

Commissioning a TPS incorporates planning and performing all measurements required to configure the fluence and dose engines. The responsible user must carefully select the appropriate detector system for each measurement, perform the measurement with low uncertainty, and correctly define and import the data into the TPS [62–64]. Most TPSs have a configuration package to process data, calculate the parameters for the fluence and dose engines, and review the results. Following commissioning the user validates its performance for an extended set of irradiation geometries that are encountered in the clinic. TPS performance testing can be an overwhelming task, considering the large number of different situations that one could check. There is a wealth of guidance and recommendations available on how to design relevant checks, which cover the cases for which a TPS is used [62,65–69]. There is also guidance on the tolerances for this testing; these being primarily dependant on the location where the dose is being evaluated [70].

Plan-Specific Quality Assurance

As part of a treatment machine or planning system QA program, a standard set of tests is typically executed and if successful, there is confidence that the equipment and software can safely be used clinically. Traditionally there has always been a secondary check on the MUs or dose being computed by the TPS. With PSQA one refers to the additional checks that are carried out to confirm that the treatment is delivered as planned for each individual patient. These tend to incorporate some type of experimental verification on the plan and this has been the role of in-vivo dosimetry, traditionally carried out using TLDs, diodes, or MOSFETS (metal oxide semiconductor field effect transistor) to measure dose at specific locations on surfaces (entry and exit doses) and from these derive an estimate of the dose at a midline in the patient [71,72]. Designing and maintaining an in-vivo dosimetry program necessitates sufficient resources in RT physics and it is time-consuming. The application of in-vivo dosimetry using a single detector to measure dose in modulated plans (IMRT or VMAT) is not straightforward because a large number of

corrections to the detector reading are needed to account for its response in fields that differ considerably from the irradiation geometry used at calibration.

The verification of treatment plans can be classified into different categories or levels. The first level is what is widely known as pretreatment verification. Here one checks that the treatment unit delivers the treatment as planned without the presence of the patient. With this approach changes in the delivered dose distribution because of changes in the patient are not checked, and any changes in data transfer or machine output at the time of patient treatment are also not checked. Pretreatment verification is carried out either by delivering the plan on a phantom using one-dimensional or two-dimensional detector systems or on the portal imager. With two-dimensional detectors and portal imagers, special software is used to evaluate and compare the dose delivered to the detector/imager against the dose calculated by the planning system.

The second level in PSQA is to perform this during patient treatment. Here one records and then reviews the changes in machine parameters (such as MLC leaf positions, gantry angle etc., saved in machine log files). The dose can be recalculated on the planning CT using the parameters from the log files. It is also possible to use transmission detectors mounted on the linac head, which record the fluence exiting the machine during treatment. In this way it is possible to also record changes in beam output during treatment and calculate the influence of this on the dose distribution. In both these cases changes in the patient anatomy during treatment are not taken into consideration.

The third level in PSQA is true in-vivo dosimetry. The dose delivered to the patient is confirmed and compared against the dose planned. There are several ways to address this. The general concept is to record the fluence through the patient during treatment on the MV portal imager and compare this with the calculated fluence on the imager (in vivo transit dosimetry). Alternatively, one could implement what is known as back-projection approach and use this information to reconstruct the dose on the planning CT or the cone-beam CT instead [73–78]. At the time of writing there are several commercial products aiming to provide solutions to PSQA based on the aforementioned or similar concepts.

Ultimately, to evaluate the success of a patient's RT treatment, it is important to know the dose delivered from the treatment and not only that the planned dose is deliverable. The integration of efficient and fast PSQA solutions in the RT chain, perhaps as part of the tools available on TPSs, is a necessity if the adaptation of treatment plans during the course of RT is to become routine practice.

REFERENCES

[1] ICRU-50. Prescribing, recording, and reporting photon beam therapy. Bethesda, MD: ICRU Publications; 1993.

[2] ICRU-78. Prescribing, recording, and reporting proton beam therapy. Bethesda, MD: ICRU Publications; 1993.

[3] ICRU-83. Prescribing, recording, and reporting photon-beam intensity-modulated radiation therapy (IMRT). Bethesda, MD: ICRU Publications; 1993.

[4] ICRU-62. Prescribing, recording, and reporting photonbeam therapy. (Supplement to ICRU Report 50). T. I. C. o. R. U. a. Measurements. Bethesda, MD: ICRU Publications; 1999.

[5] ICRU-71. Prescribing, recording, and reporting electron beam therapy. Bethesda, MD: ICRU Publications; 2004.

[6] ICRU-91. Prescribing, recording, and reporting of stereotactic treatments with small photon beams. Bethesda, MD: ICRU Publications; 2017.

[7] Bentzen SM, Constine LS, Deasy JO, et al. Quantitative analyses of normal tissue effects in the clinic (QUANTEC): an introduction to the scientific issues. Int J Radiat Oncol Biol Phys 2010;76(3):S3–9.

[8] Reft C, Alecu R, Das IJ, et al. Dosimetric considerations for patients with HIP prostheses undergoing pelvic irradiation. Report of the AAPM Radiation Therapy Committee Task Group 63. Med Phys 2003;30(6):1162–82.

[9] Hurkmans CW, Scheepers E, Springorum BG, et al. Influence of radiotherapy on the latest generation of pacemakers. Radiother Oncol 2005;76(1):93–8.

[10] Hurkmans CW, Knegjens JL, Oei BS, et al. Management of radiation oncology patients with a pacemaker or ICD: a new comprehensive practical guideline in The Netherlands. Dutch Society of Radiotherapy and Oncology (NVRO). Radiat Oncol 2012;7:198.

[11] Olch AJ, Gerig L, Li H, et al. Dosimetric effects caused by couch tops and immobilization devices: report of AAPM Task Group 176. Med Phys 2014;41(6). 061501.

[12] Keall PJ, Mageras GS, Balter JM, et al. The management of respiratory motion in radiation oncology report of AAPM Task Group 76. Med Phys 2006;33(10):3874–900.

[13] Das IJ, McGee KP, Tyagi N, et al. Role and future of MRI in radiation oncology. Br J Radiol 2019;92(1094). 20180505.

[14] Karlsson M, Ahnesjö A, Georg D, et al. Physics booklet Nr 10: Independent Dose Calculations Concepts and Models. ESTRO Physics booklets. Brussels, European Society for Therapeutic Radiology and Oncology; 2010.

[15] Aspradakis MM, Lambert GD, Steele A, et al. Elements of commissioning step-and-shoot IMRT: delivery equipment and planning system issues posed by small segment dimensions and small monitor units. Med Dosim 2005;30(4):233–42.

[16] Aspradakis MM, Byrne JP, Palmans H, et al. IPEM report 103: small field MV photon dosimetry. institute of physics and engineering in medicine. York, UK: IPEM; 2010.

[17] Ahnesjö A, Aspradakis MM. Dose calculations for external photon beams in radiotherapy. Phys Med Biol 1999;44(11):R99–155.

[18] Vassiliev ON, Wareing TA, McGhee J, et al. Validation of a new grid-based Boltzmann equation solver for dose calculation in radiotherapy with photon beams. Phys Med Biol 2010;55(3):581–98.

[19] Bush K, Gagne IM, Zavgorodni S, et al. Dosimetric validation of Acuros XB with Monte Carlo methods for photon dose calculations. Med Phys 2011;38(4):2208–21.

[20] Han T, Followill D, Mikell J, et al. Dosimetric impact of Acuros XB deterministic radiation transport algorithm for heterogeneous dose calculation in lung cancer. Med Phys 2013;40(5). 051710.

[21] Verhaegen F, Seuntjens J. Monte Carlo modelling of external radiotherapy photon beams. Phys Med Biol 2003;48(21):R107–64.

[22] Reynaert N, van der Marck S, Schaart D, et al. NCS report 16: Monte Carlo treatment planning: an introduction. Delft, The Netherlands: Netherlands Commission on Radiation Dosimetry (NCS); 2006.

[23] Seco J, Verhaegen F. Monte Carlo techniques in radiation therapy. CRC Press; 2016.

[24] Mackie TR, Bielajew AF, Rogers DWO, et al. Generation of photon energy deposition kernels using the EGS Monte Carlo code. Phys Med Biol 1988;33(1):1–20.

[25] Nyholm T, Olofsson J, Ahnesjo A, et al. Photon pencil kernel parameterisation based on beam quality index. Radiother Oncol 2006;78(3):347–51.

[26] Mohan R, Chui CS. Use of fast Fourier transforms in calculating dose distributions for irregularly shaped fields for three-dimensional treatment planning. Med Phys 1987;14(1):70–7.

[27] Boyer A, Mok E. A photon dose distribution model employing convolution calculations. Med Phys 1985;12(2):169–77.

[28] Mackie TR, Scrimger JW, Battista JJ, et al. A convolution method of calculating dose for 15-MV x rays. Med Phys 1985;12(2):188–96.

[29] Ahnesjö A, Andreo P, Brahme A, et al. Calculation and application of point spread functions for treatment planning with high energy photon beams. Acta Oncologica 1987;26(1):49–56.

[30] Ahnesjö A. Collapsed cone convolution of radiant energy for photon dose calculation in heterogeneous media. Med Phys 1989;16:577–92.

[31] Bourland JD, Chaney EL. A finite-size pencil beam model for photon dose calculations in three dimensions. Med Phys 1992;19(6):1401–12.

[32] Ulmer W, Pyyry J, Kaissl W, et al. A 3D photon superposition/convolution algorithm and its foundation on results of Monte Carlo calculations. Phys Med Biol 2005;50(8):1767–90.

[33] Tillikainen L, Helminen, H, Torsti T, et al. A 3D pencil-beam-based superposition algorithm for photon dose calculation in heterogeneous media. Phys Med Biol 2008;53(14):3821–39.

[34] Dutreix A, Bjärngard BE, Bridier A, et al. Monitor unit calculation for high energy photon beams. Leuven/Apeldoorn: Garant Publishers, N. V.; 1997.

[35] Zhu TC, Ahnesjo A, Lam KL, et al. Report of AAPM Therapy Physics Committee Task Group 74: in-air output ratio, Sc, for megavoltage photon beams. Med Phys 2009;36(11):5261–91.

[36] Stern RL, Heaton R, Fraser MW, et al. Verification of monitor unit calculations for non-IMRT clinical radiotherapy: report of AAPM Task Group 114. Med Phys 2011;38(1):504–30.

[37] Gibbons JP, Antolak JA, Followill DS, et al. Monitor unit calculations for external photon and electron beams: Report of the AAPM Therapy Physics Committee Task Group No. 71. Med Phys 2014;41(3):031501.

[38] Willoughby TR, Starkschall G, Janjan NA, et al. Evaluation and scoring of radiotherapy treatment plans using an artificial neural network. Int J Radiat Oncol Biol Phys 1996;34:923–30.

[39] Brahme A. Design principles and clinical possibilities with a new generation of radiation therapy equipment. A review. Acta Oncol 1987;26(6):403–12.

[40] Brahme A. Optimization of stationary and moving beam radiation therapy techniques. Radiother Oncol 1988;12(2):129–40.

[41] Boyer AL, Ochran TG, Nyerick CE, et al. Clinical dosimetry for implementation of a multileaf collimator. Med Phys 1992;19(5):1255–61.

[42] Boyer AL, Li S. Geometric analysis of light-field position of a multileaf collimator with curved ends. Med Phys 1997;24(5):757–62.

[43] Boyer A, Biggs P, Galvin J, et al. AAPM Report TG 50: basic applications of multileaf collimators. AAPM; 2001.

[44] Mackie TR, Holmes T, Swerdloff S, et al. Tomotherapy: A new concept for the delivery of dynamic conformal radiotherapy. Med Phys 1993;20(6):1709–19.

[45] Carol MP. A system for planning and rotational delivery of intensity-modulated fields. Int J Imaging Syst Tech 1995;6:56–61.

[46] Vaarkamp J, Adams EJ, Warrington AP, et al. A comparison of forward and inverse planned conformal, multi segment and intensity modulated radiotherapy for the treatment of prostate and pelvic nodes. Radiother Oncol 2004;73(1):65–72.

[47] Das IJ, Kase KR, Tello VM, et al. Dosimetric accuracy at low monitor unit settings. Br J Radiol 1991;64(765):808–11.

[48] Bragg CM, Conway J, Robinson MH, et al. The role of intensity-modulated radiotherapy in the treatment of parotid tumors. Int J Radiat Oncol Biol Phys 2002;52(3):729–38.

[49] Clark CH, Mubata CD, Meehan CA, et al. IMRT clinical implementation: prostate and pelvic node irradiation using Helios and a 120-leaf multileaf collimator. J Appl Clin Med Phys 2002;3(4):273–84.

[50] Pirzkall A, Carol MP, Pickett B, et al. The effect of beam energy and number of fields on photon-based IMRT for deep-seated targets. Int J Radiat Oncol Biol Phys 2002;53(2):434–42.

[51] Mackie TR. History of tomotherapy. Phys Med Biol 2006;51(13):R427–53.

[52] Otto K. Volumetric modulated arc therapy: IMRT in a single gantry arc. Med Phys 2008;35(1):310–7.

[53] Plowman PN. A review of total body irradiation. Br J Radiol Suppl 1988;22:135–44.

[54] IAEA-TRS483. Dosimetry of small static fields used in external beam radiotherapy technical report series No. 483. Vienna: International Atomic Energy Agency; 2017.

[55] Andreo P. The physics of small megavoltage photon beam dosimetry. Radiother Oncol 2018;126(2):205–13.

[56] Hogstrom KR, Mills MD, Meyer JA, et al. Dosimetric evaluation of a pencil-beam algorithm for electrons employing a two-dimensional heterogeneity correction. Int J Radiat Oncol Biol Phys 1984;10(4):561–9.

[57] Hogstrom KR. Treatment planning in electron beam therapy. Front Radiat Ther Oncol 1991;25:30–52.

[58] Neuenschwander H, Mackie TR, Reckwerdt PJ, et al. MMC–a high-performance Monte Carlo code for electron beam treatment planning. Phys Med Biol 1995;40(4):543–74.

[59] Kawrakow I, Fippel M, Friedrich K, et al. 3D electron dose calculation using a Voxel based Monte Carlo algorithm (VMC). Med Phys 1996;23(4):445–57.

[60] McKenzie AL. A simple method for matching electron beams in radiotherapy. Phys Med Biol 1998;43(12):3465–78.

[61] Paganetti H. Range uncertainties in proton therapy and the role of Monte Carlo simulations. Phys Med Biol 2012;57(11):R99–117.

[62] IAEA-TRS430. Commissioning and quality assurance of computerized planning systems for radiation treatment of cancer. Technical report series No. 430. Vienna: International Atomic Energy Agency; 2004.

[63] Das IJ, Cheng CW, Watts RJ, et al. Accelerator beam data commissioning equipment and procedures: report of the TG-106 of the Therapy Physics Committee of the AAPM. Med Phys 2008;35(9):4186–215.

[64] Low DA, Moran JM, Dempsey JF, et al. Dosimetry tools and techniques for IMRT. Med Phys 2011;38(3):1313–38.

[65] Fraass B, Doppke K, Hunt M, et al. American Association of Physicists in Medicine Radiation Therapy Committee Task Group 53: Quality assurance for clinical radiotherapy treatment planning. Med Phys 1998;25(10):1773–829.

[66] Mijnheer B, Olszewska A, Fiorino C, et al. Quality assurance of treatment planning systems - practical examples for non-IMRT photon beams. Brussels: European Society for Therapeutic Radiology and Oncology; 2004.

[67] Bruinvis IAD, Keus RB, Lenglet WJM, et al. NCS report 15: Quality assurance of 3-D treatment planning systems for external photon and electron beams. Netherlands Commission on Radiation Dosimetry; 2005.

[68] IAEA-TECDOC-1583. Commissioning of radiotherapy treatment planning systems: testing for typical external beam treatment techniques. IAEA-TECDOC. Vienna: International Atomic Energy Agency; 2008.

[69] Smilowitz JB, Das IJ, Feygelman V, et al. AAPM Medical Physics Practice Guideline 5.a.: commissioning and QA of treatment planning dose calculations—megavoltage photon and electron beams. J Appl Clin Med Phys 2016;17(1):14–35.

[70] Venselaar J, Welleweerd H, Mijnheer B, et al. Tolerances for the accuracy of photon beam dose calculations of treatment planning systems. Radiother Oncol 2001;60:191–201.

[71] Huyskens D, Bogaerts R, Verstraete J, et al. Practical guidelines for the implementation of in vivo dosimetry with diodes in external radiotherapy with photon beams (entrance dose) Brussels; 2001.

[72] Ellen Yorke E, Rodica Alecu R, Li Ding L, et al. (2005). Diode in vivo dosimetry for patients receiving external beam radiation therapy. AAPM Report 87. M. P. Publishing. Report of Task Group 62 of the Radiation Therapy Committee.

[73] Hansen VN, Evans PM, Swindell W, et al. The application of transit dosimetry to precision radiotherapy. Med Phys 1996;23(5):713–21.

[74] Kapatoes JM, Olivera GH, Ruchala KJ, et al. A feasible method for clinical delivery verification and dose reconstruction in tomotherapy. Med Phys 2001;28(4):528–42.

[75] Louwe RJ, Damen EM, van Herk M, et al. Three-dimensional dose reconstruction of breast cancer treatment using portal imaging. Med Phys 2003;30(9):2376–89.

[76] Wendling M, Louwe RJ, McDermott LN, et al. Accurate two-dimensional IMRT verification using a back-projection EPID dosimetry method. Med Phys 2006;33(2):259–73.

[77] Olaciregui-Ruiz I, Rozendaal R, Mijnheer B, et al. Automatic in vivo portal dosimetry of all treatments. Phys Med Biol 2013;58(22):8253–64.

[78] Hanson IM, Hansen VN, Olaciregui-Ruiz I, et al. Clinical implementation and rapid commissioning of an EPID based in-vivo dosimetry system. Phys Med Biol 2014;59(19):N171–9.

12

Networking, Data, Image Handling and Computing in Radiotherapy

John Sage

CHAPTER OUTLINE

INTRODUCTION

*Technology is so much fun but we can drown in our technology.
The fog of information can drive out knowledge.*

                         Daniel Boorstin

Computers permeate every aspect of modern radiotherapy. With their application we can deliver ever more intricate treatments. However, every technological innovation comes at a cost: in equipment, maintenance and added complexity. With care these costs can be kept in balance and benefits to the patient achieved.

Computing in radiotherapy has developed as computers have grown more powerful. In 1965 Gordon Moore, co-founder of the computing giant Intel, predicted that microchip complexity would increase exponentially for at least 10 years [1]. In fact, Moore's law still holds today, with processors doubling in complexity approximately every 2 years. Moore's law typifies the growth in all aspects of computing. Hard disk drive capacity nearly doubles each year whilst the cost per gigabyte nearly halves [2].

This growth has consequences for radiotherapy. The useful lifetime of any item of computer software or hardware is going to be fairly short. In the NHS, a lifetime of 5 years is used for IT equipment, compared with 10 years for a linear accelerator [3]. This growth also needs to be considered when planning for long-term needs. It will be more costly to purchase 5 years data storage immediately than it will be to buy half now and half in 2 years time, at a quarter of the cost.

History

For many decades radiotherapy was developed without computers. Isodose planning and linear accelerators both predate the use of computers. In the 1960s, the first investigations were made into using computers for radiotherapy. Such use required access to one of the small number of large 'mainframe' computers, probably at a university, because personal computers were not invented until the 1970s. The first widespread use of computers was for calculating isodose distributions, replacing laborious manual calculations. In the late 1970s, the first use was made of computed tomography (CT) data for radiotherapy planning. This required a magnetic tape reader connected to the planning system to read the CT scanner tapes.

As networking technology became available it was possible to connect computers directly together. However, CT scanners still used different file formats. In 1985, the American College of Radiology and the National Electrical Manufacturers Association created a standard for medical images called ACR-NEMA. In the third version, in 1991, the standard was developed to specify how systems should communicate directly. To mark this change a new name for the standard was used: 'Digital Imaging and Communication in Medicine', or DICOM 3.0.

Networking and computing capability have continuously driven radiotherapy development, from the first simple electronic checking of the linac beam settings in the 1980s to advanced systems which allow the real-time updating of the beam to respond to the patient position. Similarly, the use of digital imaging continues to expand with magnetic resonance (MR) imaging at point of treatment now in routine clinical use.

Such wealth of information creates a problem in how this is organised and best used. Oncology information systems manage data flow within a single centre. The next boundary to be overcome will be the pooling of information across whole populations. This will allow clinical collaboration between practitioners for rare cancers and facilitate the continuous learning systems that we are just beginning to see emerge [4].

Benefits and Hazards of Computerisation

The more advanced techniques that we practise would not be possible at all without the assistance of computers. Intensity modulated radiotherapy would be totally unfeasible without computers or data communication. Even simple techniques are enhanced by the use of computers. If data are transferred directly between computers, there is less chance of human error. The use of record and verify systems has certainly reduced the number of random human errors at the point of treatment delivery [5].

Ultimately, the hazards of computerisation relate to our increased dependence on computer systems and the faulty assumption that they are reliable. Computers and networks do fail. A radiotherapy department that is reliant on a system can be crippled if that system is the victim of component failure, a virus, or even theft.

As systems become more complicated they are harder to check for errors. It should never be assumed that the computer is correct. Furthermore, computers do not remove the risk of human error altogether. Proper use of a system relies on operators performing tasks correctly. If they do not, then incorrect information can be passed down the line and used at a later stage. Where errors do occur in computerised systems, they may affect a series of patients or a single patient for every fraction of their treatment [6].

To reduce these risks we need to reverse the assumption that the computer is reliable. Key checks should be made, during system testing and for individual treatments. Is the isocentre correct? Is the patient reference position correct? Where there are multiple data sets, has the correct one been used for the treatment? When every plan had to be calculated and delivered manually, each person involved had to fully understand the technique and the treatment. Now that the treatment can be delivered at the touch of a button, that level of understanding is critical to detect errors.

NETWORKING

Networks are commonly described as having a number of layers. In one of the simpler descriptions, the TCP/IP model, four layers are described [7]. To understand these layers we draw a comparison with the postal system, Table 12.1.

Because the network is layered in this way, any changes that occur in one layer do not affect the others, so you don't need to write a new application because you have bought a new modem.

Link Layer: Physical Infrastructure

In a very large network, such as a hospital, there will be a large number of switches, controlling and routing the flow of data in the hospital. In such a large network the computers may be organised into subnetworks, or subnets. Access between subnets is controlled by 'gateways' which can prevent unauthorised access between areas, Fig. 12.1.

Network Layer: Addressing

When you type 'www.estro.org' into a web browser, how does your computer connect to the computer that contains the homepage of the European Society for Therapeutic Radiotherapy and Oncology? Each domain name is registered to a computer address called an IP address which consists of four numbers. Your computer initially sends a request to a directory to find out the correct IP address. Then it sends a request to that IP address to retrieve the correct web page.

Inside a private network, such as a hospital, computers are still referenced using an IP address. Special ranges of numbers are reserved for use in private networks to avoid confusion with internet traffic. On many Windows computers it is possible to see the network configuration by typing the command 'ipconfig' at a command prompt.[1] If you do this, and your computer is attached to a network, you will see something like that shown in Fig. 12.2.

TABLE 12.1	The Four Network Layers of the TCP/IP Model	
Layer	**Network**	**Postal**
Link	The infrastructure of cables, switches, modems and so on which allow information to be moved from one place to another.	The infrastructure of vehicles and sorting offices which allows post to be moved around.
Network	The addressing system which allows a single computer to be identified and for data to be routed to it.	The addressing system which allows post to be directed to the correct destination.
Transport	The process of packing the data and sending it into the network. Also the process of receiving data from the network.	Taking letters to the post office to send and picking up received letters.
Application	Defining the data to be sent and interpreting any data received.	Writing and reading your post.

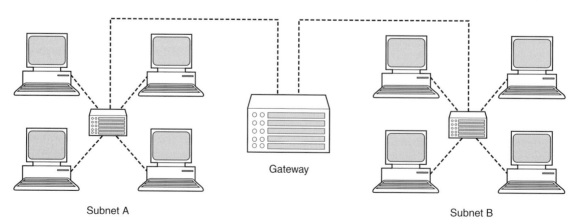

Fig. 12.1 Two subnets separated by a gateway.

Subnet A   Gateway   Subnet B

[1]To get a command prompt: click on the start button, select run, type cmd in the box and select OK.

This tells us that our computer is in the network domain hospital. nhs.uk. The first two numbers of the IP address are among those reserved for private networks. That tells us that this computer cannot be seen by the internet. The second two numbers in the IP address will be unique for this computer within the hospital. The subnet mask describes the range of IP addresses that are in our local subnet; in this case, the IP addresses 192.168.123.1 through to 192.168.123.255. The default gateway is the IP address of the computer or switch that our computer must go through to access the network outside the local subnet, such as the internet.

Transport Layer: Send and Receive

The simplest form of data transport is the 'ping', which is used for the testing of data connections. If you still have a command prompt open on your computer, type 'ping 192.168.123.1', replacing the IP address here with the IP address of your gateway, Fig. 12.3.

Your computer has just packaged a data packet and sent it into the network addressed to the gateway. On receipt, the gateway sends a return package back to your computer. The ping command is often one of the first tools used when testing a network connection. A

```
Windows IP Configuration
Ethernet adapter Local Area Connection:

  Connection-specific DNS suffix  . : hospital.nhs.uk
  IP Address . . . . . . . . . . . : 192.168.123.45
  Subnet mask. . . . . . . . . . . : 255.255.255.0
  Default Gateway  . . . . . . . . : 192.168.123.1
```

Fig. 12.2 Sample output from ipconfig.

```
Pinging 192.168.123.1 with 32 bytes of data:

Reply from 192.168.123.1: bytes=32 time<1ms TTL=255
Reply from 192.168.123.1: bytes=32 time<1ms TTL=255
Reply from 192.168.123.1: bytes=32 time<1ms TTL=255
Reply from 192.168.123.1: bytes=32 time<1ms TTL=255

Ping statistics for 192.168.123.1:
    Packets: sent = 4, Recieved = 4, Lost = 0 (0% loss)
Approximate round trip times in milli-seconds:
    Minimum = 0ms, Maximum = 0ms, Average = 0ms
```

Fig. 12.3 Sample output from ping.

successful ping proves that both the link layer and the network layer are working correctly.

There are a lot of different potential connections that a computer can make. In the example above how did the gateway know that this single data packet came from a ping request and that it should send a return message? Also, how can a computer make multiple connections of different types without them getting confused? Each computer has a whole series of network 'ports'. When a computer receives a data packet addressed to port number 7 it knows that this is a ping request and responds accordingly, whereas requests for web pages are normally addressed to port 80. Imagine having a whole series of slots outside your house and the postman sorting them out for you into bills, junk mail and so on.

Application Layer: The Program

The final layer is the program itself, which is often the hardest part. Just because you can send a letter to anywhere in the world, it doesn't mean that they will be able to understand what you have written.

Network Security

On 12th May 2017 about a third of NHS Trusts in England were disrupted by the WannaCry virus, resulting in the cancellation of thousands of patient appointments and operations [8]. Radiotherapy departments were not immune, although for many the subsequent lock down and emergency network restrictions had a greater impact than the initial attack. Because the modern radiotherapy department is so reliant on the network, it is important to protect it against various hazards. There is also a legal requirement to protect patient data and often a minimum security level which must be reached to connect to the hospital network. These are summarised in Fig. 12.4.

Most modern medical devices are network connected and this brings particular challenges. The requirement for device manufacturers to strictly control and test any change in the device design conflicts with the need to continuously update computer systems to maintain security. It is important to obtain from equipment providers detailed plans on how network security will be maintained over the equipment lifespan.

DICOM

As described previously, DICOM stands for Digital Imaging and Communication in Medicine and is produced by the National Electrical

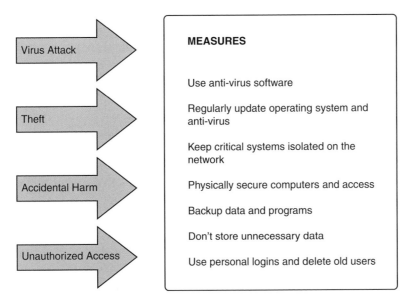

Fig. 12.4 Potential impact of network hazards and measures to mitigate them.

Manufacturers Association in the USA. DICOM is a constantly evolving standard with a number of working parties and regular releases [9].

DICOM is often mistakenly considered as a data file format. Whilst there is a file format within DICOM, it is primarily a data transfer protocol, a means to move medical images between systems. DICOM aims to be a complete specification for such transfer and specifies requirements over all the network layers.

The second common misconception about DICOM is that two DICOM-compliant devices will communicate correctly. This mistake is the root cause of a great deal of anxiety. Given the huge variety of medical imaging equipment, DICOM is not prescriptive. There is a great deal of variation possible within the standard. Where there is variation, DICOM provides us with a common language to describe the functionality of a system and check whether two systems are compatible.

DICOM Services

DICOM connections are not always about the transfer of images from one computer to another. A connection may be to print an image, send a worklist to a scanner or find patient images. Each of these possibilities is called a **service class**. Furthermore in any transaction there will be a **service class provider**, SCP, and a **service class user**, SCU. Therefore a server may offer the storage class as SCP and a number of systems may send images to it as SCU.

DICOM Communication

To establish a DICOM connection we need two critical pieces of information. Firstly, we need to know the IP address of the computer we wish to connect to. Secondly we need to know which network port the DICOM program is monitoring. Port 104 is reserved for use by DICOM programs and is normally the correct port. However, this is not always the case; a single computer may even run several DICOM servers on different ports. With these two pieces of information we are able to establish communication with the DICOM server, but this does not necessarily mean that the connection will be successful.

The security of DICOM servers varies widely. Some will communicate with any system that has the correct address and port. This makes setting the system up easy, but security will be poor. Others will make further checks. Each DICOM program has a name, called an **application entity title** or AET. Most servers will refuse a connection to a system that does not call it by the correct name. Furthermore, many servers will check the AET of the requesting system against a list of known AETs.

Upon connection, the two systems perform what is known as a 'handshake'. They swap credentials and determine whether the action which is being requested is supported and whether to continue with the action. Then information is exchanged and the association is closed.

DICOM Data Objects

One key problem in sending data between imaging systems is defining the exact meaning of the information sent. DICOM solves this through the use of a data dictionary. Each possible piece of information about the image, called a **data element**, is catalogued and given a code. The exact definition of the information for each code is contained in the standard.

Any **data object**, such as a radiotherapy plan or a CT image, will consist of a collection of data elements relevant to that object. The DICOM standard details which data elements are mandatory for a given object and which are optional. Another new term, the **service-object pair** (SOP), is used to describe the application of a particular service class to a data object. We may talk about a general **SOP class**, such as CT image storage, or even a particular **SOP instance**, one specific stored CT image.

The diagram below in Fig. 12.5 shows an example of a minimal CT object. Each row of the diagram shows the entry for each of the separate data elements. For each data element there is a two-number code which relates that element to the DICOM data dictionary. The data elements

```
0008 0008 Image Type              ORIGINAL\PRIMARY\AXIAL
0008 0016 SOP ClassVID            1.2.840.10008.5.1.4.1.1.2
0008 0018 SOP Instance VID        1.2.345.6.789.8.76.5.4321.0.10
0008 0020 Study Date              20021011
0008 0060 Modality                CT
0008 0090 Referring Physician     DR
0008 1030 Study Description       SAMPLE CT SCAN

0010 0010 Patient Name            Walter/Miller
0010 0020 Patient ID              01234

0018 0050 Slice Thickness         5
0018 0060 KVP                     130
0018 5100 Patient Posistion       HFS

0020 000d Study Instance VID      1.2.345.6.789.8.76.4.4321.0
0020 0010 Study ID                123
0020 0013 Image Number            10
0200 0020 Patient Orientation     L\P
0020 0032 Image Position Patient  -200\-500\-40
0020 0037 Image Orientation       1\1\0\0\1\0

0028 0004 Photometric Interpretation  MONOCHROME2
0028 0010 Rows                    512
0028 0011 Columns                 512
0028 0030 Pixel Spacing           0.9\0.9

7fe0 0010 Pixel Data              _
```

Fig. 12.5 A minimal stored computed tomography-digital imaging and communication in medicine object.

are grouped by the first number. In this example, group 0008 is the identity group and contains all the elements which help uniquely identify this object. Group 0010 is the patient demographics group, group 0018 is the CT parameters group and so on. The last of all of the data elements contains the actual image data itself.

One special class of data element, the **unique identifier** or UID, consists of a long numeric code. This code must be truly unique and may not be reused. In Fig. 12.5 there are three kinds of UID. The values for the SOP class UID are defined in the standard and each code describes the object. In this case, this is the code for a stored CT image. The SOP instance UID is the unique code for this object. No other DICOM object in the world may have the same UID. In this way, a DICOM server can tell if it is sent the same image twice and can disregard one of them. The study instance UID is the unique code for this study for this patient. All images in this study will contain the same study instance UID and a DICOM server can use this to correctly group images together.

DICOM Conformance

Whereas, the CT object in Fig. 12.5 is a valid CT object according to the standard, it contains very little information and would probably be rejected by many DICOM servers. This is the problem. By allowing manufacturers to choose which data elements are contained in the data object the standard creates room for incompatibility. It becomes very important for manufacturers to describe exactly how their system behaves, which data elements are important and which are ignored.

The DICOM standard specifies a common format for such descriptions, the **DICOM conformance statement**. It should be possible to determine whether two systems will be able to successfully communicate by comparing their DICOM conformance statements. In practise, these documents are quite long and an incompatibility might be difficult to spot.

RADIOTHERAPY DATA

Data Storage

Data storage essentially comprises a number of switches, which are on or off. The smallest size of data storage is one switch, called a bit, which can store a one or a zero. More bits are used to store larger numbers. If 8 bits are used then a number from 0 to 255 can be stored, called a byte. A kilobyte (kB) is equal to 1024 bytes. A megabyte (MB) is equal to 1024 kB, a gigabyte (GB) is equal to 1024 MB and a terabyte (TB) is equal to 1024 GB.

Image Quality

There is a trade-off between the quality of the image and the space it takes up. For reference, a standard CT slice uses 512 kB. To illustrate this section, a test image is used which also requires approximately 512 kB, shown in Fig. 12.6A.

Dimensions and Scale

Many images are two dimensional. We frequently also use three-dimensional data sets consisting of a series of two-dimensional images.

A CT series might comprise 50 slices at 5-mm spacing, requiring 25 MB. Time sequences can also be considered as a series of 2D frames. As the number of points increases in any dimension, so does the image size. In Fig. 12.6B the test image is shown at an eighth of the resolution. Now the image only requires 8 kB of storage, 64 times less. Much of the detail is lost at this resolution.

The bit depth describes the number of shades of grey between the maximum and minimum possible values. In medical imaging, most images are either 8-bit, with 256 levels of grey, or 16-bit, with 65,536 levels of grey. It is widely accepted that a person cannot discriminate between more than 256 shades of grey. However, a user may interrogate 16-bit images by changing the contrast window to examine different grey levels more clearly. Fig. 12.7A shows the loss in contrast from a reduced bit depth in the test image.

Compression

There are two kinds of compression. Lossless compression reduces the size of the data, generally to about half, without any alteration of the data. Lossy compression has greater ability to reduce the size of the data but at the expense of some degradation of the data as shown in Fig. 12.7B. Lossy schemes can achieve much greater compression with almost undetectable reduction in image quality. However, they are often considered inappropriate for medical applications where any subtle change might affect patient treatment.

Radiotherapy Data Types

Given the huge range of definitions found between different manufacturers, it will be easiest to consider these in the context of the range of data objects defined within DICOM. These fall into two groups: general image data types and those data types specific to radiotherapy, commonly referred to as DICOM RT.

Tomographic Images

In radiotherapy, CT images are used extensively with MRI and PET, becoming more widespread. All of these are well defined in DICOM. However, many radiotherapy systems will still only accept images with a simple transverse imaging geometry. As the use of 3D images increases, it is anticipated that manufacturers will increase the range of acceptable imaging geometries. This also includes tomographic verification images, such as cone beam CT.

Planar Images

Ideally, all planar images in radiotherapy should be presented as true RT images, described in the RT Image section following. However, many manufacturers have not implemented this and still use one of several DICOM data objects appropriate for simple planar images.

Curves, Annotations and Overlays

There is scope in DICOM to store and send any annotation that has been made on an image. Some manufacturers use these to attach additional information to an image such as anatomical outlines. Any use of

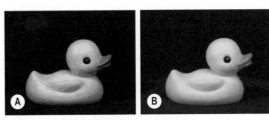

Fig. 12.7 (A) 4-Bit image showing significant degradation for only 50% space saving. (B) Compressed image taking up just 2% of the original space, but differences are visible.

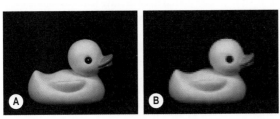

Fig. 12.6 (A) Test image. (B) At reduced resolution.

these which is more than just the simple display of annotation tends not to be transferable across manufacturers.

RT Structure Set

The RT structure set describes anatomical outlines that have been defined on tomographic data. It is used for the transfer of target volumes and organs at risk between planning systems. The structure set object specifically references the UID of each of the images on which it was defined. In this way a system can check that it does not load a structure set onto the wrong set of images.

RT Plan

The RT plan contains all the required information to deliver a radiotherapy treatment. It is possible for an RT plan to describe an external beam or a brachytherapy treatment. If the RT plan was created using target volumes from a CT dataset it will reference the UID of the RT structure set from which it was defined.

RT Dose

The RT dose object contains the result of the dose calculation. There may be a single dose object for each calculated slice or a full 3D calculation in a single object. Dose objects may also contain dose volume histograms.

RT Image

The RT image data type is used for all radiotherapy planar images. There are several differences between an RT image and a standard planar image. RT images contain much more precise details about the imaging geometry and explicitly specify the type of RT image, DRR, portal image or so on. RT images also allow the aspects of the RT plan which are relevant to that beam to be attached to the image, such as gantry angle, jaw positions and beam shaping.

RT Treatment Summary

The RT treatment summary is less widely used and is often overlooked. It contains a record of the treatment that was delivered.

Data Burden

The build-up of patient data can represent a serious problem for the radiotherapy department. Without care, it is possible for a system such as the planning system to fill up completely, with a risk of system failure, loss of data and disruption to the service. The additional build-up of data is often an unforeseen side effect of service development. For example, a patient verified using cone beam CT will have a greatly increased data use over one verified using portal images.

Measures can be taken to manage the radiotherapy data burden:

- Avoid increases in patient data for which there is no clinical benefit, such as inappropriate dose grid size or unnecessary imaging.
- Good housekeeping. Delete any patient plans or images which are not used clinically.
- Consider whether data are being stored multiple times. Identical CT data may be being stored on the CT scanner, the virtual simulator, the planning system and on a central disk.
- Assess data requirements for any new technique and ensure facilities are in place.
- Monitor the rate of data build-up and the capacity of clinical systems. Investigate any unforeseen increase in data and any system regularly greater than 80% full.
- Plan future data requirements.

With fewer datasets being stored there is also a reduced risk of patient mistreatment as a result of an incorrect data set being used.

Table 12.2 demonstrates the total data storage commitment for an example lung patient. In this example the greatest storage commitment

TABLE 12.2		Data for an Example Lung Patient	
Item	**No.**	**Format**	**Memory**
Planning CT	120	512 × 512 × 16 bit	60 MB
CT outlines	1		3 MB
Treatment plan	1		100 kB
Dose distribution	2	200 × 200 × 200 × 32 bit	61 MB
Cone beam verification	24	410 × 410 × 162 × 16 bit	1247 MB
		Total	1371 MB

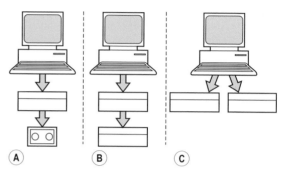

Fig. 12.8 Backup schemes. (A) Backup to tape. (B) Backup to disk. (C) Mirrored disks.

is by far the cone beam CT verification images, because of the finer resolution in the cranio-caudal axis and the number of such images acquired. With temporal images such as 4DCT and dynamic MR images this data burden will be significantly increased again.

Data Security
Backup

It is critical that the data are not lost in the event of a failure of the system on which it is stored. To achieve this, the data need to be copied to a second location. There are many ways in which this can be achieved. In Fig. 12.8A the data are written by the computer to a hard disk. Overnight, an automatic program copies the data to a digital tape. The scheme shown in Fig. 12.8B is similar except the data are copied overnight to a second hard disk drive. This has the advantage that the copies can be retrieved without any time delay. In Fig. 12.8C the data are written immediately to two separate independent disk drives. This scheme is known as drive mirroring.

It is important to ensure that backups performed by any method can actually be read. It has been known for systems to be backed up every night, but when actually require the tapes were useless. As the number of computer systems and the amount of data in a department grows, then backup can be a significant technical problem.

Archive

As patient data are acquired, computer systems may become full and old data need to be transferred to an archive to release storage capacity. Archive is very similar to backup and the two are often confused, but they fulfill very different roles. Backup is very short term in scope. Data today are stored in case of a catastrophe tomorrow. Archival is long term in scope. Archived data will need to be kept for years. It is important that sufficient records are kept to enable the data to be located in the future. Furthermore, one must have the means to read the data. It is pointless storing patient data if it can only be read by a planning system that is no longer available.

If data are archived to a physical medium such as tape or CD, then the long-term life of the medium will need to be considered. As the archive grows, the number of media being stored will grow and may take up a significant amount of space. Because disk storage is so cheap, it is feasible to create a hard disk archive, and simply purchase new disk storage when it fills up. Some systems are now being written with this in mind and have no archive facility. All of the data are available all of the time.

SOFTWARE DEVELOPMENT

Frequently, there comes a time when available products do not meet the immediate need and a centre must consider in-house developed software. Even the simplest spreadsheet can be considered as software and should be developed with care. One of the worst series of radiation therapy incidents, the Therac 25 incidents, had poor software design and testing as the root cause [10].

Detailed advice on the management and validation of software projects is available. One excellent example is 'General Principles of Software Validation; Final Guidance for Industry and FDA Staff', which is available online [11]. In particular, I recommend the section entitled 'Software is different from hardware' which details a series of reasons why care must be applied to software development. Even the most simple software program may be classed as a medical device and potentially subject to legal control. Advice is available through the MHRA [12].

A software development project can be considered as having five main areas of effort, which are shown in Fig. 12.9. Frequently, the only area of effort which has allocated resources is the actual computer programming itself, with all other effort taking place on an ad-hoc basis. This approach is inefficient as the software will need constant reworking as the specification changes during the project. This approach is also unsafe as it often leads to software coming into use without proper documentation and with only superficial testing and training. In the safer approach shown, only 20% of the effort is actually spent on computer programming.

In the specification and design work area, it is important to clearly describe the requirements for the project. This will include the functionality and any technical requirements. Important decisions such as the programming language to be used should not be left solely to the programmer as this will affect the ability of a centre to support the software in the future. This phase should also include a risk assessment of the impact of software failure and consequently any safety requirements. A framework for keeping adequate clinical safety documentation for software development is available through NHS Digital [13].

Documentation is vital to maintaining a safe software system; not just user manuals, but clear technical documentation and description

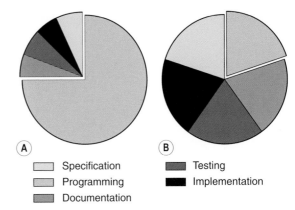

Fig. 12.9 Division of effort in software development projects. (A) What is often perceived as required. (B) A much more realistic and safe approach.

of the operation of the computer code itself. It is not sufficient for all documentation to be written retrospectively as important details can be forgotten. Testing can also be undertaken throughout software development and should be undertaken by both the programmer and a second party. The testing program should relate closely to the system specification and especially the risk assessment.

Finally, the implementation of the system needs to be planned with various 'what if' scenarios considered and all training, technical and user, undertaken in a timely manner. Ideally, the whole project will be managed by an individual or small team who will be able to sign off the project when all aspects are complete. Various software quality assurance systems exist [14,15] and should be considered for critical software projects: however the principals outlined here should be applied to all software projects large or small.

CONCLUSION

This simple introduction to the use of computers in radiotherapy will, regrettably, by the very nature of the subject be out of date almost instantly. It is important to obtain up-to-date guidance on specific aspects. The field of radiotherapy computing overlaps traditional work boundaries and there are frequently problems with IT professionals who don't fully understand the requirements of radiotherapy as much as radiotherapy professionals who don't fully understand the technicalities of IT. Out of this situation a new breed is rising, the radiotherapy computing specialist. Such people will be extremely important to ensure that we continue to reap the benefits of computerised radiotherapy.

REFERENCES

[1] Moore G. Cramming more components onto integrated circuits. Electronics Magazine 19 April 1965.

[2] Kryder's Law Walter C. *Scientific American* 2005;07–25.

[3] NHS Finance Manual, http://www.info.doh.gov.uk/doh/finman.nsf.

[4] Lustberg T, van Soest J, Jochems A, et al. Big data in radiation therapy: challenges and opportunities. Br J Radiol 2016;90(1069).

[5] Muller-Runkel R, Watkins S. Introducing a computerized record and verify system: its impact on the reduction of treatment errors. Med Dosim 1991;16(1):19–22.

[6] Patton G, et al. Facilitation of radiotherapeutic error by computerized record and verify systems. Int J Radiat Oncol Biol Phys 2003;56(1):50–7.

[7] Cerf V, Kahn R. A protocol for packet network intercommunication. IEEE Transact Commun 1974;COM-22(5):637–48.

[8] https://www.nao.org.uk/wp-content/uploads/2017/10/Investigation-WannaCry-cyber-attack-and-the-NHS.pdf.

[9] https://www.dicomstandard.org.

[10] Leveson N. Safeware: System safety and computers. *Addison-Wesley*; 1995. Available: http://sunnyday.mit.edu/papers/therac.pdf.

[11] https://www.fda.gov/downloads/medicaldevices/.../ucm085371.pdf n.d.

[12] https://digital.nhs.uk/services/solution-assurance/the-clinical-safety-team/clinical-safety-documentation. n.d.

[13] https://www.gov.uk/government/publications/medical-devices-software-applications-apps

[14] ISO/IEC 25010:2011 Systems and software engineering—Systems and software Quality Requirements and Evaluation (SQuaRE)—System and software quality models. ISO; 2011.

[15] http://www.tickitplus.org n.d.

Quality Control

John A. Mills, Phil Sharpe

INTRODUCTION

Quality control (QC) is the process of conducting measurements to demonstrate that any piece of equipment is performing to a satisfactory level. Throughout Europe, the need for such measurements to protect individuals against the dangers of ionising radiation in relation to medical exposure is set out in Article 8 of the European Commission (EC) Directive 93/47/Euratom [1]. In the United Kingdom (UK), the essential requirement for QC is specified in the statutory Ionising Regulations for Medical Exposure (IRMER) [2]. The level of performance is set out in both national and international standards as well as what professional bodies have identified as the best practice which can be achieved. For example, the International Electrotechnical Commission (IEC) Standard IEC60601 [3], which is the general standard for medical devices, contains parts which relate to the performance [4], and safety [5], of radiotherapy equipment as well as diagnostic x-ray equipment and electrical equipment. Several publications also specify performance criteria including the International Commission for Radiation Protection (ICRP) [6], the International Atomic Energy Agency [7], the American Association of Physics in Medicine (AAPM) [8] and in the UK, the Institute of Physics and Engineering in Medicine (IPEM) [9].

The hazards of radiation to normal tissue and the risk of oncogenesis [10] complicates the use of radiation in cancer treatment. From clinical experience and radiobiological studies the acceptable variation in delivered dose is estimated to be $\pm 5\%$. This puts the seriousness of the overdose of 25% because of incorrect dose measurement at Exeter in 1988 [11] into perspective. Of course in addition to inadequate QC or an absence of QC, accidents have occurred because of safety failures and human error. Systems of QC measurements endeavour to ensure safe and effective treatment.

THE QUALITY CONTROL REQUIRED

Effective QC fulfils two roles which are complementary. It demonstrates satisfactory performance or it detects a problem with the equipment which needs to be addressed. The boundary between the two is the tolerance within which performance is considered to be satisfactory.

QC historically developed to ensure that equipment can perform within a specific tolerance. The tests take place prospectively with regard to the clinical use of the equipment and may be referred to as Prospective Quality Control (PQC). PQC alone does not demonstrate that the correct treatment delivery has been achieved, and the limitations of PQC became apparent with the increasing complexity of treatment machines. As dynamic therapy was introduced, involving Multi-Leaf Collimator (MLC) shape, MLC movement, gantry rotation and even dose-rate modulation, treatment delivery by checking machine performance could not be realistically done prospectively. However, it is possible to measure the dose delivery for a specific patient treatment, a unique combination of machine operations; this is referred to as Patient-Specific Quality Control (PSQC). Not only does PSQC verify the performance of the machine, it verifies that the patient data acquisition, such as the computed tomography (CT) scanner, the dose prediction and the dose measurement, is also performing satisfactorily.

The EC Directive [1] requirements for PQC are clear and essential. These apply to the following aspects.

- **Following installation** of equipment, acceptance requires testing to ensure that the specification has been met.
- **Post repair,** it is necessary to ensure that the performance has been restored.
- **Post intervention** such as beam control adjustment to ensure performance is restored.
- **Following machine upgrade** there is a need to undertake PQC checks.
- **Following planned maintenance** there is a need to undertake PQC checks.

In addition to these the following can be added.

- **PSQC variation.**
- **Interlocks** are a major aspect which requires PQC as they ensure the safety of the treatment delivery. Beam characteristic interlocks such as flatness monitors are related to the performance of the beam and thus need to be checked in conjunction with performance measurements.

COMMITMENT TO QUALITY CONTROL

The need to be committed to QC, both patient specific and prospective, is borne out in the timescale of the detection of the 25% overdose at Exeter in 1987. Although brisk skin reactions were noticed this did not prompt a measurement check and the official report [11] states:

> ...it is seen that even a person whose treatment had started as early as mid February would not necessarily have shown any abnormal signs until about mid-May.

An under-dose may well go on for a much longer period of time such as when an approximate under-dose of 20% continued for very many years at Stoke [12] during the late 1970s and early 80s. Measurements can reveal problems much quicker than clinical indications will reveal them.

The difficult decision to be made is what to check, how often to check, how to judge measurement results and what action to take. In this respect, PSQC simplifies the complete QC process as it provides an overall assurance that a treatment is satisfactory. Although it does not eliminate the need for PQC, it removes the need to make any judgment about the clinical significance of a specific aspect of the performance of the equipment.

It is essential that the staff group responsible for the performance of equipment and the technical as opposed to the clinical delivery of the treatment embrace the QC requirements for modern radiotherapy.

SAFETY, POSITION AND DOSE

The physical dose along with its delivery to the correct location represent, in addition to safety, the three critical aspects of effective radiotherapy. In considering the various components in the radiotherapy process; data acquisition, dose prediction, treatment delivery and dose measurement, each component can be identified with both physical dose and position or a combination of both. For example, the calibration of CT number is related to dose prediction whereas movement accuracy of the scanner and processing of the image matrix is a positional aspect. PSQC provides a combined measurement, whereas PQC can be used to measure specifically a physical dose or a positional aspect.

FREQUENCY, TOLERANCES AND FAILURE TRENDS

There is no clear relationship by which the frequency of checks and the tolerances applied can be easily and systematically identified. This is in part attributed to the unknown pattern of failure which can be anything from a linear deterioration in its simplistic form to a catastrophic event unpredictable from any trend analysis. This complexity is explored in the previous edition [13].

For a linear failure trend with a recognised tolerance of ±3%, the variation in dose can be up to ±3% depending upon the period over which there is a deterioration and whether this period is greater or less than the number of days for the treatment. Although PQC can be readily used for post-repair purpose, this makes the choice of frequency for PQC difficult unless the deterioration of a performance parameter is explicitly known.

This problem is overcome with the use of PSQC as it will be required regularly, even if done on a sample basis, for example, every one in ten prostate patient treatments. It therefore provides an overview of overall treatment machine performance as well as the associated imaging, dose prediction and dose measurement performance and thus, virtually continuous confidence in the treatment being delivered.

MEASUREMENT AND UNCERTAINTY

Measurement of any parameter is unable to determine the value exactly. Instead, we make multiple measurements from which the 'Best estimate' is obtained. The variation in the multiple measurements is attributed to differences in the measurement process, measurement equipment and fluctuation of the parameter being measured. Calculation of the mean value M of the multiple measurements is the best estimate, whereas the variation in the multiple measurements is the Uncertainty of the Best estimate.

Typically, we can assume that the multiple measurements fall in a normal distribution with mean M and a standard deviation σ, see Fig. 13.1. In a normal distribution, approximately 95% of measurements will lie between $\pm 2\sigma$. Hence, there is 5% uncertainty that the true value does not lie within $\pm 2\sigma$ of the Best estimate M and this can be used to consider the significance of a measurement with regard to a Reference value R.

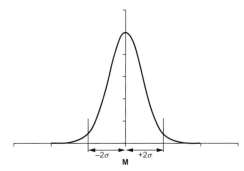

Fig. 13.1 Normal distribution of a measurement with mean M and standard deviation σ.

NULL HYPOTHESIS

This essential aspect of statistical analysis provides the method by which we can evaluate a measurement M with standard deviation σ with respect to a Reference value R. The Null Hypothesis (H_0) is that M is not different from R and the normal distribution can be used to determine with what confidence this can be assumed. In Fig. 13.2A the reference value R lies within $\pm 2\sigma$ of the Best estimate M, whereas in Fig.13.2B R lies outwith $\pm 2\sigma$ of M. This can also be stated as having 95% confidence that R belongs to M in Fig. 13.2A and therefore in Fig. 13.2B only being 5% confident that R belongs to M. Hence, at the 95% confidence level the measurement M can be judged to be within adequate agreement of R and that H_0 applies or that it is not within adequate agreement and H_0 is rejected.

COMBINING VARIANCES AND TOLERANCES

The Variance is the standard deviation squared, σ^2. The Variance therefore is attributed to differences in the measurement process, measurement equipment and fluctuation of the parameter being measured. The generalised method to determine an overall variance is to assume contributing variations are independent and combine them as in equation 13.1, known as quadrature.

$$\text{Total variance} = (\sigma_{\text{Total}})^2 = (\sigma_1)^2 + (\sigma_2)^2 + (\sigma_3)^2 + \cdots + (\sigma_n)^2 \tag{13.1}$$

As an example, let the measurement technique have a standard deviation of 0.5% and the intrinsic fluctuation of the parameter be also 0.5%. These values can be combined in quadrature to determine σ_{Total} as follows:

$$(\sigma_{\text{Total}})^2 = (0.5)^2 + (0.5)^2 = 2 \times 0.25 = 0.5 \tag{13.2}$$

This results in $\sigma_{\text{Total}} = \pm 0.707\%$ and this gives $\pm 2\sigma = \pm 1.4\%$.

It therefore follows that if a number of parameters have an associated Tolerance, the overall Tolerance can also be determined by combining the individual Tolerances in quadrature.

This can be illustrated by considering the factors used to calculate the dose delivered as shown in equation 13.3:

$$D = M.O.W.T.S.C \tag{13.3}$$

where D is the dose, M is the number of Monitor Units and the other terms: O, W, T, S and C represent output, wedge, tray and source to surface factors. C is the machine calibration factor in Gy/MU.

The assumption that the variation in the factors are independent and as suggested above should be combined in quadrature leads to the overall variance being written as:

$$\begin{aligned}(\text{Total tolerance})^2 &= (\sigma_{\text{Total}})^2 \\ &= (\sigma_O)^2 + (\sigma_W)^2 + (\sigma_T)^2 + (\sigma_S)^2 + (\sigma_C)^2\end{aligned} \tag{13.4}$$

If the aim was to deliver a Dose within a Total Tolerance of $\pm 3\%$ and the Calibration Factor C was maintained to within $\pm 1\%$ then the Tolerance on O, W, T and S would each be $\pm 1.4\%$, if they were all taken as equal. This type of consideration enables realistic tolerances to be set and, based upon known performance results, can also indicate the overall performance which can be expected.

SETTING A TOLERANCE TO ACHIEVE A PERFORMANCE LEVEL

The distribution associated with any measurement indicates that there is a 50% chance that the true value is above the mean measurement and there is a 50% chance that the true value is below the mean measurement. Hence, if the mean measurement is exactly on the tolerance value there is as much chance it is in tolerance as it is out of tolerance. In order that the measured value can be considered to be in tolerance with 95% confidence, the tolerance must be reduced by an amount related to the standard deviation of the measurement.

Hence, if a measurement M can be made with standard deviation σ_{Total} and the aim is for the performance to remain within $\pm P$, the tolerance should be set at $T = P - 2 \times \sigma_{\text{Total}}$. For example, if the performance requirement is $\pm 3.0\%$ and the measurement has a standard deviation of $\pm 0.5\%$, the Tolerance should be set to $\pm(3.0 - 2 \times 0.5)\%$ which means a tolerance of $\pm 2.0\%$.

PERFORMANCE IMPROVEMENT

Setting a Tolerance is an important aspect of maintaining performance. An overall tolerance in dose delivery is set by known clinical outcome and complications. However, it does not help to improve performance. Simply working to a tolerance range $\pm T\%$ says that it is equally good for the performance to be $-T\%$ from a target value as it is for it to be 0% or $+T\%$ from the target value. Clearly, this is not the case and it would be desirable for the performance to be within 0% of the required performance far more than not.

The Taguchi technique [14] is an example of how performance can be improved and driven towards the 0% variation from the required

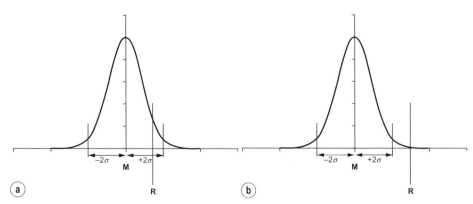

Fig. 13.2 Conceptual relationship of the mean of a measurement, M with regard to a reference value, R. 13.2a, 95% confidence M is the same as R and 13.2b, 95% confidence M is different from R.

performance. The technique uses a Loss of performance parameter based upon a quadratic sum as follows:

$$\text{Loss} = K.\left[(\sigma_{\text{Total}})^2 + (1/N.\Sigma; \sigma_n)^2\right] \qquad \textbf{(13.5)}$$

where K is a constant and for the example expressed in equation 13.4,

$$1/N.\Sigma\sigma_n = 1/5.(\sigma_O + \sigma_W + \sigma_T + \sigma_S + \sigma_O) \qquad \textbf{(13.6)}$$

which is the mean standard deviation for the parameters. This Loss parameter can be used to improve performance by intervention to reduce the variation from nominal targets.

An example from industrial production which illustrates the benefit of this technique concerns the production of Sony TV sets in Japan and the United States (US). The Japanese plant applied Taguchi whereas the US plant relied on a simple tolerance of $\pm T\%$ for colour density. A non-parametric assessment of customer satisfaction on a scale of A for Excellent to D for Unacceptable showed the striking contrast between the US and Japanese manufactured TV sets as shown in Fig. 13.3.

It can be clearly seen that whereas the Japanese satisfaction was concentrated around Excellent, for the US TV sets, the satisfaction was uniform across the colour density range. That in effect resulted in a greater number of Unacceptable responses than Excellent, the reverse of the Japanese.

Although the overall target for performance such as $\pm 5\%$ is set by clinical indications, improvement techniques such as Taguchi can provide a way that QC will improve performance.

MAINTENANCE AND CATASTROPHES

Not all aspects of equipment performance can be maintained. Catastrophes are inevitable and although these are usually because of component failure, they can also be because of human error. Although some devices and components can be replaced or action taken based upon the monitoring of a performance parameter, not everything can be maintained. The best possible provision needs to be made for such catastrophes. This provision should enable routine treatment to continue while the equipment is repaired.

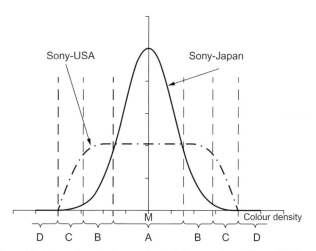

Fig. 13.3 Comparison between basic tolerance band (Sony-USA) and improvement method (Sony-Japan) production techniques.

LONG-TERM, SHORT-TERM AND IMMEDIATE MONITORING

Monitoring of performance parameters can be achieved by reviewing the data collected from QC measurements. These measurements can be used to examine trends in the performance and, if possible, used as predictors of performance deterioration, enabling the scheduling of adjustments or corrective action.

One routinely used but simple trend technique is when a double tolerance level is set against which to monitor the variation of a parameter. Let these levels be $\pm a\%$ and $\pm b\%$ where $b > a$. Results outside $\pm b\%$ are considered to require immediate attention whereas results outside of $\pm a\%$ but also within $\pm b\%$, must occur on a number of subsequent occasions in order for action to be taken.

There are three major categories of monitoring: immediate, short-term and long-term. Each method provides different but appropriate means by which to evaluate and maintain performance.

Immediate Monitoring

The immediate effect on the performance is determined from the response to changing a control parameter. Using this approach, the optimum tuning of a circuit or system can be determined. The monitoring can involve measuring parameters within the machine such as current or voltage as well as external parameters such as beam characteristics like beam uniformity and energy.

Long-Term Monitoring

Many parameters alter slowly as components age or as the performance deteriorates. To correct and compensate for the changes, including component replacement, long-term data trends provide an indication as to when action is required. This could be for a parameter which requires continuous adjustment to remain within specification or it may indicate when the end of life of a component is expected to schedule replacement and avoid treatment interruption and delays by ensuring that components are available if required and preparation is done in adequate time. As with Immediate Monitoring, the parameters may be internal, that is measured from the machine, or they could be from the beam characteristics and measured using other external equipment such as flatness or symmetry. Inevitably, data can be difficult to record, log and process. Any systems which will assist with the recording and processing of these data are valuable.

Short-Term Monitoring

In contrast to Immediate and Long-term monitoring, short-term endeavours to monitor performance of the machine during at least one treatment day. Only internal parameters of the machine are recorded during the day for subsequent processing. But these can be used in conjunction with daily measurements of the beam such as those made when the machine is run-up before treatment that day. By analysis of such data, it is again possible to identify deterioration in performance and schedule adjustments.

THE RADIOTHERAPY PROCESS

QC has a role throughout the entire radiotherapy process because of the significant technology involved at every stage. Three distinct aspects can be identified with QC: dose, position and safety. All of these aspects contribute to ensuring effective treatment delivery.

The Radiotherapy process can be considered to consist of three distinct aspects: acquisition, analysis and delivery. Any piece of equipment can be involved in any or all of the aspects. For example, the CT scanner will Acquire positional and image data and that image data will be used in the dosimetric Analysis for treatment planning as well as the Delivery verification analysis of portal dosimetry.

Acquisition

Patient information that is not determined from clinical examination and physiological and biochemical testing is almost entirely obtained through imaging. The focus of the information is the CT scan which forms the basis for dose prediction. This is supplemented by magnetic resonance imaging (MRI) and positron emission tomography (PET) imaging, the use of which relies on accurate image registration to ensure accurate target localisation and associated margins. Ultrasound can also be used on occasions.

In brachytherapy, localisation of radioactive sources or applicators is readily achieved with a C-arm radiographic device and it can also be done with CT supplemented by MRI.

Analysis

The manipulation of large CT data sets enables accurate delineation of target regions and organs at risk in a virtual environment permitting the clinical staff to make informed choices concerning the efficacy of the treatment in terms of the balance between treatment and risk to the patient.

Dose prediction remains a significant part of the analysis to determine an adequate dose distribution in the target while sparing critical tissue. With the increasing use of Intensity-Modulated radiotherapy the Analysis is an automated process also referred to as inverse planning. The automated process is governed by guidance parameters set and adjusted by operators skilled in the use of the processing software.

Delivery

The final part of the process following Acquisition and Analysis is the Treatment Delivery. The uncertainty of the first two aspects will have an impact on the final delivery. The majority of radiotherapy treatment delivery takes place with linear accelerators. However, proton treatment machines, kilovoltage machines, therapy radioisotopes, brachytherapy afterloading machines and implants and their associated equipment must also be considered.

THE NEED FOR PATIENT-SPECIFIC QUALITY CONTROL

Increased complexity in treatments such as intensity modulated arc therapy has prompted the need for more patient-specific quality control (PSQC). No longer can Prospective Quality Control (PQC) completely cover all the aspects of a treatment machine that is used for IMRT. Radiotherapy departments are becoming more focussed on the patient pathway from referral through to treatment, involving a multi-disciplinary team that combines different staff groups communicating together in a patient-led environment. Running parallel to that, QC now focusses on testing a patient's individual treatment encompassing the whole procedure from scan to plan to treat rather than individual tests for each stage.

A modern IMRT arc therapy treatment contains multiple segments, variable dose rate and varying gantry speed all combined into one or more continuous treatment arcs. The complexity of this means that from a practical point of view, the beams cannot be split into single segments or individual gantry angles to test them. Therefore, a test that can measure the sum of all these individual aspects is required.

The increased complexity of treatments has given rise to QC equipment explicitly designed for such patient-specific checks. A phantom or device that can be scanned, planned and treated using an individual patient's plan ensures a more robust QC procedure to cover all aspects of the patient pathway. The practical side of the PSQC and equipment used will be discussed further in the section titled 'practical patient-specific quality control'.

THE RADIOTHERAPY TECHNOLOGY

Consideration of the Radiotherapy process in the previous section indicates that Treatment is dependent upon the equipment used throughout the process and thus on the QC of that equipment. Detailed QC is available from several sources, for example, IPEM81 [9] for all categories of equipment used, so here we consider some general aspects and principles which should be applied.

TABLE 13.1	Six Aspects of a CT Scanner That Require Quality Control
1	Patient alignment lasers
2	Couch movement
3	Slice thickness
4	Image size
5	Image geometry
6	Hounsfield numbers for range of materials

Planning Imaging

The purpose of the QC for the CT scanner is twofold. First to ensure the alignment of the patient with respect to the scanner is appropriate and accurate, and secondly that any patient density information is appropriate for dosimetry calculations. Table 13.1 lists areas of consideration which are typical but not comprehensive.

Whereas the CT image data set forms the basis for dose prediction, the MRI and PET images aid volume localisation for target and critical organ delineation. Hence, the MRI and PET registration with the CT image data needs to be checked to ensure that geometric alignment of the MRI and PET with the CT images is accurate and that volume sizes and dimensions are not transferred inaccurately from one to the other.

C-arm radiographic devices often provide the imaging facilities essential for dose prediction in brachytherapy treatment as well as source position verification during treatment. For dose prediction, the geometric accuracy of the system needs to be checked with routine QC. In addition, the safe levels of radiation exposure and satisfactory imaging performance should also be included in a QC programme.

Virtual Simulation

The basis for accurate treatment simulation lies with the performance of the CT scanner. However, QC checks of the Virtual Simulator facility ensure that the manipulation of the CT data sets does not introduce any geometric distortions which could compromise the perception of the alignment of the treatment machine to the patient. Although it can be argued that once software is initially verified through Customer Acceptance and system commissioning, there will be no change, there is still a need for adequate QC to follow software upgrades or hardware changes. Also, because the data set originates from the CT scanner, periodic checks will verify or otherwise that the process of data handling between the systems is satisfactory.

Dose Prediction

The dose prediction accuracy is dependent upon the calculation algorithm, geometrical resolution and the application of stored electron density data to apply to CT images. As with Virtual Simulation there is a need for quality control following software and hardware upgrades as well as routinely checking the data transfer integrity with the CT scanner.

Kilovoltage Machines

Kilovoltage treatment machines require mechanical, radiation field and dosimetry checks. One fundamental aspect is the alignment of the focal spot to the mechanical alignment of collimators and applicators. Once this is accurately established and verified then accurate mechanical alignment of applicators and attachments will ensure adequate performance. Table 13.2 lists checks for an Orthovoltage kV machine which are typical but not comprehensive.

TABLE 13.2 Seven Aspects of Orthovoltage Machines That Require QC

1	Focal spot to applicator alignment
2	Applicator dimensions and orthogonality
3	Large field uniformity
4	Beam energy
5	Dose variation with tube angle
6	Dose linearity and reproducibility
7	Absolute dose

Afterloading Brachytherapy Machines

High, medium and low dose-rate machines all require QC checks for safety and performance. With this type of equipment, the mechanical aspects concern the positional accuracy of the radiation source or sources and then ensure that dummy source indicators used for planning radiographs reflect accurately the source positions. Finally, of course, measurement of the absolute dose delivered will check source activity, timer and positional accuracy in combination. Table 13.3 lists checks that are typical but not comprehensive.

TABLE 13.3 Five Aspects of Brachytherapy Machines That Require QC

1	Source position autoradiograph
2	Dummy source agreement with autoradiograph
3	Timer
4	Air kerma rate measurement
5	Absorbed dose of simulated treatment

Megavoltage Machines

Besides ensuring the satisfactory operation of safety interlocks, there are many aspects concerning the performance of these machines that require routine QC. These aspects concern mechanical and optical alignment, the performance of the radiation beam and its alignment to the optics and mechanics of the machine. The relative dose distribution within the beam normally referred to as the uniformity and symmetry, also requires checking for various orientations of the treatment gantry. Both the mechanical, optical and radiation performance checks

are prerequisites to ensuring accurate dose delivery for prospective QC. In patient-specific QC, all three components are integrated in the measurement and so are without any differentiation as to what may be causing a variation. There may be multiple energy beams to check, whether electrons, photons or protons. QC needs to be performed for all energies and modes. Table 13.4 lists checks that are typical for a linear accelerator, although not comprehensive.

TABLE 13.4 Twelve Aspects of Linear Accelerators That Require Quality Control

1	Isocentre determined by the radiation beam
2	Isocentre indicators, e.g. distance meter
3	Light field size, symmetry and x-wires
4	Patient alignment lasers
5	Radiation beam symmetry with gantry angle
6	Radiation field size
7	Radiation field alignment to optical field
8	Couch isocentric and vertical movement
9	Beam energy
10	Dose variation with gantry angle
11	Dose linearity and reproducibility
12	Absolute dose

Patient Positioning

Besides patient laser alignment systems, there are active systems which use stereotactic cameras and even kV imaging systems to monitor the position of the patient at treatment set-up and during treatment delivery. For such systems, QC is required to ensure that detected displacements are accurate and also that the relationship of the displacements to the machine reference, such as the isocentre is accurate.

Treatment Verification

Treatment verification systems monitor machine set-up parameters, patient positioning parameters and dose delivery parameters which are measured or determined from a variety of devices and techniques. Some examples are cone beam CT, portal imaging and in vivo dose measurements. Some aspects of QC are required to make sure that performance parameters crucial for satisfactory operation of these devices are checked and verified. In particular, treatment systems rely on the automatic detection of inappropriate settings before irradiation, especially with conformal and intensity-modulated techniques which make this unavoidable. The high complexity of treatment delivery now also benefits from an automated record of the treatment.

Computer Systems and Networking

Computer systems handle critical data across the entire radiotherapy process. QC of the computer systems and networks aims to verify that data transferred remains accurate. It can also identify the limitations in the system and monitor them. For example, resolution changes may occur within image sets as they are processed after acquisition. The integrity of the treatment requires that treatment data can be stored, accessed and transferred correctly.

Measurement Equipment

An important requirement for QC is that appropriate, accurate and precise measurement is used and it is essential to ensure it continues to operate satisfactorily. All equipment, from a ruler and spirit level used in mechanical checks, to calibrated ionisation chambers and electrometers used for absolute dose measurements require QC.

PRACTICAL PATIENT-SPECIFIC QUALITY CONTROL

The increased complexity of treatments involving intensity modulated arcs consisting of multiple small segments of dose per beam means each treatment can be very individual. Therefore, some form of patient-specific QC is required to ensure the treatment accuracy.

Practical Methods

The two stages within the patient process that can be used to perform patient-specific QC are:
1. Pretreatment QC: Measurements taken and processed before start of treatment.
2. On Treatment Verification: Measurements taken and processed either online during treatment or offline after treatment which is discussed in detail in Chapter 10.

There is a range of technology and techniques used in patient-specific QC. These involve absolute and relative dose measurements and predictions with comparisons between results to demonstrate the satisfactory delivery of the treatment or identify problems which need to be addressed before treatment is given. In the following sections an overview is given of these techniques and equipment.

Phantom-Based Measurements

These measurements require some form of phantom that can be imaged on the CT scanner and input into the Treatment Planning System (TPS). Patient-specific plans can then be applied to the phantom and the dose distribution calculated, a QA plan.

With the phantom set-up on the treatment machine, the treatment plan is then delivered. There must be some form of measurement device within the phantom at defined points to acquire dose measurements. These results can then be compared back to the predicted results from the planning system, thus verifying the treatment accuracy. The simplest method is the application of the treatment plan to a water equivalent uniform density block of material, for example, solid water or Perspex.

Single or multiple dose points can be measured using an ion chamber within the phantom and compared with the expected result from the planning system. A single cumulative dose point makes this method limited in respect to checking the whole plan. Multiple measurement points are better but very time consuming when done manually. There are various devices commercially available that can be used as a phantom replacement for the patient to apply the treatment plan to it.

Dosimetric Arrays

Dosimetric arrays comprise a phantom consisting of multiple dosimeters evenly spaced across either 2D or 3D planes under a set amount of build-up. The treatment plan can be delivered to the array and compared with the QA plan derived from the planning system. The most common forms of dosimeter used are small volume ion chambers or diodes.

2D Array

2D array has the advantage of being a measurement in a single plane which is generally quicker to measure than in 3D but has less resemblance to the actual plan. The array can be set on the treatment couch for fixed gantry measurements or held in a jig that rotates with the gantry for arc treatments; see Fig. 13.4.

3D Array

A 3D array enables the user to measure dose through a volume which has a closer resemblance to the original treatment plan as opposed to a

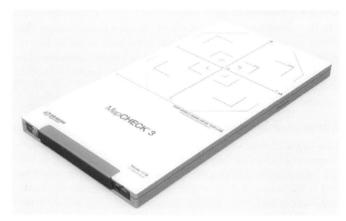

Fig. 13.4 A two-dimensional measurement array. (Courtesy of Sun Nuclear, Melbourne, FL.)

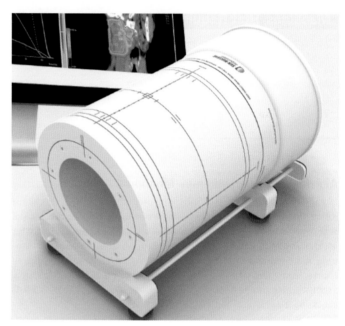

Fig. 13.5 A three-dimensional measurement array. (Courtesy of Sun Nuclear, Melbourne, FL.)

flat plane on the 2D array. The dosimeters in the 3D array shown in Fig. 13.5 are arranged in a cross structure with the device placed on the treatment couch and aligned to the machine isocentre.

The treatment is given to the array and software, usually provided by the manufacturer, and used to reconstruct the dose measured and the comparison to the QA plan made usually in the form of a Gamma Index.

Gamma Index

A series of measurement points throughout the 2D plane or 3D volume are compared with the QA plan and evaluated using a combination of dose difference and distance to agreement. The dose difference is the comparison of the dose from the QA plan to the dose measured at specific points. The distance to agreement is the shortest distance between a dose point in the QA plan and the same measured dose within the measured data. A combination of these is used within a gamma analysis or index in the form of dose deviation and spatial deviation. Each point of the dose distribution that lies within the accepted criterion, for example, 3% dose and 3-mm spatial, is classed as a pass. Each point that does not lie within the criteria is a fail. Therefore, a 95% pass rate is a common tolerance for IMRT treatment QA.

Independent Software Verification

Patient-specific QA can be performed using software to calculate doses within the patient at multiple points, either applied to the patient's original CT planning scan or geometrically calculated using the beam parameters relative to the plan isocentre and patient SSDs. This is a quicker method for patient-specific QC but is further removed from the original plan. It is a useful method of QC verification for tried and tested techniques that have been shown to have low failure rates. A suitable tolerance, for example ±3%, can be applied to these initial QA checks with the failures being sent on for a more comprehensive QC using a dosimetric array or phantom on the linear accelerator.

Secondary Treatment Planning System

For centres fortunate enough to have more than one TPS patient-specific QC can be performed by exporting the plan and CT scan to the second system and recalculating the dose distribution. The advantage of this is that the second TPS has its own independent dose algorithm which can be compared with the original plan for organs at risk and target volumes. QC should be as independent as possible from the original calculation to minimise user influence upon said test. Therefore, if possible, exporting from the record and verify system back to the second TPS also checks the original plan export, making the QC more robust.

Patient-Specific Quality Control Implementation

The implementation of IMRT is usually undertaken on one particular treatment site to risk assess the possible errors. Once this has been undertaken it can be expanded to other sites in conjunction with PSQC. The initial QC is usually done with the more complex methods of phantom or array measurements. This ensures a more complete check of the IMRT program in its infancy with a reduction in PSQC as confidence and auditing of the system is undertaken.

The increased demand for complex treatments means the equipment is in regular use, putting greater pressure on QC resources. For example, phantoms incorporating dosimetry equipment and devices acquiring measurements during treatment require robust QC to maintain their accuracy and consistency.

Regular audits of PSQC may indicate changes in the treatment process which will need further investigation to isolate the possible problem. As well as individual patient tests it is also recommended to have a standard QA plan that can be run on every treatment machine at regular intervals (e.g. monthly) to compare them to each other. This not only looks at individual machine performances but also the QC equipment itself to ensure its continuing accuracy.

Patient-specific QC has now become a common method for checking plans in the modern radiotherapy centre. With NHS targets for IMRT treatments increasing every year it becomes ever more important for a robust and independent system to be in place within the department.

GETTING THINGS IN BALANCE

QC more often than not will demonstrate adequate performance of the equipment being checked. However there are three aspects which need to be balanced when dealing with a problem:
- clinical effect because of the problem
- resources, including manpower and equipment to correct the problem
- component availability to correct the problem

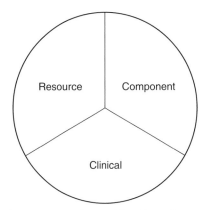

Fig. 13.6 The three aspects to be considered in equipment problems and restoring performance.

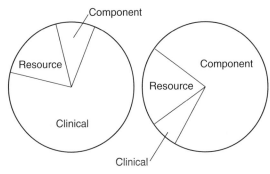

Fig. 13.7 Illustration of the contrast in split between the three aspects to be considered for two extreme equipment problems.

All problems can be considered as a balance between the three and this can assist in determining how to deal with a problem, Fig. 13.6. The clinical effect really relates to the performance of the equipment and making a judgement about how significant treating the patient with the performance compromised to a known extent will be. The resource required is the man-hours required and the skill and expertise available and required to restore the performance. The component availability relates to whether a component is affordable or available from stores or was too expensive or inappropriate to keep on the shelf at the hospital, or needs to be ordered.

The balance can be illustrated by considering two extremes. The first is high clinical impact and minimal component cost whereas the second is very high component cost coupled with insignificant clinical impact, Fig. 13.7.

On the one hand, if clinical significance is small and the resource or component availability is large, the work can be scheduled for an appropriate time such as a planned preventative maintenance (PPM) slot. However, if the clinical significance is large then an immediate repair will be appropriate.

There are no easy answers to the numerous situations between the two extremes. This has to rely on the skill, knowledge and insight of the scientists and technicians involved in the work.

QC coupled with planned maintenance forms an essential component in ensuring that safe and effective radiotherapy is achieved.

QUALITY CONTROL SCHEDULING FOR MEGAVOLTAGE MACHINES

The scheduling of routine QC should be chosen to suit local circumstances. For many types of equipment this can be accommodated within normal working hours. However, in the case of treatment machines this may not be possible because of the lack of treatment capacity and patient demand. Suitable guidance as to the frequency of tests can be found in both British Standards Institution (BSI) [5] and IPEM81 [9]. Both documents provide guidance for checks to be conducted on a monthly to a 12-monthly frequency. The BSI [5] document does not specify weekly checks; an estimate of the total annual time for the suggested checks is approximately the same. Based upon typical times for the QC, they amount to between 117 and 128 hours per year respectively, which is roughly in line with 1 to 2 hours per week and one-half day per calendar month and which requires 120 hours. If this time is taken from the normal working day, it amounts to only about a 5% loss from the typical treatment unit.

With the increasing number of treatment machines and treatment complexity in a centre, the time and resource for treatment machine QC increases and scheduling techniques are required to accommodate it. Paradoxically however, the increased treatment complexity has led to the need for patient-specific quality control (PSQC) which, in providing an overall assurance of adequate dose delivery, reduces the need for direct machine QC checks or prospective QC (PQC). If an integrated view of PQC and PSQC is taken this can lead to a reduction in the QC resource required [15].

CONCLUSION

QC and planned maintenance are a requirement of IRMER [2]. They are both often seen as an unnecessary intrusion into the routine treatment of patients. It can become very frustrating for treatment personnel when the performance of a treatment machine needs to be checked and confirmed following repair after a breakdown. It is however apparent from previous incidents that measurement of a physical parameter could have averted incorrect treatment [11], sometimes over a lengthy period before clinical indicators indicated a problem.

It is important to put the checks on performance into context. This can be done in relation to the dose distribution planned for a patient when the ICRU50 [16] criteria of a dose variation between +7% and −5% across the target is sought. The performance of the machine can compromise this because of several factors. For example, a non-uniform beam because of energy change or tilted beam because of incorrect steering could change this by ±6%. The variation of the factors used to calculate the monitor units in combination with the dose calibration of the machine could also change this by ±6%. Geometric misalignment between the radiation beam and the beam indicators can result in dose differences, particularly in regions of high dose gradient such as wedged or modulated fields. It is worth bearing in mind that, typically, within 5 mm of a radiation field's geometric edge, a 1-mm positional discrepancy can result in a dose variation of up to 10%.

A random combination of these many factors throughout the treatment cannot be guaranteed not to occur. The performance variation which might result therefore, without adequate quality control and planned maintenance, could well negate or swamp the variation expected from the dose prediction planned for the treatment.

A comprehensive system of QC for all the equipment used in radiotherapy will ensure that accurate and reproducible treatment is being delivered.

REFERENCES

[1] Council Directive 93/47/Euratom. Official J Eur Communities 1997;L180:22–7.

[2] The Ionising Radiations Regulations 2017—Statutory Instrument 1999; No. 3232. HMSO.

[3] BSI (British Standards Institution). BS EN 60601-1-1:2002. Medical electrical equipment. General requirements for safety. Collateral standard. Safety requirements for medical systems; 1998.

[4] BSI (British Standards Institution). BS EN 60976. Medical electrical equipment. Particular requirements for the safety of electron accelerators on the range 1 MeV to 50 MeV. London, UK: BSI 2007;1998.

[5] BSI (British Standards Institution). BS EN 60601-2-1. Medical electrical equipment. Medical electron accelerators. Functional performance characteristics. London, UK: BSI; 1998. p. 2007.

[6] ICRP Publication 44. Protection of the patient in radiation therapy. Oxford: Pergamon Press; 1985.

[7] Thwaites DI, Mijnheer BJ, Mills JA. Quality assurance of external beam radiotherapy. In: Podgorsak EB, editor. Radiation oncology physics; a handbook for teachers and students. Vienna, Austria: IAEA; 2005. p. 407–50.

[8] Klein EE, Hanley J. BayouthJ, Fang-Fang Y, Simon W, Dresser S, et al. Task group 142 report: quality assurance of medical accelerators. Med Phys 2009;36:4197–212. https://doi.org/10.1118/1.3190392.

[9] IPEM (Institute of Physics and Engineering in Medicine). Physics aspects of quality control in radiotherapy. IPEM report 81. 2nd ed. York, UK: IPEM; 2018.

[10] Amemiya K, Shubuya H, Yoshomura R, Okada N. The risk of radiation induced cancer in patients with squamous cell carcinoma of the head and neck and its results of treatment. Br J Radiol 2005;78:1028–33.

[11] The Exeter District Health Authority. The report of the Committee of Enquiry into overdoses administered in the Department of Radiotherapy in the period February to July 1988; 1988.

[12] West Midlands Health Authority. Second Report of the Independent Enquiry into the conduct of isocentric radiotherapy at the North Staffordshire Royal Infirmary; 1994.

[13] Mills JA. Quality Control. In: Symonds P, ed. Walter and Miller's Textbook of Radiotherapy. Oxford, UK: Elsevier; 2012. p. 211–21.

[14] Karna SK, Sahai R. An overview on Taguchi method. Int J Eng Math Sc 2012;1:11–8.

[15] Mills JA, Colligan SC. Megavoltage quality control, resources and demand: a pragmatic review. Br J Radiol 2016;89:20150709. https://doi.org/10.1259/bjr.20150709.

[16] Report 50 ICRU. Prescribing, recording and reporting photon beam therapy. International Commission on Radiation Units and Measurements; 1993.

14

Quality Management in Radiotherapy

Jill Emmerson, Karen Waite, Helen Baines

CHAPTER OUTLINE

INTRODUCTION: WHAT IS QUALITY?

There are many different, well-documented theories and approaches to quality and quality management [1] in health care. Approaches to quality have seen a shifting emphasis and have evolved from being reactive to being proactive through the following stages:

1. Inspection and remedial action
2. Identifying improvements and taking steps to prevent mistakes occurring
3. Doing things differently, that is, modernisation, including a systems approach

The current emphasis is focussed on continual improvement, safety and risk management. These changes are reflected in the history of quality in radiotherapy [2,3] (RT), such that the interpretation of quality has widened and can now be applied to every aspect of the service, incorporating many local, professional and national standards. It is not possible to cover every aspect of quality in detail in a single chapter. This chapter aims to provide an overview of quality and quality management and their significance to RT, outline the requirements of the international quality standard BS EN ISO 9001, signpost readers to further information on a number of quality initiatives and promote an integrated approach to quality management in oncology centres in the United Kingdom.

There are many different definitions and perceptions of quality and several terms associated with quality that are important to describe from the outset. Quality may be defined as fitness for purpose or conformance to requirements, but it is more than this.

Quality is the degree to which a set of inherent characteristics of an object fulfils requirements [4].

In other words, it is the degree to which a product or service satisfies the requirements of the user. Some definitions do not take costs into account. However, quality is about meeting customer requirements, stated or implied, while also keeping costs to a minimum.

Another often used term is quality control (QC) which is 'the part of quality management focused on fulfilling quality requirements' [4].

In RT, quality control does not only apply to controlling the performance of the equipment, but also to controlling the performance of RT processes.

Quality assurance (QA) refers to 'the part of quality management focused on providing confidence that quality requirements will be fulfilled' [4].

Quality assurance incorporates risk assessment, determining what might go wrong, or what is critical to get right, then planning the process and putting procedures in place to ensure that a reliable service is provided. Aspects to be included should be operational, including legislative and educational requirements; physical and technical checks to verify correct functioning of equipment; and clinical aspects, including patient care and management. This can be achieved through activities such as documentation, training and ongoing review of existing processes.

Quality management (QM) is 'management with regard to quality', where management is 'the coordinated activities to direct and control an organization' [4]. The underpinning philosophy, to get the process and the service right the first time, applies to all parts of the organisation, involving managing all functions and activities to achieve quality.

A quality system (QS) is the organisational structure, responsibilities, procedures, processes and resources which must be in place to implement quality management.

A quality management system (QMS) is part of a management system with regard to quality, where a management system is a set of interrelated or interacting elements of an organisation to establish policies and objectives and processes to achieve those objectives [4].

There are a number of documented approaches to quality, including total quality management (TQM), continuous quality improvement (CQI), the European Foundation for Quality Management model (EFQM) [5] and business process re-engineering. From these different approaches, it is possible to identify a number of recurring key themes:
- management commitment
- staff involvement
- identification of clear requirements or standards
- identification of clear processes, broken down into identifiable steps
- a focus on the prevention of problems
- recognition that quality is a continual process

The steps to achieving any quality initiative must include the following stages:
- analysis of current service
- identification of recommendations for change
- implementation of change
- evaluation of the impact of change

The main aim of quality in RT is safe and effective treatment. In addition to ensuring that all treatments are optimised, a quality system should ensure that all possible measures are taken to prevent inappropriate exposures from occurring.

HISTORY OF QUALITY IN RADIOTHERAPY

There are a number of well-documented RT incidents [6–10], which have occurred both in the United Kingdom (Table 14.1) and internationally. These have led to hundreds of patients receiving incorrect doses of radiation which, in turn, may have led to the possibility of the treatment intent being compromised or causing unnecessary and distressing acute and late side effects of treatment. Subsequent outcomes in the United Kingdom have included key reports which have contributed to the development of quality management systems in RT.

It is notable that, throughout numerous reported incidents, a number of recurring themes can be identified as contributing factors. These include:
- lack of communication, especially at staff group interfaces
- training, competency and supervision issues
- lack of up-to-date procedures, protocols and documentation
- no independent check or calibration
- inadequate identification of clear responsibilities

It is of the utmost importance that the RT community shares information and learns from past mistakes [10,11]. Departments should also search for, correct, monitor and learn from their own incidents. Departments open themselves up to risk if there are workload or time pressures or if there is an insufficiency in:
- attention to detail, alertness or awareness
- procedures or checks
- resources, for example, qualified and well-trained staff
- coordination, communication and clear responsibilities

All of these factors are encompassed by ISO 9001 and should be incorporated into a department's quality management system. These are areas that should be kept under regular review with a view to achieve continual improvement.

QUALITY MANAGEMENT SYSTEMS

A quality management system (QMS) is a set of interrelated or interacting processes which provide a framework for an organisation to

TABLE 14.1 Chronology of Quality Development in Radiotherapy in the United Kingdom

Year	Event
1988	Exeter. Overdose, 207 patients affected.
1988	Thwaites Report: detailed root cause of Exeter incident. DoH working party, chaired by Professor Bleehen, to investigate the application of quality assurance to radiotherapy to reduce the probability of incidents occurring in other centres.
1982–1991	Stoke. Underdose, 1045 patients affected.
1991	Bleehen Report: Quality assurance in radiotherapy (QART). Took the form of a quality standard and provided a formal system for managing quality in radiotherapy. It was based on the Quality Standard BS 5750, Part 2, 1987 (the predecessor of ISO 9001), a quality standard which was generic to a range of industries and services and thus, open to a degree of interpretation and translation. DoH funded two pilot sites, Bristol and Manchester: • To implement a quality system to see if it was feasible. • To prepare manuals that would serve as examples to other radiotherapy departments.
1994	Stoke: report from investigation.
1994	Sample documents from two pilot sites published and DoH recommendation for all departments to develop their own quality management system (QMS) [12].
1994	BS EN ISO 9001:1994 replaced BS5750
2000	BS EN ISO 9001:2000 replaced BS EN ISO 9001:1994. Increased emphasis on a process approach and continual improvement.
2006	Incident at Beatson Oncology Centre
2008	Redacted independent review of the circumstances surrounding a serious adverse incident [13]
2008	BS EN ISO 9001:2008 replaced BS EN ISO 9001:2000
2008	Publication of Towards Safer Radiotherapy [10]
2015	BS EN ISO 9001:2015 replaced BS EN ISO 9001:2008. Continued focus on leadership, process approach and improvement. Increased emphasis on risk management.
2016	Edinburgh: report into unintended exposure September 2015 [14]
2017	MPACE (Medical Physics and Clinical Engineering) accreditation pilot; assessment against BS 70000. See Box 14.1.

manage its activities to achieve its quality policy and quality objectives. Management system standards, such as ISO 9000 (see later), provide a model to follow in setting up and operating a quality management system. The ISO 9001:2015 requirements are based on seven quality management principles, the key elements of which are illustrated in Fig. 14.1.

1. Customer Focus

A service should understand and strive to meet and exceed the current and future needs and expectations of its customers. In RT, this would include not only external customers, such as patients and carers and health care commissioners, whose respective requirements and expectations may well be different from each other, but also internal customers, such as sections within oncology, for example, mould room and RT physics staff.

In 2017 UKAS (UK Accreditation Service) launched the pilot phase of accreditation called MPACE (Medical Physics and Clinical Engineering). The aim is to introduce a system for assessing competence for Medical Physics and Clinical Engineering departments based on the BS 70000 standard. It will go one step further than organisations that offer a certification service against a quality standard. MPACE will also assess whether a service is fit for purpose. The initiative follows the iCEPSS project (Improving Clinical Engineering and Physical Science Services) carried out by IPEM, NHS England, the Academy for Healthcare Science (AHCS) and UKAS, which started in 2013. Technical experts, stakeholders and volunteers from healthcare services are working together to establish a set of criteria for assessment considering the appropriate quality standards and the scope of the accreditation. In Radiotherapy Physics, this will initially cover treatment planning and delivery, particularly the quality assurance, calibration, maintenance and commissioning procedures as well as IT systems and medical devices. It is hoped that a national accreditation system will help the UK provide a high quality Medical Physics and Clinical Engineering service, which is important given the significant reliance that modern healthcare has on scientific and technical services.

2. Leadership

Management is responsible for creating a positive, engaging environment in which quality can flourish. The department's management team must establish a clear vision and a quality policy with linked objectives which are specific, measurable, achievable, realistic and also incorporate other initiatives, all of which must be communicated to all staff.

3. Engagement of People

All staff should be fully involved in the service and encouraged to use all of their abilities to the benefit of the department. They should be supported to achieve competence and participate in continual improvement to benefit themselves and the service.

4. Process Approach

Quality should be process driven, that is all resources and activities should be managed as a process, giving consideration to both inputs and outputs.

5. Improvement

Systems, such as audit, should be in place for continual measurement, review and improvement of a department's processes and service. Departments should be able to react to changes in internal and external parties' needs and expectations and use them as opportunities for improvement.

6. Evidence-Based Decision Making

All decisions should be evidence based, supported by appropriate data and information including key performance indicators. For example, there should be appropriate data collated to support future service planning and developments, including reflecting on previous implementations, current resources and considering risk assessment.

7. Relationship Management

Any interested party, for example, customer, supplier or partner organisation, has an effect on quality, and a healthy relationship between a

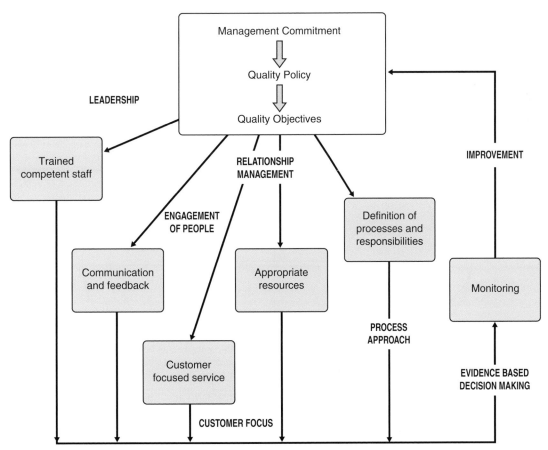

Fig. 14.1 Key quality management principles underpinning ISO 9001:2015.

department and its interested parties, both internal and external, enhances the ability of both to ensure that a high level of quality is maintained.

THE ISO 9000 STANDARD

The International Standards Organisation (ISO) provides the ISO 9000 family of documents which are an international standard code of practice for quality management systems. It is designed to be generic so that it is independent of any specific industry and therefore applicable to both manufacturing and service industries, including health care. It consists of:

- ISO 9000 Quality management systems—Fundamentals and vocabulary (last published 2015 [15])
- ISO 9001 Quality management systems—Requirements (last published 2015)
- ISO 9004 Managing for the sustained success of an organisation—A quality management approach (last published 2009 [14])

The standards themselves are subject to a review programme to ensure that they remain relevant. There were major changes when ISO 9001:2000 was introduced, whereas the publication of ISO 9001:2008 included only minor amendments. ISO 9001:2015 has an increased emphasis on leadership, improvement and risk management.

The scope of a department's QMS defines the activities included within the QMS and is determined by the department. There are variations between oncology departments: some include just RT treatment, whereas others include planning, dosimetry, medical physics, chemotherapy, clinical trials and clerical areas. ISO 9001 is the standard against which a department is assessed. It specifies the requirements a QMS must meet but not how the department should meet them.

The ISO 9001:2015 standard comprises ten clauses, listed in Box 14.2.

> **BOX 14.2   The Clauses of ISO 9001:2015**
>
> 1. Scope
> 2. Normative references
> 3. Terms and definitions
> 4. Context of the organisation
> 5. Leadership
> 6. Planning
> 7. Support
> 8. Operation
> 9. Performance evaluation
> 10. Improvement

An introduction describes the potential benefits of implementing a QMS, identifies the seven quality management principles which are reflected throughout the requirements and outlines the process approach based on the Plan-Do-Check-Act cycle, as illustrated in Fig. 14.2, as well as being risk based and forward thinking. It also identifies its relationship with other management system standards. Clause 1, Scope, states that the standard specifies requirements which an organisation's QMS should fulfil. Clause 2, Normative references, and Clause 3, Terms and definitions, give reference to the document ISO 9000:2015 [4] which is necessary for the interpretation and application of the ISO standard. The remaining clauses, 4 to 10, described subsequently, contain the requirements against which departments are assessed.

Clause 4 Context of the Organisation

Clause 4 changed in the 2015 version to begin with the importance of defining the purpose and strategy of the department. The department needs to consider internal issues, such as culture, and external issues,

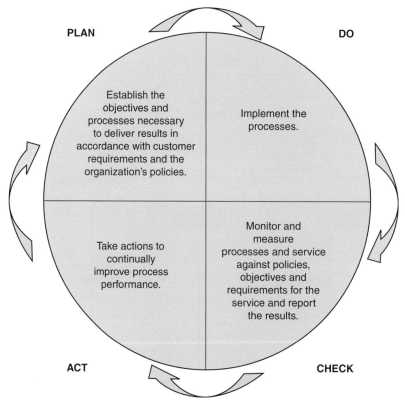

Fig. 14.2 The Plan-Do-Check-Act cycle applied to ISO 9001:2015.

such as legal requirements (Clause 4.1). It needs to determine interested parties, both internal and external such as patients, carers, suppliers and health care authorities, and what their needs and expectations are (Clause 4.2). The information determined through Clauses 4.1 and 4.2 underpins subsequent requirements, such as Clause 6, Planning. A number of methodologies are available to support this, such as a PESTLE (political, economic, social, technological, legal, environmental) analysis [16]. Given the potential wide-reaching nature of their service objectives, the department must produce a clear scope of what is and isn't covered in their QMS. This clause also requires a department to define its processes and their interactions. The 2015 version no longer requires specific procedures, instead requiring documented information throughout the requirements, with specific requirements detailed in Clause 7.5.

Clause 5 Leadership

The management team is required to demonstrate leadership and commitment, and is accountable for the effectiveness of the QMS. In addition to general requirements, such as a process approach, risk-based thinking and continual improvement, an integrated approach to the QMS requirements and the department's processes, and the availability and effective allocation of resources, there are specific requirements linked to a commitment to meeting customer requirements and enhancing customer satisfaction; establishing, maintaining and communicating a documented quality policy and objectives which reflect the vision of the department; and ensuring a clear organisational structure with well-defined responsibilities and authorities.

Clause 6 Planning

The management team is responsible for implementing a risk-based culture within the department, determining the risks and opportunities that will impact on its ability to achieve intended results. To accomplish this it needs to assess the internal and external issues that will affect it together with the needs of interested parties. Actions should be identified, communicated, implemented, monitored and evaluated for their effectiveness. Examples of risks could include not having sufficient capacity to achieve waiting time targets, or not being able to implement best practice because of obsolete equipment. Examples of opportunities might include implementing new techniques through participation in clinical trials, or networking with other departments. A department should have documented quality objectives, consistent with the quality policy, that are specific, measurable, achievable and relevant. These objectives should be monitored, communicated and updated as required. When changes to the QMS are required they should be carried out in a planned way with consideration to who is responsible, available resources, timing and any consequences which may arise.

Clause 7 Support

1. Sufficient resources are essential for an effective QMS. The management team is responsible for determining and providing adequate resources to implement, maintain, monitor and continually improve the effectiveness of the QMS and enhance customer satisfaction.
2. Examples include:
   - Human resources, for example, sufficient numbers of trained and competent staff
   - Infrastructure, for example, buildings, treatment machines, other equipment, IT and support services
   - Work environment including physical, social and psychological factors, for example, health and safety, local rules and radiation protection

- Monitoring and measurement, for example, patient satisfaction surveys or dose measuring instruments, with calibration traceable to a national standard
- Knowledge, for example, information on current legislation

There are specific requirements which cover: defining competencies: ensuring staff are aware of the quality policy and objectives, understand their role and how their performance may affect the quality management system; internal and external communication; and documented information. A department should maintain documented information as specified by ISO 9001 and as it determines what is necessary for the QMS to be effective.

This may include:
- Procedures and work instructions
- Clinical protocols
- Process flow charts
- Equipment maintenance records
- Internal audit documents
- Patient survey results
- Forms
- Data
- Reference documents

All documents within the QMS should be subject to a robust method of document control, have adequate protection from accidental changes or loss, be stored securely and be easily retrievable. It is vital to ensure that a document is identifiable, available, current and relevant to the area in which it is used. Systems should be in place to prevent previous versions from being accessed. Documentation also includes records such as patient records, training records and equipment maintenance records which provide evidence of activities performed. Departments must ensure that they incorporate any legislative, national [17] and local requirements into their documentation management processes.

Clause 8 Operation

This is the largest clause and includes requirements for providing a service from initial planning through the design, production and delivery stages to achieve consistency and meet intended requirements. A department needs to consider and review the requirements for its service including, for example, customer feedback, performance targets and legislation. Where the department processes include design and development there are specific requirements which must be met from planning the development through to validating the output. When dealing with external providers, for example, treatment machine manufacturers, departments need to establish controls to ensure that externally provided products conform to required standards and do not adversely affect the quality of their service. This may be achieved by performing quality assurance checks of the end product or checks along the pathway, for example, quality control or safety checks. General requirements relating to service delivery include the provision of controlled conditions, for example, taking actions to minimise the risk of human error. There are also requirements to ensure identification and traceability throughout, for example identification of patients and equipment, and to ensure that any changes to service provision are managed effectively. Checks must be in place at identified points of a process to detect any problems or faults and prevent errors from occurring, for example, independent treatment plan checks, and to ensure that requirements have been met. Documentation must be kept to ensure confidence in the implementation of the service and outputs must be continually be reviewed against requirements. Finally, processes must be in place for identifying any problems, such as complaints, preventing them from escalating and recording any actions taken. There should also be provision to use concessions, permitting use of a nonconforming product or service with special conditions in place, for example, off-protocol treatments.

Clause 9 Performance Evaluation

To ensure the effectiveness of its QMS, a department needs to consider what it can measure, and how, to evaluate its performance. Requirements include monitoring customer satisfaction, for example, by using surveys, complaints, compliments and user groups. Additional sources of data it could measure, monitor and analyse include clinical incidents, machine down time, waiting time data and other key performance indicators.

The department should have a programme of internal audits to demonstrate whether the QMS:

- meets the requirements of ISO 9001:2015
- meets the requirements of the department
- is implemented, effective and maintained

Documented management reviews must take place at planned intervals. The management team should review information on performance and effectiveness, for example, audit results, nonconformities and key performance indicators to determine the suitability, effectiveness and adequacy of the QMS and whether it meets the direction and requirements of the department. They should also consider provision of resources, improvement opportunities and any changes required to the QMS.

Clause 10 Improvement

Continual improvement is key to achieving departmental objectives and ensuring customer satisfaction. It can range from corrective action to innovation. Departments should take actions and opportunities that lead toward continual improvement. For example:

- Implementation of new evidence-based techniques
- Replacement of obsolete equipment
- Improvements to the environment
- Identifying the causes of incidents, nonconformities, audit findings and complaints and implementing appropriate action to prevent recurrence
- Identifying potential nonconformities and taking action to reduce the risk of occurrence

Further reading on ISO 9000 should include the standards themselves. In addition, there are many textbooks which interpret how to apply the requirements [16]. Fig. 14.3 illustrates the process of implementation of a QMS through to ongoing surveillance visits.

THE RADIOTHERAPY PROCESS

ISO 9000:2015 [4] defines a process as 'A set of interrelated or interacting activities that use inputs to deliver an intended result'. ISO 9001:2015 follows a process-based approach and requires systematic identification and management of the department's processes and the interaction between them. To adopt a process-based approach, an RT department should identify each process carried out and consider the following questions.

- What are the inputs?
- What are the outputs?
- How are they measured?
- What are the critical interfaces with other processes?
- Have responsibilities been clearly identified?

Processes are best illustrated with a diagram or flow chart. An example relating to the treatment process is shown in Fig. 14.4. It is important to remember that a process can be defined at many levels. A core process (e.g. treatment) will be made up of a number of subprocesses. Fig. 14.5 illustrates an example of the interaction between a department's core processes. For each process, consider the key elements of the ISO 9001 requirements, for example, in addition to the list already mentioned.

- Are resources allocated effectively?
- Is the work environment suitable for the task?
- Are staff trained and competent?
- Are training records up to date?
- How do you know if your customers' expectations have been fulfilled?
- How are complaints or other problems resolved?
- How could potential improvements be identified?
- What are the arrangements for ensuring calibration equipment remains within specification?
- Is identification and traceability, for example, of equipment and patients, maintained throughout the process?

AN INTEGRATED APPROACH TO QUALITY AND OTHER INITIATIVES

Quality in the National Health Service

Quality may be measured in a number of ways and there are a number of historical and current standards, measures, targets and improvement initiatives within the National Health Service (NHS), both generic and specific to cancer services. Previous examples of this include clinical governance and National Cancer Peer Review. Table 14.2 lists a number of other initiatives and documents that have contributed to the development of quality and safety in the NHS and in U.K. RT departments. Many of these complement each other or have common characteristics and should not be considered in isolation. They reflect the same principles that underpin quality management systems, together with the current NHS focus on clinical effectiveness, patient experience and safety, the three core dimensions of quality. They are all designed with the same ultimate objective—to improve the patients' experience, whether this is by, for example, improving treatment outcome, reducing waiting times, reducing the risk of incidents, improving communication with patients or improving patient facilities. Meeting such standards gives an indication that an acceptable level of quality has been achieved and allows intercomparison. Obviously, getting the right measure of quality is important. For example, waiting times measure the speed of throughput for patients but have no bearing on the standard of treatment delivered. This chapter has discussed the principles of quality management systems, but this is only part of developing and maintaining a quality service. An effective QMS should be a tool to help implement, integrate and measure any new initiative introduced into a department. In England, hospitals are regulated by the Care Quality Commission (CQC), Box 14.3, and an effective QMS will ensure an integrated approach to incorporating all the requirements addressed during a CQC inspection. The following paragraphs on risk management, clinical incidents, audit and patient-focussed care give more detail on some of the most important areas where a robust QMS can ensure smooth interfaces between different initiatives.

Risk Management

Patient and staff safety is foremost in all NHS Trusts, and risk-based thinking is a key concept throughout the ISO 9001:2015 requirements. Risk can be defined in many ways, for example 'the effect of uncertainty' [4]. Although RT is widely recognised as one of the safest specialties in health care, there is also the potential for severe patient harm when incidents do occur. There are two international documents which address managing the risks in RT. The first [9], published by the World

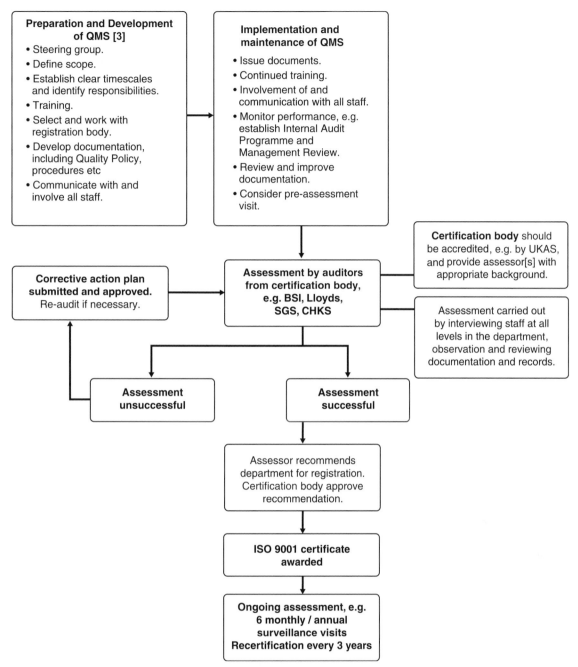

Fig. 14.3 The route to ISO 9001 registration.

Health Organisation (WHO) in 2008, reviews previous incidents and outlines a risk profile for RT, identifying ten stages in the RT pathway, the key risks associated with each stage and potential interventions to improve safety; the second [18–20], published by The European Commission in 2015, has a focus on two main approaches: proactive risk assessment and reactive analysis of events. Risk assessment includes the initial identification and evaluation of a risk, quantifying the risk by taking account of both the likelihood and the consequences, and deciding appropriate action to mitigate the risk. In simple terms, risk management aims to reduce the risks to patients thereby improving patient safety. Effective risk management should be integrated into all activities throughout the RT process, and is supported by QMS requirements such as effective communication, staff competency and

audit. Methods of risk prevention range from more effective system oriented or physical measures such as interlocks and computerisation to human oriented measures such as documented procedures and competency standards which are recognised as less effective due to their dependence on human behaviours [19]. Effective risk management should also identify latent threats which may lie dormant for months before an error actually occurs or the risk is detected.

Examples of risk management throughout the RT process include the following.

- A strict equipment maintenance programme and rigorous quality control checks (see Chapter 13).
- Active, independent checks at a number of stages within the treatment process to provide an effective error prevention system [20].

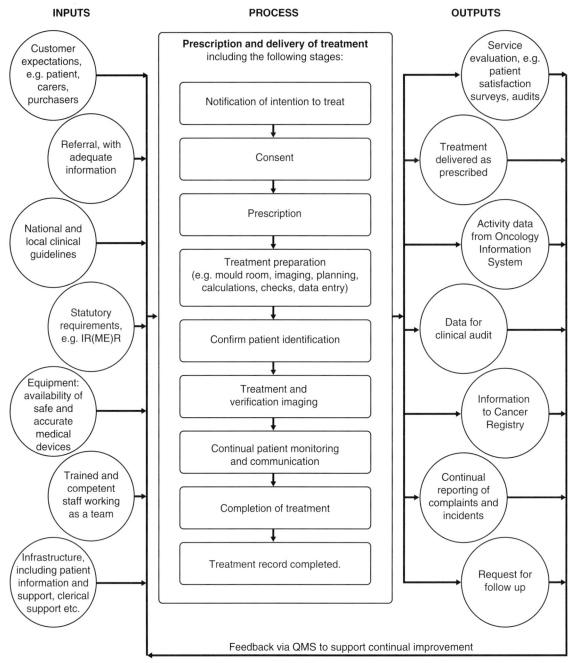

INPUTS   PROCESS   OUTPUTS

Fig. 14.4 The radiotherapy process.

- Audits of existing checking processes to ensure that they are effective, and any redundant checks eliminated.
- Reducing manual tasks, such as the transfer of data, wherever possible.
- Methods to reduce the risk of involuntary automaticity, where staff carry out checks automatically and see or hear what they expect to see, rather than what is actually written or said.
- Ensuring that a supervising member of staff is not responsible for checking a task for which they have provided supervision.
- Peer review of target volume definition [22].
- A study of incidents and near misses including prominent causes [23,24], contributory factors and the risk of accidental or unintended exposures [25].

Clinical Incidents

In 2016, NHS Improvement took over statutory patient safety functions including operating the National Reporting and Learning System (NRLS) and developing advice and guidance for the NHS on reducing risks to patients. Health organisations should be open in reporting incidents and implement local systems which are nonpunitive. There are a number of tools available for use in managing clinical incidents, such as incident decision trees [26], root cause analysis and The London Protocol for systems analysis of clinical incidents. There is a long history of incident reporting in RT both in the United Kingdom and internationally [9,21,27], including systematic incidents affecting multiple patients and random errors affecting an individual.

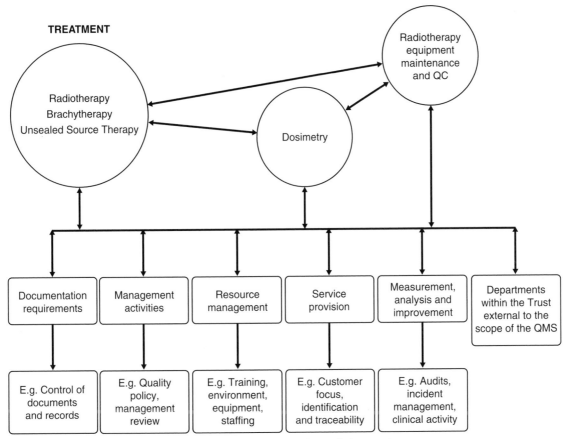

Fig. 14.5 The interaction of processes in a radiotherapy department.

Historically there has been:

- no unified approach
- no standard definitions for the terminology in use
- no defined classifications, such as level of impact, source or root cause.

This has made it difficult to compare error rates and to define any standards. Examples of current international systems include Safety in Radiation Oncology, SAFRON [28] and Radiation Oncology Safety Information System, ROSEIS [11]. A U.K. multidisciplinary working party including representation from the Royal College of Radiologists (RCR), the Institute of Physics and Engineering in Medicine (IPEM), the Society and College of Radiographers (SCoR), the British Institute of Radiology (BIR) and the National Patient Safety Agency (NPSA) was established in 2006, and in 2008 published a report [10] containing recommendations for a national system to support the reporting, analysis and learning from RT incidents. The Health Protection Agency (HPA), now Public Health England (PHE), implemented a taxonomy for severity and pathway classification dedicated to RT, and developed a U.K.-wide voluntary RT reporting system. There is now established data analysis and feedback through PHE [29,30]. The coding was extended in 2016 to include reporting and analysis of safety barriers and causative factors and in 2018 extended again to include methods of detection.

All RT departments should operate a system for defining, recording, analysing and learning from RT incidents including near misses. Local incident reporting should include a full objective description of the event, how it was detected, any identified causes and contributing factors, the severity of consequences, risk of recurrence and preventive actions to avoid future occurrence.

Major incidents are reportable under different regulations to various agencies, including:

- NHS Improvement. All patient safety incidents should be reported via the National Reporting and Learning System (NRLS).
- Care Quality Commission. Under IR[ME]R [25], any incident in which a person has been exposed to levels of ionising radiation significantly greater or lower than those generally considered to be proportionate in the circumstances.
- Health and Safety Executive (HSE). Under the Ionising Radiations Regulations 2017 [31], any incident where a person has received an overexposure as a result of work with ionising radiation carried out by that employer.
- Medicine and Healthcare Products Regulatory Agency (MHRA). Under the Medical Devices Regulations 2002, incidents and faults relating to medical equipment. Device Bulletin DB2011(01) gives further advice.
- HSE. Under the Reporting of Injuries, Diseases and Dangerous Occurrences Regulations (RIDDOR), any work-related accident resulting in death or specified injuries.

Action following an incident should be considered carefully by departments, including disclosure to the patient and Duty of Candour [32] and support for staff involved [10]. Communicating honestly and sympathetically with patients and their families is a vital component in dealing effectively with errors or mistakes. An apology can be an expression of regret and sympathy and not necessarily an admission of guilt.

Audit

Audit is a key requirement of ISO 9001:2015. It is also a recommendation or requirement of other standards, regulations and guidance such

TABLE 14.2   Overview of Quality Initiatives in Oncology and the National Health Service

Item	Year	Initiative, Publication or Requirement	Comment	Further Information (correct at April 2018)
1	2008	Towards Safer Radiotherapy	A joint report published by the British Institute of Radiology, the Institute of Physics and Engineering in Medicine, the National Patient Safety Agency, the Society and College of Radiographers and The Royal College of Radiologists. The report includes recommendations for improving safety in radiotherapy, including the implementation of an externally assessed QMS.	https://www.rcr.ac.uk/publication/towards-safer-radiotherapy
2	2008	World Health Organisation (WHO) Radiotherapy Risk Profile. Technical Manual.	This document comprises two parts, the first is an international review of patient safety measures in radiotherapy practice and the second sets out WHO's Radiotherapy Risk Profile and analyses the radiotherapy process, from patient assessment to treatment verification and monitoring.	http://www.who.int/patientsafety/activities/technical/radiotherapy_risk_profile.pdf
3	2008	High Quality Care for All. NHS Next Stage Review Final Report.	The final report from Lord Darzi's review. A review of the way the NHS delivers health care, looking at how it can become fairer, more personalised, effective and safe, setting out immediate and longer-term priorities to ensure a patient centred, high quality health service.	https://www.gov.uk/government/uploads/system/uploads/attachment_data/file/228836/7432.pdf
4	2009	Care Quality Commission (CQC)	The CQC is a public body formed from three former organisations, including the Healthcare Commission, with a role to ensure that care services, including hospitals, provide safe, effective and high-quality care.	http://www.cqc.org.uk/
5	2010	Implementing Towards Safer Radiotherapy: guidance on reporting radiotherapy errors and near misses. NPSA	Provided guidance on reporting radiotherapy errors to the National Patient Safety Agency (NPSA) and on the classification of these errors which are analysed by the HPA (now PHE). [See 21. later for updated guidance]	http://www.nrls.npsa.nhs.uk/EasySiteWeb/getresource.axd?AssetID=75031&servicetype=Attachment&type=full
6	2011	Improving Outcomes: A Strategy for Cancer	The government's commitment to improving health outcomes, including a section on providing radiotherapy services which are equitable, high quality, safe, timely, protocol-driven and quality-controlled focussed around patients' needs.	http://www.legislation.gov.uk/ukpga/2012/7/contents/enacted https://www.gov.uk/government/publications/health-and-social-care-act-2012-fact-sheets
7	2012	Health and Social Care Act (HSCA)	This recognised the need for modernisation in the NHS. Six key policy areas included clinically led commissioning and a greater voice for patients. Nine key themes included improving the quality of care.	http://www.legislation.gov.uk/ukpga/2012/7/contents/enacted https://www.gov.uk/government/publications/health-and-social-care-act-2012-fact-sheets
8	2013	Report of the Mid Staffordshire NHS Foundation Trust Public Inquiry	Referred to as the Francis Report, this details the failings in care at the Mid-Staffordshire NHS Foundation Trust.	https://www.gov.uk/government/publications/report-of-the-mid-staffordshire-nhs-foundation-trust-public-inquiry
9	2013	A promise to learn – a commitment to act, Improving the Safety of Patients in England	Known as the Berwick Report, this followed the Francis Report to address areas of improvement needed in patient safety in England.	https://www.gov.uk/government/uploads/system/uploads/attachment_data/file/226703/Berwick_Report.pdf
10	2013	National Institute for Health and Care Excellence	NICE became a non-departmental government body. It provides evidence-based guidance, develops quality standards and provides a range of information services.	https://www.nice.org.uk/
11	2014	'Hello my name is …' campaign.	A campaign founded by Dr Kate Granger, MBE, to highlight the importance of communication and patient-centred care.	https://hellomynameis.org.uk/

Continued

TABLE 14.2 Overview of Quality Initiatives in Oncology and the National Health Service—cont'd

Item	Year	Initiative, Publication or Requirement	Comment	Further Information (correct at April 2018)
12	2014	Patient Safety Collaboratives (PSC)	A national safety initiative set up to underpin a culture of safety, continuous learning and improvement. 15 regional PSC are funded and supported by NHS Improvement to facilitate improvements across the NHS.	https://improvement.nhs.uk/resources/patient-safety-collaboratives/
13	2014	Sign up to Safety	A national patient safety campaign to support organisations in ensuring harm-free care. It is designed to empower staff to highlight areas of potential risks and to report and learn from incidents	https://www.signuptosafety.org.uk/
14	2015	Culture change in the NHS	Update on the progress made since Mid Staffordshire 2013.	https://www.gov.uk/government/publications/culture-change-in-the-nhs
15	2015	The NHS Constitution for England updated.	Establishes the values and principles of the NHS, including the rights of patients, public and staff.	https://www.gov.uk/government/publications/the-nhs-constitution-for-england
16	2015	NHS Complaints guidance updated.	Advice on how patients can give feedback or make a complaint on health care services.	https://www.gov.uk/government/publications/the-nhs-constitution-for-england/how-do-i-give-feedback-or-make-a-complaint-about-an-nhs-service
17	2015	Radiation Protection No. 181. General guidelines on risk management in external beam radiotherapy. European Commission. 2015.	EU guidance on how to reduce the accidental or unintended radiation doses of patients in radiotherapy.	https://ec.europa.eu/energy/sites/ener/files/documents/RP181web.pdf
18	2015	The Q Community	A network supported by the Health Foundation and NHS Improvement to facilitate shared learning, experience and development of sustainable improvement initiatives.	https://q.health.org.uk/
19	2015	Achieving world-class cancer outcomes. A strategy for England, 2015–2020.	An independent report with 96 recommendations across the cancer pathway, including a national radiotherapy equipment replacement programme.	http://www.cancerresearchuk.org/sites/default/files/achieving_world-class_cancer_outcomes_-_a_strategy_for_england_2015-2020.pdf
20	2016	Cancer Strategy Implementation plan: Achieving World Class Cancer outcomes.	The NHS five-year plan for delivering improved cancer services in England, including prevention, diagnosis, patient experience and high quality modern services.	https://www.england.nhs.uk/wp-content/uploads/2016/05/cancer-strategy.pdf
21	2016	Development of learning from radiotherapy errors, PHE.	The introduction of additional taxonomies (causative factors and safety barriers) for the classification of radiotherapy errors.	https://www.gov.uk/government/publications/development-of-learning-from-radiotherapy-errors
22	2014	Learning from Excellence	Initiative based on the concept of learning from examples of good practice.	http://learningfromexcellence.com/
23	2016	BS70000:2017	A new British Standard for medical physics, clinical engineering and associated scientific services in health care with requirements for quality, safety and competence.	https://shop.bsigroup.com/ProductDetail/?pid=000000000030323397
24	2017	MPACE (formerly iCEPSS)	UKAS pilot for Medical Physics and Clinical Engineering accreditation scheme.	See Box 14.1 https://www.ukas.com/download/brochures/UKAS-B28-MPACE-Leaflet.pdf
25	2019	Adult External Beam Radiotherapy Services Delivered as Part of a Radiotherapy Network.	This document sets out the clinical, service and quality requirements and standards for the delivery of external beam radiotherapy to which all providers of radiotherapy must comply. It also identifies designated Networks and member departments.	https://www.england.nhs.uk/wp-content/uploads/2019/01/External-Beam-Radiotherapy-Services-Delivered-as-Part-of-a-Radiotherapy-Network-Adults.pdf Additional information on radiotherapy commissioning: https://www.england.nhs.uk/commissioning/spec-services/npc-crg/group-b/b01/

EU, European Union; *HPA*, Health Protection Agency; *iCEPSS,* Improving Clinical Engineering and Physical Science Services; *MBE*, Member of the British Empire; *MPACE*, Medical Physics and Clinical Engineering; *NHS*, National Health Service; *PHE*, Public Health England; *UKAS*, United Kingdom Accreditation Service.

BOX 14.3   Care Quality Commission (CQC)

The CQC is the independent regulator of healthcare in England. It is their role to
- Register hospitals
- Monitor, inspect and rate their services
- Take action to protect people who use the services and
- Speak with an independent voice, publishing views on major quality issues in health and social care.

They carry enforcement powers, such as fines, public warnings or closure, if standards are not being met.

Inspection visits are carried out by a team of people and take place over a number of days. An inspection is carried out by:
- Meeting and talking to people including staff in all roles and patients, both as individuals and in focus groups
- Observation, including day to day practice and the general environment
- Checking records and data.

The inspection team use Key Lines of Enquiry (KLOEs), prompts and sources of evidence to answer core questions. The 5 questions in use in 2018 are outlined below:
- **Is it safe?** Does the hospital ensure that all patients are protected from abuse and avoidable harm? For example, are medicines safely secured and medical devices compliant? Are there effective measures in place for infection control, safeguarding, duty of candour and incident reporting & learning?
- **Is it effective?** Does the hospital ensure that all patients receive the care, treatment and support they need to achieve the best possible outcomes and quality of life? Is the service provided in accordance with NICE guidance,

national guidelines, legislation, local and national audit and are outcomes monitored, e.g. with mortality reviews?
- **Is it caring?** Does the hospital ensure that all patients are treated with kindness, compassion, dignity and respect? For example, do they support patients to maintain independence and request support from other teams where needed (e.g. dementia service, pain management, alcohol liaison). Are patients involved in decision making and does the service seek patient participation and feedback?
- **Is it responsive to people's needs?** Does the hospital ensure that the care, treatment and support it provides meet the needs of all patients? For example, is there evidence of personalised care, an awareness of patients' needs & choices and are there effective systems in place to respond to concerns and complaints?
- **Is it well-led?** Do the leaders and managers provide vision, direction and energy with clear responsibilities and accountabilities and do the systems in place support the delivery of high-quality, patient-centred care? Is there evidence of good governance and of learning, improvement and innovation? Is there an open and fair culture? Is risk and performance managed effectively?

Following an inspection, informal feedback will be given at the end of the visit with a detailed report published later. For each core hospital service assessed each key question will receive a rating: Inadequate, Requires Improvement, Good or Outstanding. The service will also receive an overall rating.

Detailed information about inspections and KLOEs is available on the CQC website: http://www.cqc.org.uk/

---

as IR(ME)R [25] and Towards Safer Radiotherapy [10]. There are many definitions of audit. ISO 9000:2015 defines audit as:

A systematic, independent and documented process for obtaining objective evidence and evaluating it objectively to determine the extent to which the audit criteria are fulfilled [4]

where audit criteria are a set of policies, procedures or requirements used as a reference against which objective evidence is compared and objective evidence is data supporting the existence or verity of something [4].

Types of audit include:
- Clinical audit—typically used in the health care setting, see Box 14.4
- Internal audit—used by departments to monitor their QMS, conducted by employees of the department
- External audit—an objective check of a department's QMS, conducted by an independent external auditing organisation

All audits are cyclical in nature (Fig. 14.6) and have the same key features. Audits are a valuable tool for ensuring continual improvement. Many departments will have a clinical audit programme that is developed independently to the QMS internal audit programme. Whereas clinical audits may focus more on outcomes, for example, the effect on health or on patient experience, QMS audits aim to verify processes, particularly at the interfaces, highlight any areas of concern and identify areas for potential improvement. An integrated approach to both QMS and clinical audits could encompass a range of audit projects and provide a comprehensive audit programme.

It is important to distinguish audit from research. In the most simplistic terms, research tells us the most effective way to do things and how to achieve the best results and audit tells us if we are doing that.

Patient-Focussed Care

Patient-centred care is about an individual being able to take an active role in their health care. The National Institute for Health and Care Excellence (NICE) recommends that the patient should be given the opportunity to make informed choices about their care and treatment,

---

BOX 14.4   Clinical Audit

Clinical audit, initially termed *Medical Audit,* was introduced to the National Health Service (NHS) by the 1989 White Paper, *Working for Patients.* It has continued to evolve and is now well established in the NHS, forming a key component of the clinical governance framework.

Clinical audit is defined by the Health Quality Improvement Partnership (HQIP) as:

a quality improvement cycle that involves measurement of the effectiveness of healthcare against agreed and proven standards for high quality, and taking action to bring practice in line with these standards so as to improve the quality of care and health outcomes.

Clinical audits should be patient focussed. They can be conducted at a local level or nationwide. Health care professionals use clinical audits to measure their clinical practice against standards. It provides a framework to identify opportunities for improvement to the quality of patient care in a collaborative and systematic way. A good clinical audit will identify or confirm any problems and then lead to changes that should result in improved patient care.

At a national level, HQIP on behalf of NHS England manage and commission the National Clinical Audit and Patient Outcomes Programme (NCAPOP). The data collected from NCAPOP audits provide NHS providers with reports on compliance and performance helping to improve patient care. The National Institute for Health and Care Excellence (NICE) use the results of national clinical audits to measure compliance to NICE guidelines.

More guidance on clinical audit is available from the Health Quality Improvement Partnership (HQIP).

---

supported by health care professionals. The Mental Capacity Act 2005 exists for those unable to make such decisions.

However, patient-focussed care is not just about involving the patient themselves in their care choices, it is also about recognising the need to put the patient first. This was one of the key changes

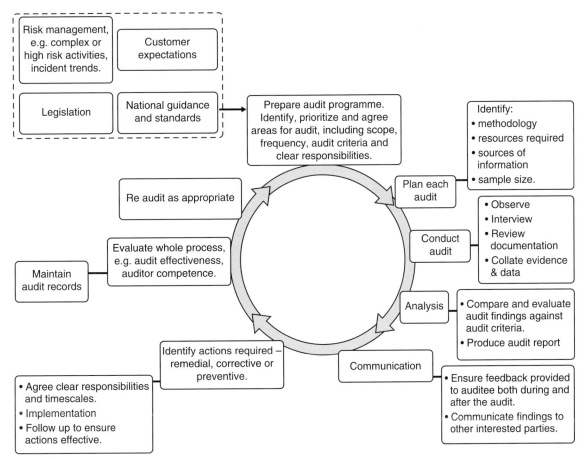

Fig. 14.6 The audit cycle.

recommended by the 2013 Francis Report, which highlighted the need for all staff to take an active role in quality management and for this to be encouraged by senior management. ISO 9001:2015 follows on this need for a culture change to promote accountability and empowerment in the organisation.

Following the Francis and Berwick Reports [33], there has been a push for NHS organisations to be more open to the public about how their services are performing. NHS England alongside the DoH, the Health and Social Care Information Service, the CQC and Public Health England developed the My NHS online tool that provides transparent performance data and encourages accountability and improvement.

There is a long history of patient and public participation in the United Kingdom, with national policies making it clear that all NHS cancer services are responsible at a local level for developing user involvement in service evaluation, planning and delivery. Patient reported outcome measures (PROMs) are about reviewing treatment in a way that is relevant to the patient by looking at quality of life and patient perceptions. In practical terms, the development of patient and carer input can be achieved in various ways including questionnaires, complaint monitoring, focus groups, interviews, websites, newsletters, workshops, user involvement training programs, suggestion boxes, facilitating support groups, patient liaison services and user councils. Patient reported experience measures are about reviewing treatment through patient feedback. A recent resource rolled out in 2013 following the Francis and Berwick Reports is the Friends and Family Test which provides feedback on patient experience data from patients on a local and national level. There is also the National Cancer Patient Experience Survey (NCPES) which started taking place annually in England from 2010.

It is important to include the patient perspective in establishing how the overall patient experience can be improved. In addition to offering the latest techniques, this may simply include adequate parking provision, a comfortable waiting area and effective communication and provision of information. In today's world, patients' expectations have increased, as too has their intolerance of failure or complications. The most common complaints concern delays, incorrect treatment and morbidity, perception of professional competence and efficiency of process.

IMPLEMENTATION OF NEW TECHNOLOGY AND NEW TECHNIQUES

The development of technology and techniques in RT continues to progress rapidly. Introducing any new development, equipment, software or change in procedure, however small, carries with it the risk of error [19] and must be managed carefully with full evaluation of safety issues and training competencies [10], and with final approval by the appropriate authority. Satisfactory management can include, for example:

- setting up specialist multidisciplinary groups to evaluate fully all implications and inviting feedback from all staff groups involved.
- visiting/liaising with other departments who already use the technique/technology.
- carrying out a full risk assessment of implementing the new technique/technology.
- developing clear guidelines as to when and how new techniques/technology may be used.
- a review of the number of staff and training needs.

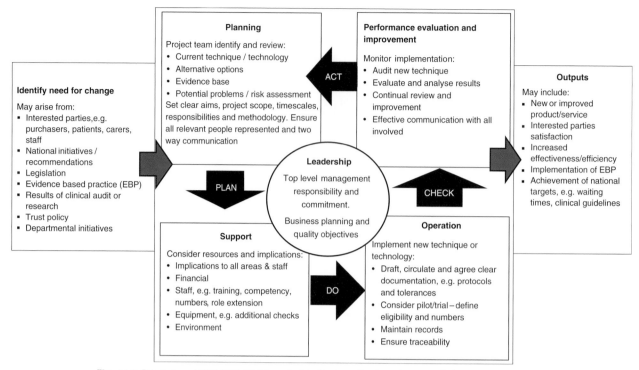

Fig. 14.7 Principles of ISO 9001:2015 applied to the introduction of new techniques or technology.

Fig. 14.7 illustrates how the principles of ISO 9001 can be applied to the safe introduction of new techniques or technology. It is vital that attention is paid to the recurrent themes identified in error reporting as outlined in this chapter. For example, provision of adequate training and assessment of competency.

CONCLUSION

The NHS has undergone many changes with a current priority being to raise the quality of care with a focus on safety, treatment effectiveness and patient experience. High quality care is a continuously moving target with the constant development of new techniques and technology together with challenges such as increased costs, staff shortages, lack of resources and increasing patient expectations. ISO 9001 has also undergone a number of changes since when it was first introduced to RT as QART in the 1990s. It is now more customer focussed, with an increased emphasis on leadership, improvement and risk management. Departments must build on the QMS framework and processes they have in place to manage both developments and challenges.

A culture of continuous improvement and a multidisciplinary approach will generate service-wide problem identification [3]. It may be argued that a QMS is costly to implement and maintain and

that there is a risk of running a system without addressing vital quality issues. However, if a system has management commitment and is run effectively, although it may not prevent disasters or eliminate human error, it will:

- reduce a department's exposure to the common elements behind disasters.
- ensure that a department has systems in place to prevent problems escalating into disaster.
- provide the tools to react quickly to put things right.
- minimise the risk of major errors and reduce the frequency of minor errors to ensure safe and effective treatment [3].

Historically, ISO 9001 has received criticism for being too generic because it is up to the organisation to set a number of its own standards. To implement a system effectively and gain the most benefit, oncology and RT departments should implement the ISO 9001 requirements in such a way as to provide a framework which ensures an integrated approach to the numerous quality standards, legislation, targets, reports, recommendations and initiatives that they are required to fulfill. A quality management system is not just about achieving certification, it is to ensure that the best possible treatments and standards of care are provided within the resources available.

REFERENCES

[1] Quality improvement made simple [Internet]. London: The Health Foundation. 2013 [cited 3 May 2018]. Available: https://health.org.uk/publication/quality-improvement-made-simple.

[2] Pawlicki T, Mundt AJ, Dunscombe P, Scalliet P. Quality and safety in radiotherapy. Boca Raton: CRC Press/Taylor & Francis Group; 2010.

[3] Kehoe T, Rugg L-J. From technical quality assurance of radiotherapy to a comprehensive quality of service management system. Radiother Oncol 1999;51(3):281–90.

[4] BS EN ISO. 9000:2015 Quality management systems — fundamentals and vocabulary. London: BSI Standards Limited; 2015.

[5] Coucke P, Boga D, Lenaerts E, Delgaudine M. From reporting incidents in a radiation therapy department to enterprise risk management (ERM) based on the European Foundation for Quality Management philosophy (EFQM). Int J Healthc Manag 2014;7(2):127–31.

[6] Applying Radiation Safety Standards in Radiotherapy. IAEA Safety Report Series no 38 [Internet]. Vienna: International Atomic Energy Agency; 2006. [cited 3 May 2018]. Available: https://www-pub.iaea.org/MTCD/publications/PDF/Pub1205_web.pdf.

[7] Valentin J. Prevention of accidental exposures to patients undergoing radiation therapy. ICRP Publication 86. Oxford. New York: Pergamon Press; 2001.

[8] Lessons learned from accidental exposures in radiotherapy. In: IAEA Safety Report Series No 17 [Internet]. Vienna: International Atomic Energy Agency; 2000. [cited 3 May 2018]. Available: http://www-pub.iaea.org/MTCD/Publications/PDF/Pub1084_web.pdf.

[9] World Health Organisation. Radiotherapy risk profile. Technical Manual [Internet]. Geneva: WHO Press; 2008. [cited 3 May 2018]. Available: http://www.who.int/patientsafety/activities/technical/radiotherapy_risk_profile.pdf.

[10] The Royal College of Radiologists, Society and College of Radiographers, Institute of Physics and Engineering in Medicine, National Patient Safety Agency, British Institute of Radiology. Towards safer radiotherapy [Internet]. London: The Royal College of Radiologists; 2018 [cited 3 May 2018]. Available: https://www.rcr.ac.uk/system/files/publication/field_publication_files/Towards_saferRT_final.pdf.

[11] ROSEIS (Radiation Oncology Safety Education Information System) [Internet]. Roseis.estro.org. [cited 10 March 2018]. Available: https://roseis.estro.org/.

[12] Department of Health. Quality assurance in radiotherapy: a quality management system for radiotherapy. London: HMSO; 1994.

[13] Toft B. Redacted Independent review of the circumstances surrounding a serious adverse incident [Internet]. 2005 [cited 3 May 2018]. Available: http://www.who.int/patientsafety/news/Radiotherapy_adverse_event_Toft_report.pdf.

[14] Unintended overexposure of a patient during radiotherapy treatment at the Edinburgh Cancer Centre, in September 2015 [Internet]. Gov.scot. 2016 [cited 3 May 2018]. Available: http://www.gov.scot/Publications/2016/07/8854.

[15] BS EN ISO 9004:2009. Managing for the sustained success of an organization—a quality management approach. London: BSI Standards Limited; 2009.

[16] Hoyle D. ISO 9000 Quality Systems Handbook; updated for the ISO9001:2015 standard. 7th ed. Abingdon: Routledge; 2017.

[17] Records Management Code of Practice for Health and Social Care 2016 [Internet]. Information Governance Alliance (IGA); 2016 [cited 9 May 2018]. Available: https://digital.nhs.uk/binaries/content/assets/legacy/pdf/n/b/records-management-cop-hsc-2016.pdf.

[18] Malicki J, Bly R, Bulot M, Godet J, Jahnen A, Krengli M, et al. Patient safety in external beam radiotherapy—guidelines on risk assessment and analysis of adverse error-events and near misses: introducing the ACCIRAD project. Radiother Oncol 2014;112(2):194–8.

[19] Radiation Protection No 181. General guidelines on risk management in external beam radiotherapy. [Internet]. Luxembourg: Publications Office; 2015 [cited 13 May 2018]. Available: https://ec.europa.eu/energy/sites/ener/files/documents/RP181web.pdf.

[20] Technical supplement to Radiation Protection n° 181. [Internet]. European Commission; 2015 [cited 10 March 2018]. Available: https://www.efrs.eu/publications/see/2015_RP_181_annexe?file=738.

[21] Holmberg O, McClean B. Preventing treatment errors in radiotherapy by identifying and evaluating near misses and actual incidents. J Radiother Pract 2002;3(01):13–25.

[22] Radiotherapy target volume definition and peer review—RCR guidance [Internet]. London: The Royal College of Radiologists; 2017. [cited 10 March 2018]. Available: https://www.rcr.ac.uk/system/files/publication/field_publication_files/bfco172_peer_review_outlining.pdf.

[23] Elnahal S, Blackford A, Smith K, Souranis A, Briner V, McNutt T, et al. Identifying predictive factors for incident reports in patients receiving radiation therapy. Int J Radiation Oncol Biol Phys 2016;94(5):993–9.

[24] Chang DW, Cheetham L, te Marvelde L, Bressel M, Kron T, Gill S, et al. Risk factors for radiotherapy incidents and impact of an online electronic reporting system. Radiother Oncol 2014;112(2):199–204.

[25] The Ionising Radiation (Medical Exposure) Regulations 2017 [Internet]. Legislation.gov.uk. 2017 [cited 4 February 2018]. Available: http://www.legislation.gov.uk/uksi/2017/1322/contents/made.

[26] Meadows S, Baker K, Butler J. The incident decision tree. Clin Risk 2005;11(2):66–8.

[27] Pawlicki T, Coffey M, Milosevic M. Incident learning systems for radiation oncology: development and value at the local, national and international level. Clin Oncol 2017;29(9):562–7.

[28] Safety in Radiation Oncology (SAFRON) [Internet]. Iaea.org; 2017. [cited 10 March 2018]. Available: https://www.iaea.org/resources/rpop/resources/databases-and-learning-systems/safron.

[29] Safer radiotherapy: error data analysis [Internet]. GOV.UK. [cited 10 March 2018]. Available: https://www.gov.uk/government/publications/safer-radiotherapy-error-data-analysis-report; 2018.

[30] Findlay Ú, Best H, Ottrey M. Improving patient safety in radiotherapy through error reporting and analysis. Radiography 2016;22:S3–S11.

[31] The Ionising Radiation Regulations 2017 [Internet]. London: HMSO; 2017 [cited 4 February 2018]. Available: http://www.legislation.gov.uk/uksi/2017/1075/pdfs/uksi_20171075_en.pdf.

[32] Regulation 20: Duty of Candour. [Internet]. CQC; 2015 [cited 16 May 2018]. Available: http://www.cqc.org.uk/sites/default/files/20150327_duty_of_candour_guidance_final.pdf.

[33] Berwick D. Improving the safety of patients in England. A promise to learn—a commitment to act. In: HSC 2901213. Department of Health and Social Care; 2013.

SECTION 2

15

Epidemiology of Cancer and Screening

Katie Spencer, David Hole[†], Paul Symonds, Eva Morris

CHAPTER OUTLINE

THE CANCER PROBLEM

In 2012, malignant tumours were responsible for over 14% of the nearly 57 million annual deaths worldwide from all causes.[1] In many countries, more than a quarter of deaths are attributable to cancer. In 2012, 7.4 million men and 6.7 million women worldwide developed a malignant tumour, and altogether 8.2 million died from the disease. Cancer has now emerged as a major public health problem in developing countries, matching its effect in industrialised nations.

Cancer rates are estimated to significantly increase from 14 million new cases globally in 2012 to almost 24 million new cases in the year 2035. This increase will mainly be as a result of steadily ageing populations in both developed and developing countries and also to current trends in smoking prevalence and the growing adoption of unhealthy lifestyles. However, there is clear evidence that healthy lifestyles and public health action by governments and health practitioners could stem this trend and prevent as many as one-third of cancers worldwide.

Lung cancer is the most common cancer worldwide, accounting for 1.8 million new cases annually; followed by cancer of the breast, with around 1.7 million cases; colorectal, 1.3 million; prostate, 1.1 million; stomach, 952,000; liver, 782,000; cervical, 528,000; oesophageal, 456,000; bladder, 429,000; malignant non-Hodgkin's lymphomas, 38,000; leukaemia, 351,000; testicular, 55,000; pancreatic, 337,000; ovarian, 238,000; kidney, 337,000; endometrial, 319,000; nervous system, 256,000; melanoma, 232,000; thyroid, 298,000; pharynx, 142,000; and Hodgkin's disease, 65,000 cases.

In developed countries, the probability of being diagnosed with cancer is more than twice as high as in developing countries. However, in rich countries, some 50% of cancer patients die of the disease whereas, in developing countries, 70% of people are diagnosed with late-stage incurable tumours, pointing to the need for much better detection programmes. The main reasons for the greater cancer burden of affluent societies are the earlier onset of the tobacco epidemic, the earlier exposure to occupational carcinogens, and the Western nutrition and lifestyle. With increasing wealth and industrialisation, however, many countries undergo rapid lifestyle changes that will greatly increase their future disease burden.

CANCER IN THE UNITED STATES

Cancer, after heart disease, is the second leading cause of death. One of every four deaths in the United States is because of cancer. It is estimated that in 2018, 1.74 million Americans would receive a new diagnosis of invasive cancer (excluding basal and squamous cell skin cancers) and over 0.6 million Americans will die of this disease.[2] The most common cancers among men are prostate, lung and colorectal, and among women are breast, lung and colorectal. For both sexes, these cancers made up over 50% of newly diagnosed cases. Age-adjusted incidence rates for all cancer sites combined have fallen slightly since 2000 with small increases in breast and endometrial cancer among women being offset by long-term decreases in lung cancer and prostate among men.

[†]Deceased.

Mortality from the four most common cancer killers: lung, breast, prostate and colorectal, has been in decline since the late 1990s. The steep decline in lung cancer rates in men and the recent slowing of an increase in rates in women are steps in the right direction and further progress will require rigorous application of strategies known to be effective in reducing tobacco use. Death rates from breast cancer are falling despite a gradual, long-term increase in the rate of new diagnoses. This has been attributed to the successful implementation of more effective adjuvant treatment and the increased use of mammography screening. However, higher rates of late-stage disease exist in some population groups such as women who lacked health insurance and recent immigrants.

Prostate cancer death rates have been declining since 1994, whereas incidence rates have fluctuated dramatically since this time. Much of the initial increase in incidence seen was as a result of the wider use of prostate-specific antigen (PSA) screening rather than a major increase in symptomatic disease. Colorectal cancer death rates have been declining since the 1970s with steeper declines beginning in the mid-1980s. This is probably as a result of improving surgical techniques and, more recently, the introduction of adjuvant treatment regimens.

Cancer in Europe

The International Agency for Research on Cancer has recently produced estimates of the number of new cancers developing and the number of deaths as a result of cancer which are likely to have occurred in 2012. Of an estimated total of 4.2 million incident cases of cancer (excluding non-melanoma skin), the most common forms were breast (552,513 cases), colorectal (499,667 cases), lung (470,039 cases), and prostate (449,761 cases). Among men, the top five cancers were prostate, lung, colorectal, bladder and stomach. Among women, the most common cancers were breast, colorectal, lung, endometrium and ovary. In terms of mortality, it is estimated there were 1.3 million cancer deaths, with the main causes being lung (387,913 deaths), colorectal (238,752 deaths), breast (137,707 deaths) and pancreas (128,045 deaths). With over 2.5 million new cancers and 1.9 million deaths each year, cancer remains one of the most important public health problems in Europe. As the European population ages, these numbers will increase even if the age-specific rates remain constant. Lung, colorectal, stomach and breast cancers account for nearly half of all cancer deaths in Europe and point very clearly to the priorities for cancer control action.

EPIDEMIOLOGY OF CANCER

Terminology

Epidemiology is the study of the occurrence, distribution and causes of disease across populations. It can be divided into three main components: descriptive, analytical and experimental.

Descriptive epidemiology is concerned with the variation in frequency (incidence or mortality) of a disease over space, time and in relation to age, sex and socioeconomic status. Analytical epidemiology is the study of the relationship between potentially causal risk factors (e.g. cigarette smoking, asbestos, ionising radiation) or their proxies, and the development of disease. Experimental epidemiology involves observing the effects of controlling relevant adverse risk factors (e.g. stopping cigarette smoking) or promoting possible preventative factors (e.g. beta-carotene).

The incidence rate of any disease is the total number of new cases occurring over a given period of time (a year) among a given number of people (usually 100,000 for cancer). This is different from the prevalence rate, which is the number of cases of a particular disease alive at a given point in time. This should be qualified by a statement as to how far back in time cancer patients are considered to be at risk from their disease—this is often taken as referring to cancers diagnosed within the previous 5 years. The mortality rate is the number of deaths attributed to the cancer in a given period of time (a year) among a given number of people (usually 100,000 for cancer).

Crude incidence or death rates are defined as the total number of cancers or deaths divided by the total population. Crude rates are of limited value because they do not take account of the differing proportions of people in particular age groups between populations. The crude rate in a particular population may exceed that of another country simply because it contains a higher proportion of elderly people. The age-standardised incidence or death rate takes account of the effect of age distribution on rates by attributing a weighting system to each of the age-specific rates. A choice of weighting systems exists—the two most common are the world standardised population and the European standardised population. When comparing cancer incidence rates in countries with very different proportions of elderly people (e.g. those in the developing world versus those in the developed world), the world standard is recommended. This is known as the world standardised rate (WSR). For comparison of countries with more similar proportions of elderly people, the European Standard is preferable. This is known as the European standardised rate (ESR).

An alternative method of expressing relative incidence or mortality is known as the standardised incidence ratio (SIR) or the standardised mortality ratio (SMR). This is an overall measure of incidence (mortality) which compares the observed number of cases (deaths) in a particular population with the expected number of cases (deaths) that would have been anticipated in a standard population (e.g. national) if the age-specific incidence (death) rates were the same. This is usually expressed as a ratio of 100 if the observed and expected rates are the same, and greater than 100 if the rate in the population of interest is higher than that for the standard (national) rate. SIRs are useful in comparing cancer incidence between socioeconomic or particular occupational groups.

SURVIVAL AND CURE IN CANCER

What do we mean by 'cure' for a cancer patient? Technically, it is when the survival for that patient is the same as that for the general population from which they originate—their 'excess' risk of death becomes zero. Thus, it makes sense to talk of 'cure' for example, of a small basal cell carcinoma treated by surgery or radiotherapy where recurrence or persistent disease is uncommon. However, for other cancers, particularly breast cancer, the possibility of local or distant recurrence remains for many years after the tumour has been successfully removed surgically. This likelihood increases substantially for larger tumours with nodal involvement and adverse histological features. Thus, survival rates are quoted as a measure of success but should be qualified by the length of follow-up, usually 5 years.

Five-year survival is often interpreted as cure. Although this is true of many tumours, it is not true of breast cancer, as suggested previously. For breast cancer, 10-, 20- or even 30-year survival figures are more appropriate end-points because of the long-term pattern of relapse and death from the disease. Survival may be with or without evidence of cancer. For this reason, the terms *disease-free survival* or *recurrence-free survival* are commonly used to define the outcome of treatment. These results require an elaborate system of clinical follow-up. Yet, it is only from painstaking analysis of this kind that we can derive a sound knowledge of both the natural history of cancer and the effects of treatment. Survival data are commonly presented plotted graphically as curves which allow the comparison of different treatments for different stages of disease over time.

In studies of patients treated for cancer, a variety of ways is used for describing their survival. Crude survival rate refers to the percentage of patients alive a given number (*n*) of years after treatment. This is not valid unless all the patients included have been followed up for at least *n* years. More often, a sizeable proportion of patients have been followed up for a shorter time than *n* years, and the life table or Kaplan-Meier method is more appropriate. This method uses information from all the patients for the time intervals for which they have been followed. Thus, someone who has been in the study for 1 year will contribute to the first-year survival estimate, those in for 2 years will contribute to the first- and second-year survival estimates, and so on. There is an underlying assumption that all patients are subject to the same time-specific probability of dying from a particular cancer whether or not they have been followed for all or part of the follow-up period of study. This method can be used for calculating survival rates for all causes of death (*overall survival rate*) or death from cancer (*cancer-specific survival rate*). Patients who die from causes other than cancer of interest (i.e. from intercurrent disease) are considered to have been withdrawn from the study at the point in time that their death occurred.

An alternative method for dealing with the problem of intercurrent deaths or mortality from natural causes of the patients studied is to examine relative or net survival. This is the ratio of the overall survival for a population with cancer to that of a comparable population (generally matched for age, sex and socioeconomic status) of people without cancer. Net survival is the method used to calculate most commonly reported publicly available cancer survival statistics.

Outcome of Palliative Care

Survival figures are essential for estimating the success of treatment aimed at cure but are of limited value in assessing the effects of palliative treatment. The main aim of palliative treatment is the relief of distressing symptoms. Palliative radiotherapy or chemotherapy may sometimes restrain tumour growth sufficiently to prolong the patient's life for a few months or sometimes years. In this case, a better measure of survival would be the median survival time. This is calculated by ranking the survival times in ascending order and choosing the middle value.

EPIDEMIOLOGY AND THE PREVENTION OF CANCER

The principal role of epidemiological studies in cancer has been the identification of risk factors, the assessment of their likelihood of being causative agents and, ultimately, whether their avoidance offers a practical solution for reducing the cancer burden. Most of the research effort has been directed at identifying factors associated with an increased risk of cancer but it is equally legitimate to try to identify factors which are associated with a decrease in risk. One, often misunderstood concept, particularly by the general media, is that the findings of epidemiological studies are indicative of causal effects. In fact, epidemiological studies will only ever identify associations.

Criteria for Causality

After individual epidemiological studies of cancer have been summarised and the quality assessed, a judgment is made concerning the strength of evidence that the agent or exposure in question is carcinogenic for humans. Several criteria are considered: a strong association (a large relative risk) is more likely to indicate causality than a weak one. Associations that are replicated in several studies of the same design or using different epidemiological approaches or under different

circumstances of exposure are more likely to represent a causal relationship than isolated observations from single studies if the risk of the disease increases with the amount of exposure, this is considered to be a strong indication of causality demonstration of a decline in risk after cessation of, or reduction in, exposure in individuals or in whole populations also supports a causal interpretation, although a carcinogen may act upon more than one target organ, the specificity of an association (an increased occurrence of cancer at one anatomical site or of one morphological type) adds plausibility to a causal relationship where an increase in exposure in a population and an increase in the incidence of a cancer are apparent. There must be a sensible latency (20+ years for solid tumours, 3+ years for blood-borne cancers) between the timings of the two increases. There is evidence from animal models of a link between the exposure and the occurrence of the cancer. There is a biological mechanism in humans for a link between the exposure and the cancer bias and confounding can be ruled out as possible explanations for the association.

It is not necessary for all of these criteria to hold for a judgment to be made that causality exists.

One current area of controversy that currently concerns public health is the impact of chronic low levels of exposure of known carcinogens. Two examples would be the impact of ionising radiation to the general population and leukaemia risk, and the effect of inhaling second-hand tobacco smoke among nonsmokers and lung cancer risk. In both cases, the first criterion listed above would not be expected to hold; the relative risks are likely to be low because the level of exposure is (relatively) low. In these circumstances, a more appropriate interpretation would be that the level of risk should be compatible with an acceptable extrapolation from the dose-response relationship observed for higher levels of exposure.

Such studies have played a major role in establishing occupational hazards in several industries (e.g. bladder cancer in aniline dye workers) and the link between lung cancer and smoking.

Epidemiology can assist in the prevention of cancer in a number of ways. First, it can show differences in the incidence of cancer in different populations and correlate them with differences in the prevalence of a potential causal factor. Secondly, it can test a hypothesis about the relationship between the occurrence of the disease to an aspect of the affected individual's constitution or exposure to some environmental factor. Thirdly, it can test the validity of a causal relationship by seeing whether the disease can be prevented or its incidence reduced by changing the prevalence of the suspected agent. A good example of the latter is the reduction in lung cancer observed among doctors since they gave up smoking cigarettes.

AETIOLOGY AND SCREENING

Lung Cancer

Tobacco

Lung cancer is currently still the largest single cause of death from any cancer in the world as well as being the most common incident cancer (excluding non-melanoma skin cancer). It was, however, a rare disease at the start of the 20th century, but exposures to new aetiological agents, particularly tobacco, and an increasing lifespan led to enormous increases in numbers of cases. Although tobacco had been used throughout the world for many centuries, the 20th century pandemic was a result of the introduction of manufactured cigarettes on a mass scale. Its addictive properties led to sustained exposure of inhaled carcinogens. Scientists in Nazi Germany conducted some of the earliest research on the links between smoking and lung cancer, but their results were generally dismissed as propaganda. In the early 1950s, case-control studies in Britain and the United States suggested a strong association. Three major cohort studies were initiated at that time—UK doctors, US veterans and the American Cancer Society volunteers—and their findings corroborated the earlier observations as well as identifying other cancers and causes of death as also being strongly linked to cigarette smoking. An increase in risk of lung cancer (relative to a nonsmoker) is consistently evident at the lowest level of daily consumption and is at least linearly related to increasing consumption.

Doll et al. reported on 50 years' worth of observations of the UK doctors study initiated in 1951. It is only now that the emergence of the full hazards for persistent smokers can be gauged as it requires a study of men whose cigarette consumption as young adults was already substantial when those who are now old were young. Men born in the 1920s in the United Kingdom may well have had the most intense early exposure as widespread military conscription of 18-year-old men, which began in 1939 and continued for decades, routinely included provision of low-cost cigarettes to the conscripts. The relative risk of lung cancer for all levels of smoking ranges from 7.5 for light smokers (<15/day) to 25.4 for heavy smokers (≥25/day) as compared with lifelong nonsmokers. These levels of risk are higher than previously observed, highlighting the fact that earlier analyses have underestimated the full effect of persistent cigarette smoking.

Smoking cessation is by far the most effective means of reducing the risk of lung cancer among active smokers. Lung cancer risk shows a steady upward trend from never-smokers, through later ages at cessation, to continuing smokers. Thus, there is substantial protection even for those who stop at 55 to 64 years, and progressively greater protection for those who stop earlier (up to 90% reduction in those stopping between 25 and 34 years).

On a global scale, the rise in cigarette consumption in developing countries such as China and India is alarming. Going on the current worldwide smoking patterns, whereby about 30% of young adults become smokers, there will be about 7 million lung cancer deaths worldwide unless there is widespread cessation. Convincing the next generation not to start smoking remains a major public health imperative.

Passive Smoking

The question as to whether involuntary smoking poses a significant risk of lung cancer has received considerable scientific interest since 1980. Involuntary (or passive) smoking is exposure to second-hand tobacco smoke, which is a mixture of exhaled mainstream smoke and sidestream smoke released from the smouldering cigarette and diluted with ambient air. Involuntary smoking involves exposure to the same numerous carcinogens and toxic substances that are present in tobacco smoke produced by active smoking, which is the principal cause of lung cancer. This implies that there will be some risk of lung cancer from exposure to second-hand tobacco smoke.

More than 50 studies, based on over 7300 nonsmoking lung cancer cases, have examined the association between involuntary smoking and the risk of lung cancer in never-smokers, especially spouses of smokers. Most showed an increased risk, especially for persons with higher exposures. In metaanalyses the excess risk of lung cancer has been identified as being of the order of 24% and this excess could not be explained by chance, potential biases or confounding. Second-hand smoke has therefore been defined as carcinogenic to humans by the International Agency for Research on Cancer (IARC) Monograph Programme (https://monographs.iarc.fr/iarc-monographs-on-the-evaluation-of-carcinogenic-risks-to-humans-38/). Interestingly, an association has also been shown between exposure to environmental tobacco smoke (ETS) in infancy and risk of lung cancer in adulthood among 60,182

lifelong nonsmokers who participated in the EPIC (European Prospective Investigation Into Cancer and Nutrition) study.

Asbestos

It has been known for many years that exposure to asbestos is a major cause of lung cancer. In 1999, a metaanalysis of 69 cohort studies found an SMR of 163 for lung cancer, but a substantial heterogeneity existed largely attributable to the different cumulative exposure to asbestos in various cohorts. These cohorts comprised workers from a variety of industries—mining, textile and manufacturing, insulation, asbestos-cement factories and shipyards—and risk was closely related to level of exposure in the different industries. Type of asbestos was also observed to be relevant, with chrysotile fibres being considered less carcinogenic than amphiboles.

Asbestos dust and cigarette smoke are both causes of lung cancer. What is less clear is the effect of the combination of the two carcinogenic agents. Initially, two hypotheses existed about the way asbestos and cigarette smoking interact. In one, it is assumed that asbestos produces the same additional risk in men who smoke cigarettes as in those who do not (additive hypothesis); in the other, it is assumed that asbestos produces an effect that is proportional to the effect of the other agent (multiplicative hypothesis). Which hypothesis is best explained by the available data remains debated.

One often quoted study by Hammond et al. estimates relative risks of 1, 5, 11 and 53 for no asbestos exposure and never smoked, asbestos exposed and never smoked, no asbestos exposure and ever smoked and exposed to both carcinogens. These results clearly favoured the multiplicative model but it has not proven to be generalisable to other studies. Indeed, a recent analysis of the Quebec chrysotile miners and millers cohort concluded that an additive model provided the best fit to their data but cautioned that there seems no good reason to believe that interactions should conform to any simple theory.

The situation with regard to mesothelioma is far simpler in that asbestos exposure is a causal factor but cigarette smoking is not. The disease is rapidly fatal, most of those affected dying within a year of diagnosis. There is a long latent period between first asbestos exposure and diagnosis of mesothelioma that is seldom less than 15 years and often exceeds 60 years. In all, 85% of deaths are among men, and the risk is highest in occupations with substantial exposure to asbestos. Shipyard workers have been a particularly susceptible group in that considerable exposures were to be found during the 1940s, 1950s and into the 1960s when ships were being repaired and the merchant fleet was being rebuilt after World War II.

Although mesothelioma is almost exclusively as a result of inhalation of asbestos fibres, this is not exclusively an occupational disease: In some areas of Turkey, environmental exposure to erionite is associated with high incidence of mesothelioma; domestic exposure and increased risk has been observed among the wives of South African Cape miners who brought home contaminated working clothes for cleaning; finally, fibre concentrations in the lungs of (nonmining) residents near the chrysotile mines in Quebec are up to 10 times higher than the average Canadian. The latter raises the critical question of whether this level of exposure represents an increased risk of the disease. The answer to this question is almost certainly yes as there appears to be no evidence that a threshold level exists below which there is no excess risk. There might exist a background level of mesothelioma occurring in the absence of exposure to asbestos, but there is no proof of this and this 'natural level' is probably lower than one case per million per year.

Radon

Underground miners exposed to radioactive radon and its decay products have been found to be at an increased risk of lung cancer. Indoor exposure to radon has been associated with a marginal increase in risk of lung cancer.

Chemoprevention

Chemoprevention is defined as the reduction of the risk of cancer development through the use of pharmaceuticals or micronutrients. There has been consistent evidence that high intake of fruit and vegetables is associated with some reduction in risk of lung cancer. Thus, it has been suggested that micronutrients and macronutrients present in our diet may act as cancer inhibiting substances. Epidemiological studies have verified that beta-carotene is inversely related to lung cancer risk and a number of randomised controlled intervention trials have been undertaken. None of these trials showed a reduction in lung cancer incidence or mortality even in high risk populations, and two of them suggested an increased risk, albeit small. Clearly, our understanding of the mechanism by which relatively short-term intake of retinoids and carotenoids affects the development of cancer in large populations is insufficient to use this approach as a specific lung cancer control procedure.

Screening

Given the high incidence of advanced disease at presentation and mortality of lung cancer, screening has been investigated as a means to improve mortality. Screening using chest x-rays and sputum cytology have not been shown to reduce lung cancer mortality. Low-dose computed tomography (CT) screening in high risk populations has been shown to reduce lung cancer mortality, although at the cost of significant false positive diagnoses and likely over-diagnosis. Ongoing studies are assessing the harms, benefits and cost effectiveness of this intervention in populations at varying levels of risk.

Colorectal Cancer

Incidence rates for cancer of the colon vary greatly across the world. The highest estimated incidence rates are in Australia and New Zealand and the lowest in Western Africa. Globally, it is one of the cancers whose incidence is increasing and it is now the third most common cancer in the world. Studies of migrants suggest that environmental factors rather than ethnic or genetic factors play a major role in its aetiology. Most studies have involved migrants moving from low-risk to high-risk areas, such as Chinese and Japanese to Hawaii or the rest of the United States, or southern Europeans to North America or Australia. In general, the risk in migrants approximates that of the new country with rates increasing with increasing duration of stay, presumably as their lifestyles merge with that of the host country.

Over time, the incidence of colon cancer has been rising, slowly in high-risk areas but more rapidly in areas where the risk was formerly low. These changes have been accompanied by changing ratios between the subsites within the bowel at which tumours occur, with left-sided tumours (of the descending and sigmoid colon and rectum) becoming more frequent.

Risk of colorectal cancer is closely related to diet and other lifestyle factors. International comparisons have suggested increased risks with increased intakes of dietary fat and a decreased intake of cereal grains and dietary fibre. Analytical studies within populations have shown a deficiency of vegetables and fruits and a sedentary lifestyle as being associated with an increased risk. However, attempts to identify independent roles for specific macronutrients have proved unsuccessful, with the exception of over-consumption of energy. Thus, dietary associations with colon cancer are characterised as typical of the Western diet, without being able to tie in any specific components. There is rapidly growing evidence, however, to link the risk of colorectal cancer to the microbiome of the intestinal tract. The microorganisms living in the gut shape their environment and the body's inflammatory response, hence influencing tumour growth and spread. As dietary and lifestyle factors can strongly influence the gut microbiotica, understanding these relationships may prove hugely informative in understanding the aetiology of this disease.

Although the vast majority of colorectal cancer cases occur sporadically in the general population, a number of specific disease groups: Crohn disease, ulcerative colitis and familial polyposis, are subject to increased risks. For example, whereas colorectal cancer in ulcerative colitis only accounts for 1% of all colorectal cancer cases, it accounts for one-sixth of all deaths in ulcerative colitis patients. The overall prevalence of colorectal cancer in any ulcerative colitis patient is estimated to be 3.7%. However, there is general agreement that the colorectal cancer risk is highest in those with extensive disease of long duration. Overall, incidence rates build to cumulative probabilities of 2% by 10 years, 8% by 20 years and 18% by 30 years.

Screening

Colorectal cancer is one of the few internal cancers that are amenable to secondary prevention, that is, prevention by detection of preclinical lesions. The precursor of advanced colorectal cancer is either an adenomatous polyp or a flat neoplastic area. To prevent premature death, people aged 50 to 74 years are the main focus of attention.

Screening programmes for the disease can take a number of forms. These can include a one-off flexible sigmoidoscopy at around the age of 55 years. Although such screening can, and does, identify cancers, its principal aim is to remove precancerous lesions and so reduce the incidence and consequently, the mortality from the disease. A large randomised trial has shown this strategy to be effective. Other screening approaches based on direct exposure to diagnostic tests include colonoscopy, CT colonography or flexible sigmoidoscopy at 5- or 10-year intervals. Such tests are, however, expensive and so potentially more cost effective programmes involve using fecal occult blood tests (FOBT) or the more sensitive faecal immunochemical tests (FIT), to limit these diagnostic tests to those people at higher risk of having some underlying relevant bowel pathology are commonly deployed. These initial screening tests detect blood in stool samples as bleeding within the gastrointestinal tract can indicate the presence of a tumour. If blood is found, then the individuals would be encouraged to undergo a diagnostic test, most commonly a colonoscopy, to determine if a tumour or other relevant pathology was present. Again, randomised trials have shown such screening to reduce colorectal cancer mortality and evaluations of national screening programmes in the United Kingdom and elsewhere suggest it has a positive impact on cancer outcomes.

Breast

Breast cancer is the most common cancer in women worldwide. Although the majority of cancers exhibit a consistently increasing rise in incidence rates with age, breast cancer is an exception and demonstrates how the frequency of a disease can be a function of duration of exposure rather than age per se. Among premenopausal women, incidence risk doubles with each decade of age. After the menopause (generally amongst women in their 50s), the incidence rate remains relatively steady (sometimes referred to as Clemmensen's hook) and thereafter starts to rise again but at a shallower gradient than is observed for premenopausal women. The examination of the shape of age-specific incidence curves can give indications as to causal factors, particularly those that change over a person's lifetime, such as hormonal factors. Thus, for breast cancer it would seem to indicate that the factors related to premenopausal breast cancer may well be different from those which cause postmenopausal breast cancer. Add to this the observation that the incidence of premenopausal breast cancer has remained stable over time whereas postmenopausal breast cancer rates have been slowly, but steadily, increasing over time, and it may well be that premenopausal and postmenopausal breast cancer should be considered as two separate diseases in aetiological terms.

Reproductive factors have been consistently related to (postmenopausal) breast cancer in that early age at first full-term pregnancy and high parity are associated with lower levels of the disease. Furthermore, risk is increased in women who have early menarche or who have late menopause. Obesity, related to various alterations in plasma levels of total and bioavailable sex steroids, is also a strong risk factor. Because circulating levels of sex steroids are regulated by a range of factors, including insulin and insulin-like growth factors, this may provide the link between many observations regarding excessive energy intake and increased risk of cancer.

The oestrogen excess hypothesis stipulates that risk depends directly on breast tissue exposure to oestrogens. Oestrogens increase breast cell proliferation and inhibit apoptosis in vitro and, in experimental animals, cause increased rates of tumour development when administered. This theory is consistent with the epidemiological evidence showing an increase in breast cancer risk in postmenopausal women who have low circulating sex hormone-binding globulin and elevated total and bioavailable oestradiol.

Two developments in the second half of the 20th century, the oral contraceptive pill and hormone replacement therapy (HRT), have impacted the risk of breast cancer. Oral contraceptives, in the form of oestrogen-progestogen combinations, were introduced in the early 1960s and rapidly found widespread use in most developed countries. Preparations of oral contraceptives have undergone substantial changes over time, reducing the potency of the oestrogens, adding in different progestogens and using biphasic and triphasic pills. A small increase in risk has been observed in current and recent users of combined oral contraceptives (a relative risk of about 1.2), but this association is unrelated to duration of use or type and dose of preparation, and 10 years after cessation of use, the excess risk disappears. Causation has not been clearly established and one suggestion has been that it could be the result of detection bias as a result the increased attention to the occurrence of breast abnormalities in women regularly visiting their doctor for contraceptive prescriptions.

HRT is used to treat the symptoms of menopause and, during the 1990s, up to one-third of all menopausal women in the United States and many European countries used HRT for some period. A small increase in breast cancer risk is correlated with longer duration of oestrogen replacement therapy use in current and recent users. The increase seems to cease several years after use has stopped. Initially, there appeared to be no difference in breast cancer risk between long-term users of all HRT and users of oestrogens alone, although two recent studies have suggested that HRT may pose a greater risk than oestrogens alone.

A second oestrogen progestogen hypothesis postulates that compared with an exposure to oestrogens alone (as in postmenopausal women not using any exogenous hormones), risk of breast cancer is increased further in women who have elevated plasma and tissue levels of oestrogens in combination with progestogens. This theory is supported by observations that postmenopausal women using oestrogen-plus-progestogen preparations for HRT have a greater increase in risk than women using oestrogens alone.

Screening

No practical strategies exist which can be recommended for the prevention of breast cancer and so considerable effort has been aimed at developing methods of early detection. Mammography can detect preclinical cancer, that is, before it is palpable or before it causes symptoms.

Tumours detected and treated at an early stage would be expected to be associated with a better survival rate than those detected symptomatically. However, as some breast cancers are characterised by early systemic dissemination, the actual effectiveness of screening is not at all clear. In this context, a number of large randomised trials were undertaken to evaluate its effectiveness on a population basis. The analysis of these trials has shown that in women aged 50 to 69 years, mammography screening can reduce mortality from breast cancer by 25% to 30%. For women in the age group 40 to 49 years, screening efficacy is significantly less.

The only true measure of success of a screening programme is an associated reduction in mortality. Survival rates can theoretically improve without extending length of life by the simple expedient of bringing forward the date of diagnosis whereas the date of death remains the same. This is known as lead-time bias. Analysis of trial data suggests that screening brings forward the date of diagnosis by an average of about 3 years, but this will vary considerably on an individual basis depending on how long the tumour remains in the screen-detectable phase. This raises a second phenomenon known as length-time bias. The argument is based on the well-founded assumption that tumours grow at varying speeds in different women. Slow-growing tumours will therefore remain in the screen-detectable window for longer than fast-growing tumours. Hence, a screening programme will tend to pick up slow-growing tumours disproportionately more than fast-growing tumours. If slow-growing tumours are also more amenable to cure, then survival rates will tend to be artificially inflated as they will tend to include a larger proportion of better prognosis tumours.

A sizeable number of developed countries have now established national or subnational screening programmes. Eligible age ranges vary, the repeat interval varies, some use single view mammography, others use two-view and independent double reading of mammograms is recommended but not always adhered to. One of the side effects of the introduction of national breast screening programmes has been the necessity to overhaul the referral and management pathway for breast cancer generally. Now, designated surgical units provide specialist expertise to manage breast cancer, particularly in those women with impalpable tumours; pathologists and oncologists with a special interest in breast cancer and clinical nurse specialists combine to form a multidisciplinary team for the management of the disease.

The effectiveness of routine national breast screening programmes has been questioned. There is general agreement that the extent of the reduction in mortality has been lower than that experienced in the trial situation. Under optimal conditions with a high compliance rate, a mortality reduction of 20% appears achievable. In reality, this may be more in the region of 10% to 15% on current data. One of the major problems in trying to assess the reduction in mortality as a result of screening now is that other factors have come into play, which were not operating at the time when the trials were being conducted. Before the late 1980s, no decline in mortality had been seen, but then a smooth downturn occurred in Europe, North America and Australia. These changes accelerated in the early 1990s but the fall occurred too soon after the widespread availability of mammography to be a consequence of it. More likely, the success of adjuvant therapy based on tamoxifen and chemotherapy was the major cause of this trend. Thus, the concurrent changes in improved adjuvant therapy, better and more focused surgical services, protocol-driven management and a better awareness of breast cancer and its symptoms among the general population make it almost impossible to isolate the contribution that breast screening is now making. However, there is no denying the fact that more women are being diagnosed with smaller tumours and consequently can safely be offered conservation surgery rather than radical mastectomy.

Stomach

On a global scale, mortality from stomach cancer is second only to lung cancer. The areas with the highest incidence rates are in Eastern Asia, the Andean regions of South America and Eastern Europe. There is marked geographical variation in incidence between countries and among different ethnic groups within the same locale. Migration studies show that the risk of cancer changes within two generations when people move from high-incidence to low-incidence areas. For example, Japanese immigrants to the United States retain their original risk, whereas subsequent generations share the incidence of the host country. No matter what level of incidence, there has been a general decline worldwide. In most European countries, it has fallen by more than 60% during the past 50 years.

Dietary risk factors include inadequate intake of fresh fruits and vegetables, high salt intake and consumption of smoked or cured meats or fish. There is good evidence that refrigeration of food also protects against this cancer by facilitating year-round consumption of fruit and vegetables and probably by reducing the need for salt as a preservative. Vitamin C, contained in vegetables and fruits and other foods of plant origin, is probably protective and so too are diets high in whole-grain cereals, carotenoids and allium compounds.

Conditions that cause an excessive rate of cell proliferation in the gastric epithelium, thus increasing the chance of fixation of replication errors induced by dietary and endogenous carcinogens, include *Helicobacter pylori* infection, gastric ulcer, atrophic gastritis and autoimmune gastritis associated with pernicious anaemia. Gastritis is associated with increased production of oxidants and reactive nitrogen intermediates, including nitric oxide. There is increased expression of the inducible isoform of nitric oxide synthase in gastritis. Gastritis and atrophy alter gastric acid secretion, elevating gastric pH, changing the gastric flora and allowing anaerobic bacteria to colonise the stomach.

Screening

About 80% of Western patients with stomach cancer present with advanced tumours. Screening for early disease by x-ray (photofluoroscopy), followed by gastroscopy and biopsy of suspicious findings, has been widely used in Japan since the 1960s. It is a costly approach to prevention and the results have been controversial. With the background incidence now falling substantially, screening has not been considered as a national priority in most other countries.

Prostate

Prostate cancer is the third most common cancer in men in the world. In the majority of developed and developing countries, prostate cancer is the most commonly diagnosed neoplasm affecting men beyond middle age. In recent times, incidence rates of prostate cancer have been influenced by the diagnosis of latent cancers whose presence has been suggested by screening of asymptomatic individuals. In the United States, for example, the introduction of screening using PSA testing has led to an enormous increase in the diagnosis of prostate cancer, making it by far the most commonly diagnosed cancer in men.

The distribution of mortality rates is less affected than incidence by the effects of early diagnosis of asymptomatic cancers and is thus a more reliable way of comparing rates of the disease. High rates are found in North America, Northern and Western Europe, Australia, New Zealand and the Caribbean. The difference between China and the United States is 26-fold and, within the United States, Black populations have higher rates than White, who in turn have rates considerably higher than populations of Asian origin.

The causes of prostate cancer are not well understood. Development of this malignancy is a multistep process associated with a long natural history. The initiation of preneoplastic lesions and microscopic cancer is probably influenced by environmental factors which implies a case for lifestyle causes and primary prevention. The strong association of race, familial and geographic patterns and the weak link of many of the risk factors proposed suggests a significant role for genetic-environmental interactions in determining patterns of disease. The role of hormones, particularly androgens, is obviously important given the impact of orchidectomy on progression. Genetic polymorphisms in the androgen receptor may be more important than any imbalance of hormones in the circulation. A diet characteristic of Asian countries, essentially a low-fat intake with consequent low body weight and an intake of relatively high levels of phytoestrogens, may provide the means of restraining the growth and progression of prostate cancer.

Screening

Secondary prevention of prostate cancer is feasible, but subject to controversy, because the capacity to detect early disease must inevitably result in the overtreatment of some individuals, with substantial costs both to individuals and to society, in exchange for decreased prostate cancer mortality. PSA testing is widely used for the early detection of prostate cancer. Elevated levels of PSA are closely, but not definitely, associated with the presence of a tumour. Using a cut-off level of 4 ng/ml for normality, 25% of patients diagnosed with prostate cancer will have levels below this value. Of men with moderately raised levels (4–10 ng/ml) 25% will have cancer but this rises to 60% when PSA levels are greater than 10 ng/ml.

To improve the sensitivity of the PSA analysis, it should be combined with a digital rectal examination. This will provide an assessment of the volume of the gland because PSA is also released into the bloodstream of patients with benign prostatic hyperplasia and other prostatic diseases. Additionally, different age-specific reference values for the cut-off threshold are of value: 2.5 ng/ml for age group 40 to 49 years and 3.5 ng/ml for age group 50 to 59 years. Any patient who asks for a PSA test should be counselled about the risks and benefits in relation to the procedure and its outcome.

Some national authorities have recommended screening for the detection of prostate cancer starting at the age of 50 for men with at least a 10-year life expectancy. Randomised studies have, however, produced conflicting results in terms of the benefits and harms of screening. Prostate cancer diagnosis has been shown to increase with screening, however, prostate-cancer specific mortality was only reduced in some studies and overall mortality was unchanged. The general expectation that the earlier detection of prostate cancer inevitably provides a unique chance for cure has to be balanced against the clear prevalence of over-diagnosing, and treating, a disease which may never become symptomatic during a man's lifetime.

Cervix

Cancer of the cervix is the second most common cancer among women worldwide with about 470,000 new cases diagnosed each year. Some 80% of cases of cervical cancer occur in developing countries where, in many regions, it is the most common cancer of women. The highest incidence rates are in South America and the Caribbean, sub-Saharan Africa, and South and Southeastern Asia.

Incidence and mortality have declined markedly in the last 40 years in Western Europe, the United States, Canada, Australia and New Zealand, mainly in relation to extensive screening programmes based on exfoliative cervical cytology, typically by means of the Papanicolaou (Pap) smear. Nevertheless, in several countries, notably the United Kingdom, Australia, New Zealand, and in Central Europe, there have been increases in risk in younger women, probably the result of changes in exposure to risk factors. These changes are most evident for adenocarcinomas, which share to some extent, the same aetiological agents of squamous cell carcinomas, but for which cytological screening is ineffective in countering the increase in risk.

Molecular studies have shown that certain human papillomavirus (HPV) types are the central cause of cervical cancer and cervical intraepithelial neoplasia (CIN), the preinvasive state. It is now clear that the well-established risk factors associated with sexual behaviour, such as multiple sexual partners and early age of starting sexual activity, simply reflect the probability of being infected with HPV. HPV DNA has been detected in virtually all cervical cancer specimens. The association of HPV with cervical cancer is equally strong for the two main histological types: squamous cell carcinoma and adenocarcinoma. Over 100 HPV types have been identified and about 40 can infect the genital tract. Fifteen of these have been classified as high risk, three as probably high risk and twelve as low risk. However, because only a small fraction of HPV-infected women will eventually develop cervical cancer, there must be other exogenous or endogenous factors which, acting in conjunction with HPV, influence the progression from cervical infection to cervical cancer. In assessing of the role of these co-factors, it should be recognised that HPV is very much the dominant effect. Cofactors which have been identified as being associated with an increased risk include high parity, smoking and long-term use of oral contraceptives.

Screening

Population-based cervical cancer screening programmes using the Pap smear were first implemented in 1949 in British Columbia. Pap smear screening programmes have since been introduced in many developed countries. The evidence supporting this is predominantly nonrandomised, being based on the trends in the incidence of, or mortality because of cervical cancer in relation to screening intensity and the risk of cervical cancer in individuals in relation to their screening history. For example, national programmes were established in Finland, Iceland and Sweden; in Denmark, programmes covered about 40% of the female population and in Norway only 5%. In Iceland, cervical cancer mortality fell by 80% between 1965 and 1982, compared with 50% in Finland, 34% in Sweden, 25% in Denmark and 10% in Norway. Similarly, cancer-registry based studies have shown a reduction in the age SIRs compared with before screening, with reductions of at least 25% in 11 of the 17 populations studied, and the largest effect occurring in the 45- to 55-year age groups.

More recently, cytological screening has been carried out using liquid-based cytology supplemented by HPV testing. In randomised studies, HPV-based screening provides 60% to 70% greater protection against invasive cervical cancer than cytology alone.

Oesophagus

Cancer of the oesophagus is the sixth most frequent cancer worldwide. About 412,000 new cases occur each year, of which over 80% are in developing countries. Although squamous cell carcinomas occur at high frequency in many developing countries, adenocarcinomas are essentially a tumour of more developed, industrialised countries. Differences between the incidence of oesophageal cancer in distinct geographical areas are more extreme than observed for any other cancer with high incidence being seen in an oesophageal cancer belt stretching from Northern Iran to North Central China, Southeast Africa and parts of South America.

Consumption of tobacco and alcohol, associated with low intake of fresh fruit, vegetables and meat, is causally associated with squamous cell carcinoma of the oesophagus worldwide. In developed countries, about 90% of the squamous cell cancers are attributable to tobacco and alcohol, with a multiplicative increase in risk when individuals are exposed to both factors. Risk factors for oesophageal cancer in developing countries vary by region, however, with oral consumption of opium by-products an important factor in the Caspian Sea area, betel chewing in Southeast Asia, drinking of scalding hot beverages, such as mate, in South America and environmental factors including nitrosamines, contamination with fungi and deficiency of vitamins A and C in parts of China.

In contrast to squamous cell carcinoma, the most important risk factor for oesophageal adenocarcinoma is gastrooesophageal reflux disease resulting in the premalignant condition, Barrett's oesophagus. Obesity is another significant risk factor with smoking playing a less significant role in adenocarcinoma. Given the strong relationship between Barrett's oesophagus and oesophageal adenocarcinoma, some countries have implemented routine surveillance for patients with known Barrett's oesophagus. Randomised data supporting this are, however, lacking.

Melanoma

There are about 232,000 new cases of melanoma worldwide each year making it the 19th most common cancer. It occurs predominantly in white-skinned populations (Caucasians) living in countries where there is high intensity ultraviolet radiation, but this malignancy afflicts to some degree all ethnic groups. Assessed in relation to skin colour, melanoma incidence falls dramatically as skin pigmentation increases and the disease is very rare in dark-skinned people. The highest incidence of melanoma occurs in Australia where the population is predominantly Caucasian, and there is an average of 6 hours of bright sunlight every day of the year and an essentially outdoors lifestyle. The lifetime risk of developing melanoma in Australia is 4% to 5% in men and 3% to 4% in women.

Dark-skinned people have a low risk of melanoma in Africa and South America; the sole of the foot, where the skin is not pigmented, is the most frequent site affected in the context of a low incidence. Asian peoples have a low risk of melanoma despite their paler skins; naevi in Asian people, although common, are predominantly of the acral-lentiginous type, which have low malignant potential. Marked increases in incidence and mortality are being observed in both sexes in many countries.

It is estimated that 80% of melanoma is caused by ultraviolet damage to sensitive skin, that is, skin that burns easily, fair or reddish skin, multiple freckles and skin that does not tan and develops naevi in response to early sunlight exposure. Prevention of melanoma is based on limitation of exposure to ultraviolet radiation, particularly in the first 20 years of life.

Ultraviolet radiation is particularly hazardous when it involves sporadic intense exposure and sunburn. Most damage caused by sunlight occurs in childhood and adolescence, making this the most important target group for prevention programmes. Established but rare risk factors include congenital naevi, immunosuppression and excessive use of solaria. Although melanoma may occur anywhere on the skin, the majority of melanoma in men is on the back, whereas in women, the majority is on the legs. The difference in site incidence is not completely explained by differential exposure to ultraviolet light.

Head and Neck

Cancers of the oral mucosa, oropharynx, larynx and hypopharynx can be considered together, because there are similarities in epidemiology, treatment and prognosis. The geographic patterns and trends in incidence for these cancers vary depending upon the anatomical subsites concerned, a phenomenon that is often explicable by the influence of risk factors, such as tobacco use and alcohol consumption. A high incidence of these cancers is observed in the Indian subcontinent, Australia, France, South America (Brazil) and Southern Africa. Cancers of the mouth and anterior two-thirds of the tongue generally predominate in developing countries, whereas pharyngeal cancers are common in developed countries and in Central and Eastern Europe.

Smoking and drinking are the major risk factors for head and neck cancer in developed countries, in the Caribbean and in South American countries. These risk factors have been shown, for laryngeal and oropharyngeal cancers, to have a joint multiplicative or synergistic effect. Smoking is estimated to be responsible for about 41% of laryngeal and oral/pharyngeal cancers in men, and 15% in women worldwide and these proportions vary among different populations. Tobacco smoking has also been found to be an important risk factor for nasopharyngeal cancer in otherwise low-risk populations whilst reverse smoking (in which the lit end of the cigarette is placed in the mouth so that an intense heat is experienced) is a risk factor for cancer of the hard palate. In the Indian subcontinent, chewing tobacco in the form of betel quid (a combination of betel leaf, slaked lime, areca-nut and tobacco with or without other condiments), bide (a locally hand-rolled cigarette of dried temburni leaf containing coarse tobacco), smoking and drinking locally brewed crude alcoholic drinks are the major causative factors. Oral snuff use is an emerging risk factor for oral cancer, particularly among young males in the United States.

Infection with Epstein-Barr virus has long been recognised as being important in the aetiology of nasopharyngeal cancer. This virus is not found in normal epithelial cells of the nasopharynx, but is present in all nasopharyngeal tumour cells, and even in dysplastic precursor lesions. More recently it has also been recognised that human papillomavirus (HPV) infection (transmitted sexually or perinatally) is associated with an increased risk of head and neck squamous cell carcinoma development, with an estimated 40% of oropharyngeal tumours attributable to HPV. Notably, HPV-related tumours carry a markedly better prognosis.

Lymphoma

Lymphoma covers a heterogeneous group of neoplasms of lymphoid tissue. Traditionally, lymphomas have been categorised as either Hodgkin's disease (HD) or non-Hodgkin's lymphoma (NHL), these distinct entities having different patterns of behaviour and response to treatment.

Geographically, NHL is most common in developed countries, although in the developing world, there are areas of moderate to high incidence in some Middle Eastern countries (Saudi Arabia, Israel) and in parts of sub-Saharan Africa. Much of the latter's high rate is because of the high incidence of Burkitt's lymphoma, an aggressive subtype of NHL.

NHL incidence rates have risen dramatically in the last 20 years, particularly in developed countries, including Western Europe, North America and Australia. In part, this reflects better diagnosis and changing classification systems, but this is by no means the complete explanation. The increasing trend is also not explained entirely because of the fact that NHL is a complication of acquired immune deficiency syndrome (AIDS) (occurring in up to 5%–10% of AIDS cases in developed countries). In contrast to incidence, mortality rates have, in general, been declining as a consequence of improvement in therapy.

In developed countries, HD incidence reaches a peak in young adults, whereas in developing countries, HD occurs mainly in children and in the elderly. In developed countries, incidence has fallen over the last 20 years.

Patients with human immunodeficiency virus (HIV)/AIDS or who have received immunosuppressant therapy have a higher risk of developing NHL. Viral infection such as HIV-1, human T-cell leukaemia virus type 1 (HTLV-1) and Epstein-Barr virus (EBV) are also associated with NHL. Infection of the stomach with *H. pylori* is associated with gastric lymphoma. There is also an increased risk of NHL among persons with a family history of lymphoma or haematological cancer.

A subtype of HD cases, the mixed cellularity type, has been linked to the EBV. Overall, around 45% of cases may be attributable to EBV. The presence of EBV in tumours seems also to be related to age and socioeconomic circumstances. EBV is involved in the aetiology of Burkitt's lymphoma, especially in cases in tropical Africa, where over 95% of tumours contain the virus. The proportion of EBV-positive tumours is much less in the sporadic cases of HD occurring in Europe and North America. The singular geographic distribution of Burkitt's lymphoma is not explicable on the basis of EBV alone; however, because infection by the virus is ubiquitous, suspicion has fallen upon intense malarial infection as predisposing to Burkitt's lymphoma in the presence of EBV infection. The risk of HD is also increased in patients with HIV infection.

Leukaemia

Leukaemias comprise about 2.5% of all incident cancers worldwide, with about 351,000 new cases occurring annually. A relatively high incidence is evident in the United States, Canada, Western Europe, Australia and New Zealand, whereas rates are generally low in most African and Asian countries with rates less than half those in the former group. The trends in overall incidence of leukaemia have generally been stable or slowly increasing. However, a substantial reduction in death rates from leukaemias, particularly in childhood, has been observed since the 1960s, thanks to advances in treatment and consequent improvement in survival.

Leukaemia has a peak in incidence in the first four years of life, which is predominantly as a result of acute lymphoblastic leukaemia (ALL), the most common paediatric malignancy, accounting for nearly 25% of all such disease. After infancy, there is a steep decline in rates of leukaemia with age, with lowest incidence being at ages 15 to 25, after which there is an exponential rise up to age 85.

The usual form of the disease in adults is acute myeloid leukaemia (AML), accounting for 70% of all cases. The more differentiated, or chronic forms of leukaemia are predominantly adult diseases, rarely occurring below the age of 30, and then increasing progressively in incidence with age. Chronic myelogenous leukaemia (CML) accounts for 15% to 20% of all case of leukaemia. For patients over 50, chronic lymphocytic leukaemia (CLL) is the dominant type of leukaemia.

The cause of most leukaemias is not known. A range of risk factors has been predominantly, although not exclusively, associated with particular leukaemia subtypes. Ionising radiation (nuclear bombs, medical procedures), and occupational exposure to benzene are associated with acute myeloid leukaemia.

Leukaemia (mainly acute myeloid) may occur in a small proportion of cancer patients treated with chlorambucil, cyclophosphamide, melphalan, thiotepa, treosulphan or etoposide, as well as certain combination chemotherapy. Leukaemia has followed induction of aplastic anaemia by the antibiotic, chloramphenicol. Certain risk factors, such as Down syndrome, have been identified for childhood leukaemia but, generally, the causes of the disease are not known. Some studies have shown a risk of childhood leukaemia with exposure to high-level residential extremely low frequency electromagnetic fields, but causality has not been established.

Infection with the virus HTLV-1 has been established as a cause of leukaemia. This virus is responsible for adult T-cell leukaemia, a disease mainly observed in tropical countries and Japan, and rarely in the United States and Europe. In experimental animals, particularly in mice, there are many retroviruses, which can cause a variety of leukaemias, but such retroviruses have not been identified in humans.

REDUCING THE RISKS OF DEVELOPING CANCER

Based largely on our current knowledge of the aetiology of cancer, it has been estimated that 40% of malignancies are preventable. To put the environmental causes of cancer in perspective, the estimated attributable fraction of the population of worldwide cancer cases they relate to has been summarised for some common cancers in Table 15.1. Similarly, Table 15.2 presents an IARC summary of human carcinogens that relate to some common cancers. The striking feature is the high proportion as a result of dietary factors and to smoking. Changing dietary habits could potentially reduce the risk of cancer, possibly by one-third. The main cancers involved are those of the stomach, colon and rectum and breast. A number of initiatives, such as the European Commission's 10-point code, have been produced to summarise ways in which the risk of cancer can be reduced.

Reducing Tobacco Smoking

Every country should give high priority to tobacco control in its fight against cancer as, unchecked, smoking will cause more than 10 million deaths from cancer (mostly lung cancer) in the next decade. Additionally, with passive smoking now implicated as a cause of lung cancer, as well as being a contributing factor in increasing coronary heart disease, the emphasis has now moved to what action public health policy makers should advocate and what legislation government should enact not only to reduce smoking but also involuntary smoking. Many countries around the world have now imposed bans on smoking in public places and working environments to protect the health of workers. One of the additional benefits of such restrictions has been a reduction in the rate of active smoking among the population at large. Further measures taken by governments around the world include making health warnings mandatory on commercial tobacco products, banning advertising of tobacco, increasing taxation, reducing tar content in

TABLE 15.1 Major Causes of Cancer

Factor	Type of Cancer	Percent (%) Population Attributable Fraction
Smoking	Lung	21
	Mouth and oropharynx	
	Oesophagus	
	Stomach	
	Cervix	
	Leukaemia	
Alcohol	Mouth and oropharynx	5
	Oesophagus	
	Breast	
Low fruit and vegetable intake	Oesophageal	5
	Stomach	
	Colorectal	
	Lung	
Indoor smoke from household use of solid fuels	Lung	<0.5
Urban air pollution	Lung	1
Overweight and obesity	Colorectal	2
	Breast	
Physical inactivity	Colorectal	2
	Breast	
Unsafe sex	Cervix	3

TABLE 15.2 International Agency for Research on Cancer Carcinogenic Agents

Cancer Site	Carcinogenic Agents With Sufficient Evidence of an Association With Cancer
Oral cavity	Alcoholic beverages
	Betel quid with tobacco
	Betel quid without tobacco
	Human papillomavirus (HPV) type 16
	Tobacco, smokeless
	Tobacco smoking
Salivary gland	X-radiation, gamma-radiation
Tonsil	HPV type 16
Pharynx	Alcoholic beverages
	Betel quid with tobacco
	HPV type 16
	Tobacco smoking
Nasopharynx	Epstein-Barr virus
	Formaldehyde
	Salted fish, Chinese-style
	Tobacco smoking
	Wood dust
Nasal cavity and paranasal sinus	Isopropyl alcohol production
	Leather dust
	Nickel compounds
	Radium-226 and its decay products
	Radium-228 and its decay products
	Tobacco smoking
	Wood dust
Larynx	Acid mists, strong inorganic
	Alcoholic beverages
	Asbestos (all forms)
	Tobacco smoking
Digestive tract, upper	Acetaldehyde associated with consumption of alcoholic beverages
Oesophagus	Acetaldehyde associated with consumption of alcoholic beverages
	Alcoholic beverages
	Betel quid with tobacco
	Betel quid without tobacco
	Tobacco, smokeless
	Tobacco smoking
	X-radiation, gamma-radiation
Stomach	*Helicobacter pylori*
	Rubber production industry
	Tobacco smoking
	X-radiation, gamma-radiation
Colon and rectum	Alcoholic beverages
	Tobacco smoking
	X-radiation, gamma-radiation
	Processed meat (consumption of)
Lung cancer	Acheson process, occupational exposures associated with aluminum production
	Arsenic and inorganic arsenic compounds
	Asbestos (all forms)
	Beryllium and beryllium compounds
	Bis(chloromethyl)ether; chloromethyl methyl ether (technical grade)
	Cadmium and cadmium compounds
	Chromium (VI) compounds
	Coal, indoor emissions from household combustion

Continued

TABLE 15.2 International Agency for Research on Cancer Carcinogenic Agents—cont'd

Cancer Site	Carcinogenic Agents With Sufficient Evidence of an Association With Cancer
	Coal gasification
	Coal-tar pitch
	Coke production
	Engine exhaust, diesel
	Hematite mining (underground)
	Iron and steel founding
	MOPP (vincristine-prednisone-nitrogen mustard-procarbazine mixture)
	Nickel compounds
	Outdoor air pollution
	Painting
	Particulate matter in outdoor air pollution
	Plutonium
	Radon-222 and its decay products
	Rubber production industry
	Silica dust, crystalline
	Soot
	Sulfur mustard
	Tobacco smoke, secondhand
	Tobacco smoking
	Welding fumes
	X-radiation, gamma-radiation
Melanoma	Solar radiation
	Ultraviolet-emitting tanning devices
	Polychlorinated biphenyls
Breast	Alcoholic beverages
	Diethylstilbestrol
	Oestrogen-progestogen contraceptives
	Oestrogen-progestogen menopausal therapy
	X-radiation, gamma-radiation
Cervix	Diethylstilbestrol (exposure in utero)
	Oestrogen-progestogen contraceptives
	Human immunodeficiency virus type 1
	HPV types 16, 18, 31, 33, 35, 39, 45, 51, 52, 56, 58, 59
	Tobacco smoking

cigarettes, regulating to enforce plain packaging of tobacco and setting up clinics for smokers to help them break the habit. As a result of these interventions and ongoing public health campaigns smoking rates are declining internationally and lung cancer incidence is falling in many countries. Worryingly, smoking rates in the Eastern Mediterranean and African regions are continuing to increase.

The rise of e-cigarettes as a means to reduce smoking remains controversial. It is unclear currently what the long-term effects of vaping are although it is very likely to be considerably safer than cigarettes. Opinion is divided between those who feel the shift towards vaping is a public health good (reducing disease both in active and passive smokers) and those who think vaping may (1) encourage smoking in younger age groups, (2) not result in the levels of cessation advertised and (3) many users of e-cigarettes will never transition completely away from tobacco (with no evidence that reducing cigarette smoking without quitting is beneficial). At an individual level, although evidence does not support e-cigarettes being more effective than other strategies for tobacco cessation, it should be considered as an option.

Modifying Alcohol Consumption

After smoking, alcohol is the second most important cause of cancer. It may be responsible in some countries for up to 10% of deaths from cancer. Cancers of the mouth, larynx, pharynx, oesophagus, liver, colorectum, breast and stomach are certainly caused in part by alcohol. For several tumours, the risk rises with the quantity consumed to more than tenfold for lifelong nondrinkers. Alcohol and tobacco smoking act as synergistic carcinogens (i.e. the combined effect is greater than that of either alone). This combination accounts for the very high incidence of these tumours in France, where they are often multifocal. Alcohol probably acts as a cocarcinogen rather than a carcinogen (i.e. it promotes rather than initiates carcinogenesis). Spirits may have a slightly stronger carcinogenic effect than other alcoholic beverages.

Any policy on moderating the consumption of alcohol has to take account of a number of facts. First, many people find it pleasurable. Secondly, moderate amounts (2–3 units/day) protect against coronary thrombosis, although heavy drinking has other undesirable social consequences (e.g. violent behaviour and road accidents). Thirdly, its carcinogenic effects are largely in conjunction with smoking tobacco. Thus, the risk of cancer induction by alcohol in nonsmokers is relatively small.

HPV Vaccination

With increasing awareness of the role of HPV in cancers of the cervix, head and neck, anus, vagina, vulva and penis a number of countries have implemented vaccination programmes. The vaccines used provide immunity to the HPV genotypes primarily responsible for cancer (16 and 18) and in some cases other additional genotypes (e.g. HPV 6 and 11 which result in genital warts). Early observational studies report reductions in high-grade cervical intraepithelial neoplasia alongside marked reductions in genital warts. Although vaccination programmes have initially been aimed at girls a number of countries are now moving to provide vaccination for all teenagers. The cost effectiveness of these programmes varies between jurisdictions and as such differing approaches exist.

Ultraviolet Light

Exposure to ultraviolet light has been increasing with the reduction of the ozone layer, caused by chemical pollution. An increase in the incidence of all forms of skin cancer can be expected. The principal culprits are the chlorofluorohydrocarbons (CFCs). These are components in, for example, aerosol sprays, refrigerants and solvents for cleaning electronic equipment. However, to put the contribution of commercial sources of CFCs into context, one volcano in Antarctica emits 100 tons of chlorine every month, substantially more than the combined output of CFCs from deodorants over the same period. Nitrogen oxides from vehicle exhaust fumes also deplete the ozone layer. International agreements have been reached, aimed at eliminating the use of CFCs.

Occupational Exposure

A wide variety of occupations are known to carry the risk of exposure to carcinogens. However, they only represent a relatively small number of cases of cancer deaths (4% in the United States). In 1987, 246 agents were classified by the International Agency for Research on Cancer as definitely (50), probably (37) or possibly (159) carcinogenic to humans. These included industrial processes, industrial chemicals, pesticides, laboratory chemicals, drugs, food ingredients, tobacco smoking and related stimulants. Drugs and industrial chemicals represent the largest risks. There are many other occupations where an agent is thought to be carcinogenic to workers but a causal link has not been established. Of these, exposure to asbestos dust, aromatic amines and the products of burning fossil fuels are the commonest.

Measures to prevent occupational exposure include labelling of products as carcinogenic, and prohibiting the marketing and use of certain substances, for example, the four aromatic amines (naphthylamine, 4-aminobiphenyl, 4-nitrodiphenyl and benzidine) and blue asbestos (crocidolite).

It is thought that preventive methods are likely to have little impact on the mortality from occupational cancers in the near future. The detection of tumours at an early stage by screening is likely to have a greater effect on mortality. Screening of urine by cytology among workers in the dyestuff and rubber industries has long been practiced.

Diet

Diet influences carcinogenesis in a variety of ways: carcinogens may be eaten; food substances may be converted to carcinogens once ingested; and dietary components may modify the ways in which the body metabolises and responds to carcinogens. The only component of food that has been found to be strongly linked to the development of cancer is aflatoxin. This is a product of the fungus *Aspergillus fumigatus*, which often contaminates damp cereals in tropical countries. It causes primary liver cancer, although the data are unclear because there is a high incidence of hepatitis B, itself associated with liver tumours, in the same group of patients.

Bracken fern containing nitrates is suspected of causing oesophageal cancer, particularly among the Japanese. Salted fish is implicated in the aetiology of nasopharyngeal cancer, possibly as a cocarcinogen with the Epstein-Barr virus.

Diet may also be indirectly related to carcinogenesis. One example is fibre, which seems to have a protective effect against colorectal cancer. A second is obesity, which is associated with an increased incidence of cancer of the breast, endometrium, colon, kidney, gallbladder and oesophagus amongst others. A third is vitamin A (retinol) and its derivatives, retinoids, which may inhibit the full malignant transformation of cells and prevent tumour formation.

Dietary measures likely to reduce the risk of cancers are:

- high-fibre diet
- reducing saturated fats
- plenty of fresh fruit and vegetables (owing to the presence of antioxidants such as vitamin E)
- maintaining a healthy body weight through a combination of diet and exercise

Ionising Radiation

The whole spectrum of sources of ionising radiations, both natural and manmade, has been calculated to contribute 1.5% of all fatal cancers. The sources of radiation exposure in the United Kingdom are shown in Table 15.3.

It is estimated that exposure to radon gas from domestic buildings may be responsible for 1% of lung cancer in Europe. Concentrations of radon gas in excess of 400 Bq/m³ (about 1 in 1000 homes) will expose the occupants to 20 mSv per year. The lifetime risk of fatal cancer from this exposure is about 10%. The carcinogenic risks of ionising radiation have been revised upwards since 1988. Current estimates of risk are two to five times higher. However, it is unclear whether these revised estimates apply to very low levels of exposure to natural background radioactivity.

The role of ionising radiation in the causation of cancer is mainly derived from occupational exposure. Early evidence came from the development of lung cancer among miners at Joachimsthal in the Czech Republic and Schneeberg in Germany. Lung disease had been known to occur among these workers since the 16th century. It was subsequently appreciated that the disease was lung cancer because of radioactive radon gas in the mines.

TABLE 15.3 Estimated Annual Dose of Ionising Radiation Received by a Member of the General Public

External terrestrial radiation	0.4 mSv
Cosmic radiation	0.3 mSv
Ingestion of naturally occurring radioactive substances	0.3 mSv
Inhalation of radon progeny	2.4 mSv
Use of ionising radiation and radioactive substances in medicine (mainly diagnostic x-rays)	1.5 mSv
Fallout from nuclear weapons testing	<0.01 mSv
Nuclear power plants	<0.01 mSv
Reactor accident in Chernobyl	<0.02 mSv
Use of radioactive materials and ionising radiation in industry, research and at home	<0.01 mSv
Occupational exposure	<0.01 mSv

The main source of evidence of the effects of ionising radiation in man are the survivors of the atomic bombs dropped on Hiroshima and Nagasaki in 1945. The incidence of acute and chronic leukaemia was significantly raised within a radius of 1.5 km from the epicentre. The highest incidence occurred 6 to 8 years afterwards. For cancers other than leukaemia, the latent period was longer (15–20 years) among victims who received 1 Gray (Gy) or more; indeed the incidence is still higher over 50 years later.

It is assumed that there is no threshold below which cancers cannot be induced by ionising radiation. Indeed, children who received only 0.01 to 0.02 Gy in utero when their mothers were irradiated had an additional 1 in 2000 risk of cancer. At low doses, the risk of developing cancer is probably proportional to dose, although much uncertainty remains.

Reducing the levels of radon gas from domestic buildings requires a number of measures. First, systematic surveys are needed to identify buildings which pose a hazard. Levels of radon gas can be reduced by alterations to the floors and installation of extractor fans.

POLLUTION

Atmospheric pollution has been suspected to be carcinogenic ever since the incidence of lung cancer was found to be higher in cities than in the country. The combustion products of coal are known to contain carcinogenic hydrocarbons. However, because the atmosphere is polluted by a wide variety of substances, often in small quantities, the assessment of carcinogenic risk is very difficult. The situation is further complicated by the contribution to atmospheric pollution of tobacco smoking. In the past, pollution probably accounted for about 1% of cancers. Atmospheric pollution in the United Kingdom is now falling with stricter rules on the burning of fossil fuels. The evidence suggests that the current burning of fossil fuels, arsenic and asbestos will contribute to much less than 1% of future cancers.

Chemoprevention

The oral cavity, lung and colon have been the commonest primary sites subject to attempts at chemoprevention. Beta-carotene, synthetic retinoids, calcium and a variety of vitamins reduce the risk of developing oral cancer. A trial of alpha-tocopherol and beta-carotene showed no protective effect against the development of lung cancer.

Among patients in China at high risk of oesophageal or stomach cancer, treatment with vitamin and mineral supplements reduced the incidence and mortality of these tumours. These populations have a 20% incidence of oesophageal dysplasia.

Trials of adjuvant tamoxifen have shown a reduction in the risk of contralateral breast cancer. Trials are ongoing to determine whether tamoxifen can prevent the disease among women at high risk on the basis of their strong family history of the disease. Antioxidants, for example, vitamins A and E, are thought to act by reducing DNA damage early in the process of carcinogenesis. It seems most likely that chemoprevention with such agents should occur early in life if they proved to be effective. The cost effectiveness of chemoprevention needs to be carefully considered. Preventive treatment may have to be continued for several decades, which may prove very expensive when compared with the numbers of lives saved.

CONCLUSION

The negative impact of cancer on individuals and communities can be greatly reduced through cancer control programmes. Although the scope of cancer control extends from prevention and screening to management of disease, rehabilitation and palliative care, successful prevention can make a huge contribution to reducing the global cancer load, and compared with the other strategies, at a relatively low cost. Because this involves changes in lifestyle for many individuals, it is critical that medical and public health professionals engage with populations in embracing healthy living as a shared goal.

FURTHER READING

Allemani C, Matsuda T, DiCarla V, Harewood R, Matz M, Niksic M, Bonaventure A, Valkov M, Johnson CJ, Esteve J, Ogunbiyi OJ, Silva GA, Chen WQ, Eser S, Engholm G, Stiller CA, Monnereau A, Woods RR, Visser O, Lim GH, Aitken J, Weir HK, Coleman MP and the CONCORD Working Group. Global Surveillance of Trends in Cancer Survival 2000-14 (CONCORD-3): Analysis of individual records for 37,513,025 patients diagnosed with one of 18 cancers from 322 population-based registries in 71 countries; Lyon: France.

Danaei G, Vander Hoorn S, Lopez AD, Murray CJL, Ezzati M. and the Comparative Risk Assessment Collaborating Group (Cancers). Causes of cancer in the world: comparative risk assessment of nine behavioural and environmental risk factors. Lancet 2005;366:1784–93.

Doll R, Peto R, Boreham J, Sutherland I. Mortality from cancer in relation to smoking: 50 years observations on British doctors. Br J Cancer 2005;92 (3):426–9.

Hammond E, Selikoff I, Seidmant H. Asbestos exposure, cigarette smoking and death rates. NYAS. December 1979.

International Agency for Research on Cancer. Global Cancer Observatory, http://gco.iarc.fr/; 2018 [accessed 01.05.18].

Siegel RL, Miller KD, Jemal A. Cancer statistics, 2018. CA Cancer J Clin 2018;68 (1):7–30.

Thomas GA, Symonds P. Radiation exposure and health effects—is it time to reassess the real consequences? Clin Oncol 2016;28:231–6.

Vineis P, Wild CP. Global cancer patterns: causes and prevention. Lancet 2014;383:549–57.

16

Biological and Pathological Introduction

John R. Goepel, Abhik Mukherjee

CHAPTER OUTLINE

INTRODUCTION

Radiotherapy is used almost exclusively for the treatment of cancer and related conditions. It is thus very important to have a reasonable understanding of this disease. This chapter contains an outline of the basic characteristics of cancer cells, and the conditions that can cause cancer. There is consideration of the natural history of untreated cancer, and of the ways that different types of cancer are named and classified.

GROWTH: PROLIFERATION, DIFFERENTIATION AND APOPTOSIS

Growth is the process of increase in size and maturity of tissues from fertilisation through to the adult. When normally controlled, the different parts of the body attain their correct size and specialist functions, and relationship to one another. Furthermore, throughout life these attributes continue despite the need for replacement and repair. This is all a reflection of accurate control of the timing and extent of cellular proliferation, cell-to-cell orientation and organisation, and differentiation. Differentiation is the process of a cell taking on a specialised function; this is usually associated with a change in its microscopic appearance. It is also usually a one-way commitment, with relative or complete loss of the ability to continue proliferating. Also important

is the ability to delete cells which are no longer needed by a process called *apoptosis* or programmed cell death. This is used in the development of the fetus, and in maintaining or adjusting the size of a structure in the adult. Apoptosis is also used to delete defective cells.

Growth Disorders

Hypertrophy is an increase in the size of an organ due to an increase in the size of its constituent cells. For example, the left ventricle of the heart becomes hypertrophic if it has to work harder because of hypertension. An inherited cause of cardiac hypertrophy is hypertrophic cardiomyopathy.

Hyperplasia is an increase in size because of an increase in the number of cells. The adrenal cortex will become hyperplastic if there is excessive adrenocorticotrophic hormone to stimulate it. However, it will return to normal if the stimulus is reduced again. Hyperplasia is also seen in other benign proliferative diseases such as in the breast, commonly, usual-type ductal hyperplasia; however, when there is atypia in the cells (atypical ductal hyperplasia), there is an increase of future malignancy, and patients may require additional follow-up.

Metaplasia is a change from one type of tissue to another. Smoking induces a change of the bronchial lining from the usual respiratory mucosa to a squamous epithelium, with resultant loss of mucus-producing and ciliated cells. It is also potentially reversible. An important metaplastic lesion in the context of cancer is Barrett's metaplasia where there is a change of oesophageal squamous mucosa to intestinal type mucosa, commonly induced by gastro-oesophageal reflux disease. It predisposes to a higher risk of oesophageal adeno-carcinoma and is managed by surveillance protocols for any developing dysplasia.

Neoplasia (literally a new growth), in contrast, is an irreversible process once initiated: it is the main subject of this chapter. It is also called cancer, or a tumour, although the latter is sometimes used to denote any swelling.

NEOPLASIA

A neoplasm can be defined as a lesion resulting from the autonomous or relatively autonomous abnormal growth of cells which persists after the initiating stimulus has been removed; that is, cell growth has escaped from normal regulatory mechanisms. The abnormality affects all aspects of cell growth and apoptosis to varying degrees. Proliferation continues unabated, irrespective of the requirements of the organ in which the neoplasm is situated. This, combined with loss of control of the normal relationships between cells, often results in the new tumour cells replacing and insinuating themselves between the adjacent normal tissues, a process called *invasion*. Loss of differentiation accompanies, and often correlates with failure of proliferation control and invasiveness. Failure of apoptosis may also be a major contribution to the survival of abnormal cells.

Benign and Malignant Neoplasms

Neoplasia is not a single disease, but rather a common pathological process with a multitude of different varieties and clinical outcomes. Neoplasms are categorised as benign or malignant mainly based on their capability of distant spread (metastases). Benign tumours remain localised, with generally, relatively little effect on the patient. In contrast, malignant tumours are locally destructive, may spread to other parts of the body, and ultimately result in the death of the patient. Fig. 16.1 and Table 16.1 show some of the differences between benign and malignant neoplasms. Further aspects of the classification of tumours are discussed later in this chapter.

The term *cancer* (Latin/Greek for 'crab') is very ancient, and there are several explanations for its usage. Some say it reflects the tenacious grip the disease has on its victim; some say that it describes the radiating prominent veins that may surround an advanced superficial tumour. Others contend that it describes the irregular infiltrative profile of some tumours, for example, of the breast. Suffice it to say that cancer is a common colloquial term that is generally applied to any malignant neoplasm.

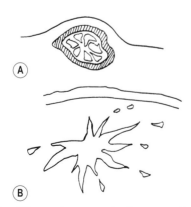

Figure 16.1 The difference between a benign tumour (A) contained by a definitive capsule and a malignant tumour (B) actively invading the tumour bed.

TABLE 16.1	Characteristics of Neoplasms	
Feature	**Benign**	**Malignant**
Growth rate	Slow	Variable, may be rapid
Margin	Encapsulated	Invasive
Local effect	Little	Destructive
Differentiation	Good	Variable, may be poor
Metastases	No	Frequently
Usual outcome	Good	Fatal

Although the behaviour of tumours, particularly malignant ones, may seem very odd, it can generally be explained by the excessive or inappropriate expression of genes that are present in all cells. The tumour continues to be dependent upon an adequate blood supply (although many acquire the capacity to induce new vessels, a process termed angiogenesis). Also, many of those which arise from hormone-dependent tissues (e.g. breast, prostate) continue to show a degree of dependence on those hormones. This can be exploited to therapeutic advantage by giving anti-hormonal therapy.

CARCINOGENESIS

The causes of cancer are numerous, and mechanisms of its production are complex, but some of the principles will be presented. There are two avenues of thought to follow: one at the molecular and genetic levels, the other concerned with causative associations. It is not always easy to relate these to each other. Underlying the mechanistic approach is the assumption that cell behaviour is controlled by the genes expressed (which ones, and how strongly), bearing in mind that these can be influenced by chemical messages relayed from outside the cell. Every cell contains the entire genetic code, but only expresses those genes appropriate to its own situation. In cancer, this has gone wrong, particularly with respect to proliferation, differentiation or apoptosis. We can generalise to say that multiple abnormalities need to have occurred between normality and cancer, and that this reflects a multi-step process. Only those cells capable of division are at risk of transforming into a neoplasm. This excludes terminally differentiated cells such as circulating red cells, the uppermost keratinised cells of the skin, and adult voluntary muscle and nerve cells.

Initiation

This describes the first step towards neoplasia. It reflects a change at the molecular level of how a cell can function, escaping in some small way from a control mechanism. Nothing can be seen microscopically at this stage. Substances that can initiate neoplasia are called *initiators* or *carcinogens* and possess the capability to cause mutations. These include either directly acting chemical initiators such as nitrogen mustard or benzoyl chloride or those which require metabolic activation, for example, polycyclic aromatic hydrocarbons.

Promotion

No more will come of the initiated cell unless it continues to divide. Further abnormalities of cell function (i.e. gene expression) arise over a period of time. Substances that enhance this process are called *promoters*, which unlike initiators may not be inherently mutagenic.

Progression

Neoplasms are clonal, that is, they are derived from a single cell. For this to happen, a cell and its progeny must acquire and sustain a growth advantage over other cells throughout succeeding cell divisions. This eventually results in visible alterations at the microscopic level. Not all the daughter cells will be identical, giving rise to differences between individual cells or subclones; this is called *pleomorphism*. In the process of evolution, a subclone of tumour cells may gain selective advantage due to their metastatic potential or resistance to therapy.

Cancer Stem Cells

Within the tumour cell population, there exists a cohort of cells that are biologically distinct in that they have the capacity to self-renew and differentiate into the tumour cell population: these are cancer stem cells (CSCs). CSCs have been characterised in a wide variety of tumours including leukaemias and skin, colon and breast cancers. CSCs may remain dormant and cause recurrence and metastases. Exterminating this population would effectively destroy the tumour as it would eliminate the root cause of the cancer. However, in other schools of thought (stochastic models), all cells are equipotent to suffer mutations, self-renew or differentiate into tumours based on both genetic and epigenetic influences, resulting in tumour heterogeneity. However, current research brings these schools of thought together; it is envisaged that there is plasticity allowing cells to transit between CSC and non-CSC states. Given these complexities, it may be more worthwhile to modulate stem cell–niche functions rather than target treatments solely to intrinsic CSC features.

Clinical Cancer

After passing through the phenomena of initiation, promotion and progression, the neoplasm finally becomes manifest as a clinically significant tumour. Unless removed, it will continue to progress with a general tendency towards further loss of growth restraint, and acquisition of the capacity to spread to other parts of the body (metastasise).

Oncogenes and Tumour Suppressor Genes

The function of a cell is critically dependent on the expression of its genes. In cancer, it has been observed that there may be both inappropriate levels of expression of otherwise normal genes, and abnormalities of genes. Although copying of the genetic code from one cell generation to another is very accurate, it is not perfect. An abnormal copy or mutation may give rise to a protein with excessive function or reduced function, or may fail to produce a protein at all, resulting in no function. Alternatively, it may be the control of the gene which is altered, so that there is increased or decreased expression resulting in excess or deficient protein product and hence function. An oncogene is an altered gene which contributes to cancer development when its expression is increased. The normally functioning counterparts of these genes (proto-oncogenes) are often concerned with control of cell proliferation. An activating mutation transforms it into an oncogene. Examples include RAS, MYC, EGFR and so on.

In contrast, tumour suppressor genes are those which, when totally absent or nonfunctioning in a cell, permit the emergence of neoplasia that is, their presence prevents neoplasia. Given that all normal cells will have two copies of each gene (one on each chromosome pair), the development of neoplasia by this means requires loss or mutation of both copies. Examples of tumour suppressor genes include Rb, p53, PTEN and so on.

It must be stressed that clinical cancer does not reflect a solitary abnormality of one of these genes, but rather the final result of a combination of several errors of function. The gradual accumulation of multiple genetic defects is typified by the progression of a benign polyp in the colon to a cancer over about 10 years. Indeed the adenoma carcinoma sequence has been characterised in great detail in the Vogelstein's model of colorectal carcinogenesis.

Defective DNA Repair Mechanisms

How is it that a cell can acquire so many abnormal genes? The explanation in several situations is that there is failure of the screening of the cell's genetic code for abnormalities, or defective repair of incidental genetic damage. The protein p53 (termed the guardian of the genome) is important in assuring the integrity of the genome, and is frequently defective in cancer cells. Similarly, the failure of DNA repair can result in much more rapid accumulation of mutations, the mutator phenotype. An inherited defect in DNA repair makes an individual prone to cancer. Accumulating DNA damage causes mutations to arise during DNA synthesis resulting in malignancies. Common known germ-line mutations that lead to an increased risk of cancer include among others defects in BRCA1/2 and the Ataxia-Telangiectasia Mutated gene (ATM) which result in defective homologous recombination and/or nonhomologous end-joining (NHEJ) processes of DNA repair and have been observed in both solid (breast, ovarian) and haemopoietic malignancies (leukaemia and lymphomas). Another common example of faulty DNA repair is exemplified by deficiencies in the DNA mismatch repair (MMR) system that normally corrects for errors in insertion, deletion and misincorporation of bases during DNA replication or damage repair. Inherited mutations in the MMR proteins (viz. MLH1, PMS2, MSH2 and MSH6) cause microsatellite instability (MSI) with an abnormal length of microsatellite repeats. This is seen in hereditary non-polyposis colorectal cancers (HNPCC or Lynch syndrome), predominantly affecting the right colon, and the Muir-Torre syndrome (MTS), which predisposes to sebaceous carcinomas of the skin. DNA mismatch repair defects are also observed in some sporadic colorectal tumours, but unlike germline defects as in HNPCC, the defect ensues from epigenetic mechanisms that reduce DNA repair gene expression, for example, methylation of the MLH1 promoter that silences MLH1.

Defective apoptotic mechanisms

Defective apoptosis has several consequences with regard to cancer. Inappropriately increased expression of BCL-2, which inhibits apoptosis, is a major reason for cell accumulation in some tumours, for example follicular lymphoma. Failure of apoptosis may contribute to survival of defective cells and also cell survival in abnormal environments such as during invasion and metastasis. Finally, many cancer treatments rely on induction of apoptosis to kill tumour cells, so these will be less effective if apoptosis is defective. The apoptotic machinery is complex and depends on the critical balance between BCL-2 and its dimerising partners, which may be pro- (e.g. with BAD) or anti-apoptotic (e.g. with BAX), as well as the concerted activity of a group of enzymes called caspases, which may suffer mutations in cancers.

Blood Vessels

The development of cancer cells into a clinically important mass requires establishing a blood supply, a process called *angiogenesis*. New capillaries form under the influence of vascular endothelial growth factors (VEGF); platelets are the main source of VEGF in the blood. VEGF may be secreted directly by tumour cells, particularly when stimulated by hypoxia, but also when tumours abnormally express a range of other oncogenes, for example epidermal growth factor receptor (EGFR) and Her2. Her2 is important in many breast cancers and is a therapeutic target for trastuzumab (Herceptin). Drugs available to target angiogenesis include the anti-VEGF antibody, bevacizumab (Avastin), often used to treat colorectal cancer whereas other small molecule tyrosine kinase inhibitors (e.g. sunitinib, sofarenib etc.) act by inhibiting VEGF receptors. Tumours also develop new lymphatic channels (*lymphangiogenesis*), detectable by lymphatic channel markers (such as D2-40/podoplanin) and in some cancers such as breast cancer, lymphovascular invasion has been shown to be the major route of metastases rather than blood vascular invasion. In general, both blood vascular and lymphovascular invasion confer poor prognosis in a wide variety of neoplasms.

Heredity and Cancer

The great majority of common tumours do not seem to have any relationship to hereditary factors. However, some rare tumours do, and have led to an understanding of tumour suppressor genes. The pioneering work of Knudson on families of patients with multiple retinoblastomas (a tumour of the eye) indicated first that there must be two genetic events (Knudson's two-hit hypotheses). In due course, it became clear that one defective gene was inherited by the patient, whereas its corresponding gene on the opposite chromosome became defective, or was lost, in some cells during the growth of the eye. With both retinoblastoma (Rb) genes now defective, the cells proceeded to neoplasia.

It is apparent that a minority of common tumours run in families because of the same sort of mechanism. For example, breast cancer kindreds may be passing on mutations in the BRCA-1 or BRCA-2 genes and may also be associated with carcinoma of the ovary or colon. In familial adenomatous polyposis, a defective APC gene results in adenomas and colon cancers, whereas as mentioned earlier, in hereditary nonpolyposis colon cancer (HNPCC), one of a number of mismatch repair genes or abnormal hypermethylation is involved, giving rise to colon cancer by a different molecular biology route. These issues are discussed in further detail in the relevant sections about breast cancer or colon cancer. An inherited risk of malignancy however, does not imply that it is certain that a cancer will arise in a particular individual.

Physical Agents

Ionising Radiation

There is no doubt that ionising radiation can cause cancer. Knowledge of radiation effects have come from evidence following exposure to the atom bomb and the Chernobyl accident, which caused an increased incidence of thyroid carcinoma and radiation-related breast cancers. Direct damage to DNA (i.e. the chemical basis of genetic information), and damage mediated via ionisation of water can result in mutation of genes. The damage is randomly scattered throughout the genetic code but can include sites critical to the development of cancer by the usual sequence of initiation, promotion and so on. Traditionally, it has been thought that radiation causes a somatic mutation in a normal cell. The earliest event is probably genomic instability. Subsequently, there is a multistep sequence of genetic events. This typically results in an interval of many years between exposure and clinical cancer. The source of radiation does not matter from the point of view of causing cancer, although it will affect the sites at risk.

Ionising radiation can lead to loss of tumour suppressor genes and activation of protooncogenes. A proto-oncogene is a normal gene which when altered by mutation becomes an oncogene that can contribute to the development of cancer. Oncogenes may also be activated as a result of point mutations. Gene amplification can lead to activation and overexpression of a proto-oncogene. It had previously been thought that mutagenesis only occurred in normal cells traversed by radiation particles. However, normal cells can undergo change without such damage by virtue of what is termed the *bystander effect*. The mechanism of this bystander effect is not clear but it could be as a result of secretion of factors (as yet unidentified) from irradiated cells that influence the survival of adjacent nonirradiated cells.

The dose at which carcinogenesis occurs may be tissue specific. Actively proliferating tissues within or adjacent to the irradiated volume (e.g. in the pelvis), and having a high capacity for proliferation not inhibited by radiation, will carry a risk of radiation-induced malignancy at lower doses than in slowly turning-over tissues such as connective tissue.

Industrial exposure. Early workers using x-rays unknowingly induced tumours, and other radiation damage, in their hands. Today, diagnostic and therapeutic radiation also carry this risk to patients and staff alike, necessitating stringent safety regulations. Some mine workers are exposed to high levels of radon, which is inhaled and may cause lung cancer (a risk increased by cigarette smoking). Radon-induced lung cancer has been linked to mutations of p53, a tumour suppressor gene. This mutation differs from those seen in lung cancer induced by smoking. Another industrial association was with the painters of luminous watch dials. These ladies pointed their brush with their lips, thereby taking in minute quantities of radium. Some of the material remained near the jaw, whereas some was absorbed and passed to bone marrow, where the alpha emissions resulted in bone necrosis, tumours and marrow failure. In all cases, there was the usual long time delay between exposure and clinical cancer.

Atomic bomb survivors have been followed up very carefully. There has been an excessive number of cases of leukaemia, mainly 7 to 12 years after exposure, and also a larger number of other cancers from about 20 years later onwards.

Ultraviolet light. The shorter wavelengths of solar ultraviolet light, UVB, are capable of damaging the DNA of various skin cells, resulting in mutations and eventually cancers. Melanin pigment protects against UV penetration to the deeper layers of cells. The common tumours, basal cell and squamous cell carcinomas, seem to result from chronic overexposure; malignant melanoma correlates better with acute and intense exposure.

Chemicals

Coal Tars, Oils and Cigarette Smoke

Percival Pott, in 1775, described carcinoma of the scrotal skin in chimney sweeps, and attributed it to the soot. Similarly, mule-spinners in mills developed tumours because of the oil that soaked their clothing and, even today, motor mechanics are at risk from lubricating oils. However, the greatest problem at present from this group of chemicals is cigarette smoke. This contains many known *carcinogenic* substances, including benzo[a]pyrene, a potent carcinogen also present in coal tars. Not only do smokers have a very greatly increased incidence of lung cancer, they also have a higher risk of cancer at several other sites, such as the bladder. Chemicals that are able to cause tumours are called *direct carcinogens*, but most require metabolism to the active chemical, so are called *procarcinogens*.

Aniline Dyes and the Rubber Industry

Workers in the chemical industry, particularly those involved in making dyes, were found to develop bladder cancer. A similar risk was noted in the rubber-processing industry. The chemical implicated, β-naphthylamine, needs to be metabolised in the kidney, thus releasing the active ingredient into the urine.

Asbestos

Many particulate minerals are now recognised as carcinogenic, including asbestos. The blue asbestos (crocidolite) particles used for insulation are easily inhaled when very small but are then retained within the lung. Over a period of decades, they may then cause tumours of the pleura (malignant mesothelioma); they also correlate with bronchial cancer, particularly if associated with smoking. Asbestos-related fatalities therefore have compensation implications for families.

Hormones

Are endogenous chemicals such as hormones carcinogenic? There is no doubt that hormone levels are important in hormonally responsive organs and their cancers. Whether the hormone is actually carcinogenic, or simply contributes to the process of carcinogenesis by promoting cell proliferation is debatable; the latter is more probable. The relationship between oestrogens and endometrial cancer is discussed in Chapter 27. Oestrogens in breast cancers and androgens in prostate cancers play major roles, and hence hormonal manipulation is an important therapeutic tool in such cancer treatment.

Viruses and Cancer

As viruses contain genetic material, and gain access to the inside of cells, they have long been suspected of having a role in carcinogenesis. This speculation has been fuelled by finding close similarity between some viral genes and oncogenes. Viruses are clearly responsible for a variety of tumours in several species, such as leukaemias in mice and cats and sarcomas in chickens. In humans, common skin warts are self-limiting benign tumours caused by a virus. Over recent years, these human papilloma (wart) viruses (HPV) have been found to be a large family of related organisms, some of which correlate closely with cancer of the uterine cervix and a subset of anal, penile, vulvar, vaginal, and oropharyngeal cancers. Similarly, Epstein-Barr virus, which is very widespread and causes infectious mononucleosis, is closely associated with tumours such as Hodgkin lymphoma, Burkitt lymphoma (a high-grade non-Hodgkin lymphoma), and nasopharyngeal carcinoma. Within mesenchymal malignancies, HHV8, the Kaposi's sarcoma-associated herpesvirus (KSHV), is associated with all varieties of KS, whether human immunodeficiency virus (HIV) related, endemic or sporadic.

Infectivity and Cancer

Some patients, or their relatives, worry that cancer may be infectious. It is possible to allay these fears and assure them that this is not the case. The association with viruses mentioned above is a rare sequel to agents widely present in the community; the cancer cannot be passed on.

Immunity and Cancer

The immune system exists to detect and eliminate foreign substances, from isolated molecules to whole organisms. This is effected by antibodies and cells, principally lymphocytes. In the development of a tumour, it is quite possible for new or inappropriate substances to be produced. From this one would predict that tumours would sometimes be antigenic, that is, provoke an immune response. This does seem to be the case. There are several examples of rare and common tumours with evidence of an immune response, generally the presence of numerous lymphocytes within and around the tumour. Tumours of the rectum and breast, melanomas and seminoma of the testis all vary in the density of tumour-infiltrating lymphocytes. Studies of patients have correlated the density of lymphocytes with survival, often showing an advantage to those with an immune response. However, the effect is not large, and is easily obscured by treatment effects.

With malignant melanoma of skin, there is slightly more evidence to suggest a significant favourable immune response in some patients. Microscopic examination sometimes shows areas of apparent regression within the primary growth. There are also some patients with advanced melanoma who respond to stimulation of their immune system against the tumour (immunotherapy).

Despite these few encouraging observations, it is obvious that the majority of clinical cancer is beyond the capability of the patient's immune system. In some cases, there is evidence that tumour cells may simply evade it. This is achieved by multiple mechanisms such as local immune evasion, induction of tolerance, and disruption of the T lymphocyte signalling pathways. In developing neoplasms, there might indeed be a selection pressure of less immunogenic apoptosis-resistant cells, a process termed immune editing. Indeed, developing immunotherapeutic approaches now seek to either stimulate immune effector mechanisms in tumours or attempt to counteract inhibitory pathways.

Immune Surveillance

The normal immune system actively seeks foreign material, apparently screening everything against its memory bank to distinguish self from nonself. This may allow the detection and elimination of some cancers before they are clinically established. For example, renal transplant patients require drugs to suppress their immune response in order for the new kidney to survive. These patients have many more skin tumours than would otherwise be expected, possibly as a result of loss of immune surveillance. Patients with AIDS suffer from a wide range of tumours, but this does not necessarily imply that loss of immune surveillance is the key event. Many patients with defects of the immune system (either as a result of disease or treatment) have an increase in tumours of lymphocytes, but this is probably a different phenomenon.

Injury and Cancer

For injury to be acceptable as a cause of cancer, three factors must be considered: the injury would need to be severe enough to have caused tissue damage, there must be evidence that the site was previously normal, and the tumour arose at the site of injury. Finally, the time interval must be long enough to be plausible, generally several years. The mechanism is presumably via a nonspecific induction of cell division as part of the repair process, rather than anything actually carcinogenic. There are a few instances that fulfill these criteria, but the usual circumstance is simply that the injury draws attention to a pre-existing tumour.

PRECANCEROUS LESIONS

There are a number of conditions in which there is an increased risk of the subsequent development of cancer. Some are disorders that are not of themselves neoplastic but carry a risk of cancer. Others are more like a halfway house in which the process of development towards cancer is recognisable as neither normal nor cancer. Some are benign tumours that may change to be malignant. In none is the development of cancer inevitable, although the risk and time scale vary greatly. Some examples include the following.

- Undescended testis is an abnormality of development: it carries a high risk of neoplasia.
- Paget's disease of bone, a condition of middle to late adult life, has a risk of osteosarcoma, a tumour otherwise seen in adolescence.
- Solar/actinic keratosis is a warty skin lesion as a result of sun exposure; it may progress to cancer.
- Leukoplakia, a whitish patch in the mouth or vulva, is a descriptive term including several conditions. Some run the risk of cancer later.
- Erythroplakia, a fiery reddish patch in the mouth, is a morphological appearance that has strong relationships to cancers in the oral cavity.
- Barrett's metaplasia, a change in the squamous epithelium of the oesophagus to intestinal type epithelium, increases the risk of dysplasia and subsequent carcinoma.
- Dysplasia may be detected at several sites (e.g. stomach, colon, urothelium), and indicates a microscopic abnormality of cells with

Benign   Malignant

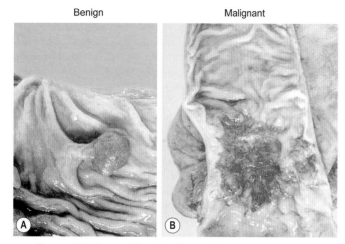

Figure 16.2 Benign (A) and malignant (B) colorectal tumours.

some, but not all, features of malignancy. Carcinoma-in-situ may be seen on a surface (e.g. cervix) or within the lumen of a duct (intraductal carcinoma of the breast). This has all the microscopic features of cancer, but the cells are still confined to their normal anatomical limits, that is, have not invaded.

- Adenomatous polyp of the large intestine (Fig. 16.2A) is a benign tumour. However, it may develop into a malignant tumour. In the condition, familial adenomatous polyposis, there are so many polyps (thousands), that malignancy (Fig. 16.2B) becomes inevitable, often at an earlier age. In addition to the malignant potential of adenomas, it is now becoming apparent that large hyperplastic polyps of the right colon, and those with a serrated morphology (sessile serrated lesions), can also progress to cancer but by a different molecular pathway.

An important consideration is that the detection of some of these conditions allows surgical intervention before cancer becomes established.

Field Change

Although an individual tumour arises from a single cell, within the vicinity of that cell there are often other cells part-way through carcinogenesis. Removal of the tumour, or its precursor lesion, may be followed by the local development of further lesions. This is regarded as a field change across the whole area. An example would be the appearance of cancer on the tongue following removal of one from the buccal mucosa. Common alterations in areas of field changes include mutations, aberrant methylation leading to reduced gene expression (e.g. DNA repair genes) and altered protein profiles.

NATURAL HISTORY AND SPREAD OF CANCER

As stated earlier, benign tumours remain localised, often separated from surrounding tissue by a capsule. The tumour has relatively little effect on the adjacent structures, unless it arises in a particularly critical site, and surgical removal is curative. In contrast, malignant tumours show a capacity to invade, frequently recur after surgery, spread to other sites and result in the death of the patient. The initial or primary site of tumour growth thus gives rise to separate secondary tumours, or metastases. Some tumours, such as basal cell carcinoma of skin have an intermediate behaviour; they invade locally but do not give rise to metastases.

In summary, spread may occur in several ways (Fig. 16.3):
- by local invasion
- by lymphatic vessels
- by blood vessels
- across cavities

Local Invasion

As the tumour invades, adjacent tissues are displaced and destroyed to be replaced by tumour. The tumour margin is ill-defined and irregular. Surgical removal therefore needs to include a generous extent of normal tissue. Failure to do so results in some tumour being left behind which proliferates and gives rise to *local recurrence*. Radiotherapy is frequently used after surgery to prevent this situation. The invasion often follows anatomical tissue planes; it may be temporarily halted by some dense structure such as bone, until this is also eroded. Certain anatomical sites may be more prone to local recurrence, such as the nonperitonealised resection margin in the lower rectum.

Functional Effects

The effects a tumour produces will depend upon the site involved; a knowledge of anatomy and physiology allows prediction of many symptoms. Thus, a tumour in the head of the pancreas will soon obstruct the bile duct, so that the patient becomes jaundiced (Fig. 16.4). A tumour of the left lung may obstruct its bronchus, with

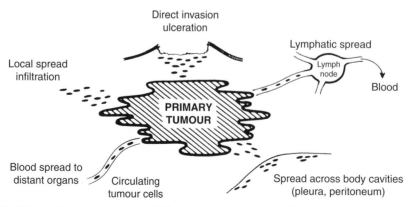

Figure 16.3 Metastasis or secondary spread. Tumours can spread by a variety of routes including local spread, spread through the lymphatics via the blood and across cavities. (Reproduced from Calman, Smyth, Tattersall. *Basic principles of cancer chemotherapy.* Macmillan; 1980. With permission of Palgrave.)

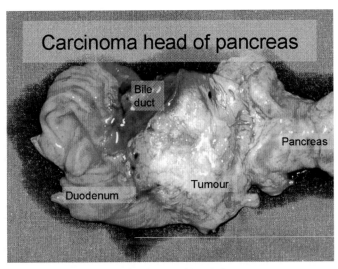

Figure 16.4 Carcinoma of head of pancreas.

resulting pneumonia from infection of retained secretions. Further local invasion of this mass will compress the recurrent laryngeal nerve and the patient's voice is altered. Further growth may obstruct the superior vena cava passing through the mediastinum, causing discoloration (cyanosis) and swelling of the face and arms (superior vena caval obstruction syndrome). If the cervical sympathetic chain is involved, this may manifest as Horner's syndrome (with droopy eyelids, less sweating on the face and constriction of the pupil).

A tumour just beneath the skin can so stretch it and impair its nutrition that it breaks down to form an ulcer. This is then liable to infection or bleeding. Pain and weakness will occur when peripheral nerves are affected, for example, Pancoast tumour at the apex of the lung invading upwards to compress nerves to the arm and hand.

The extent of local invasion dictates the extent of surgery necessary to remove it and, indeed, may render the tumour inoperable if critical structures are involved. However, the usual reason why a tumour is 'inoperable' is because of metastatic disease. Sometimes it is worth debulking the tumour, but surgery alone is insufficient to cure the patient.

Metastasis

The hallmark of tumour cells is the ability to spread to distant sites of the body (metastases). The molecular events leading to the development of metastases are thought to follow either a linear or a parallel mode of progression. The models differ in the relative timing of emergence of the metastatic precursor clone in the primary tumour, arising and disseminating late in the linear model, just before clinical detection of the primary, whereas in the parallel model, the metastatic clone is thought to evolve alongside and disseminate early from the primary. In the first model, the genetic divergence between the primary and secondary is small whereas it is substantial in the latter. In fact, the latter theory postulates that dissemination of metastasis may occur in multiple waves even before the primary tumour is clinically detectable. Different clones of metastases may even seed at different sites through different routes of spread. The major routes of metastases of tumours and clinical implications thereof are explained below:

By Lymphatic Vessels

Invasive tumours readily penetrate the thin wall of lymphatics. Then, fragments of tumour are carried downstream to lodge in one or more local lymph nodes. If the tumour cells survive this journey and proliferate in the node they form a *metastasis*, or secondary tumour. Further dissemination may proceed to other lymph nodes along the chain, for example, from pelvic to para-aortic to supraclavicular nodes. Some primary tumours remain tiny, yet have massive nodal deposits. If the node capsule is breached by tumour, the whole mass becomes fixed to surrounding structures. In some tumours such as breast cancers or melanomas, it may be possible to identify the first lymph node/s (sentinel node/s) draining the region of the cancer and evaluate whether these are involved or not, with a view to modifying the treatment plan based on the involvement status of these nodes. In other tumours such as colorectal cancer, involvement of the lymph node at the site of arterial ligation (the high-tie lymph node), forms part of the synoptic pathology report and may imply higher stage (C2 by Dukes' staging) and poorer prognosis. Knowledge of propensity of spread of tumours to some lymph node groups, may guide treatment planning. The classical dog leg field of radiation used in the treatment of testicular seminomas is based on the tenet that this field includes the lymph nodes (para-aortic and ipsilateral pelvic) most likely to be involved by this malignancy.

By Blood Vessels

Thin-walled blood vessels are similarly at risk of tumour invasion, and again, fragments of tumour float passively downstream. (Single tumour cells are generally destroyed by nonspecific defence mechanisms in the blood.) These then lodge in the next capillary bed, where they may develop into metastases. Although this can happen in any tissue, the liver, lungs and bone (Fig. 16.5) are by far the most frequent sites for secondaries.

Across Cavities (Transcoelomic)

Access to the pleura enables tumour cells to seed themselves around the pleural cavity, forming numerous further deposits or seedlings. These may be associated with secretion of fluid into the cavity, with resultant impairment of respiration. An identical process may occur in the peritoneum; the fluid accumulation is called *ascites*. Malignant cells may settle on the ovaries (Krukenberg tumours), or all over the omentum and peritoneum (Fig. 16.6). Related to this, some intracranial tumours, such as medulloblastoma of the cerebellum, may disseminate by the cerebrospinal fluid, seeding over the surface of the brain and down the spinal canal (see Chapters 30 and 33). Indeed, radiation treatment often preempts and abrogates this possibility by inclusion of spinal fields during treatment planning.

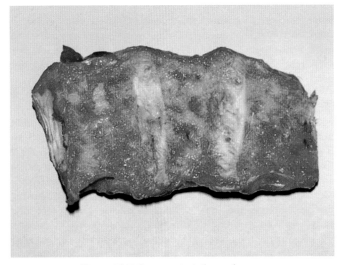

Figure 16.5 Bone metastatic carcinoma.

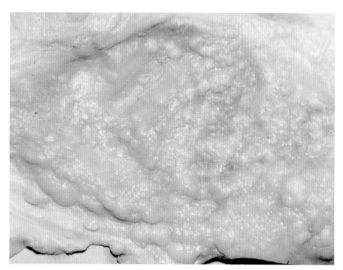

Figure 16.6 Peritoneal deposits of metastatic carcinoma.

Implantation

Occasionally, cells may be implanted in the scar by the surgeon's knife while removing a tumour, or through a pleural or abdominal paracentesis drainage site.

Functioning Tumours

Many tumour cells continue certain cell functions related to their tissue of origin but, in some, this has a profound effect on the patient. Tumours of endocrine glands typically produce an excess of their hormone. The problem is that the tumour is no longer responsive to the usual control of secretion. Thus, an adrenal cortex tumour will produce steroids despite switching off its pituitary drive, and Cushing syndrome will result.

In other circumstances, the hormone production is quite inappropriate for the tumour site. Many lung tumours produce substances that mimic the function of parathyroid hormone, antidiuretic hormone, or adrenocorticotrophic hormone. Again, it is not subject to the normal control of secretion, and the clinical consequences may be severe. Some of the other effects that tumours may have, such as profound weight loss (cancer cachexia), could be caused by tumour-derived proteolytically generated peptides.

Cause of Death from Cancer

As the word malignant implies, death is the natural consequence of untreated cancer. Sometimes the tumour will have grown locally and spread in a predictable manner. In other cases, the primary site remains undetected despite widespread metastatic deposits. Some tumours show relentless progression and run their course in a few months; others take many years, with long intervals of apparent dormancy.

Many patients with locally advanced or metastatic cancer become bedridden and die from bronchopneumonia, inanition and/or metabolic disturbance. Sometimes there may be liver failure because of numerous liver secondaries. Often the actual cause of death is unclear. It is important to consider carrying out a postmortem examination if there is reasonable doubt about the cause of death. Patients with cancer are still at risk of nonneoplastic conditions such as coronary artery disease. This is particularly likely in patients who smoke. Indeed, smoking may have given rise both to the primary tumour (e.g. in the lung, oral cavity or pharynx) and to ischaemic heart disease.

It is important to make a judgment as to whether the patient died from cancer or from an unrelated condition, because this influences cancer mortality statistics. Where a patient has remained disease free from cancer for more than 5 years, and the cause of death is said to

be cancer, this conclusion should be questioned. However, late relapses can occur after 5 years, in breast cancer, for example. Alternatively, a new primary may develop, especially in head and neck cancer.

STAGING OF CANCERS

It is of the greatest practical importance in many cases to estimate the extent of the spread of a tumour at the time of initial diagnosis. This process is called *staging*. Staging often influences the choice of treatment and can provide valuable information on prognosis. Staging may include clinical, pathological, radiological and biochemical information. This enables similar groups of patients to be compared between different oncology centres nationally and internationally. A number of staging classifications are in use. The simplest and oldest classification is as follows:

Stage 1: Tumour confined to the organ of origin
Stage 2: Local lymph nodes invaded
Stage 3: Distant nodes invaded, or local spread beyond the organ of origin
Stage 4: Blood-borne metastasis present

This classification is still used with some cancers, although often with slight modification to bring in subcategories, as with the International Federation of Gynecology and Obstetrics (FIGO) system for cervical cancer. The International Union Against Cancer (UICC) has worked towards international agreement on the staging of many tumours, coding them on the TNM system (described later).

TNM Classification

The TNM staging system provides an internationally accepted common language platform for clinicians to communicate the extent of cancer, and hence aids treatment planning, prognostication and monitoring response to treatment. This includes a succinct summary of the extent of malignancy in the patient and includes a description of the primary tumour (T), nodal spread (N) and distant metastases (M).

The mandatory parameters included are as follows:
T: size or direct extent/depth of invasion of the primary tumour
   Tx: tumour cannot be assessed
   Tis: carcinoma in situ
   T0: no evidence of tumour
   T1, T2, T3, T4: depending on increasing size or extent of the primary tumour (with T4 often signifying involvement of adjacent structures)
N: degree of involvement of regional lymph nodes
   Nx: lymph nodes cannot be assessed
   N0: no evidence of regional lymph nodes metastasis
   N1: regional lymph node metastasis present; at some sites, tumour spread to closest or limited number of regional lymph nodes
   N2: tumour spread to an extent between N1 and N3 (all sites may not have N2)
   N3: tumour spread to more distant or greater number of regional lymph nodes (N3, not for all sites)
M: presence/absence of distant metastasis
   M0: no distant metastasis
   M1: spread to distant organs (beyond lymph nodes)

Given the increase in tumour burden with the increasing value of numerical qualifiers, T1N0M0 would represent a very early cancer, whereas T4N3M1 indicates a very advanced cancer. The details of how to categorise a tumour may vary between sites; the TNM classification for breast cancer is shown in Table 26.3.

Other nonmandatory parameters that are now being increasingly used as adjuncts to the basic TNM parameters include: G (1–4) for the grade of differentiation, S (0–3) for various levels of serum tumour markers, R (0–2) for the completeness of surgical excision at margins, L

(0–1) for lympho-vascular invasion and V (0–2) for blood vascular (typically venous) invasion.

The clinical staging may differ from the pathological staging. For example, a tumour in the breast may be measured clinically as 2 cm in diameter and thus be staged as T1. However, when actually measured directly in the mastectomy specimen it might be 3 cm in maximum diameter, and thus be pathologically T2 (abbreviated as pT2). Most staging classifications are based on the clinical extent of spread. The overall stage gets a prefix p if this has been pathologically determined and y if the assessment is after chemotherapy/radiation. These designations help facilitate discussion at multidisciplinary team meetings to assess inconsistencies between clinical/radiological/pathological staging and the response to neoadjuvant treatment.

Radiological information may influence staging. For example, in carcinoma of the cervix, the presence of an obstructed kidney on ultrasound or other investigation (in the absence of a nonneoplastic cause), automatically indicates stage 3B.

The staging of testicular cancer is an example in which tumour biochemical information (the presence of serum tumour markers lactate dehydrogenase, alpha-fetoprotein and human chorionic gonadotrophin) is included. S0 signifies markers are at normal levels; S1 slightly raised markers; S2 moderately raised markers and S3 very high levels of markers.

HISTOLOGICAL GRADING: DIFFERENTIATION

In an effort to predict the future course of a tumour, an estimate is made of how malignant it is for a particular site and type of tumour. Generally speaking, the closer a tumour cell resembles its normal counterpart, that is, the better it is differentiated, the more orderly and slower its growth. Thus, histological examination allows tumour grading on the basis of the extent of differentiation. Attention is given to the nucleus (how abnormal it is and how often mitosis is observed), and the cytoplasm (the extent to which normal structures

are seen). In cancers such as breast cancer, the grading scheme also includes the proportion of cancer cells still retaining glandular/tubular differentiation (Figs. 16.7 and 16.8). In others such as pancreatic neuroendocrine tumours, the proliferative fraction, as determined by Ki67 immunohistochemistry or the mitotic count, helps determine the grade. The Ki67 index is currently based on at least 500 cells in areas of hot spots and is expressed as follows: less than 3%: grade 1, 3% to 20%: grade 2 and greater than 20%: grade 3. Mitoses are counted in 50 high power fields (hpf) in areas of high density; the cut-offs are grade 1: less than 2/10 hpf, grade 2: 2-20/10 hpf and grade 3: greater than 20/10 hpf. The final grade is determined by the worse of the Ki67 index or mitotic count. The grading system used for sarcomas, the French Federation of Cancer Centers Sarcoma Group (FNCLCC) system, incorporates necrosis as a parameter in addition to differentiation and mitoses.

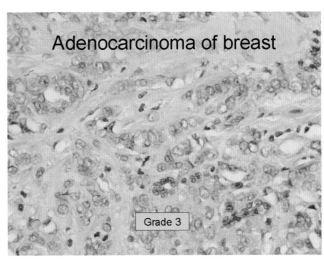

Figure 16.8 Adenocarcinoma of breast (grade 3).

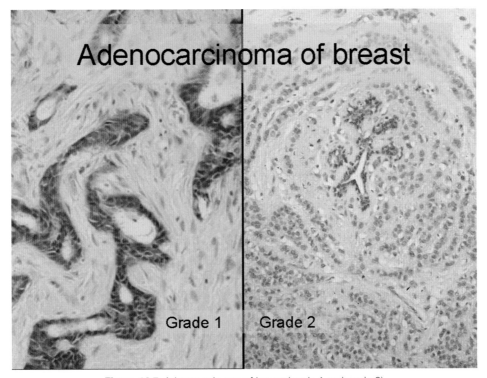

Figure 16.7 Adenocarcinoma of breast (grade 1 and grade 2).

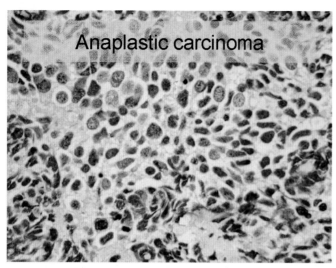

Figure 16.9 Histological features of an anaplastic carcinoma.

For most of the common tumours, the pathologist divides them into descriptive categories: well differentiated, moderately differentiated and poorly differentiated. Undifferentiated tumours lack sufficient features to allow more than a broad classification, as do anaplastic tumours (Fig.16.9) (see later under 'Classification of neoplasms').

Limitations of Grading

First, assessment of grading has an element of subjectivity and there may be a variation between pathologists in assigning pleomorphism and hence grades across different categories. Also, Ki67 assessment, where required, may be prone to errors of subjective quantification. Indeed, new technology such as digital pathology helps to overcome such errors. Biologically, some tumours show a tight correlation between histological grading and behaviour, such that treatment is guided by this information. Cancer of the bladder is one of these. However, the tumour stage is of overriding importance. Some tumours (e.g. pancreatic islet) have a high variable rate of clinical progression, but uniform histology; grading in this circumstance is misleading if attempted. Other tumours vary considerably from one microscopic field to another: in general, the outlook will depend upon the worst areas, but these could be missed without adequate sampling. Finally, the organ of origin is important: a well-differentiated cancer of the skin carries an excellent prognosis, whereas in the lung it may not.

GROWTH RATE OF CANCERS

As indicated in the section on carcinogenesis, there is usually a considerable time between initiation of a tumour and its clinical detection. Part of this time is taken by the process of becoming a cancer cell, and part by growing to a sufficient size to be found. The latter can be measured as the time taken for it to double in diameter, its doubling time. A mass 1 mm in diameter would represent about one million cells: this could result from one cell, and each of its subsequent daughter cells, dividing 20 times. A word of caution is needed before theorising further. Once a tumour exceeds about 2 mm, it is essential for it to have its own blood supply: this, together with other supporting structures, is the tumour stroma. In some tumours, the stroma is very scanty, whereas in others it constitutes the majority of the mass. (The character of the stroma also influences what the tumour feels like on palpation; most breast cancers are

hard because of abundant, dense stroma.) Thus, calculations about how many cancer cells there are in a tumour of a certain size will be incorrect if they ignore the stroma. With the advent of molecular diagnostics, which often require a minimum tumour load to be present to achieve the limit of detection, accurate assessment of the number of tumour cells in a pathology sample is becoming more important.

Another consideration is that the clinical growth of a tumour will be the result of the balance between cell proliferation and loss. It will be influenced too by the growth fraction or proportion of cancer cells actually proliferating. Many cancer cells in a tumour cease to proliferate as they differentiate, or produce nonviable daughter cells. Furthermore, if the vascularity of the stroma is inadequate there will be necrosis.

Although a cancer produces an expanding mass, this is a reflection of loss of control of growth. The actual rate at which individual cancer cells divide may be slower than comparable normal tissues. If there is a very sudden increase in the size of a tumour, it will probably reflect internal hemorrhage or fluid accumulation. (On the other hand, a slow-growing mass which begins to grow faster may have changed from benign to malignant.)

Observation of established clinical cancers has shown that doubling times vary widely, but average about 2 months. Leaving aside the question of whether this is true for the first 20 doublings to reach 1 mm size, it would require about a further 10 doublings (i.e. 20 months) to reach 1 cm diameter, at which point it might be detectable. Many tumours are 2 cm or more in diameter before they produce symptoms, so a considerable time has elapsed between the first emergence of a clone of cancer cells and the clinical disease. In comparison with that, the remainder of its course, if unchecked, is liable to be over after five or so more doublings. Metastatic deposits may be disseminated during the preclinical period, only to appear after removal of the primary. If the doubling time is considerably more than 2 months, the whole process takes on a much longer time scale.

Bearing these matters in mind, there is no fixed length of disease-free interval that equates with a cure. However, for practical purposes, 5 years disease free is tantamount to cure for many of the common tumours, with breast cancer as a notable exception. The earlier detection of a cancer at a minute size increases the possibility of removal before metastases develop, even if the tumour has been around for a long time. Prolonged postoperative survival in these patients may simply reflect earlier diagnosis rather than longer survival, a phenomenon called *lead-time bias*.

Spontaneous Regression of Cancer

Occasionally, a tumour may regress and disappear without treatment, although the original diagnosis could have been erroneous. Most of the reported cases are renal cell carcinoma, malignant melanoma and gestational choriocarcinoma. In all these instances, immunological mechanisms are thought to be responsible. Some cases of lymphoid tumours fluctuate in size, and may temporarily disappear, only to return later. In some cases of neuroblastoma, a primitive tumour of nerve cells, there is subsequent differentiation and growth ceases.

CLASSIFICATION OF NEOPLASMS

Table 16.2 lists examples of tumour nomenclature. In general, the names are built up from one part to describe the tissue type, and another to indicate its behaviour. All end in *oma* to denote a lump, a suffix almost restricted to neoplasms, although a few other terms are in use, such as hematoma for an accumulation of blood. Most malignant tumours fall into the following broad categories:

- Carcinoma
- Sarcoma
- Lymphoma

TABLE 16.2 Types of Neoplasms

Type	Benign	Malignant
Epithelial		Carcinoma
Squamous	Papilloma	Squamous cell carcinoma
Transitional	Papilloma	Transitional cell carcinoma
Basal cell	Papilloma	Basal cell carcinoma
Glandular	Adenoma	Adenocarcinoma
Mesenchymal		Sarcoma
Smooth muscle	Leiomyoma	Leiomyosarcoma
Striated muscle	Rhabdomyoma	Rhabdomyosarcoma
Fat	Lipoma	Liposarcoma
Blood vessels	Angioma	Angiosarcoma
Bone	Osteoma	Osteosarcoma
Cartilage	Chondroma	Chondrosarcoma
Hematological		Lymphoma
Lymphoid tissue		Hodgkin's lymphoma
		Non-Hodgkin's lymphoma
Plasma cell		Multiple myeloma
White blood cells		Leukaemia
Intracranial and neural		
Supporting cells		Glioma
Meninges	Meningioma	
Cerebellum		Medulloblastoma
Retina		Retinoblastoma
Sympathetic nerve	Ganglioneuroma	Neuroblastoma
Pigment cells of		
Skin or eye Gonad	Mole or nevus	Malignant melanoma
Germ cells	Dermoid cyst	Malignant teratoma
	mature	Seminoma
	teratoma	
	(Fig. 16.10)	
Placenta		
	Hydatidiform	Choriocarcinoma
	mole	

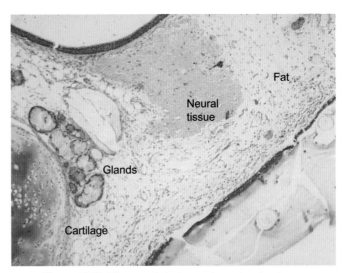

Figure 16.10 Microscopic features of a mature teratoma.

The majority of tumours arise from epithelium (surface lining cells). Benign tumours are called *papilloma* (Fig. 16.11) or *adenoma*; malignant tumours are called *carcinoma*, often with a prefix to give the cell type. Carcinoma is Greek/Latin for crab but is used in a more restricted sense than cancer and applied only to epithelial malignancy, which makes up 75% of cancer.

Squamous epithelium lines the skin, where it is called epidermis, the upper aerodigestive tract (mouth, pharynx, larynx, oesophagus), anus, vagina and cervix. It is present in the bronchi if there is metaplasia. Transitional cell epithelium (or urothelium) lines the renal pelvis, ureters and bladder.

Glandular (secretory) epithelium lines the gut from stomach to rectum, and forms the related secretory glands (salivary, pancreas, biliary tract and liver), endocrine glands (pituitary, thyroid, parathyroids and adrenals), kidneys, ovarian surface, endometrium (Fig. 16.12) and breast (Figs. 16.7 and 16.8).

Sometimes the tumour name is combined with a description of shape or function. If a cyst is formed it may be cystadenoma or cystadenocarcinoma, both of which are common in the ovary. Mucin-secreting variants would be mucinous cystadenoma.

Sarcoma denotes any tumour of mesenchymal origin (supporting structures). They are much less frequent than carcinoma. Metastasis

from sarcomas is generally blood-borne, and few give rise to lymph node secondaries (Fig. 16.13).

Lymphomas are malignant tumours of lymphoid cells; many are classified as Hodgkin lymphoma, leaving the remainder as non-Hodgkin lymphoma. Some are closely related to leukaemias (tumours of white blood cells).

There are many tumours that do not easily fit the guidelines mentioned, such as ovarian and testicular teratomas (refer to Fig. 16.14); some are shown in Table 16.2 and others are referred to elsewhere in this book under the relevant organ.

Undifferentiated Tumours

Some tumours lack obvious features to allow their identification or classification. An undifferentiated carcinoma or sarcoma cannot be ascribed to any subcategory. An anaplastic tumour could be carcinoma, lymphoma or sarcoma. Because these different categories have major therapeutic consequences, it is important to attempt a more detailed diagnosis. Simple microscopy can now be supplemented by special staining procedures, many of which involve detecting cell components with antibodies. The presence of the leukocyte common antigen (CD45), B-cell (CD20) or T-cell (CD3) markers would indicate a lymphoma, whereas finding broad spectrum cytokeratins (AE1/3, MNF116, CAM5.2) would suggest a carcinoma (Fig. 16.15). Positivity for only mesenchymal markers (smooth muscle actin, desmin) would indicate a sarcoma whereas positivity for melanocytic markers (S100, HMB45, MelanA), a malignant melanoma. Because tumours have deranged genetic function there are sometimes unexpected findings. Electron microscopy sometimes helps. There are other approaches such as cytogenetics, which depend upon finding characteristic abnormalities of the chromosomes. These are most often loss or gain of part or the whole of a chromosome, or translocations in which two chromosomes break and are rejoined with the fragments on the wrong chromosome, for example the classic t(9;22) in chronic myelogenous leukaemia.

Most oncology centres arrange for many of their patients' tumours to be reviewed before treatment. Diagnosis and classification of rare or undifferentiated tumours form a considerable part of such work.

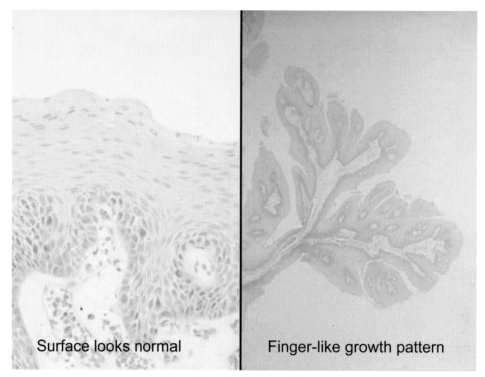

Surface looks normal   Finger-like growth pattern

Figure 16.11 Squamous papilloma.

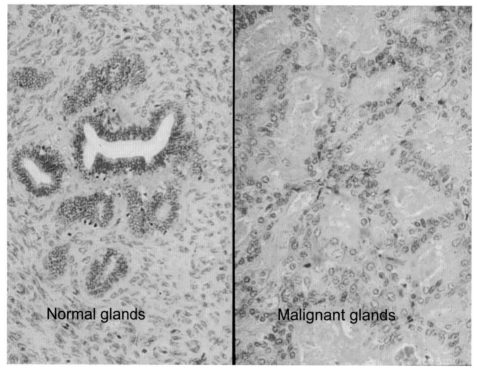

Normal glands   Malignant glands

Figure 16.12 Adenocarcinoma of endometrium.

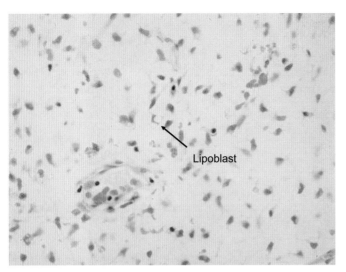

Figure 16.13 Myxoid liposarcoma.

CURRENT ADVANCES IN PATHOLOGY GUIDING PATIENT MANAGEMENT

Several pathological parameters guide patient management, for example, hormone receptor status in breast cancers (antioestrogens for ER-positive tumours and trastuzumab for HER2-positive tumours). With advances in molecular therapeutics, there is a demand for companion diagnostics to tailor therapy for patients. Examples include assessing for Ras mutations in colorectal cancers, the presence of which precludes treatment with EGFR tyrosine kinase inhibitors; ALK-EGFR mutations in nonsmall-cell lung cancers for sensitivity to EGFR inhibitors such as Erlotinib and Gefitinib; c-kit mutations in gastrointestinal mutations guiding imatinib treatment or BRAF mutations in melanomas guiding treatment with BRAF inhibitors, vemurafenib and dabrafenib. Some tests such as OncotypeDx integrate the activity of a panel of genes to figure out the risk of recurrence to guide further chemotherapy in early stage oestrogen receptor-positive breast cancer or radiation treatment in DCIS (ductal carcinoma in situ). Newer approaches such as testing for circulating tumour DNA now allow screening for early detection of cancer or its recurrence. Immunomodulation is another burgeoning field where pathology is increasingly playing a crucial role in patient selection for therapy. Apart from cancer vaccines utilising cancer antigens to activate the immune response, strategies have been developed to diminish regulatory T cells (CD25-targeted antibodies) which suppress the immune response, and use antibodies against immune-checkpoint molecules such as CTLA-4 and PD1. Immunohistochemical analysis of the programmed death receptor 1 (PD1) and its ligand (PDL-1) for example, in nonsmall-cell lung cancer, is helping to choose patients for treatment with drugs targeting PD-1 (pembrolizumab, nivolumab etc.) or PD-L1 (atezolizumab, durvalumab etc.). With the advent of next generation sequencing techniques, more and more actionable targets are being characterised and molecular pathology is proving integral to the multidisciplinary dialogue to determine prognosis and guide management.

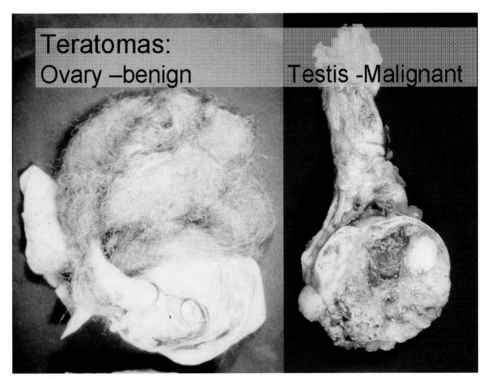

Figure 16.14 Teratomas: ovary benign, testis malignant.

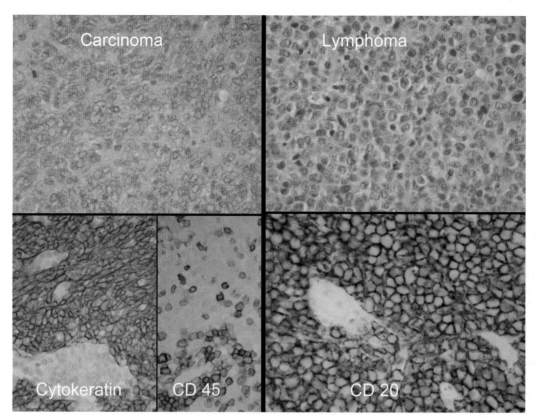

Figure 16.15 Immunocytochemistry to distinguish lymphoma from carcinoma (Carcinoma positive for cytokeratin; lymphoma for CD20. CD45 staining only tumour infiltrating lymphocytes in the carcinoma).

FURTHER READING

Batlle E, Clevers H. Cancer stem cells revisited. Nat Med 2017;23:1124–34.

Brierley JD, Gospodarowicz MK, Wittekind C, editors. The TNM classification of malignant tumours. 8th ed. Wiley-Blackwell; 2016.

Curtius K, Wright NA, Graham TA. An evolutionary perspective on field cancerization. Nat Rev Cancer 2018;18(1):19–32.

Dietel M. Molecular pathology: a requirement for precision medicine in cancer. Oncol Res Treat 2016;39(12):804–10.

Fearon ER, Vogelstein B. A genetic model for colorectal tumorigenesis. Cell 1990;61(5):759–67.

Haverkos HW. Viruses, chemicals and co-carcinogenesis. Oncogene 2004;23 (38):6492–9.

Luch A. Nature and nurture—lessons from chemical carcinogenesis. Nat Rev Cancer 2005;5(2):113–25.

Turajlic S, Swanton C. Metastasis as an evolutionary process. Science 2016;352 (6282):169–75.

Vanneman M, Dranoff G. Combining immunotherapy and targeted therapies in cancer treatment. Nat Rev Cancer 2012;12:237–51.

Williams D. Radiation carcinogenesis: lessons from Chernobyl. Oncogene 2008;27:S9–S18.

17

Molecular, Cellular and Tissue Effects of Radiotherapy

George D.D. Jones, Paul Symonds

CHAPTER OUTLINE

INTRODUCTION

One of the most often-used and successful modalities in the clinical treatment of cancer is the local eradication of a patient's tumour using radiotherapy (RT). In addition to this, external beam RT is often used in the palliation of cancer-associated symptoms, for example, to treat pain or spinal cord compression, to shrink tumour masses or to relieve bleeding. The local treatment of a patient's tumour via external beam RT is accomplished by (1) the precise and focused delivery of radiation to kill both tumour and locally metastatic cancer cells by conforming and modulating the delivered radiation dose to the target volume, and (2) by exploiting the differences in the response of tumour and normal tissue to irradiation. Through largely empirical studies, this has previously led to curative external beam RT protocols of typically around 2 to 3 gray (Gy) being delivered in daily fractions to the tumour site over 4 to 7 weeks with the exact dose and fractionation schedule depending on the clinical situation and the tolerance of the coirradiated normal tissue. Indeed, in many instances, it is the likelihood of normal tissue damage that limits the total dose that can be delivered to the tumour site. Overall, however, the exact basis for the success of RT in eliminating cancers is still poorly understood, appearing to depend on differences in intrinsic sensitivity, ability to proliferate, and repair capacity between both normal and malignant tissues.

In the last 30 years, radiobiology has gone someway to providing explanations and reasoning for these empirically derived schedules and, whereas many of the advances in RT have been realised via the optimisation of treatment delivery schedules and technologic improvements in the physical targeting of dose, biologic discoveries, particularly those investigating the molecular and cellular response to irradiation,

continue to point the way towards new and more effective methods/protocols of treatment. Indeed, there is every hope that this biologic information will improve RT efficacy, both in terms of superior targeted treatments and better patient selection.

The aim of this chapter is to describe some of the pertinent molecular and cellular principles and phenomena that underpin current radiation treatment practice, to relate this to outcomes observed in the clinic, and to provide insight into possible future developments and potential pitfalls in RT and radiobiology research. Clearly, this is a vast field, so this chapter will concentrate largely on the molecular, cellular and tissue radiobiology of low LET (linear energy transfer) x-ray irradiation. Only brief mention of other radiations such as proton irradiation will be made because this modality is covered in detail in Chapter 36 of this book.

IONISING RADIATION, FREE RADICAL GENERATION, SUBCELLULAR RADIOGENIC DAMAGE

Radiations interact with matter by transferring energy to the molecules of the absorbing material. Indeed, radiations of wavelengths less than 10^{-6} cm have sufficient photon energy to eject orbital electrons from the atoms of the absorber's molecules, leading to their ionisation. Because the most abundant molecule in a cell is water, a key product of this initial process is an ionised water molecule ($H_2O^{+\bullet}$); these radical cation species then interact with other water molecules to form hydroxyl radicals ($^{\bullet}OH$) (Fig. 17.1A). The initially ejected electrons (e^-) may possess sufficient energy themselves to cause further ionisations until their energy is dissipated and they become solvated to give an aqueous electron (e_{aq}^-) and/or combine with other species, such as protons (H$^+$) or molecular oxygen (O$_2$), to generate reducing species such as hydrogen atoms (H$^{\bullet}$) or superoxide (O$_2^{\bullet-}$). Ionising radiation is nondiscriminatory in that all molecular species in a cell are prone to being damaged. However, DNA is a key molecular target for the deleterious effects of ionising radiation in cells. $^{\bullet}$OH radicals are highly reactive and will react with the DNA bases by addition reactions, whereby the $^{\bullet}$OH radicals add to the double bonds of DNA bases to form base radical adducts and by abstraction reactions, whereby the $^{\bullet}$OH radicals abstract hydrogen atoms from the deoxyribose moieties of the DNA sugar phosphate backbone to form carbon-centred sugar radicals. Via these mechanisms, $^{\bullet}$OH radicals, together with the less reactive reducing species, are said to damage DNA via the so-called *indirect* effect (see Fig. 17.1A), whereby the initial ionisation event happens in a molecule nearby to the ultimate target molecule. Radiation can also directly ionise the DNA leading to direct damage of the DNA's

bases or sugar-phosphate backbone (R$^{+\bullet}$) (see Fig. 17.1B). However, the distinction between direct and indirect damaging effects is not always clear as electrons and radical cations produced in the DNA and DNA-associated water may lead to further ionisations/oxidations in the DNA macromolecule and its surrounding microenvironment.

Through directly and indirectly induced base radical adducts and deoxyribose radicals, radiation causes a wide range of damage in DNA, including strand breaks (both single- and double-strand breaks (DSBs)), base or sugar damage and cross-links between macromolecules (i.e. DNA–DNA or DNA–protein cross-links) (Fig. 17.2A); the frequency of these DNA lesions is shown in Table 17.1. In general, it is considered that the DNA DSB is the most responsible for the lethal effects of radiation; evidence for this is as follows:

- Under a variety of experimental conditions, it is the relative level of induced or unrepaired DSBs that best correlates with cell killing.

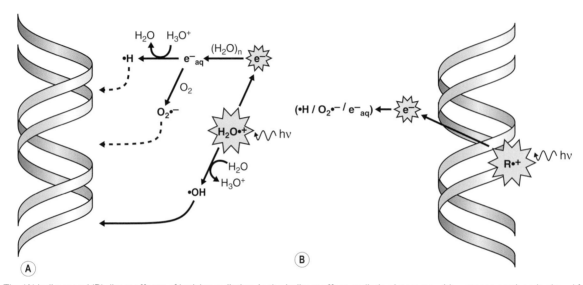

Fig. 17.1 The (A) indirect and (B) direct effects of ionising radiation. In the indirect effect, radiation interacts with water to produce hydroxyl free radicals ($^{\bullet}$OH) which, in turn, react with the DNA, producing damage. In the direct effect, the radiation interacts directly with the DNA to produce damage. Although both direct and indirect effects damage DNA, it is suggested that only indirect events happening within 2 nm of the DNA damage the DNA. Indirect effects dominate for low linear energy transfer ionising radiations. (The $^{\bullet}$ 'dot' refers to an unpaired electron of a free radical, and the dashed lines reflect the lower reactivity of the reducing species with DNA, as compared with the high reactivity of $^{\bullet}$OH.)

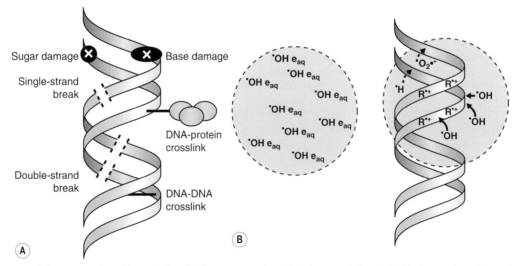

Fig. 17.2 (A) The types of damage produced by radiation. (B) The concept of multiply damaged sites (MDS) being produced by a cluster of ionisations impinging on the DNA and its local environment. Energy deposition for x-rays is not uniformly absorbed but deposited in discrete events of high energy sufficient to generate a number of ion pairs. Should this happen in pure water, it will generate locally several $^{\bullet}$OH + e$^-$ pairs; however, should these events overlap the DNA, both the direct and indirect effects will contribute to MDS formation.

TABLE 17.1 Types and Frequency of Radiation-Induced Damage

Type of Damage	Approximate Number/Gy/Cell
DNA double-strand breaks	40
DNA single-strand breaks	1000
DNA–protein cross links	150
DNA–DNA cross links	30
Base damage	2000
Sugar damage	1500

- A single DSB is lethal to yeast.
- Enzymatically produced DSBs (produced by inserting DNA restriction enzymes into cells) give the same pattern of chromosome damage and lethality as radiation.
- Microbeam irradiation has shown the cell nucleus to be the most radiation-sensitive site in the cell.
- The extreme radio-sensitivity of some mutant cell lines is because of defects in DSB repair.

However, not all DSBs are the same because the chemical nature of the strand break ends and the separation between the constituent single-strand breaks can vary considerably, as can the proximity of other types of lesions. Indeed, the influence of the proximity of induced base lesions has been shown to affect the reparability of damage and this is relevant because low LET radiations (x-rays and γ-rays) can produce multiple ionisations in localised isolated events (previously termed *spurs* and *blobs*). When these isolated events occur either close to and/or overlapping the DNA molecule (see Fig. 17.2B), several lesions may be formed within a region of a few base-pairs producing so-called *multiply damaged sites* (MDS), as described by Ward.

On a larger scale, radiation damage to chromosomes and chromatids leading to aberrations involving breakage and rejoining of chromosome/chromatid fragments (e.g. translocations and ring formations) is observed in many irradiated cells (Fig. 17.3). Because these events appear to correlate radiation-induced cell killing, such damage is considered an important aspect of the radiation-induced effects in many cells. Furthermore, chromosome damage may be a very sensitive indicator of low-dose/environmental radiation exposure in an individual.

RECOVERY, DNA DAMAGE REPAIR AND DAMAGE SIGNALLING

Recovery

Much of the DNA damage induced in cells is subject to repair (see later), with initial evidence coming from recovery studies, such as split dose and delayed plating experiments. For the former, the effect of a dose of radiation was observed to be less if it is split into two fractions delivered a few hours apart and this was attributed to the sublethal damage recovery (SLDR) or Elkind repair. For the latter, it was observed that cells irradiated in a nongrowing state, and left in this state for increasing periods of time, showed enhanced survival. This has been termed potentially lethal damage recovery (PLDR). Both SLDR and PLDR are practical definitions, in that they reflect the decrease in cell kill when RT is prolonged using lower dose rates or is fractionated (SLDR) or delivered to a tissue in a nonproliferative state (PLDR). Both are believed to have a basis in DNA repair capacity, although there is some evidence that they do not reflect the same repair processes. It has been suggested that some resistant tumours owe their resistance to substantial PLDR, although this is controversial.

Double-Strand Break Repair and Damage Signalling

One of several DNA repair pathways (Table 17.2), mostly alone but potentially in combination, repairs each of the types of radiation-induced DNA damage. Of particular significance to the deleterious biological effects of radiation is the repair of DNA DSBs. Consequently, intricate damage response pathways have evolved to repair DSBs. Two principal DSB repair pathways that employ mostly separate protein complexes have been recognised: homologous recombination repair (HRR) (Fig. 17.4A) and non-homologous end-joining (NHEJ) (see Fig. 17.4B). Briefly, DSB repair by HRR requires an undamaged template molecule that contains a homologous DNA sequence, typically on the sister chromatid found in the S and G2 phases of the cell cycle, during which the genome is being duplicated (S phase) or has been duplicated (G2 phase). This form of DNA repair is error free but takes longer than NHEJ. In contrast, NHEJ of two double-stranded DNA ends, which may occur in all phases of the cell cycle, does not require an undamaged partner and does not rely on extensive homologies between the recombining ends. It is likely that the balance between NHEJ and HRR in the removal of DSBs depends on the type and location of the lesion. Of note, however, is that NHEJ, unlike HRR, may rejoin the wrong ends to generate translocations (i.e. has reduced fidelity of repair) and may not restore the original DNA sequence if sequence information is lost from both DNA strand ends. Still, NHEJ is considered to be the dominant DSB repair pathway in mammalian cells. Further studies have uncovered additional mechanisms of DSB rejoining that use end resection and microhomology-mediated end-joining and so generate deletions. One such process is alternative NHEJ (Alt-NHEJ), which occurs predominantly when immediate NHEJ is compromised.

Both NHEJ and HR DSB repair are facilitated by the sequential recruitment and assembly of a variety of DNA repair proteins and co-factors to the sites of DNA damage in a highly choreographed process (see Figs 17.4A and B). Patterns are now emerging that allowed for the recognition of critical molecules and pathways linking DNA damage and DNA damage repair to classical outcomes of radiation exposure and pointing the way towards targets for improved outcome. Many cancers have known DNA damage repair (HHR) and/or DNA damage response (p53) deficiencies but survive high levels of treatment-induced DNA damage via alternate/back-up pathways; however the selective targeting/inhibition of these alternate/back-up pathways, via inhibitors of specific repair enzymes or response mediators, renders the cells highly sensitive. This is the concept of synthetic lethality, with for example poly ADP ribose polymerase (PARP) inhibitors of DNA single-strand break repair significantly enhancing cytotoxicity in BRCA/HRR deficient cells; several PARP inhibitors are now in clinical trials in combination with RT.

An ongoing question, which is now the focus of extensive research, is the extent to which variation in the level of expression/activity of DNA repair enzymes plus enzymes and proteins involved in downstream signalling influences the outcome of RT. Given the highly ordered nature of the described protein machines, small structural changes introduced by single amino-acid changes in individual proteins may alter the activity of the complex significantly. Indeed, there is increasing evidence that mild reductions in DNA repair capacity, assumed to be the consequence of common genetic variation in the human population (polymorphisms), affect cancer predisposition and, by inference, may modulate the response to radiation treatment as well.

Epigenetic Radiation Signalling Mechanisms

Although, traditionally, nuclear DNA has been considered to be the key target for the biological effects of ionising radiation, numerous studies

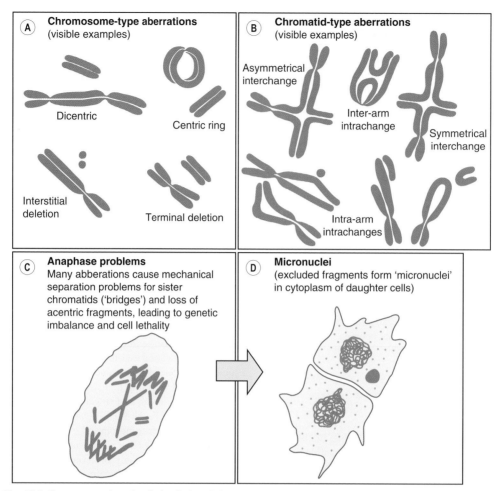

Fig. 17.3 Some examples of radiation-induced chromosomal structural changes, solid stained. (A) *Chromatid-type* aberrations—all breaks and rejoins affect both sister chromatids at the same locus. Only forms that produce acentric fragments are visible with solid staining. However, there is much hidden damage present, some of which is transmitted to future cell generations. (B) *Chromatid-type* aberrations—all breaks and rejoins affect only one of the sister chromatids at any one locus. Compared with chromosome-type changes, many more forms are visible with solid staining, but hidden damage still occurs. The observed frequencies always vary with postirradiation sampling time, so there is never a fixed yield to set against a given exposure dose. Ionising radiation can produce both types; the type recovered at first postirradiation division depends upon the duplication status of the target chromatin, with chromosome types arising from prereplicated chromatin. (C) Many forms lead to mechanical separation problems at anaphase ('intercell bridges') and acentric fragments are usually excluded from the daughter nuclei, leading to 'micronuclei' in their cytoplasm. (D) The exclusion of any visible fragment means the loss of many megabases of DNA. These bridges and fragments are the primary cause of cell lethality and genetic imbalance. (Courtesy of Dr. John Savage.)

TABLE 17.2   Pathways Involved in the Repair of DNA Damage

Repair Pathway	Type of Lesion	Involved in Radio-Sensitivity?
Base excision repair (BER)	Base damage, abasic site, single-strand base	Yes
Homologous recombination repair (HRR)	Double-strand break	Yes
Nonhomologous end joining (NHEJ)	Double-strand break	Yes
Nucleotide excision repair (NER)	Cross links, dimers, bulky adducts	?
Transcription coupled repair (TCR)	Base damage, dimers, bulky adducts	?
Mismatch repair (MMR)	Mismatched bases	?

From Steel 2002, with permission of Hodder Education.

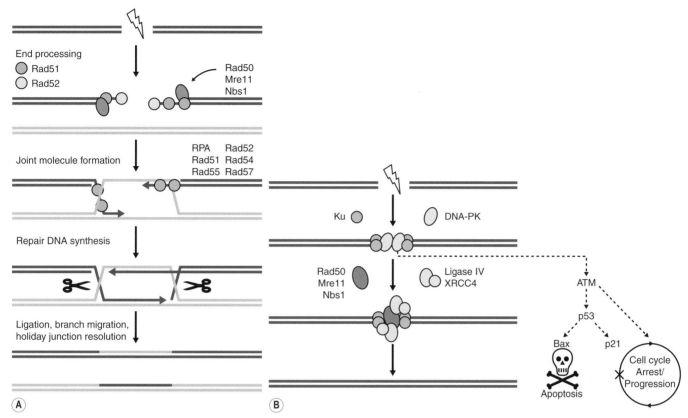

Fig. 17.4 DNA double-strand break repair; (A) homologous recombination repair (HRR) and (B) nonhomologous end-joining (NHEJ). NHEJ is potentially error prone and occasionally may rejoin the wrong ends (particularly at high doses) to give translocations. HRR uses a nondamaged homologous template and is therefore considered error free.

have revealed several nongenomic epigenetic targets that influence a cell's response to ionising radiation. Radiation-induced damage to cytoplasmic, mitochondrial and membrane structures; changes in redox balance; and protease activity have all now been suggested to mediate cellular responses to ionising radiation. These include ceramide production from plasma membrane-derived sphingomyelin and activation of numerous signalling pathways including inflammatory-type pathways, mediated by proinflammatory cytokines, for example, tumour necrosis factor α (TNF-α) and cytokine IL-1, and other cytokines and cytokine receptors, plus cell adhesion molecules and proteases/antiproteases. These responses play an important role in tissue recovery and remodelling following irradiation (see later). Another example of the epigenetic radiation-induced signalling includes expression of epidermal growth factor receptor (EGFR), which has a prosurvival effect for the cancer cell. Pharmacological inhibition of this pathway leading to cell sensitisation can be achieved with EGFR-binding antibodies or small molecule inhibitors of the EGFR tyrosine kinase, for example, gefitinib (Iressa) and erlotinib, OSI 774 (Tarceva).

Another factor to consider is the bystander effect, an intercellular signalling pathway now described in several studies. These responses appear to be cell-type dependent, and they consist of broad cellular changes including gene activation, induction of genomic instability, differentiation and changes in apoptotic potential. This appears to be mediated, at least in part, by diffusible substances, because the effect occurs when bystander cells are physically separated from the irradiated cells. Although the diffusible substance remains to be identified,

contenders include nitric oxide and/or cytokines being released to mediate membrane-dependent signalling events and possibly even exosomes; cell-derived vesicles that are present in many and perhaps all eukaryotic fluids, including blood exosomes secreted from tumour cells, which can deliver signals to surrounding cells and have been shown to regulate myofibroblast differentiation. Consequently, the entire tumour microenvironment may need to be taken into account when considering the consequences of cancer cell irradiation.

RADIATION-INDUCED CELL KILLING

As already mentioned, the objective of RT is to kill cancer cells while limiting damage to the surrounding normal tissue and this is achieved in part by exploiting the differences in the response of tumour and normal tissue to irradiation. One of the best known and most studied differences between tumour and normal tissue is the manifestation of hypoxia in tumours.

Tumour Hypoxia, Oxygen Effect and Reoxygenation

To grow, solid tumours need to develop their own blood supply through the process of angiogenesis. However, the formation of this neovasculature tends to shadow tumour growth; consequently, the nutrient and oxygen demands of a growing tumour can exceed the capacity of the host's blood supply. Furthermore, the chaotic nature of tumour vasculature coupled with the limited diffusion of oxygen in a highly proliferating tumour (see later) results in areas of chronic and sustained hypoxia and nutrient deprivation. In addition, areas of acute reversible hypoxia are also found which may be the result of physiological defects in the new vessels (leading to temporary closure of blood vessels), transient flow instability or changes in fluid pressure.

The relevance of hypoxia to the radiation treatment of cancer stems from laboratory studies that have demonstrated that cells irradiated in the absence of oxygen are considerably more resistant to the lethal effects of radiation than those irradiated in oxygen (Fig. 17.5). This is partly because of molecular oxygen reacting with the induced DNA radicals to produce chemically irreparable peroxy radicals (Fig. 17.6A). Thus, in effect, oxic cells suffer more DNA damage. The degree of sensitisation by oxygen in often quoted as an *oxygen enhancement ratio* (OER), which is the ratio of doses needed to produce a given biological effect in the presence and absence of oxygen (see Fig. 17.5). For most cells and tissues, the OER has a value of around 2.0 to 3 (*ca.* 2 at clinically relevant doses).

Numerous studies have linked hypoxia to poor RT outcome. The number of hypoxic cells has been shown to be an important factor following the irradiation of human tumours. This has been shown by direct and indirect clinical studies. One of the most important studies was by Tomlinson and Gray in 1955. They examined sections of human bronchogenic carcinoma specimens and showed that there were cords of viable cells close to blood vessels. By contrast, 150 to 180 μm from blood vessels there were areas of necrosis. The width of the viable tissue (150–180 μm) was equal to the calculated diffusion distance of oxygen from blood vessels, beyond which cells were unable to survive. They postulated that radio-resistant hypoxic cells were present within the

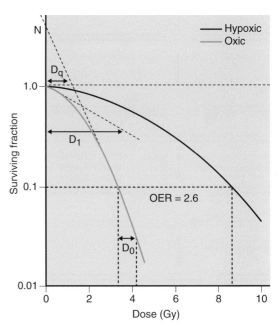

Fig. 17.5 Survival curves (and derived measures) for mammalian cells exposed to low linear energy transfer radiation under oxic or hypoxic conditions. Because the initial and final slopes depend on the presence of oxygen, the oxygen enhancement ratio is 2.5 to 3.0 for high dose-related effects (2.6 for 10% survival in the figure) but is typically less for lower dose-related effects. (From McBride, Dougherty and Milas 2002, with permission of John Wiley & Sons.)

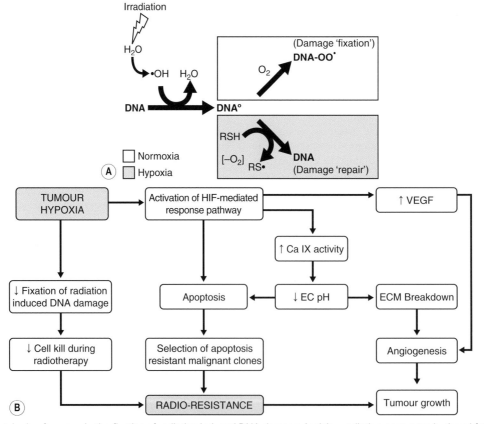

Fig. 17.6 (A) The pivotal role of oxygen in the fixation of radiation-induced DNA damage. Ionising radiation generates hydroxyl free radicals ($^{\bullet}$OH) that lead to the formation of DNA-centreed radicals (DNA$^{\bullet}$). In the presence of oxygen, this damage becomes fixed. However, under hypoxic conditions, endogenous thiols (RSH) are able chemically to repair this damage (by donating hydrogen), effectively contributing to radio-resistance. (B) Schematic diagram showing the role of hypoxia in causing radio-resistance. In addition to its physical effects on the 'fixation' of radiogenic DNA damage, hypoxia triggers specific patterns of gene expression, mediated by HIF-1α. Ca IX is pivotal in this response, causing acidification of the extracellular space, promoting extracellular matrix breakdown and apoptosis which, in turn, may provide a selective pressure favoring apoptosis-resistant subclones.

areas of necrosis. It is possible to measure oxygen tensions in accessible tumours, such as carcinoma of cervix, by directly inserting Eppendorf electrodes into the tumour. The degree of hypoxia within tumours has been correlated to clinical outcome; tumours with large areas of hypoxia tend to persist after RT, whereas those tumours that are better oxygenated are more likely to be controlled.

In addition to its effects on DNA damage, laboratory studies have shown that hypoxia can also trigger genetic mechanisms that may give tumour cells additional survival advantages. Hypoxia induces the expression of a number of genes, in particular genetic programs that are under the control of hypoxia inducible factor 1 (HIF-1). HIF-1 is recognised as a key mediator of gene expression in hypoxic tumours. The range of its downstream target genes is extensive. Some of these (i.e. vascular endothelial growth factor (VEGF), erythropoietin and TNF-α) are clearly aimed at increasing angiogenesis and oxygen delivery, so driving tumour growth. HIF-1–regulated mechanisms also control the acidity of tumour tissue and may further enhance tumour growth and radio resistance. Importantly, hypoxia can induce apoptosis by a mechanism dependent on a drop in extracellular pH. Although, intuitively, this process would be expected to reduce the tumour cell population, it can in fact provide a selective pressure for the emergence of apoptotic-resistant subclones (see Fig. 17.6B). In this way, hypoxia may select for cells with p53 mutations (because cells expressing wild-type p53 tend to undergo apoptosis more readily) and these tumours will have an antiapoptotic, more malignant phenotype. For these reasons, large areas of hypoxia may be a marker of an intrinsically more aggressive tumour; indeed, hypoxic cervical cancers have a poorer prognosis than well-oxygenated tumours when treated with surgery.

Cells that are initially hypoxic may become more oxygenated during a fractionated course of RT. Following a fraction of RT, more of the radio-sensitive aerobic cells in a tumour will be killed and the surviving fraction will be more hypoxic. If sufficient time is allowed before the next fraction of radiation, some of the tumour cells will oxygenate through the process of reoxygenation and, if this is efficient, the presence of hypoxic cells will not overtly affect the response of the tumour. However, the speed of reoxygenation varies widely, occurring within a few hours in some tumours and several days in others.

To reduce the number of hypoxic cells in a tumour, in the past, patients have been irradiated in hyperbaric oxygen chambers breathing oxygen at three atmospheres pressure. Breathing in hyperbaric oxygen has been shown to be advantageous in some tumours (locally advanced head and neck cancer) but not in others (cervical cancer). However, because of the dangers of fire, explosion and fits within the hyperbaric oxygen chamber, this treatment has fallen into disrepute.

A class of electron-affinic drugs that mimics the damage-fixating radio-sensitising effects of oxygen, the nitroimidazoles, were evaluated as radio sensitisers. It was postulated that such agents would diffuse out of the tumour blood supply and, unlike oxygen, which is rapidly metabolised by tumour cells, would be able to diffuse further and reach the more distant hypoxic cells, and thus sensitise them. The drug misonidazole produced impressive results in the treatment of mouse tumours, but neurotoxicity prevented this drug from being of clinical value in patients. Nimorazole has been shown to increase the locoregional control in patients with advanced head and neck cancer in a Danish study, but this drug is not in widespread use. However, reduction in the toxicity of the sensitising compounds and the ability to identify tumours with significant hypoxic fractions has restored faith in the potential for this approach. One potentially fruitful opportunity for further development in this area centres on the recognition that cells can react to hypoxia by switching on specific genes, that is, glucose transporter 1 (GLUT-1) and carbonic anhydrase 9 (CA 9). This will not only allow the identification of hypoxic cells but may allow the specific targeting of

hypoxic cells in gene therapy approaches. In addition, the use of drugs that are specifically activated in hypoxic areas, that is, tirapazamine (SR4233) and AQ4N, have also been studied. Intuitively, such approaches will be more beneficial to patients with hypoxic tumours, necessitating the use of biomarkers that reflect oxygenation status. Tissue biomarkers have shown utility in many studies as have markers of gene expression (see later). Further significant advances have been made in the noninvasive measurement of tumour hypoxia with positron emission tomography, magnetic resonance imaging and other imaging modalities.

The Cell Cycle and Sensitivity to Irradiation

The radio sensitivity of cells varies throughout the cell cycle. Most cells are more vulnerable in the G2/M phase of the cell cycle (because the cells have less time to repair radiation-induced damage before the cells divide) and least vulnerable in late S-phase (possibly attributed to an increased opportunity for homologous recombination). Normally, within the tumour, individual cells are in different phases of the cell cycle. If their cell division could be synchronised in some way so they would be in a sensitive phase of the cell cycle during treatment, this would increase the effectiveness of RT. Although it is possible to synchronise the population of cells in culture, it has not proved possible to do so in clinical practice. A number of drugs have been used to try to produce a cell cycle block leading to increased killing by radiation by synchronisation. A typical example is hydroxyurea, which produces a late G2/M phase block. Hydroxyurea combined with radiation has been used to treat cervical cancer without any improvement in survival.

Patterns of Cell Death After Irradiation

Historically, radiation has been considered to kill cells largely by means of a mitotic cell death in which proliferating cells undergo a general breakdown (i.e. necrosis, see later) when they attempt to divide with radiation-damaged chromosomes. This holds true for many cells but it is clear that some cells, notably those of some normal tissues, die via the morphologically distinct mechanism of apoptosis. The differences between apoptotic and necrotic cells are listed in Table 17.3. Cells lethally injured by radiation typically execute one or more divisions before dying. The number of divisions depends on the size of the radiation dose but after a dose of 2 Gy, two or three attempts to divide may be made. The progeny of these cells may all die or a proportion may survive to contribute to the reproductive (clonogenic) pool. In the *interphase death* process, whereby cells die before they divide, cells die 2 to 6 hours after irradiation. These tend to be radio-sensitive cells such as lymphocytes, spermatogonia and hair follicles and only relatively low doses of radiation are required.

Apoptosis is an important mechanism of normal tissue homeostasis and is a form of programmed cell death. It is a mechanism for eliminating cells that have sustained high levels of potentially deleterious,

TABLE 17.3 A Comparison of Some of the Morphological Features of Apoptosis and Necrosis

Necrosis	Apoptosis
Cells swell	Cells shrink
Mitochondria dilate and other organelles dissolve	Organelles retain definition for a long time
Plasma membranes rupture	Cells dissociate from surrounding cells
Nuclear changes unremarkable	Chromatin condensation and regular DNA degradation

irreversible damage. It is now recognised as being the outcome of a sequence of biochemical signals, usually requiring the involvement of p53 gene products that ultimately result in the activation of a series of enzymes (caspases) that degrade cellular proteins and DNA endonucleases that cut DNA in regularly repeated regions that are not protected by nucleosomal proteins. The latter results in the fragmentation of DNA into multiples of 80 to 100 base pairs which produces a characteristic ladder pattern when the DNA is separated in an agarose gel. The significance of this is that apoptosis is under specific genetic control and, therefore, susceptibility to radiation-induced apoptosis may be amenable to manipulation. Apoptotic cells undergo phagocytosis by neighbouring cells and inflammation is not induced. Within a few hours there is no trace of the dead cell. For this reason, apoptosis was underestimated in the past as a source of cellular loss. The frequency by which cells undergo apoptosis varies in different tumour types. For example, lymphomas have a high incidence of both spontaneous and treatment-induced apoptosis, whereas high-grade gliomas do not.

Necrosis is a pathological process that is not a component of normal tissue haemostasis and may occur in tumours because of prolonged nutrient and oxic deprivation. This involves the loss of membrane integrity and an increase in cell size with the release of lysosomal enzymes with a subsequent inflammatory response. Necrosis can follow vascular injury, changes in pattern of perfusion through the tumour or may be the mode of death of cells that lack an adequate apoptotic pathway.

Models of Radiation Cell Survival

Because radiation-induced cell killing is exponential rather than arithmetic in nature, it is traditionally illustrated as the logarithm of survival plotted against linear dose. A typical survival curve produced by low LET radiation (x- or γ-rays) is shown in Fig. 17.5. There are two components to this curve. First, there is an initial slope (designated D_1) and shoulder, then at higher doses the curve becomes steeper and straighter as survival decreases exponentially with dose. Cell killing is measured in the exponential part of the curve by using the value D_0, which is the dose sufficient to reduce the survival fraction by 37% (1/e) and in doing so the radiation induces on average one lethal event per cell. The size of the shoulder is regarded as giving an indication of the repair capacity of the cell and can be quantified by the quasi-threshold dose D_q.

There have been several mathematical models developed to describe cell survival curves, including the multitarget equation, the multitarget with single hit equation and the linear quadratic equation. The oldest, the multitarget theory, presumed that the cell contained a number of critical targets all of which have to be inactivated to bring about lethality. However, studies with human tumour cells indicate that the initial shoulder is not absolutely flat, so the simple multitarget equation is not appropriate. The linear quadratic model is a better description of cell killing, particularly at lower dose. This assumes that radiation can produce both nonrecoverable and repairable lesions. Nonrepairable damage is referred to as the alpha component (represented as αD on a logarithmic scale) and is considered induced linearly by 'single hit' mechanisms, whereas the beta component ($βD^2$) describes the quadratic cell inactivation by the accumulation and possible interaction of repairable damage induced by multiple hits. When plotting cell survival, alpha-type damage is represented by a straight line and beta damage by a curve (Fig. 17.7). The ratio of alpha-beta (α/β) is the dose at which single and multi-hit mechanisms contribute equally to cell killing; that is $αD = βD^2$.

The α/β ratio is used to define survival curve characteristics and classify cellular and tissue responses to RT. Acute/early responding tissues, which express radiation damage days or weeks after irradiation, have high α/β values of 7 to 20 Gy (typically around 10 Gy) (see

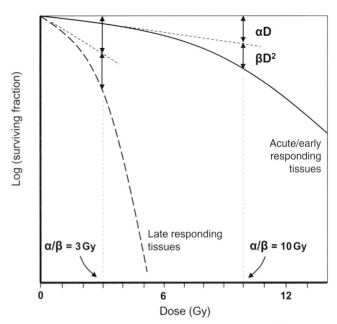

Fig. 17.7 Dose-response relationships for early- and late-responding tissues. The relationship for late-responding tissues is more curved than for early-responding tissues, which in the linear-quadratic formula translates into a larger α/β ratio for early rather than for late effects.

Fig. 17.7). Well-oxygenated tumours have even higher ratios. In contrast, late responding tissues, which express radiation damage months to years after RT, have low α/β values of between 0.5 and 6 Gy (typically ≈3 Gy). The survival curves of cells in late responding tissues are significantly more curved than those with high α/β ratios. Late responding tissues, such as the spinal cord, are much more sensitive to changes in fraction size than acute responding tissues, such as skin or the mucosa of the mouth. Generally, tumours have α/β ratios similar to acute responding tissues.

Two clinically important exceptions are breast and prostate cancer. In the case of both tumour types larger treatment doses per fraction (hypofractionation) will deliver a higher biological dose to the tumour while reducing or maintaining the same biological dose to normal tissues compared with a standard fraction of 2 Gy. The α/β ratio in prostate cancer has been estimated to be as low as 1.5. In a trial using intensity modulated RT (IMRT) (the CHHiP trial), a regimen of 60 Gy in 20 fractions was shown to produce slightly better clinical or biochemical freedom from prostate cancer recurrence at 5 years (90.6% vs 88.3%) compared with 74 Gy in 37 fractions, with a very similar incidence of late effects. A 2017 metaanalysis of three conventional versus hypofractionated noninferiority trials in 5484 men with prostate cancer has shown a statistically significant improved disease-free survival (hazard ratio 0.869 95%, confidence interval 0.66–1.07, P = .047) without any increase in late toxicity. The ultimate form of hypofractionated RT is the current PACE trial where men suffering from low/intermediate risk of prostate cancer are being treated stereotactically with a dose of 36.25 Gy given in 5 fractions in a week.

Breast cancer in many cases has a low α/β ratio. The START trials have shown a schedule of 40 Gy in 15 fractions was as effective as 50 Gy in 25 fractions with less breast shrinkage, telangiectasia, fibrosis and breast oedema.

The importance of these values is that they can be used to calculate isoeffect relationships in RT, and calculations of parameters like the biologically effective dose (BED) are important when manipulating fractionation regimens. The BED, in effect, is the dose required to produce a given biological effect when the radiation is given as an infinitely large number of very small fractions or as a single dose at extremely low-dose rate. For a given treatment, the BED can be calculated if the α/β ratio of the dose-limiting tissue and the tolerance dose for a given fractionation regimen are known. Using the BED, the relationship between tolerance dose and dose per fraction can be worked out for new fractionation regimens. Attempts to introduce biological mechanisms into the models has led to the lethal, potentially lethal damage and repair saturation models, although the actual mechanisms are rudimentary and poorly defined.

RADIATION EFFECTS IN NORMAL AND MALIGNANT TISSUE

As mentioned previously, both DNA and epigenetic sites are important initiators of radiation-induced signalling responses following exposure. Indeed, many of the effects seen at the tissue level in the clinic (i.e. recovery and remodelling) are the manifestation of these pathways. Cellular responses to irradiation include induction of early response genes (e.g. V-jun avian sarcoma virus 17 oncogene homologue (JUN), v-fos FBJ murine osteosarcoma viral oncogene homologue (FOS) and early growth response 1 (EGR1)), which can bind to specific DNA sequences to modulate the expression of other genes. Also, intermediate and late genes are induced, such as TNF-α, platelet-derived growth factor (PDGF), transforming growth factor (TGF) β and fibroblast growth factor 2 (basic) (bFGF), which are involved in premature terminal differentiation of fibroblasts by ionising radiation and therefore mediate fibrosis as a late response to RT. In addition, a growing body of evidence appears to support the hypothesis that chronic oxidative stress serves to drive the progression of radiation-induced late effects. Some of the pathways that mediate these effects are now revealed, but their importance is still the subject of current debate and the focus of continued research. What follows is a brief description of the effects of radiation at a tissue level.

Acute Responses of Normal Tissue

Following large single x-ray treatment, such as a single fraction of 10 Gy to treat bone metastasis, cytokines and proteases, products of cell signalling and from cell killing (apoptosis and necrosis) are released from the irradiated tissue and interact with normal macrophages and lymphocytes. This may bring about erythema of treated skin within hours, oedema and may be the source of nausea and vomiting associated with RT. The acute effects of RT are normally seen in tissues with a high cellular turnover rate, such as gastrointestinal mucosa, skin, bone marrow and mucosa of the upper aerodigestive tract. These effects are usually seen after 2 to 3 weeks during a fractionated course of radical RT lasting 4 to 7 weeks.

Acute reactions are as a result of cellular loss. A good model is the acute reaction in skin, especially if the patient is treated with kilovoltage radiation. After about 14 days, hair loss (epilation) occurs. This is followed by erythema. If the dose is high enough this may be followed by dry desquamation. As the skin is shed there is a serous exudate, which is referred to as moist desquamation. Healing depends on initial recovery of the skin stem cells, which usually regenerate most of their number before differentiating to restore function. This process is normally complete within a few weeks. A similar effect is seen within the mucosa of the upper aerodigestive tract. Cells are lost from the mucosa following RT leading to a characteristic radiation reaction. Initially, there is erythema of the mucosa followed by mucosal cell loss. This denuded area is covered by a white membrane containing inflammatory exudate and dead cells and is usually white in colour. In the normal mucosa, only

about 15% of stem cells are undergoing cellular division to replace normal cell loss. The majority are in the resting phase (G0) of the cell cycle. After about 10 to 12 days into a standard course of RT, virtually all surviving stem cells are dividing to replace cells loss from RT. Usually within a few weeks of completing a standard dose of RT the mucosa has healed, but if a very high dose has been given sufficiently to destroy the stem cell pool, the patient may be left with a persisting area of ulceration within the treated area.

Subacute Reactions of Normal Tissue

Some tissues, such as neural tissue, have a much longer normal turnover time than skin or oral mucosa. The effects of radiation may not be seen until several months after treatment. A typical example is Lhermitte syndrome following irradiation of the spinal cord. A few weeks after treatment the patient complains of electric shocks radiating down to fingers and toes especially if they flex their neck. This is as a result of partial temporary demyelination of the spinal cord. There is often an interval of 9 to 18 months before late effects are seen in cell populations with a slow rate of proliferation such as nervous tissue, kidney, blood vessels, subcutaneous tissue and bone or cartilage. Initially, damage to the slowly proliferating vascular endothelium was thought to be the common cellular injury linking most late effects. Undoubtedly, damage to blood vessels is important but, for example, with late demyelination of the brain there is also loss of oligodendrocytes and subsequently neurons as well as damage to small blood vessels. Similarly, in the kidney, there is loss of renal tubular cells as well as vascular injury. In late responding tissues, such as jejunal mucosa, cell loss is rapid and there may be evidence of radiation-induced cell loss within 24 hours of irradiation. By contrast, in the kidney there may be no histological evidence of cell depletion for many months after RT. If a high enough radiation dose has been given to destroy all the clonogenic tubular cells, the tubules will not regenerate. If one or more tubular clonogenic cells per nephron survives, the tubule may well regenerate over several months.

The Effect of Radiotherapy on Tissues

All tissues have different cellular populations within them and may undergo both acute and late damage. A typical example is the effects on skin and subcutaneous tissue. If the radiation dose is moderate, any acute reaction may settle without any late effects. However, if there has been marked depletion of the epidermal proliferating cell compartment, the skin may be thin (atrophic) and white owing to loss of pigment-producing cells. There may also be permanent loss of hair. The tissues of the dermis may be replaced with fibrous tissue leading to thickening of the subcutaneous tissues and loss of elasticity. The thickening of tissues around joints, such as the shoulder, may lead to marked reduction in movement. The walls of arteries may be replaced by fibrous tissue leading to narrowing of the lumen and thrombosis. This is often followed by compensating dilation of skin capillaries leading to telangiectasia of the skin. These red blood vessels on the skin surface may be very disfiguring. Ultimately, perhaps following a minor insult such a trauma or infection, the skin may necrose leading to a nonhealing ulcer.

The Tolerance of Normal Tissues

The dose that can be given to tumours is limited by the tolerance of normal tissues. The tolerance depends on the overall radiation dose, fraction size and the time between fractions. Overall treatment time and the volume irradiated are lesser factors, but the type of radiation used is also very important. Megavoltage x-rays spare the skin compared with kilovoltage (250–300 kV). Absorption in bone and cartilage is also much less with megavoltage x-rays and there is less risk of necrosis. The tolerance of organs that have rapidly proliferating cells may be quite low. The tolerance of both lungs to megavoltage RT is 20 Gy given in 15 fractions over 3 weeks. The kidney has a similar tolerance. The tolerance of the whole liver is 25 Gy given again over 3 weeks. The incidence of radiation myelitis of the spinal cord is 1% to 5% with doses of 50 to 54 Gy given in 1.8 or 2 Gy fractions.

By and large, acute reactions settle with simple medical measures (see Chapter 34). It is the late effects that are most feared as target organ damage can be severe and capacity for recovery is usually small. Such injuries are very difficult to treat surgically as the blood supply to heavily irradiated tissues is very poor. The frequency of late effects depends upon the site and the stage of the tumour. The aim of RT following lumpectomy for breast cancer is local control of the breast cancer plus a cosmetically acceptable breast. The late serious complication rate following breast irradiation should be very small (less than 0.5%). In early larynx cancer, the incidence of serious necrosis is only 1% to 2%. In a national audit in 2010 of patients treated with chemoradiotherapy or RT in UK centres in 2001–2002, for locally advanced cervix cancer, the grade 3/4 late complication rate was 8% (RT) and 10% (chemoradiotherapy). The EMBRACE trial has shown the incidence of complications from cervix RT can be reduced by the use of IMRT and image-guided brachytherapy.

Retreatment

Conventional wisdom is that heavily irradiated tissue will not tolerate a retreatment. Previous high-dose irradiation may limit the tolerance of the tissue to retreatment but, in some cases, further RT is possible. Factors governing the possibility of further therapy include the amount of cell depletion, the time elapsed since the previous treatment and the dose given and fraction size used. Clinical examination is sometimes extremely useful to decide whether the patient can be retreated. If the skin has marked late changes with extensive subcutaneous fibrosis, retreatment may well be impossible. Similarly, radiological investigations may show evidence of late radiation damage, such as pulmonary fibrosis, which may preclude further radiation treatment. Primate studies have shown a modest but significant repair of radiation damage of the spinal cord. There seems to be about a 40% recovery in radiation tolerance following a dose of 44 Gy given in 2.2 fractions by 2 years after treatment. When retreating a tumour, the volume of normal tissue should be kept to a minimum and fraction sizes should not exceed 2 Gy with a total cumulative EQD2 (equivalent dose as 2-Gy fractions) of about 100 Gy. Stereotactic retreatments may allow a higher dose to be given.

Response of Tumours to Radiation

Tumours may have numerous mitoses visible on histological examination but they only grow slowly. A classic example is the slow-growing basal cell carcinoma of skin. In this tumour, virtually all cells produced following cell division are lost by apoptosis and necrosis and only a small number of the progeny of the dividing tumour adds to the tumour mass. In most carcinomas, over 90% of cells are lost in this way and are referred to as the cell loss factor. The potential volume doubling time (i.e. the time to go from a volume of 2 to 4 cm^3) in many tumours is in the order of 60 days. Without cell loss, tumours have the potential to grow much faster than this. Mitotic count, S-phase count and bromodeoxyuridine labelling index would suggest that, in many tumours, they have a potential doubling time of 3 to 8 days. Although the growth potential of many tumours is extremely rapid, owing to the high cell loss factor, in practice they grow much more slowly.

Cell loss factor may influence the rate of tumour regression during RT. Tumours with a high spontaneous cell loss factor will regress more rapidly during therapy regardless of whether the tumour was growing

quickly or slowly before treatment. However, what will govern ultimate outcome is the number of clonogenic tumour cells surviving the radiation treatment. Classically, only one clonogenic cell needs to survive; the tumour will then regrow. Many squamous cancers have high loss fractions and regress quickly. By contrast, the cell loss factor in prostatic cancer is much smaller and these tumours shrink much more slowly after a lethal dose of radiation.

The growth fraction is the number of cells that are in cycle. In solid tumours, these are usually less than 20% of the cells. Tumours with a high growth fraction may shrink more rapidly than those with a smaller growth fraction; however, unless all clonogens are sterilised, these tumours may also rapidly regrow. Tumour growth fraction and repopulation may be increased following radiation treatment. Experiments have shown that there can be rapid regrowth of the clonogenic population of the tumour even while the tumour mass is regressing.

Overall Treatment Time

Local control in cervix cancer has been shown to decrease if overall treatment time (external beam plus brachytherapy) exceeds 56 days. This is because of repopulation of tumour cells during RT. Data, particularly from the Danish DAHANCA studies where patients with head and neck cancer were treated on 5 or 6 days in a week, have shown a dose of 0.6 Gy per day is required to compensate for tumour repopulation between fractions, including weekend breaks. Reducing overall treatment time to 3 weeks may be one reason why 40 Gy in 15 fractions in the START trial was as effective as 50 Gy in 25 fractions. Gaps in RT treatment schedules should be avoided if possible, especially in patients with rapidly proliferating tumours such as head and neck cancer.

Modification of Fractionation Patterns

Repopulation during fractionated treatment is one reason why tumours persist after RT. This may be overcome by giving two or three treatments daily. A fraction size of less than 2 Gy is normally given to reduce the late effects in tissues, although acute reactions may be enhanced. Interfraction intervals should be as long as possible, but there should be at least 6 hours between treatments. The use of fraction sizes less than 2 Gy is usually referred to as hyperfractionation, and treatment schedules shorter than standard treatments are usually called accelerated treatment. Patients with well- or moderately well-differentiated tumours seem to have the greatest capacity for repopulation during RT and seem to be the group most likely to benefit from accelerated treatment as shown in the CHART trials.

OTHER RADIATION MODALITIES

Heavy Particle Radiotherapy

Neutrons were perceived as a solution to the hypoxic cell problem as, in experimental systems, hypoxic cells were more sensitive to neutrons than conventional x- or γ-rays. However, in practice, neutron irradiation was found to be no more effective than conventional fractionated photon RT. Moreover, many trials had to be abandoned because of the severity of severe late effects associated with neutrons. This treatment is no longer used.

By contrast, treatment with protons is intuitively more promising. The relative biological effect of protons is similar to x-rays and the physical characteristics of a proton beam has potential marked depth dose advantage in the treatment of some tumours. The dose-depth curve for protons in tissue is entirely different to those of photons (x- and γ-rays). Protons increase their rate of energy deposition as they slow down with increasing penetration finally stopping and releasing an intense burst of ionisation called the *Bragg peak*. The beam has sharp edges with little side scatter, and the dose falls to zero after the Bragg peak at the end of the particles' range. By selecting proton beams of a suitable proton energy, it is possible to release most of the proton's energy within the tumour if the Bragg peak is superimposed over the tumour-bearing area.

Drug–Radiotherapy Combinations

Chemoradiotherapy (CRT, CRTx) is the combination of chemotherapy and RT to treat cancer. Chemoradiation can be concurrent (together) or sequential (one after the other). The chemotherapy component can be or include a radio-sensitising agent. Chemoradiotherapy as neoadjuvant therapy before surgery has been shown to be effective in various cancers. However, apart from the combination of traditional cytotoxic chemotherapy with RT, little progress has been made in identifying and defining optimal targeted therapy and RT combinations to improve the efficacy of cancer treatment. The National Cancer Research Institute Clinical and Translational Radiotherapy Research Working Group (CTRad) formed a Joint Working Group with representatives from academia, industry, patient groups and regulatory bodies to address this lack of progress and to publish recommendations for future clinical research. A consensus statement published by Sharma and colleagues makes recommendations to increase the number of novel drugs being successfully registered in combination with RT to improve clinical outcomes for patients with cancer. Such recommendations include pharmaceutical companies prioritising the evaluation of appropriate novel drug–RT combinations early in the clinical development plan of a drug to potentially improve response and survival rates, because there is a strong scientific rationale for the combination based on an understanding of mechanisms of action and a clear line of sight to registration for the combination based on clinical need.

FUTURE TRENDS (AND PITFALLS)

New Technologies

With many of the advances in RT having been realised via technologic improvements in the physical targeting of the radiation, work is continuing in this area to deliver superior instruments. IMRT is the latest form of three-dimensional conformal RT, designed to address a major limitation of conventionally delivered RT, namely, the inability to restrict the treatment beam to the tumour-bearing tissue. However, the move from conventional conformal RT to IMRT involves more fields and a larger volume of normal tissue being exposed to lower doses. In addition, the number of monitor units is increased by a factor of two to three, increasing the total body exposure, because of leakage radiation. Both factors will tend to increase the risk of second cancers, with IMRT estimated to approximately double the incidence of second malignancies compared with conventional RT from about 1% to 1.75% for patients surviving 10 years. The numbers may be even larger for longer survival (or for younger patients), but the ratio should remain the same. Image guided radiation therapy (IGRT) consists of a linear accelerator with an integrated three-dimensional volume imaging functionality. This allows an image of the tumour site with CT-like quality to be acquired and reconstructed immediately before treatment, with the patient already set up in the treatment position. Consequently, if the patient needs to be moved, the treatment table can be controlled remotely to do so. Alternatively, if the tumour is no longer where it was or has changed shape or size, then the treatment plan or conformal setting can be modified as appropriate. If the tumour is likely to move during treatment (for example a lung tumour during respiration) then appropriate margins can be set using sequential imaging. This allows the radiotherapist to address directly clinical concerns regarding organ

motion and deformation and uncertainties in repeating and maintaining the set-up of the patient, thereby inspiring clinical confidence in the practice of advanced radiation therapy techniques.

Before 2004, there were only two clinical proton therapy centres in the United States, at Loma Linda University in California and the Massachusetts General Hospital. These centres generated evidence supporting the use of protons for the treatment of childhood tumours and tumours of the skull base, still the only indications currently held to be secure. However, the simplicity of prostate cancer treatment (relative to paediatric cancers), the abundance of prostate cancer patients, and the concerns about the side effects of alternative therapies have contributed to the expansion of the numbers of centres offering protons, which currently stands at 26. However, active surveillance is becoming a mainstream form of management for many men with early prostate cancer creating the irony that this high investment therapy was being paid for by the treatment of men who needed no treatment at all. In addition, many competitive treatments such as stereotactic body radiation therapy (SBRT) (a very patient-friendly alternative to protons) and robot-assisted surgery diminished the use of proton radiation treatment, and thus the proton therapy share of the market. Indeed, U.S. insurers are now declining to pay for proton therapy for many indications, and some for all indications. The consequence of this is that many U.S. centres may have to close as a result of being fiscally unsustainable.

The future for proton therapy lies in smaller, more efficient, delivery units. Britain is building two proton centres based upon a review of need and represents a well-informed first step. In the future, new indications may be established among the more common cancers, perhaps postoperative breast treatment or in liver cancer, not just paediatrics. When that happens, Britain should expand its proton network cautiously, following the evidence and using newer single-room systems linked with high-performing academic cancer centres.

Molecular Studies

An important future aim of molecular/biologic studies in RT is to increase the therapeutic ratio to increase tumour control and/or to decrease late effects by predicting outcome on an individual basis to select the most appropriate treatment for each patient. Also, molecular/biologic studies should enable development of new combined-modality treatments such as RT and concurrent biological therapies or chemotherapy in a scientifically rational manner. The advent of 'Omic' technologies holds great promise for the development of molecular studies in RT. Gene expression arrays (cDNA and oligonucleotide arrays) allow investigation of large numbers of patients' genes and show variation in gene expression among tumours with similar histological features. In diffuse large B-cell lymphomas, there is a very different overall survival between two such groups using this assay. Genes expected to be good candidates for prediction of radio-sensitivity include DNA repair genes and genes related to cell cycle control, growth regulation, and differentiation. West and colleagues in Manchester, United Kingdom, have developed gene signatures reflecting tumour hypoxia. Such expression signatures have been developed for a number of cancers and have been validated in multiple cohorts and, where data are available, to predict benefit from giving hypoxia-modifying treatments with RT. Proteomic technologies may also have a role in investigation of radio-sensitivity as it can provide a more accurate indicator of protein function than gene expression arrays by taking into account posttranslational modifications.

In summary, radiobiology has reached a stage where specific molecular and cellular pathways and responses are being related to the various outcomes of RT. Such studies are exposing new potential targets for therapeutic manipulation of radiation responses. The well-established efficacy of RT, together with the accumulated knowledge of many decades of treatment, provides a robust platform from which to launch novel approaches to extend the usefulness and increase the efficacy of RT. Combined with the molecular evaluations of the probability of tumour cure and normal tissue complication, as well as the more precise delivery of dose, the future of radiobiology in RT research looks bright.

FURTHER READING

Books

Hall EJ, Giaccia AJ. Radiobiology for the radiologist. 7th ed. Philadelphia: Lippincott Williams & Wilkins; 2012.

Joiner M, van der Kogel A. Basic clinical radiobiology. 4th ed. London: Arnold; 2009.

Chapters in Books

Kiltie AE. Radiotherapy and molecular radiotherapy. In: Knowles MA, Selby PJ, editors. Introduction to the cellular and molecular biology of cancer. 4th ed. Oxford: Oxford University Press; 2005. p. 414–27.

McBride WH, Dougherty GJ, Milas L. Molecular mechanisms in radiotherapy. In: Alison M, editor. The cancer handbook. Hoboken: John Wiley & Sons; 2002. p. 1359–69.

Journal Reviews

Barcellous-Hoff MH, Park C, Wright EG. Radiation and the microenvironment tumorigenesis and therapy. Nat Rev Cancer. 2005;5:867–75.

Connell PP, Kron SJ, Weichselbaum RR. Relevance and irrelevance of DNA damage response to radiotherapy. DNA Repair (Amst). 2004;3:1245–51.

Sharma RA, et al. Clinical development of new drug-radiotherapy combinations. Nat Rev Clin Oncol. 2016;13:627–42.

Ward JF. Complexity of damage produced by ionizing radiation. Cold Spring Harb Symp Quant Biol. 2000;65:377–82.

Willers H, Dahm-Daphi J, Powell SN. Repair of radiation damage to DNA. Br J Cancer. 2004;90:1297–301.

Special Issues of Clinical Oncology

Muirhead R, Jones B, editors. Re-irradiation. Clin Oncol. 2018;30:65–136.

Symonds P, Jones D, editors. Advances in clinical radiobiology (part 2). Clin Oncol. 2014;26:241–308.

Symonds P, Jones D, editors. Advances in clinical radiobiology. Clin Oncol. 2013;25:567–624.

West C, Huddart R, editors. Biomarkers and imaging for precision radiotherapy. Clin Oncol. 2015;27:545–618.

18

Principles of Management of Patients With Cancer

Paul Symonds, Angela Duxbury

INTRODUCTION

The diagnosis of a malignancy is only the beginning of a cancer patient's journey and throughout this time decisions about how to best manage and care for patients have to be addressed. Before seeing the oncologist, the majority of cancer patients will have been given their diagnosis, most frequently in the outpatient department rather than a hospital ward. The importance of this event cannot be overemphasised and the manner of communicating this information is pivotally important.

When patients do meet their oncologist for the first time, the presence of a family member or friend can be helpful because the family member can provide emotional support, help in recall of the conversation and can ask supplementary questions. This can be important at a time when patients will be seeking to try to understand their condition and what the future may hold for them. There is little doubt that the majority of patients with cancer want as much information as possible. This often includes the elderly and the incurable. The first, sometimes initially unspoken, question is: 'Is it curable?' and after that, 'Is it treatable?' At some point, most want to know the options there are for treatment and the side effects of possible treatments. Absorbing this information can be traumatic and often patients cannot take in this complex web of information in one consultation. Support nurses, or other healthcare professionals who are present in the clinic can provide useful reinforcement and clarification of patients' questions. Often the oncologist needs to cover the ground more than twice.

This whole process involves relaying information that can severely alter a patient's view of their future and is challenging for the giver of the information as well as the patient. A useful guide in this process is the ten-step approach to giving bad news (Box 18.1). This model advocates good preparation, finding out what patients want to know, allowing denial and listening to concerns. It also recognises the importance of encouraging the ventilation of feelings and the important role played by relatives.

The most important decision at this time is whether the patient should be treated radically with cure as the aim of treatment. Radical treatment, however, may be associated with treatment-induced morbidity and, occasionally, mortality and it is therefore vital to ensure it is the appropriate route to be taking. Unfortunately, a number of patients will be unsuitable for a radical approach to treatment and palliation will be the appropriate option.

The next question is which is the best treatment modality or modalities for that particular patient. Clearly, the patient needs to have been fully investigated before such decisions can be taken and usually these investigations will have been carried out before referral to the oncologist. However, supplementary investigations may need to be carried out. These may include examination under anaesthesia, endoscopy and appropriate radiological investigations such as computed tomography (CT), magnetic resonance imaging (MRI) or isotope bone scans. Because the diagnosis of cancer has such possible dire implications, all patients should have histological proof of the diagnosis, if this is possible, especially if radical treatment is planned. To make appropriate management decisions, the clinician must take into account tumour and patient factors (listed later).

Frequently, the patient's management may have been discussed in a multidisciplinary team meeting (MDT) in which the patient's pathology and radiological investigations will have been reviewed. The decision is usually made about whether cure is possible and the appropriate treatment modality. However, only one or two of the treating team may have met the patient at this stage and decisions made at the MDT meeting may not survive the consultation with the patient and oncologist. When discussing treatment options, the patient's wishes are paramount. However, in practice, the majority of patients will accept the careful reasoned advice of their doctors. Very occasionally, patients ask for radical treatment when this is futile. Somewhat more frequently, such requests come from relatives. However, a doctor is not obliged to provide a treatment that they conscientiously feel is not in the patient's best interest.

FACTORS GOVERNING CLINICAL DECISIONS

Tumour Factors

Organ of Origin

The organ in which the cancer develops is an important factor affecting both outcome and treatment. Complete surgical removal of brain tumours is usually impossible, as a complete excision would normally damage vital parts of the brain, leading to either death or an unacceptable neurological deficit. Similarly, the brain is sensitive to ionising radiation and this limits the dose of radiotherapy (RT) that can be given. However, in other sites, such as the kidney, a complete organ can be removed with impunity.

Histological Type

Identification of the precise histological type of a tumour governs both treatment and prognosis. For instance, basal cell and squamous carcinomas arising from the epidermis of the skin have a good prognosis and the treatment is straightforward. By contrast, melanomas arising from pigment-producing cells (melanocytes) have a much more serious outlook.

Degree of Differentiation

The pathologist can grade the degree of differentiation. Well-differentiated tumours look like the tissue of origin and poorly differentiated tumours may look primitive and do not look like the tissue from which they arise. For instance, well-differentiated thyroid cancer has a good prognosis and is relatively easily treated by such measures as surgical excision and radioiodine. Anaplastic thyroid cancers rapidly spread and respond poorly to any treatment.

Tumour Staging

Where possible, tumours should be staged using the international T, N and M classifications. T stands for primary tumour stage, which is usually decided by the tumour size. N stands for the presence or absence of lymph node metastases, the usual method of spread in carcinomas and some sarcomas. M represents the presence or absence of distant metastases. In practice, other staging systems have been developed and are referred to in the preceding chapters.

Tumour Size

In general, the larger the tumour the lower is the chance of cure either by surgery or RT. It may not be possible to completely excise a large tumour. Similarly, a large tumour treated by RT contains more clonogenic tumour cells (cells capable of forming colonies of cells following RT) and an increased proportion of radio-resistant hypoxic cells. Stage Ib carcinoma of cervix is tumour confined to the cervix, but this stage is subdivided into stage Ib1 (<4 cm) and Ib2 (>4 cm). By and large, stage Ib1 tumours are treated by radical hysterectomy and stage Ib2 by chemoradiotherapy.

Locoregional Spread

Spread to regional lymph nodes usually indicates a poorer prognosis and the need for more aggressive therapy. Patients with squamous carcinoma of head and neck with spread to regional lymph nodes may be treated by a radical neck dissection along with primary RT or surgical excision of the affected organ. As spread to lymph nodes in breast cancer is often associated with occult distant spread, such patients usually receive adjuvant chemotherapy following surgery.

Distant Metastases

The presence of distant metastases may suggest that attempts to remove the primary tumour completely are futile, as is the case in lung cancer. However, such metastases may be chemo-sensitive and a high probability of cure may be possible. A typical case is testicular teratoma where high cure rates are seen following cisplatin-based chemotherapy.

Tumour Site

Tumour site may determine the treatment modality. For instance, the skin on the back of the hand or the shin does not tolerate RT well. There is an increased risk of skin necrosis at these sites compared with elsewhere in the body. Surgery is often the preferred treatment for basal cell or squamous carcinoma in these areas. However, small basal cell carcinomas on the eyelid are often better treated by RT than surgery.

Operability

Many factors must be taken into account before deciding to treat the patient by radical surgery. A patient may have other illnesses than cancer that may make the risks of surgery or anaesthesia extremely high (see later). The size of the tumour or involvement of adjacent structures may prevent complete removal of the cancer. The site of origin must also be taken into account together with the chance of complications following surgery and the functional result.

Removal of inguinal lymph nodes is an important part of the treatment of carcinoma of the vulva. However, groin wounds are slow to heal and may become infected, especially in elderly people. The high risk of complications may be a contraindication for this type of surgery in the very elderly. Functional and cosmetic results are extremely important in head and neck surgery. Before the decision is made to remove a cancer, it must be possible to reconstruct the appropriate part of the upper aerodigestive tract and guarantee reasonable function and cosmesis.

Pathological Examination of the Excised Tissue

At first, surgery may be planned as the sole method of treatment modality. However, pathological examination of the excised tissue may change this decision. If the pathologist finds that tumour extends to surgical margins, the chance of tumour recurrence is very high indeed. Postoperative RT may then be required. Radiation treatment may also be required depending on the degree of spread within the organ. The chance of microscopic spread to the pelvic lymph nodes is associated with the degree of differentiation of endometrial cancer and the degree of spread into the myometrium. Following simple hysterectomy, patients with poorly differentiated tumours and/or deep spread into the myometrium are often offered postoperative RT to reduce the chance of pelvic recurrence.

Patient Factors

Age

As a general rule, patients aged up to 75 years tolerate surgery or radical RT well. However, the biological age of the patient needs to be taken into account as well as the chronological age. A fit patient in their 80s will tolerate RT well, but younger patients with serious general medical conditions may find treatment side effects intolerable. Many elderly patients may have chronic medical problems, such as chronic obstructive airways disease or ischaemic heart disease. These comorbid conditions may increase the risks of surgery to an unacceptable degree. Similarly, they may affect outcome after RT. Patients with poor pulmonary function are not suitable for radical treatment for lung cancer. The lung may become fibrosed around the irradiated tumour. This will have no effect in a fit patient but the loss of even a small amount of lung function may cause respiratory failure in someone with chronic obstructive airways disease. Patients with ischaemic heart disease may have poor normal tissue perfusion. This may increase the number of radio-resistant hypoxic cells within the tumour and also affect the ability of normal tissue to repair damage following radiation treatment.

Performance status (Tables 18.1 and 18.2) provides a crude but very effective method for judging response to treatment, especially with chemotherapy. Poor performance status is associated with shorter life expectancy. Patients with performance status three (in bed more than 50% of the time) are often not suitable for radical treatment. A paradox

is that, although these patients have marked symptoms and the most to gain from chemotherapy, they are the group least likely to respond to this treatment. The highest response rates are seen in those with performance status zero or one.

Patient Preference

Patient's preference should be taken into account. For instance, Stage Ib carcinoma of cervix can be treated equally well by radical surgery or RT. By and large, younger and fitter patients are offered radical hysterectomy and older or more obese patients tend to be treated by RT. However, the individual patient may have a preference for one modality or the other.

Chance of Cure

Decision making is easy if the chance of cure is high. A typical case is a T1 larynx cancer, which carries a chance of cure better than 90%. The side effects of RT to the larynx are tolerable even in the very elderly. By and large, patients with a 30% or better chance of cure are offered radical treatment. In more advanced disease with a poorer outlook, a lot depends on the patient's age and fitness. For instance a T4 carcinoma of bladder carries a 10% to 25% chance of cure. A fit middle-aged man may be offered intensive chemotherapy before removal of the bladder and construction of an ileostomy, whereas the right treatment for an unfit, elderly man may be palliative RT to suppress symptoms from his bladder cancer.

Treatment Modality

Increasing use of multimodality treatment has rather blurred the once clear-cut rules for treatment by the various modalities.

Surgery

Surgery, traditionally, was important for establishing the diagnosis and finding the extent of spread of the cancer. Increasingly, diagnosis is made without operation using sophisticated imaging techniques such as in vivo nuclear magnetic resonance (NMR) spectroscopy or PET-CT scanning. Histological proof may be obtained by fine needle or Tru-cut biopsy. Radical surgery is still the treatment of choice for many adenocarcinomas, particularly arising in the stomach, colon, thyroid and kidney.

Palliative Surgery

Before palliative surgery, the risks and benefits to the patient need to be carefully measured and the patient's potential life expectancy needs to be taken into account. Surgery is particularly useful in dealing with obstruction of an organ. A classical case is the relief of large bowel obstruction by a colon cancer by a colostomy. However, palliative surgery may be inappropriate in patients with multiple small bowel obstructions. This is often the case in ovarian cancer where the risks of surgery outweigh the benefits. Advanced fungating breast tumours

TABLE 18.1 Karnofsky Performance Status Scale (allows patients to be classified as to their functional impairment)	
100	Normal, no complaints
90	Normal activity, minimal signs or symptoms
80	Normal activity with effort, some symptoms
70	Caring for self, unable to work
60	Needs occasional assistance but able to cater to most needs
50	Needs considerable assistance and frequent medical care
40	Disabled, needs special care
30	Severely disabled, needs hospital care
20	Very ill, in hospital, needs supportive care
10	Moribund
0	Dead

TABLE 18.2 Union for International Cancer Control Performance Status Scale	
Grade	
0	Able to carry out normal activity
1	Able to live at home with tolerable symptoms
2	Disabling symptoms, but less than 50% of the time in bed
3	Severely disabled, greater than 50% of the time in bed, but able to stand
4	Very ill, confined to bed

are much less common than they were 25 years ago, but surgery offers a rapid method of relieving the unpleasant odour and bleeding associated with such tumours. The pinning of the broken bone, which is often followed by palliative RT, may relieve pain following a pathological fracture.

Surgical methods. Traditional open operations are being replaced by less invasive key-hole techniques. Many patients with colon cancer are now treated laparoscopically. A telescope (laparoscope) connected to a video camera plus a light source is introduced through a small abdominal incision. The abdomen is distended by insufflating CO_2 gas. Instruments can be inserted through another small incision and are guided using the video camera. The advantage of this method is that there is less pain postoperatively and haemorrhage is reduced as smaller incisions are used and healing and recovery time are shortened. Disadvantages are a lack of depth perception through the laparoscope and a limited range of motion of the instruments introduced into the abdomen. In some cases, especially in advanced colon cancer, the operation may be converted to an open laparotomy so the surgeon can get a better view and appreciate the whole picture better. It may also be easier to mobilise and completely resect the tumour.

The current ultimate form of key hole surgery is robotic laparoscopic surgery. In Britain, the most commonly used device is the Da Vinci robot costing more than £1 million. There are two parts to the robot; the first is the patient unit which has four arms, one holds the laparoscope and the others hold surgical instruments. The control unit where the surgeon sits is remote from the patient and has a screen showing a magnified three-dimensional view of the operative field, allowing the surgeon to manipulate instruments more smoothly and with better control compared with using the human hand. Robots are increasingly used in gynaecological surgery to treat cervix and endometrial cancer and to perform radical prostatectomies. Direct evidence is lacking that this form of expensive surgery is superior because of a lack of clinical trials comparing robotic surgery with older techniques.

Radical radiotherapy. The decision to treat the patient by radical RT depends on the tumour and patient factors previously discussed. The precise regimen will depend on the potential radio-sensitivity of the tumour, the size of the treatment volume and the proximity of dose-limiting critical tissues. Seminoma of the testes is among the most radiosensitive tumours. The doses required to control small volume disease in the para-aortic lymph nodes are 25 to 30 gray (Gy) in 15 fractions over 3 weeks. By contrast, large lymph nodes containing metastatic squamous carcinoma may not be controlled by doses as high as 70 Gy given in 35 fractions over 7 weeks.

What governs radiation dose is the tolerance of the surrounding normal tissues. The small bowel is the most sensitive tissue in the abdomen and pelvis and the chance of serious small bowel damage rises steeply with doses exceeding 50 Gy given in 25 fractions over 5 weeks. Radiation damage to the spinal cord can be catastrophic, leading to permanent paralysis. In the treatment of tumours in the head and neck, oesophagus and bronchus, care must be taken to restrict the spinal cord dose to 45 to 50 Gy in 25 fractions over 5 weeks.

The side effects of radical RT may be marked. For instance, the mucositis associated with treatment of head and neck cancer may prevent the patient swallowing and may require nasogastric or percutaneous endoscopic gastrostomy (PEG) feeding. However, acute side effects are normally self-limiting and settle in a few weeks with the help of simple supportive measures. This is a probability of late radiation damage that limits the dose to the tumour. In the treatment of breast cancer, the incidence of serious late effects should be vanishingly small and certainly less than half a percent of those patients treated. As the life-threatening nature of the tumour increases, the patient and the oncologist may be persuaded to take greater chances. Serious damage is seen in the larynx following treatment for a T3 (fixed vocal cord) tumour in 1% to 3% of patients. In patients with inoperable cervical cancer, the only realistic chance of cure is chemoradiotherapy. Some of the highest complication rates associated with RT are seen following the treatment of cervical cancer. On average, 6% of patients require surgery to try to correct late damage following treatment.

Palliative Radiotherapy

Palliative treatments can make up between one-third and one-half of the workload of any department. The aim of such treatment is to relieve local symptoms in advanced cancer. An important part of the treatment is that there should be minimal upset. Treatment should be simple and a minimum number of fractions should be used. Symptomatic relief should be rapid.

Up to 80% of patients with bone metastases have significant pain relief within 3 weeks of a single radiation treatment of 8 to 10 Gy. Pain relief will be complete within half of these patients. Other important indications for palliative RT are the relief of haemoptysis, cough, dyspnoea and mediastinal obstruction in lung cancer. These symptoms can be suppressed in between 50% and 80% of patients by a course of RT lasting up to a week, with minimal side effects.

However, some symptoms require longer RT treatments. Tumours involving nerves, such as the brachial plexus (Pancoast tumours from the apex of the lung) or the lumbosacral plexus, produce pain of a very unpleasant quality that is difficult to relieve with opiate analgesia. Relief of such neuropathic pain may require 4 to 5 weeks of RT treatment. Typically, neuropathic pain from advanced rectal cancer can be relieved in two-thirds of patients with doses of 45 to 50 Gy given in 4 to 5 weeks. Radiotherapy can prolong life in some patients with incurable tumours. Randomised controlled trials have shown that the average survival of patients with glioblastomas of the brain following optimal surgery and RT is only a year. However, 6 weeks of RT increases a patient's survival by, on average, 9 months compared with treatment with surgery and best supportive care. When making the decision to offer a patient 6 weeks of RT, one needs to balance life expectancy that is taken up by the RT treatment and the associated fatigue with the survival benefit associated with a treatment which is unlikely to cure the patient. Elderly or more infirm patients are probably better treated by a simple scheme of 30 Gy given in 6 fractions, three times a week over 2 weeks rather than 60 Gy given over 30 fractions.

Radiotherapy Methods

The use of brachytherapy where gamma ray emitting sources are implanted directly into tumour or placed in body cavities such as the uterus and vagina adjacent to malignant tissue is becoming uncommon. Brachytherapy is still an essential part of radical RT regimens for cervix cancer but treatment elsewhere by interstitial sources in diseases such as prostate and head and neck is decreasing or has ceased entirely, being replaced by surgery, newer forms of RT or combinations of radiation and chemotherapy.

Traditionally external beam RT was given by square or rectangular plain or wedged fields. The majority of patients treated radically receive intensity modulated RT (IMRT). In IMRT, treatment is delivered by a linear accelerator equipped with multileaf collimators, thin tungsten columns which move independently to form shapes that fit precisely around the tumour. This allows a high dose to be given to the tumour with sparing of vulnerable normal tissue. In particular, IMRT can create concave shapes which is particularly helpful in the treatment of head and neck cancer allowing treatment of tumour-containing structures such as lymph nodes, but with sparing of the spinal cord. The majority of patients with pelvic cancers such as cervical, rectal and prostate cancer are treated with IMRT with lower doses to small and large bowel and reduced acute and late bowel damage. Breast cancer patients benefit from IMRT treatments as unwanted high-dose areas can be eliminated, and if a boost is required to the excised tumour bed, this can be included in the IMRT plan rather than a localised electron treatment at the end of photon therapy. One theoretical disadvantage of IMRT is owing to the fact that multiple beams are used and more normal tissue is irradiated, albeit at a low dose. Although this low dose irradiation does not cause increased acute side effects, it may increase the risk of second radiation-induced cancers developing 20 or more years after successful IMRT treatment.

The use of stereotactic RT which precisely delivers RT in a highly focused manner is increasing and its use is likely to increase further in the next decade. The term stereotactic means the three-dimensional localisation of a point in the body, usually relating to a fixed external reference frame or other fixation devices and requires highly accurate imaging to locate the lesion to be treated. Stereotactic treatment, sometimes called stereotactic ablative RT (SABR), when used in the treatment of small nonsmall cell lung cancer can give equivalent cure rates to those seen after surgery. The use of this modality is increasing in the treatment of prostate cancer and if phase III clinical trials fulfil the promise of phase II pilot studies, this may become the treatment of choice in prostate cancer with only five daily treatments leading to cure with a low incidence of acute and late side effects. The palliative use of SABR is increasing, especially in the treatment of cerebral metastases and it may become the treatment of choice for bone metastasis, especially vertebral lesions.

Britain now has the first of two planned proton facilities. There are established indications in the treatment of children, especially the treatment of brain tumours, owing to the sparing of normal brain in proton therapy. The indications in adults are less well defined and the majority of proton treatments in the United States are for prostate cancer, where there is no evidence of superiority of protons over other modalities. Proton therapy must be evaluated in careful well-planned clinical trials

Clinical trials. Progress in the treatment of cancer is largely dependent on well-conducted clinical trials. In the United Kingdom, the National Cancer Research Network (NCRN) requires Trusts to enter at least 12% of their cancer patients into approved trials. Clinical trials must be conducted according to good clinical practice (GCP) which is an international ethical and scientific quality standard for designing, conducting, recording and reporting trials that involve the participation of human subjects. In brief, GCP acts to ensure that the safety of patients participating in a trial is protected and the drugs or interventions developed are safe for patients in the future. The data generated in the trial must be valid and reproducible and seen by the greater public to be credible. Trial activity is backed by a raft of legislation, in particular, the set of ethical principles on human experimentation listed in the 1964 Declaration of Helsinki. Trials involving investigational medicinal products are governed by Medicines for Human Use (2004) Regulations. Radiotherapy trials are governed by either the medical devices regulations or the overarching GCP principles.

To carry out a trial, the chief investigator must secure funding and a sponsor who has overall responsibility for the proper conduct of the trial. Sponsors may be universities or National Health Service (NHS) Trust. Ethics committee and organisational research and development department approval must be obtained. Any patient entering a study must be supplied with written material about the trial and must be given time to absorb this and ask questions before signing a consent form.

Consent is commonly obtained by a GCP-trained doctor but a suitably trained nurse or radiographer can obtain informed consent.

Radiotherapy trials follow a similar pattern to medicinal product research. Phase I trials are essentially toxicity and dose-finding studies. Phase II studies are designed to evaluate efficacy. Patients in phase I studies often have very advanced cancers with limited therapeutic choices. A recent example is a Canadian study of stereotactic RT used to retreat vertebral metastases in patients who already have had conventional external beam RT.

Single fractions were associated with a greater degree of postradiotherapy vertebral body collapse when compared with fractionated treatments. This phase I study provided the data for the ongoing Canadian clinical trials SC.24 phase II trial in patients receiving initial treatment for vertebral metastases who are randomised to either 20 Gy in 5 fractions using conventional external beam RT, or 24 Gy given in 2 fractions stereotactically.

A very well-planned ongoing U.K. phase III trial is the Prostate Advances in Comparative Evidence (PACE), a randomised evaluation trial for men suffering from localised prostate cancer; it may answer the question of whether surgery is superior to RT and which is the best RT technique. In total, 1700 men will be recruited into this study. If surgery is an option, men will be randomised to either laparoscopic prostatectomy or 5 fractions of stereotactic RT. If surgery is not an option, men will be randomised to either conventional high-dose external beam RT or stereotactic treatment.

Chemotherapy

Chemotherapy can be given as the sole source of treatment when there is a high chance of cure. Only a small number of tumours are highly chemosensitive and these include the lymphomas, testicular teratoma and choriocarcinoma. Chemotherapy frequently cures children with Wilms tumours, rhabdomyosarcomas and acute lymphoblastic leukaemia. Chemotherapy may be given before RT or surgery to reduce the tumour in size. This is often referred to as neoadjuvant treatment. Increasingly, RT and chemotherapy are given together. This is of proven value in the treatment of carcinoma of cervix, squamous carcinoma of anus, carcinoma of the oesophagus and head and neck cancer. Clinical trials are continuing involving other tumour sites, particularly in lung cancer. Chemotherapy may be of palliative value only in advanced breast cancer or carcinoma of the colon but, in the treatment of small-volume disease following surgery, adjuvant chemotherapy may improve cure rates. Chemotherapy improves 10-year survival in node-positive breast cancer by about 10%. A similar survival advantage is seen following adjuvant chemotherapy in Duke's stage C colon cancer.

Support Services

During and after cancer treatment, a wide range of services to provide the patient with physical, psychological and social support should be available. The most important single individual in this process is the general practitioner. The general practitioner needs to be apprised of the patient's progress, the likely side effects of cancer treatment and what can be done at home to treat these side effects. They also need to be informed of the patient's likely prognosis. This is especially true if the treatment is palliative, because the general practitioner has a key role to play in the provision of continuing care. There is a wide range of specialist nursing services. Some have a relatively restricted role, such as stoma care nurses who provide practical advice on the management of bowel (colostomy and ileostomy) and urinary (urostomy) stomas. Increasingly, specialist nurses are attached to multidisciplinary teams in areas such as breast, gynaecological and CNS cancer. They have multiple roles in giving the patient specialist advice and psychological support. Last, but not least, is a range of national and local support services such as Macmillan Cancer Support and Marie Curie, charitable organisations headquartered in London providing nursing care support.

As well as providing advice on symptom control and emotional support for both patient and family, the nurses also have a most important liaison role. They can act as a link between the patient, the general practitioner and hospital services. District nurses play an important role in at-home care providing basic services such as bathing, dressing of wounds and giving medicines by injection.

Adequate nutrition is important following both radical and palliative RT and hospital- and community-based dieticians help with the special dietary needs of patients. Patients may also require the help of prosthetic services. For some patients, one of the most distressing side effects of chemotherapy or RT to the head is hair loss. A good quality wig may help to maintain the patient's appearance and maintain morale. Scalp-cooling devices can reduce hair loss if the chemotherapeutic agent is cleared fairly quickly from the blood. Other cosmetic prostheses that are important include replacements for eyes and sometimes ears or noses. Prosthetic limb fitters may be required to provide replacement limbs following amputation.

A patient with cancer may be the main breadwinner for the family, therefore, his or her illness may cause acute financial problems. Medical social workers and the Department for Work and Pensions may be able to provide financial support both from the State and from charitable bodies. Last, but not least, is a range of national and local support services such as Macmillan Cancer Support.

Palliative Care

In a regional oncology centre, up to 50% of the work is the treatment of advanced disease. Patients may be judged incurable from the outset and the aim of treatment is the relief of physical and psychological distress. Subsequently, patients who were thought initially to be in the curable category (such as carcinoma of breast) may develop advanced disease and may require the same type of care. Oncology centres will have developed their own systems of care to support these patients and this should interface well with their home or hospice care.

Ideally, patients should be cared for at home with the help of the general practitioner and district nurses. Macmillan specialist nurses make a significant contribution to this process and, increasingly, organisations such as Marie Curie provide hospice at home services.

Patients who have symptoms that cannot be controlled at home or when their nursing care is too complex may need admission to hospital or, ideally, to a specialist hospice. Hospices provide a more homely, less institutional and quieter environment than the noisy, busy hospital ward. The higher staff to patient ratio gives more time for patients to talk about their illnesses. The hospice team has the distinctive knowledge and skills needed to provide spiritual and emotional support for patients at this challenging time. Often, after symptoms have been controlled, patients may be able to return home perhaps to return to the hospice at a later date. Such patients while at home can be helped by attendance at the hospice day centre. As well as checking that the patient's symptoms are controlled, hospice day centres provide a social environment for patients and can allow other family members a respite from care to continue employment.

One of the main aims of a hospice is symptom control. These include pain, anorexia, nausea, vomiting, dysphasia, dyspnoea and lack of energy.

Pain Control

Up to three-quarters of patients with advanced cancer may have some degree of pain, and up to 80% of patients may have pain at multiple sites. The three most common sources of cancer pain are bone metastases, compression of nerves and soft tissue disease.

Pain has both physical and psychological dimensions. Anxiety or depression may accentuate the perception of pain and lower the pain threshold. Physical conditions such as hypercalcaemia may also physiologically increase the degree of pain. The treatment of hypercalcaemia may be a pain control measure by itself. The basis of pain control is to establish the causes of pain and, if possible, eradicate the source of pain. The patient may benefit from a single RT treatment. However, come what may, the pain should be controlled by suitable analgesia if this is possible.

Ideally, all analgesics should be given by mouth. Mild or moderate pain may respond to simple analgesics such as paracetamol or aspirin. The nonsteroidal group of analgesics, such as diclofenac, may be useful, especially for bone pain. They can, however, cause gastric irritation and should be used with caution in even mild degrees of renal failure. Codeine or dihydrocodeine are useful for moderate pain but, unlike morphine, the dose of these drugs cannot be escalated. Increasing the doses above 60 mg four times a day produces toxicity and not an increase in analgesia.

Morphine is still a standard analgesic for severe pain. In patients with normal renal and hepatic function, the metabolic half-life of morphine is two and a half hours. It therefore needs to be given no less frequently than four hourly. Morphine serum levels are stable after six half-lives, therefore, in practice, morphine doses can be escalated every 12 hours. An initial dose of oral morphine should be chosen according to the patient's age, size and the degree of pain. This may vary between 5 and 30 mg. The dose is usually given in the form of either morphine sulphate tablets or an elixir. The dose can be rapidly escalated if necessary. When pain control is achieved, the total morphine dose over 24 hours can then be added up. This is a guide for the prescription of a strong-acting analgesic such as morphine sulphate continuous tablets (MST). These tablets contain morphine in a cellulose matrix that is slowly released over a 12-hour period. If the patient has been receiving 30 mg of morphine elixir every four hours, the total morphine dosage in 24 hours is 180 mg. This can be given in the form of 90 mg of MST every 12 hours to provide sustained pain control. If the patient cannot swallow, diamorphine is a useful substitute. This is highly soluble in very small quantities of water and can be given subcutaneously either by intermittent injection or continuously using a syringe driver. Diamorphine has roughly twice the potency of morphine when given by injection and three times the potency of oral morphine. Virtually all opiates cause constipation and patients should be routinely prescribed a laxative. A common side effect is nausea, but this usually settles within 5 days.

Respiratory depression is rarely a problem but, if the patient develops significant respiratory oppression, morphine can be temporarily stopped and restarted at a lower dose. Occasionally, very high doses of morphine can cause myoclonic twitching of limbs.

About 10% to 15% of patients are intolerant to morphine because of either prolonged nausea or a dysphoric reaction. Alternative preparations are fentanyl patches, hydromorphone or oxycodone. In the treatment of neuropathic pain, tricyclic drugs, such as amitriptyline, or anticonvulsants such as gabapentin, pregabalin or sodium valproate often help symptoms. Occasionally, patients with neuropathic pain may require a nerve block. Sites where this can be carried out are in the intercostal nerves in the ribs, the brachial plexus when this is involved by an apical lung tumour, coeliac axis plexus following infiltration by a pancreatic cancer or involvement of the lumbar-sacral nerve plexus by pelvic cancer. These nerve blocks are technically very demanding. Usually a long-acting local anaesthetic is injected to check that nerve block will bring about adequate analgesia. If the pain is relieved this could be followed by a further injection using phenol or alcohol to destroy the nerve.

Dyspnoea

Shortness of breath can be more frightening than pain and sometimes more difficult to treat. Treatment of the underlying cause is often useful, such as aspirating a pleural effusion or abdominal ascites. If there is a strong anxiety component, an anxiolytic, such as diazepam, may be helpful. Morphine depresses the respiratory centre but this side effect is beneficial in reducing tumour-induced dyspnoea. As in the control of pain, the ideal route of morphine administration is by mouth but, if necessary, the patient may require diamorphine by syringe driver. As in other forms of dyspnoea, oxygen can be very helpful along with psychological support from staff.

Nausea and Vomiting

There are many causes of nausea and vomiting in advanced cancer patients. Drug-induced vomiting is one of the most common. This may also be a symptom of renal or hepatic failure. Vomiting without a headache can be a feature of raised intracranial pressure. Some 5HT3 antagonists, such as granisetron or ondansetron, are probably the most effective drugs in the treatment of RT- or chemotherapy-induced nausea and vomiting. Where nausea and vomiting are associated with a strong anxiety component, antiemetic drugs with tranquilising properties, such as prochlorperazine or haloperidol, are often useful.

Anorexia

Anorexia is often multifactorial in origin. The most common cause is the underlying malignancy. It is thought that the cancer stimulates the release of cytokines from the immune system, which induce anorexia. Anorexia though, may be attributed to treatment (RT or chemotherapy) or the physical effects of cancer, such as pain or intestinal obstruction. Dietetic advice may be helpful and a small amount of alcohol before meals may stimulate the appetite. Steroids are the most effective antianorexic agents. It is worth trying prednisolone at 30 mg over a 7-day period. If this increases appetite, the dose can be reduced to a maintenance dose of 5 to 10 mg. Progesterones, such as megestrol acetate, do improve appetite; however, they can cause ankle oedema and have been associated with an increased risk of thrombosis.

At least one-quarter of patients with advanced cancer have significant depression. Virtually all patients with advanced cancer have a feeling of sadness and a sense of loss. Antidepressant medication should be considered sooner rather than later. The selective serotonin reuptake inhibitors, such as fluoxetine or sertraline, are better tolerated than the traditional tricyclic antidepressants. They often work faster than the 3 weeks often quoted. Counselling, relaxation therapy and other measures are also useful adjuncts in the treatment of anxiety and depression.

Context of Care

It is apparent that there is a multiplicity of professionals essential to the treatment and care of patients. These individuals work across the health and social care sectors where the potential for a breakdown in communications is obvious. It is one of the challenges facing modern provision of cancer services that these groups are able to work together as a team to enable patients to be provided with a seamless service. This is now well recognised and encouraged by a host of government initiatives designed to improve cancer services across the United Kingdom.

FURTHER READING

Department of Health. The NHS cancer plan. HMSO; 2000.

Kaye P. Breaking Bad news: a ten step approach. EPL Publications; 1996.

Meredith C, Symonds P, Webster L, et al. Information needs of cancer patients in West Scotland; cross sectional survey of patients' views. Br Med J 1996;313:724–6.

National Cancer Institute, www.cancer.gov/.

National Institute for Health Research, www.ukctg.nihr.ac.uk/.

NHS Executive. Improving the quality of cancer services. HSC/021. NHS Executive; 2000.

Stead M, Cameron D, Lester N, Parmar M, Haward R, Kaplan R, et al. Strengthening clinical cancer research in the United Kingdom. Br J Cancer 2011;104:1529–34.

Chemotherapy and Hormones

Anne L. Thomas

INTRODUCTION

Chemotherapy is the use of cytotoxic (cell poisoning) drugs to control tumour growth. Over the last 30 years, there have been advances in the management of several solid tumours and haematological malignancies, such as testicular teratoma, the leukaemias, childhood cancers and choriocarcinoma. Over 70% of childhood cancers are now curable and the cure rate for teratoma is over 95%. What has been more challenging is the use of cytotoxics in the management of the common tumours, such as nonsmall cell lung cancer (NSCLC), breast cancer and bowel cancer. These tumours often present in the metastatic stage and are relatively resistant to chemotherapy. Despite intense research, chemotherapy for these tumours remains palliative in intent rather than curative. One of the major drawbacks of cytotoxic agents is that they affect all rapidly dividing cells, and do not discriminate between normal tissues and tumours, hence, the toxicity of chemotherapy. We are now entering an exciting era in oncology with new targeted and immunotherapy therapies becoming available. These novel agents are designed to exploit our increased understanding of molecular oncology and will hopefully be more successful in overcoming drug resistance and reducing the side effects of treatment.

Hormone therapy is another systemic treatment for cancer. It may involve inhibiting the production of endogenous hormones or introducing synthetic ones. There are now many different hormone preparations available and they play a vital role in the treatment of tumours, such as prostate and breast cancer.

General Indications for Chemotherapy

There are four main ways in which chemotherapy can be used in the treatment of cancer. First, it is used as the primary treatment for patients with advanced cancers for which no alternative treatment exists. This is sometimes called palliative chemotherapy and is essentially used to palliate the symptoms of cancer. Adjuvant chemotherapy is the use of cytotoxic drugs after the primary tumour has been controlled by either surgery or radiotherapy (RT). Here, the rationale is to eradicate subclinical micrometastatic disease and reduce the risk of recurrence. Examples of this would be in the treatment of bowel and breast cancer. Neoadjuvant (or primary) chemotherapy is used to debulk the primary tumour in an attempt to make the definitive treatment, for example surgery, successful. An example of this is neoadjuvant therapy of large breast primary tumours so that conservative local surgery rather than mastectomy is made possible. The fourth setting is to use chemotherapy directly into the tumour site, for example, into the blood supply of liver metastases from colorectal cancer.

Development and Testing of Anticancer Agents

Cytotoxic therapies have been discovered in a variety of ways. First, some drugs have been developed de novo based on distinct properties that should confer antitumour effects. Alternatively, a range of compounds is produced and then screened against a selection of resistant tumour cell lines. Those with significant activity are then taken forward. Once this first generation drug is discovered, then analogues with superior pharmacological properties (e.g. less toxicity, more convenient administration), are synthesised. Of course, one should not forget the past serendipitous discovery of drugs, such as cis-platin. Once an agent has been shown in its preclinical assessment to have sufficient activity against animal tumours, with acceptable toxicity, it can be considered for clinical evaluation. There are three phases of clinical assessment.

Phase I Studies

In phase I studies, the main aim is to establish the maximum tolerated dose and the safety of the agent under investigation. Such studies are often performed with the informed consent of patients for whom standard therapy has no role. The starting dose is determined by preclinical data and is usually one-tenth of the lethal dose (LD_{10}) in rodents. In phase I studies, pharmacokinetic studies (how the body handles the drug, e.g. by metabolism) and pharmacodynamic studies (assessing the impact of the drug on the physiology of the body) are conducted. Historically, phase I studies were completed in patients for whom no further standard chemotherapy options were available. Nowadays, particularly when the tumour type is rare or when the outcomes are very poor, these studies may be carried out in patients as part of their first-line treatment. This provides a much better signal read out for benefit compared with heavily pretreated patients and increases the chances of future phase II studies to be successful.

Phase II Studies

Once a drug is found to have acceptable side effects it is taken forward into phase II studies to study its efficacy in a specific tumour type. The type selected is usually ascertained from the responses to therapy seen in the cell lines and sometimes from activity demonstrated in the phase I setting. The main outcome is to achieve a response rate which is at least comparable with the standard agent in that setting. Now there is a trend to randomise some phase II studies so that either the drug can be compared with the standard or two different dose schedules could be studied. Gaining these data as early as possible in the development of a drug obviously enables the pharmaceutical company to withdraw a drug as soon as possible if activity is disappointing or, alternatively, to fast track drugs with impressive potential.

Phase III Studies

In phase III studies, the new drug is compared against the gold standard in a randomised fashion. The main endpoint is survival, but toxicity data are collected and also quality of life and health economic data. The cost effectiveness of the drug has to be assessed and deemed to be acceptable before the drug can be licensed and marketed. In this era of agents targeting specific molecular aberrations in tumours, two other types of studies are increasingly used. In umbrella studies, patients with the same type of cancer are assigned to different treatments/arms of a study based on their mutations. In basket studies, patients with a variety of cancers which share a single genomic alteration are assigned to a treatment/arm that is expected to be active. In the United Kingdom, the National Cancer Research Institute (NCRI) has a portfolio of studies that are peer reviewed and of the highest standard possible. The United Kingdom is divided geographically into research networks to coordinate the delivery of clinical studies to ensure that patients who are eligible for these studies can be referred appropriately. The rates of recruitment to clinical studies do vary network to network, but there is evidence that where centres recruit high numbers, survival outcomes for patients increase, even if they were nontrial participants. Therefore, clinical trials help raise the standard of cancer care.

Assessing Tumour Responses

It is essential that there is standardisation of how tumours are measured and responses defined so that studies can be interpreted accurately. A number of different response criteria are available, but the system used most commonly now is RECIST (Response Criteria in Solid Tumours, updated to v 1.1 in 2008). In this system, the lesions are measured in one dimension, longest diameter (LD). A complete response is defined as eradication of all known disease based on two assessments at least 4 weeks apart. A partial response (PR) represents a reduction of at least 30% in the sum of the LD of target lesions maintained for at least 4 weeks. Progressive disease (PD) represents an increase of 20% or more in the sum of LD of lesions or the development of new lesions. Stable disease (SD) occurs when the measurements are either not good enough for a PR but also not bad enough for PD.

The Evaluation of Targeted Therapies

With the advent of targeted therapies, such as antiangiogenic treatment, and epidermal growth factor inhibition, it has become apparent that there are difficulties in assessing these agents using conventional study design endpoints. This is because the classic endpoint of the maximum tolerated dose may not actually be the biologically active dose. Moreover, these agents may be cytostatic rather than cytotoxic. This means that stabilisation of disease is the best response that can be expected and the classical endpoint of reduction in tumour volume is not reached. It is therefore imperative that the actual target of these drugs is known and assays are incorporated into the study design as some 'surrogate' endpoints. An example of this would be the studies that investigated the activity of trastuzumab, the HER-2/erbB2 growth factor inhibitor, in breast cancer. Here, assays were carried out in tumour biopsies to ensure that the HER-2 receptor was indeed being targeted. It is now increasingly common for new agents to have a specific molecular diagnostic associated with them, for example, patients with lung cancer to be treated with the anaplastic lymphoma kinase (ALK) inhibitor crizotinib, must have positive ALK expression demonstrated in their tumour biopsy sample.

PRINCIPLES OF CYTOTOXIC THERAPY

To understand the rationale of cytotoxic chemotherapy, it is important to recognise the features of tumour growth. The asymmetric sigmoidal growth curve, the 'Gompertzian growth curve' (Fig. 19.1), describes the natural history of tumour growth. By the time a tumour is clinically detectable, the majority of its growth has already occurred. In the early exponential phase of growth, the rates of tumour cell growth and

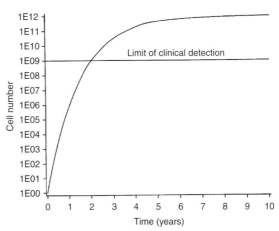

Fig. 19.1 Gompertzian growth curve.

tumour cell loss are proportional to the tumour cell burden at any point. Because most anticancer agents are more toxic to proliferating cells and most tumours are in a relatively slow phase of growth when diagnosed (i.e. they lie high and toward the plateau of the Gompertzian growth curve), it explains the limited effectiveness of chemotherapy for many cancers. The reason for tumour cytoreduction (e.g. by surgery) before chemotherapy is to bring the tumour to a lower point on the growth curve when the growth fraction of the tumour rises. The concept of moving the tumour down the Gompertzian curve underpins the rationale of adjuvant chemotherapy.

Unfortunately, it is not only the proliferating cells that must be eradicated by chemotherapy, but also the small population of clonogenic cells mainly in G_0 phase. This explains some of the inherent problems of tumour chemoresistance. Cytotoxic drugs prevent cell division by inhibiting DNA replication. Unfortunately, these agents are not specifically acting against malignant cells, and damage both normal and malignant proliferating cells. A careful balance has to be kept between toxicity to the tumour and to the patient's normal tissues. What distinguishes normal and malignant cells is the failure of the malignant cell, unlike normal cells, to recover from cytotoxic damage. It is exploitation of these differences that underpins the role of targeted therapies.

Drug Resistance

A variety of host factors influence the response to chemotherapy; these include the growth fraction of the tumour, the availability of the drug to the tumour and drug resistance. Resistance to chemotherapy may be intrinsic or acquired. Some tumours are intrinsically chemoresistant and show no response to treatment de novo. In other tumours, there is an initial response followed by relapse because of acquired resistance. Acquired resistance may have a variety of mechanisms. These include:

1. Changes in the cell membrane impeding drug transport (e.g. of methotrexate).
2. DNA repair of drug-induced lesions (e.g. caused by cisplatin).
3. Use of alternative metabolic pathways (e.g. 5-fluorouracil (5-FU)).
4. Increased production of a target enzyme (e.g. dihydrofolate reductase (DHFR), binding to methotrexate).
5. Modification of the target enzyme, enabling it to recognise the difference between true and false metabolites (e.g. 6-mercaptopurine).

The multiple drug resistance gene (*MDR1*) encodes P-glycoprotein. The latter is a membrane-associated efflux pump that is widely found in normal cells and serves to protect them from drug-induced damage. Normally, P-glycoprotein is found in very low levels; however, cancer cells can overexpress *MDR1*, so conferring resistance to a variety of chemotherapeutic agents. In addition, *p53*, the 'guardian' of the genome and an important mediator of apoptosis (programmed cell death) may be mutated and give rise to chemoresistance in a number of solid tumours.

The reasons for drug resistance are not fully understood. It is common to find that a tumour responds to a particular drug or combination of drugs for a period of time and then ceases to do so. It is thought that within many tumour populations there are genetically determined drug-resistant cells. When the chemosensitive cells have been killed, the resistant population may proliferate. Drug resistance to repeated exposure to a single agent will usually result in cross-resistance to other compounds of the same class of drugs. This is probably because of common transport mechanisms and pathways of metabolism and intracellular cytotoxic targets. However, cancer cells that have become resistant to one class of drugs may retain sensitivity to another class of drugs. Most drugs have a variety of mechanisms of drug resistance.

Some drugs which show excellent cell kill in vitro fail to do so in vivo. There may be multiple reasons for this. For example, if the tumour is in a sanctuary site, such as the central nervous system

(CNS), the drug does not cross the blood–brain barrier and is therefore ineffective. There is also evidence that some tumours exhibit drug resistance that is partly because of host factors which modify the pharmacokinetics of the anticancer agent in vivo. Chemotherapy is most effective in killing proliferating cells. Although the growth fraction is high in many chemosensitive tumours, such as the lymphomas and testicular teratomas, it is relatively low in many common tumours, for example, colorectal cancer. Finally, in parts of the tumour the blood supply tends to be poor. This not only results in an inadequate concentration of drug reaching the tumour, but also the hypoxia reduces the growth fraction.

Selection and Scheduling of Chemotherapy Agents

In an attempt to improve the curative potential of chemotherapy, agents with proven anticancer properties against a particular tumour but with different mechanisms of action and, as far as possible, non-overlapping toxicities are combined. This is known as *combination chemotherapy*. For example, in treating breast cancer, three agents: cyclophosphamide, methotrexate and 5-fluorouracil (known as CMF), all have activity against breast cancer as single agents. However, their response rate as a combination (around 40%) is two- to threefold that of their response rates as single agents. Thus, the overall response is at least additive if not synergistic.

Most schedules of chemotherapy administer the drugs on an intermittent basis to take advantage of the growth kinetics of malignant cells and normal tissues. After each pulse, the normal and malignant cell populations decline because of killing of cells in mitosis. The lowest level of the blood count is known as the nadir. However, whereas the bone marrow recovers to its previous level, the malignant cell population does not. With each subsequent course, this difference is accentuated. If the interval between pulses is too short, toxicity may prevent the delivery of further pulses on schedule; conversely, if the interval is too long, the tumour may regrow between courses. The total dose that can be administered is therefore limited by the tolerance of normal tissue, particularly the bone marrow. The crucial nadir blood count is the neutrophil value, with neutropenia being defined as an absolute neutrophil count of less than 0.5×10^9/L, or less than 1.0×10^9/L and 'falling', the interpretation of which requires some knowledge of chemotherapy regimens and expected patterns of myelosuppression. Neutropenic sepsis in patients on chemotherapy is regarded as a medical emergency and requires prompt intervention with intravenous antibiotics; failure to do this can result in death. Toxicity is often cumulative and may be irreversible. For example, the major dose-limiting toxicity of the anthracycline, doxorubicin, is cardiotoxicity.

High-Dose Chemotherapy

Higher than conventional doses of chemotherapy can be delivered if the primary organ toxicity is to the bone marrow and there is minimal toxicity to other organs. Dose intensity is recognised to be important, particularly in chemosensitive tumours. Bone marrow toxicity can be overcome by autologous bone marrow transplantation. Normal bone marrow is harvested from the patient before high-dose chemotherapy. It is then returned to the patient at the time of chemotherapy to support the bone marrow through the period of neutropenia and thrombocytopenia. Although high-dose strategies have been extremely useful in haematological malignancies, the results from similar approaches in solid tumours have been disappointing.

ROUTE OF ADMINISTRATION

The route of administration is governed by the solubility, chemical stability and local irritant properties of the agent. The simplest route, and the one that patients prefer, is the oral route. Patients can take their tablets at home with intermittent outpatient visits to monitor treatment. Unfortunately, many cytotoxic drugs are unstable and inactivated in the stomach, rendering them ineffective. Intravenous injection is the commonest route of administration of cytotoxic agents because it gives direct access to the systemic circulation. It can be done by delivery of a bolus dose or by infusion. Continuous infusions can be given (e.g. 5-FU) linked to a battery-operated pump worn around the patient's waist. The risks of intravenous administration are the introduction of infection and damage to the tissues around the site of administration if extravasation occurs.

It is possible to administer intraperitoneal chemotherapy, for example, in ovarian cancer. However, the drug absorption is variable and there are concerns about adverse effects, such as the development of adhesions. Intraarterial administration has the advantage of delivering the drug in high concentration to the tissue supplied by the artery. Its limitations are the complexity of administration and the difficulty in correctly identifying the arterial supply of the tumour. Its main use is in the infusion of chemotherapeutic agents into the hepatic artery of patients with liver metastases from colorectal cancer. Intrathecal injection is used to deliver drugs in high dose into the CNS. Many cytotoxic drugs do not cross the blood–brain barrier and are therefore unable to kill tumour cells within the CNS. Methotrexate is the agent most commonly given by this route, for example, when the meninges are involved in lymphoma.

SIDE EFFECTS OF CHEMOTHERAPY

The main normal tissues damaged by cytotoxic therapy are those with rapidly dividing cell populations: the bone marrow, the gastrointestinal epithelium, the hair and the germ cells of the testis. By contrast, there is little effect on nonproliferating tissues such as skeletal muscle and nervous tissue. The most common side effects of individual cytotoxic drugs are shown in Table 19.1. The most dramatic improvement in the management of side effects was with the development of the 5-hydroxytryptamine ($5HT_3$) antagonist antiemetics. More recently, the neurokinin-1 antagonists (NK_1), such as aprepitant, have improved the emesis of patients undergoing highly emetogenic chemotherapy. Typical antiemetic regimens are shown in Table 19.2. Other drugs that have improved drug delivery have been the recombinant growth factors for red (erythropoietin) and white (human granulocyte colony-stimulating factor, G-CSF) cells. These agents stimulate the release of progenitor cells from the bone marrow and are useful in the treatment and prevention of anaemia and neutropenia.

CLASSIFICATION OF CYTOTOXIC DRUGS

The available agents may be divided into a few broad groups on the basis of their mechanism of action:

- Alkylating agents
- Antimetabolites
- Mitotic inhibitors
- Topoisomerase inhibitors
- Miscellaneous
- Hormones

Some cytotoxic drugs act only on particular phases of the cell cycle (cell-cycle specific), whereas others act throughout the cycle (cell-cycle nonspecific).

Alkylating Agents

The main antitumour action of alkylating agents is the binding of an alkyl chemical group (R-CH2) to DNA, so inhibiting its synthesis. They also bind to RNA and other cell proteins, but these reactions are much less cytotoxic. The majority of alkylating agents have two available alkyl groups with which they can bind with DNA. Cross-linking may occur between a single strand of DNA or between two separate strands. Alkylating agents with this capacity to cross-link are called *bifunctional* and are more cytotoxic than alkylating agents with only one available alkyl group for binding to DNA.

The intravenous alkylating agents are nearly all vesicants and are an irritant to the skin and other tissues if they extravasate out of the vein. In general, they do cause nausea and vomiting but this is usually controlled with antiemetics. They all cause myelosuppression, alopecia and temporary amenorrhoea. Nitrosoureas are a group of similar drugs whose main mode of action is alkylation. Specific examples of alkylating agents and nitrosoureas with specific side effects and main uses are shown in Table 19.3.

Trabectedin is an alkylating agent that is licensed for use in soft tissue sarcoma. Its discovery is of interest; in the 1960s the National Cancer Institute carried out a wide-ranging program of screening plant and marine organism material. As part of that programme, extract from the sea squirt, *Ecteinascidia turbinata*, was found to have anticancer activity, a semisynthetic analogue, trabectedin, was synthesised to it. The compound binds to DNA binding in the minor groove and interacts with DNA repair mechanisms causing DNA double-strand breaks (DSB).

Antimetabolites

Antimetabolites are structurally similar to normal metabolites involved in nucleic acid synthesis. They are divided into three groups: folate, purine and pyrimidine antagonists. They substitute for their normal purine and pyrimidine counterparts in metabolic pathways, resulting in abnormal nuclear material that fails to function normally, or bind to enzymes, so inhibiting protein synthesis.

Folate Antagonists

Methotrexate is the classical example of an antimetabolite. A number of cofactors are necessary for the synthesis of purines and pyrimidines. The reduction of folic acid is essential for the production of these cofactors. A key reaction in this process is the reduction of dihydrofolic acid to tetrahydrofolic acid by means of an enzyme, dihydrofolate reductase (DHFR). Methotrexate is structurally similar to folic acid and has a much greater affinity for dihydrofolate reductase than does folic acid. Methotrexate therefore binds preferentially to dihydrofolate reductase and inactivates it. As a result, tetrahydrofolates cannot be made and purine and pyrimidine synthesis is inhibited. Methotrexate can be given orally, intravenously or at low dose intrathecally (Fig. 19.2).

The metabolic block on the activity of DHFR can be bypassed by administering an intermediate metabolite, folinic acid (also known as leucovorin). Folinic acid is a tetrahydrofolate which provides an alternative source for continuing nucleic acid synthesis. The cytotoxic action of methotrexate and its toxicity can be diminished by administrating folinic acid. This is termed *folinic acid rescue* and is particularly useful after high-dose methotrexate therapy has been used. The main side effects of methotrexate are on the bone marrow and on the gastrointestinal tract. The nadir of the white count is at 10 days. Anorexia, nausea and vomiting are the first symptoms, followed 4 to 6 days later by oral and pharyngeal mucositis and diarrhoea. Conjunctivitis may occur as a result of accumulation of the drug in tears. Renal failure may complicate high-dose therapy. Liver damage (ranging from elevated liver enzymes to cirrhosis) and lung injury (mainly fibrosis) may complicate prolonged therapy. Alopecia is uncommon. Methotrexate is used most commonly in non-Hodgkin's lymphoma, acute lymphoblastic leukaemia, breast cancer, and choriocarcinoma. Over the last 10 years, new antifolates have

TABLE 19.1 Side Effects of Treatment

	Alopecia	GI Toxicity	Neurotoxicity	Cardiotoxicity	Urological Toxicity	Myelotoxicity	Skin Changes	Lung Toxicity	Allergic Reactions
Cyclophosphamide	+	+			+	+			
Ifosfamide	+	+	++		++	+			
Chlorambucil		+				+	+		
Thiotepa		+				+	+		
Busulphan		+			+	+	++	+	+
Procarbazine	+	+	+			+	+	+	+
CCNU		+				+		+	
BCNU		+				+		+	
Dacarbazine		++				+	+		+
Mitoxantrone		+		+		+	+		
Temozoamide	+	+				+	+	+	
Mitomycin C		+				+	+	+	
Melphalan		+				+	+	+	+
Methotrexate		+	+			+	+		
6-Mercaptopurine		+			+	+			
Fludarabine		+			+	++		+	
5-Fluorouracil		+		+		+	+	+	
Cytosine arabinoside		+				+	+		+
Gemcitabine		+	++			++	+		
Vincristine		+	++			+			
Vinblastine		+				+			
Vinorelbine	+	+	+			+			
Paclitaxel	++	+	++			+	+		+
Docetaxel	++	++	+			++	+		+
Doxorubicin	++	++		++	++	+	+		
Epirubicin	+	+		+	+	+	+		
Actinomycin D	+	+				+	+		+
Bleomycin	+	+					+	++	++
Cisplatin		+	+		++	+			
Carboplatin		+	++		+	++			+
Oxaliplatin		+	++			+			+
Etoposide	+	+			+	+	+		+
Topotecan	+	+				+			+
Irinotecan	+	++				+			
Asparaginase		+							+
Hydroxyurea		+				+	+		

Note: +: minor toxicity; ++: moderate to high toxicity.
BCNU, Carmustine; *CCNU,* Lomustine; *GI,* gastrointestinal.

TABLE 19.2 Typical Antiemetic Regimens

Grade of Emesis	Antiemetic Protocol
Low	Metoclopramide 20 mg IV if required
	Metoclopramide 10–20 mg orally (PO) tds PRN
Moderate	5HT$_3$ antagonist PO and dexamethasone 8 mg PO then
	Metoclopramide 20 mg tds
	Dexamethasone 4 mg bd
	Both for 3 days
High	5HT$_3$ antagonist PO and dexamethasone 8 mg PO NK1 antagonist PO then
	5HT$_3$ antagonist PO for 1 day
	NK1 antagonist PO for 2 days
	Dexamethasone 4 mg bd for 3 days
	Metoclopramide 20 mg tds PRN

Second-Line Antiemetics

Acute emesis:	Give the antiemetic protocol for next grade of emesis
If already at 'high' give metoclopramide regularly, consider alternative antiemetics.	Add in aprepitant, 125 mg PO prechemotherapy and 80 mg PO for 2 days post chemotherapy.
Delayed emesis (>24 hours postchemotherapy):	Consider lengthening course of steroids, add in aprepitant and consider alternative antiemetics.
Anxiety component:	Add lorazepam, 1 mg PO or sublingually tds PRN. This can be started 1–2 days before chemotherapy.
Alternative antiemetics:	Domperidone rectally, 30–60 mg 4–8 hourly PRN. Haloperidol, 1.5 mg tds PRN. Cyclizine, 50 mg tds PRN or regularly or levomepromazine, 6 mg qds PRN.

been developed, including pemetrexed. This is a multitargeted pyrrolo-pyrimidine-based antifolate. When polyglutamated, it targets a number of folate-dependent enzymes, for example, DHFR and thymidylate synthase (TS). It has activity in a number of tumour types including NSCLC and mesothelioma.

Purine Antagonists

6-Mercaptopurine is a purine antagonist and inhibits a number of enzymes involved in the synthesis of the purine bases, adenine and guanine, which thus inhibits the synthesis of DNA. It is normally given orally and used in the treatment of leukaemia. The main toxicity is on the bone marrow (leucopoenia and thrombocytopaenia) and the liver. The nadir for white count and platelets is at 15 days.

Raised serum bilirubin is the most common feature of liver toxicity. This usually returns to normal on withdrawing the drug.

6-Thioguanine is also a purine antagonist and is an analogue of guanine. It may be given orally or intravenously but is now very rarely used in practice.

Fludarabine is a more recently developed antipurine. It is an adenosine analogue and is currently the most active single agent in the treatment of chronic lymphatic leukaemia. It is also active in the treatment of lymphomas. The main limiting side effect of fludarabine is myelosuppression which can be very severe.

Pyrimidine Antagonists

5-FU is a fluoropyrimidine that inhibits DNA synthesis by inhibiting the main enzyme in pyrimidine synthesis and thus the formation of cytosine and thymine. In addition, it is erroneously incorporated into RNA instead of uracil and inhibits RNA synthesis. 5-FU is metabolised intracellularly in a number of steps to the active fluorodeoxyuridine monophosphate (FdUMP); this then forms covalent bonds with thymidylate synthase and its cofactor 5,10-methylene tetrahydrofolate, creating a complex which inhibits the formation of thymidine from deoxyuridine monophosphate (dUMP), so inhibiting DNA synthesis (see Fig. 19.2). One problem with 5-FU is that elevated dUMP levels may overcome the inhibition of thymidylate synthase, thereby causing chemo-resistance. Specific thymidylate synthase inhibitors (e.g.

TABLE 19.3 Summary of Alkylating Agents and Nitrosoureas

Name	Route of Administration	Main Use	Nadir	Specific Side Effects
Cyclophosphami-de	PO or IV	Non-Hodgkin's lymphomas, breast, ovary, sarcomas	9–15 days	Haemorrhagic cystitis because of the urinary metabolites of the drug; treated with mesna
Ifosfamide	IV	Sarcomas	5–10 days	As above Encephalopathy nephrotoxicity
Chlorambucil	PO	Low grade lymphoma	8–15 days	GI upset
Melphalan	PO or IV	Myeloma	14–21 days	Mucositis
Thiotepa	IV	High dose therapy	28 days	Myelosuppression
Busulfan	PO	Chronic myeloid leukaemia	28 days	Lung fibrosis Prolonged myelosuppression
Procarbazine	PO	Brain tumours Hodgkin lymphoma	28+ days	CNS toxicity
CCNU (Lomustine)	PO	Brain tumours, lymphomas	28+ days	Delayed myelosuppression
BCNU (Carmustine)	IV	High dose, lymphomas	28+ days	Pulmonary fibrosis Delayed myelosuppression
DTIC dacarbazine	IV	Melanoma	21 days	Myalgia
Temozolamide	PO	Brain tumours	10–14 days	Myelosuppression
Mitomycin C	IV	Gastric, breast	14–28 days	Prolonged neutropenia

CNS, Central nervous system; *GI*, gastrointestinal; *IV*, intravenous; *PO*, orally; *PRN* as required; *tds* three times a day; *qds* four times a day

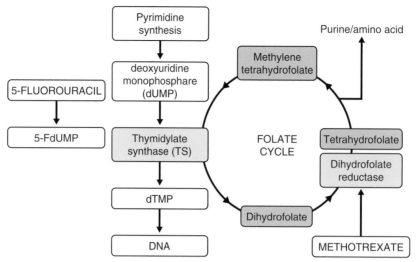

Fig. 19.2 Enzymatic pathway for 5-fluorouracil and methotrexate.

raltitrexed, have therefore been developed. Unfortunately, despite initially encouraging results, raltitrexed has not been as useful against colorectal cancer as predicted. In reality, it appears only to have a role in treating patients with cardiac problems because it has a safer cardiac profile than 5-FU.

Historically, it was only possible to give 5-FU intravenously as the oral bioavailability of 5-FU was too unpredictable. The development of the oral fluoropyrimidines, tegafur-uracil (UFT) and capecitabine, have overcome this. In particular, capecitabine is an interesting compound because it was formulated to be preferentially activated in the tumour. Capecitabine is metabolised to 5-FU in a three-step enzymatic reaction with tumour-selective generation of 5-FU through exploitation of the higher level of thymidine phosphorylase in tumour compared with normal tissue. The pharmacokinetics of orally administered capecitabine essentially mimics a continuous infusion rather than bolus 5-FU. To be able to prescribe an oral formulation of 5-FU is an enormous advantage as, understandably, patients prefer to take tablets and the potential risk of central line complications is avoided.

The main toxicities of 5-FU are to the gastrointestinal tract (diarrhoea, nausea and vomiting) and myelosuppression. The severity of the toxicity depends on the scheduling of 5-FU. For example, it is well recognised that giving 5-FU as a continuous infusion over 48 hours (de Gramont schedule) produces fewer side effects than giving the drug once every day for 5 days every month (Mayo schedule). Rarely, if a patient has genetic deficiency of the dihydropyrimidine dehydrogenase, very severe toxicity can result, including neurological effects. 5-FU is widely used in a number of tumours, especially those of the gastrointestinal tract. A recently developed compound in this class is trifluridine/tipiracil (Lonsurf) which is an oral combination drug for the treatment of metastatic colorectal cancer. It consists of trifluridine, a nucleoside analogue, and tipiracil, a thymidine phosphorylase inhibitor.

Cytosine arabinoside is an analogue of deoxycytidine. It is a competitive inhibitor of the enzyme, DNA polymerase. Its principal action is as a false nucleotide competing for the enzymes that are responsible for converting cytidine to deoxycytidine and for incorporating deoxycytidine into DNA. It can be given by intravenous or subcutaneous routes and is used mainly in acute leukaemias. The main side effects are bone marrow suppression, nausea, vomiting and diarrhoea.

Gemcitabine is a second-generation pyrimidine analogue. It is metabolised by nucleotide kinases intracellularly to the active diphosphate and triphosphate and inhibits DNA synthesis. Side effects include nausea and vomiting, myelosuppression, flu-like symptoms, rashes and oedema. Gemcitabine is the standard therapy for pancreatic tumours and also is used in NSCLC.

Mitotic Inhibitors

There are two major classes of mitotic inhibitors, the vinca alkaloids and the taxanes. The vinca alkaloids are naturally occurring or semisynthetic compounds found in the periwinkle plant (*Vinca rosea*): vincristine, vinblastine and vinorelbine. They inhibit formation of the microtubule spindle on which the chromatids line up during metaphase in mitosis and therefore prevent cell division. They are all given intravenously and, despite being similar in structure, have differing side effects. Vincristine is used in lymphomas, leukaemias and breast cancer. It is vesicant locally and neurotoxicity is the main dose-limiting toxicity. This presents in the form of a sensorimotor peripheral neuropathy (paraesthesia in fingers, muscle cramps, paralytic ileus, constipation). Vinblastine is also a sclerosant, but myelosuppression, especially thrombocytopenia, is the main dose-limiting toxicity. Neurotoxicity is less severe than with vincristine. It is used mainly in lymphoma, testicular teratoma and NSCLC. Vinorelbine is the most recently discovered vinca alkaloid and causes less alopecia and neuropathy than the older agents. It can, however, cause significant constipation. It also has the advantage of being available for intravenous and oral administration.

The taxanes are an important class of anticancer drugs in the field of oncology. Although they also have an effect on the formation of the microtubule spindle, they differ from the vinca alkaloids because they promote the assembly of the microtubule spindle and inhibit its disassembly. Paclitaxel is an extract from the bark of the Pacific yew. Initially, its development was hampered by the limited supply of the primary source and also its poor solubility in water. With the development of docetaxel, the semisynthetic analogue from the needles of the tree, the supply was no longer threatened. The most important antitumour activity of these drugs has been seen in breast and ovarian cancer although they are also used in other solid tumours such as gastrooesophageal cancer and cancer of unknown primary. The latest semisynthetic analogue to be developed is cabazitaxel which is licensed for use in men with castration-resistant prostate cancer.

All drugs are given intravenously and there has been a great deal of work involved in optimising the scheduling. Despite being closely related, there are some differences in their toxicity profiles. Both have myelosuppression as one of the major limiting side effects with the nadir occurring at days 8 to 10 postinfusion. A relatively rare but important side effect of paclitaxel is a hypersensitivity reaction with dyspnoea, urticaria and hypotension. Patients therefore receive prophylactic steroids and H2 inhibitors as premedication. Paclitaxel also produces a peripheral neuropathy characterised by sensory symptoms in a glove and stocking distribution. This can be permanent. A newcomer to the field is abraxane, a novel nanoparticle albumin-bound paclitaxel. It has fewer hypersensitivity reactions and is licensed for use in metastatic breast cancer.

Docetaxel is characterised by a unique fluid retention syndrome with the development of oedema and weight gain. As with paclitaxel, a premedication is used. Skin toxicity may occur and this produces a widespread itchy erythematous rash and nail changes characterised by discolouration, ridging and onycholysis—the nails lift up from the nail bed. Liver toxicity can occur if patients with impaired liver function are not given a dose reduction. Stomatitis and diarrhoea are more common with docetaxel. All taxanes cause alopecia.

A new approach to selectively delivering mitotic inhibitors to cancer cells has been achieved with the development of trastuzumab emtansine. This is an antibody-drug conjugate consisting of the monoclonal antibody trastuzumab (Herceptin) linked to the mitotic inhibitor emtansine (DM1). Trastuzumab is a targeted therapy (see later) that binds to the HER-2/neu receptor on cancer cells; the conjugate thereby allows delivery of the toxin (DM1) specifically to these tumour cells and kills them.

Topoisomerase Inhibitors

Topoisomerases are enzymes involved in the coiling and uncoiling of DNA. There are two types. Topoisomerase I inhibitors bind to double-stranded DNA and cause a single-strand break in DNA. The camptothecin analogues topotecan and irinotecan are topoisomerase I inhibitors. Topoisomerase II exists as alpha and beta isoenzymes. They undergo covalent bonding to complementary strands of DNA and cleave both strands. Topoisomerase II inhibitors prevent the religation of DNA cleaved by topoisomerase II and produce protein-linked breaks in DNA. Epipodophyllotoxins are examples of topoisomerase II inhibitors. The anthracyclines inhibit both type I and type II topoisomerases and therefore will be discussed in this section too.

Camptothecin was the first topoisomerase I inhibitor to be discovered. Its further development was hindered by toxicity and it was not until its analogues, topotecan and irinotecan, were developed that the usefulness of this group of drugs became apparent. Topotecan was the first camptothecin analogue approved for clinical use and is now used in ovarian cancer and small cell lung cancer. It can be given intravenously or orally with the latter being far more convenient. The major side effects are neutropenia and nausea and vomiting. Interestingly, although the neutropenia can be profound, the nadir is very short-lived and therefore is seldom complicated by sepsis.

Irinotecan is a semisynthetic derivative of camptothecin. Its active metabolite SN-38 binds to the topoisomerase I enzyme-DNA cleaved complex and prevents religation, thus causing DSB. SN-38 is mainly cleared by the liver and the drug can only be used with caution in patients with abnormal liver function. Irinotecan has a role in the treatment of colorectal cancer and is active in patients with 5-FU-resistant disease. The major side effects are diarrhoea and myelosuppression. These can occur concurrently with fatal outcome if the diarrhoea is not controlled correctly. Irinotecan is also used in the management of upper gastrointestinal malignancies.

Etoposide (VP16) is the most widely used epipodophyllotoxin. Like 5-FU, it is a good example of a schedule-dependent drug because it is more effective given over 5 days than on 1 day. It can be given orally or intravenously and the dose-limiting toxicity is bone marrow suppression. The nadir is at about 16 days. Nausea, vomiting and anorexia are relatively minor but more marked if etoposide is given orally. Alopecia is also common as is mucositis. Etoposide is used mainly in Hodgkin's disease, non-Hodgkin's lymphoma, small cell lung cancer, and testicular teratoma.

Daunorubicin, doxorubicin (Adriamycin) and epirubicin are the principal anthracycline antibiotics. They are produced from different strains of fungi (*Streptomyces*). The mechanisms of their cytotoxic action are not fully understood. These anthracyclines induce formation of topoisomerase-DNA complexes and prevent the enzyme from completing the religation of the ligation–religation reaction. In addition, they insert part of their planar structure between two adjacent base pairs (intercalation), causing single-strand breaks (SSB) and DSB. They also can undergo chemical reduction to form free radicals.

Doxorubicin and epirubicin are given intravenously and the main toxicity is to the bone marrow, gastrointestinal tract and the heart. The nadir of the white count is at 10 days. Epirubicin causes slightly less vomiting than the other two anthracyclines. Daunorubicin and doxorubicin and, to a much lesser extent, epirubicin, cause cumulative cardiotoxicity and there is a maximum recommended total dose. Acute cardiac toxicity is manifest by arrhythmias and abnormalities of electrical conduction. The chronic effect is a cardiomyopathy (pericarditis and congestive cardiac failure) and, thus, anthracyclines should be avoided if there is previous history of cardiac failure or ischaemic heart disease. Their use is widespread in lymphoma, breast cancer, sarcomas, lung cancer, Wilms' tumour and acute myelogenous leukaemia (daunorubicin).

In an attempt to improve the antitumour effect of doxorubicin, a liposomal preparation called doxil (Caelyx® in the United Kingdom) has been developed. Essentially, the doxorubicin molecule has been formulated in a fat bubble. The body's reticuloendothelial system fails to recognise the molecule as being foreign, hence the term *stealth liposome*, and therefore the drug has a longer half-life. The side effects of doxil are generally less than for doxorubicin except for the development of a hand-foot syndrome called palmar-plantar erythrodysaesthesia. It is used in breast cancer and ovarian cancer.

Miscellaneous
Platinum Analogues

The platinum drugs are widely used in a variety of tumours such as testicular teratoma and seminoma, ovarian, cervical, NSCLC and osteosarcoma. Cisplatin and carboplatin inhibit DNA synthesis in a similar way to alkylating agents. They form cross-linkages (adducts) between a pair of their chlorine atoms and the guanine molecules of opposing DNA strands (interstrand linkages) but differ in that they also bind to bases on the same DNA strand (intrastrand linkages). Both drugs are administered intravenously and are predominantly excreted in the urine. Cisplatin causes severe nausea and vomiting which can be prevented with 5-HT$_3$ antagonists and aprepitant, the NK-1 antagonist. In addition, cisplatin causes renal impairment and therefore it is essential that pre- and posttreatment hydration be used. The peripheral nerves and auditory nerves are sensitive to cisplatin and patients may develop high frequency hearing loss and peripheral neuropathy. Carboplatin has the advantage of much less emesis, ototoxicity, nephrotoxicity and neurotoxicity. The dose-limiting toxicity is to the bone marrow, particularly to platelets. Unlike the other chemotherapy agents, carboplatin is dosed depending on the renal function of the patient rather than the patient's body surface area.

Oxaliplatin is the most recent platinum analogue to be licensed. It is a third-generation platinum compound and differs from the other platinum drugs by having a large 1,2-diaminocyclohexane (DACH) ligand in its structure. It is thought that the presence of the DACH group renders the molecule nonrecognisable by the mismatch repair process. This means that the DNA repair mechanisms that are responsible for platinum resistance are not so effective. Oxaliplatin therefore is useful in tumours where cisplatin has failed and also in colorectal cancer, a tumour type not classically treated by platinum agents. Oxaliplatin does not have the nephrotoxicity associated with carboplatin, although it does have a striking neurotoxicity. Patients develop a peripheral neuropathy with cumulative drug exposure. They also develop an acute neuropathy that is characterised by cold-induced tingling (paraesthesia) in the fingertips and toes after infusion. This can also affect the throat on drinking cold drinks and the patient develops a feeling of choking. Oxaliplatin is usually administered with 5-FU chemotherapy, as in combination they are synergistic.

Nonanthracycline Antibiotics

Actinomycin D is a highly toxic drug, which is only given intravenously. It is used in the treatment of some sarcomas and causes significant myelosuppression, oral ulceration, nausea, vomiting, diarrhoea, alopecia and skin rashes.

Bleomycin intercalates with DNA strands causing SSB and DSB. It inhibits DNA synthesis and, to a lesser degree, RNA synthesis. It is usually given intravenously, although it can be given intramuscularly, subcutaneously or intrapleurally (for pleural effusions). The main toxicity is to the lung, and progressive fibrosis occurs causing nonproductive cough and dyspnoea. Respiratory complications of general anaesthesia are increased. Occasionally, patients have an immediate life-threatening anaphylactic reaction, although fever and chills are more common. Skin changes are common with pigmentation, erythema and thickening of the nail bed. There is little myelosuppression and so it is often used in combination with other agents. The main use of bleomycin is in the treatment of testicular teratoma, although it is also used in lymphoma.

Enzymes

Asparaginase is used mainly in the treatment of leukaemia. It is an enzyme that degrades asparagine, an essential amino acid for protein and nucleic acid synthesis. Tumour cells, unlike their normal counterparts, have no or little asparagine synthetase, the enzyme necessary for making asparagine. When asparagine levels fall, both protein and nucleic acid synthesis are inhibited. It is used in the treatment of acute leukaemias, and the most common side effect is a hypersensitivity reaction.

Hormones

There is a group of cancers where the mainstay of treatment is hormone therapy. These include breast, prostate, and endometrial tumours. In recent years, an increase in the understanding of the molecular biology of hormone receptors has greatly improved the treatment of these cancers, in particular breast cancer. Remissions may last for years and symptomatic benefit may be substantial, and even dramatic, during this period. Although the administration of hormones avoids the morbidities particular to surgery, RT and cytotoxic chemotherapy, side effects are seen, some of which are unacceptable (e.g. masculinising effects of androgens in women with breast cancer) and can be dangerous (e.g. cardiovascular morbidity from diethylstilboestrol for prostate cancer). A careful balance must be struck between toxicity and benefit in tumour control. There are five main areas that will be discussed:

- Antioestrogens
- Aromatase inhibitors
- Gonadotrophin-releasing hormone analogues
- Antiandrogen therapy
- Female hormones

Antioestrogens

Tamoxifen is the most important synthetic antioestrogen preparation. First, it blocks the oestrogen stimulation of breast cancer cells by competitive binding to oestrogen receptors. It also has weak oestrogenic action, raising levels of sex hormone binding globulin, which binds to freely circulating oestrogen and so reduces the amount of free oestrogen available to bind to oestrogen receptors. The binding of oestrogen to the oestrogen receptors reduces the synthesis of growth factors and stimulates the production of progesterone receptors. Tamoxifen is used in women whose breast tumour cells are found on immunohistological staining to express oestrogen or progesterone receptors. It is indicated as adjuvant therapy in early breast cancer in pre- and postmenopausal women and also in recurrent and advanced breast cancer.

The oestrogenic properties of tamoxifen are responsible for both its activity and toxicity. In general, tamoxifen is tolerated well; however, women do experience significant hot flushes and also an increase in incidence of endometrial cancer. On a more positive note, tamoxifen can prevent cardiovascular events and also osteoporosis in postmenopausal women. In an attempt to overcome the negative aspects of tamoxifen, other selective oestrogen receptor modulators (SERMS), have been developed. These include those that are tamoxifen-like including toremifene, fixed-ring compounds such as raloxifene and selective oestrogen receptor down-regulators (SERDs) such as fulvestrant. There has been a significant amount of work carried out to understand the mode of action of these compounds further and this information will inform the use of these compounds both as chemoprevention agents, and as therapy for early and advanced breast cancer.

Aromatase Inhibitors

Aromatase inhibitors play an important role in the endocrine management of adjuvant, advanced and recurrent oestrogen receptor-positive breast cancer. The earliest of these aromatase inhibitors was aminoglutethimide, a drug now considered to be outdated because of the development of selective aromatase inhibitors with superior side-effect profiles. In postmenopausal women, oestrogen synthesis occurs peripherally (e.g. adrenals and fat) as the enzyme aromatase converts androstenedione to estrone. Aromatase inhibitors block this conversion and are therefore extremely valuable drugs for postmenopausal women with breast cancer. In premenopausal women, oestrogen synthesis is governed by gonadotrophin-releasing hormone stimulating the ovary. Aromatase inhibitors are therefore only useful in premenopausal women who have been oophorectomised. There are a number of first-, second- and third-generation aromatase inhibitors available as shown in Table 19.4. Common toxicities of these drugs include nausea, headache, hot flushes and weight gain. Unlike tamoxifen, aromatase inhibitors may decrease bone density and predispose to osteoporosis. Although clear molecular differences exist between these two types of aromatase inhibitors, significant clinical differences have not been forthcoming from the studies to date. There may be some noncross resistance between the groups as switching from one to another can confer a modest improvement in outcome. A Cochrane analysis has found that in metastatic breast cancer, aromatase inhibitors show a

TABLE 19.4   Summary of Aromatase Inhibitors

Generation	Nonsteroidal	Steroidal
First	Aminogluthemide	Testolactone
Second	Fadrozole	
Third	Anastrazole	Exemestane
	Letrozole	

survival benefit compared with other endocrine therapies, although there is limited data available to identify which individual aromatase inhibitor has the greatest efficacy.

Gonadotrophin-Releasing Hormone Analogues

Downregulation of the gonadotrophin-releasing hormone (GnRH) receptors in the pituitary is achieved by the application of continuous secretion of gonadotrophin-releasing hormone analogues. These analogues of the naturally occurring hypothalamic luteinising hormone-releasing hormone (LHRH) initially cause a transient surge of gonadotrophin (LH) secretion, tumour flare. However, with continuous exposure to these analogues, the LHRH receptors in the pituitary become desensitised, resulting in reduction in the secretion of gonadotrophins. They therefore cause a medical oophorectomy in women and a medical orchidectomy in men. The advantage of this medical suppression of gonad function with GnRH analogues is that the process is reversible.

Goserelin is the most commonly used agent and is about 100 times more potent than naturally occurring GnRH. It is given as a subcutaneously injected capsule on either a monthly or 3-monthly basis for prostate cancer or premenopausal breast cancer. Obviously, the symptoms are what would be expected from sex hormone withdrawal, with menopausal symptoms in women and lack of libido in men. Gynaecomastia is uncommon. However, in general, they are very well tolerated. An alternative GnRH analogue is degarelix (Firmagon) which is a synthetic derivative of the natural GnRH hormone. It therefore competes with natural GnRH for binding to GnRH receptors in the pituitary gland and the reversible binding blocks the release of LH and FSH from the pituitary leading to a rapid suppression of testosterone. Its fast rate of action combined with lack of tumour flare are clearly advantageous.

Antiandrogen Therapy

The initial approach to treat men with prostate cancer is to reduce androgen levels with androgen deprivation therapies including antiandrogens and GnRH analogues. Flutamide is a nonsteroidal antiandrogen and is a pure androgen antagonist used in men with prostate cancer. One of its important metabolites, hydroxyflutamide, is thought to be responsible for its cellular action. It blocks the binding of dihydrotestosterone to its receptor, so inhibiting the action of androgen. It is often used in combination with GnRH analogues. The side effects include gynaecomastia and/or breast tenderness, nausea and diarrhoea and tiredness. Bicalutamide is another nonsteroidal antiandrogen that binds to androgen receptors and therefore inhibits androgen stimulation. Again, it is used in prostate cancer, usually in conjunction with a GnRH analogue to reduce a flare reaction.

Cyproterone acetate is a progestogenic antiandrogen and has two actions. First, it reduces the production of testosterone in the testis by inhibiting the secretion of the pituitary gonadotrophins. Secondly, it competes with androgen receptors, from which it displaces testosterone. Cyproterone is used in prostate cancer to suppress the tumour flare with initial GnRH analogue therapy, and when GnRH analogues are contraindicated or poorly tolerated. Side effects include liver dysfunction, impotence and fluid retention.

When men no longer respond to androgen-deprivation therapy, the disease is called castration-resistant prostate cancer. There are two further oral drugs that target the androgen pathway: abiraterone and enzalutamide. CYP171A is a member of the cytochrome P450 family and is responsible for the conversion of pregnelonone and progesterone to their 17α metabolites. In addition, it can convert 17α-hydroxypregnelonone and 17α-hydroxyprogesterone to the androgens, androstenedione and dihydroepiandrostenedione.

Abiraterone binds CYP17A1 irreversibly and prevents the formation of androgens in the adrenal gland and peripheral tissues of castrate and noncastrate men. Enzalutamide is a drug that blocks the androgen receptor in a number of ways: preventing the binding of androgen to the receptor, preventing the transfer of the androgen receptor to the nucleus and then inhibiting the association of the receptor with nuclear DNA.

Female Hormones (Oestrogens and Progestogens)

Synthetic rather than naturally occurring oestrogens (these are metabolised in the liver), such as diethylstilboestrol, are sometimes used in the treatment of prostate cancer. The side effects from these agents are significant, in particular, risk of cardiovascular disease and nausea and vomiting. With the advent of the antiandrogens, the use of these hormones is now declining.

Progestogens, such as medroxyprogesterone and megestrol, are occasionally used in the treatment of advanced breast cancer and also in endometrial cancer. Their mechanism of action is not completely understood but probably the most important effect is the antioestrogenic action, and less importantly, the direct cytotoxic action. Side effects include weight gain, fluid retention, increased blood clotting and risk of thrombosis and vaginal bleeding.

Targeted Therapies

The real highlight in oncological research over the last 10 years has been the incorporation of targeted therapies into clinical practice. There has been a phenomenal increase in the understanding of the cellular and molecular events in carcinogenesis. By focusing on the differences between normal and malignant tissue, we can target pathways and receptors unique to cancer cells, thus avoiding the blunderbuss of universal killing of dividing cells by conventional cytotoxics. Molecular events that distinguish malignant from normal cells are activation of oncogenes (e.g. ras, erbB2), inactivation of tumour suppressor genes (e.g. p53) and activation of immortality genes (e.g. telomerase). At the cellular level, for a tumour cell to grow and divide it needs its own blood supply (angiogenesis), and the ability to migrate through local tissue (tumour invasion and migration).

Leading the way in this field was the development of imatinib. Nearly all patients (90%) with chronic myeloid leukaemia have a specific genetic abnormality called the Philadelphia chromosome. This is a genetic mutation where reciprocal translocation between chromosomes 9 and 22 result in the production of the oncogene Bcr-Abl. Investigators developed the agent imatinib mesylate (STI571) which specifically inhibits the receptor kinase of BCR-ABL. The results of the clinical trials were truly impressive; complete haematological responses were seen in patients with chronic myeloid leukaemia who failed to respond to conventional agents. Moreover, not only is imatinib an oral drug, the patients had mild side effects, particularly when compared with their previous cytotoxic-induced toxicity. Results of this kind were really unprecedented in oncology and warranted the accelerated approval of imatinib for clinical use. The development of imatinib therefore represents a paradigm for the development of targeted therapies. Currently there are 35 kinase inhibitors which have been approved for cancer therapy with hundreds in development. In addition, there are 27 monoclonal antibodies licensed for use in cancer therapy. Key groups of targeted therapies include:

- Epidermal growth factor receptor (EGFR) inhibitors
- RAS-RAF-ERK (MAPK) and PI3 kinase inhibitors
- Vascular endothelial growth factor (VEGF) inhibitors
- Protease inhibitors
- PARP inhibitors
- CDK4/6 inhibitors

Epidermal Growth Factor Receptor

Epidermal growth factor receptor (EGFR) (ERBB1) and ERBB2 (HER-2) are overexpressed or amplified in many malignancies including NSCLC, breast, head and neck, pancreas and colorectal cancers. Licensed anti-EGFR therapies include monoclonal antibodies (cetuximab, panitumumab, trastuzumab and pertuzumab) and oral small molecule inhibitors of thymidine kinase (TK) activity (gefitinib, erlotinib and lapatinib).

Trastuzumab (Herceptin) is a humanised anti-HER-2 (ERBB2) monoclonal antibody that has been approved for monotherapy or combination therapy (with paclitaxel) for women with HER-2 over-expressing breast cancer and HER-2-positive gastric cancer. Pertuzumab (Perjeta) is a monoclonal antibody used in combination with trastuzumab and docetaxel for the treatment of metastatic HER-2-positive breast cancer It is the first-in-class HER dimerisation inhibitor which means it inhibits the dimerisation of HER-2 with other HER receptors, thereby preventing the signalling pathway in the cell and subsequent proliferation. Cetuximab (Erbitux) is a chimeric immunoglobin (Ig) G1 antibody and is licensed for use in combination with irinotecan-containing chemotherapy in patients with metastatic colorectal cancer with wild-type-RAS mutation status. This treatment is complicated by a unique rash which is acneiform—indeed there is a suggestion that the rash may actually be a predictive biomarker of response to cetuximab. Other side effects include diarrhoea and infusion reactions. Panitumumab (Vectibix) is a fully human IgG2 monoclonal antibody that binds to the ectodomain of EGFR. It is also licensed for use in RAS wild-type colorectal cancer.

Gefitinib (Iressa) is a tyrosine kinase inhibitor (TKI) which blocks the binding of the adenosine triphosphate to the intracellular domain of EGFR. Only patients with activating EGFR mutations respond well to the drug, and therefore gefitinib is only approved for use in metastatic NSCLC with activating mutations of the EGFR-TK. The most common side effects seen with gefitinib are rash, diarrhoea and fatigue. Erlotinib (Tarceva) is another EGFR TKI and is licensed for use in NSCLC and pancreas cancer. Lapatinib (Tykerb) is a dual-specific TKI targeting both EGFR and HER-2. It is licensed for use in combination with capecitabine chemotherapy in patients with metastatic breast cancer who have progressed after trastuzumab and other chemotherapy. Afatinib (Gilotrif) is an inhibitor of EGFR and erbB-2 (HER-2) and is used in patients with EGFR mutation-positive NSCLC. Osimertinib (Tagrisso) is a third-generation EGFR TKI which is used to treat locally advanced or metastatic NSCLC, with a T790M mutation in EGFR. This mutation may be de novo or acquired following first-line treatment with other TKIs, such as gefitinib and afatinib.

Signalling Through RAS-RAF-ERK (MAPK) and PI3K-AKT

Both these pathways are major downstream signals for the EGFR family members and RAS-regulated pathways interact at multiple points, including with the PI3K-AKT-mTOR pathway, and with c-MYC. The PI3K-Akt-mTOR pathway is activated in many cancers, therefore is a good target for therapy. Temsirolimus (Torisel) is the first-in-class mTOR inhibitor licensed for use in metastatic renal cancer. It is administered intravenously, unlike everolimus (Afinitor) which is an oral mTOR inhibitor used in renal cell cancer, breast cancer and some neuroendocrine tumours. Both compounds are relatively well tolerated with pneumonitis, asthenia, rash, anaemia, nausea, anorexia, and hyperglycaemia being documented but not usually severe.

It has not been possible to develop a drug to target RAS; however the BRAF protein kinase, which is downstream in the pathway, has been successfully directly targeted with the oral small molecule inhibitors vemurafenib (Zelboraf) and dabrafenib (Tafinlar). Overall, 6% of human cancers contain activating mutations in BRAF13 and like RAS mutations, BRAF mutations are very oncogenic. Just as RAS-mutated cells are dependent on MEK, it is also the case that cells with the activating BRAF mutation, V600E, are dependent on MEK and, thus, ERK signalling for cell survival and proliferation. Vemurafenib and dabrafenib and the MEK inhibitor, trametinib (Mekinist), are now approved for the treatment of BRAF-mutated melanoma, clinically validating the possibility of targeting the RAS/RAF/MEK pathway to achieve meaningful benefit for patients.

Vascular Endothelial Growth Factor Signalling Pathway

Angiogenesis is known to be pivotal in tumour progression and metastasis and because VEGF is the driving force behind angiogenesis, it is not surprising that it has been the target of many approaches. Agents have been developed that target the VEGF ligand, blocking its interaction with the VEGF receptors (bevacizumab) and agents that directly block the receptor (TKIs such as sunitinib). Bevacizumab (Avastin) is a recombinant humanised monoclonal antibody to VEGF-A. It is licensed for use in metastatic colorectal, breast, NSCLC and renal cancer. The side effect profile of bevacizumab includes hypertension, a class effect of VEGF inhibitors, thromboembolic events (both arterial and venous) and gastrointestinal perforation. Aflibercept (Zaltrap) is a recombinant fusion protein consisting of VEGF-binding portions from the extracellular domains of human VEGF receptors 1 and 2 that are fused to the Fc portion of the human IgG1 immunoglobulin. It is used in the treatment of metastatic colorectal cancer and has a similar side effect profile to Avastin but with more neutropenia demonstrated.

Because VEGF mediates its angiogenic effect through several TK receptors, many VEGF TKIs have been tested. Sorafenib (Nexavar) is licensed for use in renal cell and hepatocellular cancer, and sunitinib (Sutent) is licensed for use in renal cell cancer and gastrointestinal stromal tumour (GIST). Numerous other TKIs are in clinical studies. Some are highly selective, targeting only specific VEGF receptors, whereas others are more promiscuous and target other kinases such as platelet-derived growth factor (PDGF) and EGFR. Despite being targeted therapies, these drugs do have significant side effects including neutropenia, fatigue, rashes, diarrhoea and stomatitis.

Proteasome Inhibitors

Proteasome inhibitors, exemplified by bortezomib (Velcade), prevent degradation of various proteins in the proteasome. Bortezomib was the first selective proteasome inhibitor and is licensed in patients with refractory or relapsed multiple myeloma (MM). It is believed to be effective in myeloma by interfering with normal function of the NFkB signalling pathway, thus reducing tumour cell replication and angiogenesis, and promoting apoptosis. Other drugs in the class include carfilzomib (Kyprolis) and ixazomib (Ninlaro). Both are used to treat myeloma and the latter is the first orally available proteasome inhibitor.

Poly(ADP-Ribose) Polymerase Inhibitors

DNA damage and its repair, or lack of, are responsible for the formation of mutations, which cause nearly all cancers. Healthy cells defend themselves against the potential negative effects of DNA damage through the DNA damage response (DDR). In this process, DNA damage is recognised, the cell cycle pauses, and DNA repair mechanisms start with the result of genomic integrity and fidelity. Poly(ADP-ribose) polymerases (PARPs) are critical enzymes in repairing DNA damage, specifically SSB. If SSB are not repaired before DNA is replicated then DSB occur during that process which result in cell death. Therefore, PARP inhibitors have for some time been studied as anticancer therapies. However, it was only with the application of the genetic concept of synthetic lethality that real progress was made in getting the agents into the clinic. This concept is based on the idea that a defect in either one of two genes has little effect on the cell, but a simultaneous combination of defects in both genes results in death. Thus for example, tumour cells with inactivating mutation of the BRCA DNA-repair genes, which in itself is not lethal, will be killed if they are also exposed to PARP inhibitors. So far, three agents, olaparib (Lynparza), rucaparib (Rubraca) and niraparib (Zejula) have been licensed for use in BRCA-mutant ovarian and breast cancer. Generally, the agents are well tolerated; nausea and fatigue are relatively common with grade 3 and 4 events being seen more rarely. Patients are therefore able to take them for prolonged periods, unlike many cytotoxic agents, although the accumulation of a number of grade 2 toxicities may lead to dosing interruptions.

CDK4/6 Inhibitors

Even before the publication of Hanahan and Weinberg's seminal paper 'The hallmarks of cancer', targeting the cell cycle was a key anticancer strategy. Only recently with the development of CDK4/6 inhibitors has this approach come to fruition. CDK4 and CDK6 are cyclin-dependent kinases that control the transition between the G1 and S phases of the cell cycle. CDK4/6 activity is usually deregulated and overactive in cancer cells. A major target of CDK4 and CDK6 during cell-cycle progression is the retinoblastoma protein (Rb). When Rb is phosphorylated, its growth-suppressive properties are inactivated. Selective CDK4/6 inhibitors 'turn off' these kinases and dephosphorylate Rb, resulting in a block of cell-cycle progression in mid-G1. This causes cell-cycle arrest and prevents the proliferation of cancer cells. Oestrogen receptor-positive breast cancer is particularly dependent upon CDK4 for proliferation. Therefore, the combination of a CDK4/6 inhibitor and antioestrogen therapy works synergistically in oestrogen receptor-positive breast cancer. Palbociclib (Ibrance) and ribociclib (Kisqali) are both licensed for use in oestrogen receptor-positive metastatic breast cancer in combination with aromatase inhibitors. Toxicities are manageable although patients need to be carefully monitored for neutropenia, liver dysfunction and QTc prolongation.

Immunotherapy

In recent years there has been an explosion of activity in the area of immunotherapy. Some extraordinary responses to these therapies have been realised in tumour types such as melanoma, renal cell and NSCLC. Essentially, the main premise of immunotherapy approaches in cancer treatment is to stimulate the patient's immune system to attack the tumour. This can be achieved by immunising the patient with a cancer vaccine, administering therapeutic antibodies or with the greatest recent success, manipulating immune checkpoints and pathways.

Therapeutic Antibodies

In addition to the antibodies discussed in the previous section, rituximab (MabThera) is a chimeric monoclonal antibody targeting the CD20 antigen found on normal B cells and B-cell lymphomas. It is licensed for use for follicular lymphoma, diffuse large B-cell lymphoma and chronic lymphocytic leukaemia and has remarkably improved the outlook for these patients. It can be administered either as monotherapy or in combination with chemotherapy such as the CHOP regimen. Iodine-131 tositumomab (Bexxar) and 90Y ibritumomab tiuxetan (Zevalin) are both radiolabelled CD20 targeted antibodies. They are licensed for use in some refractory lymphomas but their costs are prohibitive.

Alemtuzumab (previously known as CAMPATH) is a humanised monoclonal antibody targeting the CD52 antigen found on B lymphocytes. It has been licensed for use for patients with B-cell chronic lymphocytic leukaemia who are unable to receive the chemotherapy drug,

fludarabine. It is associated with significant haematological toxicity, especially neutropenia.

Lenolidamide is an immunomodulating drug that is licensed for patients with advanced MM. It is a potent analogue of thalidomide and works in a number of ways: inhibiting proliferation of certain haematopoietic tumour cells (including MM plasma tumour cells and those with deletions of chromosome 5), enhancing T cell and natural killer (NK) cell-mediated immunity, inhibiting angiogenesis, and inhibiting production of proinflammatory cytokines (e.g. TNF-α and IL6) by monocytes. In studies, the most concerning side effects of treatment were venous thromboembolic events and myelosuppression. Not surprising there is also a significant risk of teratogenicity and therefore patients or their partners must not get pregnant while on treatment.

Immune Checkpoint Inhibitors

The two key targets for manipulating the immune checkpoint mechanism are cytotoxic T-lymphocyte-associated molecule-4 (CTLA-4) and programmed cell death receptor-1 (PD-1) or programmed cell death ligand-1 (PD-L1). Ipilimumab (Yervoy), was the first-in-class anti-CTLA-4 antibody to be licensed for the treatment of melanoma, NSCLC, small cell lung cancer, bladder cancer and metastatic hormone-refractory prostate cancer. Some exceptional responses were seen, especially in melanoma, although there was quite marked variation in response. In addition, unique side effects were seen because of nonspecific immunological activation—immune-related adverse events (irAEs). These include skin, gastrointestinal, liver and endocrine toxicities, often requiring specific management strategies, not usually adopted in more typical cytotoxic reactions. For some, the irAEs were fatal and for others, the adverse event persisted even when the causative agent was stopped. Complete new algorithms have had to be developed to manage these compounds safely, for example, using high dose steroids and then infliximab for the treatment of immune-related colitis.

Antibodies that disrupt the PD-1 pathway include those that target PD-1, nivolumab (Opdivo) and pembrolizumab (Keytruda), and those that target PD-L1, atezolizumab (Tecentriq) and avelumab (Bavencio). Because of durable responses and reduced toxicity, these agents are licensed for use in urothelial cancer, NSCLC, Merkel cell carcinoma and head and neck squamous cancer. Interestingly in 2017, pembrolizumab was licensed for use by the US Food and Drug Administration, not based on a specific tumour type, but rather a specific genetic alteration–mismatch repair deficiency or microsatellite instability. Generally speaking, these agents are less toxic than CTLA-4 inhibitors; however, there is a lag phase before response which on average is 2 months. Therefore, to use these drugs safely, patients need to be well enough to tolerate this wait. Also when monitoring responses, the standard RECIST criteria can be misleading as occasionally there can be pseudo-progression seen on CT scans. This is borne out by the fact that in one analysis of patients with melanoma on ipilimumab surviving 4 years or more, 25% had never achieved more than progression of disease as measured by RECIST.

Currently in the field of immunotherapy, clinical studies are ongoing, studying agents such as bispecific antibodies which combine recognition of antigen-binding sites on tumour cells with engagement of effector immune cells. There are more antibody-drug conjugates in development and of course numerous combination studies trying to combine immunotherapies with cytotoxics, RT and also different class immunotherapies. Combinations are particularly challenging because of the adverse event profiles and establishing safe but biologically effective doses when the adverse event may arise later in the course of treatment and outside the stand window of testing in a classical phase I study. Major enthusiasm at the moment is around the utility of chimeric antigen receptor (CAR) T cells. Typically, these are synthetically engineered T cell receptors with an extracellular domain that recognises a tumour cell antigen, and an intracellular domain that activates T cells. In practice, T cells are removed from the patient, genetically engineered and reinfused. To date, some significant clinical results have been seen using this technique in patients with haematological malignancies, for example anti-CD19 CAR T cells have been approved for treatment in lymphoma (axicabtagene ciloleucel marketed as Yescarta) and tisagenlecleucel (Kymriah) in B-cell acute lymphoblastic leukaemia. Translating these successes into the management of solid tumours remains the subject of much ongoing research.

There is no doubt that major progress has occurred in the management of patients with anticancer agents. This is both in the supportive care of patients undergoing toxic treatment and the development of innovative therapies. We cannot however afford to be complacent. Even with extraordinary early responses with immunotherapy, eventually the hope of cure is thwarted by development of resistance. Precision medicine approaches are again limited by resistance pathways, tumour heterogeneity and the availability of drugs which have been licensed on the basis of a tissue biopsy rather than genetic aberration. Toxic effects can be very burdensome to patients and finally, the cost of these drugs is prohibitive. In the next decade we will continue to see great innovation, but we need to ensure that these approaches are affordable and continue to benefit patients. Making cancer a chronic disease that is treatable rather than a fatal disease is acceptable as long as the therapy is acceptable for the quality of life of patients.

FURTHER READING

Brock A, Huang S. Precision oncology: between vaguely right and precisely wrong. Cancer Res 2017;77(23):6473–9.

Brufsky A. Long-term management of patients with hormone receptor-positive metastatic breast cancer: concepts for sequential and combination endocrine-based therapies. Cancer Treat Rev. 2017;59:22–32.

Corona SP, Ravelli A, Cretella D, Cappelletti M, Zanotti L, Dester M Gobbi A, Petronini P, Generali P. CDK4/6 inhibitors in HER2-positive breast cancer. Crit. Rev. Oncol/Hematol. 2017;112:208–14.

Devita VT, Lawrence TS, Rosenberg SA, Depinho RA, Weinberg RA. Cancer principles and practice of oncology. 10th ed. Philadelphia: Lippincott Williams; 2016.

Downing A, Morris EJA, Corrigan N, Sebag-Montefiore D, Finan PJ, Thomas JD, Chapman M, Hamilton R, Campbell H, Cameron D, Kaplan R, Parmar M, Stephens R, Seymour M, Gregory W, Selby P. High hospital research participation and improved colorectal cancer survival outcomes: a population-based study. Gut. 2017;66:89–96.

Eisenhauer EA, Therasse P, Bogaerts J, Schwartz LH, Sargent D, Ford R, Dancey J, Arbuck S, Gwyther S, Mooney M, Rubinstein L, Shankar L, Dodd L, Kaplan R, Lacombe D, Verweij J. New response evaluation criteria in solid tumours: revised RECIST guideline (version 1.1). Eur J Cancer. 2009;45:228–47.

Gougis P, Wassermann J, Spano JP, Keynan N, Funck-Brentano C, Salem JE. Clinical pharmacology of anti-angiogenic drugs in oncology. Crit Rev Oncol Hematol. 2017;119:75–93.

Ke X, Shen L. Molecular targeted therapy of cancer: The progress and future prospect. Front Lab. Med. 2017;1:69–75.

Editorial Lancet Oncology. Calling time on the immunotherapy gold rush. Lancet Oncol. 2017;18:981.

Komura K, Sweeney J, Inamoto T, Ibuki N, Azuma H, Kantoff P. Current treatment strategies for advanced prostate cancer. Int J Urol. 2017.

Lopez JS, Banerji U. Combine and conquer: challenges for targeted therapy combinations in early phase trials. Nat Rev Clin Oncol. 2017;14(1):57–66.

Manasanch EE, Orlowski RZ. Proteasome inhibitors in cancer therapy. Nat Rev Clin Oncol. 2017;14:417–33.

Ohmoto A, Yachida S. Current status of poly(ADP-ribose) polymerase inhibitors and future directions. Oncotargets Therapy. 2017;10:5195–208.

Perry MC. The chemotherapy source book. 5th ed. Philadelphia: Lippincott Williams & Wilkins; 2012.

Velasquez M, Bonifant C, Gottschalk S. Redirecting T cells to hematological malignancies with bispecific antibodies. Blood 2018;131(1):30–8.

Wang X, Huang S, Zhang Y, Zhu L, Wu X. The application and mechanism of PD pathway blockade for cancer therapy. Postgrad Med J. 2018;94:53–60.

Wu P. Small-molecule kinase inhibitors: an analysis of FDA-approved drugs. Drug Discovery Today. 2016;21(1):5–10.

Younes A, Ansell S, Fowler N, Wilson W, de Vos S, Seymour J, Advani R, Forero A, Morschhauser F, Kersten MJ, Tobiani K, Zinzani PI, Zucca E, Abramson J, Vose J. The landscape of new drugs in lymphoma. Nat Rev Clin Oncol. 2017;14:335–46.

Zheng H-C. The molecular mechanisms of chemoresistance in cancers. Oncotarget. 2017;8(35):59950–64.

20

Skin and Lip Cancer

Charles Kelly, Paul Symonds,
Cliff Lawrence

CHAPTER OUTLINE

INTRODUCTION

Skin cancer is the most common human cancer. It can be divided broadly into two types. These are melanoma and nonmelanoma. Keratinocyte-derived skin cancers are a group made up of squamous and basal cell carcinoma. A further group of much less common skin tumours, arising from the skin appendages, are primary cutaneous lymphoma, Kaposi's sarcoma and Merkel cell tumours.

Keratinocyte skin tumours and basal cell carcinoma, in particular, are the most common skin cancers. Their true numbers are often underreported because they do not have to be counted as new cancers in many cancer registries.

Basal cell carcinomas are very common and relatively benign. However, melanomas and squamous cell carcinoma of the skin carry a significant mortality, as do much less common Merkel cell tumours, skin lymphomas and Kaposi's sarcoma (KS). In 2016 (CRUK 2018), the incidence of malignant melanoma in the United Kingdom was 15,906 new cases with 2285 deaths. By comparison, there were 142,101 new cases of nonmelanomatous skin cancer (NMSC) and 1319 deaths.

The incidence of both melanoma and keratinocyte skin cancers is increasing decade by decade, and further increases can be expected as the population ages.

KERATINOCYTE SKIN TUMOURS

Keratinocyte skin tumours are the most common form of skin cancer and develop from epidermal keratinocytes. The incidence of both squamous cell carcinoma (SCC) and basal cell carcinoma (BCC) is related to increased life-time sun exposure.

Aetiology

The following factors can all be involved in the development of keratinocyte skin tumours, but these skin cancers are all more common in white skin. Skin pigmentation protects from the development of these tumours, so that, at one extreme, albinos have a much-increased risk of skin cancer, whereas NMSC is rare in people with black skin.

Ultraviolet Radiation

Excessive exposure to ultraviolet B (UVB) from sunlight and ultraviolet A (UVA) from sunbeds has been implicated as an aetiological factor. BCCs are common in Caucasians living in Australia and the United States. It is estimated there will be 2 million new BCCs diagnosed in the United States in 2018. The incidence is highest in the southern and southwestern states.

Premalignant Skin Lesions

Lesions such as actinic keratosis (Fig. 20.1) or Bowen's disease (Fig. 20.2) are known for their potential to develop into SCC. These lesions are found on sun-exposed parts of the body. Bowen's disease is squamous carcinoma in situ and, in about 5% of cases, develops into invasive squamous cancer. Actinic keratoses do carry an increased risk of developing SCC but only a small minority, approximately 1 in 1000, go on to become skin cancers.

Topical Carcinogens

Direct skin contact with chemicals such as tar, pitch or nonsolvent refined mineral oils are a potential cause of SCC.

Ingested Carcinogens

These are becoming less common but, previously, it was relatively common to include arsenic in proprietary 'tonics'. Arsenic can cause multiple skin tumours, both SCCs and basal cell, as well as premalignant skin changes (Fig. 20.3).

Psoralen Ultraviolet A Treatment for Psoriasis

Psoralen UVA (PUVA) (Fig. 20.4) is an effective treatment for psoriasis, where a drug (a psoralen), is given before exposing the patient to UVA. However, this treatment does increase the chance of development of a keratinocyte origin tumour, particularly a squamous cancer. Risk increases with the cumulative dose of UVA.

Immunosuppression

This is most commonly seen now in patients who have had organ transplants, and the normal ratio of SCC to BCC is reversed, with SCC becoming more common than BCC. Twenty years after a kidney transplant 50% of patients listed in the Oxford transplant register had either a squamous or basal cell skin tumour.

Basal Cell Naevus Syndrome (Gorlin Syndrome)

Basal cell naevus syndrome (BCNS) is an uncommon autosomal dominant genetic abnormality having a familial syndrome, with patients at increased risk of developing multiple BCCs at a relatively young age.

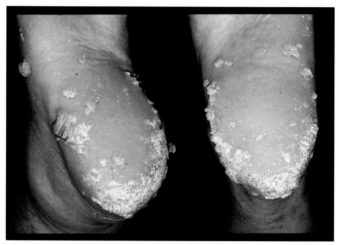

Figure 20.3 These thick keratoses developed following the ingestion of arsenic as a constituent of a 'tonic'.

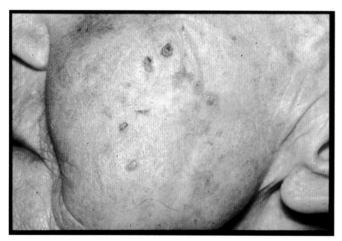

Figure 20.1 Actinic keratosis with a background of sun-damaged skin.

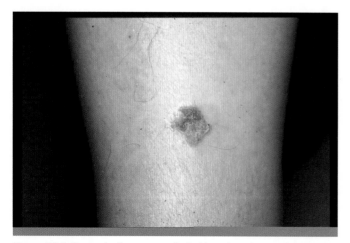

Figure 20.2 Bowen's disease on a limb. Note the colour and the superficiality of the lesion.

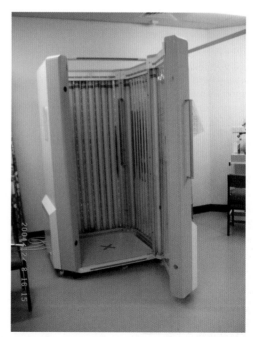

Figure 20.4 This is a typical ultraviolet A generating machine used in psoralen ultraviolet A (PUVA) treatments. Note the tubes used to produce the UVA.

There are also other skeletal and skin abnormalities, such as tiny pinpoint lesions on the palms known as palmar pitting (Fig. 20.5), dental cysts, frontal bossing, bifid ribs and calcification of the falx. These other abnormalities may well be picked up by chance when the patient is being investigated for other problems. Radiotherapy (RT) is contraindicated in patients with the syndrome, as it is thought that giving RT can initiate the development of BCCs. Medulloblastoma is also more common in patients with BCNS. It is important to exclude BCNS before RT is given to children with medulloblastoma because of the risk of radiation-induced multiple BCCs at the treatment site.

Xeroderma Pigmentosa

Xeroderma pigmentosa (Fig. 20.6) is a very rare, autosomal recessive genetic condition in which there is defective repair of DNA after damage by UV exposure. These patients can develop SCC or BCC of the skin, or Bowen's disease in childhood, after minimal sun exposure. Although very uncommon, xeroderma pigmentosa has provided great insight into the mechanism of skin cancer development.

Chronic Trauma

Forms of chronic ulceration (Fig. 20.7), direct thermal damage, or previous burn scars can all predispose to the development of SCC of skin.

Age

These skin cancers are essentially a disease of the elderly, reflecting accumulated UV skin damage. As the population ages, the incidence of skin cancer is steadily increasing.

Ionising Radiation

In the early days of RT, a variety of benign skin diseases were treated by ionising radiation. Many years after treatment, basal cell or squamous lesions appeared in the irradiated skin. The maximum effects were seen in children treated for ringworm.

Basal Cell Carcinoma

BCC is the most common skin cancer in white populations, being three to four times as common as SCC of the skin. As the name suggests, these tumours arise from cells in the basal cell layer of the epidermis. They are more common in the elderly. Because the main cause of these tumours is UV exposure, they are more common on sun-exposed sites (Fig. 20.8A).

There are several clinical subtypes, the most characteristic being nodular BCC (see Fig. 20.8B). This presents as a characteristic pearly papule or nodule, classically with the rolled translucent edge and telangiectasia. The centre of this lesion often ulcerates and becomes crusted. The lesion may appear as if it is about to heal, but then can progress into further cycles of growth, breakdown, crusting and regression. These lesions will not, however, disappear without active treatment.

There are other clinical subtypes as well as the classical nodular BCC including: superficial, micronodular, sclerosing, infiltrating and pigmented variants. Diagnosis of these variants may be difficult without a biopsy. It is rare for a BCC to metastasise but it can occur and is more frequent with longstanding large lesions, which have often been neglected for years.

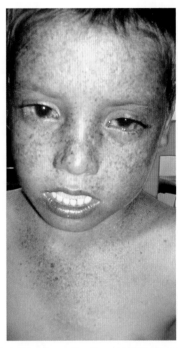

Figure 20.6 This patient shows the characteristic signs of skin damage at an early age, found in xeroderma pigmentosa. There are also cataracts present, which can also be found in this condition.

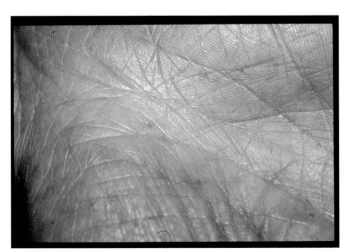

Figure 20.5 This shows the very subtle palmar pitting found in Gorlin syndrome.

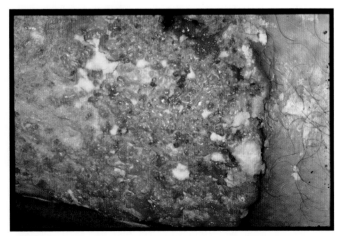

Figure 20.7 Marjolin ulcer. Here, a carcinoma has developed in a long-standing area of damaged skin on the leg.

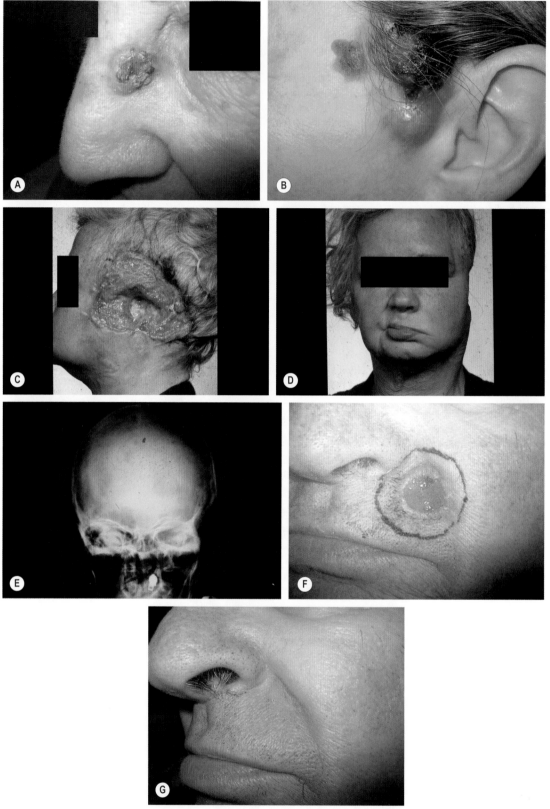

Figure 20.8 (A) This is a typical basal cell carcinoma (BCC), with a pearly appearance to the edge, and central ulceration. (B) Nodular BCC. (C–E) This is an advanced BCC. Note the local soft tissue destruction (C), the left 7th nerve palsy (D) and the bone loss because of erosion by this tumour (E). (F, G) A typical example of a BCC at the left nasolabial fold before and 6 weeks after being treated with radiotherapy.

The most common site for BCC is in a butterfly distribution in the central face. Elsewhere, tumours are more common on sun-exposed areas of skin. If untreated, tumours invade deep tissues, including bone, leading to extensive ulceration and deformity over several years in patients who have not sought medical help (see Fig. 20.8C–E).

A typical example of a BCC at the left nasolabial fold before and 6 weeks after being treated with RT is shown in Fig. 20.8F and G.

Squamous Cell Carcinoma of the Skin

SCC is the second most common skin cancer after BCC, and the incidence of this tumour is rising as a result of increased exposure to UV radiation because there seems to be a direct association between development of these tumours and hours of sun exposure. These tumours can enlarge and cause local destruction and metastasise, initially to regional nodes, which should be checked clinically when the patient first presents.

Following treatment for SCC, a full 5-year follow-up is required as they can recur locally or in lymph nodes or even with distant metastases. This is in contrast to BCCs where patients can be discharged from follow-up as soon as the treatment side effects have settled.

Well-differentiated SCCs produce keratin and the presence of keratin on the surface of a tumour is the characteristic feature of SCC. The best example of this is SCC producing a keratin horn, although these can also result from a benign cause, such as actinic keratosis or a viral wart. Poorly differentiated, and hence more aggressive SCCs are often less distinctive and present as a nodule or ulcer (Fig. 20.9A). SCC may develop within Bowen's disease or actinic keratosis.

A typical SCC before and 4 weeks after RT is shown in Fig. 20.9A and B.

Cancer of the Lip

Cancer of the lip is predominantly a malignancy affecting elderly males. The lower lip is affected more frequently than the upper lip by a factor of 10. Almost all lower lip cancers are SCCs. It is rare to find a BCCs on the lip vermilion, but they can arise from skin immediately adjacent. BCC develops most commonly on the skin close to the upper rather than the lower lip.

These malignancies are more common in fair skinned, weather-beaten outdoor workers. Sun exposure is one important factor but there may be others, such as pipe smoking, as cumulative UV exposure does not always correlate with some of the higher risk occupational groups prone to developing this cancer. As with squamous carcinoma of the skin, transplant patients are at a higher risk of developing lip SCC.

Clinically, premalignant changes leading to carcinoma of the lip may precede the development of a mass or ulcer within the lip. This then enlarges, involving more of the lip. Spread to the submental or submandibular nodes is possible, especially with larger or more poorly differentiated lesions, but spread to other neck nodes early on is uncommon. Classically, 5% of lip cancers have palpable nodes at diagnosis and 5% subsequently develop nodal metastases after successful treatment of the primary.

Management of Cancer of the Lip

Initially, a pathological diagnosis needs to be made with an incisional biopsy. The treatment options can be discussed with the patient. For early tumours involving only the vermilion of the lip, the tumour can be removed with a lip shave and the oral mucosa advanced to replace the area removed. Superficial early tumours may be associated with other areas of premalignant change. This technique allows for these areas of premalignant change to be removed at the same time and sent for histological evaluation to exclude other areas of carcinoma in situ or frank invasive change. With larger lesions, the tumour can be removed surgically using a "V" or "W" incision. Here, the amount of functional tissue loss may make RT more appropriate.

Radiotherapy is given using either an iridium implant or electron beam, using wax and lead behind the lip to protect the rest of the mouth and take advantage of the backscatter effect. Dose/fractionation regimens used include 55 gray (Gy) in 20 fractions or 66 Gy in 33 fractions. The cosmetic result is usually very good, as the lip has an excellent blood supply and healing usually occurs quickly and completely. Because electron treatments are highly effective, iridium implantation is now rarely indicated.

Keratoacanthoma

Keratoacanthomas are benign but can be very difficult to distinguish from SCC of the skin. They present as a rapidly growing nodule with a central keratin plug. The central plug detaches, and the residual lesion resolves (Fig. 20.10A and B). Keratoacanthomas are problematic in that they cannot be differentiated from SCC of skin by biopsy alone and, in the growth phase, the pathologist will usually call them a SCC. As a result, although benign, they are often excised, to avoid missing a rapidly growing squamous cell cancer.

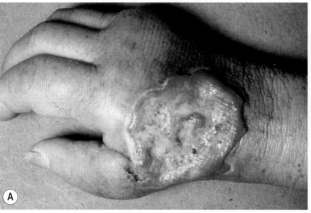
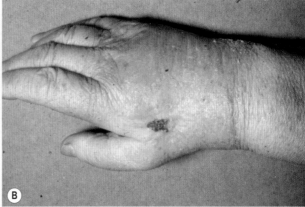

Figure 20.9 (A) This shows an extensive squamous cell carcinoma of the back of the hand before radiotherapy (RT), and (B) four weeks after treatment.

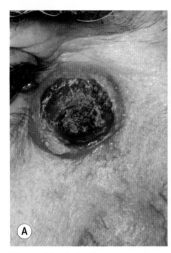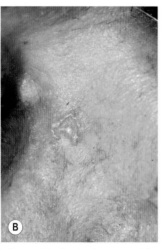

Figure 20.10 (A) Keratoacanthoma in its rapidly developing stage. The central keratin plug is obvious. This lesion has developed in a matter of a few weeks. (B) Keratoacanthoma in its healing stage. This is the same lesion as in Fig. 20.10(A), 3 months later. The keratin plug was discharged spontaneously and complete healing rapidly ensued.

Treatment of Nonmelanoma Skin Cancer

As can be seen from the list later, there are several ways to treat keratinocyte skin tumours.

There have been few randomised studies of different treatment modalities for BCC and SCC primary treatment, but Mohs micrographic surgery (MMS) gives the lowest short- and long-term recurrence rate for BCC and probably for SCC. One of the few randomised control trials in the treatment of skin cancer, which was carried out in The Netherlands, has shown a lower, but not statistically significant, rate of recurrence after MMS compared with conventional excision. Operative costs were higher for Mohs methodology.

Patients with these tumours should be seen in the multidisciplinary skin cancer clinic where a treatment plan can be formulated for the individual patient. Often, the decision as to which treatment is given is based not on the historical evidence of the efficacy of that particular treatment, but on the size and site of the skin lesion, the age, fitness and wishes of the patient, and the local resources and distances from the local hospital and cancer centre. In general, surgery or RT are equally effective in eradicating these tumours. Radiotherapy is often avoided in younger patients on the basis that long-term cosmesis is usually better with surgery. As time passes, the surgical scar becomes less obvious, whereas the hypopigmentation produced by RT can become more prominent.

Curettage and Electrolysis

This is the simplest approach, but is usually only suitable for small, previously untreated, well-defined BCCs of less than 10-mm in diameter on noncritical sites (Fig. 20.11A–D).

Cryosurgery With Liquid Nitrogen

This technique is used more for BCCs than SCCs. For 2 to 3 days after treatment there can be oedema, blister formation, sloughing and crust formation. It has the advantage of being able to be done in the outpatient clinic and can be useful in the frail elderly patient, where surgery is best avoided, and when the patient does not wish to travel to their local RT centre (Fig. 20.12).

Surgical Excision

Pathological evidence of complete removal is the main advantage of surgical excision, but for some morphoeic BCCs this may give a false

reassurance with subsequent recurrence. For these tumours, MMS gives a higher rate of complete excision. The main disadvantage of surgical excision is that, in some sites, primary skin closure may be impossible and flap closure or skin grafting is required. The cosmetic results may be poor, especially in areas such as the tip of the nose.

Laser Ablation

Laser ablation is rarely if ever used. It is in effect using the laser as a cutting tool to remove the tissue, similar to surgical excision. The defect left is usually allowed to heal by secondary intention. Confirmation of complete excision may be more difficult with this technique than surgical excision because of the tissue distortion produced by the heat artifact at the excision margins.

Photodynamic Therapy

In photodynamic therapy, a cream containing a porphyrin precursor is placed on the skin. This is metabolised by the tumour to porphyrin. The porphyrin is then activated by exposure to red light and, in the process, free radicals are produced which destroy the tumour. It is partially effective and still being developed. Photodynamic therapy is mainly reserved for large superficial truncal BCCs.

Mohs' Micrographic Surgery

MMS uses repeated excisions at the tumour site until there is no histological evidence of any remaining tumour. It gives the highest cure rate but is also resource intensive. The interval between excisions depends on whether frozen sections or fixed tissue are examined by the pathologist. Frozen sections enable the surgeon to do several excision stages in 1 day. Inevitably, the time taken to fix and examine paraffin embedded sections results in the excision stages being spread over several days (Fig. 20.13A–G).

Imiquimod

Imiquimod is a cream that can be applied on "low risk" BCCs as an alternative to surgery or RT. It is a form of local immunotherapy that releases interferons into the skin. In a UK multicentre trial comparing 5% imiquimod applied for 6 or 12 weeks, or surgical excision, by 5 years the local control rate was 97.7% for those receiving surgery compared with 82.5% for imiquimod.

Medical Treatment of Basal Cell Carcinomas

Vismodegib is an inhibitor of the smoothen homologue oncogene (SMO) which is part of the hedgehog signaling pathway responsible for the uncontrolled proliferation of basal cells in BCCs. Vismodegib is an oral preparation that is indicated for the treatment of locally advanced BCC unsuitable for surgery and/or RT, including people suffering from Gorlin syndrome or metastases. Metastases from basal cell tumours are rare. Two phase II studies gave similar results with durable responses. In the ERIVANCE study, the complete response rate (CR) was 20.6% with a partial response (PR) rate of 22.2%. In the STEVIE trial, the CR rate was 33.4% with a PR rate of 35.1%. The median duration of response was 23 months for local advanced lesions and 13.9 months for metastasis.

Patients, predominantly elderly, often find the side effects of vismodegib (altered or decreased taste, decreased appetite, fatigue, muscle and joint pain) intolerable and ask to discontinue the medication. In the United Kingdom, the National Institute for Health and Care Excellence (NICE) has not recommended vismodegib and permission for its use has been withdrawn "because of the uncertainty in the evidence and because it is not cost effective"

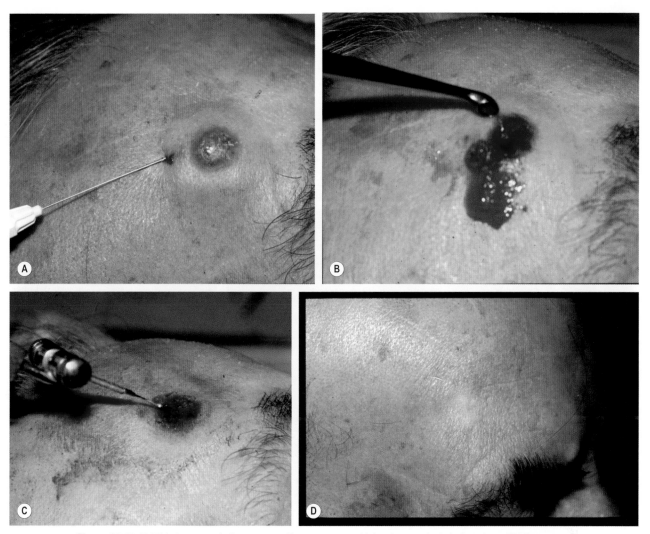

Figure 20.11 (A) This is an area being prepared for curettage, with local anaesthetic being given. (B) The tumour is then curetted out. (C) Further curettage is then performed at the tumour's base. (D) This shows the result at 2 years, following curettage.

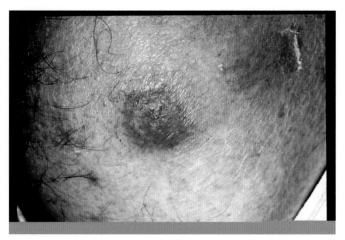

Figure 20.12 This is the appearance of an area of skin, 1 week after cryosurgery.

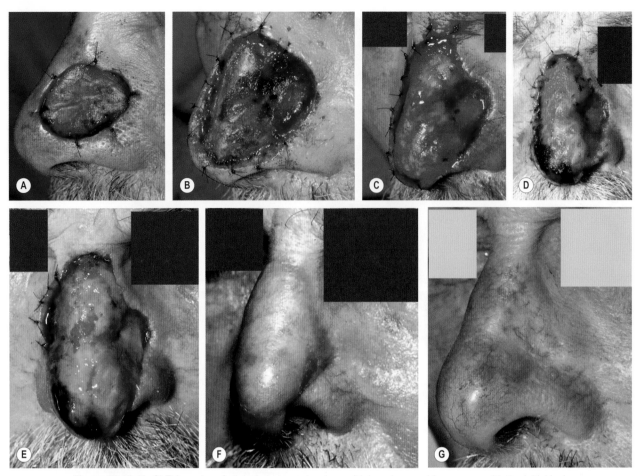

Figure 20.13 (A–G) This series of clinical photographs shows Mohs micrographic surgery, with the initial incision, the further wider excisions and the final result.

(https://www.nice.org.uk/guidance/TA489/chapter/1-recommendations). Pembrolizimab, with or without vismodegib, is being tested in the same patient population.

Radiotherapy for Keratinocyte Skin Cancers

Radiotherapy is particularly useful in treating tumours of the central face, around the nose and eyes, where surgical treatment may give a relatively poor cosmetic result or more loss of function than with RT. There is a relative contraindication for giving RT to certain sites, such as the pinna, with its underlying cartilage; the back of the hand with its tendons lying superficially; and the anterior shin where there is a relative lack of underlying subcutaneous tissue. Even these sites can be treated in appropriate patients if due consideration is given to the skin condition, site of treatment and treatment volume, total dose and fractionation.

In giving RT around the eye, treating the lateral upper eyelid may cause damage to the lacrimal gland and ducts, leading to a permanently dry eye and, in treating lesions at the medial canthus, the lacrimal drainage system can be occluded. However, if the lacrimal duct is uninvolved by cancer and is patent before RT begins, it is more likely than not to remain patent after RT.

The RT dose used for treating skin malignancies varies from centre to centre and dose/fractionation schedules have developed empirically

TABLE 20.1 Examples of Superficial Radiotherapy Fractionation Regimens for Treating Basal Cell Carcinoma and Squamous Cell Carcinoma of the Skin

Total Dose (Gy)	Number of Fractions	Fraction Interval
18	1	-
28	2	7 weeks apart
35	5	Daily (if <4 cm field size)
45	10	Daily (if >4 cm field size)

over the years. In general, the more fractions used, the better the late cosmetic result (Table 20.1). As well as efficacy in curing the tumour, other factors, such as the late cosmetic effects and convenience to the patient are important. Some elderly, frail patients will trade off the cosmetic outcome against convenience if they can visit the RT treatment centre for fewer visits, without compromising the probability of cure.

Radiotherapy can be given to these skin cancers using either superficial x-ray beams, usually in the range 50 to 120 kV, or with electron beams. The latter are used where rapid fall off of the depth dose is required to spare underlying normal tissue. If the skin tumour overlies cartilage or bone, low voltage x-rays are absorbed disproportionately, owing to the high atomic number of bone compared with soft tissue, and the risk of radio-necrosis is much greater than following treatment with electrons.

Electron Beam Treatment

Sites where the use of electron therapy beams may be indicated in preference to superficial x-ray beams include the pinna, nasolabial fold or the back of the hand. In the latter site, the use of an electron beam may reduce damage to the underlying tendon sheaths.

Electron beams are also used to irradiate larger areas of skin, either treating larger single epithelial skin tumours or when treating skin lymphomas. As can be seen in Figs 20.14 and 20.15, superficial x-ray beams lose energy exponentially through matter (see Fig. 20.14) and electron

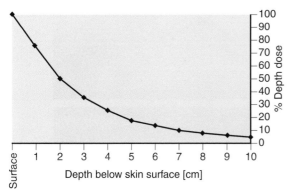

Figure 20.14 This shows the exponential fall-off of dose at depth as a superficial x-ray beam penetrates tissue.

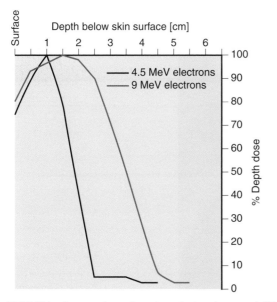

Figure 20.15 This diagram shows how two electron beams of different energies interact with matter, delivering different doses at depth, depending on their energy.

beams reach a peak (at a depth proportional to the energy of the beam) and then fall off rapidly, delivering very little radiation at depth (see Fig. 20.15).

When using an electron beam on superficial tumors, the aim is to have the tumour within the 85% isodose (see Fig. 20.15) and to achieve this for some tumours, bolus may be needed to increase surface dose. Electron beams have a larger penumbra and have a different beam profile to superficial x-ray beams. Low energy electron beams as used in treating skin tumours show isodoses coming together at depth, and this requires that a larger margin of normal tissue is included at set-up, for example 1.5 cm instead of 1 cm.

Electron Backscatter

Electron beams also have the advantage of being able to use the physical phenomenon of backscatter (Fig. 20.16A). If electrons encounter lead, a proportion will be scattered back toward the direction of the incident beam, and by placing wax in front of the lead, some of the backscatter electrons will be absorbed in the wax. By choosing the thickness of the lead and the wax carefully, the degree of backscatter can be modified. This allows greater homogeneity within the treated area. However, the amount of backscatter is difficult to measure and its contribution to irradiating the tumour volume changes with every individual patient set-up. Electrons are scattered in many directions, not just at 180 degrees to the incident beam, and may contribute to dose outside the treatment volume, and so by placing wax in front of the lead, some of these backscattered electrons will be absorbed in the wax. Backscatter therefore has both positive and negative potential effects (see Fig. 20.16B–F illustrate an SCC of pinna treated by electrons).

One of the most common treatment sites for the use of backscatter to clinical advantage is when a cancer of the lower lip is treated with electrons. Wax and lead are put behind the lip. The lead helps to protect the oral cavity from the electron radiation beam. By varying the thickness of the wax for each individual patient, depending on how thick the lip and tumour are and, consequently, how wide the target volume needs to be, the degree of backscatter can be modified, giving greater homogeneity in dose across the tumour.

Fig. 20.16G–L show a wax and lead block being used for a lower lip cancer with the area to be treated marked out in Fig. 20.16I.

Superficial X-Ray Treatment

Most small BCCs on the face can easily be treated using x-ray energies of 90 to 120 kV. A lead cut-out is placed around the lesion with a margin of 5 mm if a BCC, and 10 mm if an SCC (Fig. 20.17A and B). If the lesion is an irregular shape, then a lead cut-out may need to be specifically made, tracing the area to be treated with adequate margin onto a piece of lead, which is then cut out. If the treated site is close to the eyes, then an external or internal eye shield is used to keep radiation dose to the eye to a minimum (Fig. 20.18).

Each fraction takes only a few minutes to deliver and the patient should be warned that the reaction will start with erythema, followed by ulceration, over which a crust forms. Healing takes place underneath this crust, which detaches a few weeks after treatment. If it is detached prematurely, or is inadvertently knocked off, a second or even a third crust can form.

After the acute reaction has settled down, late changes may develop with the possibility of hypopigmentation and telangiectasia.

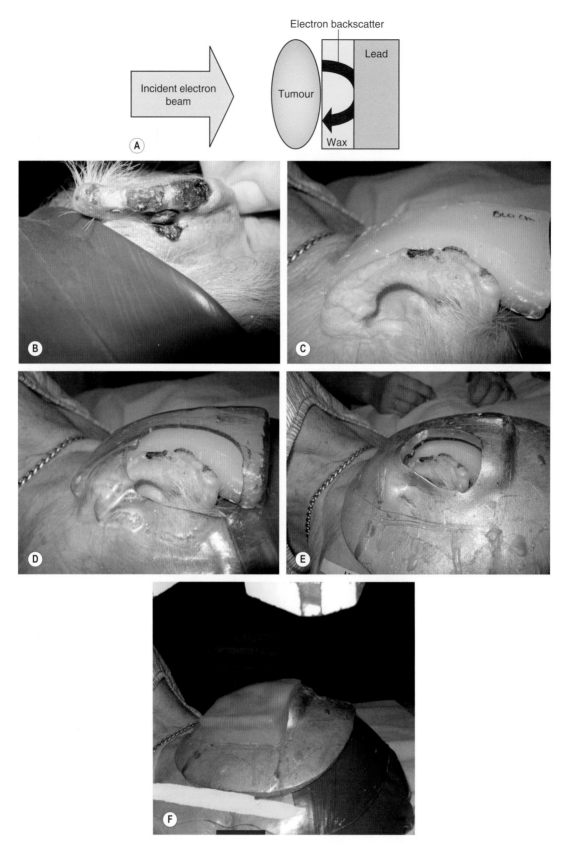

Figure 20.16 (A) Here is a simplified diagrammatic representation of the electron backscatter effect. By choosing different thicknesses of the lead and wax used, both the amount of backscatter and how many backscatter electrons are absorbed by the wax can be controlled, improving the homogeneity of dose over the tumour volume. (B–F) Here, use is made of the electron backscatter effect in treating a squamous cell carcinoma on the pinna of the ear. (B) The lesion. (C) Wax and lead are then placed behind the ear, in the thicknesses required for maximal affect. (D) A Perspex cut-out is then placed over the ear giving the treated electron field volume. An alloy cut-out is then placed over this. (E) to tailor the electron beam to the treatment volume. (F) Finally, more wax bolus is applied to increase the percentage depth dose at the skin surface.

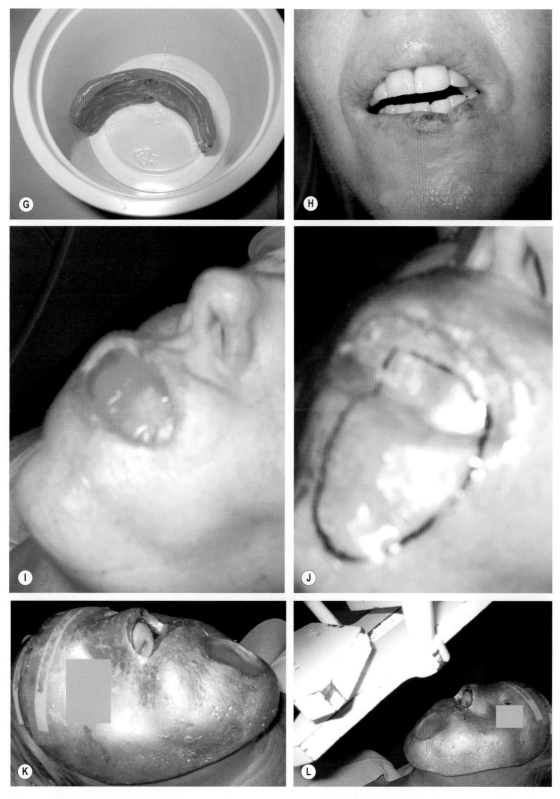

Figure 20.16—Cont'd (G–L) The process of treating a lower lip cancer with electrons. A wax and lead insert is first made, the treatment volume marked out with it inserted and then, a Perspex mask is fitted over this. An alloy cut-out is then placed on top. In this case, it is large, not to protect the whole face, but because it is less likely to fall off during treatment. Further wax is used to increase the surface electron dose at the lip. Finally, the treatment reaction on the last day of treatment after 55 Gy in 20 fractions is shown.

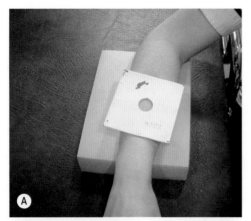

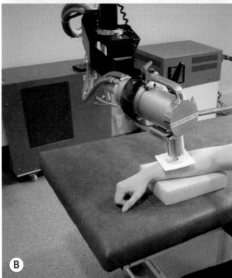

Figure 20.17 (A) This is a typical example of a lead cut-out used in treating small skin tumours with a superficial x-ray machine. (B) This shows a superficial x-ray machine being set up with a volunteer.

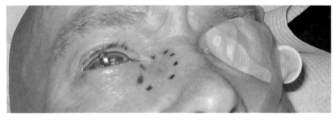

Figure 20.18 If eye shields are required, either an external shield as shown covers this patient's left eye, or an internal gold shield can be inserted under the eyelid after anaesthetising the conjunctiva with local anaesthetic, as shown with the right eye.

COMPARISON OF OUTCOME FOR DIFFERENT MODALITIES IN THE TREATMENT OF BASAL CELL CARCINOMAS

In 2018, Drucker and colleagues published a systematic review and metaanalysis of 40 randomised and 5 nonrandomised trials comparing different modalities used to treat basal cell lesions. Estimated recurrence rates were excision (3.8%), MMS (3.8%), curettage and diathermy (6.9%) and external beam RT (3.5%). Recurrence rates were higher for

cryotherapy (22.3%), curettage and cryotherapy (19.3%), imiquimod (14.1%) and dynamic phototherapy using Methyl- aminolevulinic acid (18.8%) or amino- aminolevulinic acid (16.6%).

MELANOMA

The incidence of melanoma is rising worldwide, but successful public education programmes have reduced mortality in countries such as Australia.

Aetiology

Melanoma is much more common in white races and is related to UV radiation exposure. There is evidence that episodes of sunburn before the age of 15 increase the risk of developing melanoma.

Approximately 50% of melanomas arise in preexisting moles and 50% on otherwise normal skin.

Subtypes of Melanoma

As with other skin tumours, there are several types of melanoma.

Superficial Spreading

Superficial spreading (Fig. 20.19) is the most common, representing 60% to 70% of all cases. It appears as a flat, pigmented lesion which may be related to a naevus. As the name implies, it initially grows outwards before invading downwards. Consequently, patients may present with a better prognosis if they seek help while the lesion is still in its horizontal or "radial" growth phase, which may last for many months or even years.

Nodular Melanoma

Nodular melanoma (Fig. 20.20) is less common, making up 15% to 20% of all cases. It appears clinically as a papule or nodule, usually pigmented, which represents the malignancy in vertical growth phase from early in its natural history. This gives a worse prognosis at presentation. The clinical course is more rapid than with superficial spreading lesions.

Lentigo Maligna Melanoma

Lentigo maligna melanoma (Fig. 20.21) makes up 5% to 15% of melanomas. It is most commonly found in the skin of the nose or the cheek in the elderly and develops within a premalignant pigmented lesion known as lentigo melanoma (Fig. 20.22), which can be present for several years. This lesion eventually enlarges, undergoes malignant change and may develop a central pigmented nodule.

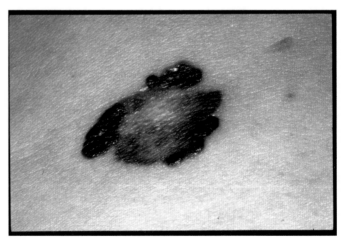

Figure 20.19 Superficial spreading melanoma.

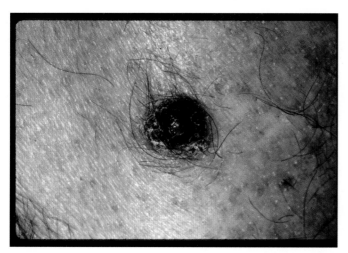

Figure 20.20 Nodular melanoma.

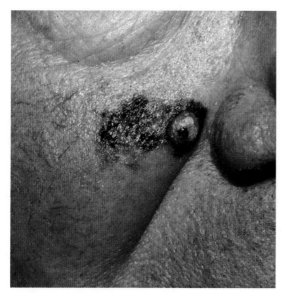

Figure 20.21 Lentigo maligna melanoma.

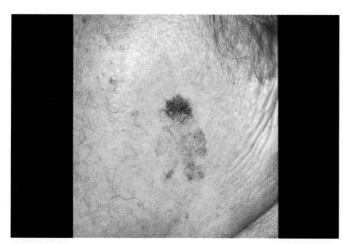

Figure 20.22 Lentigo maligna, from which lentigo maligna melanoma can develop.

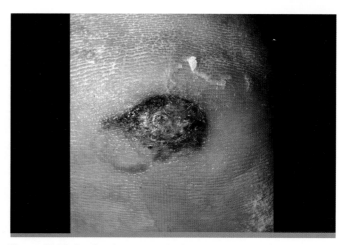

Figure 20.23 Acral melanoma on the heel.

Acral Lentiginous Melanoma

Acral lentiginous melanoma (Fig. 20.23) is much less common, comprising only 5% to 10% of melanomas, and is seen more frequently in pigmented skin. It can occur on the palms, sole of the foot, or characteristically, beneath nails. There may be a relatively long radial growth phase. In some cases of subungual melanoma, suspicion may be raised by extension of the pigmentation onto the skin of the proximal nail fold (Hutchinson's sign).

Note that not all melanoma presents as pigmented lesions and a nonpigmented "amelanotic melanoma" (Fig. 20.24A) can cause diagnostic confusion until it is biopsied.

Diagnosis

Clinically, there should be suspicion that a melanoma may be developing. There are three cardinal features to look out for when considering the possibility of malignant change in an existing mole:

- Increase in diameter.
- Change of colour.
- Change in shape, that is, becoming asymmetrical or developing border irregularity.

This is the basis of the ABCDE method: Asymmetry, Border, Colour, Diameter, Evolving—changing in size, shape or colour.

Moles greater than 6 mm are more likely to be malignant. Dermatoscopic examination using an amplified illuminated image is a helpful adjunct to clinical examination.

Melanoma TNM Staging

The TNM 2018 Classification of Malignant Tumors, 8th edition was introduced at the beginning of 2018, but some multidisciplinary teams are using both the 7th edition 2009, and the 8th edition. As can be seen in the new 8th edition, mitotic rate is not now used in staging T1 melanomas and Clark level has not been used in either the 7th or 8th edition for prognostic purposes (Tables 20.2 and 20.3).

These classifications can be gathered together into stage groupings, so that each stage can bring together several TNM classes (Table 20.4).

Stage and Prognosis

In summary, the stage and subsequent prognosis depend on tumour thickness and the presence or absence of ulceration. The finding of nodal spread shows the melanoma has already metastasised and ultimate survival depends on the number of nodes involved by melanoma and the quantity of tumour in the lymph nodes (macroscopic or microscopic). Distant spread to liver, lungs or brain carries a grave prognosis

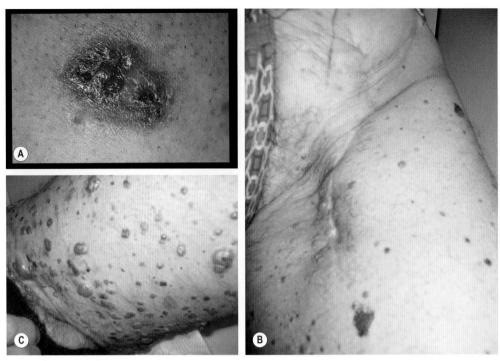

Figure 20.24 (A) This shows an amelanotic melanoma, which is not markedly pigmented. (B) Malignant melanoma in transit metastases. (C) The same patient 4 months later.

TABLE 20.2 Depth of Skin Invasion Described by Clark Level

Clark Level	
I	Melanoma confined to epidermis
II	Papillary dermis invaded
III	Invasion to the papillary-reticular dermis junction
IV	Reticular dermis invaded
V	Subcutaneous fat invaded

TABLE 20.3 The 2009 7th Edition TNM Staging System for Malignant Melanoma

pT1a	≤1.0 mm, without ulceration and mitosis $<1/mm^2$
pT1b	≤1.0 mm, with ulceration or mitosis $\geq 1/mm^2$
pT2a	1.01–2.0 mm, no ulceration present
pT2b	1.01–2.0 mm, ulceration present
pT3a	2.01–4.0 mm, no ulceration present
pT3b	2.01–4.0 mm, ulceration present
pT4a	>4 mm, no ulceration present
pT4b	>4 mm, ulceration present
N1a	1 node involved, microscopically positive
N1b	1 node involved, macroscopically positive
N2a	2–3 nodes involved, microscopically positive
N2b	2–3 nodes involved, macroscopically positive
N2c	Satellite lesions or in-transit metastases *without* nodal involvement
N3	>4 nodes involved or matted node mass
	Or satellite lesions or in-transit metastases *with* nodal involvement
M1a	Skin, subcutaneous tissue, lymph nodes beyond the regional lymph nodes
M1b	Lung metastases
M1c	Any other site or any metastasis with elevated lactic dehydrogenase

Modified from TNM Classification of Malignant Tumors, 7th edition.

TABLE 20.4 2009 7th Edition TNM Clinical Pathological Staging Prognostic Groups

Stage IA	T1a
Stage IB	T1b/T2a
Stage IIA	T2b/T3a
Stage IIB	T3b/T4a
Stage IIC	T4b
All of the above are N0	
Stage IIIA	T1a-4a + N1a/2a
Stage IIIB	T1a-4a + N1b/2b/2c or T1b-4b + N1a/N2a/N2c
Stage IIIC	T1b-4b + N1b/2b/2c or any T + N3
Stage IV	Any T or any N + M1

Modified from TNM 2018 Classification of Malignant Tumors, 7th edition.

with average survival times of 3 to 12 months depending on the metastatic site. Patients with metastases confined to the skin can often have a surprisingly long survival time.

An approximate measure of prognosis against stage at presentation for both the American Joint Committee on Cancer (AJCC) 7th and 8th editions are shown in Table 20.5 for stages I to III. For stage IV, there has always been a tail to the survival curve and today it would level out at just under 20% survival, but the present survival figures and prognostic forecasting is almost certainly obsolete, being based on patient information from the era before the introduction of targeted agents and immunotherapy. We are going through a seismic change in melanoma treatment, possibly even curing some patients with metastatic disease, who were previously incurable. The survival graphs have not had enough time to incorporate these changes as yet, and the real-world situation may well not be reflected in older survival graphs. More detailed but older prognostic data can be found in Balch et al. for AJCC 7th edition and Gershenwald et al. for AJCC 8th edition.

Melanoma TNM Classification AJCC 8th Edition January 2018

T Category	Criteria /Thickness	Criteria/Ulceration Status
TX	Primary tumor thickness cannot be assessed (e.g. diagnosis by curettage)	Not applicable
T0	No evidence of primary tumor (e.g. unknown primary or completely regressed melanoma)	Not applicable
Tis	Melanoma *in situ*	Not applicable
T1	≤1.0 mm	Unknown or unspecified
T1a	<0.8 mm	Without ulceration
T1b	<0.8 mm	With ulceration
T1b	0.8–1.0 mm	With or without ulceration
T2	>1.0–2.0 mm	Unknown or unspecified
T2a	>1.0–2.0 mm	Without ulceration
T2b	>1.0–2.0 mm	With ulceration
T3	>2.0–4.0 mm	Unknown or unspecified
T3a	>2.0–4.0 mm	Without ulceration
T3b	>2.0–4.0 mm	With ulceration
T4	>4.0 mm	Unknown or unspecified
T4a	>4.0 mm	Without ulceration
T4b	>4.0 mm	With ulceration

EXTENT OF REGIONAL LYMPH NODE AND/OR LYMPHATIC METASTASIS

N Category	Number of tumor-involved regional lymph nodes	Presence of in-transit, satellite, and/or microsatellite metastases
NX	Regional nodes not assessed (e.g. SLN biopsy not performed, regional nodes previously removed for another reason) **Exception:** pathological N category is not required for T1 melanomas, use cN.	No
N0	No regional metastases detected	No
N1	One tumor-involved node or in-transit, satellite, and/or microsatellite metastases with no tumor-involved nodes	One tumor-involved node or in-transit, satellite, and/or microsatellite metastases with no tumor-involved nodes
N1a	One clinically occult (i.e. detected by SLN biopsy)	No
N1b	One clinically detected	No
N1c	No regional lymph node disease	Yes
N2	Two or three tumor-involved nodes or in-transit, satellite, and/or microsatellite metastases with one tumor-involved node	Two or three tumor-involved nodes or in-transit, satellite, and/or microsatellite metastases with one tumor-involved node
N2a	Two or three clinically occult (i.e. detected by SLN biopsy)	No
N2b	Two or three, at least one of which was clinically detected	No
N2c	One clinically occult or clinically detected	Yes
N3	Four or more tumor-involved nodes or in-transit, satellite, and/or microsatellite metastases with two or more tumor-involved nodes, or any number of matted nodes without or with in-transit, satellite, and/or microsatellite metastases	Four or more tumor-involved nodes or in-transit, satellite, and/or microsatellite metastases with two or more tumor-involved nodes, or any number of matted nodes without or with in-transit, satellite, and/or microsatellite metastases
N3a	Four or more clinically occult (i.e. detected by SLN biopsy)	No
N3b	Four or more, at least one of which was clinically detected, or presence of any number of matted nodes	No
N3c	Two or more clinically occult or clinically detected and/or presence of any number of matted nodes	Yes

M CRITERIA

M Category	Anatomic Site	LDH Level
cM0	No evidence of distant metastasis	Not applicable
cM1	Evidence of distant metastasis	Any
cM1a	Distant metastasis to skin, soft tissue including muscle, and/or nonregional lymph node	Not recorded or unspecified
cM1a(0)	Distant metastasis to skin, soft tissue including muscle, and/or nonregional lymph node	Not elevated
cM1a(1)	Distant metastasis to skin, soft tissue including muscle, and/or nonregional lymph node	Elevated
cM1b	Distant metastasis to lung with or without M1a sites of disease	Not recorded or unspecified
cM1b(0)	Distant metastasis to lung with or without M1a sites of disease	Not elevated
cM1b(1)	Distant metastasis to lung with or without M1a sites of disease	Elevated
cM1c	Distant metastasis to non-CNS visceral sites with or without M1a or M1b sites of disease	Not recorded or unspecified
cM1c(0)	Distant metastasis to non-CNS visceral sites with or without M1a or M1b sites of disease	Not elevated
cM1c(1)	Distant metastasis to non-CNS visceral sites with or without M1a or M1b sites of disease	Elevated

M CRITERIA		
M Category	Anatomic Site	LDH Level
cM1d	Distant metastasis to CNS with or without M1a, M1b, or M1c sites of disease	Not recorded or unspecified
cM1d(0)	Distant metastasis to CNS with or without M1a, M1b, or M1c sites of disease	Not elevated
cM1d(1)	Distant metastasis to CNS with or without M1a, M1b, or M1c sites of disease	Elevated
pM1	Evidence of distant metastasis, microscopically proven	Any
pM1a	Distant metastasis to skin, soft tissue including muscle, and/or nonregional lymph node, microscopically proven	Not recorded or unspecified
pM1a(0)	Distant metastasis to skin, soft tissue including muscle, and/or nonregional lymph node, microscopically proven	Not elevated
pM1a(1)	Distant metastasis to skin, soft tissue including muscle, and/or nonregional lymph node, microscopically proven	Elevated
pM1b	Distant metastasis to lung with or without M1a sites of disease, microscopically proven	Not recorded or unspecified
pM1b(0)	Distant metastasis to lung with or without M1a sites of disease, microscopically proven	Not elevated
pM1b(1)	Distant metastasis to lung with or without M1a sites of disease, microscopically proven	Elevated
pM1c	Distant metastasis to non-CNS visceral sites with or without M1a or M1b sites of disease, microscopically proven	Not recorded or unspecified
pM1c(0)	Distant metastasis to non-CNS visceral sites with or without M1a or M1b sites of disease, microscopically proven	Not elevated
pM1c(1)	Distant metastasis to non-CNS visceral sites with or without M1a or M1b sites of disease, microscopically proven	Elevated
pM1d	Distant metastasis to CNS with or without M1a, M1b, or M1c sites of disease, microscopically proven	Not recorded or unspecified
pM1d(0)	Distant metastasis to CNS with or without M1a, M1b, or M1c sites of disease, microscopically proven	Not elevated
pM1d(1)	Distant metastasis to CNS with or without M1a, M1b, or M1c sites of disease, microscopically proven	Elevated

fixes for M category: (0) LDH not elevated, (1) LDH elevated.
suffix is used if LDH is not recorded or is unspecified.

Clinical Stage Groups

When T is...	And N is...	And M is...	Then the stage group is...
Tis	N0	M0	0
T1a	N0	M0	IA
T1b	N0	M0	IB
T2a	N0	M0	IB
T2b	N0	M0	IIA
T3a	N0	M0	IIA
T3b	N0	M0	IIB
T4a	N0	M0	IIB
T4b	N0	M0	IIC
Any T, Tis	≥N1	M0	III
Any T	Any N	M1	IV

Pathological Stage Groups

When T is...	And N is...	And M is...	Then the stage group is...
Tis	N0	M0	0
T1a	N0	M0	IA
T1b	N0	M0	IA
T2a	N0	M0	IB
T2b	N0	M0	IIA
T3a	N0	M0	IIA
T3b	N0	M0	IIB
T4a	N0	M0	IIB
T4b	N0	M0	IIC
T0	N1b, N1c	M0	IIIB
T0	N2b/c, N3b/c	M0	IIIC
T1a/b, T2a	N1a, N2a	M0	IIIA
T1a/b, T2a	N1b/c, N2b	M0	IIIB
T2b, T3a	N1a/b/c, N2a/b	M0	IIIB
T1a/b, T2a/b, T3a	N2c, N3a/b/c	M0	IIIC
T3b, T4a	Any N ≥ N1	M0	IIIC
T4b	N1a/b/c, N2a/b/c	M0	IIIC
T4b	N3a/b/c	M0	IIID
Any T, Tis	Any N	M1	IV

Management of Melanoma

It is important to have a high level of suspicion if there is any change in a pigmented skin lesion. Change in size or shape, degree or homogeneity of pigmentation, ulceration or bleeding in a pigmented lesion should lead to referral to the local melanoma screening clinic.

A suspicious mole should be excised with a margin of 2 mm. Shaving a suspected melanoma is contraindicated because this will not allow the true Breslow thickness to be measured and results in incomplete excision. The pathology report should give the depth of invasion in millimetres (the Breslow thickness) and state whether ulceration and/or regression are present or not, and whether excision is complete. These are all prognostic factors. If regression is present then this may obscure the dermoepidermal junction and the given Breslow depth may be an underestimate.

If melanoma is discovered, the patient should then undergo a definitive wider local excision. If the tumour was 1 mm Breslow thickness or less, another lateral excision margin of 1 cm is taken, down to the deep fascia. Tumours greater than 1.0 mm thick are normally excised with a 2-cm lateral margin down to deep fascia.

Thicker, more advanced melanomas carry a higher risk of occult positive lymph nodes. Prophylactic node dissection to identify those with occult metastases has not improved survival and is associated with a high potential complication rate, including wound infection and lymphoedema. Patients who require node dissection can be identified by the sentinel biopsy technique. Trials are still being performed on the technique of sentinel lymph node biopsy (SLNB), where the first node that drains the area of the primary tumour is identified by injecting both a blue dye and a radioactive marker close to the site of the primary tumour bed. The theory that underlies the concept of SLNB suggests that these markers are then taken up by the local lymphatics and identify the first or sentinel draining node. This node is then sampled surgically and, if tumour free,

TABLE 20.5 Five-Year Survival Rates for Stage Groups		
Melanoma Stage	5-Year Survival %[a]	5-Year Survival %[b]
IA	98	99
IB	93	97
IIA	80	94
IIB	70	87
IIC	56	82
IIIA	78	93
IIIB	60	83
IIIC	43	69
IIID	N/A	32

[a]Balch CM, Gershenwald JE, Soong S, et al. Final version of 2009 AJCC melanoma staging and classification. J Clin Oncol. 2009;27(36):6199–206.
[b]Gershenwald JE, Scolyer RA. Melanoma staging: American Joint Committee on Cancer (AJCC) 8th Edition and Beyond. Ann Surg Oncol. 2018;25:2105–10 and correction https://doi.org/10.1245/s10434-018-6689-x.

then it is thought it is unlikely there is tumour in further nodes and the patient will therefore not require a nodal block dissection. If the sentinel node is positive, then block dissection is required. No survival advantage has been shown so far for SLNB compared with removing nodes if and when they are found by clinical examination. Even SLNB is associated with some surgical complications.

There has been only one randomised trial with an endpoint of melanoma-specific survival following SLNB. In this trial, 2001 patients were randomised to either observation or SLNB after wide local excision. Both the interim and final results were negative with 10-year melanoma-specific survival rate of 81.4% in the sentinel node group and 78.3% in the nodal observation group ($P = .18$).

If the sentinel node contained malignant cells in the past, the surgeon proceeded to a full dissection of the lymph node compartment. Following the publication of two recent randomised clinical trials of immediate lymph node dissection following SLNB or observation, a more selective approach has been advocated. In the German DeCOG-SLT trial containing 473 patients, there was no difference in 3-year distant metastases-free survival following ultrasound based follow-up (77%) compared with immediate lymph node dissection (74%).

Similar results were seen in the larger American MSLT-II trail containing 1934 patients. The 3-year melanoma-specific survival was the same in 86% in both the observation arm and the immediate lymph node dissection group.

The current U.S. consensus is that the surgeon should only proceed to immediate lymph node dissection if there are palpable lymph nodes at the time of sentinel node biopsy. Although no survival advantage has been demonstrated from SLNB, Kudchadkar and colleagues consider it to be the standard of care in the United States. In the United Kingdom, the advice is more nuanced. NICE currently recommend discussing the advantages and disadvantages (including surgically induced lymphoedema) with the patient. In clinical practice a decade ago, observation was the standard of care in the United Kingdom, but in the intervening years nearly all U.K. centres now perform SLNB.

SLNB currently is largely a staging tool, but with the increasing role of adjuvant immunotherapy, it may have a greater role to play.

Adjuvant Treatment for Melanoma

Melanoma is largely resistant to standard cytotoxic chemotherapy. There is no role for adjuvant cytotoxic chemotherapy to destroy

micrometastases because it used to treat patients with colorectal or breast cancer. There is, however, rapidly emerging evidence that drugs that stimulate the patient's own immune system can improve survival in patients with a high risk of recurrence after surgery. Immune check points are negative regulators of the immune response. One of the immune check points most successfully targeted is the PD-1 receptor found on the surface of T lymphocytes. In health, PD-1 acts to regulate excessive immune responses and this is manipulated by tumours to evade immunological action against the cancer. Antibodies that block the PD-L1/PD-1 (programmed cell-death ligand 1or 2) reduce tumour down regulation of the antitumour immune response and increase the cytotoxic response of antitumour-specific T cells. The most common anti-PD-1 drugs in current clinical use are pembrolizumab and nivolumab. A more toxic antibody is ipilimumab which is a human monoclonal antibody against cytotoxic T cell-associated protein (CTLA-4).

To date, there have been several trials of immunotherapy as adjuvant treatment showing a survival advantage with this treatment. In the European Organisation for Research and Treatment of Cancer (EORTC) 1325 trial, pembrolizumab was compared with a placebo in patients with fully resected stage III disease. The 1-year recurrence free survival was 74.5% in the pembrolizumab group compared with 61% in those receiving a placebo. In the CheckMate 238 study, patients with completely resected stage IIIb/IIIc or stage 1V disease were randomised to receive either ipilimumab or nivolumab. The 12-month recurrence-free survival was 70.5% in the nivolumab group compared with 60.8% in the ipilimumab group. Toxicity was considerably greater in the ipilimumab group.

There is little data at present to indicate superiority of pembrolizumab over nivolumab as adjuvant treatment. Nivolumab and Pembrolizumab are now available in the UK through the Cancer Drugs Fund for use as adjuvant treatment. Further data is still being gathered for full NICE approval. Pembrolizumab has been authorised for adjuvant use in the United States.

Another approach to adjuvant therapy is to take advantage of a mutation in the BRAF oncogene that can be therapeutically exploited. Between 40% to 50% of melanomas have a mutation in the BRAF oncogene. This encodes a protein (activated threonine kinase) which is important for melanoma cell proliferation. Combining a BRAF pathway inhibitor (dabrafenib) with an inhibitor (trametinib) of another growth pathway, Mek, in patients with completely resected stage III melanoma exhibiting either a BRAF V600 E or 600 K mutation produced superior 3-year relapse-free survival compared with a placebo. In the past, single-agent BRAF inhibition only did not produce better survival. The 3-year relapse-free survival was 58% in the combination arm compared with 39% in the placebo group ($P = .001$).

The development of adjuvant regimes is a rapidly changing field. In the future, decisions for individual patients will depend on the results or well-conducted clinical trials and individual tumour markers such as mutations and the level of PD-1 expression.

Interferon, which was formerly widely used in the United States as an adjuvant treatment, may still have a role in the treatment of deep, ulcerated melanoma without nodal metastases (stage IIB disease), but its use will probably be overtaken in the future by immunotherapy.

MANAGEMENT OF RECURRENT OR METASTATIC MELANOMA

Any evidence of further local, regional or metastatic melanoma requires that the patient be restaged to define the extent of the recurrence. If there is only local recurrence at the primary site, further surgery should be considered. This may be appropriate even if there is other locoregional or metastatic disease present to achieve local control.

If regional lymph nodes are involved, a nodal block dissection may be indicated, depending on the extent and fixity of the nodal disease, the extent of other disease and patient factors such as performance status, frailty, comorbidities present and the potential functional loss and changes in quality of life (both positive and negative) that extensive surgery may bring. In selected cases, adjuvant RT may improve local control after surgery as after nodal dissection for primary disease.

In-transit metastases may present in a limb (Fig. 20.24B and C). These represent disease in cutaneous lymphatics between the primary site and local draining nodes. They can erupt and involve widespread areas of skin as small erythematous or pigmented macules and nodules. In-transit metastases can be very problematic and distressing to the patient, especially if they break down or coalesce into larger masses. Patients who develop this condition can be referred to one of a few specialised units around the United Kingdom which offer isolated limb perfusion (ILP): a technique in which the circulation in a limb is isolated and chemotherapy is given to the limb alone, without significant amounts of drug entering the general circulation. This technique can give considerable palliative benefit and, in some patients, a complete response may be achieved with all the nodules and papules disappearing. If in-transit metastasis affects the skin of the trunk, then the area cannot be isolated and systemic chemotherapy is required.

Patients may develop blood-borne metastasis, most commonly in the liver, lungs, brain or bone. Radiotherapy is useful for brain and bone and cutaneous metastases. Malignant melanoma is often said to be "radio-resistant" and it is true that melanoma cells can sustain more sublethal damage than other cancer cell lines, but this can be countered by using regimens using a higher dose per fraction and treating less frequently, for example, treating three times per week rather than five times per week. Cutaneous metastasis can be treated by relatively small electron fields, restricting both field size on the skin and the depth treated.

Chemotherapy using dimethyl triazeno imidazole carboxamide (DTIC), also known as dacarbazine, was previously the standard treatment for visceral soft-tissue metastasis, although the response rate is only about 15%. It is now not used, having been replaced by immunotherapy and biologically targeted agents. Ipilimumab is an antibody which blocks cytotoxic T lymphocyte-associated antigen 4, present on cytotoxic T lymphocytes and results in an active immune response to melanoma cells. Vemurafenib is a B-raf enzyme inhibitor which can cause cell death in melanomas which show a V600E B-raf mutation. This mutation is characterised by glutamic acid replacing valine at position 600 on the B-raf protein. Vemurafenib is only effective in melanomas with this mutation. Other drugs with similar mechanisms of action are also being developed.

In patients with metastatic disease, especially those without BRAF mutations, immunotherapy offers the possibility of increased survival. Ipilimumab was the first systemic treatment to show prolonged survival of patients with metastatic disease entered into randomised clinical trials. A pooled analysis of 12 studies of patients with advanced melanoma showed a 3-year survival of 26% and a survival up to 10 years in about 20% of all patients.

Ipilimumab was associated with considerable toxicity. Skin rashes were seen in 47% to 68% of patients. The most important toxicities were colitis leading to diarrhoea with a grade 3/4 incidence in 8% to 23%, and hepatitis with a grade 3/4 incidence in 3% to 7% of patients. The newer anti-PD-1 inhibitors, nivolumab and pembrolizumab, have shown superior overall survival, and progression-free survival with less toxicity than ipilimumab.

In the KEYNOTE-006 trial, the overall survival at 33 months was 50% in the pembrolizumab group compared with 39% in the ipilimumab group. Combining ipilimumab with anti-PD-1 drug offers only a slight survival advantage but with markedly increased toxicity. In the CheckMate 067 trial, at 36 months the overall survival rate was 58% in patients treated with both ipilimumab and nivolumab, 52% in patients receiving nivolumab alone and 34% in the ipilimumab only group. Grade 3/4 treatment-related adverse effects were seen in 59% of the combination group, 21% in those receiving only nivolumab and 28% in the ipilimumab only group.

The long-term survival figures of these trials are not yet known but a feature of immunotherapy for metastatic melanoma is a number of patients, perhaps 20% to 30%, who appear tumour free up to 10 years after treatment; only time will tell if they have been cured of metastatic disease.

SIDE EFFECTS OF IMMUNOTHERAPY

The introduction of immune system altering agents has also brought a wide range of novel side effects or adverse events not seen previously with chemotherapy. Immune agents can affect almost all visceral organs, causing the common muscle aches and pains of myositis, immune-based hepatitis, colitis, carditis, pneumonitis and several forms of endocrinopathy, and several forms of endocrinopathy, including commonly, hypothyroidism and the rare but potentially fatal, sudden onset type 1 diabetes or pituitary failure. The side effects, especially immune hepatitis and the endocrinopathies, can develop several weeks after starting treatment and in some cases even after immunotherapy has been discontinued. Careful, recurrent assessment of patients on immunotherapy is therefore essential.

ROLE OF RADIOTHERAPY IN MALIGNANT MELANOMA

Melanoma is classically described as radio-resistant. Standard palliative doses bring about pain relief in at least a third of those with bone metastases using, for example 20 Gy in 4 fractions, or a single 8-Gy fraction. Stereotactic RT, also known as stereotactic radiosurgery (SRS), in which brain metastases are treated individually with a very narrow margin, can bring about useful shrinkage in brain metastases, and more and more patients are being treated with this modality instead of with whole brain RT (WBRT). With the latter dose, fractionation is usually 30 Gy in 10 fractions or 6 fractions treated on alternate days using 6-MV beam energy, but with SRS, single doses of up to 21 Gy can be given to individual brain metastases, depending on volume in cubic centimetres (cc) and the number of metastases to be treated. If more than three metastases are to be treated, then fractionated schedules using 21 Gy in 3 fractions or 25 Gy in 5 fractions are used again; depending on the number and volume in cc of the metastases to be treated, there are also studies ongoing of using SRS with WBRT and with immunotherapy, based on the theory that SRS should cause melanoma cell breakdown exposing more antigen for an enhanced immune response.

In Australia, the experience has been that although surgery is the treatment of choice for lentigo maligna (melanoma in situ), RT has a role to play in those patients in whom surgery would be difficult or contraindicated owing to comorbidities, impact on function or cosmesis and in those who failed surgery with positive excision margins. There is an ongoing Australia and New Zealand Melanoma Trials Group study (RADICALS) comparing imiquimod versus RT in this group of patients.

There is clear evidence from another Australian trial (ANZMTG 01.2/TROG 02.01) that "in field" recurrences can be reduced in patients with a high risk of local recurrence in the nodal area after lymphadenectomy. After a median follow-up of 73 months, 23/109 relapses occurred in field following postoperative RT (48 Gy in 20 fractions) compared with 39/108 in those randomised to observation only (P = .023). Overall survival, however, did not differ between the two groups. Although RT does reduce local recurrence, this effect may be dwarfed by the increase in survival seen in adjuvant immunotherapy trials. In the United Kingdom, the evidence that nivolomab has a survival benefit in the adjuvant setting has already started a movement away from adjuvant RT to systemic therapy in the adjuvant setting, because adjuvant RT to groin and axilla only improves local control without improving survival.

Studies are in progress of combined RT with pembrolizumab in patients with metastatic disease. Abscopal effects have been seen with disease regression outside the radiation field in patients whose tumours had progressed when receiving anti-PD-1 therapy only.

CUTANEOUS LYMPHOMAS

Primary cutaneous lymphomas are uncommon tumours. The majority are T-cell lymphomas with less than 25% being B cell. They are more common in males. At present, their aetiology is unknown, but a viral association has been suggested.

Within the primary cutaneous T-cell lymphomas, mycosis fungoides is the most common type and usually presents in men over 60 years of age. There is a range of clinical presentation varying from erythematous cutaneous patches, which may show very slow progression, to thickened plaques or nodular tumours, over several years (Fig. 20.25).

The development of lymphadenopathy or visceral organ involvement worsens prognosis markedly and the development of large abnormal circulating T cells, the so-called Sézary cells, in the peripheral blood in association with lymphadenopathy and erythroderma is diagnostic of Sézary syndrome. Patients with this condition are also at greater risk of developing other SCCs of the skin and internal malignancies, especially lung cancer.

There is a wide range of treatments for cutaneous T-cell lymphomas. Topical chemotherapy with nitrogen mustard, carmustine or PUVA all have high response rates for early disease. For thicker plaques, total skin electron therapy is effective (Fig. 20.26A–E). Systemic

chemotherapy is indicated for more advanced disease. There are studies in progress evaluating immunotherapy with interferon or interleukin, monoclonal antibody therapy, photopheresis and new combination chemotherapy regimens.

Primary cutaneous B-cell lymphomas are rare and include a wide variety of subtypes including, for example, primary cutaneous follicular centre cell lymphoma and marginal zone B-cell lymphoma. In general, these lymphomas have a more indolent course. They are more likely to be managed by local RT presenting as a solitary mass, or systemic chemotherapy if they have spread. Secondary cutaneous lymphomas may also affect the skin.

MERKEL CELL TUMOURS

These tumours represent neuroendocrine carcinoma of the skin. They tend to affect the elderly, often presenting as a painless nodule in the head and neck or on a limb. They may respond well to initial treatment but go on to recur locally or to develop metastatic spread. They are treated with wide local excision where possible, with postoperative RT, or RT alone, if inoperable. Chemotherapy is used for advanced local or recurrent disease, using agents similar to those used in small cell lung cancer, such as carboplatin and etoposide combination. Initially, tumours may respond to chemotherapy but almost inevitably recur. The main differential diagnosis of Merkel cell tumours is small cell carcinoma, which has metastasised to the skin. Cytokeratin 20 is useful in differentiating between these two possibilities histologically. Avelumab, an anti-PD-L1 monoclonal antibody, has recently been approved for first line treatment in Merkel cell cancer.

SKIN SARCOMA

Primary sarcomas of the structures of the skin or subcutaneous tissues are uncommon but may present as a diagnostic problem. They often have no defining clinical characteristics and most often present as a skin or subcutaneous nodule. These tumours can arise from a range of connective tissue cell precursors, including vascular nerve and muscle tissues with a wide arange of pathological types and subtypes, often not easy to diagnose even with adequate histological material.

The most important pathological diagnosis is to decide if the tumour is benign or malignant, with the potential to recur or metastasise. If the tumour is benign and has been excised completely, then no further intervention is required.

True malignant sarcomas affecting the skin, for example angiosarcoma, can carry a poor prognosis. These vascular malignancies (Fig. 20.27A) present with an erythematous or vascular nodule, which can then ulcerate or go on to form several other nodules. They can metastasise early, and wide surgical excision is the treatment of choice. They are also associated with developing in areas of postmastectomy lymphoedema, either in the chest wall or arm, often a decade after initial surgery. This phenomenon is known as the Stewart-Treves syndrome.

Other malignant variants of sarcoma which can develop from skin structures include malignant fibrous histiocytoma, malignant peripheral nerve sheath tumours and clear cell sarcoma, which is a malignancy derived from melanocytes. These are all uncommon and initial treatment for all is wide surgical excision.

As well as the skin sarcomas with true metastatic potential, there are also connective tissue tumours that can affect the skin, showing local invasion and having the potential for local recurrence if inadequately excised. Metastases are very rare. The most common example in this

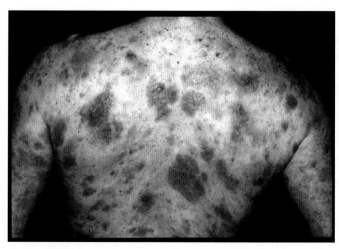

Figure 20.25 Mycosis fungoides, with patches, plaques and nodules.

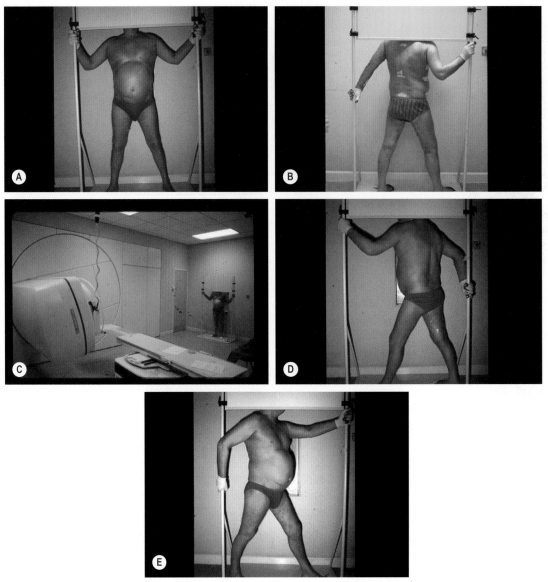

Figure 20.26 (A–E) Total skin electrons being used to treat cutaneous lymphoma.

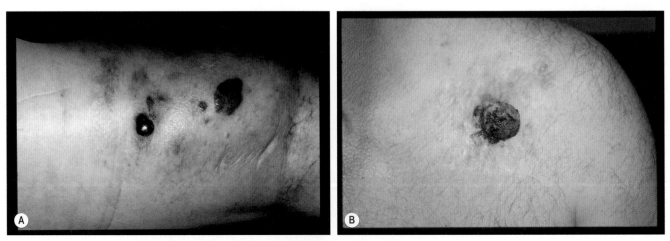

Figure 20.27 (A) Angiosarcoma. (B) Dermatofibromasarcoma protuberans.

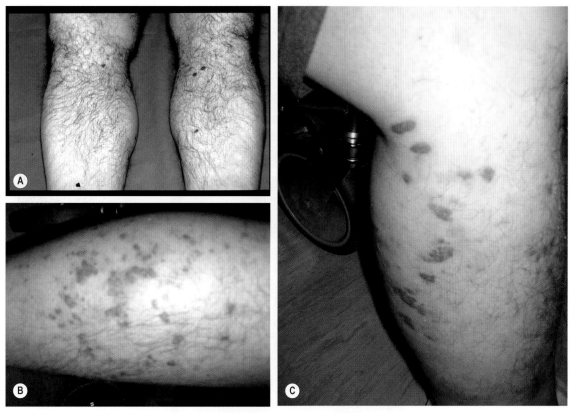

Figure 20.28 (A–C) Kaposi sarcoma.

group would be dermatofibrosarcoma protuberans (see Fig. 20.27B). These tumours can be difficult to diagnose pathologically, especially in their early stages, when histologically they may appear to be benign. They have a long natural history, with local recurrences stretching over years. The can de-differentiate and become more aggressive clinically, and histologically more malignant. If this occurs, there is a greater risk of metastasis.

KAPOSI SARCOMA

This is a particular form of vascular sarcoma which is derived from endothelial cells. It has become much more prevalent with the increased incidence of acquired immune deficiency syndrome (AIDS). KS has several variants including: classical KS, and epidemic KS, both associated with human herpes virus type 8. There are also types associated with immunosuppressive treatment and African KS.

Before the AIDS epidemic, classical KS was a rare disease, affecting elderly males, usually of Italian or East European Jewish descent, who developed the pigmented patches and nodules around the lower leg or ankle (Fig. 20.28A–C). These tumours develop slowly, but patients are at risk of developing a second malignancy, often non-Hodgkin's lymphoma. Most patients are treated with relatively low doses of RT, such as 8 Gy in a single fraction, which may be repeated.

Epidemic KS develops in approximately 20% to 25% of patients with AIDS, although there was a much higher incidence in AIDS patients when the epidemic first started. Since the introduction of highly active antiretroviral treatment (HAART), the incidence of age-related KS has been reduced. Patients with this variant are more likely to develop disseminated disease. Chemotherapy is used to treat KS using agents such as liposomal doxorubicin or a taxane. These tumours can be exquisitely sensitive to RT: great care must be taken in treating sites such as the oral mucosa or considerable morbidity can be caused. There have been a variety of dose schedules used, all giving relatively low total doses for the management of this condition, such as a single 6-Gy fraction, using a low-energy electron beam, for single or a few cutaneous lesions, or 12 Gy in three fractions. There is a suggestion that using slightly higher fractionated doses, such as 20 to 30 Gy in 10 to 15 fractions may produce a longer lasting response for individual lesions.

SKIN APPENDAGE TUMOURS

These are also known as adnexal tumours. They arise from skin structures including the hair follicle, sebaceous glands or sweat glands. There is a wide range of benign skin appendage tumours which occasionally undergo malignant transformation. They most often appear as smooth nondistinctive masses which are diagnosed not by their clinical appearance, but on biopsy histopathology. There are multiple pathological subtypes (Fig. 20.29A and B).

Sebaceous carcinoma is an example of an uncommon potentially metastatic skin appendage tumour. These classically occur on the eyelid, diagnosed on biopsy. Surgery is the treatment of choice. Sweat gland carcinoma gives a similar indistinct clinical picture. These tumours usually present as an odd-looking BCC or SCC, with the diagnosis again not being made until excision biopsy has been done. Surgery is again the treatment of choice.

Paget's disease of the breast or nipple is a malignant condition in or around the skin of the nipple. It can also occur outwith the

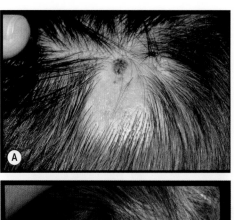

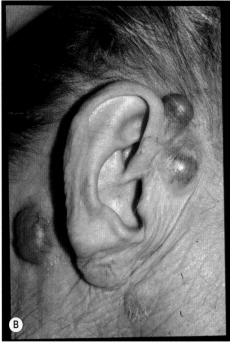

Figure 20.29 Skin appendage tumours. (A) A sebaceous naevus with an associated basal cell carcinoma. (B) A multiple cylindroma, with a typically noncharacteristic appearance.

breast, when it is known as extra mammary Paget's disease, with the most common extra mammary site being the vulva. This condition is thought to arise from epithelial cells in an apocrine duct, looks like eczema. It can give rise to pruritus and ulceration and may spread to local regional nodes and even metastasise systemically.

FURTHER READING

Balch CM, Gershenwald JE, Soong S, et al. Final version of 2009 AJCC Melanoma Staging and Classification. J Clin Oncol 2009;27(36):6199–206.

Burmeister BH, Henderson MA, Ainslie J, et al. Adjuvant radiotherapy versus observation alone for patients at risk of lymph-node field relapse after therapeutic lymphadenectomy for melanoma: a randomized trial. Lancet Oncol 2012;13(6):589–97.

Burmeister BH, Mark Smithers B, Burmeister E, et al. A prospective phase II study of adjuvant postoperative radiation therapy following nodal surgery in malignant melanoma: Trans Tasman Radiation Oncology Group (TROG) study 96.06. Radiother Oncol 2006;812:136–42.

Chang AS, et al. Pembrolizumab for advanced basal cell carcinoma: an investigator initiated, proof-of-concept study. Jam Acad Dermatol 2019 Feb 80;2:565–6.

Chapman PB, Hauschild A, Robert C. improved survival with vemurafenib in melanoma with BRAF V600E mutation. N Engl J Med 2011;364:2507–16.

Drucker AA, Adam GP, Rofeberg V, et al. Treatments of primary basal cell carcinoma of skin; a systematic review and network meta–analysis. Ann Intern Med 2018;169:456–66.

Eggermont A, Blank C, Mandala M, et al. Adjuvant pembrolizumab versus placebo in resected stage 111 melanoma. N Engl J Med 2018;378:1789–801.

Faries MB, Thompson JF, Cochran AJ, et al. Completion dissection or observation for sentinel-node metastasis in melanoma. N Engl J Med 2017;376:2211–22.

Fogarty GB, Hong A, Economides A, et al. Experience in treating lentigo maligna with definitive radiotherapy. Derm Res Pract 2018. Article ID 7439807.

Frampton JE, Basset-Seguin N. Vismodegib: a review in advanced basal cell carcinoma. Drugs 2018;78:1145–56.

Gershenwald JE, Scolyer RA. Melanoma staging: American Joint Committee on Cancer (AJCC) 8th edition and beyond. Ann Surg Oncol 2018;25. 2105-2110 and correction, https://doi.org/10.1245/s10434-018-6689-x.

Henderson MA, Burmeister BH, Ainslie J, et al. Adjuvant lymph-node field radiotherapy versus observation only in patients with melanoma at high risk of further lymph-node field relapse after lymphadenectomy (ANZMTG 01.02/TROG 02.01): 6 year follow up of a phase 3 trial. Lancet Oncol 2015;16:1049–60.

Hersh E, Weber J, Powderly J, et al. Long-term survival of patients (pts) with advanced melanoma treated with ipilimumab with or without dacarbazine. J Clin Oncol 2009;27. 15s (suppl; abstr 9038).

Hodi FS, O'Day SJ, McDermott DF, et al. Improved survival with ipilimumab in patients with metastatic melanoma. N Engl J Med 2010;363:711–22.

Kamath P Darwin E, Arora H, et al. A review on imiquimod therapy and discussion on optimal management of basal cell carcinomas. Clinical Drug Invest 2018;38:883–99.

Kaufman HL Russell JS, Hamid O, et al. Updated efficacy of avelumab in patients with previously treated metastatic Merkel cell carcinoma after ≥1 year of follow-up: JAVELIN Merkel 200, a phase 2 clinical trial. J Immunother Cancer 2018;6:7–14.

Kudchadkar RR, Michielin O, van Akkooi A. Practice changing developments in stage 111 melanoma: surgery, adjuvant targeted therapy and immunotherapy. ASCO Educational Book; asco.org/edbook; 2018. p. 759–62.

Leiter U, Stadler R, Mauch M, et al. Complete lymph node dissection versus no dissection in patients with sentinel lymph node positive biopsy positive melanoma (De-COG-SLT): a multicentre, randomised phase 3 trial. Lancet Oncol 2016;17:757–67.

Locke J, Karimpour S, Young G, et al. Radiotherapy for epithelial skin cancer. Int J Radiat Oncol Biol Phys 2001;51:748–55.

Long GV, Hauschild A, Santinami M, et al. Adjuvant dabrafenib plus trametinib in stage 111 BRAF-mutated melanoma. N Engl J Med 2017;377:1813–23.

Maity A, Mick R Huang A, et al. A phase 1 trial of pembrolizumab with hypofractionated radiotherapy in patients with metastatic solid cancer. Br J Cancer 2018;119:1200–7.

Marsden JR, Newton-Bishop JA, Burrows L. BAD guidelines revised. U.K. guidelines for the management of cutaneous melanoma. British J Derm 2010;163:238–56.

Morrison WH, Garden AS, Ang KK. Radiation therapy for non melanoma skin carcinomas. Clin Plast Surg 1997;24:718–29.

Morton DL, Thompson JF, Cochran AJ, et al. MSLT group sentinel node biopsy or observation in melanoma. N Engl J Med 2014;370:1307–817.

Ott MJ, Tanabe KK, Gadd MA, et al. Multimodality treatment of Merkel cell carcinoma. Arch Surg 1999;134:388–93.

Petit JY, Avril MF, Margulis A, et al. Evaluation of cosmetic results of a randomized trial comparing surgery and radiotherapy in the treatment of basal cell carcinoma of the face. Plast Reconstr Surg 2000;105:2544–51.

Robert C, Schacter J, Long G, et al. KEYNOTE-006 investigators. Pembrolizumab versus ipilimumab in advanced melanoma. N Engl J Med 2015;372:2521–32.

Shadendorf D, et al. Pooled Analysis of Long-Term Survival Data From Phase II and Phase III Trials of Ipilimumab in Unresectable or Metastatic Melanoma. J Clin Oncol 2015 Jun 10;33(17):1889–94.

Stelzer KJ, Griffin TW. A randomised prospective trial of radiation therapy for AIDS-associated Kaposi's sarcoma. Int J Radiat Oncol Biol Phys 1993;27:1057–61.

Thompson JF, Scolyer RA, Kefford RF. Cutaneous melanoma. Lancet 2005;365:687–701.

Tsao H, Atkins MB, Sober AJ. Management of cutaneous melanoma. N Engl J Med 2004;351:998–1012.

Weber J, Mandala M, Del Vecchio M, et al. Adjuvant nivolamab versus ipilimumab in resected stage III or IV melanoma. N Engl J Med 2017;377:1824–35.

Wolchok JD, Chiarion-Silini V, Gonzalez R, et al. Overall survival with combined nivolumab and ipilimumab in advanced melanoma. N Engl J Med 2017;377:1345–56.

21

Head and Neck Cancer—General Principles

Christopher D. Scrase

INTRODUCTION

Head and neck cancer is a rather inaccurate term for describing cancers of the upper aerodigestive tract because tumours of the facial skin and the brain are not conventionally included. They are a diverse group, comprising oral cancers, as well as those of the oropharynx, larynx, nasopharynx and hypopharynx; also the paranasal sinuses, salivary glands and ear (Fig. 21.1). Worldwide, there are more than 500,000 cases per annum. In England and Wales the overall incidence is approximately 11 cases per 100,000 per year, although there are regional variations, giving rise to about 12,000 new cases per annum. The incidence is increasing at present (see the Aetiology section of this chapter). Although the treatment for these areas is often highly specialised, the areas also have many features in common with regard to investigation, diagnosis and management. Perhaps more than any other anatomical site, the concept of a multidisciplinary team working is paramount in head and neck cancer and it is essential that the team members are involved as early as possible to provide the best outcome in terms of tumour control, maintaining function and acceptable cosmesis. Radiotherapy (RT) and chemotherapy, are now widely used, either as primary therapy or postoperative treatments.

DEMOGRAPHICS

Head and neck cancers make up 3% to 4% of all new cancers in the United Kingdom. Overall, 70% of all head and neck cancers in the United Kingdom occur in men and 30% occur in women. Between 1993 and 1995, and 2013 and 2015 age-standardised incidence rates of head and neck cancer increased by 22%. For females over the same period, incidence rates increased by 40%. The majority of head and neck cancers present beyond the 5th decade, reflecting cell DNA damage accumulating over time with an average age of onset of 60 years. Cancers of the head and neck are more commonly found in people from the lower social classes and this is multifactorial with higher incidences of smoking and alcoholism, late presentation, poor oral hygiene, inadequate diet, etc. These cancers are linked to delayed diagnosis and worse outcome.

AETIOLOGY

Of head and neck cancers in the United Kingdom, 46% to 88% are preventable. The most important risk factor in the development of head and neck cancers is tobacco. Smoking or chewing tobacco is associated with 85% to 90% of head and neck malignancies. Alcohol intake has

Head and Neck Cancer (C00–C14, C30–C12) 2010–2012
Distribution of Cases Diagnosed By Anatomical Site, UK

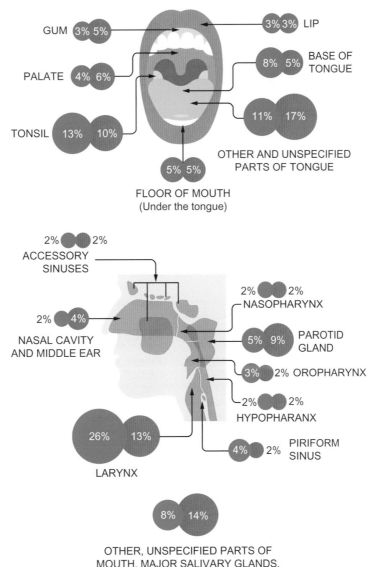

Fig. 21.1 Head and neck cancer (C00–C14, C30–C12) 2010 to 2012. Distribution of cases diagnosed by anatomical site, United Kingdom. (From Cancer Research UK. https://www.cancerresearchuk.org/health-profes sional/cancer-statistics/statistics-by-cancer-type/head-and-neck-cancers/incidence?_GA=2.213863444. 1088329562.1547202121-885388111.1547202121#HEADING-FOUR. With permission.)

also been shown to cause an increase in this group of cancers. There is also a synergistic effect of combining alcohol and tobacco with regard to developing cancers in this site. There is a clear increase in the incidence of second malignancy of the head and neck and other sites (lung, oesophagus) in persistent smokers.

Other risk factors in head and neck cancers have been suggested including poor oral hygiene, dental disease and trauma from badly fitted dentures, although direct causation has not been demonstrated. Viral infections have also been investigated for a role in the aetiology of head and neck cancers. There is a very strong association with Epstein-Barr virus infection and nasopharyngeal cancer. There is an increasing incidence of human papilloma virus

(HPV) associated oropharyngeal tumours world-wide. Such tumours develop in younger patients and have an inherently better prognosis. Immunosuppression is known to be a risk factor for malignancy and this includes cancers of the head and neck. Syphilis is a recognised risk factor too, and of significance given the resurgence of cases.

Premalignant conditions also exist, which predispose for the development of head and neck cancers. These are most commonly seen in the oral cavity and include leucoplakia (white patches), which carry an approximately 5% risk of progressing to invasive malignancy and, more sinisterly, erythroplakia. Regular specialist follow-up is therefore essential. Lichen planus with dysplastic features can also become malignant and requires monitoring.

Radiation exposure is also a risk factor for developing head and neck cancers. A previous history of RT treatment should be sought in newly diagnosed patients. Radiation exposure will also have an impact on any future RT treatment options.

PREVENTION AND EARLY DIAGNOSIS

When diagnosed early, head and neck cancer has quite a good chance for cure, but at present there is no established screening programme. It has been shown that targeted education in the primary sector with general practitioners and dentists has had some impact on early referral for oral cancers. This is important as patients presenting with advanced disease have a poorer prognosis.

Tobacco cessation is also an important factor in preventing head and neck cancers. The prevalence of cigarette smoking has fallen by nearly 50% in men and women over the last 40 years. The sex gap in cigarette smoking prevalence has also narrowed in recent years. (Fig. 21.2). Aggressive treatment of premalignant conditions is important in reducing the incidence of invasive cancer. One can envisage, in time, a positive impact on HPV-related cancers in nonsmokers subsequent to the HPV vaccination programme.

TUMOUR TYPES

The majority (>90%) of cancers of the head and neck are squamous cell carcinomas (SCCs) arising from mucosal cells. They are usually graded into well, moderately or poorly differentiated on the basis of their histological assessment (mitoses, pleomorphism). Poorly differentiated tumours tend to metastasise to lymph nodes more frequently than well-differentiated lesions. The remainder are made up of small numbers of adenocarcinoma, lymphoma (these are treated by a different team in most institutions), sarcoma, melanoma and various salivary gland tumours (muco-epidermoid, adenoid cystic, acinic tumours).

It is essential that a histological diagnosis is confirmed before treatment to ensure the correct management and that a specialist head and neck pathologist is part of the multidisciplinary team.

PRESENTATION

The majority of cases of head and neck cancer present symptomatically. The symptoms therefore depend on the primary site and the adjacent structures that may be involved. This may be a visible lesion in the oral cavity—leucoplakia, erythroplakia or nonhealing ulcer—or may relate to a swelling or mass in the oropharynx, hypopharynx or larynx. There may be hoarseness, difficulty swallowing, discomfort or pain on eating, referred aural pain, trismus or cranial nerve palsies. The onset of these symptoms is an indication for urgent referral to a head and neck department. More nonspecific symptoms of weight loss, anorexia or generalised discomfort can also be seen in this group of patients.

A common presentation of head and neck cancer is with lymph node metastases in the neck. The histology may be confirmed by fine needle aspiration (FNA) or biopsy. A thorough search for a potential primary tumour is required, aided in recent years with functional imaging (fluorodeoxyglucose-positron emission tomography-computed tomography 'FDG-PET-CT'). Two metaanalyses have indicated sensitivities of 88.3% to 97% and specificities of 68% to 74.9% in detecting unknown primaries.

INVESTIGATION

Patients presenting with possible head and neck cancer should be referred urgently to a specialist head and neck oncology team. The work-up requires confirmation of the histological diagnosis and full examination of the aerodigestive tract for accurate staging and to exclude second primary lesions. Cross-sectional imaging with CT or magnetic resonance imaging (MRI) with contrast enhancement is also

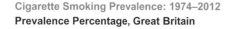

Cigarette Smoking Prevalence: 1974–2012
Prevalence Percentage, Great Britain

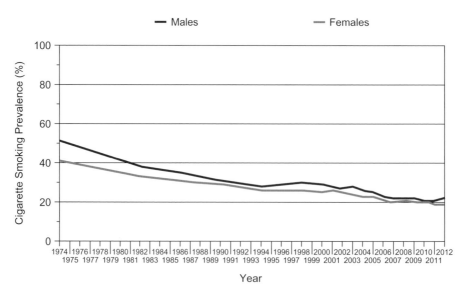

Fig. 21.2 Cigarette smoking prevalence: 1974 to 2012. Prevalence percentage, Great Britain. (From Cancer Research UK. Data for 1974–2011:Office for National Statistics. General Lifestyle Survey, 2011. Available from: https://webarchive.nationalarchives.gov.uk/20160106020741/http://www.ons.gov.uk/ons/rel/ghs/general-lifestyle-survey/2011/index.html. Data for 2012 onwards: Office for National Statistics. Opinions and Lifestyle Survey. Available from: https://www.ons.gov.uk/peoplepopulationandcommunity/healthandsocialcare/healthandlifeexpectancies/compendium/opinionsandlifestylesurvey/2015-03-19.)

essential for staging purposes detailing the anatomical extent of the primary lesion and any nodal involvement. CT provides more limited soft tissue resolution than MRI and often the two modalities are complimentary. Imaging of the chest with chest x-ray or CT is required to exclude pulmonary metastases especially in those patients with more advanced local disease or a synchronous lung primary. There may be a synchronous primary in 2% to 5% of head and neck cancer patients and these are often tobacco related. The incidence of distant metastases is reported to be between 5% and 30% and the majority is in the lung, although very occasionally bone or liver secondaries are found. The occurrence of metastases correlates with the increasing stage of the primary tumour and the number, size and bilaterality of lymph node involvement at presentation. PET using 18 FDG combined with CT for anatomical data is invaluable now in assisting in identifying potential primary sites in the head and neck territory in patients who present with malignant neck nodes from an otherwise unknown primary. As such, true unknown primaries of the head and neck territory are comparatively rare these days.

All head and neck cancer patients should be discussed in a multidisciplinary meeting at the time of diagnosis and staging to determine the optimum treatment. The choice is usually between radical surgery with or without postoperative RT (or chemoradiotherapy), or primary radical RT (or concurrent chemoradiation), with possible neck dissection for residual disease. The decision is usually determined by the site of the primary tumour, the size of the primary tumour and consequent functional morbidity, evidence of lymph node involvement and patients' co-morbidity or individual preference. Before embarking on any radical treatment options, there are a number of preparatory steps that need to be assessed.

NUTRITION

Head and neck cancer patients have many reasons to be malnourished before diagnosis of their malignancy. Many have a background of excessive alcohol intake and the tumour may have resulted in impaired swallowing function or caused oral discomfort. The success of any radical treatment is compromised by inadequate nutrition and morbidity is also increased. It is essential that all head and neck cancer patients have assessment by a specialist dietician, and speech and language therapist (SALT) before any treatment. They may require enteral feeding before treatment and will certainly need it following reconstructive surgery. Patients receiving radical RT will usually have a course of treatment over many weeks and will develop mucositis and dysphagia in the acute phase. Nasogastric tube or percutaneous gastrostomy should be actively considered in all patients, especially those with large treatment volumes and is essential for patients being considered for concurrent chemoradiation where the acute toxicity is invariably increased. It is also important for the dietetic and SALT input to continue regularly throughout the treatment course—patients need to be weighed weekly because outcome data show ongoing weight loss to be a negative prognostic factor—and into the recovery phase following treatment, which may last many weeks. Close monitoring with a rehabilitation focus should therefore continue during the follow-up period until tube feeding is no longer required and patients have returned to sufficient oral intake and proven maintained weight.

DENTITION

Patients receiving radical RT for head and neck cancers will often have treatment volumes involving part or all of the mandible and the salivary glands. Following RT, these patients are often left with some xerostomia even with parotid-sparing RT approaches. Saliva has a protective role in

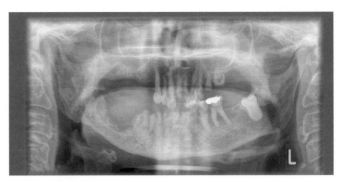

Fig. 21.3 Orthopantomogram of mandible showing osteoradionecrosis on right side.

neutralising oral acids and reducing dental caries. Tooth decay and dental problems can be increased postradiotherapy. Patients need to have a full dental assessment before RT. The ideal is for review by a restorative dentist or maxillofacial team to remove teeth if required. Any problem teeth should be removed and, because this typical patient population has often neglected their oral hygiene, many end up with a dental clearance. Dental extractions should be done a minimum of 2 weeks before commencing RT. Edentulous patients should be reviewed to ensure dentures are well fitting and will not aggravate their RT reaction by movement.

When taking consent from patients for RT, they must be counselled about the risks of dental problems following the treatment and, in particular, osteoradionecrosis (ORN) of the mandible, which can develop spontaneously but is more likely after dental procedures, particularly extractions (Fig. 21.3). Patients need to be encouraged to use fluoride mouthwash or gel daily and to have regular dental check-ups; if dental work is considered necessary, it should be performed by specialist hospital dental teams in view of the high risk of complications.

INDICATIONS FOR RADIOTHERAPY

Definitive Radiotherapy

The chief aim in using RT in head and neck cancer is organ preservation. In early laryngeal cancer, equivalent cure rates are attainable with radical RT and laryngectomy, but the former has the clear advantage of normal voice preservation. In some sites, RT is the only option or preferred option because of the inaccessible nature of the primary, for example, nasopharyngeal cancer.

Postoperative Radiotherapy

The purpose of postoperative RT is to improve locoregional control. It has recently been estimated that cancer-specific and overall survival at 5 years might be improved by about 10% with postoperative RT.

There are a number of indications for postoperative RT (Table 21.1). In some cases postoperative RT is mandatory; in other situations the real benefit to the patient is less clear.

Postoperative RT should ideally commence within 6 weeks of surgery as evidence suggests an inferior outcome if started later than this.

Palliative Radiotherapy

As a general rule, RT should be used with curative intent and with standard curative doses. On occasion, however, patients will not be fit to undergo any form of radical RT, and RT can provide useful symptom relief using a shorter schedule and limited irradiation volume.

TABLE 21.1   Indications for Postoperative Radiotherapy

Positive (involved) resection margins
Extracapsular lymph node spread
Close resection margins, i.e. <5 mm
Invasion of soft tissues
≥2 nodes involved
>1 positive nodal group (i.e. level)
Involved node >3 cm in diameter
Vascular invasion
Perineural invasion
Poor differentiation
Stage III/IV
Multicentric primary
Oral cavity/oropharynx tumours with involved nodes at level IV/V
Carcinoma in situ/dysplasia at resection 'margin/"field changes"'

Guidelines for cervical nodal irradiation in squamous cell carcinoma of the head and neck.

Reproduced with kind permission of Dr. M. Henk and the CHART steering committee.

RADIOTHERAPY PLANNING

Once RT has been decided as the treatment modality for head and neck patients, there are a number of steps required before commencing. Patients need to be informed of all possible side effects (see Toxicity of Treatment) and to give consent.

Immobilisation

The next step is to consider immobilisation. Tumours in the head and neck may be relatively small compared with other anatomical sites, and they are also often adjacent to several critical normal structures. It is therefore essential for accurate treatment delivery that patients have good quality reproducible immobilisation. In general, this involves an individual shell to cover the head, neck and sometimes, the shoulders. These shells are commonly typically thermoplastic devices and are created specifically for the patient during the planning phase. The patient then has subsequent imaging in the mask. Mould room staff who make the shell also require information about the patient's position (usually supine) and the orientation of the neck. This is important and is determined by the site one intends to irradiate and needs consideration of the primary beam orientation; an extended neck position would be required for treatment of the parotid bed and middle/inner ear to facilitate the exiting dose below the contralateral eye. It is also necessary to consider whether the patient requires a mouth bite or tongue depressor. A mouth bite is used to push the tongue out of the treatment volume, for example, maxillary antral tumours. A tongue depressor is used to push the tongue into the treatment volume, for example, oral tongue tumours. Centres vary in their use of these devices because of issues of patient comfort and consistency in placement.

The most important issue of any immobilisation device is to know what the reproducibility of set-up is for any particular patient. All centres should know the accuracy of their set-up because this is the information required for determining the margin from clinical target volume (CTV) to planning target volume (PTV). In practice, an accuracy of 3 mm can be expected with existing devices, although this can be reduced further with on-line imaging (see later).

TARGET VOLUMES

Definitive Radiotherapy

When RT (with or without chemotherapy) is the definitive treatment, a gross tumour volume (GTV) will be present and a planning CT scan will allow it to be delineated combined with information from the examination under anaesthesia (EUA), histology and other diagnostic imaging. Help from a specialist radiologist is recommended. The CTV is to account for microscopic spread. Overtly involved nodes should be included in a separate nodal CTV. Occult lymph node metastases occur in up to 20% to 30% of the N0 neck patients, so prophylactic irradiation is required for many head and neck tumours and is delineated as a separate CTV. Some centres differentiate between high-risk nodes and those at a lower risk and define those by separate nodal CTVs and prescribed doses of irradiation. The sites where prophylactic nodal irradiation is not considered is early glottic cancer (T1/T2 disease) (Table 21.2). The likelihood of nodal involvement has been widely studied and it is clear that the probability increases with site of primary, size of primary and differentiation.

The regions of the neck have been divided into levels to allow international consensus on the lymph node anatomy (Fig. 21.4):

- Level I contains the submental and submandibular lymph nodes.
- Level II contains the upper jugular lymph nodes, which are above the hyoid bone.
- Level III contains the mid-jugular lymph nodes, which are between the hyoid bone and the cricoid cartilage.
- Level IV contains the lower jugular lymph nodes beginning below the cricoid.
- Level V contains the lymph nodes of the posterior triangle.
- Level VI contains the pretracheal lymph nodes.

The levels included in the treatment of any particular primary site depend on the anatomical drainage and knowledge of patterns of lymph node spread. Lymph node maps for the N0 neck have been compiled to aid the planning of RT. In unilateral structures (parotid, buccal

TABLE 21.2   Indications for Nodal Irradiation by Tumour Site

Location of Primary Tumour	APPROPRIATE NODE LEVELS TO BE TREATED	
	Stage N0–N1	Stage N2b
Oral cavity	I, II, and III (+ IV for anterior tongue tumours)	I, II, III, IV and V[a]
Oropharynx	II[b], III, and IV (+ retropharyngeal nodes for posterior pharyngeal wall tumours)	I, II, III, IV, V and retropharyngeal nodes
Hypopharynx	II[b], III, and IV (+ IV for oesophageal extension)	I, II, III, IV, V and retropharyngeal nodes (+ IV for oesophageal extension)
Larynx[c]	II[b], III, and IV (+ VI for transglottic and subglottic tumours)	(I), II, III, IV and V (+ VI for transglottic and subglottic tumours)
Nasopharynx	II, III, IV, V, and retropharyngeal nodes	II, III, IV, V, and retropharyngeal nodes

[a]May be omitted if only levels I–III are involved.
[b]Nodes in level IIb could be omitted for N0 patients.
[c]T1 glottic cancer excluded.
From Gregoire 2000 R+0.

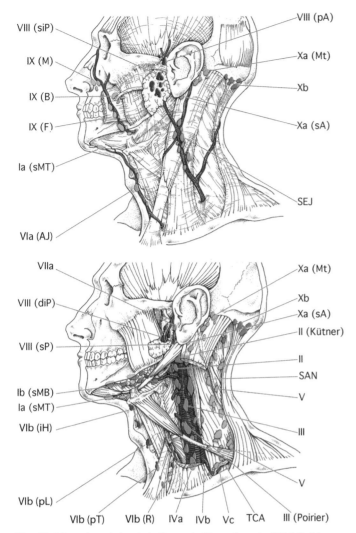

Fig. 21.4 Lymph node levels in the neck. (From Gregoire 2014 R+0.)

mucosa, lateral floor of mouth), it is possible to treat the primary site and ipsilateral neck nodes but, in midline structures, bilateral treatment is required because the lymph drainage may be to either side of the neck. Ipsilateral irradiation has obvious advantages in terms of normal tissue irradiation (and thus toxicity reduction) and compliments intensity modulated RT (IMRT) (see later).

Postoperative Radiotherapy

The principles discussed in the previous section on definitive RT are applicable in the postoperative setting, but there are some important additional points to note.

As a general rule, the whole surgical bed where the tumour is located should be included in the postoperative irradiated volume. With CT planning, it often becomes apparent that changes within the subcutaneous tissues will give volumes at risk that are bigger than anticipated and a pragmatic view must be taken on what to include in the lower risk target volume.

Unless there is gross residual disease or where RT is planned for the primary site following a neck dissection, a GTV will not be apparent on the planning CT scan. It is often helpful to coregister any diagnostic scans with the planning CT scan in determining more precisely the preoperative GTVs to arrive at a meaningful CTV.

Debate continues on whether to irradiate the neck postoperatively when it is planned to irradiate the primary site and there is no nodal

disease identified in the neck dissection specimen. The additional morbidity of irradiating the lower neck to intermediate prophylactic doses is relatively low compared with the rest of the neck, whereas recurrence in those not irradiated is difficult if not impossible to salvage. The decision must rest with the treating clinician, but a factor in that decision-making process will be the adequacy of the neck dissection.

The retropharyngeal nodes are not routinely sampled in a neck dissection. Depending on the tumour site (and hence risk of involvement), these should be included if the rest of the neck is to be irradiated postoperatively.

RADIOTHERAPY TECHNIQUE

Conformal Radiotherapy

In the past, conventional planning for head and neck RT has involved orthogonal films taken in the simulator with fields defined directly. With developments in RT planning, it became possible to shape beams to shield normal structures and thereby reduce toxicity. A CT scan with the patient located in the immobilisation device is a prerequisite to the process. The GTV and CTV(s) are defined directly on the CT. Structures to be avoided, including the spinal cord, are then outlined separately. The volumes are then used for planning purposes. This approach remains the basis for much small volume irradiation (e.g. early larynx). Most RT in the head and neck territory in the United Kingdom is undertaken now using IMRT.

Intensity Modulated and Image Guided Radiotherapy in Head and Neck Cancers

Developments in computer and the multileaf collimator (MLC) technology have facilitated the establishment of IMRT as the standard of care for most head and neck cancer treatment. It has significant advantages in the many subsites within the head and neck territory because of the high degree of conformality that may be achieved and thus normal tissue sparing.

Image guided RT (IGRT) is distinct from IMRT. The technique of IGRT is intended to ensure the target volume as defined at the outset of treatment is treated consistently throughout the course of RT. Organs move and patients move, although immobilisation techniques should ensure that patient movement is less than 3 mm in the head and neck region. IGRT then has as its purpose to correct for motion and set-up errors by imaging the treatment area on a daily basis. It has other advantages as will be seen later.

What Is Intensity Modulated Radiotherapy?

Any radical RT technique aims to treat tumour tissue while minimising the exposure of healthy adjacent normal tissue. In the head and neck region, it is self-evident that there are many normal tissues that potentially need not be treated. The clinical target volume is often complex with structures nearby which, if damaged, could result in catastrophic sequelae, for example, binocular blindness and myelopathy. Two-dimensional techniques use parallel-opposed fields to minimise these risks by the 'shrinking-field' technique (Fig. 21.5).

CT delineation of target volumes has facilitated the use of three-dimensional conformal RT (3D CRT). By defining a CTV and a margin for set-up error to give the PTV, the resulting field with blocks or MLCs will achieve improved conformality and potentially reduced normal tissue dose (Fig. 21.6).

IMRT uses the computer control of the MLC to produce either a finite or infinite number of subfields within each field to improve target volume coverage. In essence, in a single beam's eye view, the target volume is seen as a three-dimensional structure and is treated as such.

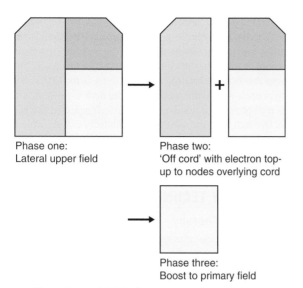

Phase one:
Lateral upper field

Phase two:
'Off cord' with electron top-up to nodes overlying cord

Phase three:
Boost to primary field

Fig. 21.5 Three-phase shrinking field treatment.

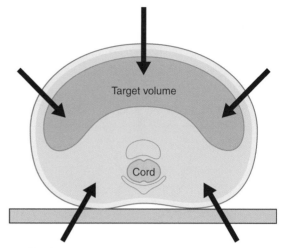

Fig. 21.7 Treating a target volume with normal tissue in the concavity.

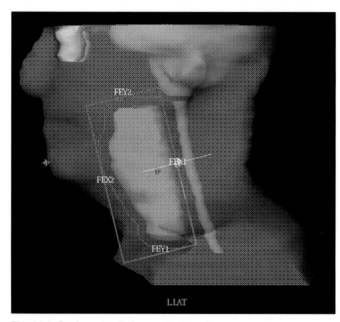

Fig. 21.6 Conformal radiotherapy treatment.

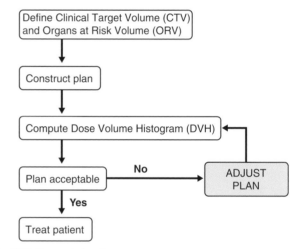

Fig. 21.8 Forward planning.

Photographers will be able to relate this to the concept of depth of field. The net effect of such complex beam modulation (Fig. 21.7) is the ability to treat concave target volumes with normal tissues in the concavity. It is self-evident why, therefore, IMRT has become so well established in the head and neck territory.

Treatment Planning in Intensity Modulated Radiotherapy

Conventional (forward) planning techniques cannot be used with IMRT (Fig. 21.8). In other words, it is not possible to define a target volume and expect the planner to work out the modulation of each beam (or beam profile) to achieve the desired conformality. Instead, computer technology has assumed that role driven by the planner, aided by various inputted parameters (or planning constraints). Planning then when using IMRT requires a different approach; instead of a plan being arrived at by a manual iterative process (often itself reliant on the experience of the planner), parameters including the intended

target volume dose to a specified volume and maximum and median/mean doses allowed to normal tissues are specified at the outset. This is a process known as *inverse* planning.

It is evident that the process of inverse planning requires absolute clarity of target volume definition (Fig. 21.9). This is not a minor issue because arriving at definitions, particularly in the head and neck area, is through a process of integration of all planning data. This will include any pretreatment visual inspection and imaging, operative findings, pathology results, postoperative and planning scans and knowledge of patterns of spread. Clearly, this approach should be applied to all RT where accurate target-volume definition is necessary, that is, curative RT, but the ability of IMRT to achieve a high degree of conformality makes this crucial. International updated consensus guidelines from Gregoire et al. (2014) exist for the definition and delineation of the nodes in the cervical chain, which should lead to uniformity between centres and within centres amongst treating teams. More recently, guidelines have been published for the primary tumour and selection of associated CTV (Gregoire et al., 2018). Adherence to these guidelines should dispel any remaining concerns of geographical misses that were raised at the outset of IMRT.

The process of inverse planning requires as much clarity on normal tissue volume definition as that of the clinical target volume. In the head and neck region, these organs at risk (OAR) would include the spinal cord, brainstem, brain, optic pathway, cochlea and salivary tissues depending on the primary site of irradiation. Failure to delineate these accurately could mean that they are irradiated unintentionally beyond conventional tolerance limits because IMRT achieves its goal of improved conformality, in simple terms, by moving the dose elsewhere. Guidelines now exist that comprehensively describe these normal tissues and should result in consistency. Normal tissues, once delineated, require a specification of dose. These constraints may be specified in terms of maximum doses (e.g. spinal cord) or dose-volume constraints (e.g. parotid glands) and will be determined on the functional unit arrangement (i.e. parallel vs series). The QUANTEC data published by Marks et al. in 2010 details the dose limits and risks if exceeded and is an invaluable resource.

It is because IMRT achieves its goal through shifting dose that some structures that would not have been irradiated using conventional techniques need delineation. For example, in the treatment of oropharyngeal tumours, the oral cavity will receive modest doses of radiation. By specifying a limit of dose there, it is possible to minimise the impact of irradiation on the oral mucosa. In addition, it is helpful to treat the patient in such circumstances in an extended neck position to move the oral cavity out of the primary beam array. Fictitious structures (dummy organs) might need to be drawn to keep doses out of areas that would never normally be irradiated and/or to try to improve conformality of target volume coverage and are useful tools for the planner. The end result is an array of volumes for the planner to use (Fig. 21.10). This process is time consuming but is a prerequisite to successful IMRT. Software programs exist that speed this process through the use of stored templates of normal structures with built-in elasticity to morph to the individual patient's anatomy and body profile.

The Scope of Intensity Modulated Radiotherapy in Head and Neck Tumours

The improvement in conformality in head and neck tumours with IMRT has two important fundamental benefits. First, it facilitates the coverage of complex and especially concave target volumes. Second, it can achieve avoidance of dose-limiting normal tissues.

It is perhaps the avoidance function that is more useful in head and neck tumours. The parallel-opposed technique does, as the name suggests, treat everything in its path. Mucosa and salivary glands that need not necessarily be treated can now be spared by this approach (Fig. 21.11). The net effect is reduced toxicity. This has perhaps been best explored in relation to reducing xerostomia through sparing of one or both parotid glands as seen in the PARSPORT study. In addition, however, is the improved tolerability of some of the more intense schedules that have emerged as superior in the management of head and neck tumours; that is, altered fractionation and concurrent chemoradiotherapy.

An improvement in conformality, however, also facilitates comprehensive coverage of the target volume as defined, as well as dose escalation. With conventional, even three-dimensional CRT approaches, some compromise in target volume coverage may have been necessary if normal tissue tolerance had been reached. The obvious example is in the treatment of cervical nodes overlying the spinal cord. Typically, these would be treated with electrons of a specified energy. IMRT treats this concave volume to the specified dose with sparing of the underlying cord without the need for electron applicators. In other sites, such as the paranasal territory, some of the target volume may be at risk of complete sparing with non-IMRT techniques because of the complex inter-relationship of normal tissue and tumour volumes (Figs 21.12 and 21.13). Dose escalation can be used at areas of greatest risk of recurrence, for example, gross residual primary tumour and nodes with extracapsular spread.

INVERSE PLANNING

- Define CTV and ORVs
- Define C(P)TV and (P)ORV constraints
- Define beam geometry
- Optimise beam intensives
- Compute delivery sequence → TREAT PATIENT

Fig. 21.9 Inverse planning.

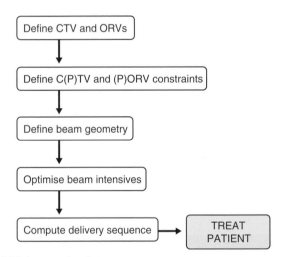
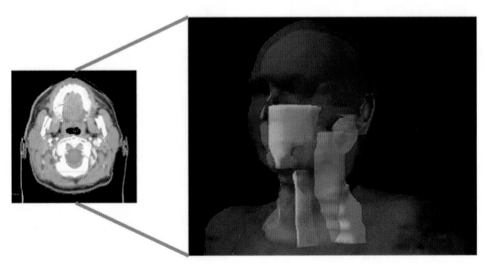

Fig. 21.10 The array of volumes with which the planner can work.

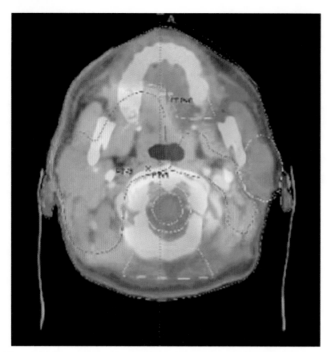

Fig. 21.11 The scope of intensity modulated radiotherapy in sparing the parotid and mucosa.

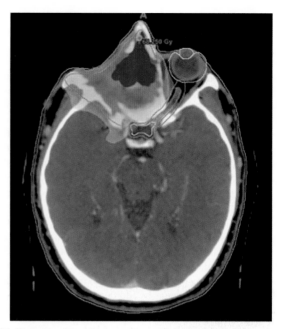

Fig. 21.13 Achievable with intensity modulated radiotherapy tumor volume irradiated with out treating left eye.

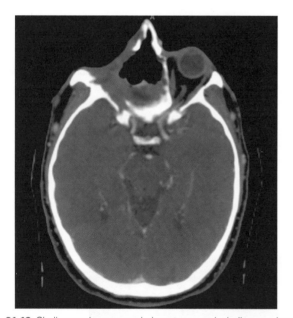

Fig. 21.12 Challenges in paranasal sinus tumours including sparing the one remaining eye.

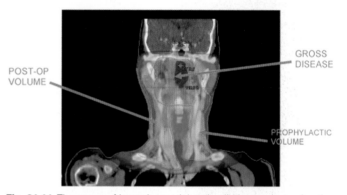

Fig. 21.14 The scope of intensity modulated radiotherapy in sparing the parotid and delivering dose according to risk of disease.

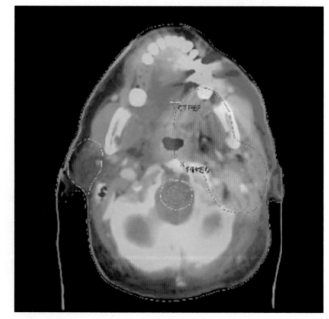

Fig. 21.15 The scope of intensity modulated radiotherapy in treating high risk areas with the synchronous boost technique.

Dose escalation with IMRT needs consideration of radiobiological principles. A single phase technique is used throughout the whole volume (Fig. 21.14) with different doses specified according to areas of variable risk, for example, gross disease, high-risk (e.g. involved nodes postexcision) and low-risk territories (e.g. elective nodes in contralateral neck). Not only is the total dose modified according to perceived risk but so is the dose per fraction. A higher than conventional dose per fraction will have a higher cell kill effect and is important in the area that is dose escalated. This approach is called the synchronous or simultaneous integrated boost (SIB) technique (Fig. 21.15) and is well

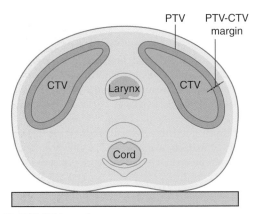

Fig. 21.16 PTV–CTV margins.

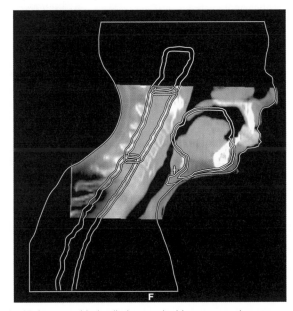

Fig. 21.17 Image-guided radiotherapy; in this case cone beam computed tomography.

established as an approach in IMRT of the head and neck. Care is clearly required in the volume of normal tissue exposed to this as higher than expected morbidity may result because of the negating effect on normal tissue damage. In areas to receive prophylactic irradiation, the total dose needs to be modified upwards to compensate for the longer elective treatment (e.g. 54 gray (Gy) in 30 fractions rather than 50 Gy in 25 fractions; see later section) to compensate for repopulation.

It is no wonder that IMRT has become the standard of care for most head and neck cancers.

Image-guided Radiotherapy

Patients with head and neck tumours need a high degree of reproducibility and this is generally achieved through good immobilisation techniques. These immobilisation devices cannot achieve complete immobility and it is for that reason that a CTV–PTV margin exists even in IMRT (Fig. 21.16). IGRT seeks to reduce this margin by daily imaging. In the case of head and neck cancer bony and soft tissue landmarks the iso-center can be adjusted on a daily basis. This on-line approach of volumetric imaging and correction before the treatment itself then facilitates a reduction in that CTV–PTV margin. IMRT then seeks to achieve conformality to the CTV, IGRT with a reduction in the PTV margin required (Fig. 21.17). A further advantage of IGRT is in treatment adaptation. For head and neck cancer by using axial imaging, it is possible to see the impact of treatment on the disease and where appropriate to modify the plan so that high-dose target volumes can be reduced if there has been a good response. The complimentary approach is where treatment results in a change in body profile, that is, through weight loss, which can impact on received doses and can be clinically significant. Hot spots, if evident, can be addressed through replanning (Fig. 21.18).

DOSE AND FRACTIONATION

Definitive Radiotherapy

The conventional schedule for RT to head and neck cancer involves the delivery of 70 Gy in 2 Gy fractions over 7 weeks, treating 5 days per week. Shorter schedules remain useful for small-volume treatments: 50 Gy in 16 fractions over 3 weeks or 55 Gy in 20 fractions over 4 weeks.

The Danish Head and Neck Cancer Group (DAHANCA) compared six fractions per week with the standard five (still using 2 Gy per fraction). In total 66 to 68 Gy was given in either 6.5 or 5.5 weeks. They

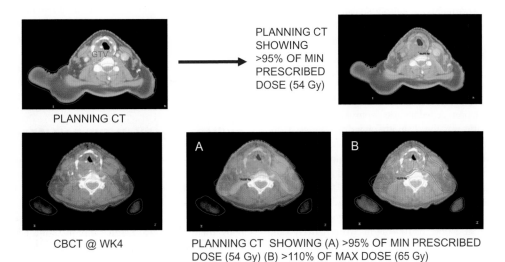

Fig. 21.18 Adaptive radiotherapy.

showed improved 5-year local control in the moderately accelerated group of 68% versus 56% for standard therapy without chemotherapy. The extra treatment was either given on Saturday, or the patients were treated twice on Friday (with ≥6 hour gap).

Another schedule is to use a concomitant boost to the primary site during the conventional RT. This provides the first phase of treatment (primary disease plus involved nodes and microscopic spread) in the morning and then later the same day a second smaller boost dose is given to the phase 2 volume, involving the gross disease only. The dose is 1.8 Gy daily with a 1.5 Gy boost for the last 12 treatments, a total dose of 72 Gy in 42 fractions given over 6 weeks. This accelerates the overall treatment time.

A recent metaanalysis of fractionation schedules has concluded that there is a survival benefit with altered fractionation. The largest survival benefit (8.2% at 5 years) was evident with hyperfractionation, not dissimilar to the benefits seen with concurrent chemoradiation. Accelerated schedules resulted in a lesser survival gain, although such a schedule would be easier to implement in the clinic than hyperfractionation. To some extent this debate on fractionation has been superseded by the accelerated hypofractionated schedules (i.e. dose per fraction slightly higher than 2 Gy) used in IMRT, at least in the United Kingdom: 65 to 66 Gy in 30 fractions over 6.5 weeks would be considered an accepted schedule with reduced doses to areas of less risk of disease.

Postoperative Radiotherapy

Doses to sites of gross residual disease, that is, the primary and involved nodes, are treated to doses similar to the definitive setting (70 Gy when using 2-Gy fractions). More typically, where this is true, adjuvant therapy doses of 66 Gy in 33 fractions would be recommended in the presence of high-risk pathological findings (extracapsular spread and/or positive/close margins). Lower doses equivalent to 50 to 54 Gy in 2-Gy fractions would be given to lower areas of risk of microscopic disease.

CHEMOTHERAPY IN HEAD AND NECK CANCER

There has been much work done looking into chemotherapy agents in head and neck cancer. Many drugs have been shown to have some response in squamous cell cancers of the head and neck, in particular, the platinum compounds, 5-fluorouracil, methotrexate, bleomycin, vinca alkaloids and, more recently, the taxanes. However, the most compelling data is in the use of chemotherapy given concurrently with RT.

Concurrent Chemotherapy and Definitive Radiotherapy

The accepted standard treatment for radical nonsurgical therapy is concurrent cisplatin chemotherapy with radical RT at least in those patients younger than 70 years of age. The evidence for this comes from Pignon's original metaanalysis updated in 2009, which showed a small but significant survival advantage to the combined treatment, but only if the chemotherapy was given concurrently. This benefit was not seen in induction or adjuvant schedules. The overall survival benefit for any chemoradiation schedule was approximately 4% but increased to 8% if cisplatin was the chemotherapy drug chosen. Concomitant chemotherapy is given simultaneously with radiation therapy to improve local and distant control. The mechanisms for action include the elimination of micrometastases and increased sensitivity to the RT.

The standard schedule for concurrent chemoradiotherapy for head and neck cancer involves cisplatin given intravenously on days 1, 22 and 43 of the RT at a dose of 100 mg/m^2. Alternatively (and increasingly in the United Kingdom), the cisplatin is being delivered using the weekly schedule of 40 mg/m^2 for 6 weeks. There is anecdotal evidence that this regimen is better tolerated than the 3-weekly schedule, particularly in the head and neck cancer population, although this is still being debated. Patients require a satisfactory full blood count and adequate renal function throughout. Nutritional support is essential and a feeding tube is advised in all patients undergoing combination treatment. Acute toxicity is usually more severe in these patients and should be looked for and managed aggressively.

Although cisplatin remains the gold standard agent for concurrent chemotherapy, cetuximab, a monoclonal antibody to the epidermal growth factor receptor (EGFR), when given concurrently with RT, has been shown to improve progression-free and overall survival without the added burden of traditional sensitising chemotherapy. It is generally reserved for fit patients in whom all forms of platin-based chemotherapy treatment are contraindicated.

Given the excellent prognosis with HPV-positive head and neck cancers, studies are underway to evaluate the safety of de-escalating treatment, especially regarding cisplatin substitution or avoidance of concurrent chemoradiation completely.

Concurrent Chemotherapy and Postoperative Radiotherapy

A previous section has outlined the range of indications for postoperative RT. Some situations would be considered particularly adverse for locoregional recurrence and, in these cases, consideration should be given to concurrent chemoradiation postoperatively. Two trials by Cooper and Bernier and a consensus view have suggested that such patients would be those with positive primary resection margins, and those with pathologically involved nodes with extracapsular spread.

Induction Chemotherapy

Neoadjuvant or induction chemotherapy has been used to downstage a primary tumour before definitive surgery or RT, and to decrease the incidence of distant metastases. In the Pignon metaanalysis of chemotherapy with RT in head and neck cancer, there was evidence that organ preservation was increased in patients receiving chemotherapy followed by radical RT compared with primary surgery for advanced but resectable laryngeal cancer. Although the original metaanalysis did not show any real survival benefit, a more recent review on updated data has shown that induction schedules may convey a survival advantage of up to 2% to 3%. The majority of these studies used the previous standard induction chemotherapy schedule of cisplatin and 5-fluorouracil (PF). The debate on the role of induction chemotherapy has been ignited with the publication of two key trials using the triplet of docetaxel, cisplatin and 5-fluorouracil, and further ones since reviewed in a metaanalysis that has shown progression-free and overall survival and distant failure rate benefits over PF. To date however, the only widely accepted setting for which induction chemotherapy has consensus value is in laryngeal preservation in patients with resectable but locally advanced disease.

CHEMOTHERAPY IN THE PALLIATIVE SETTING

Chemotherapy is used for palliation in patients with recurrent or metastatic head and neck cancer. If patients have not received prior treatment with chemotherapy, then cisplatin and 5-fluorouracil could be considered as first-line treatment or a more outpatient equivalent, such as carboplatin and capecitabine, could be considered. Monoclonal antibody therapy against EGFR with platinum-based chemotherapy is active and has been shown to improve median overall survival compared with standard chemotherapy alone.

TOXICITY OF TREATMENT

Radiotherapy for head and neck cancer has many side effects that must be effectively communicated to the patient before embarking on treatment. A detailed explanation is essential not only for informed consent but also to improve compliance with the full course of treatment to give the best chance of a successful outcome. As with RT to any part of the body, the side effects (apart from fatigue) relate to structures within the radiation field. They can be divided into acute (early) or late side effects. Reactions will, to some extent, be site specific and are discussed in more detail in Chapter 22. However, it is useful to consider the principles here.

Acute Toxicity

Mucositis will develop in the treatment volume for all patients with head and neck cancer and can be severe and disabling. It may be mild (grade 1/2) but is often severe (grade 3) (Fig. 21.19), especially in those receiving concurrent chemotherapy, which may lead to a break in treatment. Grade 4 mucositis (frank ulceration) should not be allowed to develop. Management includes analgesia using the pain ladder. Opiates may be required at some stage. Topical agents may be used initially and alongside systemic analgesia. Patients must have their weight monitored and nutritional supplements considered. The majority of patients will have a level of discomfort that requires opiate-level analgesia. This can be administered in oral preparations (solutions, syrups, etc.) or delivered via feeding tube if present. It can often become difficult for patients to tolerate oral medications, particularly in the latter stages of treatment, but the development of transdermal delivery systems for opiates can be an excellent alternative in head and neck cancer patients where swallowing is often difficult or uncomfortable and, in the main, transdermal delivery has avoided the need for subcutaneous infusions of an opiate, which were occasionally required in the past for patients with severe symptoms.

Dysphagia secondary to mucositis, loss of taste, loss of appetite and thickened secretions lead to weight loss in head and neck cancer patients. This should be predicted before treatment and a feeding tube considered in all patients with large treatment volumes, especially those to be treated by chemoradiotherapy. If patients without a tube are struggling and losing weight, a tube may need to be inserted during treatment—this will usually involve a radiologically placed gastrostomy. Prophylactic tube insertion is usually more satisfactory and allows early feeding to be initiated before the patient develops difficulties.

Thickened secretions can be alleviated with carbocisteine, which has a systemic mode of action and acute xerostomia, managed symptomatically.

A skin reaction is seen in any treated area and develops as the treatment progresses. The skin changes from mild redness (Figs 21.20 and 21.21) to brisk erythema to desquamation; initially, dry changes and peeling but progressing to moist desquamation (Fig. 21.22). A skin-care regimen should include washing with lukewarm water and unperfumed soap, avoiding shaving until treatment is completed and applying regular moisturising cream. Once skin is broken then a barrier product should be used. The optimal regimen is unclear and is often centre specific. Patients should be reviewed regularly posttreatment to monitor the resolution of skin and mucosal reactions.

Fatigue is seen in many patients receiving radical RT. It has been shown that maintaining a level of gentle activity is the best way to overcome the asthenia during therapy. In head and neck cancer patients, especially those receiving chemoradiotherapy, it is usual to monitor the haemoglobin during RT and transfusing patients as required to keep the level greater than 12 g/dl. There is evidence that RT is less effective in patients with anaemia, although no good evidence exists that correcting anaemia improves outcomes. Indeed, a review of five key trials using erythropoietin (EPO) found a worse outcome in the treated groups. The conclusion was that EPO should not be

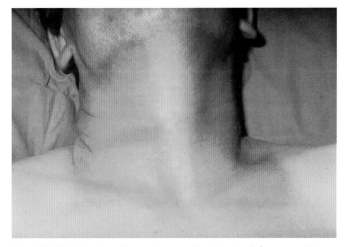

Fig. 21.20 Marked erythema in a patient treated for nasopharynx cancer (neck).

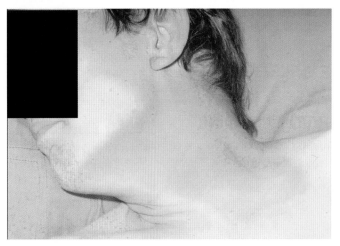

Fig. 21.21 Marked erythema in a patient treated for nasopharynx cancer (face).

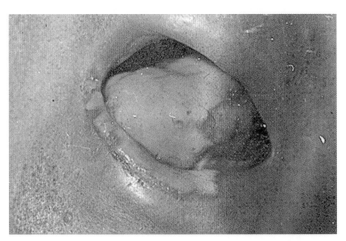

Fig. 21.19 Acute side effects of radiotherapy: acute mucositis.

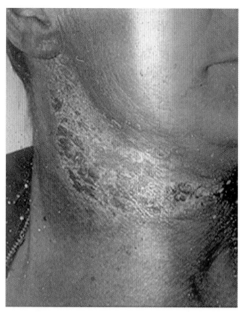

Fig. 21.22 Acute side effects of radiotherapy: skin erythema with associated dry desquamation.

administered as an addition to RT outside of the study setting myelosuppression can occur and can be life-threatening.

Late Toxicity

Skin pigmentation/atrophy can be seen in patients treated with head and neck RT as a result of the doses received by the skin. Skin sparing is achieved where possible as a result of the use of megavoltage RT and modern designs of shells that minimise the bolus effect. Bolus can be used if there is evidence of skin involvement in a tumour, that is, impending fungation.

Alopecia can occur and may be outside of the primary irradiated area because of the IMRT delivery technique (rotational IMRT). Patients should be warned of the possibility.

Xerostomia is a common late side effect of RT to the head and neck. It most commonly arises because of RT to the parotid gland, although the submandibular and sublingual glands can also be included. The risk of xerostomia increases with increasing dose. The initial symptom may become apparent from as early as the first week of therapy, and irreversible damage to the gland will arise with modest doses. It can be a most distressing side effect for patients and efforts to minimise the dose to one or both salivary glands should be routine during RT planning, given the compelling trial data that first demonstrated the value of IMRT in head and neck cancer. If it develops, patients should be offered artificial saliva preparations

and advised to use fluoride mouthwashes regularly. Dental check-ups are essential.

ORN is the breakdown of bone in an area treated with RT (See Fig. 21.3). It is seen in the mandible most often in head and neck cancer patients and can be triggered by dental extractions. It may mimic local recurrence of a tumour. ORN is difficult to manage as further surgery can exacerbate the problem. The best management is prevention, which means dental treatment before RT and aggressive dental hygiene post-radiation treatment. The ability of IMRT to conform and the avoidance of high doses to the mandible unless integral to the target volume, should also reduce the risk of ORN. Patients must be educated about the risk of dental work after RT and seeking specialist advice for any treatment required. It should be performed under general anaesthetic and with antibiotic cover.

Myelitis secondary to RT is a rare but recognised side effect from head and neck RT. There has been considerable debate over what constitutes a safe dose of radiation to the spinal cord. This is complicated because of many variables including volume treated, fraction size and total dose. Different series have described different maximal doses. A safe total dose is 44 to 46 Gy, although consensus is that doses up to 50 Gy in 2 Gy per fraction is acceptable and is clarified in the QUANTEC series. As discussed earlier, IMRT facilitates coverage of volumes with sparing of the spinal cord in the concavity, obviating many of the historical challenges of tumours close to the spinal cord. Some patients may develop Lhermitte's syndrome secondary to early transient myelitis. In Lhermitte's syndrome, patients complain of tingling or electric shocks in the legs. This can be provoked by flexing the neck. These symptoms begin about 6 weeks following the RT and may last a few months. Progression to late damage is rare, but is still observed with IMRT.

FUTURE DEVELOPMENTS

Immunotherapy

Reference has already been made earlier to molecularly targeted agents and specifically to monoclonal antibodies that competitively bind to EGFR. More recently interest has grown in targeted therapies that act on the immune system. Head and neck SCCs are associated with multiple alterations in the immune system, potentially resulting in depressed antitumour immunity. These alterations include expression of immune checkpoint molecules. Therapies that overcome these immune checkpoints and restore immune function have demonstrated activity in such cancers. Two checkpoint inhibitors, pembrolizumab and nivolumab, have established efficacy in recurrent/metastatic disease as seen in Ferris and Seiwert. These agents are currently being evaluated in the curative setting alongside standard therapies. It remains to be seen whether this will result in the additions of substitutions to standard therapies of conventional chemoradiotherapy.

FURTHER READING

Ang KK, et al. Randomised trial of addressing risk features and time factors of surgery plus radiotherapy in advanced head-and-neck cancer. Int J Radiat Oncol Biol Phys 2001;51:571–8.

Bernier J, et al. Postoperative irradiation with or without concomitant chemotherapy for locally advanced head and neck cancer. N Engl J Med 2004;350:1945–52.

Bernier J, et al. Defining risk levels in locally advanced head and neck cancers: a comparative analysis of concurrent postoperative radiation plus chemotherapy trials of the EORTC (#22931) and RTOG (#9501). Head Neck 2005;27:843–50.

Blanchard P, et al. Taxane-cisplatin-fluorouracil as induction chemotherapy in locally advanced head and neck cancers: an individual patient data meta-analysis of chemotherapy in head and neck cancer group. J Clin Oncol 2013;31(23):2854–60.

Blanchard P, et al. Meta-analysis of chemotherapy in head and neck cancer (MACH-NC): an update on 100 randomized trials and 19, 248 patients, on behalf of MACH-NC group. Ann Oncol 2016;27(Suppl 6). v1328-vi350.

Bonner JA, et al. Radiotherapy plus cetuximab for squamous-cell carcinoma of the head and neck. N Engl J Med 2006;23:1125–35.

Bourhis J, et al. Hyperfractionated or accelerated radiotherapy in head and neck cancer: a meta-analysis. Lancet 2006;368:844–54.

Brouwer CL, et al. CT-based delineation of organs at risk in the head and neck region: DAHANCA, EORTC, GORTEC, HKNPCSG, NCIC CTG, NRG Oncology and TROG consensus guidelines. Radiother Oncol 2015;117:83–90.

Budach W, et al. A meta-analysis of hyperfractionated and accelerated radiotherapy and combined chemotherapy and radiotherapy regimens in unresectable locally advanced squamous cell carcinoma of the head and neck. BMC Cancer 2006;6:28.

Cooper J, et al. Postoperative concurrent radiotherapy and chemotherapy for high-risk squamous-cell carcinoma of the head and neck. N Engl J Med 2004;350:1937–44.

Ferris RL, et al. Nivolumab for recurrent squamous-cell carcinoma of the head and neck. N Engl J Med 2016;375(19):1856–67.

Fletcher GH. Elective irradiation of subclinical disease in cancers of the head and neck. Cancer 1972;29:1450–4.

Fu KK, et al. A radiation therapy oncology group (RTOG) phase III randomized study to compare hyperfractionation and two variants of accelerated fractionation to standard fractionation for head and neck squamous cell carcinomas: First report of RTOG 9003. Int J Radiat Oncol Biol Phys 2000;48:7–16.

Gregoire V, et al. Selection and delineation of lymph node target volumes in head and neck conformal radiotherapy. Proposal for standardizing terminology and procedure based on surgical experience. Radiother Oncol 2000;56:135–50.

Gregoire V, et al. CT-based delineation of lymph node levels and related CTVs in the node-negative neck: DAHANCA, EORTC, GORTEC, NCIC, RTOG consensus guidelines. Radiother Oncol 2003;69:227–36.

Gregoire V, et al. Proposal for the delineation of the nodal CTV in the node-positive and the post-operative neck. Radiother Oncol 2006;79:15–20.

Gregoire V, et al. Delineation of the neck node levels for head and neck tumours: a 2013 update. DAHANCA, EORTC, HKNPCSG, NCIC CTG, NCRI, RTOG, TROG consensus guidelines. Radiother Oncol 2014;110:172–81.

Gregoire V, et al. Delineation of the primary clinical target volumes (CTV-P) in laryngeal, hypopharyngeal, oropharyngeal and oral cavity squamous cell carcinoma: AIRO, CACA, DAHANCA, EORTC, GEORCC, GORTEC, HKNPCSG, HNCIG, IAG-KHT, LPRHHT, NCIC CRG, NCRI, NRG Oncology, PHNS, SBRT, SOMERA, SRO, SSHNO, TROG consensus guidelines. Radiother Oncol 2018;126:3–24.

Institute of Physics and Engineering in Medicine. Report 96 Guidance for the Clinical Implementation of Intensity Modulated Radiation Therapy. IPEM; 2008.

Jackson A, et al. The lessons of QUANTEC: recommendations for reporting and gathering data on dose-volume dependencies of treatment outcome. Int J Radiat Oncol Biol Phys 2010;76(3 Suppl.).

Lambin P, et al. Erythropoietin as an adjuvant treatment with (chemo) radiation therapy for head and neck cancer. Cochrane Database of Systematic Reviews 2009;(3):CD006158. https://doi.org/10.1002/14651858.CD006158.pub2.

Lengelé B, et al. Anatomical bases for the radiological delineation of lymph node areas. Major collecting trunks, head and neck. Radiother Oncol 2007;85:146–55.

Marks LB, et al. Use of normal tissue complication probability models in the clinic. Int J Radiat Oncol Biol Phys 2010;76(3):S10–9.

Moharti BK, et al. Short course palliative radiotherapy of 20Gy in 5 fractions for advanced and incurable head and neck cancer: AIIMS study. Radiother Oncol 2004;71:275–80.

Nguyen NT, et al. 0-7-21 hypofractionated palliative radiotherapy in head and neck cancers. Br J Radiol 2015;88(1049). 20140646.

Nutting CM, et al. Parotid-sparing intensity modulated versus conventional radiotherapy in head and neck cancer (PARSPORT): a phase 3 multicentre randomized controlled trial. Lancet Oncol 2011;12:127–36.

Overgaard J, et al. Five compared with six fractions per week of conventional radiotherapy of squamous-cell carcinoma of head and neck: DAHANCA 6&7 randomised controlled trial. Lancet 2003;362:933–40.

Peters LJ, et al. Evaluation of the dose for postoperative radiation therapy of head and neck cancer: first report of a prospective randomized trial. Int J Radiat Oncol Biol Phys 1993;26:3–11.

Pignon JP, et al. Chemotherapy added to locoregional treatment for head and neck squamous-cell carcinoma: three meta-analyses of updated individual data. Lancet 2000;355:949–50.

Pignon JP, et al. Meta-analyses of chemotherapy in head and neck cancer (MACH-NC): an update. Int J Radiat Oncol Biol Phys 2007;69(Suppl. 2): S112–4.

Pignon JP, et al. Meta-analysis of chemotherapy in head and neck cancer (MACH-NC): an update on 93 randomised trials and 17,346 patients. Radiother Oncol 2009;92(1):4–14.

Posner MR, et al. (TAX324 Study Group). Cisplatin and fluorouracil alone or with docetaxel in head and neck cancer. N Engl J Med 2007;357:1705–15.

Royal College of Radiologists. Radiotherapy Dose Fractionation. 3rd ed, London: RCR 2019; p 40–45.

Seiwert TY, et al. Safety and clinical efficacy of pembrolizumab for treatment of recurrent or metastatic squamous cell carcinoma of the head and neck (KEYNOTE-012): an open-label, multicenter, phase 1b trial. Lancet Oncol 2016;17(7):956–65.

Szyszko TA, et al. PET/CT and PET/MRI in head and neck malignancy. Clin Radiol 2018;73:60–9.

Vermorken JB, et al. (EORTC 24971/TAX 323) Study. Cisplatin, fluorouracil, and docetaxel in unresectable head and neck cancer. N Engl J Med 2007;357:1695–704.

Vermorken JB, et al. Platinum-based chemotherapy plus cetuximab in head and neck cancer. N Engl J Med 2008;359:1116–27.

22

Sino-Nasal, Oral, Larynx and Pharynx Cancers

Christopher D. Scrase, Paul Symonds

CHAPTER OUTLINE

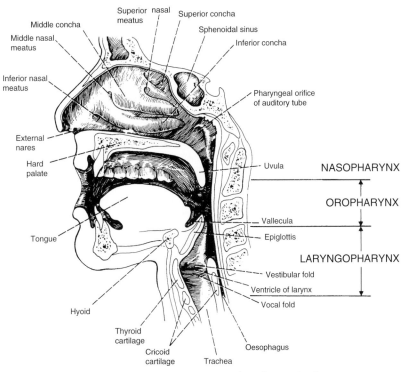

Fig. 22.1 Section of the pharynx, from front to back.

This chapter reviews each anatomical subtype of the head and neck region.

NASOPHARYNX

Anatomy

The nasopharynx is cuboidal in shape and comprises the most superior of the three pharyngeal structures. As such it has a direct communication with the nasal cavity anteriorly and oropharynx inferiorly (Fig. 22.1).

Anterior Wall

The anterior wall comprises the posterior choanae and nasal cavity.

Posterior Wall

The posterior wall is formed by the tissues of the prevertebral space adjacent to the first and second cervical vertebrae.

Lateral Walls

The pharyngobasilar fascia forms the lateral and posterior walls. Within this is the opening of the eustachian tube and, more posteriorly, a deep recess called the fossa of Rosenmüller (lateral nasopharyngeal recess) (Fig. 22.2).

Superior Wall

Strictly, the roof slopes in an anterior to posterior direction abutting the base of skull. The sphenoid sinus lies superiorly and the superior component of Waldeyer's ring, the most prominent in childhood, is located here. There is a depression in the mucosa in the midline known as the pharyngeal bursa which sometimes extends into the basiocciput.

Inferior Wall

The inferior wall is, in reality, an imaginary horizontal line running from the lower border of the soft palate to the posterior pharyngeal wall.

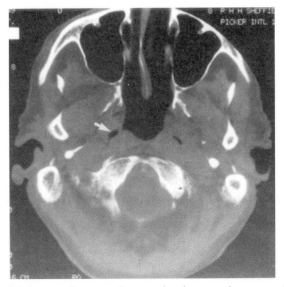

Fig. 22.2 Computed tomography scan showing normal anatomy of the nasopharynx. The fossa of Rosenmüller (pharyngeal recess) is arrowed. (Courtesy of Dr .R. Nakielny, Sheffield.)

Incidence of Nasopharyngeal Tumours

Cancer of nasopharynx (NPC) is rare in the United Kingdom with an annual incidence rate of 0.39 per 100,000 population. By contrast, NPC is far more common in patients of Southern Chinese, North African and Alaskan origin. The incidence in the Hong Kong population is between 20 and 30 per 100,000 a year. It is also more common in men than women (3:1) with a median age at presentation of 50 years.

Staging System for Nasopharyngeal Tumours

The staging system is based on the International TNM System updated most recently to version 8:

T1	Tumour confined to the nasopharynx or extends to the oropharynx and/or nasal cavity
T2	Tumour with parapharyngeal space extension and/or infiltration of the medial pterygoid, lateral pterygoid and/or prevertebral muscles
T3	Tumour that invades bony structures of the skull base, cervical vertebra, pterygoid structures and/or paranasal sinuses
T4	Tumour with intracranial extension and/or involvement of cranial nerves, infratemporal fossa, hypopharynx, orbit or masticator space
N1	Unilateral metastases in cervical lymph node(s) and/or unilateral or bilateral metastases in retropharyngeal lymph nodes, ≤6 cm above the caudal border of the cricoid cartilage
N2	Bilateral lymph node(s) ≤6 cm above the caudal border of the cricoid cartilage
N3	Any lymph node >6 cm and/or extension below the caudal border of the cricoid cartilage

Stage grouping

Stage 1	T1N0M0
Stage 2	T2N0M0
	T1N1M0
	T2N1M0
Stage 3	T1N2M0
	T2N2M0
	T3N0M0
	T3N1M0
	T3N2M0
Stage 4A	T4N0M0
	T4N1M0
	T4N2M0
	Any T N3M0
Stage 4B	Any T, Any N M1

Aetiology, Pathology and Lymphatic Spread

Squamous cell carcinomas SCCs comprise the commonest histological type. They may be subdivided into well- to poorly differentiated types, those with a heavy lymphatic infiltrate (lymphoepithelioma), transitional cell tumours and keratinising and nonkeratinising types. The World Health Organization (WHO) usefully classifies nasopharyngeal tumours as follows:

Type 1	Well-differentiated keratinising type SCC (KSCC)
Type 2	Moderately differentiated nonkeratinising type (NKDC)
Type 3	Undifferentiated type typically with an extensive lymphocytic infiltrate (NKUC)

The presence of keratin (i.e. type 1) is associated with local infiltration, whereas type 3 tumours tend to disseminate widely. The WHO III subtype is the most common form of NPC in endemic areas and differs from squamous type of NPC in its association with the Epstein-Barr virus (EBV) and sensitivity to chemotherapy and radiotherapy (RT)

NPC is thus associated with infection with the EBV. EBV DNA is incorporated into the tumour genome. Infection with EBV is common and is the cause of glandular fever. In Hong Kong, almost all children aged 10 years have been infected by the virus. Even in Hong Kong, only a small minority develop NPC. Genetic and dietary factors seem important in tumour development. Genetic alterations include deletion of chromosomal regions at 1p, 14q, 16p and amplification of 4q and 12q. Dietary factors are also important, including eating salt-dried fish (containing carcinogenic nitrosamines) and lack of fresh fruit and vegetables (lack of antioxidants).

Although SCCs form the majority of nasopharyngeal cancers, other pathologies are recognised in this region. These include adenocarcinoma, adenoid cystic carcinoma and lymphoma. Treatment may vary by tumour type according to the propensity for nodal spread and response to radiation, although the principles of technique as described here can still broadly be applied.

It is because of the rich lymphatic supply that these tumours commonly spread and, indeed, present with neck nodes. This spread may be bilateral, but the distribution is dissimilar to other head and neck SCCs and is reflected in the TNM classification outlined earlier. It has been found that 70% to 90% of cases have nodes at some point. Levels 1A/B are rarely involved, whereas levels 2 and 5 (the postcervical chain) can be considered the first echelon nodes for this tumour site.

Nasopharyngeal cancers have a high propensity for distal haematogenous spread and, as a consequence, distal failure.

Signs and Symptoms

The first presenting symptom is often painless node enlargement confirmed on examination. These are often bilateral in their distribution and, as mentioned earlier, typically involve the posterior cervical chain.

Other common symptoms include nasal obstruction and epistaxis through expansion into the nasal cavity and auditory disturbances, especially unilateral deafness and recurrent otitis media. Examination findings may confirm a mass in the postnasal space and cranial nerve palsies especially of II to VI through direct expansion through bone and via nerve foramina, and IX to XII through compression from Rouviere's node. This node is the most superior of the retropharyngeal node chain and overlies the transverse process of C1.

Patients may report headaches, although other symptoms or signs will usually be readily apparent.

Diagnosis and Staging

The diagnosis may be strongly suspected on clinical grounds alone from the above findings especially on nasendoscopic examination, but histological confirmation of any nasopharyngeal mass will be required. Patients should be assessed with rigid and fibreoptic nasendoscopy. Further locoregional staging, best with magnetic resonance imaging (MRI), is mandatory. A computed tomography (CT) scan, although adequate, does not afford the same degree of information, particularly in the base of skull region.

In the context of neck nodes where a primary is not readily apparent, especially when it lies posteriorly in the upper neck, the finding of EBV genomic material most reliably detected using in situ hybridisation is usually indicative of a clinically inapparent nasopharyngeal primary and treatment should be along the lines of such tumours.

Because nasopharyngeal cancers have a high propensity for systemic spread, a work-up for distal disease is essential. As such, haematological and biochemical screens and a CT scan of the chest, abdomen and pelvis should be undertaken. A positron emission tomography (PET)-CT scan may be useful, especially for patients with a suspected occult primary in the nasopharynx.

Treatment

The relative inaccessible nature of the primary tumour and frequent involvement of Rouviere's node dictates that radiation therapy is the main modality for treatment. In addition, and unlike other head and neck SCCs, the presence of substantial neck nodes should not lead to initial surgical excision as they generally respond well to radiation therapy. Any nodes that have failed to respond adequately or at recurrence can, provided the primary disease is controlled, then be managed by an appropriate neck dissection.

Before radiation therapy, a thorough dental assessment is mandatory with essential treatment performed as necessary.

Small tumours of the nasopharynx (T1-T2N0M0) can be adequately treated with radiation alone. A dose of 70 Gray (Gy) in 35 fractions or the biological equivalent should be given to the primary site and grossly involved nodes. The majority of nasopharyngeal tumours will, given their advanced staging and comorbidity permitting, be managed with concurrent chemoradiation. The nasopharynx is the one head and neck site where concurrent chemoradiation has been more readily adopted internationally due in part to the Intergroup 0099 Study. This study compared concurrent chemoradiation and adjuvant chemotherapy with RT alone and showed a significant advantage in survival with the combined modality approach. The control arm was particularly inferior, however, when compared with other studies. Further studies and a recent meta-analysis specifically of nasopharyngeal cancers have, however, supported the concurrent chemoradiation approach. The roles of neoadjuvant and adjuvant chemotherapy are more controversial and subject to ongoing evaluation. Neoadjuvant chemotherapy improves disease-free, but not overall survival. The most frequently used concurrent regimen is cisplatin, 100 mg/m^2 on days 1, 22 and 43 of RT and results in an improvement in overall survival of 6% at 5 years compared with RT alone.

Radiation Technique

The technique of Ho formed the basis of the two-dimensional approach to treating nasopharyngeal carcinoma. Treatment fields were vast but adapted according to local staging. Determination of the primary clinical target volume is now very much individualised based on all clinical information and using intensity-modulated RT (IMRT) facilitates comprehensive coverage while sparing radio-sensitive neuronal structures and the salivary glands. The pattern of spread outlined earlier dictates that the whole cervical lymphatic chain should be outlined and treated as routine, although doses prescribed will be determined by whether they are overtly involved and proximal to the primary site or more distal and clinically uninvolved. In other words, even in early cases, at least prophylactic doses of radiation should be given to all nodes. Guidelines with international consensus have recently been published by Lee et al Radiotherapy and Oncology 2018. which should lead to standardisation and optimisation of volume definitions.

A full head and neck immobilisation device is mandatory with the shoulders kept well down. A tongue depressor may be used, although sparing of some of the oral cavity and thus minor salivary glands can be achieved with IMRT. The consensus guidelines suggest tight (5-mm) margins to the primary gross tumour volume (GTV) as the high dose margin, and lesser doses to the remainder of the nasopharynx. The clinical tumour volume (CTV) will need to include all areas of potential spread including into the base of skull and the nerve root foramina. There are many normal tissues to be delineated to optimise sparing including the brainstem, optic nerves and chiasm. The doses recommended are 70 Gy in 33-35 fractions given five times a week or 65 Gy in 30 fractions, both using 6-MV photons (see Figs 22.3–22.8).

Complications

The significant volumes of normal tissue ordinarily irradiated can give rise to a range of long-term sequelae. IMRT facilitates salivary gland sparing and whilst not avoiding chronic xerostomia completely, significantly reduces this without compromising irradiation of adjacent lymph nodes. IMRT also facilitates sparing of other normal tissues enabling risk reduction of late damage.

High doses of radiation may be delivered to elements of the mandible. As a consequence, treatment risks, osteoradionecrosis (ORN), and preventive measures beyond meticulous radiation technique should be adopted. Moreover, the proximity of the pterygoid muscles to the primary target volume will give rise to trismus, and jaw exercises should be encouraged to minimise this.

Endocrine failure as a result of irradiation of the pituitary and thyroid glands, although relatively easy to treat, is a not uncommon outcome in long-term survivors and should be actively sought through routine testing in the follow-up of these patients.

Advanced tumours with extension into the skull base introduce additional tissues exposed to the high doses of radiation that will be necessary to achieve local control. Aspects of the temporal lobes, optic nerves and chiasm, middle and inner ear will be irradiated and, as a consequence, are at risk of late neurological damage. Careful attention to tolerance doses as determined by the QUANTEC data (Chapter 21) should minimise this risk.

Follow-up

Patients should be assessed clinically with endoscopic examination and neck palpation. There is no consensus on the best mode of radiological assessment to determine the completeness of response to treatment. MRI and/or PET-CT scans may have added value.

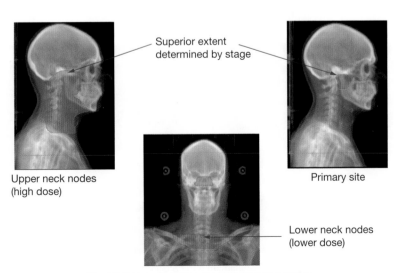

Superior extent determined by stage

Upper neck nodes (high dose)

Primary site

Lower neck nodes (lower dose)

Fig. 22.3 Volume delineation: primary and nodes.

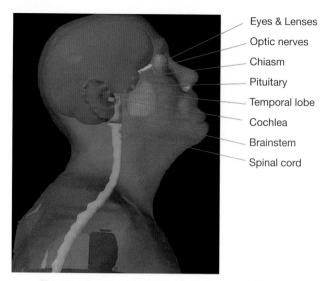

Eyes & Lenses
Optic nerves
Chiasm
Pituitary
Temporal lobe
Cochlea
Brainstem
Spinal cord

Fig. 22.4 Primary site and proximity to normal tissues.

Results

Effective treatment of early (stage 1–2) tumours of the nasopharynx should give rise to 5-year overall survival rates of 80% to 90%. More

advanced tumours, when treated optimally, will result in 5-year survival rates of the order of 50% to 70%.

Late recurrences are recognised, suggesting that follow-up beyond 5 years might be prudent and/or advising patients and primary care practitioners of this so that patients can be re-referred without delay. Recurrent disease may, on occasion, be amenable to re-irradiation as long as volumes to be treated are relatively small and the patient is prepared to accept the additional risks associated with such an approach. Surgery may be used for small disease in the nasopharynx and for nodal relapses.

NOSE AND NASAL CAVITY

Anatomy

The external nose is like the tip of an iceberg with a complex array of passageways and air cavities within it that form the nasal cavity and paranasal sinuses. The hair-bearing entrance that forms the vestibule and the mucociliary escalator provides an important initial defence against the inhalation of germs (Fig. 22.9).

The nasal vestibule lies within the aperture of the nostril. It is bounded laterally by cartilage that forms the nasal ala, medially by cartilage that forms the columella and inferiorly by the most anterior portion of the floor of the nose. Importantly, this area is lined by squamous epithelium as an extension from the outside skin.

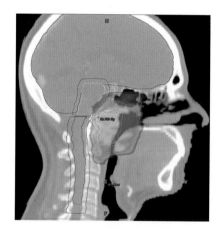

Dose distribution (50 Gy minimum and 65 Gy in 30 fractions maximum) to primary site in axial plane

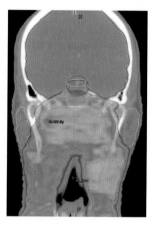

Dose distribution (50 Gy minimum and 65 Gy in 30 fractions maximum) to primary site and involved nodes in coronal plane

Fig. 22.5 Dose distribution to upper neck.

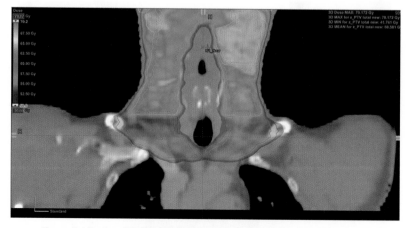

Dose distribution (50 Gy minimum and 65 Gy maximum in 30 fractions) to lower neck in coronal plane

Fig. 22.6 Dose distribution to lower neck.

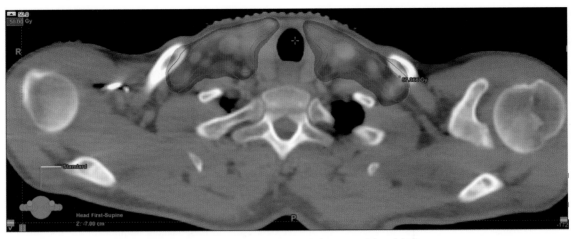

Dose distribution (50 Gy minimum) to lower neck in axial plan

Fig. 22.7 Dose distribution in axial plane to lower neck.

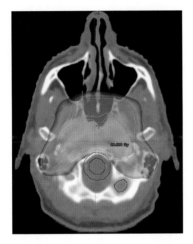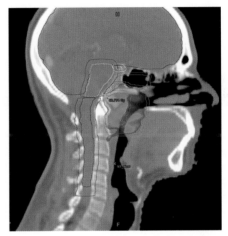

Dose distribution (50 Gy minimum and 65 Gy maximum in 30 fractions) to nasopharynx and adjacent structures

Dose distribution (60 Gy minimum) to primary site with integrated boost to GTV of 65 Gy in 30 fractions

Fig. 22.8 Dose distributions.

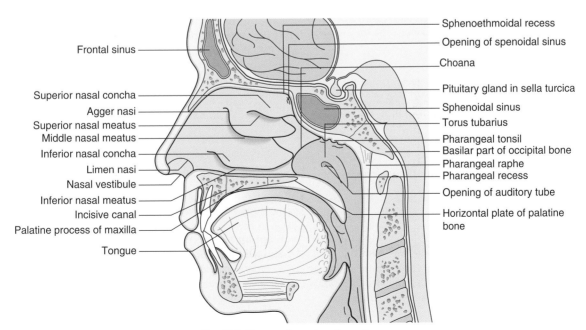

Frontal sinus

Superior nasal concha
Agger nasi
Superior nasal meatus
Middle nasal meatus
Inferior nasal concha
Limen nasi
Nasal vestibule
Inferior nasal meatus
Incisive canal
Palatine process of maxilla
Tongue

Sphenoethmoidal recess
Opening of spenoidal sinus
Choana
Pituitary gland in sella turcica
Sphenoidal sinus
Torus tubarius
Pharangeal tonsil
Basilar part of occipital bone
Pharangeal raphe
Pharangeal recess
Opening of auditory tube
Horizontal plate of palatine bone

Fig. 22.9 Nose and nasal cavity anatomy.

The nasal cavity or nasal fossa proper lies between the maxillary sinus inferiorly, and the eyes and ethmoidal sinus superiorly. It is divided into two by a midline cartilaginous septum.

Superior Wall

The superior wall is comprised of the cribriform plate of the ethmoidal sinus. The olfactory apparatus that lies here provides us with our sense of smell.

Inferior Wall

Broader than the superior wall, the inferior wall is formed from the hard palate.

Anterior Wall

The nasal bones and cartilage that form the external nose give rise to the anterior wall.

Posterior Wall

The posterior border of the hard palate and maxillary sinus gives an open passage into the nasopharynx.

Lateral Wall

Three turbinates overlie the lateral wall, which itself is formed from the medial walls of the maxillary sinus inferiorly, and the ethmoid sinus superiorly.

Incidence

Many cancer registries combine nasal, paranasal and middle ear tumours together when reporting incidence, as all three types are rare. The incidence of all three types combined is 1:100,000 per annum. About two-thirds of all cases arise in the sinuses giving a true incidence of nasal cancer of about 0.3:100,000. The nasal vestibule is the most common site of origin. Men who have worked in the chromium industry (Glasgow/Teeside, England) or nickel refining (South Wales) are at increased risk of developing this rare cancer. Chromate-induced cancers are often accompanied by a septal perforation.

Staging System

The system used for the nasal cavity is identical to that for ethmoidal sinus tumours in view of the anatomical relationship of these two structures. The reader is referred to the later section on paranasal sinus tumours for fuller details, but the following summarises the T classification as applicable here.

T1	Tumour restricted to one subsite of the nasal cavity with or without bony invasion
T2	Tumour involves two subsites in a single site or extends to involve an adjacent site within the nasoethmoidal complex, with or without bony invasion
T3	As ethmoid sinus
T4A	As ethmoid sinus
T4B	As ethmoid sinus

Aetiology, Pathology and Lymphatic Spread

The normal lining of the nasal cavity is pseudostratified columnar ciliated epithelium except for the vestibule, as mentioned earlier, that comprises squamous epithelium with sweat and sebaceous glands.

The aetiology of true nasal cavity tumours is not dissimilar to that of the paranasal sinuses with many environmental factors being implicated. Smoking is associated with the commonest histological subtype seen. Such SCCs arise most commonly at the lateral wall.

Other histologies comprise the remaining 20% and include adenocarcinoma, adenoid cystic carcinoma, melanoma, lymphoma, plasmacytoma and sarcoma. Inverted papillomas, themselves rare, can transform or coexist with SCC. Olfactory neuroblastomas (esthesioneuroblastomas) arise from the olfactory tissue at the level of the cribriform plate. Basal cell carcinomas can arise in the vestibule.

The lymphatic drainage of the nasal cavity can be usefully divided into two. The main part of the nasal cavity drains via the nasopharynx to the retropharyngeal nodes and upper deep cervical nodes (levels 2A and 2B). The lower anterior portion drains to the submandibular (level 1B), parotid (preauricular) and jugulodigastric (level 2A) nodes. The nasal vestibule itself includes, additionally, the buccinator node as part of the facial lymphatic complex.

Signs and Symptoms

Unlike paranasal sinus tumours, these tumours tend to present comparatively early with obstructive symptoms and epistaxis. However, symptoms of benign disease can blur the presence of malignancy, and SCCs of the lateral wall may, on further investigation, be a late manifestation of maxillary sinus disease. Inspection of the nasal cavity will typically reveal a fleshy outgrowth.

Diagnosis and Staging

Biopsy of the suspected lesion is required. A polypoidal lesion may be snared off and may give rise to an unsuspected tumour when examined pathologically. It may be necessary to perform a lateral rhinotomy to obtain adequate exposure and surgical evaluation of lesions within the nasal cavity.

Except for the small tumour of vestibule, which can usually be demarcated in the clinic, tumours of the nasal fossa proper require thorough staging with CT and/or MRI. Care must be taken in interpreting benign secretions from malignant infiltration of soft tissue and bone invasion as this may impact on the degree of surgery.

Certain tumour types, for example adenoid cystic as well as lymphoma, will require exclusion of distal involvement as this may dictate local management.

Treatment

Small tumours of the vestibule can be managed by either surgery or RT. The choice will in part be based on the expected cosmetic outcome.

More advanced tumours of the vestibule or those of the nasal fossa proper will usually require surgical clearance often followed by RT, especially if it is a SCC in view of the propensity for bone invasion. Lymphomas and plasmacytomas can be managed by primary RT at appropriate doses with or without the addition of chemotherapy.

Inoperable nasal cavity tumours should be managed by combined chemoradiation according to the co-morbidity of the patient.

Radiotherapy Technique

Tumours of the vestibule and low anterior nasal fossa tumours may be treated by a direct anterior appositional electron beam or with photons. Given the relatively superficial nature of such tumours, some bolus material is likely to ensure adequate surface dose. Consideration will need to be given to transmission of dose through air spaces.

More advanced tumours and those within the nasal fossa proper frequently require an approach similar to that used for maxillary sinus tumours using IMRT and doses up to 65 Gy in 30 fractions.

CT planning for all but the most superficial tumours facilitates accurate tumour definition and normal tissue avoidance. The true CTV may extend much more posteriorly than initially envisaged and therefore needs to be considered to minimise late relapse as a result of target volume selection.

As with all head and neck tumours, good immobilisation is required. A mouth-bite may be used to move the tongue away from the treatment volume (Figs 22.10–22.14).

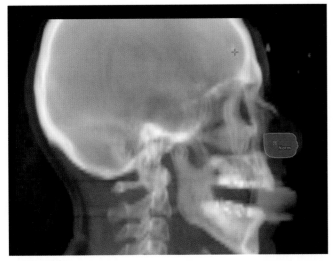

Fig. 22.10 Gross tumour volume in the case of a low nasal cavity tumour superimposed upon a digitally reconstructed radiograph.

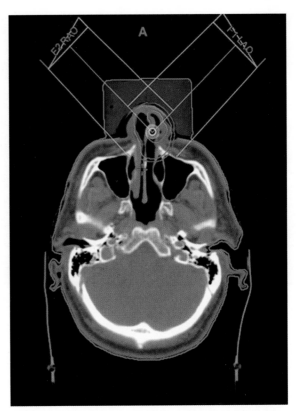

Fig. 22.12 Anterior wedged pair arrangement. Note Gross Tumour Volume (GTV), Clinical Tumour Volume (CTV) and Planning Tumour Volume (PTV) are all defined.

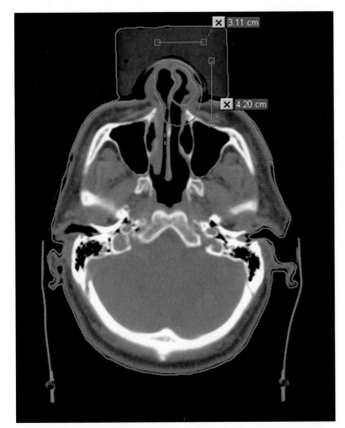

Fig. 22.11 Clinical target volume with gross target volume defined on axial computed tomography slice. Note bolus material.

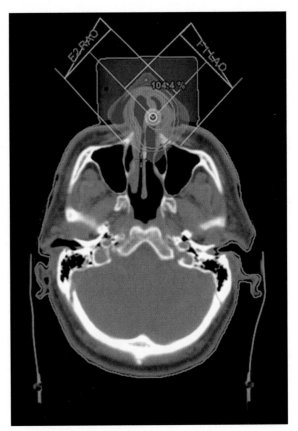

Fig. 22.13 Resulting dose distribution in the axial plane (alternatively patient could be treated with IMRT).

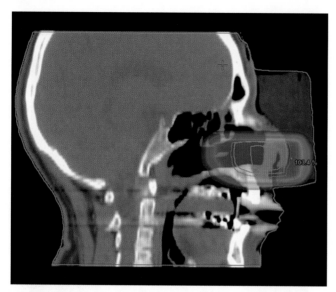

Fig. 22.14 Resulting dose distribution in the sagittal plane shown at midline.

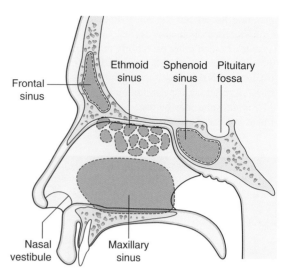

Fig. 22.15 Paranasal sinus anatomy.

Complications

Superficial tumours will inevitably manifest acute skin reactions that usually heal promptly. In the longer term, atrophy of the nasal cartilage may result in some loss of the original nasal profile.

Deeper tumours managed with techniques similar to that used for paranasal sinus tumours may be complicated by damage to the normal tissues in the vicinity. Atrophy of the nasal lining will result in dryness and a tendency towards the development of crusts. Regular use of a saline spray helps to address this. Epiphora will result if there is stenosis of the nasolacrimal duct.

Results

The diversity of pathologies at this site and the relative rarity even of SCC of the nasal cavity give rise to only limited outcome data. Nonetheless, early SCC of the vestibule can be expected to result in cure rates of the order of 80% to 90% at 5 years. More advanced tumours of the vestibule and fossa proper will give rise to cure rates of the order of 40% to 60%. Olfactory neuroblastomas carry a better prognosis, whereas patients with mucosal melanomas generally fare badly.

PARANASAL SINUS TUMOURS

Anatomy

The paranasal sinuses comprise four pairs of linked hollow cavities within the anterior and mid-portions of the skull that link to the nasal cavity (Fig. 22.15). They are named according to the bone within which they lie. The purpose of the paranasal sinuses is to lighten the bone and give resonance to the voice.

Maxillary Sinuses

Lying under the eyes, these sinuses are pyramidal in shape. The base of the pyramid forms the lateral wall of the nasal cavity with the apex extending towards the zygomatic process. The superior aspect comprises the floor of the orbit and the ethmoidal sinus, whereas the inferior extent is that of the alveolar process and typically lies just below the floor of the nasal cavity. The infraorbital nerve traverses the roof of the sinus whereas the first and second molar teeth typically project into the

sinus floor. The posterior wall abuts the infratemporal and pterygopalatine fossae. The maxillary sinus drains via the ostium maxillare beneath the middle concha.

Frontal Sinus

Lying over the eyes in the frontal bones, these sinuses only reach full size after puberty. They drain into the nasal cavity through the middle meatus beneath the middle concha via the frontonasal duct.

Ethmoid Sinus

Lying either side of the upper part of the nasal cavity and between the orbits, these sinuses are grouped into three portions: the anterior and middle drain into the nasal cavity via the middle meatus, and the posterior drains via the superior meatus beneath the superior concha. A thin bony lamina (the lamina papyracea) separates the sinus from the orbital and nasal cavities. The optic nerve lies posteriorly to the sinus and the anterior cranial fossa lies superiorly.

Sphenoid Sinus

Lying deep in the skull base beneath the pituitary gland, this sinus, which also develops mainly after puberty, drains into the nasal cavity via the sphenoethmoidal recess above the superior concha of the nasal cavity. The nasopharynx lies inferiorly and the nasal cavity anteriorly to the sinus, whereas the optic nerve and cavernous sinuses lie laterally.

Incidence of Paranasal Sinus Tumours

These tumours are rare with a crude incidence of less than 1/100,000 people per year. Most tumours arise in the maxillary sinus, less commonly, in the ethmoid sinus. Tumours arising de novo in the frontal and sphenoidal sinuses are especially rare. Frequently, multiple sinuses are involved at presentation.

Staging System for Paranasal Sinus Tumours

The TNM system (8th edition) as described here is only applicable to maxillary sinus tumours. The ethmoidal sinuses are classified separately. There is no formal system that applies to tumours of the sphenoidal and frontal sinuses. The N component is as elsewhere for head and neck SCCs.

	Maxillary Sinus	Ethmoidal Sinus
T1	Mucosa only with no erosion or destruction of bone	One subsite with or without bony invasion
T2	Bone erosion/destruction including extension into hard palate and/or middle meatus except extension to posterior wall of maxillary sinus and pterygoid plates	Two subsites with or without bony invasion
T3	Bone erosion/destruction of the posterior wall of maxillary sinus, involvement of the subcutaneous tissues, floor or medial wall of the orbit, pterygoid fossa and ethmoid sinuses	Involvement of the medial wall or floor of the orbit, maxillary sinus, palate or cribriform plate
T4A	Involvement of the anterior orbital contents, skin of the cheek, pterygoid plates, infra-temporal fossa, cribriform plate, sphenoidal or frontal sinuses	Involvement of the anterior orbital contents, skin of the cheek, infra-temporal fossa, cribriform plate, sphenoidal or frontal sinuses
T4B	Involvement of the orbital apex, dura, brain, middle cranial fossa, cranial nerves (excluding the second division of the Vth cranial nerve), nasopharynx or clivus	As maxillary sinus

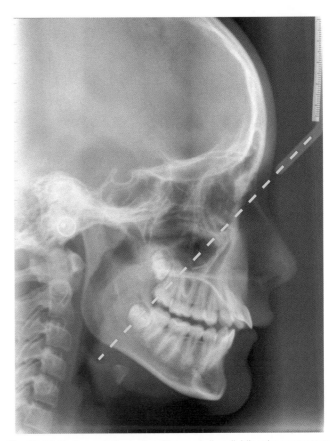

Fig. 22.16 Radiograph illustrating Ohngren's line dividing the suprastructure and infrastructure of the paranasal sinuses.

Although it does not form part of the TNM staging system, division of maxillary sinus lesions into those arising from the infrastructure, that is, anteroinferiorly, from lesions arising from the suprastructure which lie superoposteriorly, is potentially useful. This division arises from a theoretical line drawn from the medial canthus to the angle of the mandible in a lateral plane (Ohngren's line) (Fig. 22.16).

Aetiology, Pathology and Lymphatic Spread

The healthy sinuses are lined with ciliated columnar epithelium. SCCs comprise the commonest histological subtype and, as with other head and neck SCCs, are associated with smoking and, to a lesser extent, excess alcohol. Adenocarcinomas, particularly of the ethmoid sinus, occur and are associated with hard wood furniture manufacturers. Other tumour types include adenoid cystic carcinoma, melanoma and lymphoma.

The lymph system is remarkably sparse and, as such, tumours can be quite advanced without involved nodes. The corollary is that it is rare to present with neck nodes from an unsuspected primary located in the paranasal sinuses. Lymphatic drainage is typically towards the retropharyngeal (Rouviere's node) and upper deep cervical nodes (level II) unless the tumour is particularly anteriorly placed when the buccinator (now referred to as level IX) and level I nodes are at risk as well.

Signs and Symptoms

The complex anatomical relationship with neighboring structures is reflected in the diverse presenting features of these tumours. On the other hand, the air cavities permit substantial expansion and, as such, these tumours often present late, the early symptoms blurring with benign inflammatory disease.

Maxillary sinus tumours present with symptoms and signs related to the mode of expansion of the tumour: inferiorly, pain related to teeth

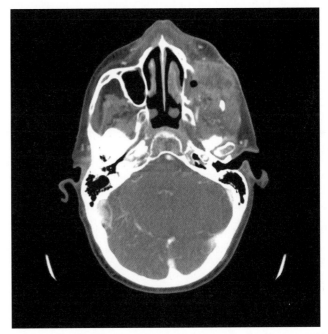

Fig. 22.17 Extensive tumour of the left paranasal sinus territory with extension into subcutaneous tissues and infratemporal fossa.

and ulceration may manifest, whereas inferoposteriorly, there is trismus (Fig. 22.17), superiorly, proptosis and diplopia; medially, there may be nasal stuffiness with discharge, which may not necessarily be bloody; anteriorly and laterally, a soft tissue mass may emerge in the

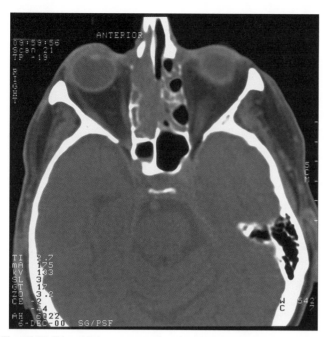

Fig. 22.18 Ethmoid sinus tumour showing close proximity to optic nerve and chiasm.

cheek. If the infraorbital nerve is involved, there will be numbness of the cheek and upper lip.

Ethmoidal sinus tumours frequently present with nasal obstruction. There may, in addition, be a discharge, which again may not be blood-stained. Less commonly, there may be bone expansion overlying the superior aspect of the nose (Fig. 22.18). Loss of smell is often overlooked and may indicate tumour.

Bearing in mind the rarity of primary tumours of the sphenoidal sinus, these will typically present with deep-seated pain, often referred to the vertex of the skull, and there may be associated cranial nerve palsies. Frontal sinus tumours may simply present with bony swelling.

Diagnosis and Staging

Initial assessment in the clinic should comprise a thorough examination including the use of a nasal speculum and upper airway endoscopy. The oral cavity must be inspected. A mass may be readily apparent and a sample taken for histological assessment. An examination under anaesthesia will invariably be required.

Plain x-rays may demonstrate bony erosion but a CT and MRI scan will ultimately both be required to define this more precisely as well as locoregional staging generally. CT scanning gives excellent bony detail whereas MRI scanning gives better distinction of tumour from adjacent soft tissues. Care must be exercised in the interpretation of signal changes on MRI which may reflect inflammatory disease (which often coexists). An orthopantomogram (OPG) will assist in the assessment of tooth preservation.

Treatment

Surgical options include endoscopic resection, craniofacial resection and maxillectomy with or without orbital exenteration or a combination of both. The type of surgery will be determined by the site, tumour type, stage of the tumour and the surgical intent. As a general rule though, surgery and postoperative RT will be indicated for tumours of the maxillary and ethmoidal sinuses except for the rare T1 lesion with complete clearance. Surgery will comprise a partial or total maxillectomy (depending on location and extent), ethmoidectomy and/or sphenoidectomy. Vascularised flap reconstruction is now favoured over obturating the cavity left

with a prosthesis, as the quality of life appears improved in such patients and the early concerns of lack of direct viewing of the cavity has been superseded by more advanced imaging in follow-up.

Where RT comprises definitive therapy, it may be given concurrently with chemotherapy and/or following neoadjuvant chemotherapy. The role of neoadjuvant chemotherapy is unclear but may be a pragmatic solution to generate tumour shrinkage before RT. On occasions, surgery may follow RT in advanced tumours where there has been a good response.

Radiotherapy when given postoperatively is delivered to the operative bed comprising the original location of the tumour and known and potential areas of spread. In the definitive setting, the volume irradiated will be determined by all staging information available to the clinician.

Radiotherapy Technique

An immobilisation device should be used. Care should be taken in achieving the optimal head position. In practice, it is often best for the plane of the floor of the orbit to be perpendicular to the treatment couch. A tongue depressor may be used and facilitates movement of the tongue inferiorly *away* from the treatment volume. A full head and neck shell over the shoulders should be used.

The volume definition has been outlined earlier in the chapter. Volumes should be delineated on a contrast-enhanced planning CT scan. Rarely is it necessary to include the neck nodes as a clinical target volume but the retropharyngeal nodes should be included as routine. Coregistration of images is invaluable in the process of volume delineation. Intensity modulated RT is the standard of care, given its ability to improve target-volume coverage and sparing of adjacent normal tissues (Figs 20.19–22.22).

The doses used will be determined by treatment intent. Gross disease postoperatively and when used in the definitive setting will demand a higher dose (i.e. 65 Gy in 30 fractions) with consideration to irradiation of critical normal tissues, even with IMRT techniques.

Complications

The biggest risk with treatment of paranasal sinus tumours is lack of local control, given the generally advanced nature at presentation. On the other hand, those patients who do survive long term or are cured are at risk of treatment-related sequelae.

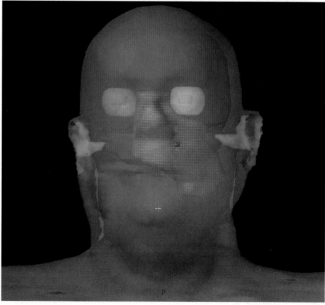

Fig. 22.19 Typical paranasal sinus volume viewed anteriorly.

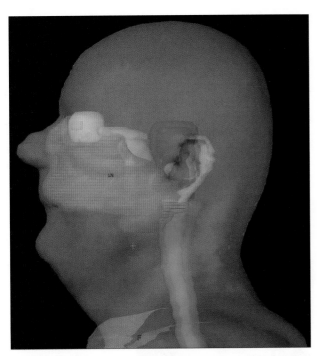

Fig. 22.20 Typical paranasal sinus volume viewed laterally.

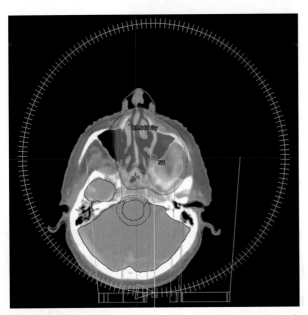

Fig. 22.21 Dose distribution (50 Gy minimum 60 Gy maximum in 30 fractions) to post-operative target volume in axial plane.

Late sequelae following surgery relate to fibrosis within the operated bed, potentially exacerbated by RT and issues related to any prosthesis if still used. Some degree of nasal crusting is inevitable and epiphora may occur.

Radiotherapy with or without surgery will invariably result in some xerostomia as a result of the irradiation of the ipsilateral parotid gland although some sparing is possible with IMRT. It is for that reason that any teeth remaining following resection should be in healthy condition. Trismus may result and should be actively managed with appropriate jaw exercises. Binocular blindness is a rare but catastrophic complication of maxillary sinus irradiation. Pituitary failure may emerge in long-term survivors.

Given the complex relationship of tumour and normal tissues, particularly the optic chiasm, it is no wonder that IMRT has become established as standard of care, although mature follow-up data are awaited.

Follow-up

Follow-up is required to monitor for recurrence and manage any long-term sequelae. Cavities should be inspected by endoscope. Imaging with MRI and/or PET/CT has offset early reservations of the reconstructive approach obscuring direct inspection of cavities.

Results

Overall, paranasal sinus tumours lead to a 25% to 30% 5-year survival. Tumours within the infrastructure and where there is good clearance by surgery, give rise to more favourable outcomes of the order of 50% 5-year survival.

LIP AND ORAL CAVITY CARCINOMA

Anatomy

Cancers of the lip arise from the vermilion (external) border.

The anatomical sites conventionally regarded as constituting the oral cavity are buccal mucosa, upper and lower alveolus, retromolar trigone, hard palate, tongue (anterior two-thirds: anterior to the circumvallate papillae) and the floor of the mouth.

Incidence of Oral Cavity Carcinoma

The oral tongue and then the floor of mouth are the commonest subsites. Overall, they are still a rare group of cancers making up less than 1% of cancer deaths. The United Kingdom incidence of mouth cancer is increasing: from 1992 to 1995 there were 8 cases per 100,000 people. That figure increased to 13 per 100,000 from 2012 to 2014. Although mouth cancer is more common in men, the ratio has fallen to 2:1 with the increasing prevalence of smoking and alcohol use in women.

Staging System for Oral Cavity and Lip Carcinoma (TNM, 8th Edition)

There are changes from the 7th edition TNM insofar as depth of invasion has been shown to be an independent prognostic factor with depths of 4 to 5 mm being an important threshold for the risk of nodal involvement. Clinicians are expected to estimate the depth of invasion (DOI) from palpation. Extrinsic muscle invasion has been removed from T4 status as it has been difficult for histopathologists to define, and it lacked specificity.

T1	Tumour ≤2 cm and depth of invasion (DOI) ≤5 mm
T2	Tumour ≤2 cm and DOI >5 mm or size 2–4 cm and DOI ≤10 mm
T3	Tumour >2 cm and ≤4 cm with DOI >10 mm or tumour >4 cm and DOI ≤10 mm
T4a	Tumour >4 cm and DOI >10 mm or tumour-invading adjacent structures, e.g. through cortical bone of the mandible or maxilla or involving the maxillary sinus of skin of face
T4b	Tumour invades masticator space, pterygoid plates, or skull base and/or encases internal carotid artery
N1	Single ipsilateral node ≤3 cm diameter and extranodal extension (ENE)–ve
N2A	Single ipsilateral node >3 cm ≤6 cm and ENE–ve
N2B	Multiple ipsilateral nodes ≤6 cm and ENE–ve
N2C	Bilateral or contralateral nodes ≤6 cm and ENE–ve
N3A	Any node >6 cm and ENE–ve
N3B	Any N and clinically overt ENE + ve

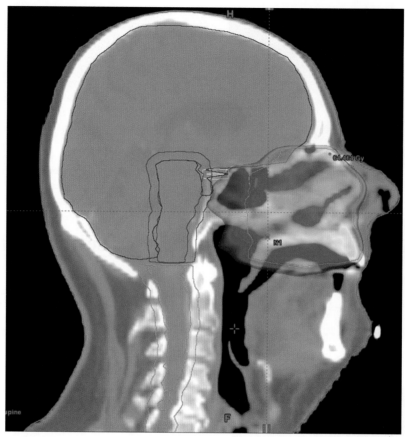

Fig. 22.22 Dose distribution (50 Gy minimum 60 Gy maximum in 30 fractions) to target volume in sagittal plane in midline. Note proximity to optic chiasm.

Aetiology, Pathology and Lymphatic Spread

Whereas tumours that occur within the oral cavity share with the majority of other upper aerodigestive tract tumours the etiological factors of exposure to alcohol and tobacco, tumours of the lip tend to be seen in patients with much exposure to sunlight, particularly smokers. Alcohol seems to be less important in the aetiology of cancers of this site. Other risk factors for oral cavity cancers include local trauma (e.g. badly fitted dentures) and leucoplakia. There is an association with betel nut, chewed in many cultures and also with syphilis, which is still prevalent in some parts of the world.

Cancers of the lip are almost always SCCs and over 90% of the oral cavity cancers are too. A small proportion of oral cavity tumours are adenocarcinomas or arise from the minor salivary glands of the oral cavity.

Nodal involvement in cancers of the lip occurs rarely (<5% of all cases at presentation) but the incidence is higher with large, poorly differentiated tumours or those at the angle of the mouth (Fig. 22.23). The neck nodes can be a site of potential relapse and therefore must be included in follow-up assessment. Nodal disease can be salvaged surgically or can be anticipated by sentinel node biopsy.

In oral cavity cancers, spread may be local to adjacent structures including the mandible. Nodal involvement is usually primarily to the submental and submandibular glands followed by the upper deep cervical nodes, that is, levels 1A, 1B and 2, although disease can spread directly to levels 3 and 4, so-called *skip* nodes (Fig. 22.24). Midline tumours may develop bilateral nodal spread. Retropharyngeal nodes are rarely involved in this group of cancers.

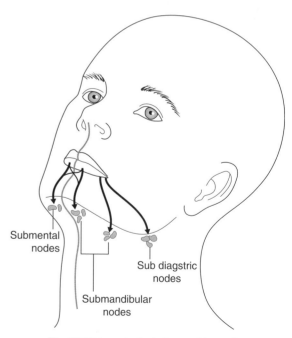

Submental nodes

Sub diagstric nodes

Submandibular nodes

Fig. 22.23 Lymphatic drainage of lower lip.

Signs and Symptoms

Lip cancers present in a similar manner to skin tumours with visible lesions over the lip. There may be a nonhealing ulcer or persistent scabbing. The lesions may be ulcerative or exophytic. There

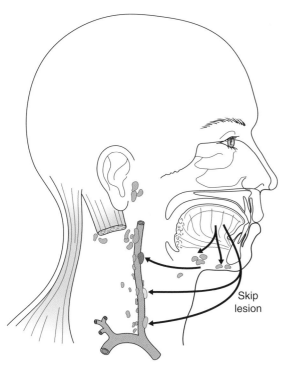

Fig. 22.24 Skip lesion.

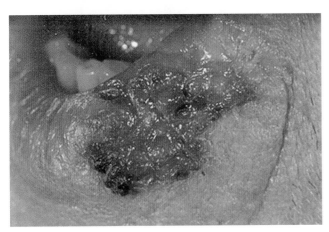

Fig. 22.25 Small-cell carcinoma of lip.

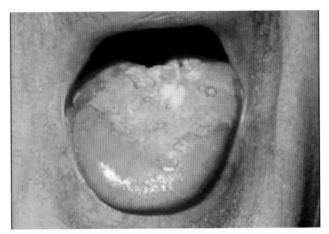

Fig. 22.26 Extensive carcinoma of dorsum of tongue.

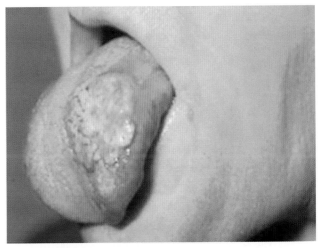

Fig. 22.27 Tumour on left lateral edge of tongue.

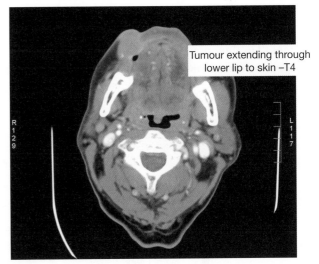

Fig. 22.28 Carcinoma of buccal mucosa.

can be discomfort or bleeding associated with the area and occasionally infiltration of adjacent skin or the underlying oral mucosa (Fig. 22.25).

Oral cavity cancers also commonly present with ulcerated lesions. They are often detected at dental check-up and can be associated with leucoplakia or erythroplakia. Local pain can be a symptom and, in more advanced tumours, may radiate to the ear on the involved side (Figs 22.26 and 22.27).

Diagnosis and Staging

Patients should be referred to a specialist head and neck team for full assessment. Local examination should be performed including full inspection of the oral cavity (Figs 22.26 and 22.27) and nasendoscopy to examine the rest of the aerodigestive tract. Imaging is required for any tumours in the anterior part of the oral cavity to exclude mandibular involvement (Figs 22.28 and 22.29). It also assists in the assessment of dentition before any planned RT. For oral cavity tumours, CT or preferably MRI of the primary site is required to determine depth of invasion or involvement of adjacent structures (Figs 22.30, 22.31, 22.36 and 22.37) and, as with any head and neck cancer, imaging of the neck nodes and chest is required to exclude distant spread.

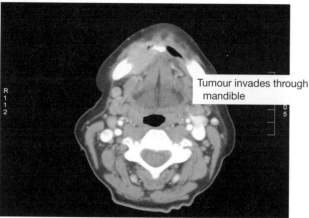

Fig. 22.29 Carcinoma of lower alveolus.

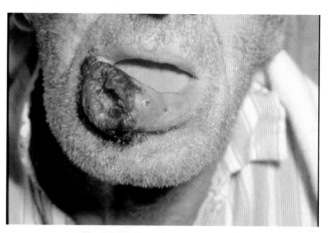

Fig. 22.32 Extensive lip carcinoma.

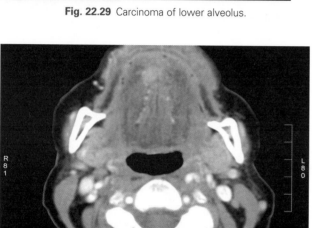

Fig. 22.30 Carcinoma of anterior floor of mouth.

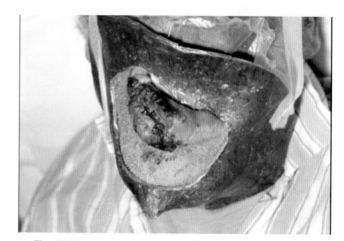

Fig. 22.33 Lead cut-out and gum shield for 300-kV treatment.

A biopsy of the lesion is required and can be done in the clinic or as part of an examination under anaesthetic if more detailed information about tumour extent is required.

Treatment Lip Cancers

Most lip cancers occur on the lower lip and, because of their conspicuous position, the majority of these tumours present relatively early, and so are regularly curable. Both surgery and RT are treatment options, and the choice between the two often comes down to deciding which will give the better cosmetic/functional result. Very small superficial lesions can be treated by a lip shave, as long as an adequate deep margin is obtained. This will give a very good cosmetic result.

For larger lesions, surgery using a variety of surgical approaches, the choice of which is dependent on the size and location of the lesion and the needs for reconstruction is preferred, although there is still a place for RT using external beam with/without brachytherapy if available.

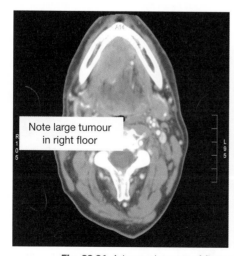

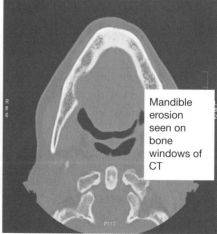

Fig. 22.31 Advanced cancer of floor of mouth. *CT*, Computed tomography.

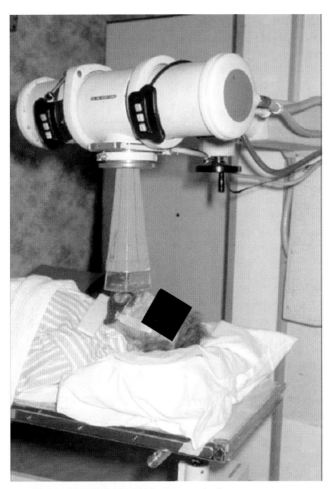

Fig. 22.34 300-kV treatment for lip cancer.

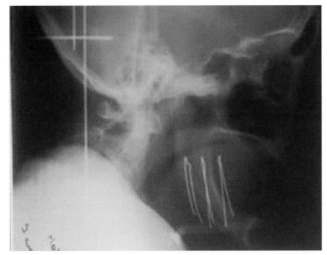

Fig. 22.35 Lateral radiograph showing three iridium hairpin insertions in an early tongue tumour. This effective treatment is rarely now used in the UK as both operator and nurses are irradiated by the iridium sources.

Radiotherapy Technique

For small tumours, the technique will be similar to that used for skin tumours. A margin of at least 1 cm is required around the disease as assessed by inspection and palpation to arrive at a suitable CTV.

An individualised lead cut-out, and an internal gum shield will usually be used (Figs 22.32–22.34). This arrangement facilitates

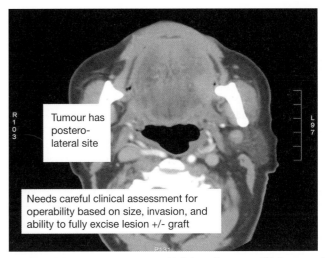

Fig. 22.36 CT showing carcinoma of left lateral tongue. *CT*, Computed tomography.

Tumour has postero-lateral site

Needs careful clinical assessment for operability based on size, invasion, and ability to fully excise lesion +/- graft

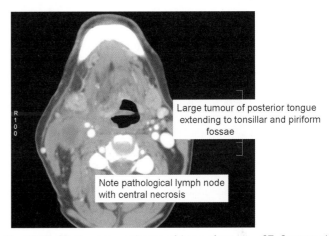

Fig. 22.37 CT showing carcinoma of base of tongue. *CT*, Computed tomography.

Large tumour of posterior tongue extending to tonsillar and piriform fossae

Note pathological lymph node with central necrosis

appropriate sparing of the adjacent tissues including the unaffected (usually upper) lip and the deeper tissues of the oral cavity. These lesions are usually exophytic, so electrons will often be preferred or othovoltage if available and, because the energy chosen is likely to be less than 12 MeV, a few millimetres of wax should be placed over the lesion to ensure maximum dose at the tumour surface. The gum shield will require wax on its anterior surface to absorb any backscatter electrons that could potentially enhance the dose to the treated volume. Care will need to be exercised in the degree of underlying bone irradiated that cannot be shielded by the gum shield.

Dose schedules for SCCs of the lip are similar to those for skin cancers and the reader is referred elsewhere. Longer fractionation schedules give better long-term cosmesis than a few large fractions and are preferred. Usual treatment regimens for these tumours range from 50 to 55 Gy in 15 to 20 fractions, treating daily.

Cancers of Oral Cavity

Whereas at many other head and neck sites primary RT (or, increasingly, chemoradiotherapy) is becoming more usual as first-line treatment, this is not so for oral cavity tumours, where primary surgery retains its place as the preferred management of at least operable disease. High-level evidence to support the use of surgery here is scant, but other evidence does support this approach.

The surgery for oral cavity cancers depends on the extent of the primary. Small T1 and T2 lesions may be suitable for simple excision which may be left to heal or closed with a split-skin graft or free flap. Larger lesions or those with more extensive invasion may require hemimandibulectomy with or without removal of part of the mandible and reconstruction with myocutaneous flaps.

Radiotherapy remains an integral part of many patients' treatments, as postoperative adjuvant treatment has been established as an important part of the overall management of many of these tumours. In recent years, evidence has accumulated of the value of adding chemotherapy to RT schedules in high-risk patients.

Selection criteria for giving postoperative RT or chemoradiotherapy are widely agreed, even if the evidence level for some of these indications is not high. The reader is referred to the earlier chapter 21 on these criteria.

Radiotherapy Technique

An immobilisation device is used and should include fixation of the shoulders even if it is not intended to irradiate the neck nodes comprehensively. An intraoral device may be used. For tongue tumours, it has as its purpose to move the tongue into the treatment volume and, as a consequence, achieve physical sparing of some of the palate. There is then sparing of some of the minor salivary tissue. For buccal tumours, its intention is different: here, it is helpful to move the tongue *away* from the irradiated mucosa and thereby lessen the toxicity.

Volumes should be defined on a planning CT scan with co-registration of any imaging undertaken preoperatively. A fundamental decision is whether to treat the neck bilaterally. This decision should be based on the anticipated risk of contralateral spread and will vary according to tumour site within the oral cavity and the nodal burden assessed at surgery. For well-lateralised tumours, an ipsilateral approach will often suffice. Relapse in the contralateral neck can potentially be salvaged later.

Postoperatively, the surgical tumour bed and nodes are included even if node negative, although this remains an area of debate. For most oral cancers seen in UK practice, there is a low risk of involvement of the retropharyngeal nodes so they can be excluded from the CTV unless there is extensive node involvement pathologically. Where there is involvement of the mandible, the whole of that hemi-mandible should be included in the initial CTV.

An IMRT approach enables comprehensive coverage of the operated primary site and lymph nodes and sparing of clinically significant normal tissues.

The doses of radiation used will be dictated by the surgical findings and follow the principles outlined in Chapter 21.

Complications

Acute reactions with RT to the oral cavity include the usual effects on the skin and mucosa but should be self-limiting. The effect on nutrition can be profound and should be managed aggressively if not proactively.

Late effects will be determined in part by the site of irradiation. Sparing of salivary tissue should be possible and as such, xerostomia should be minimised. Taste and a heightened intraoral sensitivity may result. Fibrosis of the neck may result although the relative impact of surgery and RT is poorly documented. Mucosal ulceration may occur but usually heals with conservative measures, that is, antimicrobial mouthwashes. Osteoradionecrosis (see Fig. 22.2) can be minimised by meticulous dental hygiene before and following RT. The least amount of mandible should be irradiated while ensuring complete coverage of the volume at risk. Hot spots in the treatment plan should be avoided, particularly overlying the mandible.

Follow-up

Patients should be assessed for recurrence including in the neck and especially if not treated initially and any late effects. Inspection of the primary site is often comparatively straight forward notwithstanding any reconstructive approaches to aid function.

Results of Treatment

Lip Cancer

As mentioned previously, the majority of these tumours present relatively early and if treated with radical RT (or surgery) have an excellent chance of cure. T1 and T2 lesions would be cured in 90% to 100% of patients. Larger or more advanced tumours have a worse prognosis.

Oral Cavity Cancers

The same rules apply for these cancers as others in the head and neck. Small, early cancers have a better prognosis than those with invasion into adjacent structures or nodal involvement. T1 and small T2 lesions of the oral cavity may be cured by surgery alone and the overall survival is 85% to 95%. This can fall to as low as 50% for T4 tumours or those with extensive nodal disease.

OROPHARYNGEAL CARCINOMA

Anatomy

The oropharynx comprises the tonsil, the base of tongue, otherwise known as the posterior one-third of the tongue, and the undersurface of the soft palate. It is continuous with the nasopharynx superiorly, the hypopharynx inferiorly and the oral cavity anteriorly. The major components of Waldeyer's ring lie within the oropharynx: only the superior component lies within the nasopharynx. The function of the oropharynx is multifactorial: swallowing and respiration, including protection of the airway, phonation, taste and immune surveillance.

Anterior Wall

There is no true anterior wall as the oropharynx communicates directly with the oral cavity. The anterior tonsillar pillar divides the oral cavity from the oropharynx whereas the circumvallate papillae (sulcus terminalis) on the surface of the tongue, divide the oral tongue from the base of tongue.

Posterior Wall

The posterior wall is formed by the tissues of the prevertebral space adjacent to C2 and C3 and constitutes the posterior pharyngeal wall.

Lateral Wall

The palatoglossal (anterior pillar) and palatopharyngeal (posterior pillar) arches, the faucial tonsil (the tonsil) and a small component of the pharyngeal wall constitute the lateral wall of the oropharynx. The parapharyngeal space lies more lateral still. The internal and external carotid arteries, internal jugular vein, superior cervical ganglion and retropharyngeal nodes lie within this area.

Superior Wall

The superior wall is composed anteriorly of the undersurface of the soft palate. Otherwise, there is a direct opening into the nasopharynx.

Inferior Wall

The hyoid bone constitutes the anatomical boundary between the oropharynx and hypopharynx. The vallecula, which is a trough that lies between the tongue base and the epiglottis, lies within this area. Lingual tonsillar tissue gives the inferior component of Waldeyer's ring.

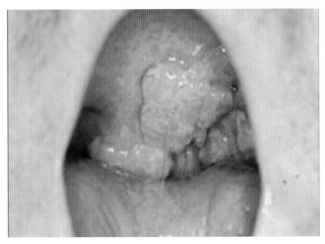

Fig. 22.38 Advanced tonsillar cancer involving soft palate.

Incidence of Oropharyngeal Tumours

Cancers of the oropharynx are increasingly common in the developed world. Incidence has tripled in men from 2.0 to 5.8 per 100,000 and doubled in women from 0.8 to 1.7 between 1995 and 2011. This has been in part attributed to human papilloma virus (HPV)-related oropharyngeal carcinomas, which tend to occur in younger patients, although in the United Kingdom at least a similar increase has occurred in non-HPV positive oropharyngeal cancers.

Of oropharyngeal cancers, the most common are tonsillar ($\approx$60%) (Fig 22.38) followed by 25% in the base of the tongue and 10% in the soft palate.

Staging System of Oropharyngeal Tumours

Staging has been updated in the latest version of the TNM system (8th edition) to reflect the inherently better prognosis of HPV + ve tumours.

T0	No evidence of primary tumour
T1	Tumour $\leq$2 cm in greatest dimension
T2	Tumour >2 cm but $\leq$4 cm in greatest dimension
T3	Tumour >4 cm in greatest dimension or extension to lingual surface of epiglottis
T4	Tumour invades the larynx, deep/extrinsic muscle of tongue, medial pterygoid, hard palate or mandible or beyond

For HPV–ve tumours, the T staging is subdivided into T4A and T4B.

T4A	Tumour invades the larynx, deep/extrinsic muscle of tongue, medial pterygoid, hard palate or mandible
T4B	Tumour invades lateral pterygoid muscle, pterygoid plates, lateral nasopharynx, or skull base or encases carotid artery

For nodal status, the differences between HPV + ve and HPV–ve SCC tumours are even more striking.

HPV + ve tumours: clinical staging

cN0	No regional lymph node metastases
cN1	One or more ipsilateral lymph nodes, none larger than 6 cm
cN2	Contralateral or bilateral lymph nodes, none larger than 6 cm
cN3	Lymph nodes >6 cm

HPV + ve pathological staging

pN0	No regional lymph node metastases
pN1	Metastases in 4 or fewer lymph nodes
pN2	Metastases in more than 4 lymph nodes

For HPV–ve tumours, this follows the same approach as described with oral cavity tumours with extracapsular extension of nodes that have a significant impact on upstaging.

Aetiology, Pathology and Lymphatic Spread

As with other head and neck cancers, tobacco and alcohol consumption are the most significant risk factors for developing cancers in this region. There are no specific genetic risk factors for this type of tumour. There is a specific group of oropharyngeal carcinomas in younger (often nonsmoker) patients, which are found to be associated with HPV. Although there appears to be distinct histopathological appearances with less differentiation and basaloid-type cells, some argue that such is the positive influence of the HPV status, that description of the morphological subtype of SCC might be misleading. The presence of HPV can be confirmed by immunochemical staining for the virus associated protein p16. Moreover reviews of the outcomes of these specific tumours compared with the typical SCCs indicate an improved prognosis. The intrinsic better prognosis and higher chemo-radiosensitivity of HPV positive tumours is also directing treatment strategies towards treatment deintensification, including omission of concurrent chemotherapy or a reduction in total RT dose.

Histologically, almost all oropharyngeal carcinomas are the squamous cell cancers prevalent in the head and neck region. One variant of SCC of the oropharynx is the lymphoepithelioma. Histologically, it is lymphocyte predominant and may mimic lymphoma. Lymphoepithelioma may arise in the base of tongue, tonsils or nasopharynx. It is a very radiosensitive variant of SCC. Other cancers in this area include minor salivary gland carcinomas and lymphoma. Mention has already been made of Waldeyer's ring. It is a site of extra-nodal non-Hodgkin's lymphoma (NHL) and the tonsil is the commonest primary extranodal site of head and neck NHL.

The oropharynx has a rich lymphatic supply; 60% of oropharyngeal cancers have nodal involvement at presentation. In tonsillar tumours, this is predominantly unilateral spread unless the primary crosses the midline and is important when determining volumes to irradiate. Tonsillar cancers drain to the adjacent jugulodigastric or subdigastric node (the so-called *tonsillar node*) within level 2 and then to the remainder of the deep cervical nodes of level 2 and 3. The remainder of oropharyngeal cancers are midline structures and therefore can drain to bilateral nodes. Tumours of the soft palate and posterior pharyngeal wall drain to the retropharyngeal nodes and upper deep cervical lymph nodes, that is, level 2. Base of tongue tumours commonly spread to the mid- and upper-cervical nodes, that is, levels 2 and 3.

Signs and Symptoms

Cancers in this region commonly present with sore throat or painful swallowing. Tumours in the tonsillar region or posterior oropharynx may present with earache because of extension into the parapharyngeal space or the sensation of a lump in the throat. Tumour or ulceration in the oropharynx can usually be visualised in the clinic via nasendoscopy. A fine needle aspiration (FNA) or biopsy can often be taken at the time.

As with many head and neck cancers, the presentation may be via a neck mass from secondary lymph nodes. In this case, the primary may be identified from tonsillectomy or targeted biopsies guided by PET-CT.

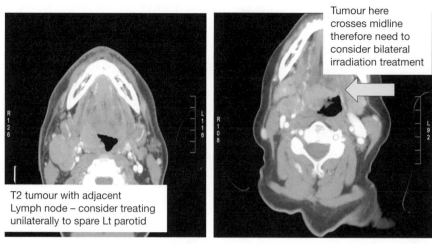

Tumour here crosses midline therefore need to consider bilateral irradiation treatment

T2 tumour with adjacent Lymph node – consider treating unilaterally to spare Lt parotid

Fig. 22.39 CT scan showing carcinoma of tonsil. *CT*, Computed tomography.

Diagnosis and Staging

Patients with a history of persistent sore throat should be referred urgently to the ear-nose-throat (ENT) clinic. Patients may also be referred urgently for persistent tonsillar swelling or neck lymphadenopathy.

A full history should be undertaken. The importance of co-morbidities may determine the preferred treatment modality. This is particularly the case in patients who are heavy smokers or have a history of alcohol intake.

A full ENT examination is performed in the clinic. This allows delineation of the primary. It should include fibreoptic examination to look for synchronous tumours. The neck should be clinically examined for palpable lymph nodes.

Radiological assessment of the primary is essential to complete the staging. This is usually a CT or MRI scan noting the pros and cons of each approach referenced earlier (Fig. 22.39). This may also reveal pathological lymphadenopathy not identified clinically. Imaging of the chest is also essential for exclusion of metastatic spread or synchronous primary tumours of the lung.

Treatment

Currently, management of primary tumours of the oropharynx is largely nonsurgical and in contrast to most oral cavity tumours. Chemoradiation is the standard-of-care for the younger and healthier patients, and RT alone for the less robust, typically using an altered fractionation schedule.

Management of neck disease, especially in those with more advanced disease has been strongly debated over the years: Data now favour nonsurgical treatment and follow-up with PET-CT, with surgery reserved for those patients with an incomplete or equivocal response on imaging at 12 weeks or later posttreatment, especially in HPV-positive patients. Neck dissection, thus, might be preferred in patients with bulky nodes who are HPV–ve.

Radiation Technique

Patients are treated in an immobilisation device that includes the head and shoulders. The patient is treated supine. The neck will typically be in a comfortably extended position as this then moves some of the oral cavity out of the primary beam. A tongue depressor is not usually used.

A planning CT scan coregistered with diagnostic scans facilitates precise volume definition (Fig 22.40). The primary CTV must include reasonable margins to account for microscopic spread. These margins have recently been refined and agreed by consensus. In practice, the GTV is defined on optimal datasets and grown volumetrically with

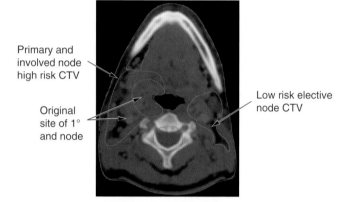

Primary and involved node high risk CTV

Low risk elective node CTV

Original site of 1° and node

Fig. 22.40 Volume definitions in this case for a tonsil that has in this case been excised in which case primary GTV and primary CTV has been interpolated from pre-op images (in this case three dose levels have been selected).

high-dose margin for the CTV of the order of 5 mm only, and lower dose larger margins of 10 mm, excluding any air or bone unless affected. This approach means that the older approach of anatomically determined volumes are no longer required and would be expected to reduce the morbidity of treatment. The selection of lymph nodes is based on the known pattern of spread of these tumours. A well-lateralised early tumour of the tonsil rarely spreads to the contralateral lymph nodes and, as such, affords useful sparing of the contralateral salivary tissues (Figs 22.41–22.47). Where a neck dissection has been carried out, this additional information allows for appropriate doses to be specified according to the risk of disease, that is, nodes with extracapsular spread would be irradiated to a high dose.

Tonsillar Tumours

Small ipsilateral primary tumours with a node-negative neck can be treated with a small volume treatment, which includes the primary site and level 1B and 2 cervical lymph nodes. Level 2 nodes are divided into 2A and 2B, with those nodes (those nodes that sit anterior to the internal jugular vein are considered as level 2A and could be irradiated alongside level 1B in such cases.

The relatively small volumes of irradiation mean that shorter fractionation schedules, such as 55 Gy in 20 daily fractions using 6-MV photons, are reasonable. The plan would need to spare organs at risk (OARs) such as the spinal cord and brainstem.

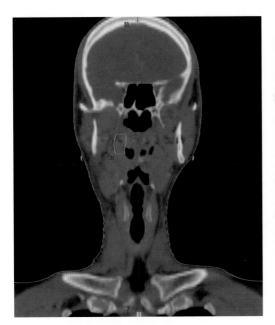
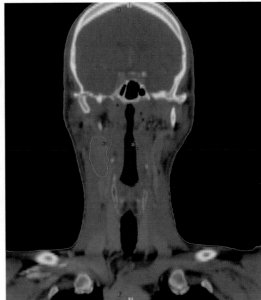

Oropharyngeal primary (tonsil)   Involved level 2/3 node

Fig. 22.41 Primary and involved node superimposed upon digitally reconstructed radiograph.

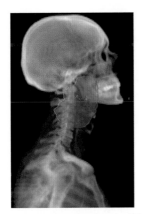

Primary and involved node CTV

Fig. 22.42 High dose CTV.

Large Tonsillar Tumours and Other Oropharyngeal Tumours

Larger tumours of the tonsil that approach or cross the midline, which have spread locally to the base of tongue or are node-positive, should be treated with a volume that encompasses the primary and bilateral upper cervical neck nodes.

Other oropharyngeal tumours, (i.e. base of tongue, postpharyngeal wall and soft palate), usually require a similar bilateral approach because of the high risk of contralateral lymph node involvement.

Fractionation schedules used in this situation are typically 65 Gy in 30 fractions over 6 weeks. Concurrent chemotherapy, certainly in younger, fitter patients, forms an important component of this treatment. Indeed, the strongest evidence for concurrent chemoradiotherapy originates from oropharyngeal tumours.

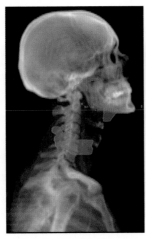
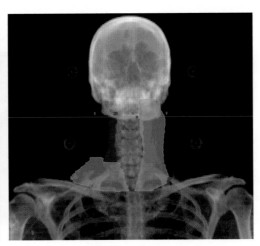

High risk ipsilateral CTV   Low risk ipsilateral and contralateral neck

Fig. 22.43 High risk and low risk CTVs superimposed on digital reconstructed radiographs.

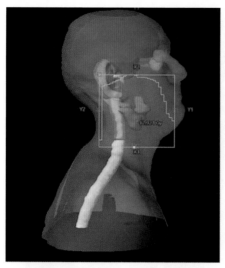

Fig. 22.44 Field arrangement for upper neck (non-IMRT).

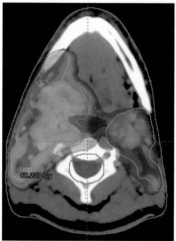

Dose distribution (50 Gy minimum)
of all three CTVs in axial plane

Fig. 22.45 IMRT dose distribution (50 Gy minimum) of all three CTVs in axial plane. Note adjusted doses to these CTVs (65 Gy, 60 Gy and 54 Gy).

Complications

Acute reactions in the oropharynx are predictable. Mucositis will compromise nutrition and should be managed aggressively. In practice, this often means that these patients have feeding tubes sited before therapy (percutaneous endoscopic gastrostomy tube [PEG] or radiologically inserted gastrostomy tube [RIG]) and opiate analgesia. Acute xerostomia and the often copious mucous production should be managed symptomatically. Skin reactions and reversible alopecia will occur in the irradiated volume.

Chronic xerostomia has been a common side effect of wide-field RT as used here. There is now level one evidence that sparing at least one parotid gland with IMRT techniques results in an improvement in the quality of life of these patients and thus should be routinely applied. Trismus may result from high-dose RT to the pterygoid muscles and should be spared as far as clinically appropriate. Active stretching exercises can also help to alleviate this.

Follow-up

Patients will require follow-up imaging using PET-CT in the vast majority of cases to detect and manage residual disease early. Ordinarily, this would be conducted at 12 weeks and repeated if there are equivocal lesions, which the multidisciplinary team would favour observing.

Results

HPV association has a markedly positive impact on prognosis. Most patients with early stage disease do well with 5-year survival rates of 75% to 90%. For more advanced disease, the survival curves diverge such that HPV–ve disease cases plummet to 30% to 60% whereas HPV + ve cases still fare very well, with 5-year survival rates being maintained even with more advanced disease. It is no wonder that there is ongoing debate about treatment de-intensification in HPV + ve patients and treatment intensification in HPV–ve patients.

LARYNX

Anatomy

The larynx is a cartilaginous frame held in position by intrinsic muscles and ligaments. The anterior and lateral part of this box is formed by the thyroid cartilage. The cricoid cartilage is below the thyroid

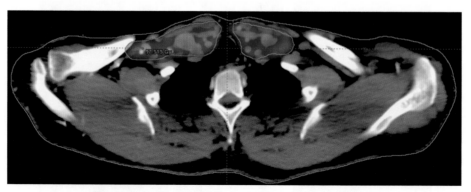

Fig. 22.46 IMRT dose distribution in lower neck in axial plane.

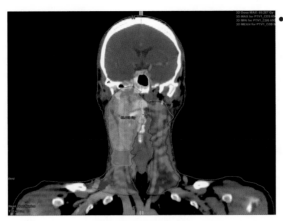

● Note sparing of contralateral parotid and avoidance of level 5 nodes

Fig. 22.47 IMRT dose distribution in a coronal plane.

cartilage forming a complete ring around the larynx just below the vocal cords.

The larynx is divided into three areas: The supraglottis, glottis and subglottis (Fig. 22.48). The structures of the supraglottis are the epiglottis, the aryepiglottic folds, the arytenoids, the ventricular bands (often called the false cords) and the ventricular cavities. The true glottis is the area by the vocal cords. The subglottic area is the area beneath the vocal cords and above the trachea.

Incidence of Laryngeal Cancer

In 2011, there were 2360 cases of laryngeal cancer in the United Kingdom, which makes the larynx the most common site for head and neck cancer overall, but numbers are falling. The male:female ratio is 4.5:1. In some parts of France, Spain and Italy, the incidence of laryngeal cancer can be up to six times more common. Unlike the United Kingdom, where true glottis is the most common site, the supraglottic area is the most common site for laryngeal tumours in southern Europe. Typically, 60% to 70% of tumours begin in the glottis, 25% of cases are supraglottic, 2% only are true subglottic cancer and the remainder are transglottic tumours, in which the precise site of origin cannot be determined.

Staging System for Laryngeal Cancer (TNM, 8th Edition)

Although the nodal status follows the principle described elsewhere for HPV−ve tumours, the T status is described according to which element of the larynx the tumour is considered to arise from.

(1) Supraglottic larynx

T – Primary tumour	
T1	Tumour limited to one subsite of supraglottis with normal vocal cord mobility
T2	Tumour invades mucosa of more than one adjacent subsite of supraglottis or glottis or region outside the supraglottis (e.g. mucosa of base of tongue, vallecula, medial wall of piriform sinus) without fixation of the larynx
T3	Tumour limited to larynx with vocal cord fixation and/or invades any of the following: postcricoid area, preepiglottic space, paraglottic space, and/or inner cortex of thyroid cartilage
T4A	Tumour invades through outer cortex of thyroid cartilage and/or extends beyond the larynx
T4B	Tumour invades prevertebral space, encases carotid artery, or mediastinal structures

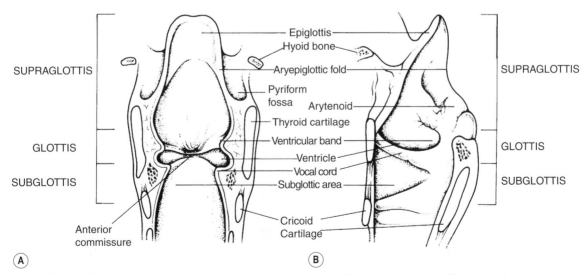

Fig. 22.48 Landmarks of the normal larynx and pharynx from (A) the posterior and (B) the lateral aspect. (Redrawn from Robinson, Surgery, 7th Edition, Longmans.)

(2) Intrinsic larynx: glottis

T – Primary tumour

T1	Tumour limited to the vocal cord with normal mobility
	A = one vocal cord
	B = both vocal cords
T2	Tumour extends to supraglottis and/or subglottis and/or with impaired vocal cord mobility
T3	Tumour limited to the larynx with vocal cord fixation and/or invasion of paraglottic space and/or inner cortex of the thyroid cartilage
T4A	Tumour invades through the outer cortex of the thyroid cartilage and/or invades tissues beyond the larynx
T4B	Tumour invades prevertebral space, encases carotid artery or invades mediastinal structures

(3) Subglottis

T – Primary tumour

T1	Tumour limited to the subglottis
T2	Tumour extends to vocal cord(s) with normal or impaired mobility
T3	Tumour limited to larynx with vocal cord fixation and/or invasion of paraglottic space and/or inner cortex of the thyroid cartilage
T4A	Tumour invades cricoid or thyroid cartilage and/or invades tissues beyond the larynx
T4B	Tumour invades prevertebral space, encases carotid artery or invades mediastinal structures

Aetiology, Pathology and Lymphatic Spread

As with many head and neck cancers, laryngeal tumours tend to develop in smokers. In contrast with oropharyngeal cancer, HPV infection is not a major cause. The higher incidence of supraglottic cancer in parts of Europe may be caused by the type of alcoholic drink consumed and the use of dark rather than blond tobacco. The true glottis has a poor lymphatic supply and tumours arising from the true vocal cord are relatively slow to metastasise to regional lymph nodes. This is even true of T3 glottic cancers. But supraglottic carcinoma of the larynx spreads far more readily to the lymph nodes within the neck. The incidence of lymph node spread from even T1 and T2 lesions ranges between 27% and 40%, and for T3/T4 lesions the rate of lymph node metastasis is 55% to 65%.

Initially, lymphatic spread is upwards to the jugulodigastric lymph nodes immediately beneath the angle of the jaw (level 2). Tumours also commonly spread to the mid-jugular lymph nodes (level 3). Over 95% of laryngeal tumours are invasive squamous carcinoma. Although usually well differentiated, some tumours, especially of the supraglottic region, can be poorly differentiated and are more likely to spread to lymph nodes. A common variant of well-differentiated squamous cancer is a verrucous carcinoma. This tumour contains a large amount of keratin and has a heaped-up warty appearance. Sometimes, invasive cancer can be preceded by carcinoma in situ of the epithelium of the vocal cords. However, this usually transforms into invasive cancer within 1 to 2 years of detection.

Signs and Symptoms

The first symptom in more than 90% of patients with true glottic cancer is hoarseness. Comparatively small tumours of the vocal cords can cause marked changes in the voice and there is National Health Service (NHS) guidance for early referral to exclude cancer. Advanced tumours of the vocal cords may narrow the airway, especially if a vocal cord is paralysed, leading to stridor. This is a whistling noise when the patient breathes and is an oncological emergency. Untreated, the patient will develop progressive dyspnoea and can suffocate. For this reason, patients with stridor should be immediately referred for consideration of an emergency tracheostomy or urgent laser debulking.

Hoarseness is less common as a symptom for early supraglottic cancer. Most patients complain initially of either a sore throat or a foreign-body-like sensation in the upper larynx, which they often describe as either caused by a fish bone or a piece of silver paper. Hoarseness only develops when the tumour reaches the vocal cord. More advanced tumours may have pain referred to the ear and patients may occasionally cough up blood (haemoptysis).

Diagnosis and Staging

Many laryngeal cancers are visible during a flexible fibre-optic examination. As well as visualising the larynx, the neck should be carefully palpated for lymph nodes, especially in the jugulodigastric area.

Patients should then have an examination under anaesthetic when histology is often acquired using rigid fibreoptic endoscopes to inform the staging, which is so critical to subsequent management. The mobility of the vocal cords should be assessed with the patient conscious and anaesthetised. CT and MRI scanning will give further information about the degree of spread, as these imaging modalities may show small impalpable lymph nodes in the neck or subglottic spread, or disease in the mediastinum and should be undertaken in all but the earliest cases of laryngeal cancer (Figs 22.49 and 22.50).

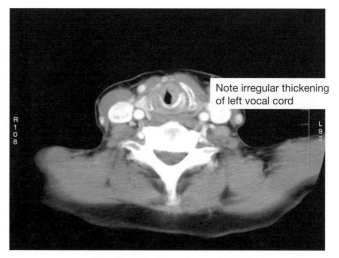

Fig. 22.49 Early carcinoma larynx.

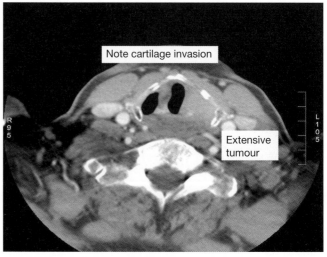

Fig. 22.50 T4 carcinoma larynx.

Most patients with laryngeal cancer smoke. Smoking can affect the cardiovascular and respiratory systems. If the patient has chronic obstructive airways disease (COPD) or ischaemic heart disease, this may alter management decisions. Such patients may only be fit for less radical treatments and surgery, or chemoradiotherapy may be contraindicated.

Treatment

Early Laryngeal Tumours T1, T2 (Fig 22.51)

Either RT or transoral laser microsurgery or open partial laryngeal surgery may be employed as initial therapy for early laryngeal tumours. In the United Kingdom, RT with surgical salvage (total laryngectomy) or laser microsurgery and RT as salvage are the commonest approaches with comparable efficacy. Treatment selection will, in part, be determined by tumour factors, for example, distinctiveness of margin of tumour, location on cord, as well as patient preference.

GLOTTIC CANCERS (FIGS 22.52–22.56)

The larynx is a mobile structure and, although the vocal cord occupies about 1 cm only, the radiation volume should be at least 4 × 4 cm to allow for vocal cord movement during respiration and swallowing, thus encompassing a CTV and ITV. This is determined on a planning CT scan. The vocal cords are easily determined as they sit about 1 cm below the thyroid cartilage promontory. The anterior commissure sits just under the skin and bolus material may be required to ensure adequate dose coverage. This is one of the few head and neck sites where non-IMRT approaches are still routine in the United Kingdom. Opposed fields or anterior oblique fields with margins to ensure coverage of the planning tumour volume (PTV) are determined and typically give rise to field sizes of 5 × 5 cm or even 6 × 6 cm (Figs 22.53–22.56). Dosage schemes in use nationally and internationally range from 50 Gy in 16 fractions over 3 weeks to 66 Gy in 33 fractions over 6 ½ weeks using 6-MV photons. The British Institute of Radiology short versus long trial compared a 3-week schedule against a 6-week schedule and showed that, if anything, the complication rate was higher among patients treated over 6 weeks. Many centres give a slightly higher dose for T2 tumours (52.5 Gy in 16 fractions for T1, 55 Gy for T2 in 20 fractions, or 60 Gy in 30 fractions for T1 carcinomas, and 60 Gy in 25 fractions for T2 tumours).

Early Supraglottic Carcinomas of Larynx T1, T2 N0

Owing to the fact that supraglottic larynx tumours are more likely to spread to lymph nodes in the neck, most centres advocate prophylactic irradiation of the jugular chain even if there are no palpable lymph nodes or lymph nodes detectable on MRI scanning. Many oncologists incorporate at least the jugulodigastric lymph node within the irradiated volume for part or all of the treatment. Therefore the typical treatment volume for an early supraglottic larynx cancer is slightly longer to enable irradiation albeit prophylactically of the level 2 and 3 nodes (Fig. 22.53). Somewhat higher doses are often given to treat supraglottic compared with glottic cancer. In the United States, doses of 70 Gy in 7 weeks are frequently prescribed. In the United Kingdom, schedules vary between 50 Gy in 16 fractions to 66 Gy in 33 fractions.

Complications of Treatment for Early Laryngeal Cancer

Most patients develop a brisk radiation mucositis towards the end of treatment, but this usually resolves within a month. A small number of patients develop persisting laryngeal oedema. This is more common in supraglottic cancers where the incidence can be as high as 25% and more common among heavy smokers. Treatment is by advising cessation of smoking, taking antibiotics if there is evidence of infection, and corticosteroids. Persistent severe laryngeal oedema may be a reason for tracheostomy. Patients with persisting oedema should be carefully examined for persisting recurrent tumour. Laryngeal necrosis is rare with an incidence of less than 1%.

Bulky T2 and T3 Glottic and Supraglottic Tumours (Fig 22.64)

Most of these tumours can be well managed with larynx-preservation approaches. In all cases, nodal irradiation, even if given with prophylactic intent, will be required and is enabled with an IMRT through a synchronous boost technique. In node-negative cases, levels 2 to 4 should be irradiated. If the patient is node positive, the levels 1 to 5 should be treated and level 1B included if level 2 is diseased. Concurrent chemotherapy improves outcomes as evidenced in the meta-analysis (see Chapter 21). As such, concurrent chemotherapy would be considered standard of care in fit patients.

Induction chemotherapy followed by RT has had an established role in laryngeal preservation based on the early work of the Veterans Affairs Laryngeal Cancer Study Group, although later work of the Radiation Therapy Oncology Group (RTOG) demonstrated the superiority

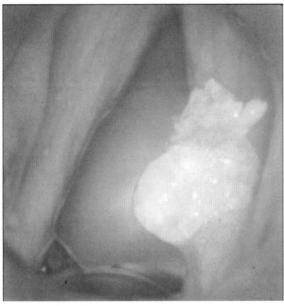

Fig. 22.51 Early (T1) carcinoma of vocal cord.

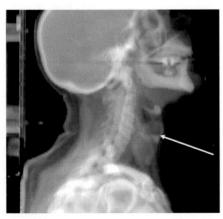

"Figure of eight" sign depicts anterior border of true cord

Fig. 22.52 Landmarks for early laryngeal cancer on a digitally reconstructed radiograph.

Early intrinsic glottic laryngeal cancer

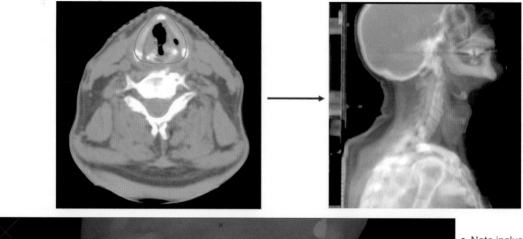

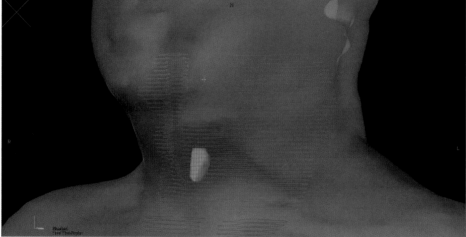

- Note inclusion of levels 2 and 3/4 nodes in CTV in contrast to an early intrinsic laryngeal cancer

Early supraglottic cancer

Fig. 22.53 Compare supraglottic volume that requires inclusion of at risk lymph nodes with volume used to treat early intrinsic glottic tumours.

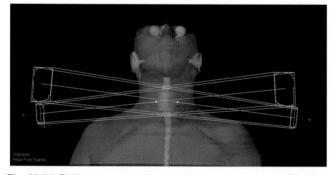

Fig. 22.54 Field arrangement for early glottic tumour (non IMRT). Note that, in this case, the two fields are noncoplanar so that they exit above the shoulders.

in terms of laryngeal preservation with concurrent chemoradiotherapy. That said, there is continued interest in the neoadjuvant approach, especially given the superiority of the triplet regimen, docetaxel-cisplatin-fluorouracil (TPF), (see Chapter 21).

T4 Laryngeal Cancers

Patients with tumour that extends through the thyroid cartilage or into the base of tongue do not do well with laryngeal preservation approaches. Similarly, patients with a poorly functioning larynx are better managed with a total laryngectomy if fit enough.

Patients with inoperable disease may be considered for neoadjuvant chemotherapy followed by concurrent chemoradiotherapy, recognising the toxicity of such an approach.

Postoperative Radiotherapy

Incomplete excision of laryngeal tumour with positive surgical margins is an absolute indication for RT treatment. Laryngeal cancers can spread out of the larynx either by infiltration through the thyroid cartilage or through the thyrocricoid membrane into the soft tissues of the neck, that is, pT4 disease. Such spread, again, is an indication for postoperative therapy, as is extracapsular nodal spread. In cases of involved margins at the primary site and extracapsular spread, concurrent chemotherapy would also be offered. The other indications for postoperative RT are considered in Chapter 21.

The tracheostomy opening is a potential site for recurrence, especially if the patient has had an emergency tracheostomy or if there is subglottic tumour. The tracheal stoma should be included in all or part of the treatment. The radiation reaction though, can be brisk around the tracheostomy, with soreness, desquamation and occasionally bleeding after doses as low as 40 Gy in 20 fractions and the delivered dose might need some reduction to that delivered elsewhere in the neck.

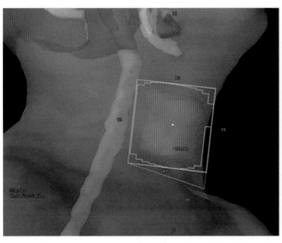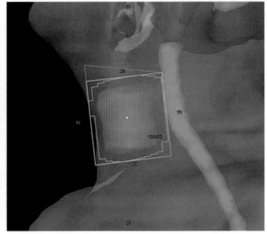

RIGHT FIELD   LEFT FIELD

Fig. 22.55 Beam's eye view of fields for early glottic tumour.

Typical dose distributions for glottic and supraglottic laryngeal cancer

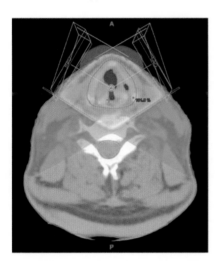

- Note use of wax to ensure that the anterior commissure is adequately covered

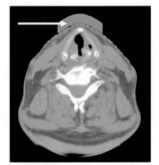

Dose distribution using two anterior oblique fields with thick ends anteriorly

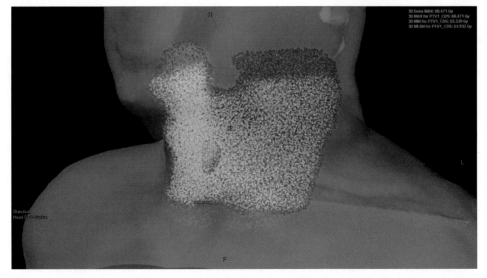

Dose cloud (minimum 50 Gy) for supraglottic case demonstrating dose painting to nodes according to estimated risk

Fig. 22.56 Typical dose distributions for early glottic and supraglottic tumours.

Results of Treatment

Early Laryngeal Cancers

Local control rates for T1A glottic tumours are around 90% to 93%. For T1B tumours this drops slightly to 85% to 89% and for T2 tumours, marginally less again.

Local control rates for T1N0 supraglottic tumours range from 77% to 100% whereas for T2N0, this falls slightly to 62% to 83%.

Advanced Laryngeal Cancers

It is possible to get 65% 5-year survival with RT alone in selected T3 glottic cancers. In the past, more advanced transglottic T3 lesions had between a 40% to 50% survival if treated by RT alone rising to about 65% if treated by laryngectomy with postoperative RT if required. The results of RT alone are significantly improved by the administration of concomitant cisplatin chemotherapy, with 4-year survivors with T4 disease exceeding 50%.

HYPOPHARYNGEAL CARCINOMA

Anatomy

The hypopharynx extends posterolaterally in relation to the larynx, at the level of the hyoid bone to about the lower level of the cricoid cartilage (Fig. 22.65). The hypopharynx comprises the piriform fossa, the postcricoid region and the posterior pharyngeal wall and, therefore, cancers of these three regions comprise the hypopharyngeal carcinomas. The piriform fossae (or sinuses) are pear-shaped channels that run alongside the larynx and are adjacent to the inner aspect of the thyroid cartilage. The postcricoid region is behind the larynx and runs from the arytenoids to the inferior border of the cricoid cartilage. The posterior pharyngeal wall links the floor of the vallecula to the cricoid cartilage (Fig. 22.66).

Incidence of Hypopharyngeal Tumours

Cancers of the hypopharynx are uncommon with an age-standardised incidence rate of 0.63 per 100,000 population. Most arise in the piriform sinuses. These tumours mainly occur in the fifth to seventh decades and are approximately three to four times more common in men than women.

Staging System of Hypopharyngeal Tumours (TNM, 8th Edition)

T1	Tumour limited to one subsite of the hypopharynx and/or measuring ≤2 cm in greatest dimension
T2	Tumour involves more than one subsite of the hypopharynx or an adjacent site, does not fix the hemilarynx and/or measures >2 cm but not >4 cm in greatest dimension
T3	Tumour measures >4 cm in largest dimension or fixes the hemilarynx, or extends into oesophageal mucosa
T4a	Tumour invades thyroid/cricoid cartilage, hyoid bone, thyroid gland, oesophageal muscle or central compartment soft tissue
T4b	Tumour invades prevertebral fascia, encases carotid artery or invades mediastinal structures

Regional lymph nodes are staged as per other head and neck sites.

Aetiology, Pathology and Lymphatic Spread

As with other head and neck cancers, tobacco and alcohol consumption are the most significant risk factors for developing cancers in this region. There are no specific genetic risk factors for this type of tumour. The postcricoid cancers may be associated with iron deficiency anaemia as part of the Plummer-Vinson syndrome.

Tumours of the hypopharynx are rare in the United Kingdom but are more common in parts of Europe. Piriform fossa tumours are more prevalent in the Mediterranean regions whereas postcricoid tumours are commoner in parts of Northern Europe.

Histologically, almost all hypopharyngeal carcinomas are SCCs, prevalent in the head and neck region.

The hypopharynx has an extensive lymphatic supply (Fig. 22.67). The majority of piriform fossae cancers have nodal involvement at presentation. There is early spread to the upper and mid-deep cervical nodes (levels 2 and 3), but the drainage can include all levels including the supraclavicular nodes. Spread can be bilateral. The posterior pharyngeal wall drains to the retropharyngeal nodes and deep cervical lymph nodes. The postcricoid region drains to levels 3 and 4 and the paratracheal nodes (level 6). The extensive nodal drainage generally needs to be considered in RT planning.

Signs and Symptoms

Cancers in this region commonly present at an advanced state with sore throat, which may radiate to the ear, or with painful or difficulty swallowing. There may be hoarseness or haemoptysis. Tumour or ulceration in the hypopharynx can usually be visualised in the clinic via nasendoscopy and FNA, or biopsy taken if required.

Many present, however, with a neck mass from secondary lymph nodes.

Diagnosis and Staging

Patients with a history of persistent sore throat should be referred urgently to the ENT clinic. Patients may also be referred urgently for the other symptoms listed above or because of the presence of neck lymphadenopathy.

A full ENT examination is performed in the clinic. This allows delineation of the primary and facilitates exclusion of synchronous tumours. Examination should include fibreoptic examination. The neck should be clinically examined for palpable lymph nodes. Patients should have an examination under anaesthesia to assess the extent of the primary and for a biopsy to confirm the tissue diagnosis. Radiological assessment of the primary is essential for full locoregional staging (Fig. 22.68). This may also reveal pathological lymphadenopathy not identified clinically. Ideally, this assessment this should be undertaken before biopsy to avoid any artefact that may lead to over-staging, and may be CT or MRI, or both. Imaging of the chest is also essential for exclusion of metastatic spread or synchronous primary tumours of the lung. PET-CT is now recommended in advanced cases and will help to determine the upper and lower extent of disease.

Early consideration of co-morbidity factors and performance status should occur to tailor subsequent treatment.

Treatment

Given the advanced nature of most cases, surgery followed by RT (with/-without chemotherapy) is the standard of care in fit, motivated patients. Surgery is thus considered the optimal initial treatment for bulky or T4 tumours in this region and usually involves pharyngolaryngectomy. In other instances, the aim of organ preservation via treatment with induction chemotherapy followed by RT or concurrent chemoradiotherapy could be considered; that said, many of these patients present malnourished, and a period of nutritional support is often required before embarking on intensive treatment. Even then, up to 25% of patients may not be suitable for any curative treatment.

Radiotherapy Technique

Patients are treated in the supine position and immobilised in the usual fashion. The shoulders should be held well down as the primary target volume sits relatively low in the neck and would be clipped by the radiation beam affecting delivered dose. A planning CT scan facilitates delineation of the primary tumour and nodes. The intimate relationship between areas of the hypopharynx means that primary CTVs are generally quite large themselves. In addition, hypopharyngeal tumours have a high propensity for submucosal spread, and as such, CTV margins need to take that into consideration, especially in the inferior extent. The choice of nodes to include in the irradiation volume, that is, the nodal CTV, is based on the previous discussion, although in practice, all the nodes in the neck are irradiated. The exception would be small tumours of the piriform fossa, that is, T1 and low volume T2 with no clinical or radiological evidence of node involvement. In this case, the primary site and immediate draining nodes, that is, levels 2 and 3 alone, could be irradiated alone prophylatically.

Radiotherapy prescriptions will follow the principles in Chapter 21. The large volumes characteristic of these tumour sites do not lend themselves to short fractionation schedules as used in early laryngeal disease, and thus, 65 Gy in 30 fractions over 6 weeks would be standard. Concurrent treatment with platinum will generally be an essential component of treatment (Figs 22.57–22.63).

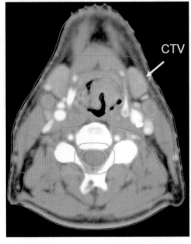

- In this example, the epiglottis is involved and there are bilaterally involved nodes.

Fig. 22.57 Volume definition. *CTV*

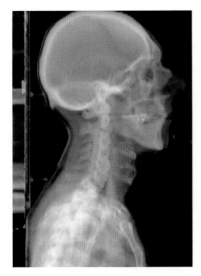

PRIMARY

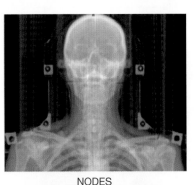

NODES

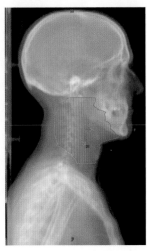

Fig. 22.58 Primary and involved nodes GTVs superimposed on sagittal digitally reconstructed radiographs.

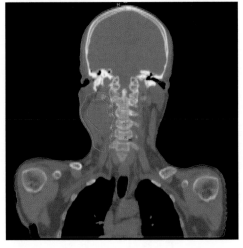

Upper involved neck volume in coronal plane

Upper neck node volume superimposed on digital reconstructed radiograph

Fig. 22.59 CTV to high dose volume ie involved nodes and primary site.

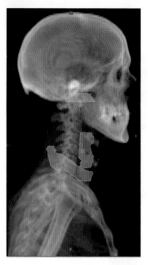

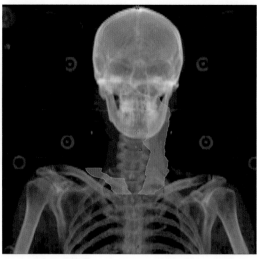

- In this example there is a large cluster of nodes on the ipsilateral side to the hypopharyngeal primary

CTV of nodes adjacent to large nodes that were involved and thus considered at higher risk

CTV of contralateral nodes considered at lower risk

Fig. 22.60 CTVs to lower risk territories both on the ipsilateral and contralateral side.

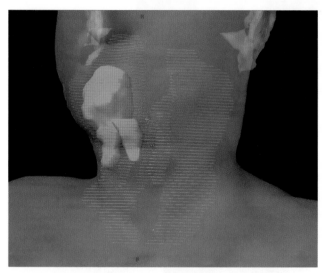

Fig. 22.61 All clinical target volumes combined.

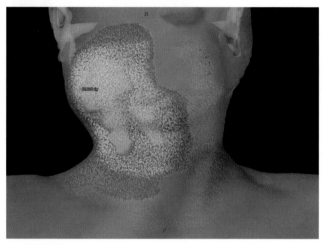

Fig. 22.63 Dose cloud (minimum 50 Gy) to the whole target volume bilaterally.

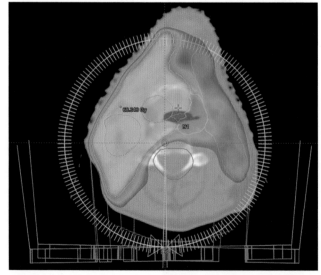

Fig. 22.62 Dose distribution (minimum 50 Gy-maximum 65 Gy in 30 fractions) in representative axial slice with primary and involved nodes.

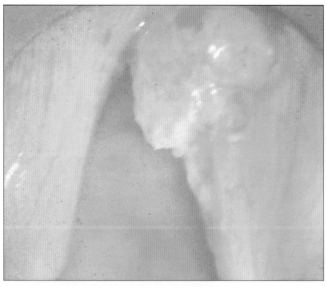

Fig. 22.64 T3 carcinoma of larynx with a fixed cord.

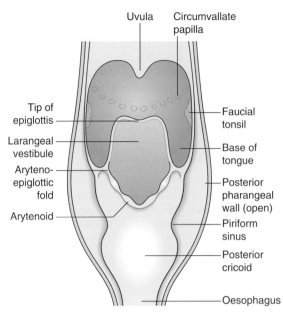

Fig. 22.65 Hypopharyngeal carcinoma anatomy.

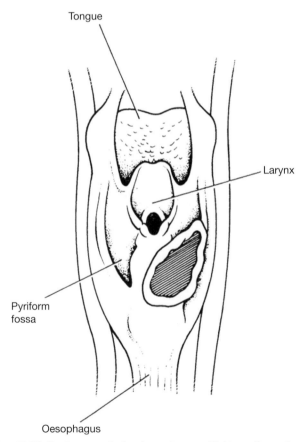

Fig. 22.66 Carcinoma of the hypopharynx (right pyriform fossa). (Reproduced with permission from Macfarlane. Textbook of Surgery, 7th Edition. London: Churchill Livingstone.)

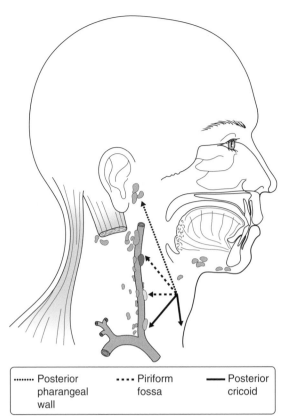

| ········· Posterior pharangeal wall | - - - Piriform fossa | —— Posterior cricoid |

Fig. 22.67 Hypopharynx lymphatic supply.

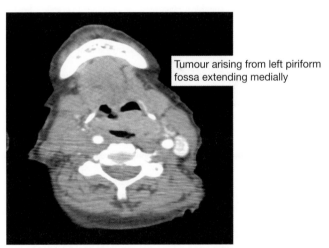

Tumour arising from left piriform fossa extending medially

Fig. 22.68 Carcinoma of piriform fossa.

Complications

Treatment results in a predictable acute reaction of mucositis, which should be managed as discussed earlier. If patients have not undergone a pharyngolaryngectomy (and hence a stoma), they are at risk of aspiration pneumonia, and this should be managed aggressively.

Late complications at this site will include some degree of xerostomia because of the need to extend the volume superiorly, although some sparing will be possible with IMRT. Some patients have permanent dysphagia, either secondary to strictures or late damage to nerves and muscles, leading to uncoordinated swallowing. Sparing of some of the constrictor apparatus may be possible again with IMRT to offset this.

Follow-up

Given that most patients present with advanced disease, a high index of suspicion should remain of residual/recurrent disease. Patients should be supported nutritionally and any late effects managed expectantly. Follow-up imaging will depend on treatment goals.

Results

Overall, the prognosis with hypopharyngeal carcinoma is poor with an overall 5-year survival rate of 30% reflecting the late presentation of most cases. Most patients succumb to distal metastases, intercurrent illness, or second primaries if locoregional control has been attained. The outcome for tumours diagnosed at an earlier stage is predictably more favourable: treatment of T1 lesions can give rise to local control rates of greater than 85%, but with T2 and T3 lesions, the control falls to less than 60% translating into 5-year survival rates of about 35%.

For very advanced hypopharyngeal tumours, standard therapy is surgery and postoperative (chemo-) radiation, although the clinician may opt, with the patient, to manage the condition palliatively in the light of an anticipated poor outcome (10% 5-year survival) and the significant morbidity and mortality from treatment.

FURTHER READING

Alpert TE, et al. Radiotherapy for the clinically negative neck in supraglottic laryngeal cancer. Cancer J 2004;10:335–8.

Al-Sarraf M, et al. Chemoradiotherapy versus radiotherapy in patients with advanced nasopharyngeal cancer: phase III randomized Intergroup study 0099. J Clin Oncol 1998;16:1310–7.

Baujat B, et al. Chemotherapy in locally advanced nasopharyngeal carcinoma: an individual patient data meta-analysis of eight randomized trials and 1753 patients. Int J Radiat Oncol Biol Phys 2006;64:47–66.

Bernier J, et al. Post-operative irradiation with or without concomitant chemotherapy for locally advanced head and neck cancer. N Engl J Med 2004;350:1945–52.

Byers RM, et al. Selective neck dissections for squamous cell carcinoma of the upper aerodigestive tract: patterns of regional failure. Head Neck 1999;21:499–505.

Candela FC, et al. Patterns of cervical node metastases from squamous carcinoma of the oropharynx and hypopharynx. Head Neck 1990;12:197–203.

Chen SW, et al. Hypopharyngeal cancer treatment based on definitive radiotherapy: who is suitable for laryngeal preservation? J Laryngol Otol Oct 2007;12:1–7.

Claus F, et al. An implementation strategy for IMRT of ethmoid sinus cancer with bilateral sparing of the optic pathways. Int J Radiat Oncol Biol Phys 2001;51:318–31.

Cooper JS, et al. Postoperative concurrent radiotherapy and chemotherapy for high-risk squamous cell carcinoma of the head and neck. N Engl J Med 2004;350:1937–44.

Dirix P, et al. Intensity-modulated radiotherapy for sinonasal cancer: improved outcome compared to conventional radiotherapy. Int J Radiat Oncol Biol Phys 2010;78:998–1004.

Duthoy W, et al. Postoperative intensity-modulated radiotherapy in sinonasal carcinoma. Cancer 2005;104:71–82.

The Department of Veterans Affairs Laryngeal Cancer Study Group. Induction chemotherapy plus radiation compared with surgery plus radiation in patients with advanced laryngeal cancer. N Engl J Med 1991;324:1685–90.

Forastiere AA, et al. Concurrent chemotherapy and radiotherapy for organ preservation in advanced laryngeal cancer. N Engl J Med 2003;349:2091–8.

Forastiere AA, et al. Long-term results of RTOG 91-11: a comparison of three nonsurgical strategies to preserve the larynx in patients with locally advanced larynx cancer. J Clin Oncol 2013;31:845–52.

Garden AS, et al. Early squamous cell carcinoma of the hypopharynx: outcomes of treatment with radiation alone to the primary disease. Head Neck 1996;18:317–22.

Gowda RV, et al. Three weeks radiotherapy for T1 glottic cancer: the Christie and Royal Marsden Hospital Experience. Radiother Oncol 2003;68:105–11.

Gregoire V, et al. Delineation of the neck node levels for head and neck tumours: A 2013 update. DAHANCA, EORTC, HKNPCSG, NCIC CTG, NCRI, RTOG, TROG consensus guidelines. Radiother Oncol 2014;110:172–81.

Gregoire V, et al. Delineation of the primary clinical target volumes (CTV-P) in laryngeal, hypopharyngeal, oropharyngeal and oral cavity squamous cell carcinoma: AIRO, CACA, DAHANCA, EORTC, GEORCC, GORTEC, HKNPCSG, HNCIG, IAG-KHT, LPRHHT, NCIC CRG, NCRI, NRG Oncology, PHNS, SBRT, SOMERA, SRO, SSHNO, TROG consensus guidelines. Radiother Oncol 2018;126:3–24.

Jackson SM, et al. Cancer of the tonsil: results of ipsilateral radiation treatment. Radiother Oncol 1999;51:123–8.

Jones AS, et al. The treatment of early laryngeal cancers (T1–T2N0): surgery or irradiation? Head Neck 2004;26:127–35.

Lee AW, et al. Preliminary results of trial NPC-0501 evaluating the therapeutic gain from concurrent-adjuvant to induction-concurrent chemoradiotherapy, changing from fluorouracil to capecitabine, and changing from accelerated radiotherapy fractionation in patients with locally advanced nasopharyngeal carcinoma. Cancer 2015;121:1328–38.

Lee AW, et al. International guideline for the delineation of the clinical target volumes (CTV) for nasopharyngeal carcinoma. Radiotherapy and Oncology 2018;126:25–36.

Lee MS, et al. Treatment results and prognostic factors in locally advanced hypopharyngeal cancer. Acta Otolaryngol 2007;22:1–7.

Lydiatt W, et al. Major changes in head and neck staging for 2018. Accessed on line: www.asco.org/edbook.

Kam MK, et al. Prospective randomized study of intensity-modulated radiotherapy on salivary gland function in early-stage nasopharyngeal carcinoma patients. J Clin Oncol 2007;25:4873–9.

Mahenna H, et al. PET-CT Surveillance versus neck dissection in advanced head and neck cancer. N Engl J Med 2016;374:1444–54.

O'Sullivan B, et al. The benefits and pitfalls of ipsilateral radiotherapy in carcinoma of the tonsillar region. Int J Radiat Oncol Biol Phys 2001;51:332–43.

Orus C, et al. Initial treatment of the early stages (I, II) of supraglottic squamous cell carcinoma: partial laryngectomy versus radiotherapy. Eur Arch Otorhinologol 2000;257:512–6.

Parsons TJ, et al. Squamous cell carcinoma of the oropharynx: surgery, radiation therapy, or both. Cancer 2002;94:2967–80.

Schache AG, et al. HPV-related oropharyngeal cancer in the United Kingdom: an evolution in understanding of disease etiology. Cancer Res 2016;76(22):6598–606.

Scola B, et al. Management of cancer of the supraglottis. Otolaryngol Head Neck Surg 2001;124:195–8.

Shah JP, et al. The patterns of cervical lymph node metastases from squamous carcinoma of the oral cavity. Cancer 1990;66:109–13.

Varghese C, et al. Predictors of neck node control in radically irradiated squamous cell carcinoma of the oropharynx and laryngopharynx. Head Neck 1993;15:105–8.

Wang H-Y, et al. A new prognostic histopathologic classification of nasopharyngeal carcinoma. Chin J Cancer 2016;35:41.

Wendt CD, et al. Primary radiotherapy in the treatment of stage I and II tongue cancers: importance of the proportion therapy delivered with interstitial therapy. Int J Radiat Oncol Biol Phys 1990;18:1529–30.

Westra WH. The pathology of HPV-related head and neck cancer: Implications for the diagnostic pathologist. Semin Diagn Pathol 2015;32(1):42–53.

23

Thyroid Cancer

Charles Kelly, Paul Symonds

CHAPTER OUTLINE

INTRODUCTION AND EPIDEMIOLOGY

Thyroid cancer is a spectrum of tumours characterised by different biology and clinical behaviour. The presence of a micropapillary carcinoma of thyroid may have little impact on life expectancy, whereas anaplastic thyroid cancer is often lethal. Although this disease is uncommon, representing only about 1% of all cancers, thyroid cancer is the most frequently occurring endocrine malignancy and incidence of papillary thyroid cancer is increasing. This rise in part is as a result of the increased use of thyroid ultrasound and most of the increase is because of the diagnosis of lower risk tumour types. In spite of the increase in incidence, there has been no increase in mortality. The incidence worldwide has more than doubled since 1973 with the highest incidence in women in the United States and Israel with an annual incidence of 14.5 per 100,000. In the United Kingdom in 2015, there were 3542 new cases, but only 382 deaths because of thyroid cancer. In the United States it is estimated that there will be 53,990 new cases in 2018, but owing to the high chance of cure, 765,547 people were living after treatment for thyroid cancer. Differentiated thyroid cancer is highly curable (about 95% or more 5-year survival) and can also affect children and young adults. All suspected and confirmed thyroid cancers should be discussed at a thyroid cancer multidisciplinary meeting. Comprehensive, updated international guidelines are available. 'Guidelines for the Management of Thyroid Cancer', 2014, by the British Thyroid Association and the Royal College of Physicians and 'Revised American Thyroid Association Guidelines', 2016, are available and summarised in Mitchell et al. (see Further Reading).

In general, prognosis is very good with differentiated thyroid cancer, with approximately 95% 10-year survival rates; however, 10% to 15% of patients will develop distant metastases. Lifelong follow-up is now advised to maintain optimum endocrine status as well as to monitor for recurrence.

ANATOMY

The thyroid gland is situated in the anterior part of the neck just above the clavicle and sternum (Fig. 23.1A and B). The gland consists of a right and left lobe joined by an isthmus which crosses the trachea at the second and third cartilaginous rings. The average weight of the thyroid gland is 20 g. The parathyroid glands lie on the posterior surface of both thyroid lobes and the recurrent laryngeal nerves are in a cleft between the trachea and the oesophagus. Lymphatic drainage from the thyroid can be to nodes superior to the thyroid gland and lateral to the gland and the paratracheal region.

AETIOLOGICAL FACTORS

Differentiated thyroid cancer shows two age-related peaks of incidence, one before the age of 40 years and one after age 60 years. The condition is approximately three times more common in women than in men. Exposure to ionising radiation in childhood, either therapeutic, such as radiotherapy (RT) for Hodgkin's disease, or associated with environmental exposure, increases the risk of developing thyroid cancer. Following exposure to fallout (particularly radioiodine) following the Chernobyl nuclear reactor fire in 1986, there has been a marked increase in well-differentiated thyroid cancer in Russia, Ukraine and Belarus in children and young people, with over 5000 new cases reported. The mortality from the accident has been low, with less than 50 deaths and a projected 30-year mortality of 1%. There is, however, no proven relationship between the development of thyroid cancer and administration of iodine-131 for the treatment of hyperthyroidism.

Other medical conditions that affect the thyroid have also been linked to an increased risk of developing thyroid cancer, namely, endemic goitre, which occurs in areas where there is low natural iodine,

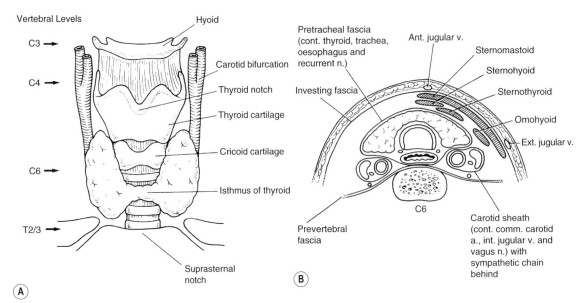

Fig. 23.1 (A) Structures palpable on the anterior aspect of the neck, together with corresponding vertebral levels. (B) Transverse section of the neck through C6 showing the relations of the thyroid gland. (Reproduced with permission from Ellis. Clinical anatomy. 5th ed. Oxford: Wiley-Blackwell; 1975.)

Hashimoto's thyroiditis, a past history of thyroid adenoma or a family history of thyroid adenoma or cancer. Some genetic conditions which increase the risk of thyroid cancer include Gardner syndrome, Cowden's syndrome, familial adenomatous polyposis and the multiple endocrine neoplasia syndromes.

Thyroid cancer initiation and progression is supposed to be through accumulation of genetic and epigenetic events. These include point mutations of BRAF (predominantly papillary) and RAS (N,H,K-Ras predominantly follicular) genes and chromosomal rearrangements, RET/PTC (papillary, particularly radiation-induced), PAX8/PPARγ (follicular); abnormal miRNA (microRNA) with gene methylation problems also plays its part. These events are described in the 2014 "Thyroid Cancer Genome Atlas". All cancers are now being detected on fine-needle aspiration cytology (FNAC). This avoids diagnostic lobectomies for indeterminate and benign nodules in the future, protecting patients from unnecessary surgery as well as allowing one-stage total thyroidectomy for cancer patients (rather than lobectomy followed by total thyroidectomy in Thy3 cases); in addition, it provides cost savings. P53 mutations are thought to be a late event in progression from differentiated to anaplastic thyroid cancer in a high proportion of cases. The increased knowledge about the molecular alterations underlying the development of thyroid cancer has led to the development of targeted therapies, particularly tyrosine kinase inhibitors active against signalling pathways, especially those associated with the RET oncogene.

PRESENTATION, DIAGNOSIS AND PATIENT PATHWAY

The most common presenting feature of thyroid cancer is a painless lower neck lump in the thyroid area which may or may not have been noted to have increased in size. In more advanced cases, patients may complain of a lump on the side of the neck because of the spread to lymph nodes, hoarseness or change in voice, suggesting recurrent laryngeal nerve involvement, stridor or, rarely, dysphagia. Patients presenting with a thyroid nodule are more likely to have malignancy if the nodule is fixed, there are palpable lymph nodes, vocal cord palsy is

present, or there is a past history of Hashimoto's thyroiditis, previous neck irradiation or a family history of thyroid cancer. Malignancy is also more common if a patient is younger than 20 years of age or older than 60 years.

A rapid enlargement of the mass or a rapid development of symptoms, suggesting compression of other structures, may be because of a more rapidly growing anaplastic carcinoma or lymphoma.

In the first instance, the patient should be referred to an ear-nose-throat (ENT) physician or general surgeon with a particular interest and experience in managing thyroid cancer. A history of the development of the mass and any relevant personal past history or family history of thyroid problems are important. Examination is undertaken to define whether the mass is solitary or multiple, whether it is tender, which might suggest a benign cause, and whether the mass is fixed to the skin or to underlying structures in the neck. Any enlarged lymph nodes within the neck are noted. Development of stridor is a medical emergency, demanding urgent hospital admission, for management of airway compromise.

Ultrasound and FNAC are essential for neck masses suspected of being a thyroid cancer. Ultrasound guidance may help in obtaining the aspiration cytology and can help to distinguish solid from cystic masses in the neck. It can differentiate between solitary and multiple nodules, help to detect involved lymph nodes (if needed by guided FNAC) and can provide sonographic features, suggesting probable malignancy in some cases. Ultrasound grading of thyroid nodules shows U1, normal tissue; U2, benign; U3, indeterminate or equivocal; U4, suspicious; and U5, malignant. The last three are indications for FNAC.

Follicular cancers cannot be differentiated from adenomas on FNAC alone as evidence of invasion is required and lobectomy is usually necessary. If FNAC is not helpful, it should be repeated and, if it is still inconclusive, thyroid lobectomy should be performed to obtain enough tissue for diagnosis. There are no indications for an incisional biopsy of the thyroid, which might compromise future therapeutic interventions, but if thyroid lymphoma is suspected, an ultrasound-guided core biopsy may be indicated.

Radioactive iodine scans can rarely help differentiate nonfunctioning "cold" nodules within the thyroid, which may represent a malignancy, from "hot" nodules which rarely contain a cancer; usually these scans are not helpful with diagnosis and are much more useful in the postoperative period for diagnosing residual disease or early recurrence.

Computed tomography (CT) and magnetic resonance imaging (MRI) scans are not routinely required but can help show the local extent of spread, detailing involvement of lymph nodes and other neck structures.

Thyroid function tests are usually normal in patients with thyroid cancer; calcium, phosphate and thyroglobulin can be sampled for baseline measurement, but thyroglobulin level is not useful in the preoperative phase. If there is any suspicion that the thyroid tumour may be a medullary cancer, then the calcitonin level is checked.

Staging performed using the TNM system, 7th edition, American Joint Committee on Cancer (AJCC) is summarised in Table 23.1. All anaplastic carcinomas are considered T4 tumours. In 2017, AJCC revised the TNM staging in the 8th edition, Table 23.2, which came into use on 1 January 2018, largely because of the marked increase in the diagnosis of small (>2 cm) papillary thyroid cancers in the United States in the last 20 years and a revised view of the prognostic significance of spread to the strap muscles. The AJCC also increased cutoff for age as an adverse prognostic factor from 45 to 55 years. In 2015, the British and American Thyroid Associations agreed on guidelines listing postoperative risk stratifications according to the degree of local invasion, presence of local and distant spread and the aggressiveness of histology. These groupings are listed subsequently:

Low risk: No metastases. Complete surgical resection, no local invasion, low-risk histology.

Intermediate risk: Microscopic invasion of tumour into soft tissue outside of thyroid. Cervical lymph node metastases. High-risk histology (e.g. poorly differentiated elements) or angioinvasion.

High risk: Extra-thyroid invasion, incomplete R2 surgical resection, distant metastases.

In this transitional phase, following the introduction of AJCC 8th edition, some MDTs (Multi-disciplinary team meeting) continue to use the 7th edition, some use the 8th edition and others use both; hence the inclusion of both in this chapter, but more and more centres will move to using the 8th edition.

One major disadvantage of the TNM system is that the presence of positive nodes does not necessarily give a worse prognosis, consequently making this staging system less useful in the practical setting than at other cancer sites.

In addition to the TNM system, there are other risk categorisation systems, used less in the United Kingdom, including AMES, based on *age*, distant *metastasis*, tumour *extent* and tumour *size*.

This system defines high-risk patients as follows.
- Distant metastasis present.
- Men younger than 40 years or women younger than 50 years with either extra-thyroid capsule spread or tumour size larger than 5 cm. Low-risk patients are described as follows.
- Men aged 40 years or younger (women aged 50 years or younger).
- If older, primary tumour smaller than 5 cm *and* confined to thyroid.

Another system which gives prognostic information is the MACIS scoring scheme (metastases, age, completeness of resection, invasion and size) developed at the Mayo Clinic.

DIFFERENTIATED THYROID CANCER

These tumours are divided into papillary and follicular thyroid cancers and are distinguished by their behavior, as they are sensitive to thyroid stimulating hormone (TSH), take up iodine and can produce thyroglobulin. All three of these factors are used in their management.

TABLE 23.1 TNM Staging System: AJCC 7th Edition (2010)

Thyroid Cancer: TNM Classification

T1 Tumour ≤2 cm, confined to thyroid
   T1a ≤1 cm
   T1b 1–2 cm
T2 Tumour >2–4 cm, confined to thyroid
T3 Tumour >4 cm with minimal extra-thyroid extension
T4 Tumour extending beyond the thyroid capsule
   T4a Subcutaneous tissue, larynx, trachea, recurrent laryngeal (RL) nerve, oesophagus
   T4b Prevertebral fascia, mediastinal vessels, carotid artery

N: Regional Lymph Nodes
NX Regional lymph nodes cannot be assessed
N0 No regional lymph node involvement
N1 Regional lymph node involvement
   N1a Level VI
   N1b Other regional nodes

M: Distant Metastasis
M0 No distant metastasis
M1 Distant metastasis present

Staging Grouping: TNM Classification
Separate stage groupings are recommended for papillary or follicular (differentiated), medullary and anaplastic (undifferentiated) carcinoma.

Papillary or Follicular (Differentiated); <45 Years of Age
Stage I Any T, Any N M0
Stage II Any T, Any N M1

Papillary or Follicular (Differentiated); ≥45 Years of Age
Stage I T1 N0 M0
Stage II T2 N0 M0
Stage III T1 N1a M0; T2 N1a M0; T3 N0 M0; T3 N1a M0
Stage IVA T1 N1b M0; T2 N1b M0; T3 N1b M0
   T4a N0 M0; T4a N1a M0; T4a N1b M0
Stage IVB T4b Any N M0
Stage IVC Any T, Any N M1

Medullary Carcinoma (All Age Groups)
Stage I T1 N0 M0
Stage II T2 N0 M0; T3 N0 M0
Stage III T1 N1a M0; T2 N1a M0; T3 N1a M0
Stage IVA T1 N1b M0; T2 N1b M0; T3 N1b M0; T4a N0 M0; T4a N1a M0; T4a N1b M0
Stage IVB T4b Any N M0
Stage IVC Any T Any N M1

Anaplastic Carcinoma (All Anaplastic Carcinomas Are Considered Stage IV)
Stage IVA T4a Any N M0
Stage IVB T4b Any N M0
Stage IVC Any T, Any N M1

It should be remembered that, in general, differentiated thyroid cancer carries a very good prognosis, with 20-year survival of over 85% in those patients who do not develop distant metastasis.

Papillary thyroid cancer is the most common type of thyroid cancer, accounting for almost 80% of all cases, and its incidence is increasing

TABLE 23.2 TNM Staging System: AJCC 8th Edition (2018)

Thyroid Cancer: TNM Classification

T: Primary tumour, including papillary, follicular, poorly differentiated, Hurthle cell and anaplastic carcinomas.

TX Primary tumour cannot be assessed

T0 No evidence of primary tumour

T1 Tumour 2 cm or less in greatest dimension, limited to the thyroid

T1a Tumour 1 cm or less in greatest dimension, limited to the thyroid

T1b Tumour more than 1 cm but not more than 2 cm in greatest dimension, limited to the thyroid

T2 Tumour more than 2 cm but not more than 4 cm in greatest dimension, limited to the thyroid

T3a Tumour more than 4 cm in greatest dimension, limited to the thyroid

T3b Tumour of any size with gross extrathyroidal extension invading strap muscles (sternohyoid, sternothyroid or omohyoid muscles)

T4a Tumour extends beyond the thyroid capsule and invades any of the following: subcutaneous soft tissues, larynx, trachea, oesophagus, recurrent laryngeal nerve

T4b Tumour invades prevertebral fascia, mediastinal vessels or encases carotid artery

N: Regional Lymph Nodes

NX Regional lymph nodes cannot be assessed

N0 No regional lymph node metastasis

N1 Regional lymph node metastasis

N1a Metastasis in Level VI: pretracheal, paratracheal and prelaryngeal/Delphian lymph nodes; or upper/superior mediastinum

N1b Metastasis in other unilateral, bilateral or contralateral cervical (Levels I, II, III, IV or V) or retropharyngeal

M: Distant Metastasis

M0 No distant metastasis

M1 Distant metastasis

Staging Grouping: TNM Classification

Separate stage groupings are recommended for papillary or follicular (differentiated), medullary and anaplastic (undifferentiated) carcinoma.

Papillary or follicular (differentiated); <55 years of age
Stage I Any T, Any N M0
Stage II Any T, Any N M1

Papillary or follicular (differentiated); ≥55 years of age
Stage I T1a,T1b,T2 N0 M0
Stage II T3 N0 M0; T1,T2,T3 N1 M0
Stage III T4a Any N M0
Stage IVA T4b Any N M0
Stage IVB Any T Any N M1

Medullary
Stage I T1a, T1b N0 M0
Stage II T2, T3 N0 M0
Stage III T1, T2, T3 N1a M0
Stage IVA T1, T2, T3 N1b M0; T4a Any N M0
Stage IVB T4b Any N M0
Stage IVC Any T, Any N M1

Anaplastic
Stage IVA T1,T2,T3a N0 M0
Stage IVB T1,T2,T3a N1 M0; T3b,T4a,T4b N0,N1 M0
Stage IVC Any T, Any N M1

worldwide. These tumours are also derived from the follicular cells of the thyroid, and may show psammoma bodies, small flecks of calcification, on microscopy. The distinctive feature of these tumours is that they have characteristic nuclei (Orphan Annie appearance) and seem to grow in branching stalks (the so-called papillae). These tumours are often multifocal, and they can show more local extension and cervical node involvement and less tendency to haematogenous spread when compared with follicular cancers. Papillary carcinoma is three times more common in women than men with a peak incidence in the 3rd to 4th decade of life.

Follicular thyroid cancer makes up about 10% of thyroid malignancy. It generally affects a slightly older age group than papillary cancer and tends to involve the neck nodes less. Follicular carcinomas are often solitary within the thyroid gland and have a marked tendency to invade the vascular channels and to spread via the bloodstream to distant sites.

Management of Differentiated Thyroid Cancer

The aims of treatment are the removal of all thyroid cancer and any remaining normal thyroid tissue by surgery and radioiodine treatment and the suppression of TSH by triiodothyronine (T3) or thyroxine (T4). Successful treatment should result in an undetectable thyroglobulin level and no clinical, radiological or radioiodine uptake scan evidence of thyroid cancer.

Surgery

Surgery is required for all thyroid cancer, if operable, with the exception of lymphoma. If differentiated thyroid carcinoma greater than 4 cm in size is confirmed, total thyroidectomy, or near total thyroidectomy, with preservation of the recurrent laryngeal nerves and at least some of the parathyroid glands, should be carried out depending on diagnostic findings. Total lobectomy alone is indicated in tumours smaller than 1 cm if differentiated, or in very low-risk tumours. Surgery should be individualised and based on clinical, sonographic, staging and cytology findings. Patients with suspected thyroid cancer should have a preoperative ultrasound scan and a CT or MRI scan.

Nomenclature currently used for diagnostic categorisation is the Thy 1, Thy 2 etc. system and can be found in the Guidelines for the Management of Thyroid Cancer in Adults published by the British Thyroid Association and the Royal College of Physicians of London. This system can be summarised as shown in Table 23.3.

Total thyroidectomy or near total thyroidectomy is required for follicular or papillary carcinoma greater than 4 cm, familial papillary micro-cancers, multifocal cancers and in patients who have had

TABLE 23.3 British Thyroid Association Coding System

Thy1	Nondiagnostic; FNAC needs repeating
Thy2	Nonneoplastic; two diagnostic tests with benign results 3–6 months apart are needed to exclude malignancy
Thy3 F	Follicular lesion; lobectomy required with completion thyroidectomy if malignant histology
Thy3 A	Atypia present; repeat ultrasound and FNAC; consider diagnostic hemi-thyroidectomy
Thy4	Abnormal, suspicious but not diagnostic of any histological form of thyroid cancer; treatment required depending on histology
Thy5	Diagnostic of thyroid malignancy; surgery required for differentiated thyroid cancer; other management may be more appropriate if other forms of malignancy

FNAC, Fine-needle aspiration cytology.

previous neck radiation. During this procedure, at least one parathyroid gland is left behind, but, even then, approximately one-third of patients will develop temporary symptomatic hypocalcaemia.

Although there are no prospective randomised trials comparing outcomes with different operations, the UK National Multidisciplinary guidelines now suggest that for papillary and follicular differentiated thyroid cancer, hemi-thyroidectomy is adequate treatment if the tumour is less than 4 cm in size, the patient is younger than 45 years of age, there is no extra-thyroid or extra-capsular spread and there is no angioinvasion, nodal involvement or metastatic spread. If any of these features are present or pathology shows the more aggressive Hurthle cell histology, then total or near total thyroidectomy should be undertaken.

Level VI nodal dissection should be done if level VI or any lateral cervical nodes are involved, and positive lateral cervical nodes need a selective neck dissection including levels II to V. Removal of single nodes is inadequate treatment. There is no indication for prophylactic cervical node dissection if there is no evidence of cervical node involvement.

After surgery, patients will require suppressive doses of thyroxine and will need calcium levels checked and calcium supplements, if required. Thyroglobulin, used as a marker for differentiated thyroid cancer recurrence, should be checked regularly, at least 6 weeks postsurgery.

Radioiodine Ablation

Radioiodine ablation is recommended following surgery in many patients as it helps monitoring by measuring thyroglobulin and might reduce recurrence and improve survival in high- and intermediate-risk patients with differentiated thyroid cancer by destroying any remaining microscopic foci of thyroid carcinoma cells. It destroys any remaining normal thyroid tissue and any rise in serum thyroglobulin following ablation should only suggest tumour recurrence, thereby helping earlier detection and treatment of recurrent disease. If there is a large thyroid remnant remaining, further surgery may be appropriate. The indications for using radioiodine have been described in the latest guidelines, Table 23.4.

In some centres, the patient undergoes a postoperative radioiodine uptake scan using iodine-123 to show any thyroid-derived tissue

TABLE 23.4 Indications for Radioiodine (Iodine-131) After Total Thyroidectomy

Clinical Presentation	
Patients who require iodine-131 ablation	Gross extra-thyroid extension Metastases Large tumour >4 cm
Patients who should be considered and discussed in thyroid MDT (Multi-disciplinary team meeting)	Tumour size 1–4 cm Extra-thyroidal extension Multiple lymph nodes involved Large lymph nodes present Extracapsular nodal involvement Unfavourable histology, e.g. poorly differentiated or tall cell Widely invasive histology
No iodine-131 required if all present	Papillary or follicular Minimally invasive No angio-invasion No extra-thyroid extension Tumour <1 cm but can be unifocal or multifocal

remaining. Iodine-131 is generally avoided so as not to interfere with the later ablation dose. This is followed by radioiodine remnant ablation where the patient is given a dose of 1.1 or 3.7 GBq of iodine-131 in the first instance. In the recent past, T4 or usually T3 was withdrawn before radioiodine to ensure TSH levels were greater than 30 µ/L to enhance the uptake of iodine-131, but now Thyrogen, recombinant TSH (rhTSH), can be used instead, so T3 or T4 withdrawal is unnecessary. Patients are admitted for treatment to a side room or cubicle with its own washing and toilet facilities. Thyrogen is given on days 1 and 2 of the treatment, and radioiodine is given on day 3 as an oral capsule. Patients then usually spend a further 1 to 2 days in isolation while radioactivity falls.

Patients are discharged home when total body radioactivity has fallen below the permitted levels. The dose rate from the patient in millisieverts (mSv) is measured at 1 meter on each day of their hospital stay following administration of radioiodine; these points are plotted on a graph and future levels over the next few days are extrapolated.

Typical permissible doses are as follows: patients are allowed home using private transport when the dose rate from the patient has fallen to 40 mSv/hour. Use of public transport is only permitted when the dose emitted by the patient has fallen to 20 mSv. Patients are advised to avoid public gatherings such as going to the cinema or church, close contact with family members or journeys on public transport lasting longer than an hour until a level of 7.5 mSv/hour has been reached. Patients should not have close contact with children or pregnant women or go to work until the extrapolated level is 1.5 mSv/hour. Pregnancy is a contraindication to the use of iodine-131

There is a school of thought particularly in the United States that questions the use of postoperative radioiodine in patients with low-risk disease. The necessity for radioiodine in this group of patients is being tested in the current UK trial "iodine or not" (IoN), which is ongoing. Following the result of the UK HiLo trial (2012) which showed equivalence of efficacy of low-dose radioiodine (1.1 GBq) with high-dose radioiodine (3.7 GBq) as ablation treatment with fewer adverse effects, an ablation dose of 1.1 GBq may be given in patients with T1-T3 disease and no residual microscopic residual disease instead of the traditional dose of 3.7 GBq.

Those patients who are having repeat treatment with radioiodine or who have recurrent or metastatic disease receive a dose of 5.5 GBq.

All patients who have had a total thyroidectomy require thyroid hormone replacement and can recommence replacement with either T4 or T3. T4 has the advantage of being given as a once-daily tablet and gives more optimal suppression of TSH. The initial dose of T4 is usually 200 µg daily, which is altered depending on TSH measurements. As the half-life of T3 is shorter than T4, it is easier to stop and then restart while the patient is undergoing scanning or radioiodine treatment. The aim of thyroid replacement is twofold. The first is to replace the natural hormone produced by the gland and the second is to suppress the patient's TSH. This is produced in the pituitary gland and can stimulate well-differentiated tumours as well as any thyroid remnant. The target TSH level for suppression is less than 0.1 mU/L.

The patient has a further radioiodine diagnostic scan 4 to 6 months after ablation and, if any residual thyroid tissue still remains, the patient may require further treatment doses. If the 6-month challenge scan shows no evidence of any remnant of thyroid tissue, the patient does not require further radioiodine diagnostic (RAIS) scans and can be monitored clinically and by thyroglobulin level. Regular RAIS scans are being replaced in low-risk cancers by thyroglobulin assessment only after Thyrogen injections and neck ultrasound (± FNAC).

If radioiodine uptake scans are required, the patient must discontinue thyroxine 4 weeks before the scan. T3 can then be substituted for 2 weeks and discontinued 2 weeks before the scan. Many patients understandably complain of lethargy and other symptoms of severe hypothyroidism during this period when their replacement thyroid hormone is removed. These symptoms can be countered by the use of Thyrogen, which does not interfere with the challenge scan and allows the patient to continue with T4 treatment.

Iodine-131 therapy can cause some discomfort and swelling in the neck. This can be treated by a short course of steroids. Sialoadenitis (inflammation of the salivary glands) can occur because of the preferential iodine uptake by these glands. Radiation cystitis from excretion of radioiodine is also possible, but both of these are uncommon. Replacement thyroxine is restarted 2 days after any radioiodine diagnostic (if no further treatment is planned), remnant ablation or treatment scan. Before any radioactive iodine is given, pregnancy should be excluded and patients advised to avoid pregnancy for one year after iodine-131 ablation or treatment. The usual dose for ablation is 3.7 GBq.

There is a small dose-related risk of developing leukaemia following treatment with radioiodine. This risk increases with cumulative doses greater than 18.5 GBq and if the patient also has external beam RT (EBRT) to the neck. Patients who receive cumulative injections of iodine-131 do have a higher risk of developing second malignancies, for example, bladder and salivary gland, as a consequence of the treatment. The total dose should be kept to less than 40 GBq in any individual patient and, as with any radiation, the total cumulative dose should be kept as low as possible.

Thyroglobulin

Monitoring serum thyroglobulin level after radioiodine ablation is a sensitive marker for recurrence, especially if the level rises after thyroxine replacement is withdrawn or Thyrogen is used to raise the TSH level to above 30 mU/L. It is important to know if antibodies to thyroglobulin are present as this may compromise the test ($\leq$25% of patients). Thyroglobulin levels are considered unreliable within 3 months of thyroidectomy. During follow-up, one difficult diagnostic situation that can arise is the patient who develops rising levels of serum thyroglobulin with no positive radioactive iodine scan, but having a rising or persistently raised thyroglobulin level requires further investigations with CT, MRI or positron emission tomography (PET-CT) scanning, which may show suspected recurrent disease which does not take up iodine but can be treated with surgery or RT or newer targeted treatment. Empirical treatment with iodine-131 followed by a scan a few days later may show disease not seen on a normal uptake scan and was not infrequently used in the past. If the thyroglobulin level is slightly elevated but not rising, a watch and wait policy can be undertaken as it can spontaneously disappear over time.

An exciting possibility is that radiosensitivity can be restored if tumours become refractory to radioiodine treatment. Radioiodine is absorbed into the tumour via the sodium iodine support pathway (NIS). In resistant tumours there are areas in the tumour which are less differentiated and have lost NIS expression. The NIS pathway may be restored by the use of a redifferentiated agent such as MEK inhibitor, selumetinib. This concept is being tested in the ongoing UK SEL-I-METRY trial.

Management of Hypocalcaemia

Transient hypocalcaemia is relatively common after thyroidectomy, with 30% of patients needing some form of calcium supplementation. This drops to only 2% of patients requiring supplements at 3 months. Calcium levels can be checked postoperatively and calcium supplements started and titrated, as required, with the addition of α-calcidol if no improvement is seen in serum calcium level with calcium supplements alone. Patients need to continue to be monitored for serum calcium level until this has stabilised.

Management of Locoregional Recurrence

Up to 20% of patients may develop locoregional recurrence, usually signalled by a rising thyroglobulin or clinically recurrent disease detectable on ultrasound (or rarely other cross-sectional imaging) or palpable in the neck. These patients may remain curable, with appropriate intervention. If operable, surgery should be considered as the first salvage procedure offered. Postoperatively, or if the recurrence is inoperable and a radioiodine uptake scan is positive, further radioiodine therapy is appropriate. These patients obviously require further close monitoring, with clinical examination, thyroglobulin levels and further radioiodine ultrasound or other scans. If the locoregional recurrence is inoperable, or salvage surgery has been incomplete and the recurrent tumour does not take up radioiodine, then EBRT is an option.

Metastatic Disease

Metastatic disease will develop in 10% to 15% of patients, usually to the lungs or bones. These metastatic sites may show radioiodine uptake and respond to radioactive iodine therapy doses. Usually, higher radioiodine doses are given for metastatic disease than for initial ablation, for example, 5 GBq. Even with initial iodine uptake, these metastatic sites may become radioiodine uptake negative. In recent years, palliative molecular targeted therapy with sorafenib, sunitinib and so on have been shown to improve progression-free survival in these iodine refractory cases and are preferred over toxic chemotherapy which is rarely effective. These small-molecule drugs are simple tablets which inhibit receptor tyrosine-serine-threonine protein kinase and pathways inside the cell via specific cancer cell membrane receptors. This prevents tumour growth, invasion and spread and increases cell death (apoptosis). Further palliative treatment consists of local RT to sites of bony pain, with orthopaedic intervention.

Overall, the prognosis in differentiated thyroid cancer is generally good with 10-year survival figures for papillary cancer being over 90% and for follicular tumours over 85%. Prognosis is worse in the elderly or in very young patients; men have a worse prognosis than women. Extra-thyroid invasion, vascular invasion, metastases at diagnosis and large size of primary tumour are all bad prognostic features. Surprisingly, lymph node metastases in the neck at the time of diagnosis have less effect on long-term survival if completely resected.

Survival of patients with metastatic well-differentiated thyroid cancer can be surprisingly good. In one series from the Royal Marsden Hospital London, 54% of patients with disease confined to the lungs were alive and free of disease 10 years after radioiodine treatment. No patients with bone involvement which is difficult to eradicate with radioiodine alone survived longer than 8 years. The group of patients with distant metastases who have the best prognosis are those who are female, under 45 years of age and have small miliary metastasis in the lungs which take up radioiodine. A French series reported a 15-year survival of 89% in this subgroup of patients.

MEDULLARY THYROID CANCER

Derived from parafollicular C cells, which produce calcitonin, these cancers are part of a familial endocrine cancer syndrome in 25% of the patients who develop medullary thyroid cancer (MTC). MTC is sporadic, without a familial component in 75% of cases. Not all patients with the inherited form give a positive family history as the condition can skip generations. These familial syndromes can be broadly divided into three types.

Familial MTC can occur by itself and is inherited in an autosomal dominant pattern and is associated with a mutation in the RET proto-oncogene. If this mutation is present, then almost 100% of patients will develop MTC. If it occurs by itself without other endocrine neoplasia, the thyroid cancer may behave in a more indolent manner than when it appears as a part of the multiple endocrine neoplasia (MEN) syndromes. MTC is also a component of the familial syndromes- MEN 2A- (also known as Sipple syndrome) and MEN 2B. Patients may develop pheochromocytoma in both MEN 2A and 2B, hyperparathyroidism in MEN 2A- and ganglioneuromatosis in MEN 2B. MTC may occur relatively early in MEN 2B and be more aggressive.

Patients with any of these syndromes should be offered prophylactic thyroidectomy while still young, before MTC develops. As this condition is potentially inheritable, patients and family members should be offered RET mutation genetic testing with the local clinical genetics service after appropriate counselling, detailing the implications of positive or negative test results, for them and their relatives.

Diagnosis in this type of thyroid cancer can be made with FNAC. An elevated serum calcitonin helps confirm the diagnosis. Patients presenting with these tumours require screening for the other potential components of these familial syndromes, with CT and/or MRI of the neck, chest and abdomen. These cases, because of their rarity, should be treated by specialist teams including a surgeon, endocrinologist, geneticist, oncologist and so on in cancer centres.

In those patients who present with this thyroid cancer, the majority will have positive neck nodes at presentation and so require total thyroidectomy with selective radical neck dissection. Radical surgery with total thyroidectomy, removal of any regional deposits and level VI lymph node clearance is key to effective treatment, so adjuvant RT is rarely indicated. Serum calcitonin levels are used postoperatively for monitoring potential recurrence. Monitoring can be improved by using a pentagastrin-stimulated calcitonin evaluation. Radioactive iodine has no effect in these tumours. If serum calcitonin can be brought down to undetectable levels, which may take several months after surgery, the recurrence rate at 5 years is only 5%, so cure is possible with effective surgery. Those patients who continue to have raised calcitonin need further assessment for residual or metastatic disease.

If recurrent medullary cancer presents, then further surgery should be used, if possible. If surgery is not possible, high-dose EBRT may be considered in selected cases. In recent years, targeted therapy with vandetanib and sorafenib is showing some benefit in progression-free survival. Palliative chemotherapy, using a variety of agents in combination, has also been tried, but shown to be not very effective.

ANAPLASTIC THYROID CANCER

Anaplastic tumours are less common, making up less than 5% of thyroid malignancies, but are in general-aggressive and carry a much worse prognosis than differentiated thyroid cancer. Anaplastic carcinoma develops from the follicular cells, and up to 20% of patients have a history of having a differentiated thyroid cancer. This rare tumour occurs in older patients (mean age at diagnosis is 65 years) who present with a rapidly growing mass in the neck. The trachea and oesophagus are frequently involved at an early stage, leading to dysphagia, dyspnoea and, later, stridor. The voice may be hoarse because of infiltration of the laryngeal nerves and subsequent vocal cord palsies. Neck node involvement and metastatic spread, usually to the lung, are relatively common, with metastases being present at initial presentation in up to 50% of patients. Diagnosis is done with FNAC, core biopsy or very rarely, open biopsy, and CT scans and neck ultrasound help show extent of disease.

Patients usually have advanced disease at presentation and tend to be older and more frail than other thyroid cancer patients. In a small minority, surgery with total thyroidectomy and radical neck dissection may be possible. In the majority, surgery is either impossible or inappropriate, and management is with EBRT with or without concurrent chemotherapy. Anaplastic thyroid cancers, however, can show a variable radiosensitivity with some tumours continuing to enlarge, even while undergoing RT.

Palliative chemotherapy with Adriamycin, with or without cisplatin, is also used. Median survival for this condition is usually between 6 and 9 months from diagnosis.

THYROID LYMPHOMA

Thyroid lymphomas are non-Hodgkin's B-cell lymphomas of varying grade and can be associated with Hashimoto's thyroiditis. They usually present as an enlarging thyroid mass. Core biopsy is often required in addition to FNAC to determine the grade and type of lymphoma. The majority are high-grade diffuse large B-cell lymphomas although low-grade tumours do occur. Once a diagnosis of lymphoma has been made, staging is as for other extra-nodal sites for lymphoma, with CT scan covering all the potential nodal and extra-nodal lymphoma sites, and marrow examination. Treatment is usually postoperative chemotherapy and RT or RT only to the neck, with excellent long-term survival.

THYROID SARCOMA

Thyroid sarcomas are uncommon, but can be difficult to distinguish from anaplastic thyroid cancer or sarcomatoid variants of differentiated thyroid cancers. As they are radioiodine insensitive, treatment is with surgery and EBRT.

HURTHLE CELL CARCINOMA

These tumours consist of eosinophilic Hurthle cells and have been thought to be a variant of follicular carcinoma and stage for stage behave as such; however, some professionals believe it is more aggressive than the other differentiated forms, with a higher incidence of recurrence and metastatic spread and a reduced 5-year survival because it does not usually take up radioiodine (10% of cases).

EXTERNAL BEAM RADIOTHERAPY FOR THYROID CANCER

EBRT, although not used frequently, does have a role in all histological types of thyroid cancer. Its main role is in differentiated thyroid cancer (DTC), anaplastic thyroid cancer (ATC) and lymphoma. In MTC it has a limited but defined role. In DTC according to UK British Thyroid Association (BTA) Guidelines (2014), the indications are as follows.

As Adjuvant Treatment

With gross evidence of local tumour invasion at surgery, presumed to have significant macro- or microscopic residual disease, particularly if the residual tumour fails to concentrate sufficient amounts of radio-iodine, including:

1. Extensive pT4 disease in patients over 60 years of age with extensive extra-nodal spread after optimal surgery, even in the absence of evident residual disease.
2. Use of high-dose EBRT as part of primary treatment for:
   1. Unresectable tumours that do not concentrate radioactive iodine; and/or
   2. Unresectable bulky tumours in addition to radioactive iodine treatment.

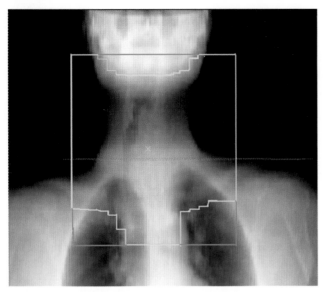

Fig. 23.2 Anterior field defined on virtual simulator, shielding defined with MLCs (Multi-leaf collimators).

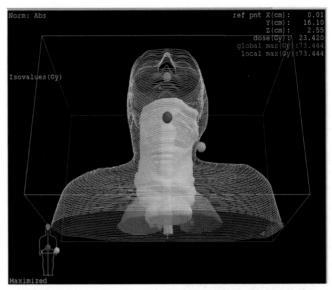

Fig. 23.3 Anterior view of PTV (Planning Target Volume).

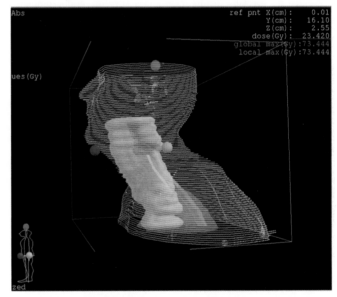

Fig. 23.4 Lateral view of PTV.

Palliative High Dose

High-dose palliative EBRT for recurrent neck disease uncontrolled by surgery and iodine-131 therapy.

Low Dose Palliation

- Spinal cord compression
- Stridor
- Superior vena cava obstruction
- Cerebral metastases with or without surgery
- Solitary or limited number of bone metastases along with surgery etc. if appropriate
- Dysphagia
- Bleeding tumour and so on

If palliative high-dose treatment is to be given, a polyfoam or Orfit head support, or similar, can be made for patient immobilisation. Localisation and treatment plan generation are done with a planning CT scan, with the patient planned and treated in a supine position, and the cervical spine as straight as possible. For large anterior and posterior parallel-opposed fields used for phase I of radical/adjuvant treatment, or in palliative treatments, the fields may be defined on a conventional simulator or virtual simulator (Fig. 23.2).

The anatomical boundaries for the planning treatment volume are:
- Tip of the mastoid process, superiorly
- The carina, inferiorly
- Laterally to include the supraclavicular fossae (Figs 23.3 and 23.4)

This volume includes the thyroid bed and adjacent relevant lymph node drainage areas. The length of cervical and upper thoracic spinal cord should be noted as an organ at risk. This technique is appropriate for many ATC (Anaplastic thyroid cancer) with poor prognosis in frail patients with the dose most commonly used being 30 Gy/10 fractions for palliative treatment.

For radical or adjuvant treatment, especially for DTC and MTC, patients should now be treated with intensity modulated radiotherapy (IMRT) techniques. This allows more accurate dose distribution and the reduction of dose to organs at risk. It also allows for much greater dose homogeneity superiorly and inferiorly, where the treatment volume may markedly change shape, improving dose distributions for thyroid cancer (Fig. 23.10). It is now standard in centres in the United Kingdom and elsewhere for high-dose radical or adjuvant therapy for DTC, MTC and some good performance status ATC.

IMRT can achieve steep dose gradients between high-dose PTV (Planning Target Volume) (See Figs 23.3 to 23.9) and nearby normal tissues. This allows improved protection of organs at risk (OARs) such as spinal cord and parotids, pharyngeal constrictors etc. while achieving dose escalation to tumour-bearing target volumes. The planning process is called inverse planning. Here the primary high-dose volume (e.g. CTV1 (first Clinical Target Volume) intended dose 60–66 Gy), prophylactic dose volumes (e.g. CTV2 (second- smaller Clinical Target Volume), delineating microscopic lymph node areas according to published consensus guidelines; intended dose 54 Gy) and OARs (spinal cord dose constraint 46 Gy, parotid median <24 Gy etc.) are outlined. The planning system, then by several iterations, finds out the best acceptable plan to meet these constraints. This produces superior and more optimal dose distribution and fewer early and late side effects and better quality of life because of improved OAR sparing, confirmed

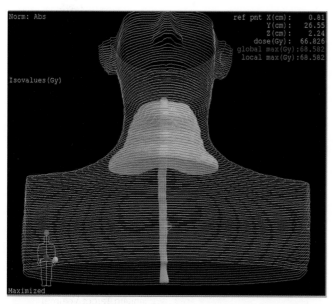

Fig. 23.5 Phase II anterior view of PTV.

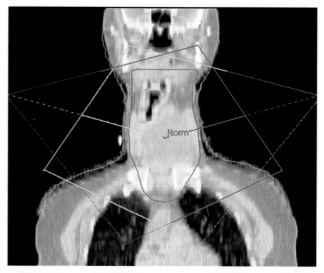

Fig. 23.8 Couch rotation to avoid field entry through shoulders.

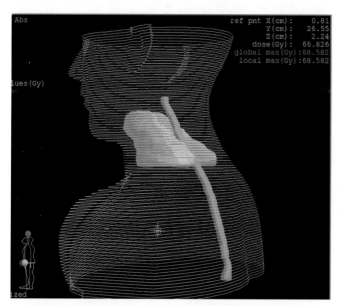

Fig. 23.6 Phase II lateral view of PTV.

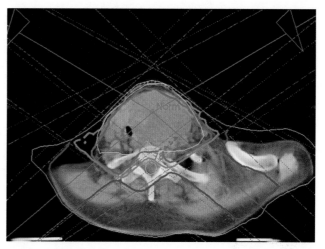

Fig. 23.9 Four-field technique, cord dose 78%.

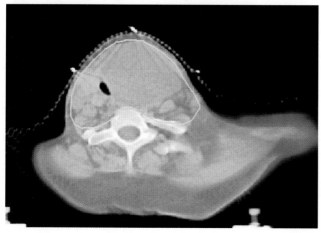

Fig. 23.7 Concave PTV.

by published trials. Ongoing studies are looking at potentially better local control and survival because of dose escalation.

IMRT is a complex technique which relies on trained staff and is also more time intensive. IMRT can also be used to create plans delivering a concomitant boost to specific areas for dose escalation without extending treatment time.

It is ideally suited for head and neck, thyroid, prostate cancers and others (Figs 23.11 to 23.13).

Historically, thyroid cancers were treated with a single anterior high-energy electron field (20–30 MeV). Appropriate bolus was attached to the anterior immobilisation shell (Fig. 23.14). In addition, although being a reasonable technique for treating thyroid tissue in the neck and sparing spinal cord dose, the disadvantage with this technique is that the upper mediastinum cannot be adequately treated, the dose distribution is not optimal and cosmesis is poor because of the high skin electron dose, making IMRT a more favourable technique.

A minority of patients suffering from anaplastic cancers with good performance status (0–2), no distant metastases and a higher life expectancy may be treated with 60 to 66 Gy using techniques described previously, with or without concurrent chemotherapy, as definitive or neoadjuvant and adjuvant treatments along with surgery. However,

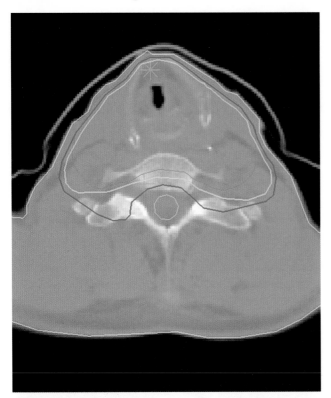

Fig. 23.10 Intensity modulated radiotherapy five-field inverse plan.

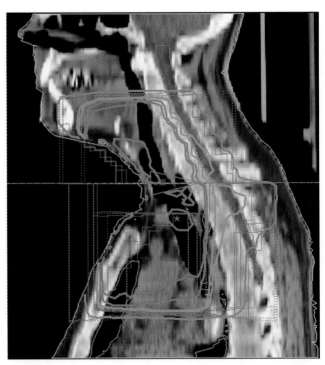

Fig. 23.12 Lateral isodose maps showing dose distribution of intensity modulated radiotherapy boost to nodal disease. Red = 100%, orange = 50%, blue = 20%.

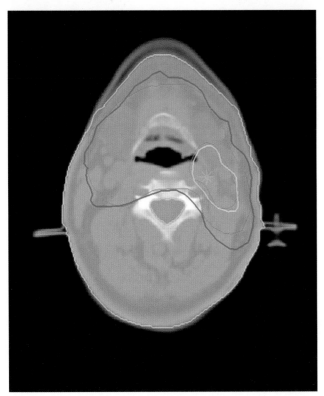

Fig. 23.11 Intensity modulated radiotherapy boost to nodal disease.

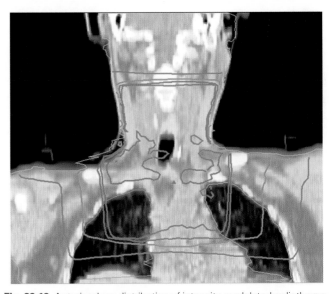

Fig. 23.13 Anterior dose distribution of intensity modulated radiotherapy boost to nodal disease.

the majority are treated by simpler palliative techniques. Parallel-opposed anterior and posterior fields are used with doses of 30 Gy given in 10 fractions, but if a large irregular volume is to be treated , an IMRT plan is preferred, which gives better dose distribution and allows OAR blocks to be used, even in the palliative situation. The apices of the lungs are usually shielded by multileaf collimators or lead blocks. For palliation of symptoms for metastatic or recurrent cancers, 30 Gy/10 fractions, or 20 Gy/5 fractions or 8 Gy/1 fraction can be used depending on the clinical situation, frailty and prognosis for the patient.

Radiotherapy for Thyroid Lymphoma

Radiotherapy is usually given after four cycles of chemotherapy, using for example, the rituximab-cyclophosphamide, doxorubicin, vincristine and prednisone (R-CHOP) chemotherapy regimen. The

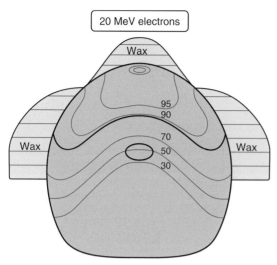

Fig. 23.14 A 20-MeV electron field.

anatomical PTV is as for other thyroid tumours, but nowadays only the volume on presentation with a margin (involved field) is usually preferred. The dose is usually about 30 to 40 Gy in 15 to 20 fractions for diffuse high-grade lymphomas after chemotherapy. The lower dose

is preferred for complete responders. A planned IMRT set-up is optimal, 24 to 30 Gy are used in daily 2 Gy/fraction; without any chemotherapy, 35 Gy in 20 fractions are used. The maximum acceptable spinal cord dose is no more than 40 Gy, and IMRT will allow doses well below this.

FOLLOW-UP POLICY FOR THYROID CANCER PATIENTS

It is now regarded as good practice to follow patients who have developed differentiated thyroid cancer for life. This is because long-term survival is the rule, but patients are still at risk of developing late curable locoregional recurrence or treatable metastatic disease. These patients also require management of the TSH suppression; long-term suppression can have cardiac effects, increased risk of osteoporosis and potential calcium metabolism problems. They are also followed because they have a small risk of developing second malignancies related to radioiodine treatment. At each visit, patients are examined clinically and blood samples are taken for thyroid function tests, thyroglobulin and thyroglobulin antibody and a calcium screen if appropriate. Arrangements can be made for ultrasound and other imaging and radioiodine uptake scans.

FURTHER READING

Hay ID, Bergstralh EJ, Goellner JR, et al. Predicting outcome in papillary thyroid carcinoma: development of a reliable prognostic score in a cohort of 1779 patients treated surgically at one institution during 1940 through 1989. Surgery 1993;114:1050–8.

Haugen BRM, Alexander EK, Bible KC, et al. American Thyroid Association management guidelines for adult patients with thyroid nodules and differentiated thyroid cancer. Thyroid 2016;26:1–133.

James BC, Mitchell JM, Jeon HD, et al. An update in international trends in incidence rates of thyroid cancer 1973–2007, Cancer Causes Control 2018;29:465–73. Available: https://seer.cancer.gov/statfacts/html/thro.html.

Mallick U, Harmer C, Yap B, et al. Ablation with low-dose radioiodine and thyrotropin alfa in thyroid cancer. N Engl J Med 2012;366:1674–85.

Mallick U, Reed N. Clin Oncol 2017;29:276–7 special edition on thyroid cancer. May 2017;275-328.

McLeod DSA, Sawka AM, Cooper DS. Controversies in primary treatment of low risk papillary thyroid cancer. Lancet Oncol 2013;381:1046–57.

Mitchell AL, Gandhi A, Scott-Coombes D, et al. Management of thyroid cancer: United Kingdom National Multidisciplinary Guidelines. J Laryngol Otol 2016;130(Suppl. S2):S150–60.

Perros P, Colley S, Boelaert K, et al. British Thyroid Association. Guidelines for the management of thyroid cancer. Third edition. Clin Endocrinol 2014;81 (Suppl. 1):1–122.

The Cancer Genome Atlas Research Network. Integrated genomic characterization of papillary thyroid carcinoma. Cell 2014;159:676–90.

24

Gastrointestinal Cancer

Somnath Mukherjee, Maria Hawkins

CANCER OF THE OESOPHAGUS

Epidemiology

Oesophageal cancer is the eighth most common cancer worldwide (456,000 in 2012) and the sixth most common cause of death (400,000). Cancer of the oesophagus has high mortality (mortality to incidence 0.88) and marked geographic variation. Globally, the incidence is highest in Eastern Asia and Southern Africa in men, and Eastern and Southern Africa in women. Squamous cell carcinomas (SCCs) are most common in Southeastern and Central Asia (79% of the total global SCC cases); the highest burden of adenocarcinoma (AC) was found in Northern and Western Europe, North America and Oceania (46% of the total global AC cases). Men had substantially higher incidence than women, especially in the case of AC (male:female ratio AC: 4.4; SCC: 2.7).

Within Europe (2012), the highest world age-standardised (AS) incidence rates for oesophageal cancer are in The Netherlands for men and the United Kingdom for women. Within the western population, an increasing incidence of adenocarcinomas of the oesophagus and cardia has been observed. Variation in incidence and mortality between countries may reflect diversity of aetiological factors, use of screening and the access to healthcare.

In the United Kingdom, an excess of 9200 new cases are diagnosed per year with an annual death rate of around 8000. The peak age of diagnosis is 80 to 89 years. The incidence in males has increased by 10% in the last two decades (between 1993–1995 and 2013–2015), whereas the incidence in females has decreased by 9% in the same period. The largest increase in incidence has been in males in the age group 60 to 69 years (21%).

Aetiology and Pathology

The most common histological subtypes are SCC and AC, accounting for more than 90% of tumours. More recently, based on whole genome sequencing, mutational signatures have defined aetiologically distinct subgroups of oesophageal adenocarcinoma: the DNA damage repair (DDR) impaired (18%), the mutagenic (53%) and G;C > A/T dominant (29%) (Secrier et al., 2016) The DDR impaired and mutagenic subgroups have potentially actionable mutations, as can be targeted with DNA-damaging therapy (e.g. poly ADP ribose polymerase [PARP] inhibitors, radiotherapy [RT]) and immunotherapy, respectively.

Risk Factors for Squamous Cell Carcinomas

Alcohol and tobacco make up the largest risk factors for oesophageal SCC in the western world. The relative risk is reported as 6.2 for smokers who do not consume alcohol. Smokers who have significant intakes of alcohol have a 10- to 25-fold increased risk of SCC. Equally, chewing tobacco and betel leaves, as practised in Southern Asia contributes to the excess risk seen in these regions. Nitrosamines, N-nitroso compounds, aromatic amines and polycyclic hydrocarbons found in alcohol and tobacco, alone or in combination, contribute to the carcinogenic effect.

Patients with iron deficiency anaemia and a diet low in riboflavin (Plummer-Vinson, also called Paterson Brown-Kelly syndrome) are at a higher risk of upper digestive tract SCCs. Tylosis, a hereditary condition characterised by hyperkeratosis of the palms and soles and papilloma of the oesophagus, is associated with a one in three chance of developing oesophageal cancer below the age of 50 years. Long-standing achalasia cardia is associated with a 5% risk of oesophageal squamous carcinoma. Patients with a history of previous cancer of the aerodigestive tract have a 2% to 4% incidence of oesophageal cancer. A higher incidence of SCCs was observed in individuals exposed to ionising radiation.

Risk Factors for Adenocarcinoma
Gastrooesophageal Reflux Disease
Gastrooesophageal reflux disease is commonly referred to as GORD or GERD. Acid and bile reflux result in intestinal metaplasia of the oesophageal squamous epithelium. The area of metaplastic change looks red on endoscopy, whereas the normal oesophagus has a pearly appearance. This change is called Barrett's oesophagus. Obesity and smoking contribute to these changes. The probable morphological sequence is metaplasia → dysplasia → carcinoma, accompanied by a series of genetic events resulting in invasive cancer. The incidence of AC developing in Barrett's oesophagus is 0.5% to 1% per year. Chemoprevention, using a combination of high dose esomeprazole and aspirin has been shown to reduce the incidence of oesophageal cancer in patients with Barrett's oesophagus. (Jankowski et al., 2018)

Obesity
Risk of AC of the oesophagus increases with increasing body mass index with up to threefold increases reported in very obese cohorts.

Alcohol and Tobacco
The association between alcohol and tobacco and oesophageal AC is less robust than for squamous cancer, but several large studies show that there is a moderate increased risk of AC of the oesophagus and the cardia of the stomach.

Anatomy
The oesophagus is a flattened muscular tube of 18 to 26 cm in length with diameters varying from 1.6 to 2.5 cm. The oesophagus starts at the pharyngooesophageal junction at the level of C5–6 vertebral interspace and ends at the oesophagogastric junction at the level of T11 vertebra. It is traditionally divided into three segments: cervical, thoracic and abdominal. The cervical segment is about 4 to 5 cm long and extends from the pharyngooesophageal junction (vertebral level C7, distance on endoscopy at about 15 cm) to the thoracic inlet (vertebral level T3, endoscopically at about 18 cm). The thoracic oesophagus extends from the thoracic inlet to the diaphragmatic opening, also called hiatus (vertebral level T9–10, endoscopically at about 37 cm), and is about 20 cm long. The thoracic oesophagus is divided into three segments (upper to T5/carina/24 cm on endoscopy; mid to 32 cm; lower to diaphragmatic opening). The abdominal segment is short, varying from 1 to 2.5 cm, extending from the hiatus to the oesophagogastric junction. The oesophagus moves with respiration and during swallowing, and movement is more prominent in the region of the gastrooesophageal junctional; this has implications for RT planning.

The lymphatic drainage is of importance to the surgeon and the oncologist. A dense lymphatic network is found in the submucosa, which travels a variable distance longitudinally before penetrating the muscle layer and draining into the periooesophageal lymph nodes. This may explain the extensive intramural spread of the cancer beneath an intact mucosa, and tumour-free margins may not necessarily mean complete tumour resection. The lymphatic drainage of the proximal oesophagus is towards the deep cervical chain and thoracic duct. The distal oesophagus drains into the lower mediastinal, left gastric and coeliac axis nodes.

The oesophageal wall is composed of four layers: the innermost non-keratinised squamous epithelium; the mucosa, submucosal connective tissue, muscularis propria with inner circular and outer longitudinal layers; and finally, the adventitial layer. The myenteric or Auerbach's plexus of nerves responsible for coordinating swallowing is located between the inner circular and outer longitudinal layers. The oesophagus has no mesentery or serosal lining, which may explain the relatively easy spread of oesophageal cancer into the surrounding tissues.

Clinical Manifestations
Dysphagia and weight loss are the most common initial symptoms in over 90% of patients. Odynophagia (pain during swallowing) is seen in about 50% of patients. Epigastric pains, haematemesis, regurgitation of undigested food and aspiration pneumonia are less common, but recognised symptoms. Cough from a tracheobronchial fistula, hoarse voice, superior vena caval obstruction and haemoptysis are less frequent. Pleural effusions and ascites, and bone pain secondary to metastases can occur. Anorexia and right upper quadrant discomfort/pain may suggest liver metastases. Clinical examination should be directed at any presence of obvious metastatic disease, such as neck or supraclavicular lymph nodes, hepatomegaly, pleural effusions and ascites.

A thorough nutritional assessment by a specialist oncology dietician at baseline and at regular intervals while on treatment is mandatory.

Diagnostic Evaluation
Any patient who presents with recent onset dysphagia and weight loss should be investigated for a possible oesophageal cancer. Many major

TABLE 24.1   TNM Staging (8th edition) Oesophageal Cancer

T: Primary Tumour

Tx Primary cannot be assessed

T0 No evidence of primary tumour

Tis Carcinoma in situ/high-grade dysplasia

T1 Tumour invades lamina propria, muscularis mucosae or submucosa

    T1a Tumour invades lamina propria muscularis mucosae

    T1b Tumour invades submucosa

T2 Tumour invades muscularis propria

T3 Tumour invades adventitia

T4 Tumour invades adjacent structures

    T4a Tumour invades pleura, pericardium, azygos vein, diaphragm or pericardium

    T4b Tumour invades other adjacent structures such as aorta, vertebral body or trachea

N: Regional Nodes

Nx Regional nodes cannot be assessed

N0 No regional lymph node metastasis

N1 Metastases in 1–2 regional lymph nodes

N2 Metastases in 3–6 regional lymph nodes

N3 Metastases in 7 or more regional lymph nodes

M: Distant Metastasis

M0 No distant metastasis

M1 Distant Metastasis

TNM, 8th edition, AJCC, 2017.

centres have a fast track dysphagia endoscopy service available to minimise the delay in the diagnosis of the cancer. Oesophageal tumours are staged using the 8th edition of the UICC/AJCC staging system (see Table 24.1).

In the majority of cases, upper gastrointestinal (GI) endoscopy visualises the tumour and its distance from the incisor teeth. The endoscopist should also define the lower extent of the tumour (if the lumen is traversable) and evaluate the oesophagogastric junction. Multiple biopsies should be taken to maximise the yield. Any associated Barrett's segment, its length and relation to the invasive cancer should be noted.

In patients who are fit for curative treatment, the first step is a multi-slice computed tomography (CT) scan of the chest and abdomen to exclude obvious metastatic disease. CT has poor sensitivity in predicting the T or N stage. The sensitivity and specificity of CT for T4 disease are 25% and 94% respectively, and for coeliac node involvement are 30% and 90% respectively.

In patients with localised disease, further evaluation with fluorodeoxyglucose-positron emission tomography (FDG-PET)-CT and endoscopic ultrasound (EUS) is recommended. EUS is useful in evaluating the local T and N stage and has improved the preoperative staging of oesophageal cancer. FDG-PET is primarily undertaken to rule out metastatic disease, and based on a metaanalysis, sensitivity and specificity for detection of distant disease is 71% and 93% respectively.

In patients with hoarseness of voice or haemoptysis/unexplained cough, bronchoscopy is recommended to rule out recurrent laryngeal nerve involvement or tracheobronchial fistula. Endobronchial ultrasound (EBUS) may be required in selective cases to rule out involvement of respiratory tract.

Therapy

General Principles

Dietary assessment and nutritional support are an essential component of management. Many patients are symptomatic at diagnosis, and life expectancy is limited in patients with advanced disease; specialist nurses and the palliative care team play a vital role in patient management and should be involved early. For patients undergoing chemotherapy, monitoring of blood count, liver and renal function is mandatory.

Surgery

Surgery is the treatment of choice for all T stages of resectable oesophageal AC. In all but T1/2 N0 disease, surgery is combined with neoadjuvant chemotherapy, neoadjuvant chemoradiotherapy (CRT) or perioperative chemotherapy. For SCC, both surgery (with neoadjuvant chemotherapy or CRT for all but T1/2N0 disease) and definitive chemoradiotherapy (dCRT) should be discussed as options. The surgery involves resection of the primary tumour with an adequate margin along with regional lymph nodes. Two standard surgical techniques have been described for surgical resection of oesophageal cancers: transthoracic (Ivor-Lewis technique) and transhiatal. The aim is complete resection. The margin status and the extent of nodal burden are powerful prognostic indicators for relapse-free survival.

Radical Radiotherapy

External beam radiation alone or as part of combined modality treatment has been evaluated in both SCC and AC of the oesophagus. Radical radiation treatment alone for treatment of clinically localised oesophageal cancer is not generally recommended in the curative setting. Both local and distant failure rates remain high despite higher doses of radiation, and 5-year survival is reported to be less than 5%. It is therefore infrequently used.

Definitive Chemoradiation

This is an option for all patients with SCC and in patients with AC who are not considered candidates for surgery. Chemoradiation protocols typically use cisplatin and 5-fluorouracil (5-FU) (or its oral derivative capecitabine) with fractionated external beam radiation to a dose of 50 to 60 gray (Gy). In two phase III trials in SCCs, definitive chemoradiation gave comparable median survival figures of around 15 to 19 months with a 25% to 40% 2-year survival. In the United Kingdom, the chemoradiotherapy with or without cetuximab in patients with oesophageal cancer (SCOPE 1) trial (Crosby et al. 2013) randomised a conventional dCRT regimen (4 cycles of cisplatin and capecitabine, with cycles 3 and 4 being concurrent with radiation, 50 Gy in 25 fractions) to the same regimen with the addition of the epidermal growth factor receptor (EGFR) antagonist, cetuximab. Nearly three-quarters of the patients had SCC. Although the trial failed to show benefit of adding cetuximab, it demonstrated unprecedented survival in patient treated with dCRT (median overall survival [OS] of 34.5 months; 95% confidence interval [CI] 24.7–42.3 months) with a 3-year OS of 47.2% (95% CI 38.2–55.7). Treatment failure at 24 weeks was highly predictive of OS (median OS 8.3 vs. 42.3 months). The SCOPE regimen has become the standard of care in the United Kingdom. Weekly carboplatin/paclitaxel as the chemotherapy component of dCRT is gaining popularity and has been reported in some retrospective series to demonstrate similar efficacy with less toxicity than the conventional cisplatin-fluoropyrimidine-based dCRT regimen and is currently being tested in clinical trial.

Typical treatment regimen:

Four cycles of: cisplatin 60 mg/m^2, day 1 and capecitabine 625 mg/m^2 twice daily, days 1 to 21.

Concomitant radiotherapy (RT) (given with cycles 3 and 4): 50 Gy in 25 fractions.

Neoadjuvant Chemoradiation

Weekly paclitaxel-carboplatin-based preoperative chemoradiation is now considered as the standard of care both in Europe and in the United States; within the United Kingdom, both neoadjuvant chemoradiation (nCRT) as well as neoadjuvant chemotherapy (see later) are considered acceptable standards of care. The use of nCRT is based on the results of the randomised phase III CROSS trial (van Hagen et al., 2012) which showed a significant survival advantage for nCRT over surgery alone (49.4 months vs. 24 months, hazard ratio [HR] 0.657, $P = .003$), with no increase in postoperative mortality. A longterm follow-up paper demonstrated that the benefit was particularly pronounced for participants with SCC (median OS 81.6 months vs. 21.1 months, HR 0.48, $P = .008$).

Typical treatment regimen:

Five weekly cycles of: carboplatin AUC2 and paclitaxel 50 mg/m^2.

Concomitant RT: 41.4 Gy in 23 fractions or 45 Gy/25 fractions.

Adjuvant Radiation or Chemoradiation

There are no prospective randomised trial data to support the routine use of adjuvant chemoradiation in resected oesophageal cancer. Single institute series have shown some improvement in local control (LC) rates and progression-free survival, but this could be caused by the inherent bias in the studies that the patients were fit enough to receive the adjuvant treatment.

Palliative Radiotherapy

Palliative RT is recommended for local pain, bleeding, dysphagia or LC. Brachytherapy is rarely used.

Radiation Therapy Techniques

External Beam Radiation

Radical treatment: RT is delivered preferably using intensity modulated radiotherapy (IMRT), typically using 6-MV photons. Four-dimensional CT planning is recommended for tumours of lower oesophagus and gastrooesophageal junction (GOJ) because of tumour motion (Figs. 24.1 and 24.2). The tumour, including involved nodes, are outlined based on the information from the staging CT scan, PET-CT scan and endoscopic ultrasound. EUS can detect submucosal spread and gives a more accurate extent of the disease. Clinical target volume (CTV) is derived using a margin of 2 cm in the superior-inferior direction along the course of the oesophagus and 1 cm in the circumferential direction, editing out uninvolved organs at risk (heart, lung, large vessels, bone). Planning target volume (PTV) includes a margin of 1 cm in superior-inferior direction and 0.5 cm circumferentially. Where four-dimensional CT is used, an internal target volume (ITV) is generated taking into account tumour motion during respiratory cycle, and a smaller margin (about 0.5 cm, depending on institutional setup errors) is applied to generate PTV.

Palliative treatment: Gross tumour with 1.5 to 2 cm margin is identified as PTV. Parallel-opposed fields (anterior/posterior) can be used for palliative RT. Beam energy: 6 to 15 MV photons.

Dose options are single fraction (8–10 Gy) or fractionated RT (typically 20 Gy/5 fractions; 30 Gy/10 fractions; 36 Gy/12 fractions) using 6 to 15 MV photons.

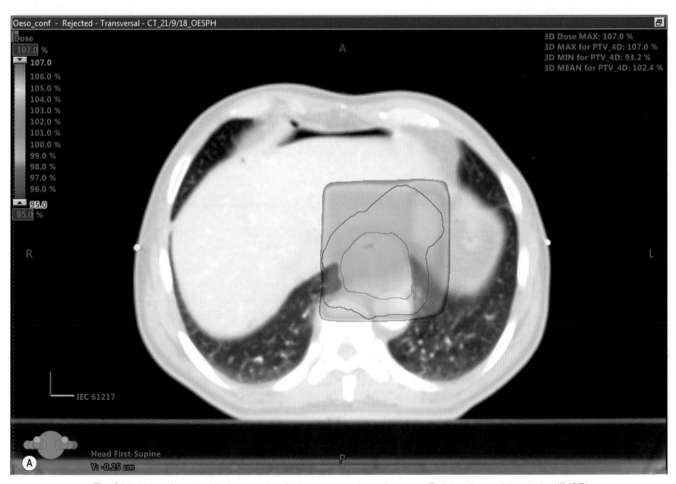

Fig. 24.1 (A) conformal radiotherapy plan for lower oesophageal cancer. (B) Intensity modulated plan (IMRT/Rapid Arc) for lower oesophageal cancer. (C) Dose-volume histogram showing comparative PTV coverage, lung and heart doses. (From Aitken and Hawkins 2014. With permission.)

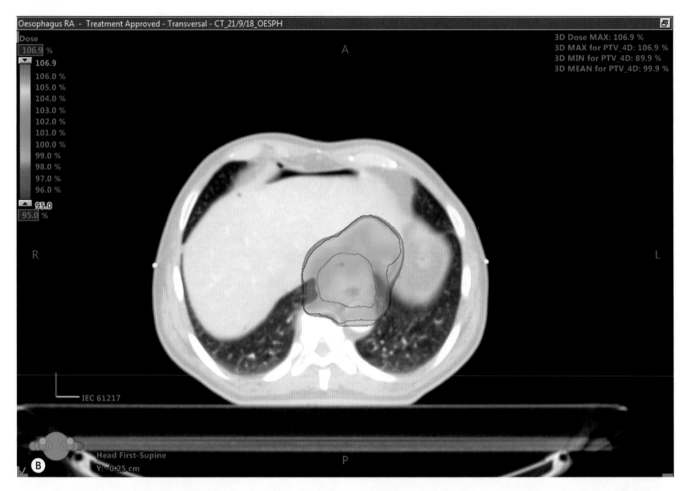

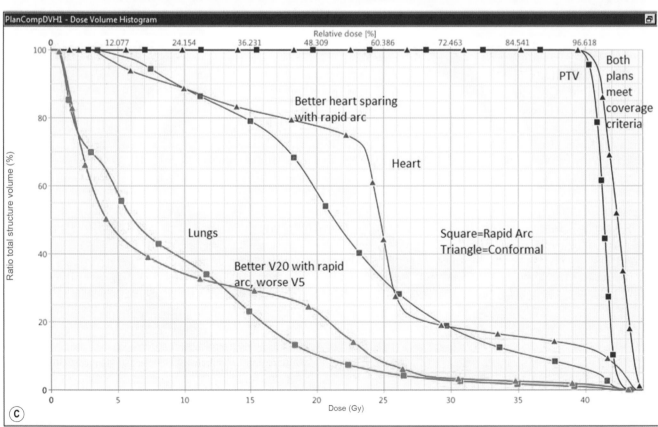

Fig. 24.1, cont'd

Chemotherapy

Neoadjuvant Chemotherapy

Preoperative chemotherapy with cisplatin and 5-FU (two cycles) has been the standard of care in the United Kingdom for patients with resectable oesophageal cancer. Updated results from the MRC OE-2 trial of preoperative chemotherapy in patients undergoing curative surgery showed 5-year OS rates of 23% in the combined modality arm compared with 17% in the surgery alone arm. The MRC OE-05 study compared four cycles of epirubicin, cisplatin and capecitabine (ECX) chemotherapy with two cycles of cisplatin and 5-FU, and failed to show OS advantage for the more intensive regimen. (Alderson et al. 2017)

Where neoadjuvant chemotherapy is being offered, two cycles of platinum-fluoropyrimidine therefore remains a standard of care for patients with oesophageal cancer and type 1 gastrooesophageal junctional tumours (although 5-FU is often replaced by capecitabine in current clinical practice). Neoadjuvant CRT (CROSS regimen) is also an option as discussed earlier, and the choice between neoadjuvant chemotherapy versus CRT continues to be debated. The randomised phase III ESOPEC trial is comparing the CROSS regimen with FLOT4 (docetaxel, oxaliplatin, 5-FU, leucovorin) in patients with oesophageal AC. The Neo-Aegis trial is comparing CROSS with perioperative ECX/EOX (epirubicin, oxaliplatin, capecitabine) chemotherapy in patients with AC of the oesophagus and GOJ.

Palliative Chemotherapy

Palliative chemotherapy for oesophagus and GOJ cancer is similar to gastric cancer and is discussed together subsequently.

Other Treatments

Endoluminal techniques have been used for the treatment of Barrett's metaplasia and dysplasia These include circumferential radiofrequency ablation, endoscopic mucosal resection (EMR) and photodynamic therapy. EMR for early invasive mucosal lesions is fast gaining acceptance as a local curative treatment and is best performed in experienced centres. EMR is indicated for superficial lesions, that is, high-grade dysplasia and moderately to well-differentiated carcinomas limited to lamina propria only. Endoscopic submucosal dissection (ESD) may be preferred for tumours larger than 15 mm, poorly lifting tumours or tumours with risk of submucosal invasion (European Society for Gastro-Intestinal Endoscopy guidelines).

Palliative treatment options are tailored to the individual patient and are best discussed in a multidisciplinary setting along with the palliative care team. Oesophageal stenting provides palliation of dysphagia. Endoscopic laser treatment may be suitable for bulky endoluminal squamous tumours. Palliative radiation and chemotherapy are other alternative options for symptomatic benefit.

Oesophagogastric Junctional Tumours

ACs of the oesophagogastric junction have been divided into three subtypes as proposed by Siewert and Stein. Type 1 junctional tumours primarily arise from the distal oesophagus and involve the junction; type 2 junctional tumours straddle the junction; and type 3 tumours are predominantly in the cardia of the stomach, involving the junction. Type 1 and 2 junctional AC is treated using oesophagus protocols. Type 3 junctional tumours are thought to behave like gastric AC, and therefore, are treated using gastric protocols.

Summary

Management of oesophageal cancer has evolved over the past few decades. Treatment decisions should be made within a multidisciplinary team setting. Careful staging and selection of patients for curative treatments are vital and surgery should be performed in high-volume specialist centres for best outcome. Combined modality treatments remain the standard of care in curative setting for all patients with oesophageal cancer except those with very early tumours.

CANCER OF THE STOMACH

Anatomy

The stomach begins at the oesophagogastric junction and ends at the pylorus. It is divided into three parts: cardia (fundus), body and pyloric antrum. The blood supply of the stomach is derived from the branches of the coeliac axis. The regional lymphatics drain into the coeliac axis nodes, splenic hilar, porta hepatis and gastroduodenal and suprapancreatic nodal groups. Venous drainage is primarily through the portal venous system into the liver.

Epidemiology

There is a considerable variation in the worldwide incidence of gastric cancer. The highest incidence is seen in Eastern Asia, South America and Eastern Europe (http://globocan.iarc.fr/old/FactSheets/cancers/stomach-new.asp). The incidence in Western Europe is in decline. However, the incidence of tumours of the cardia and oesophagogastric junction has increased. The incidence of stomach cancer has been declining in the United Kingdom since 1930 and has halved since the 1990s. Cancer Research United Kingdom (CRUK) reported 6740 new cases in the United Kingdom in 2015 making this the 17th most common cancer. The incidence is projected to fall further by 17% between the years 2014 and 2035 and to 11 cases per 100,000 people by 2035.

Aetiology

Environmental and genetic factors play a role in the pathogenesis of gastric cancer. Carcinogens implicated in the aetiology include nitrates and nitrites in food and a diet which is high in processed meat and salt and low in fruits and vegetables, smoking and industrial dust exposure. The role of alcohol remains uncertain. Increased risk has been reported with a specific strain of *Helicobacter pylori* (CAG+ve) especially in noncardia lesions, and infection with *H. pylori* has been implicated in around one in three stomach cancers. Pernicious anaemia and previous subtotal gastrectomy for benign conditions, and villous adenomas are thought to be associated with increased risk of gastric cancer after a long period of latency.

Genetic factors include mutations in specific genes, CDH1 and p53. CDH1 encodes for E-cadherin and mutations in this gene are associated with hereditary diffuse gastric cancer. Another familial gastric cancer syndrome is associated with p53 mutations. Gastric cancer is also a component of Li-Fraumeni syndrome, hereditary nonpolyposis colorectal cancer (HNPCC), Peutz-Jegher polyposis, BRCA-2 mutations and juvenile polyposis.

Pathology

AC constitutes 95% of the gastric cancers. They are classified into intestinal and diffuse types (Lauren's classification system). The intestinal type is more common in older patients, high-risk groups and men. The diffuse type is more commonly seen in women and younger patients and carries a poorer prognosis. Other histological types of gastric malignancies include carcinoids, lymphomas and gastrointestinal stromal tumours (GISTs). GISTs are the most common mesenchymal tumours of the gastrointestinal tract.

More recently, comprehensive molecular characterisation has classified gastric AC into 4 different subtypes, The Cancer Genome Atlas (TCGA) research network: (1) Epstein-Barr virus (EPV) positive (characterised by recurrent *PIK3CA* mutations, extreme DNA hypermethylation, and amplification of *JAK2*, *PD-L1* and *PD-L2*); (2) microsatellite unstable tumours characterised by high mutation rates; (3) genomically stable tumours which are enriched for the diffuse histological variant; and (4) tumours with chromosomal instability (CIN), which show marked aneuploidy and focal amplification of receptor tyrosine kinases. These molecular subtypes provide rationale for targeted therapy for distinct populations of gastric cancer patients.

Clinical Features

The most common presenting symptoms are anaemia, weight loss, anorexia, haematemesis, melena, upper abdominal pain/discomfort, nausea/vomiting. Occult bleeding is more common than overt haematemesis. Possible clinical findings include anaemia, abdominal mass, left supraclavicular lymphadenopathy, and ascites.

Staging

The initial investigations often include an endoscopy. Gastroscopy and biopsy will confirm the diagnosis in the majority of patients. Multiple biopsies increase the sensitivity and yield. The TNM staging system is used for staging gastric cancer. Endoscopic ultrasound is of value in proximal cardia and junctional tumours to assess operability. Cross-sectional imaging with a spiral CT is the first step to exclude overt metastatic disease. CT is not a sensitive tool for detecting peritoneal spread, therefore, laparoscopy is mandatory before surgery to detect any occult peritoneal spread. Laparoscopy may also help in identifying tumours in the lesser sac, on the surface of the liver and nodal disease. FDG-PET imaging may identify metastases not clearly seen on CT, but 25% to 30% of primary gastric cancers are not FDG avid (especially the diffuse type) (See Table 24.2).

Management

The optimal management of gastric cancer should take place within a multidisciplinary setting. The radical treatment options are surgery

TABLE 24.2 TNM (8th Edition) Stomach Cancer

T: Primary Tumour

Tx Primary cannot be assessed

T0 No evidence of primary tumour

Tis Carcinoma in situ: intraepithelial tumour without invasion of the lamina propria, high-grade dysplasia

T1 Tumour invades lamina propria, muscularis mucosae or submucosa

    T1a Tumour invades lamina propria or muscularis mucosae

    T1b Tumour invades submucosa

T2 Tumour invades muscularis propria

T3 Tumour invades subserosa

T4 Tumour perforates serosa or invades adjacent structures

    T4a Tumour perforates serosa

    T4b Tumour invades adjacent structures

N: Regional Nodes

Nx Regional nodes cannot be assessed

N0 No regional lymph node metastasis

N1 Metastases in 1–2 regional lymph nodes

N2 Metastases in 3–6 regional lymph nodes

N3 Metastases in 7 or more regional lymph nodes

    N3a Metastases in 7–15 regional lymph nodes

    N3b Metastases in 16 or more regional lymph nodes

M: Distant Metastasis

M0 No distant metastasis

M1 Distant metastasis

TNM, 8th edition, AJCC, 2017.

with perioperative chemotherapy (in Europe) or adjuvant chemoradiation (in the United States). For advanced disease, palliative chemotherapy may be offered for survival benefit and radiation for symptomatic benefit where appropriate. As with oesophageal cancer, involvement of a dietician and palliative care is very important in this disease.

Surgery

The goal of surgery is complete resection. However, only 25% to 30% of patients with gastric cancer may be suitable for potentially curative surgery. Distal tumours can be treated with partial gastrectomy if suitable margins can be obtained; however, proximal tumours usually require a total gastrectomy. The extent of lymphadenectomy—D1 (perigastric nodes) versus more extensive D2 lymphadenectomy (D2 or D3)—is a matter of debate; however, in the United Kingdom, a D2 lymphadenectomy is recommended (NICE guidance). More extensive radical lymphadenectomy has not shown to be of survival benefit but increases morbidity.

Surgery may be the only treatment needed for early lesions (T1N0M0) and endoscopic therapy may be used for very early lesions confined to the mucosa. However, in the majority of patients treated with a curative intent, a combined modality approach is necessary.

The common sites of relapse following a curative resection are locoregional (lymph nodes, gastric bed and anastomosis) and metastatic (liver and peritoneal seeding).

Palliative gastrectomy or gastric bypass procedure can be offered for patients with obstructive symptoms, bleeding or intractable pain.

Perioperative Chemotherapy/Chemoradiotherapy for Gastric Cancer

General principles: A variety of approaches are considered standards of care in different parts of the world. Perioperative chemotherapy is the standard of care in Europe, postoperative chemotherapy in the Far East, and postoperative CRT is preferred in the United States. Each of these approaches are discussed next.

Perioperative (Neoadjuvant and Adjuvant) Chemotherapy

The relapse rate is high for patients who have had gastrectomy for stages T2 and beyond. This is thought to be mainly because of the locoregional failure (LRF) and micrometastatic disease present at diagnosis. Various adjuvant treatments have been explored to improve the survival. Perioperative chemotherapy with epirubicin/cisplatin/5-FU has been shown to improve the disease-free and OS in patients with resectable gastric cancer. The U.K. Medical Research Council (MRC) MAGIC trial randomised over 500 patients to either surgery alone or three cycles of preoperative ECF (epirubicin 50 mg/m^2, cisplatin 60 mg/m^2, day 1 and infused 5-FU 200 mg/m^2 for 21 days) followed by surgery and then three more cycles of postoperative ECF. Both progression-free and OS were superior in the combined modality arm. Five-year survival rates were 23% in the surgery alone arm and 36% in the perioperative chemotherapy arm. In the United Kingdom, following the publication of this trial, perioperative chemotherapy has become the standard of care for patients with curable and resectable gastric cancers. The addition of bevacizumab to chemotherapy failed to show additional benefit. (NCRI ST03) More recently, a randomised phase III study comparing perioperative ECX (epirubicin, cisplatin and capecitabine) with perioperative FLOT4 (docetaxel, oxaliplatin, 5-FU, leucovorin) in AC of GOJ and stomach has been reported in abstract form only. The study reported a significant survival advantage for FLOT4 (3-year OS 57% vs. 48%), and this is set to become a new standard of care for operable cancers of the GOJ and stomach. (Al-Batran et al. 2017)

Ongoing trials: The Australian TOPGEAR trial (NCT01924819) is comparing perioperative ECF/ECX chemotherapy with/without preoperative chemoradiation for resectable gastric cancer.

Adjuvant Chemotherapy

Compared with the prominent use of perioperative chemotherapy in Europe, adjuvant chemotherapy is widely used in East Asia, including Japan and Korea. The ACTS-GC study (Japan) has confirmed the benefit of adjuvant single agent S1 chemotherapy for 1 year over surgery alone in a randomised phase III trial involving over 1000 patients (OS 71.7% vs. 61.1%; HR 0.67, 95% CI [0.54, 0.83]). The CLASSIC trial (South Korea, Taiwan, China) recruited a similar number of patients and showed a survival benefit for six cycles of adjuvant oxaliplatin and capecitabine over surgery alone (78% vs. 69%; HR 0.66, $P = .0015$). Adjuvant chemotherapy therefore remains the standard of care in East Asia.

Adjuvant Chemoradiation

In North America, adjuvant chemoradiation is offered for patients with resected gastric cancer based on the results of the Intergroup 0116 randomised trial comparing surgery alone with surgery followed by postoperative chemoradiation with 5-FU and folinic acid (FA). The adjuvant chemoradiation improved the median progression-free survival (19 vs. 30 months $P < .0001$) and OS (26 vs. 35 months $P < .006$). It is felt that a significant proportion of patients may have had suboptimal lymph node dissection and the postoperative chemoradiation may have compensated for the inadequate surgery. Although adjuvant chemoradiation remains the standard of care in North America, more recently, the benefit from this approach has been called into question. The Korean ARTIST trial ($n = 458$) compared the addition of CRT with platinum-fluoropyrimidine adjuvant therapy alone. There was no OS benefit, although in a subgroup analysis, 3-year disease-free survival was improved in node-positive patients who received chemoradiation (77.5% vs. 72.3%, $P = .04$). The Dutch CRITICS trial compared perioperative ECX chemotherapy versus preoperative ECX and postoperative CRT in patients with cancer of the stomach and GOJ treated with D1/D2 gastrectomy. The trial failed to show any advantage for postoperative CRT (40.8% vs. 40.9%, $P = .99$).

Radiation Techniques

The postoperative radiation target volumes are generated based on the tumour site in the stomach and the known pattern of LRF and need to be tailored to the individual patient's T stage and type of surgery. The CTV includes the gastric/tumour bed, gastric remnant, anastomosis, duodenal stump (where present), nodal stations along the lesser and greater curvature of the stomach, gastroduodenal, coeliac axis, suprapancreatic and retropancreatic nodes, porta hepatis and splenic groups. Additional nodal groups are included based on site of tumour. A margin of 1 cm in all directions (except posteriorly where a 0.5 cm margin is used) generates PTV. IMRT is recommended. Typical recommended dose constraints for organs at risk are as follows: kidneys—at least three-quarters of one kidney should receive less than 20 Gy; heart—no more than 30% to receive more than 40 Gy; spinal cord—maximum dose 45 Gy; liver—mean liver dose less than 30 Gy. The standard dose fractionation is 45 Gy in 25 fractions over 5 weeks. The concomitant chemotherapy options include single agent capecitabine (825 mg/m^2 2 times daily [bd], on days of radiotherapy only, as in ARTIST trial) or cisplatin/capecitabine combination (weekly cisplatin 20 mg/m^2 with capecitabine 575 mg/m^2 bd on days of radiotherapy only as in the CRITICS trial). The patient needs to be monitored carefully with weekly full blood counts, biochemistry, dietetic assessment including weight and adequate measures for gastrointestinal toxicity (nausea, vomiting and diarrhoea).

Palliative Treatments in Advanced/Metastatic Gastric Cancer

Palliative Chemotherapy

First line chemotherapy as follows: platinum- and fluoropyrimidine-based regimens are now considered to be the standard option for systemic chemotherapy for patients with advanced/metastatic oesophagogastric AC. Cisplatin with 5-FU (or capecitabine) (CF/CX) with/without epirubicin (ECF/ECX) or docetaxel (DCF) are regimens with response rates of 35% to 45% and a median OS of around 9 to 12 months. The REAL-2 study comparing cisplatin versus oxaliplatin and intravenous (iv) 5-FU versus oral capecitabine showed that the four regimens are of similar efficacy. (Cunningham et al. 2008). A docetaxel-based regimen, DCF (docetaxel, cisplatin and 5-FU) and irinotecan with cisplatin produces similar median survival figures of around 9 months. In unselected population, addition of targeted therapy with EGFR inhibitors (panitumumab in REAL3 trial) or vascular endothelial growth factor (VEGF) inhibitors (bevacizumab in AVAGAST trial) have failed to show survival benefit over conventional chemotherapy alone in first-line trials. In patients with HER-2 + ve gastric cancer, addition of trastuzumab to cisplatin + fluoropyrimidine chemotherapy has been shown to improve both overall and progression-free survival. (Bang et al., 2010) In the ToGA trial, the subgroup of patients with HER-2 + ve (FISH + ve or IHC 3 + ve) gastric cancers had 4.2 months improvement in OS with the addition of trastuzumab to chemotherapy (16 months vs. 11.8 months, HR 0.65, 95% CI 0.51–0.83).

Second and subsequent line chemotherapy: Single agent docetaxel provides modest survival benefit in the second-line setting (median OS 5.2 months [95% CI 4.1–5.9] vs. 3.6 months HR (0.67) in the active symptom control group [hazard ratio 0–67, 95% CI 0.49–0.92; $P = ·01$]). (Ford et al. 2014) Patients in the docetaxel arm reported improvement in disease-related symptoms (pain, nausea) and quality of life. The RAINBOW trial, a double-blind, phase III, randomised trial, demonstrated that the addition of the monoclonal antibody ramucirumab (VEGFR-2 inhibitor) to paclitaxel resulted in a significant survival advantage compared with single agent paclitaxel, with a median OS of 9.6 months ([95% CI: 8.5–10.8] vs. 7.4 months [95% CI: 6.3–8.4], HR = 0.807 [95% CI: 0.678–0.962], $P = .017$). In the phase III REGARD trial, ramucirumab monotherapy significantly improved survival compared with placebo (HR = 0.776, 95% CI: 0.603–0.998, $P = .047$).

Palliative Radiotherapy

In selected patients, palliative RT (8–10 Gy in a single fraction or 20 Gy in five fractions, parallel opposed fields, using 4–15 MV photons) may help to palliate pain, bleeding and obstructive symptoms.

Summary

Management of gastric cancer has improved over the last decade. Most patients with resectable gastric AC are likely to need a combined modality approach for best results. Future directions in systemic therapy include integrating the newer targeted molecules into existing protocols.

PANCREAS

Anatomy

The pancreas lies in the retroperitoneal space transversely along its long axis in the upper abdomen at the level of the first two lumbar vertebrae. It is divided into head, body and tail. The pancreas is closely related to the surrounding structures including the stomach, duodenum and jejunum, lesser sac, kidneys, transverse colon, liver, spleen and vascular structures including the coeliac axis, superior mesenteric vessels and the splenic and portal vein. Pancreatic cancer often locally infiltrates these structures. The pancreatic duct joins the bile duct to form the common bile duct which opens into the second part of the duodenum through the major papilla. Pancreatic tumours originating from the head can compress the common bile duct resulting in obstructive jaundice. The pancreas has a complex and extensive lymphatic drainage into the superior and inferior pancreaticoduodenal, coeliac axis, superior mesenteric and porta hepatis nodes. The tumour cells can also spread along the perineural pathways.

Incidence and Epidemiology

CRUK reports that 9921 new cases were diagnosed in the United Kingdom in 2015. The incidence of pancreatic cancer has been steadily rising in the United Kingdom through the decades with an 11% rise in the last decade; it is projected to rise by 6% between 2014 to 2035, with a projected incidence of 21 new cases per 100,000 per annum in 2035. Pancreatic cancer is the 11th most common cancer in the United Kingdom. The mortality rate mirrors the incidence because of the poor prognosis. The causes of this cancer are largely unknown. The only known association is with smoking, although the association is much less than seen with lung cancer. There is a doubling of incidence of this cancer in cigarette smokers. Exposure to organic chemicals is thought to increase the risk. Hereditary pancreatic cancer syndromes account for less than 10% of the cancers and include hereditary pancreatitis, familial melanoma, BRCA-2, familial adenomatous polyposis (FAP), HNPCC, Peutz-Jegher's and ataxia telangiectasia syndromes. There is an association between diabetes mellitus and pancreatic cancer.

Pathology

Some 90% of tumours in the pancreas are AC; 65% arise from the head of the pancreas. Neuroendocrine tumours, cystadenomas and cystadenocarcinomas are uncommon and have a better prognosis. The tumour spread is through local invasion into adjacent organs, in particular, perineural invasion through splanchnic nerves causing back pain. Lymphatic spread is common into regional and para-aortic lymph nodes. Tumours often metastasise to the liver and peritoneum. More than 80% of the patients with pancreatic cancer present with either locally advanced or metastatic cancer which is not amenable for curative treatments.

More recently, based on molecular (mutational, transcriptomic) signatures, several subtypes of pancreatic cancer have been proposed. RNA expression analysis defined four subtypes: (1) squamous; (2) pancreatic progenitor; (3) immunogenic; and (4) aberrantly differentiated endocrine exocrine (ADEX) that correlate with histopathological characteristics. (Bailey et al. 2016) These various subtypes identify opportunities for therapeutic intervention.

Clinical Features

The majority of the early symptoms are nonspecific, therefore, most patients present with advanced disease. The common presenting symptoms are obstructive jaundice, weight loss, anorexia, back pain and fatigue. Back pain may be present in more than 50% of patients caused by deep perineural invasion. Classically, this pain is referred between the shoulder blades and is partially relieved by sitting up and leaning forward. Back pain is usually considered to be a sign of inoperability. Less commonly, patients can present with new onset diabetes as a result of pancreatic insufficiency. Rarely, the cancer may be found following a bout of acute pancreatitis.

Clinical examination may reveal jaundice, evidence of weight loss, palpable supraclavicular nodes (Virchow's node) and umbilical nodule (Sister Mary Joseph's nodule). Superficial thrombophlebitis is a paraneoplastic feature. The liver may be enlarged and there may be epigastric fullness/mass on palpation. Venous thromboembolism is a common association of pancreatic cancer (associated with >10% of cases).

Diagnostic Evaluation and Imaging

A full blood count may reveal anaemia, and biochemical tests confirm obstructive jaundice. CA19.9, a serum tumour marker, is raised in 60% to 90% of patients with pancreatic cancer.

Endoscopic retrograde cholangiopancreatography (ERCP) is an extremely useful investigation for evaluating the ampulla, obtaining cytological specimens and also for biliary drainage. Multislice contrast enhanced dual-phase CT with three-dimensional reconstruction is extremely useful to define the relationship of the tumour to the vessels and surrounding structures, and for detection of metastatic disease. Endoscopic ultrasound by an experienced endoscopist will help in detecting small lesions, any nodal involvement and, more importantly, venous involvement. Endoscopic ultrasound-guided fine needle aspiration (EUS FNA) may increase the diagnostic sensitivity to near 100% and has been shown to be reliable for presurgical work-up. Laparoscopy is helpful in detecting unsuspected peritoneal disease because up to 30% of patients with locally advanced pancreatic cancer have occult microscopic peritoneal disease. FDG-PET is an important imaging modality in nonmetastatic pancreatic cancer, particularly in those due to undergo resection. The PET-PANC study assessed the benefit of PET-CT in 589 patients with suspected pancreatic cancer. Patients underwent multidetector CT scan as standard of care and then a subsequent PET-CT as the experimental investigation. (Ghaneh et al. 2018) Sensitivity (92.7% vs. 88.5%) and specificity (75.8% vs. 70.6%) for the diagnosis of pancreatic cancer was superior with PET-CT. PET-CT significantly improved diagnostic accuracy in all scenarios ($P < .0002$). PET-CT influenced management in 45% of patients and stopped resection in 20% of patients who were due to have surgery. However, the benefit of PET/CT was limited in patients with chronic pancreatitis or pancreatic tumours other than AC. PET-CT should be considered as standard of care for apparently localised pancreatic cancer, particularly where resection is planned. In selected patients, magnetic resonance imaging/magnetic resonance cholangiopancreaticogram (MRI/MRCP) may offer a better definition of local and vascular anatomy before surgery (See Table 24.3).

Therapy

Surgery

Less than 20% of patients have potentially surgically resectable lesions. Standard surgical treatment is pancreatico-duodenectomy pioneered by Whipple and his team in 1935. Distal body and tail of the pancreas tumours may require en bloc resection of the spleen along with the pancreas. The overall 5-year survival following surgical resection is 5% to 20%. For best results, surgery should be performed in high volume centres with specialist experience. In the absence of distant metastases, features which make a tumour unresectable are based on: (1) arterial involvement: tumour involvement/encasement of the superior mesenteric artery (SMA) or coeliac axis greater than 180 degrees or involvement of the first jejunal branch of SMA, (2) venous involvement: unreconstructable portal vein (PV)/superior mesenteric vein (SMV) or tumour contact with proximal jejunal branch of SMV, or (3) invasion of adjacent organs (kidney, adrenal, and colon). Tumours are considered to be borderline resectable if (1)

TABLE 24.3 TNM Staging (8th edition) Pancreatic Cancer

T: Primary Tumour

Tx Primary cannot be assessed

T0 No evidence of primary tumour

Tis Carcinoma in situ (includes PanIN I-III Classification)

T1 Tumour 2 cm or less in greatest dimension

    T1a Tumour 0.5 cm or less in greatest dimension

    T1b Tumour greater than 0.5 cm and less than 1 cm in greatest dimension

    T1c Tumour greater than 1 cm but no more than 2 cm in greatest dimension

T2 Tumour more than 2 cm but no more than 4 cm in greatest dimension

T3 Tumour more than 4 cm in greatest dimension

T4 Tumour involves coeliac axis, superior mesenteric artery and/or common hepatic artery

N: Regional Nodes

Nx Regional nodes cannot be assessed

N0 No regional lymph node metastasis

N1 Metastases in 1–3 regional lymph nodes

N2 Metastases in 4 or more regional lymph nodes

M: Distant Metastasis

M0 No distant metastasis

M1 Distant Metastasis

TNM, 8th edition, AJCC, 2017.

arterial involvement: SMA contact of 180 degrees (or less) or contact with common hepatic artery without extension to coeliac axis or hepatic artery bifurcation, (2) venous involvement: contact with the SMV or PV of more than 180 degrees but suitable vessel proximal and distal to the site of involvement allowing for safe and complete resection and vein reconstruction. Patterns of failure after surgical resection without any adjuvant therapy are well described; 50% to 85% of patients have local relapse, 25% to 35% have peritoneal recurrences and 25% to 90% have liver metastases. Tumour stage, grade and resection margin status are the best predictors for survival after potentially curative surgery.

Adjuvant Therapy

Adjuvant (postoperative) chemotherapy to reduce the risk of cancer recurrence is considered standard of care in Europe. The ESPAC-1 trial was the first study that confirmed the benefits of adjuvant chemotherapy (5-FU/FA), reporting a survival of 20.1 months (vs. 15.5 months in patients not receiving chemotherapy, $P = .0009$). The study also found adjuvant CRT to be detrimental (15.9 months vs. 17.9 months, $P = .05$). The CONKO-001 study demonstrated benefits of adjuvant gemcitabine (OS 22.8 months vs. 20.2 months, $P = .01$). The ESPAC-3 trial showed that both 5-FU/FA and gemcitabine in the adjuvant setting have similar outcomes; however gemcitabine was less toxic. The ESPAC-4 trial demonstrated OS benefit for the combination of gemcitabine and capecitabine over gemcitabine alone (28 months vs. 25.5 months, $P = .032$). (Neoptolemos et al. 2017) However, subgroup analysis shows that significant benefit is largely confined to patients who have R0 resection. More recently, a randomised phase III trial demonstrating the benefit of modified oxaliplatin, leucovorin, irinotecan and fluorouracil (mFOLFIRINOX) over single agent gemcitabine has been reported in abstract form only. (ASCO, 2018) In the Unicancer GI PRODIGE 24/CCTG PA.6 trial, 473 participants were included,

and with a median follow up of 30.5 months, the median OS was 54.4 months in the mFOLFIRINOX arm vs. 34.8 months in the gemcitabine arm (HR 0.66, 95% CI 0.49–0.89). The randomised phase III APACT study, evaluating the role of nab-paclitaxel in combination with gemcitabine in the adjuvant setting, is yet to be reported.

The standard of care in North America is postoperative adjuvant CRT with 5-FU. This was based on one randomised study by the Gastrointestinal Tumor Study Group (GITSG) in the 1980s and subsequent nonrandomised single institute prospective studies. Compared with historical controls, there seems to be a survival benefit with adjuvant chemoradiation, the overall median survival improved from 11 to 15 months to around 18 to 23 months; however, benefits of CRT over and above chemotherapy alone are not known. The ongoing Radiation Therapy Oncology Group (RTOG) 0848 trial is randomising patients to 6 cycles of adjuvant gemcitabine chemotherapy with or without consolidation of capecitabine-based CRT.

Neoadjuvant Therapy

OS in resectable pancreatic cancer remains poor, and 40% to 60% of patients have positive resection margin, with corresponding poor outcome. There has been a growing interest in the use of neoadjuvant treatment in pancreatic cancer with a view to treating micro-metastatic disease, sparing surgery in patients with bad tumour biology and reducing the risk of positive margins.

Several metaanalyses suggest that preoperative treatment may downstage locally advanced and borderline resectable tumours and improve resectability and overall survival; however down-staging a truly unresectable tumour is rare. (Zhan et al. 2017) The role of neoadjuvant treatment in resectable pancreatic cancer is not clear, and one German randomised trial closed early and failed to show any survival benefit (Golcher et al, 2015). The benefit of the neoadjuvant approach is most likely to be in the borderline resectable patients and this approach is being investigated as part of well-designed randomised clinical trials.

Management of Locally Advanced Pancreatic Cancer

Chemotherapy (see the Palliative chemotherapy section later) is considered as the standard of care for locally advanced pancreatic cancer (LAPC). Trials of upfront CRT versus chemotherapy alone have shown conflicting results and one large randomised trial of chemotherapy alone versus induction chemotherapy followed by consolidation CRT (the LAP07 study) failed to show benefit for addition of CRT, median OS being 16.5 months and 15.2 months respectively ($P = .83$). (Hammel et al. 2016) However, CRT was associated with a decrease in local progression (32% vs. 46%, $P = .03$) and no increase in grade 3–4 toxicity, except for nausea. Outside clinical trials, CRT is currently considered for patients with prominent local symptoms, or as consolidation following 4 to 6 months of chemotherapy. (Balaban et al. 2016) Where CRT is being considered, capecitabine is the preferred radio-sensitiser based on the SCALOP trial which compared radio sensitisation with capecitabine to gemcitabine (Mukherjee et al. 2013). Capecitabine is given at a dose of 830 mg/m^2 twice a day on the days of treatment. IMRT and IGRT including four-dimensional CT techniques help to optimise the tumour dose distribution while minimising the radiation dose to the normal tissue.

Stereotactic B Radiotherapy (SBRT) is being increasingly used as an alternative to CRT. Whereas previous studies using 1 to 3 fraction treatment had reported high incidence of grade 3–4 GI toxicity, a more recent study using 5-fraction regimens has reported early and late grade 3+ toxicity of 2% and 11% (Herman et al. 2015). A systemic review of 19 prospective and retrospective SBRT studies has shown 1-year survival of 51.6%, and a 1-year LC of 72.3%. (Petrelli et al. 2017)

External Beam Radiation Techniques

In patients with locally advanced pancreatic cancer, the target volumes are defined using the information from the imaging studies available (EUS, CT, PET-CT, MRI) (Fig. 24.2). IGRT (four-dimensional CT) is preferable. Gross tumour volume (GTV) is defined as tumour and any lymph nodes > 1 cm in short axis diameter (or smaller nodes that are metabolically active on PET-CT). Prophylactic nodal irradiation of noninvolved nodes is not advocated. Where four-dimensional CT is available, a composite GTV is created to account for tumour motion during multiple phases of respiration. For CRT, clinical target volume (CTV) is created by a 5-mm expansion of the GTV/composite GTV, and the CTV is then edited off the GI tract. Planning target volume (PTV): four-dimensional CT is the preferred option and when available, a 5-mm expansion around CTV defines PTV. When four-dimensional CT is not available, it is defined as CTV with a 10-mm expansion for anterior-posterior and lateral margin and a 15-mm expansion for superior-inferior margin. Intensity modulated radiotherapy is preferred, typically using 6-MV photons, to deliver 50.4 to 54 Gy in 1.8-Gy fractions.

For SBRT, four-dimensional CT, organ compression (and/or other motion management strategies including active breathing control/fiducial placement) are essential for treatment delivery. PTV is generated by direct expansion of the GTV/composite GTV by 3 to −5 mm. A typical dose-fractionation scheme is 33 to 35 Gy in 5 fractions, typically using 6-MV photons. Dose volume histograms for each of the organs at risk (liver, kidneys, GI tract, spinal cord) should be critically evaluated before accepting the final plan, in particular, the dose to the GI tract if often critical.

Palliative Chemotherapy

Single agent gemcitabine has long been the standard of care for patients with inoperable or metastatic pancreatic AC, with a median survival of about 6 months. More recently FOLFIRINOX (5-FU, FA, irinotecan, oxaliplatin) has demonstrated superior median survival in metastatic pancreatic AC (11.1 months vs. 6.8 months in the gemcitabine group, HR 0.57, $P < .001$). (Conroy et al., 2011) The combination of gemcitabine with nab-paclitaxel has also demonstrated a superior OS (8.5 months vs. 6.7 months in the gemcitabine group, HR 0.72, $P < .001$). (Von Hoff et al., 2013) However, grade 3/4 toxicity was higher with combination. Both gemcitabine/nab-paclitaxel and FOLFIRINOX are considered standard treatment options for fit patients with metastatic pancreatic cancer and many clinicians have moved to using these combinations for LAPC although there are no randomised trials in this setting.

Second-line chemotherapy:

Not many patients are suitable for second-line chemotherapy. Survival benefit from second line chemotherapy is 1 to 2 months and must be carefully weighed against toxicity and quality of life.

In patients who have received gemcitabine/gemcitabine combination, an oxaliplatin-based regimen may be appropriate. Alternatively, a combination of liposomal irinotecan with 5-FU may be used.

Supportive Care for Symptom Palliation

Endoscopic biliary stenting of a resectable pancreatic tumour for the release of jaundice is as good as surgical bypass to relieve jaundice. The duodenal obstruction can be relieved by expandable stents. Pain

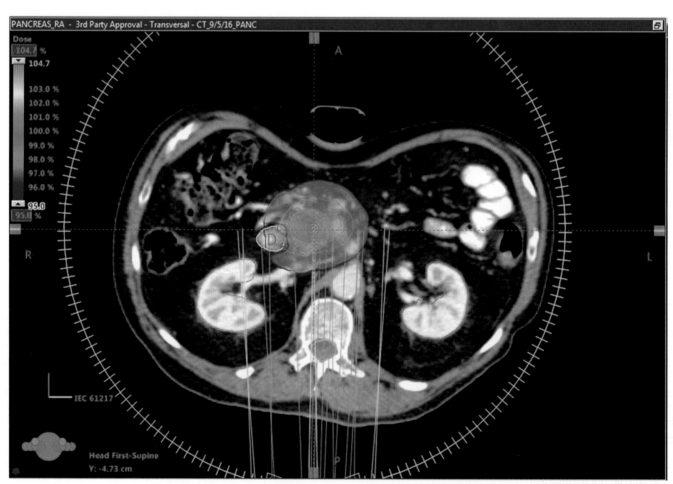

Fig. 24.2 IMRT plan for cancer head of pancreas showing duodenal sparing.

relief is important for the palliation of pancreatic cancer. Severe pain can be caused by infiltration of the coeliac plexus and this can be relieved by destruction of the plexus by an injection of alcohol which can be carried out either under x-ray control or CT guidance.

HEPATOCELLULAR CARCINOMA

Epidemiology

Hepatocellular carcinoma (HCC) is a global problem; in males it is the second cause of cancer deaths worldwide with 83% occurring in poorly developed countries. An estimated 782,500 new liver cancer cases and 745,500 deaths occurred worldwide during 2012, with China alone accounting for half of the cases. The prognosis for liver cancer is very poor (with an overall ratio of mortality to incidence of 0.95), therefore, the geographical patterns in incidence and mortality are analogous. HCC has a strong male preponderance with a ratio of male:female being 2:4 and its occurrence increases with age, reaching a peak at age 70 years.

A risk factor can be identified in 90% of HCC with the most frequent factors being chronic viral hepatitis (types B and C), cirrhosis caused by alcohol intake and aflatoxin exposure. All etiologic forms of cirrhosis are associated with increased tumour risk factors, with one-third of cirrhotic patients developing HCC during their lifetime. (Pineda et al. 2009)

Symptomatology

Because most cases occur in patients who already have chronic liver disease, often there are no specific symptoms of worsening of symptoms as a result of underlying disease. Decompensation of disease because of the presence of HCC can be seen and it can manifest with encephalopathy, variceal bleeding or ascites. There could be jaundice, ascites and bruising right upper quadrant pain, or other GI symptoms such as loss of appetite, nausea, vomiting, diarrhoea, unintentional weight loss and tiredness. Metastatic disease can also cause symptoms: bone pain for example, because of bone metastases. The physical findings usually reflect the underlying liver disease. Laboratory examination is usually nonspecific and reflects the degree of underlying cirrhosis.

Diagnostics and Classification

Noninvasive diagnosis criteria (Bruix et al. 2001) for HCC are based on a combination of imaging and laboratory findings, which are hallmarks for HCC (arterial hypervascularity and venous/late-phase washout) and depend on the nodule size. A biopsy is only required if the radiological hallmarks of HCC are not seen or systemic treatment is considered. A triphasic CT scan and/or MRI are often the initial diagnosis manoeuvre. The serum alpha-fetoprotein is often elevated in patients with HCC but does not correlate with other clinical features such as stage, size or prognosis.

Clinical staging drives treatment options for HCC and ultimately influences OS and consists of the following factors: liver function and performance status; the ability to deliver optimal liver-directed therapy; and cancer biology.

The liver function is key for deriving prognosis with Child-Pugh classification (Child and Turcotte 1964) being the most commonly used. The Child-Pugh score combines clinical findings (encephalopathy and ascites) with laboratory findings (bilirubin, albumin and prothrombin time) to classify the patients in three categories, with grade A having the more favourable outcome and considered suitable for surgery or more aggressive therapies. (Child and Turcotte 1964)

Classically, the disease has been classified using tumour numbers, size and overall disease volume as a surrogate for biology. Combining these criteria with the underlying liver function have been used to provide clinical guidance to aid treatment selection.

General Management Principles

The mainstay of therapy is surgical resection; however, the majority of patients are not eligible for surgery because HCC is diagnosed late in its course. Options of treatment are determined by both extent of tumour and the severity of underlying liver disease. The approaches of treatment in HCC are constantly evolving with new treatment and indications being adopted rapidly; however, therapeutic approaches often vary depending on the available expertise. For inoperable patients, locoregional treatments should be considered.

Surgical Therapy

Potentially curative partial hepatectomy is the preferred treatment for HCC in patients with adequate liver functional reserve. The ideal candidate for resection has a solitary HCC (≤ 5 cm) that is confined to the liver and shows no imaging evidence of invasion of the hepatic vasculature, no evidence of portal hypertension, and well-preserved hepatic function (normal bilirubin and platelet count >100,000). Long-term relapse-free survival rates average 40%, and 5-year survival rates as high as 90% are reported in selected candidates. A large number of patients are considered unresectable because of poor liver function rather than tumour size; these patients will be considered for liver transplantation. Invasion of the major portal vein, hepatic vein or adjacent organs (gallbladder) are not suitable for resection.

Liver Transplantation

Orthotopic liver transplantation (OLT) is a suitable option for patients with liver disease (usually cirrhosis) who would not tolerate liver resection, and who have a solitary HCC 5 cm (or smaller) in diameter, or up to three separate lesions, none of which is larger than 3 cm, no evidence of gross vascular invasion, and no regional nodal or distant metastases.

When these selection criteria are strictly applied, excellent overall 3- to 4-year actuarial (75%–85%) and recurrence-free survival rates (83%–92%) can be achieved, although these series represent highly selected cases.

Locoregional Treatments

Although the mainstay of therapy is surgical resection, the majority of patients are not eligible because of tumour extent or underlying liver dysfunction.

Several other treatment modalities are available, including:

1. Ablative methods: Radiofrequency ablation (RFA), microwave ablation, cryo or ethanol ablation, radiation therapy and stereotactic RT. Local ablation with radiofrequency or percutaneous ethanol injections (PEI) are considered as the standard of care for patients with BCLC-A tumours not suitable for surgery. PEI delivered with a "single-session" multipronged needle has resulted in a complete response of 80% to 90% in tumours smaller than 4 cm. RFA is the most widely used alternative to PEI. Several randomised controlled studies have shown that RFA has a better LC than PEI (2-year local recurrence rate 2%–18% vs. 11%–45%, respectively) mainly in Asian studies. The EASL guidelines (European Association for Study of, European Organisation for, and Treatment of 2012) recommend that RFA should be used in tumours smaller than 5 cm, with PEI to be used when RFA is not technically possible. For lesions less than 3 cm, away from blood vessels and ducts and BCLCO, the complete response for both RFA and PEI is greater than 90% and they are considered competitive approaches to resection. Surgery is preferred, if feasible, as the benefits of RFA over surgery have not yet been proved prospectively.

Microwave and cryoablation are still under investigation. Microwave ablation is a promising technique with encouraging response rates in tumour up to 5 cm in size.

2. Transarterial chemoembolisation (TACE) and radioembolisation.

Arterially directed therapies involve the infusion of particles via a catheter into the arterial branch of the hepatic artery, feeding the portion of the liver where the tumour is located. This is made possible by the dual blood supply to the liver and the hypervascular nature of HCC. The following arterial directed therapies are currently in use: transarterial bland embolisation (TAE), TA chemoembolisation (TACE), TACE with drug-eluting beads (DEB-TACE) and TA radioembolisation with yttrium-90 microspheres (TARE). The principles of these therapies are to cause ischaemia by eliminating or minimising the blood flow to the tumour, ultimately causing tumour necrosis.

TACE has shown survival benefit, and more than 50% of the patients achieve an objective response.

Systemic Therapy and Molecularly Targeted Agents

The results with systemic therapy in HCC are poor. The knowledge of molecular events has permitted development of targeted therapies. In 2008, sorafenib was the first agent to have been proven to improve median survival versus placebo in western patients, 10.7 versus 7.9 months and eastern populations, 6.5 versus 4.2 months. Regorafenib has also been shown to improve survival after progression on sorafenib.

Radiation Therapy

Liver-directed external beam radiation was historically limited by the lack of precise tumour imaging to target or on treatment, older RT techniques, and the inability to quantify and assess the dose received by a given volume of tissue. The entire liver was often treated with radiation, therefore, low doses of RT were used, which resulted in a low likelihood of tumour cure or control. Consequently, RT was primarily limited to the palliative setting.

The development of improved treatment planning and dose delivery methods, such as three-dimensional conformal radiation therapy and IMRT, volumetric imaging on treatment and motion management techniques provided a mechanism not only to target hepatic lesions while sparing uninvolved hepatic parenchyma but also to precisely measure the radiation dose delivered to both the tumour volume and the surrounding normal tissue. RT is not limited by the location of the lesion and can be safely delivered to lesions in a variety of locations, including in the dome of the liver.

The use of liver-directed RT significantly increased with the development of SBRT. SBRT uses multiple conformal beams to deliver high doses of RT with rapid-dose fall-off beyond the target volume (See Fig. 24.3). Although the complete mechanism underlying SBRT-induced cell death is still a topic of research, the high radiation doses in SBRT are thought to result in an ablative effect on the tumour through vascular injury, in addition to the DNA damage and cell death seen in conventionally fractionated RT. Given the highly conformal nature of SBRT, precise tumour definition and dose delivery are imperative. In addition to sophisticated treatment-planning software systems, SBRT also depends on accurate target identification, precise and reproducible patient immobilisation and assessment of target and organ motion. LC was reviewed in five studies that treated a total of 394 patients. The median follow-up was 18 months (IQ range 11–29 months). The 1-, 2-, and 3-year actuarial LC rates were 93%, 89% and 86%, respectively.

Charged particle therapies have also been employed in the treatment of hepatic tumours. Unlike photon-based RT, which has an exponential dose fall-off, particle-based therapy (such as proton therapy) has an extremely rapid dose fall-off at the end of its range. Consequently, tumours can be treated more effectively with less toxicity by charged particles than by photons, even in the cirrhotic liver with limited hepatic functional reserve. Hong et al. (2016) reported on 92 patients with unresectable HCC or intrahepatic cholangiocarcinoma (IHCC) treated with moderately hypofractionated proton therapy with larger tumours. The median tumour size was approximately 6 cm with a dose prescribed of 58 GyE in 15 fractions. After a median follow-up of 19.5 months, the 1-year LC of 97% was reported; this translated into a 22.5-month median OS. A systematic review of charged particles versus protons (Qi et al. 2015) included 73 cohorts from 70 noncomparative observational studies. Pooled OS was significantly higher at 1, 3 and 5 years for protons than for conventional RT (relative risk [RR] 1.68, 95% CI 1.22–2.31, $P < .001$; RR 3.46, 95% CI: 1.72–3.51, $P < .001$; RR 25.9, 95% CI: 1.64–408.5, $P = .02$, respectively). LC was also significantly higher for patients treated with protons than for CRT ($P = .013$ and $P < .001$, respectively).

Principles of Radiation Delivery

A. Immobilisation and motion management

In general for conformal RT and conventional fractionation a larger margin for internal target coverage is accepted and the set-up errors are usually larger to account for uncertainties in tumour localisation (Fig. 24.4). These are accepted as multiple fractions average dose errors need to consider the inaccurate organ localisation.

SBRT relies on the delivery of accurate high doses to the target and errors in localisation could result in increased normal tissue toxicity and geometric tumour miss. Therefore the use of techniques or devices to localise the radiation to the tumour, minimise margins and optimise on-treatment quality assurance is very important. Immobilisation devices are needed to ensure that patients remain in a consistent, reproducible position throughout treatment. There is no universal agreed standard for liver SBRT, but recommendations from groups with experience in SBRT are available. The primary motion with liver RT is respiratory motion which can be controlled with fixed immobilisation including abdominal compression, breath hold and/or tracking. For immobilisation, vacuum bag systems or fixed body immobilisers can be used. The AAPM suggests a cut-off of 5 mm after which respiratory management is recommended. The options can be categorised into three types: (1) nongated ITV reduction strategies, (2) active or passive breath-hold techniques, and/or (3) surrogate markers (e.g. fiducial markers or radio-opaque lipiodol). A simple margin expansion to account for ITV is then applied based on a four-dimensional CT scan, fluoroscopy and/or cine MRI to capture the full range of motion. These are categorised as ITV methods, or motion encompassing methods. An additional margin for set-up motion is added for PTV with recommendations ranging between 2 and 5 mm.

B. Localisation

At simulation, intravenous (IV) contrast is considered standard in HCC. Information from the diagnostic triphasic dynamic contrast enhanced CT is particularly useful for tumour visualisation. MRI is integral to localisation, especially in cirrhotic patients or those who are unable to tolerate IV contrast. The addition of oral contrast is useful to identify GI structures in the vicinity of the tumour.

C. Dose selection and toxicity

HCCs are radiosensitive and radiation yields excellent local tumour control rates.

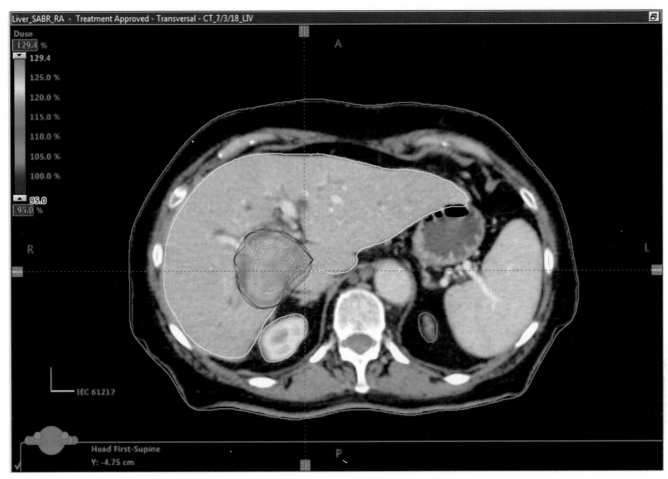

Fig. 24.3 Stereotactic Ablative Radiotherapy (SBRT) of liver tumour.

Schedules of 33 to 60 Gy in 3 to 5 fractions, biologically effective dose (BED) 60 to 180 Gy10 have been used. Actuarial local rates at 1, 2 and 3 years for lesions treated with BED of 100 Gy or less were 94%, 89% and 86%, respectively. Similar LC rates (92%, 89%, and 86%) were seen in lesions treated with BED greater than 100 Gy10 (log-rank $P = .972$) (Fig. 24.3) (Ohri et al. 2018). These suggest that there might not be a dose-response relationship within the range of reported doses. It would be reasonable to use 40 to 50 Gy in 5 fractions to achieve an LC of greater than 90% at 2 years. The normal tissue dose constraints are becoming better described as experience with SBRT is increasing.

Radiation-induced liver disease (RILD), which can present in both classic and nonclassic forms, is perhaps the most feared complication of liver irradiation; however, severe toxicity after SBRT is reported in less than 10% in Child-Pugh A patients. The risks are higher in patients with underlying cirrhosis. Predictors of toxicity to RT include baseline Child-Pugh scores and higher normal liver doses (e.g. mean dose, effective liver dose, doses to 700–900 cc) are associated with liver function decline 3 months post-SBRT. Lower baseline platelet count and portal vein thrombus were also associated with an increased risk.

Normal tissue complication probability models are now able to predict the risk of classic RILD associated with a given radiation treatment plan.

D. Treatment delivery

Daily on-line treatment verification is crucial for accurate delivery of RT. The verification should be appropriate to the type of RT delivered and equipment used. Volumetric imaging (such as on board cone-beam CT) or tracking of fiducial markers can be used. Alignment solely on bony anatomy should not be applied as it may lead to errors in set-up. Attention should be given to the organ function of the patient with assessment of status during RT.

FUTURE PERSPECTIVES

The treatment of hepatocellular carcinoma has evolved considerably in the past decade. A multidisciplinary approach and liver function optimisation in every patient have made it possible to offer an option for treatment and disease control and survival extension at any stage of presentation. Prevention is still key in this disease, therefore, promotion of a healthy lifestyle, including decreasing alcohol and prevention of metabolic syndrome are important. Sequencing and combination of locoregional treatments need to be investigated systematically in prospective trials, and combinations of locally ablative treatments with systemic treatments need to be tested. Effective adjuvant therapies are needed after curative local treatment. The incorporation of RT in standard of care with high level evidence is urgently needed.

Biliary Tract Cancers

Biliary tract cancers (BTCs) are uncommon cancers comprising cholangiocarcinoma (divided in 3 disease subtypes: intrahepatic, perihilar and extrahepatic), gallbladder and ampullary cancers. They account for around 3% of all GI cancers globally. The overall incidence of cholangiocarcinoma has increased progressively worldwide over the past four decades and increased mortality was seen in the United States and Europe, representing an area of unmet need.

The incidence of cholangiocarcinoma in England in 2013 was reported to be 1965 cases and mortality of 2161, with a total of 7606 cases diagnosed and 7743 deaths in the 2010 to 2013 period (http://www.ammf.org.uk/wp-content/uploads/2015/06/Rare_and_less_common_cancers_For-AMMF-web_0-1.pdf accessed 23/11/2017). This is the first time cholangiocarcinoma information has been reported separately from hepatocellular carcinoma (previously pooled as "liver cancer"). In 2015, Public Health England's National Cancer Intelligence Network (NCIN) reported that the 5-year survival was less than 5% and 1-year survival was less than 30% for patients diagnosed in 2008 and in 2012, respectively.

Cholangiocarcinomas are aggressive tumours. Most patients have advanced stage disease at presentation and management requires a multidisciplinary approach. Surgery is the only potentially curative treatment modality for cholangiocarcinoma, but only a minority of patients (<35%) have disease that is amenable to surgical resection with curative intent. Achieving clear resection margins is critical to a better outcome, with median disease-free survival durations of 12 to 36 months reported. An even smaller subset of patients, typically with hilar cholangiocarcinoma are candidates for liver transplantation following neoadjuvant chemoradiation. However, transplantation for cholangiocarcinoma is not available in the United Kingdom.

The current standard of care for patients with advanced disease was established by the ABC-02 trial, a combination chemotherapy with cisplatin and gemcitabine (CisGem). (Valle et al. 2010) Other treatment options include participation in a clinical trial, RT and best supportive care, as appropriate.

To date, no new agents have emerged as contenders to the CisGem chemotherapy backbone. Studies so far have mostly included patients with different anatomical and histological subtypes of disease grouped together under the broad definition of BTC by necessity (patient numbers). Targeted therapies that emerged following the publication of the International Cancer Gene Consortium data are negative to date.

Potential targeted therapies are currently undergoing investigation in the molecular pathways currently known to be activated in these cancers.

Cell metabolism: isocitrate dehydrogenase (IDH)-mutated advanced intrahepatic cholangiocarcinoma is a subgroup in whom IDH-inhibitors are being tested (e.g. dasatinib).

Currently, there are no molecular markers that are available to use for prognosis or selecting treatment, although IDH-1 and fibroblast growth factor receptor (FGFR) fusion rearrangements look like the initial most likely candidates in patients with intrahepatic cholangiocarcinomas.

The optimal strategy for patients with locally advanced/unresectable (i.e. nonmetastatic) disease has not been determined. The evidence regarding the use of RT in cholangiocarcinoma is scarce. A PRISMA systematic review of the role of RT in primary liver undertaken by Hawkins et al. in 2014 (Aitken and Hawkins 2014), concluded that: "SBRT is a promising technique in the locally advanced setting, with the dual advantages of enabling dose escalation whilst minimising time off systemic therapy and requires further investigation."

Published reports describing RT response are generally of nonrandomised, single institution experiences that are subject to selection bias. Patients with better performance status may receive higher radiation doses. Reports of patients receiving EBRT for bile duct carcinoma have suggested that doses of 40 to 45 Gy result in improved survival outcomes compared with lower doses. These data have been superseded and now doses of more than 80 Gy are recommended. Tao et al. (2016) reported a retrospective analysis of 79 patients with inoperable, locally advanced intrahepatic cholangiocarcinoma and the impact of radiation dose on outcomes. Patients treated to a biologic equivalent dose of 80.5 Gy, achieved remarkable levels of long-term LC, OS, and progression-free survival (78%, 58%, and 39%, respectively, at 3 years). Most (89%) patients had received previous systemic treatment. The median OS time after diagnosis was 30 months; 3-year OS rate was 44%. Radiation dose was the single most important prognostic factor; higher doses correlated with an improved LC rate and OS. Additionally a single-arm phase II hypofractionated proton beam study also demonstrated high LC rates in cholangiocarcinoma (2-year LC and OS rates were 94.1% and 46.5%, respectively), with minimal toxicity (7.7% grade 3).

The principles of RT delivery follow HCC principles (see previously).

In the postoperative setting, nodal positive and R1 tumours might benefit from adjuvant CRT. SWOG S0809, a phase II intergroup trial of adjuvant capecitabine and gemcitabine followed by RT and concurrent capecitabine in extrahepatic cholangiocarcinoma and gallbladder carcinoma (Ben-Josef et al. 2015) was a phase II multicentre study that met the primary objectives. A total of 79 eligible patients were treated (86% completed). For all patients, 2-year survival was 65% (95% CI, 53% to 74%); it was 67% and 60% in R0.

Principles of Radiotherapy

Delineation of the CTV should be based on review of the preoperative scans, postoperative scans, clips or markers placed by the surgeon, and surgery summary notes. Review and discussion of the targets with the surgeon is strongly recommended. CTV will include the tumour bed and retropancreatic, Coeliac and portal vein nodes with a possible boost to and areas of positive margins (best estimate). Radiation doses of 45 Gy in 25 fractions and 55 Gy in 25 fractions are delivered as a simultaneous integrated boost with concurrent capecitabine.

CANCER OF THE COLON AND RECTUM

Epidemiology

Malignancies of the colon and rectum constitute the third commonest form of cancer in the United Kingdom with an annual incidence of 41,700 new cases in 2013 to 2015 (http://www.cancerresearchuk.org/health-professional/cancer-statistics/statistics-by-cancer-type/bowel-cancer#heading-Zero). One in 14 men and 1 in 19 women will be diagnosed with bowel cancer during their lifetime. Incidence rates for bowel cancer are projected to fall by 11% in the United Kingdom between 2014 and 2035 to 74 cases per 100,000 people by 2035. In Europe, approximately 477,000 new cases of bowel cancer were estimated to have been diagnosed in 2012. The UK incidence rate is the 20th highest in Europe for males and the 17th highest for females. The age-specific incidence rises markedly over the age of 60 years, whereas less than 1% of all cases occur in patients under the age of 40 years.

Aetiology

The majority of rectal cancers develop via the chromosomal instability pathways. About 13% are caused by deficient mismatch repair (dMMR).

1. Familial clustering

    Approximately 20% of cases of colorectal cancer are associated with a familial history, and first-degree relatives of patients with invasive colorectal cancer or colorectal adenomas are at increased risk of colorectal cancer. There are well-defined inherited syndromes such as Lynch syndrome (also known as HNPCC) and familial adenomatous polyposis). It is therefore recommended that all patients with colorectal cancer to have a family history investigated and a risk assessment undertaken. A screening colonoscopy every 6 years is recommended for most individuals without a personal history of colorectal cancer and with one first-degree relative with colorectal cancer diagnosed before the age of 50 years, or two first-degree relatives with colorectal cancer diagnosed at any age (Galiatsatos and Foulkes, 2006).

2. Environmental factors

    It is likely that rectal cancer has a different aetiology than colon cancer (https://www.wcrf.org/int/research-we-fund/continuous-update-project-findings-reports/colorectal-bowel-cancer) with high body mass index, body or abdominal fatness, low levels of physical activity, metabolic syndrome and type II diabetes being seen as risk factors. Some data suggest that these are also associated with a poor prognosis. Risk is also increased by excessive consumption of meat (red or processed) and alcohol (moderate/high intake), longstanding ulcerative colitis or Crohn affecting the rectum.

Histopathology and Clinical Features

The vast majority of colorectal cancers are ACs. Macroscopically, they present as an endoluminal mass that protrude into the lumen and originate from mucosa. The mass could be exophytic or polypoid and bleeding may be seen in ulcerated, friable or necrotic lesions. They typically show glandular differentiation, mucin formation and stain positively for carcinoembryonic antigen (CEA). Small cell carcinomas, lymphomas, melanomas and adenosquamous carcinomas have been reported.

More recently, a consensus molecular subtype classification based on gene expression data, has been described (Consensus Molecular Subtypes, CMS 1–4) (Guinney et al. 2015).

Usually, patients will present with symptoms of rectal bleeding, altered bowel habits, or weight loss and are diagnosed by colonoscopy. Asymptomatic patients are diagnosed during routine screening colonoscopy or an imaging performed for other reasons. Rarely, bulky lesions may present with overt bowel obstruction.

Total mesorectal excision (TME) is the procedure used in the treatment of colorectal cancer in which a significant length of the bowel around the tumour is removed. The procedure is mainly used in mid and lower rectal tumours where it is essential to remove the rectum along with the mesorectum up to the level of the levators.

For mesorectal resections, histopathological examination should include a photographic record of the surgical specimen; assessment is a strong quality-control measure. The classification has three grades based on the completeness of the removal of the mesorectum and/or plane of surgical excision and impacts on both local recurrence and survival. The status of the circumferential resection margin (CRM) (i.e. ≤ 1 mm) and TME quality are surrogates for good oncological outcomes. At least 12 lymph nodes should be examined. The RCP minimum dataset for a colorectal surgery histopathology report should be used (https://www.rcpath.org/asset/E94CE4A2-D722-44A7-84B9D68294134CFC).

Pretreatment Staging Evaluations

The aim of pretreatment evaluation is to assess the presence or absence of distant metastatic disease (with CT chest, abdomen and pelvis, and CT-PET and or MRI [liver] as appropriate), to determine the tumour location and its local extent. An accurate assessment is necessary for rectal cancer with pelvic MRI and/or endorectal USS is required. High-quality pelvic MRI is the most accurate investigation to define locoregional clinical staging. By detecting extramural vascular invasion (EMVI), and determining the T substage and distance to the CRM, MRI can also predict the risks of local recurrence, and should be carried out in select patients for the respective preoperative management and to define the extent of surgery. A specialist and dedicated multidisciplinary team of surgeons, medical oncologist, radiation oncologist, gastroenterologist, radiologist and pathologist should discuss all relevant cases of colorectal cancer.

Staging Systems

Colon and rectal cancers are staged using the tumour, node and metastasis (TNM) staging system from the joint American Joint Committee on Cancer (AJCC)/Union for International Cancer Control (UICC); the current (8th edition, implemented in 2018) version is presented in the Table 24.4. The prefixes p and yp used in the TNM staging system denote pathologic staging and pathological staging following neoadjuvant therapy respectively.

TABLE 24.4 TNM Staging (8th edition) Colon and Rectal Cancer

T: Primary Tumour

Tx Primary cannot be assessed

T0 No evidence of primary tumour

Tis Carcinoma in situ: invasion of lamina propria

T1 Tumour invades submucosa

T2 Tumour invades muscularis propria

T3 Tumour invades subserosa or into nonperitonealised pericolic or perirectal tissue

T4 Tumour directly invades other organs or structures and/or perforates visceral peritoneum

    T4a Tumour perforates visceral peritoneum

    T4b Tumour directly invades other organs or structures

N: Regional Nodes

Nx Regional nodes cannot be assessed

N0 No regional lymph node metastasis

N1 Metastases in 1–3 regional lymph nodes

    N1a Metastasis in 1 regional lymph node

    N1b Metastasis in 2–3 regional lymph nodes

    N1c Tumour deposit(s), i.e. satellites, in the subserosa or in the nonperitonealised pericolic or perirectal soft tissue *without* regional lymph node metastasis

N2 Metastases in 4 or more regional lymph nodes

    N2a Metastasis in 4–6 regional lymph nodes

    N2b Metastasis in 7 or more regional lymph nodes

M: Distant Metastasis

M0 No distant metastasis

M1 Distant metastasis

    M1a Metastasis confined to organ (liver, lung, ovary, nonregional lymph node(s)) without peritoneal metastases

    M1b Metastasis in more than one organ

    M1c Metastasis to the peritoneum with or without other organ involvement

TNM, 8th edition, AJCC, 2017.

Colon Cancer—Treatment Principles

Surgery

Surgery is still the main treatment modality. The aim of surgery is excision of the primary tumour with wide excision margins. The tumour spreads to the lymph nodes located in the mesentery close to the vascular supply for that portion of colon. This portion of node-bearing mesentery is excised along with the bowel. Continuity of the bowel is usually re-established by a direct anastomosis, either between excised segments of colon or the colon and the terminal ileum.

Adjuvant Chemotherapy

Adjuvant chemotherapy is of proven benefit for patients with node-positive colon cancer. Six months of 5-FU and FA chemotherapy given to such patients is estimated to reduce the risk of death by 30%, which translates into a 10% to 13% absolute improvement in survival. Two randomised controlled trials have confirmed that the addition of oxaliplatin to 5-FU and FA improves 3-year survival by an additional 7%. Patients with Duke's B tumours have derived less benefit from adjuvant chemotherapy. Trials, such as the British QUASAR trial, have shown only a 3.6% increase in 5-year survival in this group of patients. However, Duke's B is a heterogeneous group of patients and multivariate analysis of patterns of relapse has shown that patients with T4 tumours, tumour perforation, lymphovascular invasion and poor differentiation are most likely to derive benefit from chemotherapy. The Xeloda in Adjuvant Colon Cancer Therapy (X-ACT) trial has shown that oral capecitabine is at least as effective as 5-FU and FA. Orally administered capecitabine is an alternative treatment for patients who may not be able to tolerate oxaliplatin-based regimens. Currently, irinotecan-based regimens have not been shown to give an advantage in an adjuvant setting, therefore are not currently recommended. A shorter course of chemotherapy (3 months) may be selected as a treatment for some patients with colon cancer. The International Duration Evaluation of Adjuvant therapy (IDEA) pooled analysis compared 3 with 6 months of adjuvant chemotherapy for stage III colon cancer. The overarching goal was to reduce chemotherapy-related toxicity, mainly oxaliplatin-induced neuropathy. Patients were classified into low-risk and high-risk groups, suggesting that low-risk patients may be offered only 3 months of treatment (Qian et al. 2017).

Management of Advanced Colorectal Cancer

The median survival for patients with metastatic colorectal cancer has improved vastly over the past few decades. Combination chemotherapy with targeted therapy has improved the median survival beyond 2 years. Patients with resectable liver metastases have an overall 5-year survival of 25% to 30% following hepatic resection and perioperative chemotherapy.

Chemotherapy for Advanced Disease

Oxaliplatin or irinotecan in combination with a fluoropyrimidines (5-FU or the oral prodrug, capecitabine) is the backbone of treatment for advanced/metastatic colorectal cancer. Given as single agent, fluoropyrimidines have a response rate in the order of 20%. The DNA topoisomerase 1 inhibitor, irinotecan, used in combination with 5-FU and FA (FOLFIRI) yields a response rate of 39%; oxaliplatin with 5-FU and FA (FOLFOX4) has a response rate of 51%, used in first-line therapy. The consecutive use of both regimens (used in either sequence) extends OS to 18 months. One Italian phase III study has shown that the chemotherapy triplet (FOLFOXIRI) to be superior to FOLFIRI in the first-line setting (22.6 months vs. 16.7 months, HR 0.7, $P = .03$) (Falcone et al., 2007). The chemotherapy triplet is currently recommended for BRAF mutant patients (who have a partticularly poor prognosis) (E. Van Cutsem et al., 2016). In clinical practice, chemotherapy is frequently combined with targeted agents, both in the first- and second-line setting.

Targeted (Biological) Therapies

Anti-VEGF therapy: Bevacizumab, which binds circulating VEGF-A, has demonstrated improved efficacy (OS, PFS, response) in combination with single agent 5-FU as well as a 5-FU-irinotecan combination (Kabbinavar et al., 2008) in combination with 5-FU-oxaliplatin; the benefit was seen in terms of PFS only (Saltz et al. 2008).

Anti-EGFR therapy: Cetuximab and panitumumab are active in combination with irinotecan-5-FU or oxaliplatin-5-FU chemotherapy in the first-line setting in patients who do not harbour *RAS* mutations (exons 3 and 4 of *KRAS,* and exons 2, 3 and 4 of *NRAS*). In *RAS* wild-type population, OS of 23 months has been demonstrated with cetuximab and FOLFIRI combination (Van Cutsem et al. 2011) and an updated analysis of the PRIME study has shown a survival benefit of combining panitumumab with FOLFOX4 (median OS 23.9 months) (Douillard et al. 2014).

Biological agents are indicated for most patients in the first-line setting unless contraindicated. An anti-EGFR therapy may be preferred in the first line (over anti-VEGF therapy) in *KRAS* wild-type patients based on the FIRE3 study which demonstrated an OS benefit for the former combination (FOLFIRI plus cetuximab, 28.7 months vs. FOLFIRI plus bevacizumab, 25 months, HR 0.77, $P = .017$) (Heinemann et al. 2014).

Biological agent combinations in second-line setting:

Where bevacizumab has not been used in first line (typically *KRAS* wild-type patients treated with FOLFIRI-cetuximab as first-line combination), it can be used in combination with FOLFOX4 in the second-line setting, because it has demonstrated OS benefit over FOLFOX4 alone (12.9 months vs. 10.8 months, HR 0.75, $P = .001$) (Giantonio et al. 2007). Where bevacizumab has been used in first line (typically in combination with FOLFOX4 for *KRAS* mutant patients), aflibercept (Van Cutsem et al. 2012) or ramucirumab (Tabernero et al. 2015) may be used in combination with FOLFIRI.

Third-Line Options

Both regorafenib and trifluridine/tipiracil are available for fit patients who have progressed on fluoropyrimidines, oxaliplatin, irinotecan, bevacizumab and in case of KRAS WT, anti-EGFR antibodies.

Radiotherapy and Colon Cancer

There are very few studies that investigated the role of CRT in colon cancer. A single phase III randomised controlled study evaluating adjuvant radiation therapy in patients with locally advanced colon cancers (T3N1, T3N2 and T4anyN) showed similar OS in patients receiving chemotherapy and radiation compared with those treated with chemotherapy alone, but with higher toxicity in patients receiving radiation therapy. Unfortunately, this study was closed because of poor accrual. There are some institutional retrospective reports suggesting a R0 resection rate of 92% to 100%, increased down staging and a possible reduction in locoregional recurrence following preoperative chemoradiotherapy. The RT doses range between 45 to 50.4 Gy in 25 to 28 fractions with concurrent fluoropyrimidines. The RT fields reflect the tumour location (e.g. sigmoid, descending/ascending colon and proximity to other normal structures). IMRT/VMAT are preferred, and daily volumetric imaging is recommended to aid localisation during treatment delivery. In the palliative setting, either a single fraction of 8 Gy or up to 30 Gy in 10 fractions may be used as a palliative procedure in colon cancer to stop bleeding and aid reduce pain; however this depends on the clinical setting.

Follow-Up

Follow-up protocols for patients with colonic cancer vary across institutions but, in all cases, the patient will undergo endoscopic examination to rule out any local recurrence or new primary lesions. Patients should also have imaging of the liver, either by CT or as part of their follow-up protocol as per NICE guidance.

Rectal Cancer—Treatment Principles

The determination of an optimal treatment plan for an individual patient with rectal cancer involves a multidisciplinary approach and incorporates patient preferences. Once the intent of the treatment has been decided (radical or palliative) the consideration of the likelihood of maintaining bowel function and preservation of genitourinary functions needs to be made.

The sequencing of multimodality therapy needs to be carefully considered especially in patients that present with synchronous metastatic disease that entertain a curative intent.

A risk-adapted approach is recommended for rectal cancer (Glynne-Jones et al. 2017).

The quality of primary surgery for rectal cancer is of key importance in reducing local recurrence rates. Historically, 5-year local recurrence rates of 20% were common, which led to an interest in offering neoadjuvant RT to reduce the risk of local recurrence.

Specialist colorectal surgeons have been trained in the technique of total mesorectal excision. This technique involves removal of the entire rectum and associated mesorectal fat and reduces the risk of local recurrence at 5 years from 20% to 6%. It has also been shown that the single most important factor for predicting disease recurrence is the circumferential resection margin. The circumferential resection margin is said to be clear if there is no evidence of tumour from either the primary site, or in an associated lymph node that extends to within 1 mm of the inked resection margin around the circumference of the excision specimen. Patients at high risk of local recurrence are typically offered long-course postoperative RT, typically a dose of 45 Gy in 25 fractions over 5 weeks.

Because TME surgery is now the gold standard for surgical excision, and recurrence rates have fallen to 5% to 6%, the role of preoperative RT has been brought into question. A recent study from The Netherlands reported after a median follow-up of just over 2 years that the local recurrence rate was 2.4% for patients who received preoperative RT before TME surgery, compared with an 8.2% recurrence rate in patients receiving no preoperative RT. The MRC CR07 study was a large prospective study in which patients with operable rectal cancers were randomised to either receive short-course preoperative RT or primary surgery followed by long-course postoperative RT if the circumferential resection margin was positive. Local recurrence after short-course RT was 4.4% at 3 years compared with 10.6% ($P < .0001$) for postoperative CRT.

Advances in pelvic imaging, specifically endoscopic ultrasound and MRI of the pelvis, can provide excellent soft tissue definition in perirectal tissues and visualise tumour penetration through the mesorectal fascia. Such patients may then be correctly selected for long-course preoperative RT, to downstage the tumour before surgery.

Patients who are offered long-course RT receive concomitant chemotherapy with either infusional 5-FU at 200 mg/m^2/day continuous schedule OR oral capecitabine, 825 mg/m^2 bid for the duration of RT. In more locally advanced tumours, neoadjuvant chemotherapy could be considered as a total neoadjuvant therapy (TNT) approach; however, there are controversies over published data and outcomes of randomised trials are still warranted. Palliative RT can be very helpful in patients with advanced rectal tumours with symptoms of bleeding or intractable pelvic pain. A short course of treatment (20–30 Gy in 5–10 fractions) is often used for such patients.

Radiotherapy Technique

Patient set-up: The patient is immobilised supine with feet and popliteal fossa support (e.g. Combifix). Ideally, the bladder should be comfortably full at the time of simulation (>150 ml) and the same instructions for bladder filling should be used during treatment as used for simulation. Anal marker can be placed at the anal verge. Intravenous contrast for visualisation of the pelvic vessels is recommended. Oral contrast does aid delineation of small bowel and can be used (e.g. gastrografin 10–20 ml in 1 litre of water taken 40–60 minutes before planning CT). CT slices should not be more that 3-mm thickness and the true pelvis should be imaged (approximately lumbar vertebrae 5 to at least 4 cm below the anal verge/or anal marker).

Rectal tumours are ideal for CT-planned conformal RT because even small reductions in target volume can significantly reduce the volume of irradiated small bowel. MRI imaging complements CT, defining further the extent of the primary tumour and any nodal spread. Oral contrast to outline the small bowel plus IV contrast to highlight vessels are strongly recommended.

Scan from L5 to 4 cm below the anal marker; recommended slice thickness is 2.5 mm or greater.

The target volume definitions are given subsequently.

GTV: Gross tumour—Primary tumour plus the regional lymph nodes thought to be involved by radiological criteria plus areas of extramural vascular invasion. All normal rectal wall between areas of macroscopic disease should be included as part of the GTV.

CTVA: GTV with a 1-cm margin in all directions; editing to remove all areas of bony structures (pelvic side wall) and muscle as anatomical barriers, sacral hollows not to be edited out.

CTVB: Elective nodal irradiation includes the mesorectal nodes within the mesorectum and presacral and internal iliac nodes (see Table 24.6 for nodal definition). An international consensus has made recommendations of nodal areas to further include depending on the tumour location and stage (Valentini et al. 2016).

CTVF (final CTV): A combination of CTVA and CTVB, modified at the clinician's discretion.

PTV: CTVF + 1-cm margin in all directions.

The anatomical boundaries for the CTVB are as follows:

Superior limit: S⅔ interspace for mid- and lower-third rectal cancers. There should be a 2-cm margin above the most superior limit of the GTV. The CTVB margin may have to extend above S⅔ to achieve this 2-cm margin from the GTV.

Inferior limit: CTVB inferior limit is 1 cm inferior to CTVA or the puborectalis muscle, if there is no involvement of the puborectalis (whichever is inferior). If there is involvement of puborectalis or sphincter or levator ani, then the lower limit for CTVB would be the ischiorectal fossa.

Lateral limit: No internal iliac node involvement—medial aspect of the obturator internus, internal iliac node involvement present—limit is bony pelvic sidewall.

Anterior limit: 1 cm anterior to the anterior mesorectal fascia or 7 mm anterior to the internal iliac artery (whichever is anterior).

Posterior limit: Anterior margin of the sacrum.

Organs at Risk

The following OARs must be delineated (RTOG normal pelvic atlas for male https://www.rtog.org/LinkClick.aspx?fileticket054g99vNGps%3d&tabid=354 and female https://www.rtog.org/LinkClick.aspx?fileticket=P5eAjYB90Ow%3d&tabid=355 provides pictorial guidance):

small bowel, bladder and right and left femoral heads. Small bowel contouring should include all individual small bowel loops to at least 20 mm above the superior extent of both PTVs. It may be helpful to initially delineate the large bowel ± endometrium to exclude these from subsequent delineation of the small bowel.

Technique and Dose

The potential benefit of IMRT in locally advanced rectal cancer is because of its highly conformal dose distribution to the PTV especially if the CTV was defined using elective nodal boundaries, allowing dose reduction to the small bowel and other organs at risk. The clinical benefit has not been validated in randomised studies; however IMRT has been adopted especially in phase I and II studies and when dose escalation is considered. In a metaanalysis of six studies including a total of 859 patients, of which 98.7% received neoadjuvant CRT, IMRT reduced grade 2 or higher acute overall GI toxicity, diarrhoea and proctitis with ORs of 0.38, 0.32 and 0.60, respectively (all $P < .05$), compared with three-dimensional CRT. IMRT also reduced acute grade 3 (or higher) proctitis compared with three-dimensional CRT (OR, 0.24; $P = .03$). No significant heterogeneity or publication bias was detected in the studies selected.

Dose. Short-course preoperative RT: 25 Gy in 5 fractions over 1 week (6–8 MV photons), 45 Gy in 25 × 1.8-Gy fractions, 5 ×/week with concurrent fluoropyrimidines.

Long-course postoperative RT: 45 to 50.4 Gy in 25 to 28 fractions over 5 weeks (68 MV photons) with concurrent IV infusional 5-FU or oral capecitabine chemotherapy.

If there is a clinical indication, such as patient wishing to avoid primary surgery, or post-TEM >50 >54 Gy in 28 to 30 fractions, ×1.8-Gy fractions, 5 ×/week is an alternative.

Palliative RT: 20 to 30 Gy in 5 to 10 fractions.

Daily volumetric imaging is recommended if IMRT is used.

Treatment toxicity. During treatment, patients may experience cystitis, proctitis and lethargy. The dose-limiting structure for long-term toxicity is the small bowel, with the associated risk of fibrosis, stricturing and obstruction. The risk of small bowel toxicity is directly related to the volume of irradiated small bowel. With careful planning, the risk of significant small bowel toxicity can be reduced to around 5%. Other long-term toxicities that need to be considered are impotence in male patients, loss of fertility and insufficiency fractures.

Follow-Up

Patients with rectal cancer require regular endoscopic follow-up to look for local recurrence and the development of new tumours. In most protocols, regular pelvic MRI combined with CT chest, abdomen and pelvis are undertaken at intervals of 3 to 6 months.

ANAL CANCER

Epidemiology and Aetiology

Anal cancer constitutes 1% of all malignancies of the bowel, with 1400 new cases being diagnosed each year in the United Kingdom (https://www.cancerresearchuk.org/health-professional/cancer-statistics/statistics-by-cancer-type/anal-cancer/incidence#heading-Zero). Anal cancer is associated with human papilloma virus (HPV) infection, a history of receptive anal intercourse or sexually transmitted disease. Immunosuppression after organ transplantation of HIV, haematologic malignancies and previous cervix malignancies are also associated with increased risk of developing the cancer; smoking also plays a role. The association with HPV type 16 and 18 (HPV-16, HPV-18) infections is especially strong.

High-grade anal intraepithelial neoplasia (AIN) is associated with HPV infections and is thought to be a precursor for invasive carcinomas; the treatment of high-grade AIN might prevent the development of anal cancer. HPV immunisation uses the 4-valent of 9-valent vaccine in boys and girls and one of the goals of vaccination is cancer prevention.

Anatomy

The anus is defined as extending from the rectum to the skin of the perianal region. The superior margin is the palpable upper border of the anal sphincter and puborectalis muscle. Inferiorly, it extends to skin within a 5-cm radius of the anal verge.

There is a transition in the histological type of epithelium lining the anus. Perianal skin is squamous epithelium, which turns to a transitional type epithelium at the dentate line, and then into the glandular mucosal lining of the rectum.

The anus has a dense lymphatic supply via three main routes. The upper canal drains to perirectal and superior hemorrhoidal nodes. The area round the dentate line drains to hypogastric and obturator nodes. The anal verge and perianal skin drains to superficial inguinal nodes.

Histopathology

Approximately 80% of anal tumours are SCCs (Fig. 24.3). The recognised subtypes are keratinising large cell, nonkeratinising (transitional cell) and basaloid. ACs occur in 10% of cases, and tend to arise from the glandular mucosa of the upper anal canal. Other tumour types include lymphomas, melanomas, small cell carcinomas and sarcomas.

Clinical Features

The symptoms often are nonspecific and common symptoms include anal pain and bleeding, pruritus, a mass in the anal region or discharge. Occasionally, tumours may affect the sphincter mechanism and cause incontinence. On examination, patients may present with ulcerated or exophytic lesions, and inguinal lymphadenopathy may be present. Associated features, such as anal warts or leucoplakia, may be present. Inguinal lymph node metastases are noted in 15% of patients and surgical series show that pelvic nodal spread is present in about 30% of patients at presentation. Systemic metastatic spread is observed in less than 5% of patients at the time of initial diagnosis. Increasing tumour size and depth of penetration into the anal wall increase the risk of nodal metastases.

Diagnostic Work-Up and Staging

Patents are staged using the UICC/AJCC staging scheme (See Table 24.5). Full history digital rectal and physical examination including risk factor assessment is followed by an examination under anaesthetic to assess the extent of the tumour and to obtain a biopsy for histological confirmation of the diagnosis. One third of patients present with enlarged inguinal lymph nodes. These should always be biopsied, as 50% of enlarged lymph nodes are reactive, usually caused by infection associated with the primary tumour. MRI of the pelvis provides improved soft tissue definition of the primary tumour and pelvic lymph nodes. CT scan of the chest, abdomen and pelvis completes the staging. PET scanning has been reported to be useful in the evaluation of pelvic lymph nodes, even in patients who have normal lymph nodes on CT imaging. A metaanalysis of 17 clinical studies calculated the pooled specificity and sensitivity for detection of lymph node involvement by PET CT at 93% and 76%, respectively. The use of PET CT can either downstage/upstage the patients and has produced treatment plan modifications between 12% and 59% of patients by either changes in radiation dose or fields. However, the PET CT is not considered a replacement for pelvic MRI and CT. Gynaecologic examination

TABLE 24.5 Staging

TNM Staging (8th Edition) Anal Canal Cancer

T: Primary Tumour

Tx Primary cannot be assessed

T0 No evidence of primary tumour

Tis Carcinoma in situ, Bowen disease, high-grade squamous intraepithelial lesion (HSIL), anal intraepithelial neoplasia II–III (AIN II–III)

T1 Tumour 2 cm or less in greatest dimension

T2 Tumour more than 2 cm but no more than 5 cm in greatest dimension

T3 Tumour more than 5 cm in greatest dimension

T4 Tumour of any size invades adjacent organ(s), e.g. vagina, urethra, bladder

N: Regional Nodes

Nx Regional nodes cannot be assessed

N0 No regional lymph node metastasis

N1 Metastases in regional lymph node(s)

  N1a Metastases in inguinal, mesorectal and/or internal iliac nodes

  N1b Metastases in external iliac nodes

  N1c Metastases in external iliac and in inguinal, mesorectal and/or internal iliac nodes

M: Distant Metastasis

M0 No distant metastasis

M1 Distant metastasis

TNM, 8th edition, AJCC, 2017.

including colposcopy is suggested for female patients because of the association of the anal cancer and HPV.

HIV testing on patients should be undertaken if the status is unknown, as patients with undiagnosed HIV and low CD4 counts and tend to tolerate chemoradiation poorly.

Treatment

Definitive Chemoradiation

Three trials performed between 1987 and 1994 determined concurrent mitomycin C (MMC), 5-FU and RT (MF-CRT) as the standard of care. ACT1 was performed in the United Kingdom and randomised 585 patients to RT alone or MF-CRT, and significantly reduced LRF from 59% to 36%. This benefit was maintained after a median follow-up of 13 years, with a significant reduction in the risk of relapse or death.

A parallel European Organisation for Research and Treatment of Cancer (EORTC) trial of 110 patients with locally advanced disease also showed a significant reduction in the risk of LRF. A RTOG trial ($n = 310$) demonstrated a significant reduction in LRF colostomy-free survival with MF-CRT compared with 5-FU and RT (F-CRT). All trials used crude RT schedules and a significant treatment gap between the first phase of RT and a subsequent boost.

Three further phase III trials were performed between 1998 and 2008. The RTOG 9811 trial (Ajani et al. 2008; Gunderson et al. 2013) of 641 patients found that neoadjuvant and concomitant cisplatin 5-FU resulted in inferior LRF, colostomy-free survival (CFS) and OS when compared with MF-CRT. In the United Kingdom, the largest trial, ACT2 (James et al. 2013) enrolled 940 patients and used a two-phase RT schedule. There was no evidence of a difference in the complete response rate for concurrent cisplatin compared with mitomycin C, and no improvement in PFS with the addition of two cycles of maintenance 5-FU cisplatin. Subset analysis did not show any benefit in subsets based on established prognostic factors. However, the cancer outcomes were improved compared with ACT1 and the continuous RT schedule may have contributed to this finding. The ACCORD 03 trial enrolled 307 patients and showed no benefit from the addition of neoadjuvant cisplatin 5-FU chemotherapy. It also compared two doses of boost (15 vs. 20–25 Gy) after whole pelvic irradiation. A nonsignificant 5% improvement in LC was seen, although one-third of patients had early stage disease. These three trials did not demonstrate any benefit from the use of cisplatin concurrently, neoadjuvantly or as adjuvant therapy.

Radiotherapy Treatment Principles (Fig. 24.4)

The RT techniques used in previous phase III trials were relatively simple and resulted in substantial irradiation of the surrounding normal tissues (Fig. 24.4). ACT2 used a shrinking field technique, treating the whole pelvis with 30.6 Gy, followed by a reduced treatment volume to all sites of macroscopic disease, giving 19.8 Gy using a generous margin and without a planned gap in treatment. Significant improvement in RT treatment can be achieved with the use of IMRT. This also allows the use of altered doses to the gross tumour volume and sparing of normal tissues. The use of IMRT in future trials is supported by the RTOG 0529 single arm phase II trial led by Kachnic et al. (2013). In the United Kingdom, we have developed guidance for the multicentre introduction of IMRT (Muirhead et al. 2014) www.analimrtguidance.co.uk and many UK centres have now implemented IMRT in routine clinical practice. Although long-term effects are not yet fully characterised, IMRT has been increasingly adopted by the radiation oncology community and should no longer be considered investigational for the treatment of anal cancer.

Target volume—external beam radiotherapy. The CTV includes the primary tumour, first station nodes (pararectal, hypogastric and obturator nodes) and presacral and internal iliac nodes. In patients with positive inguinal nodes, the inguinal nodal areas must also be included in the treatment field.

Patient simulation and immobilisation. Patients are positioned supine with immobilisation for popliteal fossa or feet, a comfortably full bladder, and the use of IV contrast to aid delineation of pelvic vessels is indicated.

Before pretreatment scan, the clinician will assess the diagnostic imaging and ascertain whether the primary tumour is adequately bolused by the surrounding buttocks, that is, 5 mm of tissue surrounding main tumour, and consideration of tailored wax or sheet bolus should be given. The distal point of macroscopic disease or anal verge should be delineated with a radio-opaque marker before imaging, whichever is more inferior. All patients must be scanned with a comfortably full bladder using a local bladder-filling protocol.

Target definition. The primary tumour should be visualised with the aid of the diagnostic MRI and CT. A 10- to 15-mm margin to the gross tumour should be considered depending on the stage.

The elective nodes (Table 24.6) should include inguinal, mesorectum nodes, internal and external iliacs and presacral space. If the tumour stage is early and there are no mesorectal nodes, only the lower 50 mm of the mesorectum should be irradiated.

For organs at risk, see guidance for rectal cancer; in addition, consider defining the external genitalia. For male genitalia, it should include the penis and scrotum out laterally to the inguinal creases. In woman, it should include the clitoris, labia majora and minora, out to the inguinal creases. Superior border in both sexes should lie midway through the symphysis pubis.

Online volumetric imaging should be performed days 1 to 5 and weekly thereafter, as a minimum.

The optimal dose and schedule for anal cancer is still under evaluation. The dose recommended for the elective nodes is 40 Gy in 28

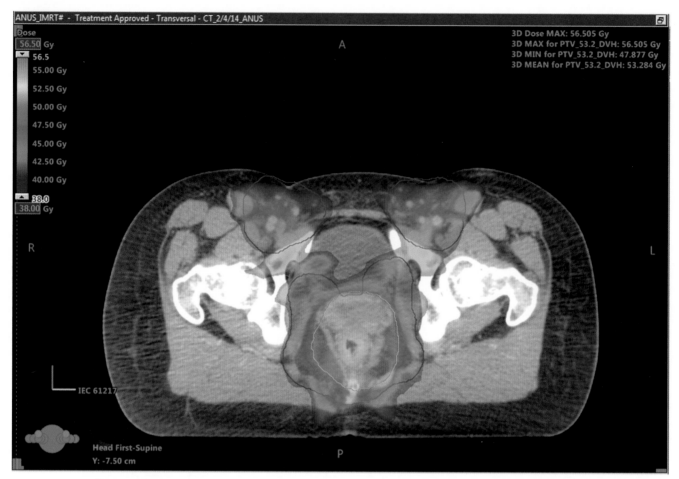

Fig. 24.4 IMRT plan for locally advanced anal cancer showing showing dose painted primary tumour and regional nodes.

fractions over 5.5 weeks; however, a minimum dose of 30.6 Gy in 1.8-Gy per fraction to 36 Gy for negative nodes is acceptable, with tumour and involved nodes receiving doses between 50.4 and 53.2 Gy in 28 fractions over 5.5 weeks.

Systemic chemotherapy should be prescribed concurrently in all patients that are considered fit for standard treatment.

Accepted regimens are:
- Mitomycin, 12 mg/m^2 on day 1 with 5-FU 1000 mg/m^2 on days 1 to 4 and 29 to 32.
- Mitomycin, 12 mg/m^2 on day 1 with capecitabine 825 mg/m^2 bd on days of RT.

Dose reductions in fluoropyrimidines should be considered if patients are elderly or the renal function is impaired.

Treatment-Related Toxicity

In general, IMRT treatments are well tolerated with patients rarely needing admission for symptom control or skin toxicity. Female patients should be considered for vaginal dilators and counselled about vaginal stenosis and infertility risk.

Follow-Up

Assessing the response to primary CRT: A clinical assessment of response by physical examination is typically performed from 6 to 8 weeks following the completion of therapy. There is considerable controversy regarding the optimal time to assess response posttreatment.

SCCs regress slowly and continue to decrease in size for up to 26 weeks following therapy. For patients with a clinical complete response, re-evaluation every 3 to 6 months with DRE, anoscopy and inguinal node palpation is recommended for 5 years. Based upon the results from the ACT II trial, patients with persistent disease can be watched for up to 6 months following completion of treatment as long as there is no progressive disease during this period of follow-up.

Role of Surgery

Surgical therapy is reserved for patients with recurrent or persistent disease after CRT. Although prognosis is poor overall, an APR offers the potential for long-term survival.

Recurrent disease: Post-CRT, local recurrences can be successfully salvaged with surgery, but locally recurrent anal SCC can be a difficult clinical problem that is associated with profound morbidity and long-term disease control in about 25% to 40% of cases.

Palliative Treatment

Metastatic disease after locoregional treatment may develop in 10% to 20% of patients. The most common site for spread is liver; however, lung, bone, lymph nodes and skin metastases have been reported. Cisplatin- and fluoropyrimidine-based chemotherapy produces response rates of around 50% with a median survival of 12 months. Palliative RT can be offered for patients with symptomatic nodal, bone or skin metastases.

TABLE 24.6 Anatomical Boundaries for Pelvic Lymph Nodes

	Superior	Inferior	Lateral	Medial	Anterior	Posterior
Internal iliac nodes	20 mm above the inferior aspect of sacroiliac joint or 15 mm above the most anterior site of gross tumour, whichever is most superior.	The point of levator ani insertion into the obturator fascia and obturator internus.	In the upper pelvis, the iliopsoas muscle. In the lower pelvis, the obturator internus muscle.	In the upper pelvis, 7 mm medial to internal iliac vessels. In the lower pelvis, the mesorectum and presacral space.	In the upper pelvis, 7 mm anterior to the internal iliac vessels. In the lower pelvis, the obturator internus muscle or bone.	The bony pelvis.
External iliac nodes	See superior border of internal iliac.	The inguinal lymph nodes.	The iliopsoas muscle.	In the upper pelvis, 7 mm medial to the external iliac vessels. In the lower pelvis 10 mm inside the bladder or small bowel.	7 mm anterior to the external iliac vessels encompassing all visible benign lymph nodes.	The internal iliac lymph node group.
Inguinal nodes	The external iliac nodal group.	At the inferior slice demonstrating the lesser trochanter.	The medial edge of sartorius or iliopsoas.	To include all visible lymph nodes or lymphocoeles. The spermatic cord in men. The medial third to half of the pectineus or adductor longus muscle in women.	Approximately 5 mm in from the skin surface.	The pectineus, adductor longus and iliopsoas.
Mesorectal nodes	The level of the recto-sigmoid junction, best identified where the superior rectal artery turns anteriorly.	The ano-rectal junction approximately where the levator ani inserts into the sphincter complex.	The medial edges of the mesorectal fascia and levator ani.		10 mm anterior to the mesorectum into the anterior organs. (Penile bulb/prostate and seminal vesicles/bladder in males; bladder/vagina/cervix and uterus in females.)	The sacrum or coccyx
Presacral nodes	See superior border of internal iliac.	The edge of the coccyx.	Sacroiliac joints.		10 mm anterior to the anterior sacral border encompassing any lymph nodes or presacral vessels.	The sacrum
Obturator nodes	Superiorly 3–5 mm above the obturator canal where the obturator artery is sometimes visible.	The obturator canal where the obturator artery has exited the pelvis.	The obturator internus muscle.	Medial: 10 mm into the bladder.	The anterior extent of the obturator internus muscle.	The internal iliac lymph node group.

Prognosis

Male sex and positive lymph nodes are independent prognostic factors for higher locoregional failure, anal cancer death and lower survival in both United Kingdom and United States multivariate analysis. P16 positivity and or HPV negativity are an independent prognostic factor for OS.

Gastrointestinal Stromal Tumours

Gastrointestinal stromal tumours (GISTS) are the most common mesenchymal tumours of the GI tract. However, they are rare tumours and account for less than 3% of all GI tumours and 5% of all soft tissue sarcomas. GISTS are defined as c-KIT-positive mesenchymal tumours arising from anywhere in the GI tract or abdomen. The median age at presentation is around 60 years. GISTS are uncommon before the age of 40 years and extremely rare in children. They occur equally in both males and females. The most common site is stomach (60%–70%) followed by small bowel (20%–30%). GISTS are thought to arise from the precursors of the interstitial cells of Cajal (ICC), the pacemaker cells which initiate and control peristalsis. Mutations within the KIT and PDGFRA genes are common and have prognostic and predictive value.

GISTS can present as incidental masses in the abdomen. The common presenting complaints include GI bleeding (50%), abdominal pain (20% to 50%) and feeling of a mass. The most frequent sites of metastases are liver (65%) and omentum (often without ascites) (21%). Risk stratification for relapse is assessed using tumour site, size and mitotic index.

In view of the rarity of GISTS, they should be managed by an experienced multidisciplinary team within a specialist cancer centre. Surgery remains the primary treatment for operable tumours. The response rates to chemotherapy are very low. The systemic treatment has been revolutionised by the discovery of KIT tyrosine kinase inhibitor, imatinib, which is effective in 85% of the patients with metastatic GISTS. Sunitnib, another multitargeted tyrosine kinase inhibitor is licensed for second-line use in patients who have progressed or are intolerant to imatinib. Imatinib has been shown to improve both the progression free and OS in the adjuvant setting in resected high-risk GISTS.

REFERENCES (OESOPHAGOGASTRIC)

Al-Batran S-E, Homann N, Schmalenberg H, Kopp H-G, Haag GM, Luley KB, et al. Perioperative chemotherapy with docetaxel, oxaliplatin, and fluorouracil/leucovorin (FLOT) versus epirubicin, cisplatin, and fluorouracil or capecitabine (ECF/ECX) for resectable gastric or gastroesophageal junction (GEJ) adenocarcinoma (FLOT4-AIO): a multicenter, randomized phase 3 trial. J Clin Oncol 2017;35(15_suppl):4004. 4004.

Alderson D, Cunningham D, Nankivell M, Blazeby JM, Griffin SM, Crellin A, et al. Neoadjuvant cisplatin and fluorouracil versus epirubicin, cisplatin, and capecitabine followed by resection in patients with oesophageal adenocarcinoma (UK MRC OE05): an open-label, randomised phase 3 trial. Lancet Oncol. 2017;18(9):1249–1260.

Bang Y-J, Van Cutsem E, Feyereislova A, Chung HC, Shen L, Sawaki A, et al. Trastuzumab in combination with chemotherapy versus chemotherapy alone for treatment of HER2-positive advanced gastric or gastro-oesophageal junction cancer (ToGA): a phase 3, open-label, randomised controlled trial. Lancet 2010;376(9742):687–97.

Crosby T, Hurt CN, Falk S, Gollins S, Mukherjee S, Staffurth J, et al. Chemoradiotherapy with or without cetuximab in patients with oesophageal cancer (SCOPE1): a multicentre, phase 2/3 randomised trial. Lancet Oncol 2013;14(7).

Cunningham D, Starling N, Rao S, Iveson T, Nicolson M, Coxon F, et al. Upper Gastrointestinal Clinical Studies Group of the National Cancer Research Institute of the United Kingdom. Capecitabine and oxaliplatin for advanced esophagogastric cancer. N Engl J Med 2008;358(1):36–46. https://doi.org/10.1056/NEJMoa073149.

Ford HER, Marshall A, Bridgewater JA, Janowitz T, Coxon FY, Wadsley J, et al. COUGAR-02 Investigators. Docetaxel versus active symptom control for refractory oesophagogastric adenocarcinoma (COUGAR-02): an open-label, phase 3 randomised controlled trial. Lancet Oncol 2014;15(1):78–86.

Secrier ML, De Silva N, Eldridge MD, Contino G, Bornschein J, et al. Mutational signatures in esophageal adenocarcinoma define etiologically distinct subgroups with therapeutic relevance on behalf of the Oesophageal Cancer Clinical and Molecular Stratification (OCCAMS) Consortium 13 Europe PMC Funders Group. Nat Genet 2016;48(10):1131–41.

van Hagen P, Hulshof MCCM, van Lanschot JJB, Steyerberg EW, Henegouwen M van B, Wijnhoven BPL, et al. Preoperative chemoradiotherapy for esophageal or junctional cancer. N Engl J Med 2012;366(22):2074–84.

REFERENCES (PANCREAS)

Bailey P, Chang DK, Nones K, Johns AL, Patch AM, Gingras MC, et al. Genomic analyses identify molecular subtypes of pancreatic cancer. Nature 2016;531 (7592):47–52.

Balaban EP, Mangu PB, Khorana AA, Shah MA, Mukherjee S, Crane CH, et al. Locally advanced, unresectable pancreatic cancer: American Society of Clinical Oncology clinical practice guideline. J Clin Oncol 2016;34(22).

Conroy T, Ychou M, Bouché O, Guimbaud R, Bécouarn Y, Adenis A, et al. Folfirinox versus gemcitabine for metastatic pancreatic cancer. N Engl J Med 2011;364.

Ghaneh P, Hanson R, Titman A, Lancaster G, Plumpton C, Lloyd-Williams H, et al. PET-PANC: multicentre prospective diagnostic accuracy and health economic analysis study of the impact of combined modality 18fluorine-2-fluoro-2-deoxy-d-glucose positron emission tomography with computed tomography scanning in the diagnosis and management of pancreatic cancer. Health Technol Assess 2018;22(7):1–114.

Golcher H, Brunner TB, Witzigmann H, Marti L, Bechstein W-O, Bruns C, et al. Neoadjuvant chemoradiation therapy with gemcitabine/cisplatin and surgery versus immediate surgery in resectable pancreatic cancer. Results of the first prospective randomized phase II trial. Strahlenther Onkol 2015;191:7–16.

Hammel P, Huguet F, Van Laethem JL, Goldstein D, Glimelius B, Artru P, et al. Effect of chemoradiotherapy vs chemotherapy on survival in patients with locally advanced pancreatic cancer controlled after 4 months of gemcitabine with or without erlotinib the LAP07 randomized clinical trial. JAMA 2016;315(17):1844–53.

Herman JM, Chang DT, Goodman KA, Dholakia AS, Raman SP, Hacker-Prietz A, et al. Phase 2 multi-institutional trial evaluating gemcitabine and stereotactic body radiotherapy for patients with locally advanced unresectable pancreatic adenocarcinoma. Cancer 2015;121(7):1128–37.

Mukherjee S, Hurt CN, Bridgewater J, Falk S, Cummins S, Wasan H, et al. Gemcitabine-based or capecitabine-based chemoradiotherapy for locally advanced pancreatic cancer (SCALOP): a multicentre, randomised, phase 2 trial. Lancet Oncol 2013;14(4).

Neoptolemos JP, Palmer DH, Ghaneh P, Psarelli EE, Valle JW, Halloran CM, et al. Comparison of adjuvant gemcitabine and capecitabine with gemcitabine monotherapy in patients with resected pancreatic cancer (ESPAC-4): a multicentre, open-label, randomised, phase 3 trial. Lancet 2017;389(10073):1011–24.

Petrelli F, Comito T, Ghidini A, Torri V, Scorsetti M, Barni S. Stereotactic body radiation therapy for locally advanced pancreatic cancer: a systematic review and pooled analysis of 19 trials. Int J Radiat Oncol Biol Phys 2017;97 (2):313–22.

Von Hoff DD, Ervin T, Arena FP, Chiorean EG, Infante J, Moore M, et al. increased survival in pancreatic cancer with nab-paclitaxel plus gemcitabine. N Engl J Med 2013;369(18):1691–703.

Zhan H-X, Xu J-W, Wu D, Wu Z-Y, Wang L, Hu S-Y, et al. Neoadjuvant therapy in pancreatic cancer: a systematic review and metaanalysis of prospective studies. Cancer Med. https://doi.org/10.1002/cam4.1071.

REFERENCES (HEPATO-BILIARY, COLO-RECTAL AND ANAL CANCER)

Aitken KL, Hawkins MA. The role of radiotherapy and chemoradiation in the management of primary liver tumours. Clin Oncol (R Coll Radiol) 2014;26(9):569–80.

Ajani JA, Winter KA, Gunderson LL, Pedersen J, Benson 3rd AB, Thomas Jr CR, Mayer RJ, Haddock MG, Rich TA, Willett C. Fluorouracil, mitomycin, and radiotherapy vs fluorouracil, cisplatin, and radiotherapy for carcinoma of the anal canal: a randomized controlled trial. JAMA 2008;299:1914–21.

Ben-Josef E, Guthrie KA, El-Khoueiry AB, Corless CL, Zalupski MM, Lowy AM, Thomas Jr CR, Alberts SR, Dawson LA, Micetich KC, Thomas MB, Siegel AB, Blanke CD. SWOG S0809: a phase II intergroup trial of adjuvant capecitabine and gemcitabine followed by radiotherapy and concurrent capecitabine in extrahepatic cholangiocarcinoma and gallbladder carcinoma. J Clin Oncol 2015;33:2617–22.

Bruix J, Sherman M, Llovet M, Beaugrand M, LencioniR, Burroughs AK, Christensen E, Pagliaro L, Colombo M, Rodes J, Easl Panel of Experts on

HCC. Clinical management of hepatocellular carcinoma. Conclusions of the Barcelona-2000 EASL conference. European Association for the Study of the Liver. J Hepatol 2001;35:421–30.

Child CG, Turcotte JG. Surgery and portal hypertension. Major Probl Clin Surg 1964;1:1–85.

European Association for Study of, Liver, Research European Organisation for, and Cancer Treatment of. EASL-EORTC clinical practice guidelines: management of hepatocellular carcinoma. Eur J Cancer 2012;48:599–641.

Galiatsatos P, Foulkes WD. Familial adenomatous polyposis. Am J Gastroenterol 2006;101:385–98.

Glynne-Jones RL, Wyrwicz E, Tiret G, Brown C, Rodel A, Cervantes D, et al. Esmo Guidelines Committee. Rectal cancer: ESMO clinical practice guidelines for diagnosis, treatment and follow-up. Ann Oncol 2017;28: iv22–40.

Gunderson LLJ, Moughan JA, Ajani JE, Pedersen KA, Winter AB, Benson CR, Thomas RJ, Mayer MG, Haddock TA, Rich, Willett CG. Rich, and. Willett, CG. Anal carcinoma: impact of TNM category of disease on survival, disease relapse, and colostomy failure in US Gastrointestinal Intergroup RTOG 98-11 phase 3 trial. Int J Radiat Oncol Biol Phys 2013;87:638–45.

Hong TS, J Y, Wo BY, Yeap E, Ben-Josef EI, McDonnell LS, Blaszkowsky EL, Kwak JN, Allen JW, Clark L, Goyal JE, Murphy MM, Javle JA, Wolfgang LC, Drapek RS, Arellano HJ, Mamon JT, Mullen SS, Yoon KK, Tanabe CR, Ferrone DP, Ryan TF, DeLaney CH, Crane, Zhu AX. Multi-institutional phase II study of high-dose hypofractionated proton beam therapy in patients with localized, unresectable hepatocellular carcinoma and intrahepatic cholangiocarcinoma. J Clin Oncol 2016;34:460–8.

James RD, Glynne-Jones HM, Meadows D, Cunningham AS, Myint MP, Saunders T, Maughan A, McDonald S, Essapen M, Leslie S, Falk C, Wilson S, Gollins R, Begum J, Ledermann L, Kadalayil, Sebag-Montefiore D. Mitomycin or cisplatin chemoradiation with or without maintenance chemotherapy for treatment of squamous-cell carcinoma of the anus (ACT II): a randomised, phase 3, open-label, 2 × 2 factorial trial. Lancet Oncol 2013;14:516–24.

Jankowski JAZ, de Caestecker J, Love SB, et al. Esomeprazole and aspirin in Barrett's oesophagus (AspECT): a randomised factorial trial. Lancet. 2018 Aug 4;392(10145):400–8. Epub 2018 Jul 26.

Kachnic LA, Winter K, Myerson RJ, Goodyear MD, Willins J, Esthappan J, Haddock MG, Rotman M, Parikh PJ, Safran H, Willett CG. RTOG 0529: a phase 2 evaluation of dose-painted intensity modulated radiation therapy in combination with 5-fluorouracil and mitomycin-C for the reduction of acute morbidity in carcinoma of the anal canal. Int J Radiat Oncol Biol Phys 2013;86:27–33.

Muirhead R, Adams RA, Gilbert DC, Glynne-Jones R, Harrison M, Sebag-Montefiore M, et al. Anal cancer: developing an intensity-modulated radiotherapy solution for ACT2 fractionation. Clin Oncol (R Coll Radiol) 2014;26:720–1.

Ohri N, Tome WA, Mendez Romero A, Miften M, Ten Haken RK, Dawson LA, et al. Local control after stereotactic body radiation therapy for liver tumors. Int J Radiat Oncol Biol Phys 2018;.

Pineda JA, Aguilar-Guisado M, Rivero A, Giron-Gonzalez JA, Ruiz-Morales J, Merino D, Rios-Villegas MJ, Macias J, Lopez-Cortes LF, Camacho A, Merchante N, Del Valle J. Infecciosas Grupo para el Estudio de las Hepatitis Viricas de la Sociedad Andaluza de Enfermedades. Natural history of compensated hepatitis C virus-related cirrhosis in HIV-infected patients. Clin Infect Dis 2009;49:1274–82.

Qi WX, Fu S, Zhang Q, Guo XM. Charged particle therapy versus photon therapy for patients with hepatocellular carcinoma: a systematic review and meta-analysis. Radiother Oncol 2015;114:289–95.

Qian S, Sobrero A, Shields AF, Kerr R, Iveson T. Prospective pooled analysis of six phase III trials investigating duration of adjuvant (adjuv) oxaliplatin-based therapy (3 vs 6 months) for patients (pts) with stage III colon cancer (CC): the IDEA (International Duration Evaluation of Adjuvant chemotherapy) collaboration. Chicago: J Clin Oncol; 2017.

Tao R, Krishnan S, Bhosale PR, Javle MM, Aloia TA, Shroff RT, Kaseb AO, Bishop AJ, Swanick CW, Koay EJ, Thames HD, Hong TS, Das P, Crane CH. Ablative radiotherapy doses lead to a substantial prolongation of survival in patients with inoperable intrahepatic cholangiocarcinoma: a retrospective dose response analysis. J Clin Oncol 2016;34:219–26.

Valentini V, Gambacorta MA, Barbaro B, Chiloiro G, Coco C, Das P, Fanfani F, Joye I, Kachnic L, Maingon P, Marijnen C, Ngan S, Haustermans K. International consensus guidelines on clinical target volume delineation in rectal cancer. Radiother Oncol 2016;120:195–201.

Valle J, Wasan H, Palmer DH, Cunningham D, Anthoney A, Maraveyas A, Madhusudan S, Iveson T, Hughes S, Pereira SP, Roughton M, Bridgewater J, Trial Investigators ABC. Cisplatin plus gemcitabine versus gemcitabine for biliary tract cancer. N Engl J Med 2010;362:1273–81.

25

Tumours of the Thorax

Michael Snee

CHAPTER OUTLINE

LUNG CANCER

Lung cancer is the second most common cancer in the United Kingdom and because of the high mortality rate is the most common cause of death from cancer with 35,895 deaths in 2014 (Cancer Research UK). Most of these deaths are preventable because smoking causes around 85% of cases.

As a result of the long induction period from exposure to carcinogen until the development of cancer, the incidence of lung cancer today reflects smoking habits of the population in previous decades. The incidence of lung cancer in men in Britain has been falling since 1990 but is rising in women because they took up smoking later than men. Similarly the incidence of cancer in the undeveloped countries continues to rise in parallel with the increasing prevalence of smoking. Other proven causes of lung cancer include ionising irradiation and asbestos. Exposure to diesel fumes and a diet low in fruit and vegetables are probable causes of lung cancer.

However, only 10% to 15% of smokers eventually develop lung cancer. There is probably interplay between genetic susceptibility of the disease and exposure to carcinogens.

Pathology

There are three main types of lung cancer, with the percentage of cases in the United States in the years 2010 to 2014 shown in parentheses: small cell (13%), adenocarcinoma (47%) and squamous carcinoma (23%); the latter two grouped together with other less common lung cancers such as large cell carcinoma (1.6%), and adenoid cystic carcinoma in the term, nonsmall cell lung cancer (NSCLC) (National Cancer Institute). However, with the development of new noncytotoxic cancer treatments directed against specific molecular targets, the genetic type of cancer and whether it expresses the programmed death ligand is becoming much more important than the morphology of lung cancer. The incidence of squamous and small cell lung cancer (SCLC) is falling and that of adenocarcinoma is rising. Mesothelioma, a cancer of the pleura, which is almost always caused by exposure to asbestos, is increasing in incidence, again reflecting the induction period from exposure to the development of disease.

Symptoms

Primary

Lung cancer is often advanced by the time patients develop symptoms because these are predominantly because of proximal spread to the mediastinum, causing central chest pain, dysphagia and hoarseness (attributed to compression of the oesophagus and recurrent laryngeal nerve, respectively) or growth into a main or lobar bronchus causing cough, haemoptysis, breathlessness and infection. A pleural or pericardial effusion may also cause dyspnoea. Direct extension into the chest wall causes pain. If the tumour is in the apex of the lung and infiltrates into the brachial plexus, Pancoast syndrome develops. This results in pain or sensory loss of the C7/8 T1 dermatomes and wasting of the small muscles of the hand.

Secondary Spread

Unfortunately, up to 25% of patients present with symptoms of metastatic disease beyond the thorax. Common sites of metastases are bone (producing pain), brain (producing fits, headaches and hemiparesis), liver and adrenals.

Paraneoplastic Syndromes

Tumours may produce proteins that have hormonal activity producing various biochemical abnormalities. Recognised syndromes include hyponatremia secondary to antidiuretic hormone secretion (almost always produced by small cell carcinoma), hypercalcaemia as a result of parathyroid hormone like protein (almost always produced by squamous cell carcinoma) and Cushing syndrome as a result of adrenocorticotropic hormone (ACTH). Antigens expressed by the tumour may lead to cross-tissue reactivity and syndromes suggestive of autoimmune disease.

Diagnosis and Staging

Patients presenting with the above symptoms require a clinical examination, particularly focusing on the chest, including palpation of the supraclavicular fossa, which is a common site for lymph node metastases. Investigation then proceeds with a full blood count and biochemical tests of renal and liver function. Thereafter, radiology includes a chest x-ray and a computed tomography (CT) scan of the chest and upper abdomen. This latter examination provides the stage and will, in most cases, demonstrate the site, which can most easily be biopsied to confirm the diagnosis. If the tumour is seen to involve a lobar bronchus, bronchoscopy may be required whereas if metastases are identified then it is often advisable to biopsy one of the affected organs to confirm both the diagnosis and stage of the cancer. If the only site of disease is the periphery of the lung, a CT-guided biopsy is required for pathological diagnosis. However, this test is associated with a small risk of pneumothorax and haemoptysis, which rarely can be fatal. Therefore, if the patient has poor pulmonary function such that performing a biopsy poses an unacceptable risk to the patient or the lesion is inaccessible to biopsy, a clinical diagnosis based on imaging is acceptable.

Patients who have no evidence of metastases beyond the chest need further staging before undergoing curative treatment (surgery or radiotherapy (RT)). In most cases, a positron emission tomography (PET) scan is required. The basis of PET scanning is the increased metabolic activity of cancer which avidly takes up glucose. Following administration of 18-fluorodeoxy-D-glucose (^{18}F-FDG), there is emission of positrons from tumour-bearing areas. The PET scan is usually combined with a CT scan taken on a hybrid machine, a PET/CT scanner, so that the areas of high uptake can be coregistered with the anatomy provided by the CT. Lesions that have PET activity equal to or less than the mediastinal blood pool are deemed negative and those with higher activity, positive. PET scanning will demonstrate metastases that were not previously identified in up to 20% of cases of confirmed lung cancer. In a patient with a small peripheral lesion, PET can help characterise the lesion; malignant lesions tend to be positive, and benign negative. Algorithms have been developed to estimate the probability of malignancy based on patient demographics, growth, PET and CT characteristics. The PET scan is also useful for demonstrating spread to local lymph nodes in the hilum and mediastinum. However, such PET abnormalities should usually be confirmed, if possible, by ultrasound guided biopsy, either by a bronchoscope or oesophagoscope, as benign conditions such as sarcoidosis and infection can produce significant ^{18}F-FDG uptake in lymph nodes. Fig. 25.1 shows the CT and PET scans of a patient with early stage lung cancer and Fig. 25.2 shows a patient with mediastinal nodal involvement that was confirmed by Endobronchial Ultrasound (EBUS).

If diagnostic material is not obtained by endoscopy, then the mediastinal lymph nodes can be surgically sampled by mediastinoscopy. In this procedure a small incision is made above the suprasternal notch and the mediastinoscope is carefully inserted by dissection in front of the trachea and lymph nodes are removed for pathological examination. Magnetic resonance imaging (MRI) can be used in specific situations such as Pancoast tumours to determine the extent of invasion of adjacent structures such as vertebrae or the neurovascular bundle that would determine the extent of surgery. MRI is the best test for demonstrating brain metastases and should be performed if the patient has demonstrated spread to the lymph nodes and is being considered for curative treatment. In most patients with signs or symptoms of spread to the brain, a contrast enhanced CT is adequate to confirm the diagnosis, although if the examination is equivocal and/or the patient is being considered for ablative therapy to the brain, an MRI should be performed.

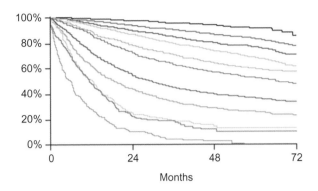

Proposed	Events / N	MST	24 Month	60 Month
IA1	68 / 781	NR	97%	92%
IA2	505 / 3105	NR	94%	83%
IA3	546 / 2417	NR	90%	77%
IB	560 / 1928	NR	87%	68%
IIA	215 / 585	NR	79%	60%
IIB	605 / 1453	66.0	72%	53%
IIIA	2052 / 3200	29.3	55%	36%
IIIB	1551 / 2140	19.0	44%	26%
IIIC	831 / 986	12.6	24%	13%
IVA	336 / 484	11.5	23%	10%
IVB	328 / 398	6.0	10%	0%

Fig. 25.1 Survival by tumour stage for Non Small Cell Lung Cancer (NSCLC).

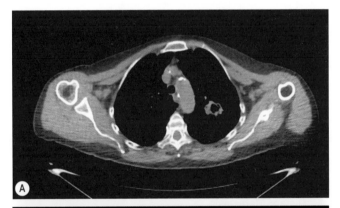

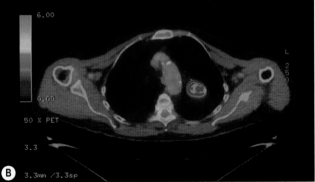

Fig. 25.2 CT scan (A) and PET scan (B) of patient with a carcinoma of left upper lobe.

Staging

The NSCLC staging system is based on the TNM (tumour, node, metastases) scheme and divides patients into prognostic groups for treatment.

The eighth edition of this classification is shown in Table 25.1 and the survival by stage of NSCLC in Fig. 25.3 which illustrates the major impact stage has on outcome.

Screening

Because of the poor prognosis of lung cancer, mainly as a result of the advanced stage at presentation, screening has been proposed to reduce the mortality of lung cancer. Using a chest x-ray to detect lung cancer before it produces symptoms has proved unsuccessful. However, a large North American trial involving over 50,000 subjects aged 55 to 74 years, with a significant smoking history, showed that screening with CT both reduced mortality from lung cancer and overall mortality. This latter finding is extremely important and is unique in cancer screening where studies of other sites have only shown a reduction in cancer-specific mortality. A reduction in overall mortality is the gold standard for the evaluation of a screening program as it excludes a significant detriment from overdiagnosis. That is, detecting cancers that would never produce illness during the patient's lifetime and diagnosing these asymptomatic cancers would merely expose the subject to the hazards of treatment such as surgery, RT and chemotherapy, without any improvement in survival. Despite the incontrovertible evidence of benefit, at the time of writing, screening for lung cancer has not been introduced in the United Kingdom.

TABLE 25.1   TNM Staging Classification (8th Edition)

Proposed T, N and M Descriptors for the 8th Edition of TNM Classification for Lung Cancer

T: Primary Tumour

Tx Primary tumour cannot be assessed or tumour proven by presence of malignant cells in sputum or bronchial washings but not visualised by imaging or bronchoscopy

T0 No evidence of primary tumour

T1s Carcinoma in situ

T1 Tumour ≤ 3 cm in greatest dimension surrounded by lung or visceral pleura without bronchoscopic evidence of invasion more proximal than the lobar bronchus (i.e. not in the main bronchus)[a]

    T1a (mi) Minimally invasive adenocarcinoma[b]

    T1a Tumour ≤ 1 cm in greatest dimension[a]

    T1b Tumour >1 cm but ≤ 2 cm in greatest dimension[a]

    T1c Tumour >2 cm but ≤ 3 cm or in greatest dimension[a]

T2 Tumour >3 cm but ≤ 5 cm or tumour with any of the following features[c]:

    – Involves main branchus regardless of distance from the carina but without involvement of the carina

    – Invades visceral pleura

    – Associated with atelectasis or obstructive pneumonitis that extends to the hilar region, involving part or all of the lung

    T2a Tumour >3 cm but ≤ 4 cm in greatest dimension

    T2b Tumour >4 cm but ≤ 5 cm in greatest dimension

T3 Tumour >5 cm but ≤ 7 cm in greatest dimension or associated with separate tumour nodule(s) in the same lobe as the primary tumour or directly invades any of the following structures: chest wall (including the parietal pleura and superior sulcus tumours), phrenic nerve, parietal pericardium

T4 Tumour >7 cm in greatest dimension or associated with separate tumour nodule(s) in a different ipsilateral lobe than that of the primary tumour or invades any of the following structures: diaphragm, mediastinum, heart, great vessels, trachea, recurrent laryngeal nerve, oesophagus, vertebral body, and carina

N: Regional Lymph Node Involvement

Nx Regional lymph nodes cannot be assessed

N0 No regional lymph node metastasis

N1 Metastasis in ipsilateral peribronchial and/or ipsilateral hilar lymph nodes and intrapulmonary nodes, including involvement by direct extension

N2 Metastasis in ipsilateral mediastinal and/or subcarinal lymph node(s)

N3 Metastasis in contralateral mediastinal, contralateral hilar, ipsilateral or contralateral scalene or supraclavicular lymph node(s)

M: Distant Metastasis

M0 No distant metastasis

M1 Distant metastasis present

    M1a Separate tumour nodule(s) in a contralateral lobe; tumour with pleural or pericardial nodul(s) or malignant pleural or pericardial effusion[d]

    M1b Single extrathoracic metastasis[e]

    M1c Multiple extrathoracic metastases in one or more organs

[a]The uncommon superficial spreading tumour of any size with its invasive component limited to the bronchial wall, which may extend proximal to the main bronchus, is also classified as T1a.

[b]Solitary adenocarcinoma ≤ 3 cm with a predominantly lepidic pattern and ≤ 5 mm invasion in any one focus.

[c]T2 tumours with these features are classified as T2a if ≤ 4 cm in greatest dimension or if size cannot be determined and T2b if >4 cm but ≤ 5 cm in greatest dimension.

[d]Most pleural (pericardial) effusions with lung cancer are as a result of tumour. In a few patients, however, multiple microscopic examinations of pleural (pericardial) fluid are negative for tumour and the fluid is nonbloody and not an exudate. When these elements and clinical judgment dictate that the effusion is not related to the tumour, the effusion should be excluded as a staging descriptor.

[e]This includes involvement of a single distant (nonregional) lymph node.

Source: Goldstraw, P., Chansky, K., Crowley, J., Rami-Porta, R., Asamura, H., et al. (2016). The IASLC lung cancer staging project: Proposals for revision of the TNM stage groupings in the forthcoming (eighth) edition of the TNM classification for lung cancer. *Journal of Thoracic Oncology*, 11(1), 39–51.

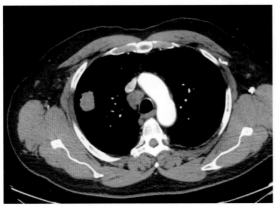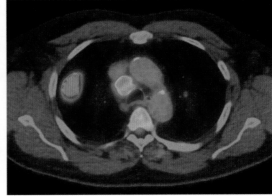

Fig. 25.3 CT scan and PET scan of a patient with a carcinoma of right upper lobe and spread to the mediastinum.

Management of Nonsmall Cell Lung Cancer

Curative Treatment

. *Surgery.* In patients with early stage disease (I and II) surgery is usually offered. However, this is associated with significant risks to the patient with an overall 90-day mortality of 3% and depending on pulmonary reserve and the extent of surgery, a long-term risk of dyspnoea. The mortality and morbidity increase sharply in patients with impaired cardiopulmonary reserve. Therefore, before surgery the patient requires careful assessment with cardiopulmonary function (e.g. spirometry, measurement of transfer factor, echocardiography) and if these tests are significantly below normal (typically <40% predicted), a cardiopulmonary exercise test is advised before proceeding with thoracotomy. The most common operation is lobectomy with pneumonectomy being performed in less than 10% of patients because of the high mortality (≤8%) and risk of disabling breathlessness following surgery. Procedures removing less than the lobe such as segmentectomy or wedge resection can be considered in patients with poor pulmonary function, but these operations are associated with higher rate of local recurrence than full lobectomy.

Radical radiotherapy. RT is used to cure patients where surgery is contraindicated because of local spread (e.g. infiltration of mediastinum, trachea or great blood vessels) and/or the patient is not fit for surgery because of comorbidity. Thoracic RT is particularly challenging because the tumour is a moving target within an area surrounded by critical and radiosensitive tissues, such as lung parenchyma, heart and spinal cord. In addition, because of the low electron density of lung, the planning system must be able to accurately model photon absorption both within the lung and at air tissue interfaces to ensure the tumour is not underdosed or surrounding critical normal organs are not overdosed. However, in recent years two developments have enabled RT to be planned and delivered more accurately and precisely. Firstly, four-dimensional CT scanning enables tumour motion because of respiration and heartbeat to be measured and allowed for in the planning process. A four-dimensional CT combines a conventional CT simulator with a device to measure the movement of the patient's chest so that the CT images taken whilst the patient breathes normally can be sorted into several (typically 10) bins conforming to various phases of the respiratory cycle from full inspiration through to full expiration. Secondly, modern linear accelerators are equipped with on-board cone beam CT including four-dimensional CT so that the tumour can be accurately imaged with the patient in the treatment position, and if necessary, adjustments made before RT is delivered.

Technique. Patients should be CT planned, lying supine, arms abducted and elbows flexed in an immobilisation device that incorporates hand bars for the patient to grip. To ensure consistency of position and patient comfort, a vac bag is used in most centres, combined with lateral and sagittal lasers aligned with tattoos to ensure a consistent position between planning and treatment and minimise movement in all planes as well as rotation between fractions. If the patient is unable to abduct their arms, or in the case of an apical (Pancoast) tumour, then consistency of position is achieved with the aid of an Orfit shell. The patient is usually instructed to breathe normally. In some centres, breath hold techniques and/or abdominal compression are used to reduce respiratory motion, but many patients, particularly those with pulmonary diseases, which often co-exist with lung cancer, are unable to do this.

A four-dimensional CT scan is performed from the level of the larynx to the bottom of L2. Contrast is used for central tumours to accurately contour lymph nodes and normal structures such as heart and blood vessels. If there is collapse or consolidation of the whole or part of the lung, contrast can help delineate tumour from uninflated lung. The tumour, including any spread to contiguous hilar lymph nodes, is carefully delineated on the mid-respiration phase (usually 40% exhale) to produce an internal target volume (ITV). This is then reviewed on all phases of respiration (usually 10 studies from full inspiration to full expiration) to ensure that the tumour and its movement is encompassed by the ITV. Lymph nodes deemed not to be involved with tumour are not contoured or treated, as this increases the ITV and thus side effects without any long-term benefit. The ITV is then expanded usually by 5 to 8 mm in all directions to allow for microscopic spread of the cancer to produce a clinical target volume (CTV). If mediastinal lymph nodes are deemed to be involved, then the adjacent mediastinal envelope in the lateral direction is included in the CTV. A combined CTV encompassing both tumour and lymph node is then manually edited to conform to areas where the tumour abuts tissue planes such as pleura or bone, as generally microscopic spread does not occur beyond such planes. The CTV is then expanded by an appropriate margin depending on the individual centre's protocol for managing day-to-day movement of patients (typically this is 5 mm in all directions) to produce a PTV. Finally, normal structures such as lungs, spinal cord, heart and oesophagus are contoured to calculate the dose to these organs. It is vital that patients receiving radical RT undergo regular onboard imaging during the course of RT. For stereotactic ablative radiotherapy (SABR), this is performed before each fraction and in cases where respiratory motion is large, a four-dimensional cone beam CT is invaluable to ensure treatment is delivered accurately. For

TABLE 25.2   Planning Dose Constraints for Stereotactic Ablative Radiotherapy

Planning Dose Constraints

OAR	Volume (cm³)	3# Tolerance	3# Minor Deviation	5# Tolerance	5# Minor Deviation	8# Tolerance	8# Minor Deviation
Spinal cord[a]	0.01	18 Gy	18–22 Gy	25 Gy	25–28 Gy	25 Gy	25–28 Gy
Oesophagus[a]	0.1	24 Gy	24–27 Gy	27 Gy	27–28.5 Gy	27 Gy	27–28.5 Gy
Brachial plexus[a]	0.1	24 Gy	24–26 Gy	27 Gy	27–29 Gy	27 Gy	27–29 Gy
Heart[a]	0.1	24 Gy	24–26 Gy	27 Gy	27–29 Gy	50 Gy	50–60 Gy
Trachea, bronchus[a]	0.1	30 Gy	30–32 Gy	32 Gy	32–35 Gy	32 Gy	32–35 Gy
Lungs-GTV		V20 < 10%	N/A	V20 < 10%	N/A	V20 < 10%	N/A
		V12.5 < 15%		V12.5 < 15%		V12.5 < 15%	

[a]Taken from ROSEL study.
GTV, Gross tumour volume; *Gy*, gray; *OAR*, Organs at risk.
Reproduced by kind permission of UK SABR consortium.

conventional RT, imaging needs to be individualised depending on the location of the tumour and adjacent critical organs. If there is significant collapse of all or part of the lung, then imaging should be performed before each fraction as the lung can re-expand in response to therapy in which case replanning is usually required.

Planning. The best dose distribution, that is, good coverage of the tumour with the lowest dose to critical normal organs, is obtained by employing intensity-modulated RT (IMRT). This requires careful contouring of normal organs and complex planning software that can both accurately model electron transfer and optimise the dose distribution to ensure the PTV is not underdosed and normal organs not overdosed. However in the specialised situation of SABR, significant inhomogeneity is allowed within the PTV with hot spots up to 140% being acceptable, although normal tissue tolerances must not be exceeded; otherwise serious or even fatal side effects can result. Various techniques of IMRT are used, including step and shoot, or more commonly, arc therapy, where the output and shape of the beam are continually modulated as the treatment head rotates around the patient. The beam energy is usually 6 MV or less to reduce the effect of secondary buildup at the lung tumour interface. Generally, two dosage protocols are used depending on the indication for RT. If the patient has a peripheral tumour less than 5 cm and is unable to have surgery because of cardiac or respiratory comorbidity, then SABR is used to deliver treatment using large fractions of radiation. In this technique, a continuous arc or up to 8 beams are used to deliver the prescribed dose to an isodose encompassing the tumour. The common dose prescriptions and normal tissue tolerances are shown in Table 25.2. These doses are highly potent (in excess of 100 gray (Gy) given in 2 Gy per fraction) and meticulous planning and treatment setup are vital to avoid toxicity. Recent studies have shown that SABR is superior to conventionally fractionated RT in terms of side effects, and in one study, local control. However, at present, state of knowledge SABR cannot be used for central tumours that arise in or are close to lobar bronchi and/or are in close proximity to major blood vessels and heart, as the doses used in SABR can result in severe morbidity that can be fatal. Thus, for central tumours, an IMRT technique is used to deliver conventionally fractionated (2–2.75 Gy per fraction) RT. If the patient has involvement of lymph nodes, then this is often combined with the concurrent administration of chemotherapy. Treatment plans for early and late stage lung cancer are shown in Figs 25.4 and 25.5 (these are the same patients shown in Figs 25.1 and 25.2).

Combined treatment chemoradiation. In cases of locally advanced NSCLC, that is, with spread to lymph nodes or other central structures such as mediastinum or great blood vessels, then combining chemotherapy concurrently with the delivery of radiation produces superior survival results compared with giving treatments sequentially. However, concurrent chemoradiation produces significant morbidity and an overall mortality rate of 3%, and therefore should only be used in patients of good performance status (0 or 1) and adequate organ (particularly heart and lung) function. The drugs used are usually cisplatin and etoposide as these drugs can be given at full doses with radical (60 Gy or more) radiation. Carboplatin can be used either as a single agent or combined with paclitaxel (in NSCLC), as a less toxic alternative to cisplatin, but the evidence of benefit is not as convincing as for cisplatin.

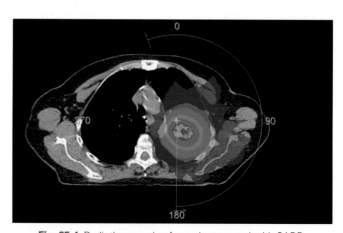

Fig. 25.4 Radiotherapy plan for patient treated with SABR.

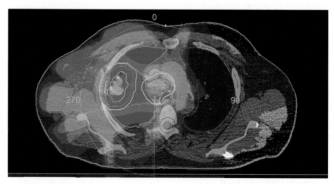

Fig. 25.5 Radiotherapy plan for patient with chemo-radiation.

Combined modality treatment

Surgery, radiotherapy and chemotherapy. For selected cases, there is some evidence that a combined approach of surgery and RT and chemotherapy (trimodality therapy) is best. This can be given electively when RT, usually with concurrent chemotherapy, is delivered before surgery in cases of locally advanced lung cancer with either spread to the mediastinal lymph nodes or adjacent soft tissue as in Pancoast tumours. This approach is associated with significant postoperative mortality and requires close cooperation with the operative and oncology teams to ensure that only suitable patients are treated and that the treatment program is delivered without unplanned gaps. In this regime two cycles of chemotherapy are combined with a course of RT at a subradical dose of 45 Gy in 25 fractions and surgery performed within 3 to 5 weeks of completion of radiation.

Adjuvant therapy. In cases where the resected tumour is found on postoperative histology to have spread to the lymph nodes, adjuvant platinum-based chemotherapy is offered with the aim of sterilising occult metastatic disease. However, the overall benefit is relatively small with an improvement in 5-year survival of less than 5%, and side effects are significant. Postoperative RT is considered if the tumour was thought to be incompletely resected either by the surgeon or the pathologist. The evidence of benefit for postoperative RT is limited and it should never be used without careful selection, as a meta-analysis of clinical trials (albeit using obsolete techniques and in unselected patients) showed an excess mortality of up to 20% for postoperative RT. Therefore postoperative treatment requires careful planning to ensure the dose to the remaining lung is kept to a minimum. The placement of clips by the surgeon at sites where the cancer is seen invading structures beyond the limit of resection can help define the clinical target volume.

Tolerances. In the thorax, the radiotherapist is confronted with several critical organs that can be affected by radiation with serious, sometimes fatal, consequences including the lungs, heart, oesophagus, spinal cord and brachial plexus along with a cancer that requires a high dose to be sterilised. Specific tolerances have been developed by empirical study over many years, and in particular, the heart is now considered a critical structure where excess radiation has been associated with early death following thoracic RT. The tolerances for the various organs, with the commonly used RT doses used for curative treatment are given in Box 25.1. These planning doses are a guide and it is important to remember that patients with pulmonary disease will have reduced tolerance. However, consistent information of the interplay of patient factors, that is, preexisting cardiopulmonary function with radiation, is somewhat sparse and inconsistent. However, patients with impaired performance status (2 or worse) should generally not be given concurrent chemoradiation and those with impaired pulmonary function indices (spirometry and transfer factor) of less than 40% of normal, corrected for age and sex, and particularly those with pulmonary fibrosis, should only be treated after careful consideration. Full information about the possible consequences (particularly breathlessness and death) of radiation should be provided. Patients will usually opt for treatment, despite the risks, as the outlook for even early-stage untreated lung cancer is very poor.

Doses. There is no good evidence that for conventionally fractionated radiation, a dose in excess of 60 Gy (or equivalent) given as a sole modality or combined with chemotherapy is beneficial to patients. This does not mean that most lung cancers are sterilised with 60 Gy but simply that controlled trials of doses greater than 60 Gy have either shown no benefit or in some cases, actual inferior results, probably due the higher dose producing greater mortality. This is not true for the hypofractionated regimes used in SABR where doses in excess of 100 Gy can be safely delivered.

BOX 25.1 Planning Dose Constraints for Radical Radiotherapy Conventionally Fractionated, Total Dose 60–66 Gy in 30–33 Fractions or 55 Gy in 20 Fractions

Lung

These constraints are a guide, and important clinical considerations should be taken into account such as pulmonary function and alternative forms of treatment.

Mean Lung Dose

>20 Gy (considered unacceptable), 18–20 Gy high risk of pneumonitis, 15–18 Gy moderate risk, <15 Gy low risk.

DV 20 Gy (% volume of lung minus PTV receiving 20 Gy)

>40% very high risk of pneumonitis only acceptable with specific consent, 35%–40% very high risk, 30%–35% high risk, 20%–30% moderate risk, <20% low risk.

Oesophagus

No more than 12 cm should receive total dose.

Spinal Cord

60–66 Gy @ 2 Gy per fraction: 50 Gy @2 Gy per fraction up to 54 Gy is deemed acceptable if the tumour is close to cord and the patient at risk of spinal cord compression if treatment fails.

55 Gy @ 2.75 Gy per fraction: 42 Gy, 50 Gy is deemed acceptable if the tumour is close to cord and the patient at risk of spinal cord compression if treatment fails.

Brachial Plexus

No more than 0.5 cc, should receive 60 Gy for 60–66 Gy in 30–33 fractions or 53 Gy for 55 Gy in 20 fractions.

Heart

No more than one-third should receive total dose.

However, the studies that evaluated 60 Gy often employed dose prescriptions that did not correct for the reduced electron density within the lung or used what now would be considered obsolete planning systems. Therefore, the dose actually delivered may well have been considerably greater than 60 Gy and so many centres will prescribe 66 Gy in 33 fractions to allow for this factor. In the United Kingdom, a commonly used dose for radical treatment of lung is 55 Gy in 20 fractions. A continuous hyperfractionated accelerated radiotherapy (CHART) dose of 54 Gy in 3 daily fractions delivered (without a break) over 12 days showed superiority over 60 Gy in 30 daily fractions and is still used in some centres. However, because of the increasing use of SABR for small peripheral cancers and chemoradition for large central tumours, plus the logistical difficulties of delivering RT during weekends, the CHART scheme is being employed less frequently.

Acute reactions. General fatigue and oesophagitis are common. Oesophagitis is managed with antacids (sometimes combined with a local anesthetic) and analgesics; soluble paracetamol is used initially, but there should be a low tolerance for administering opiates to maintain hydration and nutrition. Patients should be advised to adopt a bland diet avoiding extremes of temperature. In severe cases, meals may have to be liquidised and oral nutritional supplements prescribed; in such cases a dietician can be very helpful. With conventionally fractionated RT, significant skin reactions are rare. However, palliative RT and some SABR plans will give an appreciable dose to the skin resulting in erythema and indeed in some cases moist desquamations. The radiation plan should be reviewed before treatment and patients warned about the possibility of radiation dermatitis and instructed on appropriate skin care.

Late reactions. Some degree of pneumonitis and fibrosis is an inevitable consequence of radical RT, and it is important that other specialists are aware of this complication because it can be radiologically misdiagnosed as local recurrence. The severity of this side effect depends on radiation and patient factors as mentioned above. It is important that patients and their medical attendants are also aware that this complication can develop in the months following RT to ensure that early and aggressive treatment is given. Patients present with dry cough, fever and shortness of breath. A chest x-ray may show a hazy appearance in the irradiated area. Therapy is supportive, including oxygen and high-dose steroids. Although there is no evidence of benefit, antibiotics are also often coprescribed. There is no satisfactory treatment for neurological complications of RT and every effort should be made (even in the case of palliative RT) to avoid exceeding the radiation tolerance of the spinal cord and brachial plexus. Oesophageal stricture and pericardial effusion are seen in the longer term, but with modern RT planning these problems should occur in less than 5% of patients. Long-term cardiac morbidity and mortality is the subject of active research and it is now clear that radiation-induced cardiac dysfunction can be misdiagnosed as pneumonitis and may be responsible for excess mortality in the year following radical RT. Treatment is again supportive with the prescription of medication for cardiac failure.

Palliative radiotherapy. Patients who are not candidates for radical treatment by virtue of advanced stage of disease or poor performance status can benefit from palliative RT. The extent of the tumour and symptoms determine the treatment volume. Generally, large fields are used for palliation to encompass the tumour and adjacent areas of likely spread/subclinical extension to avoid marginal recurrence or the need for retreatment during the patient's lifetime. However, it is acceptable to treat part of the gross tumour to avoid significant toxicity (particularly oesophgitis), especially in a patient with poor performance status. Thus in a patient with a peripheral primary and mediastinal disease, radiation is usually directed solely at the latter site. The patient is simulated and treated supine, usually hands by side; however in cases where the tumour extends to the chest wall, one or both arms need to be abducted out of the fields. Simple parallel field arrangements are used, but the tolerance of the spinal cord must not be exceeded, as some patients can survive long enough to be at risk of radiation myelitis. Therefore, oblique fields and/or shielding may be required, which can also be employed to reduce the dose to the oesophagus and lung parenchyma. It is often helpful to delineate a gross tumour volume, expand this by 1.5 cm in all directions, and then utilise isocentric fields to encompass this volume, and where possible shield normal tissue. Field sizes of up to 15×10 cm are typically used, but no more than 10 cm of oesophagus should receive the prescribed dose to avoid inducing severe and prolonged dysphagia. The doses used for palliative treatment were established by a series of British Medical Research Council (MRC) trials published between 1991 and 1996 that also produced evidence of the effectiveness of palliative RT for the common symptoms of lung cancer: haemoptysis will be relieved in most (up to 90%) patients, and cough and pain will improve in over half of patients treated. The doses employed are 10 Gy single fraction (for patients of poor performance status), 17 Gy in 2 fractions a week apart, 20 Gy in 5 fractions or 36–39 Gy in 12 or 13 fractions, depending on the extent of both intra- and extra-thoracic disease. For fit patients, even those with advanced disease, a higher dose improves survival at the cost of increased side effects, particularly oesophagitis.

Other than a single fraction of 10 Gy and 20 Gy fractionated, all these doses exceed cord tolerance. In the modern era, it unacceptable to subject patients to the risk of developing radiation myelitis, so every department should have in place protocols to limit the dose to the cord. This may require formal CT planning, particularly if doses in excess of 30 Gy are employed. Retreatment is challenging as usually the spinal cord will have previously received a dose close to tolerance. However, if oblique fields can be employed to avoid the spinal cord, palliative doses up to 30 Gy can be delivered. A review of seven studies involving a total of 159 patients suggests similar levels of palliation as reported in first-line studies can be achieved.

Bone metastases. Bone pain and pathological fracture are common complications of lung cancer. An 8-Gy single fraction delivered in a parallel pair or direct field can improve pain.

Brain metastases. Brain metastases are common in lung cancer with up to half of patients with advanced disease developing intracerebral disease, and as a consequence, suffering from the disabling symptoms of headache, ataxia, hemiparesis and fits. Dexamethasone is used to reduce cerebral oedema and improvement in symptoms is often seen within a few days. A large clinical trial has shown that the addition of palliative whole brain irradiation to steroid therapy is of no benefit. However, patients of good performance status, with disease controlled elsewhere and limited volume of disease, can be treated with ablative therapy, which has been shown, in contradistinction to whole brain radiation, to improve quality of life. Surgery or radiosurgery (using the gamma knife or specially adapted linear accelerator) can be used to ablate brain metastases. Generally, up to three metastases can be treated in one session with low morbidity, and because of the noninvasive nature and day case administration, this form of RT is increasingly being preferred over surgery. The value of adjuvant whole brain RT (30 Gy in 10 fractions) following ablative treatment to treat microscopic disease is being increasingly questioned as to whether this prophylactic therapy reduces the rate of intracranial relapse because no overall survival benefit is found and radiation-induced lethargy, alopecia and cognitive impairment are significant side effects. Therefore the practice of many centres is to monitor patients following ablative therapy with three monthly MRI scans and offer further ablative therapy to new metastases as they arise.

Systemic Treatment for Nonsmall Cell Lung Cancer

Three types of systemic treatment can be offered to patients of good performance status with advanced (stage III and IV) NSCLC: chemotherapy, targeted therapy and immune therapy.

Chemotherapy

It is now firmly established that the quality and quantity of life of patients with metastatic NSCLC may be improved by the judicious use of a platinum agent combined with one other drug: gemcitabine, paclitaxel, docetaxel or vinorelbine (doublets). A metaanalysis has shown a modest increase in survival of 3 months with platinum doublets compared with best supportive care. Clinical trials have shown that overall, for all types of NSCLC combined, no particular doublet was superior, with response rates of around 25%, a similar median survival of 8 to 10 months and 1-year survival of 30% to 40%. A metaanalysis showed cisplatin doublets produced a statistically significant better response rate and marginally better survival when compared with carboplatin-based combinations for all indications. However, in the palliative setting, this difference was almost imperceptible, and given the palliative nature of this type of chemotherapy, the toxicity, particularly nausea and vomiting and hearing loss caused by cisplatin, most clinicians prefer a carboplatin combination for the palliative treatment of NSCLC. The addition of a third drug did not increase response rates or survival. However, a large trial compared cisplatin platinum combined with either gemcitabine or the anti-folate drug, pemetrexed. The trial was designed to compare the results by histological type. The results showed a clear advantage for the pemetrexed combination for adenocarcinoma, whereas gemcitabine was superior for squamous carcinoma. A further trial has shown that in cases of adenocarcinoma, continuing the pemetrexed as a single agent following the combination therapy (providing the tumour does not progress on doublet therapy) improves survival. In the second-line setting, docetaxel as a single agent for squamous carcinoma or combined with nintedanib, a drug that inhibits the development of blood vessels in adenocarcinoma, has shown to produce a survival benefit. However, docetaxel produces significant toxicity and is now being replaced by drugs which enhance immunity.

Targeted Therapy

A large number of mutations can be detected in lung cancer cells. Specific therapies have been developed to target some of these mutations. At the time of writing, two mutations have been identified for which established (licensed) therapies have been developed. These are epidermal growth factor (EGFR) and anaplastic lymphatic kinase (ALK). These mutations are uncommon, found in about 10% and 5% respectively of patients with NSCLC. These mutations are almost exclusively found in adenocarcinoma and are more prevalent in nonsmokers and Asian patients. The drugs targeted at EGFR include afatinib, erlotinib and gefitinib. These drugs are superior to chemotherapy both in efficacy (response rate) and side effects. This is a fast-developing field, and new drugs that can be effective when the patient relapses during initial anti-EGFR therapy (often because of the development of a further mutation) are under investigation. These drugs include osimertinib which has proven activity in patients who have developed the T790 mutation. The first drug targeting the ALK gene was crizotinib, but more recently, other drugs that are active following crizotinib include ceritinib, alectinib, brigatinib and lorlatinib. It is likely because of the proven activity of these drugs following progression on crizotinib therapy that they will be increasingly used as initial treatment.

Immune Therapy

For cancer to progress, it needs to overcome the immune response of the host (patient).

Some of the mechanisms by which a cancer achieves this have recently been identified. In particular, lung cancer cells have shown to express a ligand that suppresses the activities of killer T cells which would normally kill cancer cells, a process known as programmed death.

Therapies have been developed which block this action of the cancer cell by binding with the ligand or receptor and thus effectively reactivating the body's own immunity against the cancer. These drugs are particularly effective where a high percentage of tumour cells express the ligand. In such cases, drugs such as pembrolizumab have been proven to be superior to chemotherapy in the first-line setting. In patients with a relatively low expression of Programmed Death Ligand (PDL), chemotherapy is used first. However pembrolizumab and similar drugs such as nivolumab are superior to second-line chemotherapy following initial cytotoxic treatment. Occasionally, even in patients with widespread metastases, a sustained response to immune therapy is seen. The dramatic effect of these drugs in the advanced disease has led to trials being devised to test the value of immune therapy in the early disease setting, particularly combining immune therapy with RT. Initial results of these trials are promising with durvalumab, an anti-PDL agent, improving progression-free survival by 11 months when given after chemoradiotherapy for NSCLC.

Small Cell Lung Cancer
Natural History

There is a tendency for this cancer disease to disseminate widely and rapidly, with 80% of patients presenting with metastatic disease and often with a short history of symptoms of a few weeks before diagnosis.

Spread is local, via the lymphatics and haematogenous systems. There is a high prevalence of paraneoplastic conditions.

Staging and Diagnosis

The investigation and staging for SCLC are generally the same as for NSCLC with the aim of establishing the diagnosis and determining if the patient has disease limited to the chest that can be irradiated without exceeding normal tissue tolerance. The TNM system is now used for SCLC. However, it is still useful to classify patients as having limited-stage disease, that is, if the disease is confined to one hemithorax and adjacent supraclavicular lymph nodes or as extensive stage, if the disease has spread beyond the chest and regional lymph nodes. The former group of patients can be assessed with further tests that may include PET scanning with a view to curative treatment with chemotherapy and RT. The latter group can only be offered palliative treatment.

Prognostic factors include performance status, age and abnormal biochemistry.

Management

Chemotherapy. Combination chemotherapy produces a response in over 60% of patients with extensive disease. Responders experience improvement in quality of life and survival. However a significant proportion of patients present in very poor clinical condition with advanced organ failure and only supportive care is appropriate in this situation. In those patients who receive chemotherapy, the duration of response is short and the overall median survival is around 8 months. Several chemotherapy regimens exist and most are equivalent in terms of response; therefore in the palliative situation, a combination of carboplatin and etoposide (CE) is the standard therapy as this regime is generally well tolerated. Single-agent therapy has been tried, but because of lower response rates leading to uncontrolled symptoms, palliation and survival were inferior to combination chemotherapy.

Usually four to six cycles of chemotherapy are sufficient. More prolonged, alternating regimens or dose-intensive chemotherapy has been found to be of no benefit.

Retreatment with chemotherapy on relapse can be considered if the patient remains of good performance status, particularly if several months have elapsed since initial treatment. The regimes used for retreatment are the combination of cyclophosphamide, Adriamycin and vincristine (CAV) or topotecan as a single agent. If the disease-free interval is greater than 6 months, retreatment with CE can be of benefit. Responses, however, are of short duration. Patients who do not respond to first-line therapy and those who have relapse within 3 months of treatment are unlikely to respond to further chemotherapy.

Radiotherapy. Radiotherapy to the thorax, given sequentially or concurrently, has been shown to improve the survival of patients with limited-stage SCLC. The best results are obtained if the RT is given concurrently with chemotherapy; using this approach 5-year survival of 20% can be obtained. However, patients need to be of good performance status and the disease of such a volume that it can be treated to an adequate dose without risking severe or even fatal pneumonitis. If concurrent chemoradiation is not feasible, then sequential RT can be used, providing the patient responds to initial chemotherapy. A recent trial showed similar results using either 66 Gy in 33 daily fractions or 45 Gy in 30 fractions bi-daily when combined concurrently with cisplatin and etoposide. Radiation doses of similar biological potency are used for sequential treatment. The technique of RT is the same as that employed for NSCLC.

Prophylactic cranial irradiation. Brain metastases are a common problem in SCLC and without prophylactic irradiation develop in approximately 20% and 50% of patients with limited and extensive disease, respectively. Prophylactic cranial irradiation (PCI) reduces the incidence of brain metastases and improves the survival of patients with limited SCLC who have successfully undergone chemotherapy and thoracic RT. No benefit has been found for giving a dose higher than 25 Gy in 10 fractions. PCI is given after chemotherapy to avoid radiosensitisation by cytotoxic chemotherapy and to limit its use to those patients who have responded to chemotherapy and therefore are most likely to benefit from this treatment.

Technique: The patient's head is immobilised with an Orfit mask in the supine position and a planning CT performed. A parallel pair technique is used comprising of two opposed lateral fields. The orbits, most of the parotid glands and oral cavity can be shielded with multileaf collimators. This approach is better than using head rotation to conform to the traditional anatomical line drawn from the outer margin of the orbit, outer canthus and through the lower tragus used to set up the fields, as this arrangement often under-doses the middle cranial fossa and provides inadequate shielding of the parotid glands. Both fields are irradiated daily. The dose is prescribed to the midpoint intersection of both beams.

However, a dose of this order is known to cause significant side effects in NSCLC and there is some evidence that patients with SCLC suffer long- and short-term central nervous system sequelae from cranial irradiation. Therefore, techniques of radiation that reduce the dose to the hippocampus have been developed to reduce these serious side effects and at present are the subjects of clinical trials.

Although PCI also reduces the incidence of brain metastases in patients with extensive stage SCLC who respond to chemotherapy, the effect on overall survival is small and somewhat uncertain, and because of side effects and the generally poor survival, patients with advanced SCLC must be carefully counseled before being prescribed PCI. The benefit of thoracic radiation in patients with extensive disease is also uncertain, but in patients who respond well to chemotherapy, it can be considered. A dose of 30 Gy in 10 fractions is appropriate.

Toxicity. Common acute side effects are headache, tiredness, nausea and reversible alopecia. These can be treated with steroids or other antiemetics. In the 12 weeks following PCI postirradiation, somnolence, cognitive impairment and lethargy are common complaints. These are self-limiting, however, and do not predict late neurotoxicity. Patients with SCLC have a limited life span so the true incidence of late neurological damage is not known.

The role of surgery. Less than 10% of patients have stage 1 (T1, T2) disease and, occasionally, these patients have surgical resection to remove an undiagnosed pulmonary nodule. Small retrospective studies suggest that these patients may do well if standard chemotherapy and RT follow treatment. There is no evidence that patients with more advanced disease, T3 or N2 benefit from surgical treatment.

Neuroendocrine Tumours

Pulmonary carcinoid tumours are rare, accounting for only 1% of all lung tumours, but the lung is the primary site of 25% of all carcinoid tumours. The biological aggressiveness of carcinoid tumours is variable but most are well differentiated and rarely metastasise. These tumours are found in main, lobar or segmented bronchi and present with cough, haemoptysis or local obstructive symptoms. Surgery is the treatment of choice. Unlike bronchial carcinoma, carcinoid tumours do not exhibit extensive submucosal spread and therefore surgical techniques such as sleeve resection that enable significant volumes of lung to be preserved can be performed without compromising local control and are particularly useful for tumours originating in main bronchi. Five-year survival rates in excess of 90% have been reported following resection.

By contrast, patients with histologically atypical carcinoids (poorly differentiated, pleomorphic cells, increased mitosis and necrotic areas)

have a much higher risk of metastases to organs such as liver, bones, adrenals and central nervous system and therefore a poorer survival. However the disease often runs an indolent course, with patients surviving for many years with metastatic disease: the median survival from diagnosis is around 10 years. As well as conventional imaging, such as CT scanning, radiolabelled octreotide (octreoscans) can be useful in establishing the extent of disease. Carcinoids may produce excess catecholamines and kinins leading to the carcinoid syndrome which is characterised by facial flushing (often provoked by stress or alcohol), diarrhoea and, in the long term, fibrosis and incompetence of the right-sided heart valves. Such patients have raised levels of catecholamine metabolites in urine such as 3-methoxy-4-hydroxy mandelic acid (UMA) and hydroxyindole acetic acid (HIAA). Treatment of patients with locally advanced disease or metastatic disease is palliative. Somatostatin analogs such as octreotide and lanreotide block the release of catecholamines and can improve the symptoms of carcinoid syndrome in 80% of cases. Radionuclide treatment can help if the tumour takes up compounds such as radiolabelled octreotide. Radiotherapy is used for palliation for chest symptoms as well as metastatic disease.

No chemotherapy combination has clearly been shown to be beneficial in this disease. The cytotoxic combinations used are those prescribed for small cell carcinoma, that is, cisplatin or carboplatin combined with etoposide, although response rates are low, generally less than 20%. However, everolimus (an immunosuppressant originally developed to prevent rejection following organ transplantation) has been found to improve survival in patients with advanced neuroendocrine tumours and is now probably the systemic treatment of choice.

Mesothelioma

Mesothelioma is a malignant tumour of the pleura and the majority of cases are caused by exposure to asbestos.

There are two main types of asbestos fibres: serpentiles (white asbestos) and amphiboles (blue asbestos). White asbestos fibres are pliable, curly and easily broken down in the lung releasing magnesium, iron and silica. About 90% of industry used this type and, fortunately, it is rarely associated with mesothelioma. Blue asbestos fibres, however, are rigid and nonpliable. Lung phagocytes repeatedly attempt to break down these fibres and eliminate them. It is thought that this chronic inflammatory response leads to eventual mesothelial cell proliferation, mutation and malignancy. This may explain the long latency period of 20 to 40 years from first exposure to asbestos and development of this tumour. Asbestos was commonly used for insulation in buildings and homes, building ships, and car parts. It is estimated that the risk of development of this disease is greatest in men born around 1945 to 1950, of whom, it is anticipated that 1 in 150 will die of mesothelioma.

In Turkey, there is a high incidence of mesothelioma. At first this was thought to be as a result of asbestos-like mineral fibres in the soil. However, these nonasbestos-related tumours are hereditary in nature and have been found to be associated with carriage of an autosomal dominant gene.

Natural History

The majority of patients will progress rapidly and succumb to their illness within 12 months, although occasionally patients may remain stable for some time with or without treatment.

Most patients present with a pleural effusion but in the later stages of the illness, the tumour encases and constricts the lung and invades the chest and mediastinum, causing pain, dyspnoea and sometimes dysphagia. Fig. 25.6 shows a CT scan of a patient with advanced mesothelioma. Night sweats are seen in advanced disease. Although metastases are commonly found at postmortem, disease beyond thorax rarely causes symptoms during the patient's lifetime.

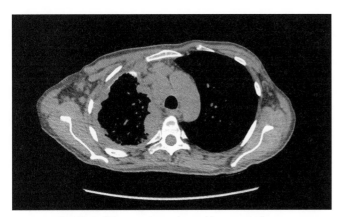

Fig. 25.6 CT scan of a patient with mesothelioma.

Prognostic groups are based on the following factors: patient age, sex, weight loss and performance status, tumour histology and clinical stage, values of haemoglobin, leucocyte ($>8.3 \times 10^9$/L) and platelet count ($>400 \times 10^9$/L) at presentation.

There are several different staging systems but they are mostly based on surgical staging and therefore are of no value for the majority of patients.

Initial Assessment and Treatment

A CT is used to establish a provisional diagnosis and there should be a low threshold for performing this imaging in cases of persistent pleural effusion, particularly in patients who have been exposed to asbestos. The next step is to establish a diagnosis and provide optimum control of any pleural effusion. Although the diagnosis can be suggested by cytology, confirmation by histology is usually required. This is usually done with a thoracoscopy, where the scope is introduced into the pleural space and abnormal tissue is biopsied and the effusion drained. Control of the effusion is by the introduction of talc into the pleural space, which causes inflammation of the pleural surfaces, which then fuse together, preventing reaccumulation of fluid. If the lung does not re-expand, the placement of a permanent drain provides drainage. This procedure can be performed under general anaesthetic or in a conscious patient with sedation.

Surgery

Apart from thoracoscopy as outlined above, there is no established role for surgery in mesothelioma. A trial of debulking surgery showed a small improvement in the time to recurrence of pleural effusion, but no improvement in survival. Radical surgery involving removal of the lung and pleura (radical pleuro-pneumonectomy) has high mortality, approaching 10%, and has largely been abandoned in the United Kingdom following the results of the Mesothelioma and Radical Surgery (MARS) trial which showed no benefit of trimodality therapy (chemotherapy, surgery and RT) compared with the standard approach of chemotherapy. To avoid the mortality of a pneumonectomy, the lesser procedure of pleurectomy has been developed and is proposed as a treatment for mesothelioma. However there is no good evidence that it is of benefit and the procedure is at present being evaluated in the United Kingdom based on the MARS 2 randomised trial. However, the vast majority of patients either are not fit for surgery and or have disease that is amenable to resection.

Radiotherapy

RT has a limited role in mesothelioma. Although in the past, irradiation was used prophylactically to prevent disease developing in scars from surgical intervention, recent randomised trials of postoperative RT have shown no benefit. The frequency of surgical scar recurrence in these trials was much lower than that historically observed, probably because minimally invasive techniques are used, and possibly because of the increasing use of chemotherapy. RT can produce palliation of pain, particularly where the disease infiltrates the chest wall, but unfortunately, although initial benefit is seen, recurrence of pain is common. Administering RT to the hemithorax following pneumonectomy or pleurectomy to delay local progression is extremely difficult to achieve without exceeding lung tolerance, and deaths as a result of radiation pneumonitis have been reported following pneumonectomy and RT. Therefore this form of wide-field RT for mesothelioma cannot be justified outside a clinical trial.

Chemotherapy

Chemotherapy is the only treatment for mesothelioma that has shown proven benefit in terms of quality and quantity of life. The evidence is indirect in that the trials that have established the value of chemotherapy randomised patients between single-agent cisplatin and a combination with an antifolate drug, either pemetrexed or raltitrexed. Both trials showed an improvement in survival for the combination implying that chemotherapy is superior to supportive care. A UK trial compared chemotherapy with supportive care and showed no significant benefit. However, the drugs used in this study (vinorelbine or the combination of mitomycin, vinblastine and cisplatin) were probably suboptimal and most clinicians would offer fit patients with mesothelioma the option of palliative chemotherapy. There is no standard line-second line option for mesothelioma.

Thymoma

Thymoma presents as a mediastinal mass. It is well-known for associated paraneoplastic syndromes such as myasthenia gravis and red cell aplasia. These syndromes can persist following complete resection of the tumour. Thymoma has an unpredictable clinical behavior, which does not correlate with the pathological findings and may recur after many years.

Symptoms

Thymoma can present as an incidental finding on x-ray or symptoms of a paraneoplastic syndrome. Spread occurs via the lymphatics or by the haematogenous route.

Diagnosis

Investigations should concentrate on identifying the extent of disease in the anterior mediastinal and possible areas of spread followed by biopsy.

Pathology and Natural History

Thymomas can be classified as epithelial or lymphocytic. Mixed and spindle forms also exist. The tumour can behave unpredictably regardless of the pathological appearance. Differentiation between benign and malignant disease is determined by the presence of gross invasion of adjacent structures, metastasis or microscopic evidence of capsular invasion.

Management

Surgical resection is the treatment of choice. Locally invasive, large or unresectable tumours should be treated with multimodality therapy.

The tumour is chemosensitive and over half of patients will respond to cisplatin-based regimens. Chemotherapy can be used for locally advanced disease, followed by, if feasible, surgery and postoperative RT (50 Gy), or if the tumour is not resectable, by RT alone. Local recurrence may occur late, often 5 or more years after initial surgery, and is frequently associated with more undifferentiated histology. The treatment is similar to initial presentation. In view of the propensity for late recurrence, 10-year survival figures are considered more reliable.

CONCLUSION

Tumours of the thorax and in particular, lung cancer, remain a common cause of disability and death. Although the outcome is generally poor, there has been progress in the last two decades through the judicious use of newer RT techniques where both locally advanced and localised tumours can be treated aggressively with IMRT and SABR, respectively. Minimally invasive surgery has also contributed to the increase in survival that has been seen in recent years. The systemic treatment of lung cancer has undergone a revolution in the last decade with the introduction of a bewildering array of drugs targeting specific molecular abnormalities seen in lung cancer. The sad fact remains that the majority of cases could be prevented and the priority for dealing with lung cancer is the introduction of measures to reduce and preferably abolish tobacco consumption.

FURTHER READING

Baldwin DR, Callister MEJ. What is the optimum screening policy for the early detection of lung cancer? Clin Oncol 2016;28:672–81.

Harris C, Meek D, Gilligan D, et al. Assessment and optimisation of lung cancer patients for treatment with curative intent. Clin Oncol 2016;28:682–94.

Ireland RH, Tahir BA, Wild JM, Lee CE. Functional image- guided radiotherapy planning for normal lung avoidance. Clin Oncol 2016;28:695–707.

Bradley JD, Paulus R, Komaki R, et al. Standard dose versus high dose conformal radiotherapy with concurrent and consolidation carboplatin plus paclitaxel with or without cetuximab for patients with stage111A or 11B non -small cell lung cancer (RTOG 0617): a randomised two by two factorial phase 3 study. Lancet Oncol 2015;16:187–99.

Medical Research Council lung cancer working party. Randomised trial of palliative two fraction versus more intensive 13 fraction radiotherapy for patients with inoperable non-small cell lung cancer and good performance status. Clin Oncol 1996;8:167–75.

Paz-Ares L, Luft A, Vincente A, et al. Pembrolizumab plus chemotherapy for squamous non-small cell lung cancer. N Eng J Med 2018;379:2040–51.

Woolf DK, Slotman BJ, Faivre-Finn C. The current role of radiotherapy in the treatment of small cell lung cancer. Clin Oncol 2016;38:712–9.

Schild SE, Sio TT, Daniels TB. Prophylactic cranial radiation for extensive small cell lung cancer. J Oncol Pract 2017;13:732–8.

Lehman JM, Mary ME, Massion PP. Immunotherapy and targeted therapy for small cell lung cancer: There is hope. Curr Oncol Rep 2017;19(49):1–9.

Waller DA, Dawson AG. Randomized trials in malignant pleural mesothelioma surgery-mistakes made and lessons learned. Ann Transl Med 2017;5:240 1–6.

De Gooijer CJ, Baas P, Burgers JA. Current chemotherapy strategies in malignant pleural mesothelioma. Transl Lung Cancer Res 2018;7(5):574–83.

Willman J, Rimner A. The expanded role of radiation therapy for thymic malignancies. J Thorac Dis 2018;10(Suppl 21):S2555–64.

26

Breast Cancer

Ian Kunkler

CHAPTER OUTLINE

ANATOMY

Most of the breast tissue extends from the edge of the sternum to the anterior axillary line and from the second or third to the sixth or seventh costal edge. It overlies the second to the sixth ribs. Breast tissue can be found beyond these areas as high as the clavicle and laterally to the edge of the latissimus dorsi muscle.

The mammary glands are composed of approximately 12 lobes, separated by fibrous tissue and surrounded by fat. Each lobe consists of multiple ductulo-lobular units lined by two layers of cells. The luminal layer is made up of epithelial cells and the outer layer of contractile myoepithelial cells.

Lymphatic Drainage

The principal lymphatic drainage of the breast (Fig.26.1) is to the axillary nodes lying between the second and third intercostal spaces. Additional drainage occurs to the supraclavicular nodes through the pectoralis major and to the internal mammary chain adjacent to the sternum.

PATHOLOGY

Epidemiology

Worldwide, breast cancer is the most common form of malignancy in women. The International Agency for Research on Cancer estimates that the incidence in 2018 is 2.1 million cases per year with 562,500 in European women. In 2014–2016 in the United Kingdom there were on average 55,123 new cases of breast cancer and in 2016 11,563 deaths. One in 8 women in the United Kingdom will develop breast cancer during their lifetime and 1 in 870 men. Nearly half (48%) of breast cancer is diagnosed in women 65 years of age and older. The incidence is highest in the United Kingdom in women aged 80 years or older. Since the early 1990s, the incidence of breast cancer has risen by about one-fifth (19%). It has risen in females and is stable in males. The incidence in the United Kingdom is estimated to rise by 2% between 2014 and 2035 to 210 cases per 100,000 women by 2035. Half the global burden of breast cancers occurs in less developed regions. Breast cancer is the most common cause of cancer death in women with in excess of 626,600 deaths worldwide and 150,700 in Europe in 2018. Unfortunately, mortality from breast cancer in less developed regions is continuing to rise, in part because of lack of access to modern diagnostic facilities and treatment.

Female breast cancer is rare below the age of 30 years. The incidence rises rapidly during the reproductive years. The incidence of breast cancer in younger women (<45 years) is lower but rates are rising. After the age of 50 years, the incidence rises at a lower rate. Male breast cancer is rare in the United Kingdom (390 cases in 2014), accounting for only 1% of breast cancer cases.

Encouragingly, the mortality of breast cancer is declining in the European Union and the United States, mostly attributed to breast screening and better systemic therapy. In England and Wales, 78% of women diagnosed with breast cancer survive for 10 or more years and about two-thirds (65%) survive for 20 years or more.

In the United Kingdom there were about 7900 new cases of ductal carcinoma in situ (DCIS), a preinvasive form of breast cancer, in 2015. Approximately one-half of cases of DCIS each year in the United Kingdom occur in women aged 60 years or older. The incidence of DCIS continues to rise, in part because of the development of breast screening programmes.

Aetiology

The aetiology of breast cancer is not fully understood, but a number of predisposing factors have been identified.

Genetic Factors

High-risk mutations. It is estimated that up to 10% of breast cancers have a genetic basis. Mutations in high penetrance genes (BRCA1/2) and others explain the concentration of cases in high-risk families. Abnormal amplification and mutations of both oncogenes and antioncogenes are involved in the pathogenesis and progression of breast cancer.

Nearly 25% of breast cancer cases are related to family history. The sisters and daughters of a woman with breast cancer have a threefold increased risk of developing the disease. The risk of breast cancer for a woman whose sister is affected is doubled. Women who have a first-degree relative with breast cancer have a 1.75 higher risk. In women with two or more first-degree relatives with breast cancer, there is a 2.5-fold increased risk of breast cancer. Women with

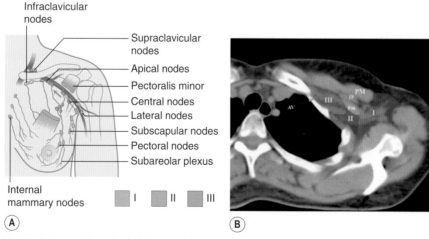

Fig. 26.1 (A) Diagram of lymphatic drainage of the breast. (B) Transverse computed tomography scan of the left axilla (patient with arms up) both showing the position of levels I to III axillary lymph nodes. *AV*, Axillary vessels; *Pm*, pectoralis minor; *PM*, pectoralis major; *IP*, interpectoral nodes. (From Barrett A, Dobbs J, Morris S, Roques T. Practical radiotherapy planning. 4th ed. London: Hodder Arnold; 2009. With permission.)

premenopausal or bilateral breast cancer are at a particularly high risk. At least five germline mutations predispose to breast cancer. These include mutations in BRCA1, BRCA2, p53, PTEN and ATM. BRCA1 and BRCA2 mutations confer the highest level of risk of breast cancer and also predispose to ovarian cancer. Approximately 5% to 10% of all breast cancers and 20% to 25% of all hereditary breast cancers are caused by BRCA1/2 mutations. Germline mutations in p53 give rise to the Li-Fraumeni syndrome (childhood sarcomas, brain tumours and early onset breast cancer), and mutations in PTEN give rise to Cowden's disease.

The mode of inheritance is usually autosomal dominant with incomplete penetrance. Note that the genetic susceptibility can be passed on by both males and females. Most cases of breast cancer with a genetic basis will have occurred by the age of 65 years. Those at substantial risk include women with:

- Three first- or second-degree relatives with breast or ovarian cancer.
- One first-degree relative with bilateral breast cancer.
- Two first- or second-degree relatives with breast cancer diagnosed under the age of 60 years or ovarian cancer at any age on the same side of the family.

First-degree relatives are mother, sister or daughter. Second-degree relatives are grandmother, granddaughter, aunt or niece. Other features in the family history that increase the risk of breast cancer include male breast cancer and paternal history of breast cancer (two or more relatives on the father's side of the family). Specialist advice should be sought on eligibility of patients or their relatives for genetic counselling and testing.

Low-penetrance breast cancer susceptibility genes. In sporadic cases there are many low-penetrance "modifier" genes associated with breast cancer. Normally, the variants in these genes are common in the general population. Genome-wide association studies have identified more than 70 variants. Each variant may be associated with a small increased risk for breast cancer in an individual. Modifier genes are found in a number of pathways including steroid metabolism, DNA damage response, immunomodulation and detoxification of environmental carcinogens.

Acquired

Benign breast disease. A number of benign conditions (e.g. fibroadenomas, palpable cysts) in the breast increase the risk of breast cancer, although the effect is small. Overall, the risk of breast cancer is raised four- to tenfold for women with previous benign breast disease.

Risk factors for breast cancer

Menstruation. The epithelium of the breast proliferates during ovulatory cycles. This may be because of the stimulus of either progesterone or oestrogen. This proliferation causes temporary growth of the milk-secreting glandular tissue in preparation for possible pregnancy. If the menarche starts before the age of 12 years, the risk of breast cancer is nearly double that of women who begin to menstruate after the age of 13 years. If menstruation continues above the age of 55 years, the risk of breast cancer is doubled compared with a normal menopause at 45 years. Early menarche and late menopause almost certainly confer an increased risk of breast cancer by prolonging the period in which both breasts are exposed to high levels of oestradiol (and possibly progesterone). Each 1-year delay in menopause increases the risk of breast cancer by 3%.

Oral contraceptive pill and hormonal replacement therapy. The role of the ovarian oestrogens in the genesis of breast cancer is strongly suspected. Oral contraceptives suppress the production of oestradiol and progesterone. Reductions in oestrogen levels may protect against breast cancer. Oral oestrogens, either as the contraceptive pill or as hormone replacement therapy (HRT), may accelerate the development of breast cancer. The relative risk of breast cancer for HRT is 1.66 for current users compared with those that have never used it. Combined therapy for periods of 5 years or more confers a higher risk. The risk of breast cancer falls substantially after 2 years of stopping HRT. Oral contraceptives do not increase the risk of breast cancer if they have been stopped for more than 10 years.

Pregnancy. The risk of breast cancer in a woman rises with her age at first pregnancy. It is three times higher in women who have their first baby over the age of 30 years, compared with those under the age of 18 years.

Lactation. Women who have breast-fed their children are slightly less prone to breast cancer.

Age at first full-term pregnancy. Pregnancy itself seems to have a protective role.

Mammographic density. The density of the breast on mammography is a strong factor in determining breast cancer risk. Breast density is influenced by both genetic and nongenetic factors.

Diet and lifestyle. Risk factors for breast cancer at critical times of exposure interact and impact on the normal transformation of the breast, either directly or by modulating the hormonal regulatory environment.

Nutrition and lifestyle may be principally responsible for large variations in breast cancer between countries and marked changes in these rates between migrating populations. Asian women, for example, experience much higher rates of breast cancer after moving to the United States.

Dietary fat, whose effects are mediated by oestrogens, is thought to be a key risk factor for breast cancer. An increased intake of calories, sugar, alcohol and saturated fats increases the risk of developing breast cancer. Consumption of alcohol increases the incidence of breast cancer in both pre- and postmenopausal women. An intake of 35 to 44 grams of alcohol per day can increase the risk of breast cancer by 32%. The association between smoking and breast cancer is controversial but the risk of breast cancer is increased (relative risk (RR) 1.54) for women who drink and smoke. There is accumulating evidence that women who start smoking at an early age are at increased risk of breast cancer. Active smoking before a first full-time pregnancy is especially harmful.

Physical exercise. Physical exercise also appears to have a protective effect against breast cancer in postmenopausal women. The protective effects of physical activity are likely to be through changes in sex hormone levels, immune function, adiposity and insulin-related hormones. Being physically active can change the levels of some hormones, including oestrogen and insulin. Physical activity can lower levels of oestrogen and insulin. High levels of insulin stimulate the production of insulin-like growth factors, which increase breast cancer risk by stimulating cell turnover. Women who do the most activity have a 12% lower risk of developing breast cancer compared with the least active women. The more activity a woman does, the more she can reduce her risk of breast cancer. The risk of breast cancer falls by 5% for every 2 hours a week a woman spends doing moderate to vigorous activity. Even moderate exercise has a protective effect.

Ionising radiation. The breast is one of the tissues most sensitive to the induction of malignancy by ionising radiation. Exposure to ionising radiation increases the risk of breast cancer. This is true of women who underwent low-dose breast irradiation for benign mastitis. There is a linear relationship between dose and incidence of breast cancer up to 4 gray (Gy). Beyond this, the incidence plateaus. It has been calculated that one extra breast cancer per year after 10 years may be caused by radiation from a single mammogram among 2 million women over the age of 50 years. The risk of breast cancer is well validated for women irradiated under the age of 40 years with a relative risk of 1.1 to 2.7 at

1 Gy. Women irradiated in their teenage years by mantle radiotherapy (RT) for Hodgkin's disease, where the mediastinal fields commonly treat the medial part of both breasts, have an increased risk of breast cancer by a factor of 1 in 7 if aged 20 to 29 years when treated by mantle RT, and then rising to 50% at the age of 50 years for girls treated before age 20 years.

Children irradiated by the atomic bombs dropped on Nagasaki and Hiroshima showed an increased risk of breast cancer with dose.

Ductal and Lobular Carcinoma In Situ

Premalignant in situ carcinoma may occur confined to the lobules (lobular carcinoma in situ [LCIS]) or ducts (ductal carcinoma in situ [DCIS]) without evidence of penetration on light microscopy of the basement membrane. DCIS occurs in 25% of breast cancers. With the advent of breast screening, the diagnosis of DCIS has increased three to four times and now accounts for 20% of screen-detected cancers. Some 90% of DCIS is confined to one segment of the breast. DCIS is a heterogeneous disease based on histology, genetic alterations and clinical course. Inactivation of the tumour suppression gene, e-cadherin, is associated with the development of LCIS. Loss of the tumour suppressor gene, p53, is associated with the development of poorly differentiated DCIS. Most of the genetic alterations seen in DCIS are also seen in invasive cancer which often accompanies DCIS. DCIS is categorised as low grade, intermediate grade or high grade based on combinations of architecture, cell morphology and the presence of necrosis. There are two principal histological groups: comedo and non-comedo type. The most common noncomedo types are solid, cribriform, papillary and micropapillary.

The pathway of development of low- and intermediate-grade DCIS is thought to differ from high-grade disease. Low-grade DCIS shows a loss in 17q chromosome, whereas high-grade DCIS often shows a 17q gain.

More than 90% of cases of DCIS present asymptomatically with malignant calcifications at screening mammography. Mammography commonly underestimates the extent of the disease. Magnetic resonance imaging (MRI) is more effective at detecting multifocality. Other presentations are Paget's disease of the nipple, nipple discharge or a lump. Core biopsy is able to establish a diagnosis in 90% of screen-detected cases. DCIS is associated with a substantial risk of progression to invasive carcinoma, with a mean delay of about 7 years. LCIS is associated with an increased risk of tumour in both breasts, particularly infiltrating ductal carcinoma.

Invasive Breast Cancer

Malignant tumours mainly arise from the glandular epithelium (adenocarcinomas). Breast cancers are classified as of no special type or of special type. The majority (80%) are of no special type. The histological types of breast cancer are shown in Table 26.1.

TABLE 26.1 Classification of Invasive Breast Cancer
1. No special type
2. Special type
a. Tubular
b. Mucoid
c. Cribriform
d. Papillary
e. Medullary
f. Classic lobular

Invasive cancers have traditionally been classified by their microscopic appearance and by histological grade. Grading is based on nuclear pleomorphism, degree of glandular formation and frequency of mitoses. The Bloom and Richardson system of grades 1, 2 and 3 from least to most malignant is widely adopted. Grading yields useful prognostic information. Both disease-free survival and overall survival are shorter for high-grade cancers.

If in excess of 25% of the main tumour mass contains noninvasive (in situ) disease, and in situ disease is present in the adjacent breast tissue, the tumour is described as having an *extensive in situ component*. Such patients are at risk of developing invasive cancer elsewhere in the breast and are not suitable for breast conservation.

Lymphatic or vascular invasion within the tumour confers an increased risk of local and distant recurrence.

Inflammatory carcinomas are typified by an enlarged warm breast, often associated with an ill-defined underlying mass. Histologically, there is tumour infiltration of the subdermal lymphatics and the prognosis is poor. In contrast, medullary carcinoma is slow growing and has a much better prognosis.

Lobular invasive carcinomas are often bilateral (40%) and multicentric. Paget disease of the nipple is commonly associated with an underlying ductal adenocarcinoma.

MOLECULAR CLASSIFICATION OF BREAST CANCER

There are at least four different molecular subtypes of breast cancer: luminal-A, luminal-B, HER2 enriched and basal-like. These subtypes can be determined on formalin-fixed paraffin-embedded samples either using a multigene assay, or indirectly reconstructed with immunochemically measured steroid receptors: oestrogen receptor (ER), progesterone receptor (PgR) and HER2 status in addition to proliferation status assessed by Ki67. Luminal-A subtype is ER- or PgR-positive or both, HER2-negative and low Ki67. Luminal-B–like subtype is ER-positive or both, HER2-negative, high Ki467 or PgR low or has a high-risk molecular signature. HER subtype, non-luminal is HER2 positive and ER and PgR negative or luminal, HER2-positive and ER- and PgR-positive or both. Basal-like subtype is HER2-negative and ER- and PgR-negative (triple negative).

MULTIDISCIPLINARY MANAGEMENT OF BREAST CANCER

Breast cancer is heterogeneous and potentially a curable disease. It has a very long natural history with recurrence being common, even many years after primary treatment. Over the last few decades there has been a reduction in the intensity of locoregional and systemic therapy with the focus on increasing personalisation of treatment. The net effects have been improvements in survival for both early and advanced disease. Patients with suspected breast cancer or recurrent disease should be referred to a specialist breast unit for assessment and treatment. Their management plan (sequence and timing of staging investigations, pathology, imaging and selection of therapy) should be formulated within a multidisciplinary team (surgeons, medical and clinical oncologists, radiologists, pathologists and specialist nurses). Patients undergoing surgery should be discussed by the team before and after surgery to decide on the best policy for the individual patient. Comorbidities, quality of life and the patient's wishes should be taken into account. Practice should be evidence based and recorded in national/local written protocols and standards, against which compliance should be regularly audited.

DIAGNOSIS

The patient may notice a lump herself on routine or casual self-examination. Sometimes it is detected as part of clinical examination for other reasons or as a result of routine examination in hospital. With the introduction of the National Health Service (NHS) breast-screening programme by mammography (Fig. 26.2) in the United Kingdom in 1988, asymptomatic breast cancer is being more frequently diagnosed among women routinely screened. All eligible women aged 50 to 70 years are invited for screening every 3 years. The coverage (percent of women in the population who are eligible for screening at a particular point who have a recorded result in the last 3 years) was 74.9% in England in 2018 and remains above the standard of 70%. Of the women who had cancer detected, 41.2% (7543) had small invasive cancers less than 15 mm diameter (which would be difficult to detect clinically). Detection rates were highest in women aged over 70 years (14.6 women per 1000 screened) and lower in women aged 45 to 49 years (6.2 women with cancer per 1000 women screened). Breast screening is considered to achieve a 20% relative risk reduction of breast cancer mortality. It is estimated that, assuming the reduction in mortality continued for 10 years after breast screening ended, for every 235 women invited to screening, one breast cancer death would be prevented (i.e. 43 breast cancer deaths per 10,000 women invited to screening). Overdiagnosis is difficult to estimate (i.e. where women have their cancer treated by surgery, RT and systemic therapy but it is unknown whether or not the cancer would have become clinically overt during their lifetime). The best estimate of overdiagnosis in the screened population is about 11% (defined as excess incidence in the screened population as a proportion of the long-term suspected incidence).

In addition, some women experience pain on mammography. About 4% of women screened are recalled for further mammography and sometimes biopsy. The vast majority (99%) of patients with screened-detected breast cancer will have surgery, 70% postoperative RT, 70% endocrine therapy and 25% chemotherapy. Each treatment has its attendant morbidities, including adverse psychological effects. Clear explanation is required for patients about the risks and benefits of breast screening.

Features suggestive of malignancy on mammography are small microcalcifications, stellate opacities with "legs" extending into the surrounding tissues (Fig. 26.3) or distortion of architecture. The sensitivity of mammography is reduced in dense breasts seen in younger women. Mammography may also show enlarged nodes in the axilla. About 15% of cancers are not detected by mammography, and nearly 4% are neither palpable nor visible on mammography.

Clinical Assessment

Triple assessment is required (history and examination; breast imaging (usually mammography and ultrasound) and core biopsy of suspicious lesions). A full history is required, including details of breast-related symptoms, particularly breast pain, nipple discharge, changes noted in the skin (erythema, dimpling) or shape of the breast, indrawing or distortion of the nipple, axillary lumps and systemic symptoms of weight loss, anorexia, nausea, vomiting, bone pain, breathlessness, headache or motor or sensory disturbance. A full menstrual history should be taken including onset of menarche, menopause, parity, age of first pregnancy, breast/bottle feeding and use of the contraceptive pill and hormone replacement therapy.

Breast Ultrasound

Ultrasound of the breast has an important role in helping to distinguish benign from malignant lesions, particularly when mammography is normal or equivocal. Malignant tumours tend to show an irregular echo poor pattern compared with the smooth outline of a benign fibroadenoma (Fig. 26.4A, B). Colour Doppler ultrasound may show changes caused by increased tumour vasculature both in primary tumours and in lymph nodes.

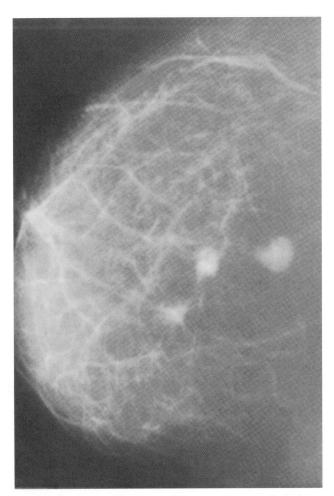

Fig. 26.3 Mammogram showing three spiculated tumours in the breast. (Courtesy Dr. R. Peck, Sheffield.)

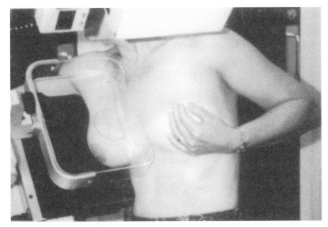

Fig. 26.2 Patient undergoing mammography. (Courtesy the Rotherham Breast Screening service.)

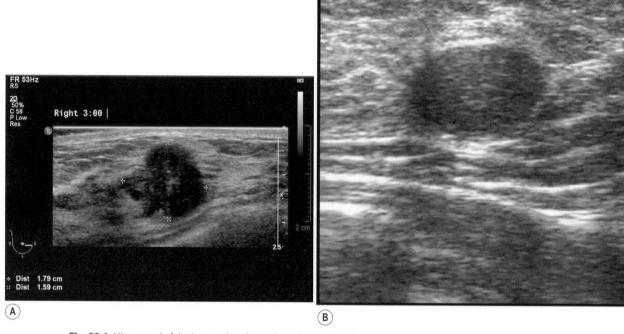

Fig. 26.4 Ultrasound of the breast showing an irregular mass lesion characteristic of a cancer (A) compared with well-defined margins of benign fibroadenoma (B). (From Dixon JM, editor. ABC of breast diseases. 4th ed. Oxford: Wiley Blackwell; 2012. With permission.)

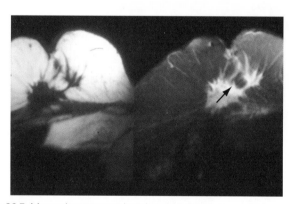

Fig. 26.5 Magnetic resonance imaging scan showing recurrent cancer in the breast. (Courtesy Prof J.M. Dixon, Edinburgh Breast Unit.)

Magnetic Resonance Imaging

MRI may have an important role in the assessment of (1) the local extent of the primary tumour and of (2) multifocality in younger women where the density of the breast is often a limiting factor to the resolution of mammography. MRI may show 10% to 30% additional invasive cancer in patients presenting with a unifocal lesion. However, MRI may lead to an overestimation of the size of lesions, potentially resulting in unnecessary mastectomies. MRI results in false positive findings in 10% to 15% of patients. Biopsy should be considered where a lesion appears on MRI alone. MRI may also show recurrent cancer in the breast (Fig. 26.5).

Positron Emission Tomography

Positron emission tomography (PET) normally does not have a role in the staging of most cases of breast cancer. PET scanning is based on the uptake of fluorine-18. Its resolution is only 5 to 6 mm so it cannot identify very small lesions. PET may generate false positives with metabolic uptake in inflammatory or other nonmalignant conditions. Its advantages are that it may show responses to systemic therapy earlier than computed togography (CT) or MRI and may show regional or distant metastases (e.g. bone metastases) not detected on other imaging. In addition, it may provide clarity where other imaging is equivocal.

Obtaining a Histological Diagnosis

It is important to obtain a histological diagnosis of breast cancer to confirm suspicious clinical or radiological features. If the tumour is palpable (usually $\geq$1 cm), core biopsy under local anaesthetic is recommended or stereotactic image-guided core biopsy for impalpable lesions. Tumour from core biopsy should be stained for ER and PgR status and for epidermal growth factor receptor 2 (HER2) status. Fine needle aspiration cytology (FNAC) does not make a reliable distinction between invasive and in situ disease, but it is helpful in the diagnosis and treatment of breast cysts.

STAGING

Staging is important to assess the local, regional and metastatic spread of breast cancer because management may differ significantly depending on the extent of the disease. Staging involves clinical, radiological and laboratory assessment. The simplest clinical staging system that is still in use is shown in Table 26.2. However, the TNM classification of the International Union Against Cancer (Table 26.3) has gained widespread acceptance.

TABLE 26.2 Clinical Staging of Breast Cancer

Stage	Clinical Findings
I	Freely movable (on underlying muscle); no suspicious nodes
II	As stage I but mobile axillary node(s) on the same side
III	Primary more extensive than stage I, e.g. skin invaded wide of the primary mass or fixation to muscle. Axillary nodes, if present, are fixed; or supraclavicular nodes involved
IV	Extension beyond the ipsilateral chest wall area, e.g. opposite breast or axilla; or distant metastase,s

Staging Investigations

For patients with T1–2, N0, M0 disease, a full blood count, liver biochemistry and chest radiograph are recommended. For patients with (1) T3 or T4 tumours, (2) N1–3 or MI, or (3) T0–2, N0 disease with symptoms that could be caused by metastatic disease (e.g. unexplained bone pain or weight loss), CT scan of chest and abdomen and a bone scan are recommended. MRI of the breast may help where breast cancer is not detected on mammography or ultrasound.

All patients with locally recurrent disease following mastectomy (Figs 26.6 and 26.7) or breast-conserving therapy, or with regional or metastatic recurrence require a CT scan.

TABLE 26.3 TNM Classification of Breast Cancer (8th edition)

Stage T Primary Tumour	Clinical Findings
TX	Primary tumour cannot be assessed
T0	No evidence of primary tumour
TiS	Carcinoma in situ
TiS (DCIS)	Ductal carcinoma in situ (DCIS)
TiS (LCIS)	Lobular carcinoma in situ (LCIS)
TiS (Paget's)	Paget's disease of the nipple not associated with invasive carcinoma and/or (Paget's) carcinoma in situ (DCIS and/or LCIS) in the underlying breast parenchyma. Carcinomas in the breast parenchyma associated with Paget disease are categorised based on the size and characteristics of the parenchymal disease, although the presence of Paget disease should still be noted
T1	Tumour ≤2 cm in greatest dimension
T1mi	Microinvasion ≤0.1 cm in greatest dimension
T1a	>0.1 cm but <0.5 cm in greatest dimension
T1b	>0..5 cm but <1 cm in greatest dimension
T1c	>1 cm but <2 cm in greatest dimension
T2	>2 cm but <5 cm in greatest dimension
T3	>5 cm in greatest dimension
T4	Tumour of any size with direct extension to chest wall and/or to skin (ulceration or skin nodules)
T4a	Extension to chest wall (does not include pectoralis muscle invasion only)
T4b	Ulceration, ipsilateral satellite skin nodules or skin oedema (including peau d'orange)
T4c	Inflammatory carcinoma
Regional Lymph Nodes	
NX	Regional lymph nodes cannot be assessed (e.g. previously removed)
N0	No regional lymph node metastases
N1	Metastases in ipsilateral level I, II axillary lymph nodes
N2	Metastases in ipsilateral level I, II axillary lymph node(s) that are clinically fixed or matted; or in clinically detected[a] ipsilateral internal mammary lymph node(s) in the absence of clinically evident axillary lymph node metastasis
N2a	Metastasis in axillary lymph node(s) fixed to one another (matted) or to other structures
N2b	Metastasis only in clinically detected[a] internal mammary lymph node(s) and in the absence of clinically detected axillary lymph node metastasis
N3	Metastasis in ipsilateral infraclavicular (level III axillary) lymph node(s) with or without level I, II axillary lymph node involvement; or metastasis in ipsilateral supraclavicular lymph node(s) with or without axillary or internal mammary lymph node involvement
N3a	Metastasis in infraclavicular lymph node(s)
N3b	Metastasis in internal mammary and axillary lymph nodes
N3c	Metastasis in supraclavicular lymph node(s)

Continued

MANAGEMENT OF DUCTAL CARCINOMA IN SITU

With adequate therapy, 99% of patients will survive following treatment. Where the prognosis is good, the morbidities associated with particular treatments (particularly from RT) need to be carefully weighed against the benefits of treatment. A palpable mass should undergo core biopsy. Impalpable malignant calcifications should be biopsied by stereotactic wire localisation. Paget's disease of the nipple should undergo punch biopsy. Microdochectomy or total ductal excision should follow smear of nipple discharge for malignant cells. Treatment will depend on presentation but will usually involve breast-conserving surgery with or without postoperative RT or mastectomy.

TABLE 26.3	TNM Classification of Breast Cancer (8th edition)—cont'd
Stage T Primary Tumour	**Clinical Findings**
M Distant Metastasis	
M0	No distant metastases
M1	Distant metastases
pTNM Pathological Classification	
pT: Primary Tumour The pathological classification requires the examination of the primary carcinoma with no gross tumour at the margins of resection. A case can be classified pT if there is only a microscopic tumour in a margin. The pT categories correspond to the T categories.	Note: When classifying pT, the tumour size is a measurement of the invasive component. If there is a large in situ component (e.g. 4 cm) and a small invasive component (e.g. .5 cm), the tumour is coded pT1a.
pN: Regional Lymph Nodes The pathological classification requires the resection and examination of at least the low axillary lymph nodes (level I). Such a resection will ordinarily include 6 or more lymph nodes. If the lymph nodes are negative, but the number ordinarily examined is not met, classify as pN0.	
pNX	Regional lymph nodes cannot be assessed (e.g. previously removed, or not removed for pathological study) pN0 No regional lymph node metastasis[b]
pN0	No regional lymph node metastasis [b]
pN1 larger than 2.0 mm	Micrometastases; or metastases in 1–3 axillary ipsilateral lymph nodes; and/or in internal mammary nodes with metastases detected by sentinel lymph node biopsy but not clinically detected [b]
pN1mi	Micrometastases (>2 mm and/or >200 cells, but none>)
pN1a	Metastasis in 1–3 axillary lymph node(s), including at least one larger than 2 mm in greatest dimension
pN1b	Internal mammary lymph nodes
pN1c	Metastasis in 1–3 axillary lymph nodes and internal mammary lymph nodes
pN2 pN2a Metastasis in 4–9 axillary lymph nodes, including at least one that is larger than 2 mm	Metastasis in 4–9 ipsilateral axillary lymph nodes, or in clinically detected [b] ipsilateral internal mammary lymph node(s) in the absence of axillary lymph node metastasis
pN2b pN3	Metastasis in clinically detected internal mammary lymph node(s), in the absence of axillary lymph node metastasis
pN3a	Metastasis in 10 or more ipsilateral axillary lymph nodes (at least one larger than 2 mm) or metastasis in infraclavicular lymph nodes
pN3b	Metastasis in clinically detected [b] internal ipsilateral mammary lymph node(s) in the presence of positive axillary lymph node(s); or metastasis in more than three axillary lymph nodes and in internal mammary lymph nodes with microscopic or macroscopic metastasis detected by sentinel lymph node biopsy but not clinically detected
pN3c	Metastasis in ipsilateral supraclavicular lymph node(s)
Posttreatment ypN: Posttreatment yp "N" should be evaluated as for clinical (pretreatment) "N" methods (see Section on Regional Lymph Nodes). The	

Continued

TABLE 26.3 TNM Classification of Breast Cancer (8th edition)—cont'd

Stage T Primary Tumour	Clinical Findings
modifier "sn" is used only if a sentinel node evaluation was performed after treatment. If no subscript is attached, it is assumed that the axillary nodal evaluation was by axillary node dissection. The X classification will be used (ypNX) if no yp posttreatment sn or axillary dissection was performed. N categories are the same as those used for pN.	

^aClinically detected is defined as detected by clinical examination or by imaging studies (excluding lymphoscintigraphy) and having characteristics highly suspicious for malignancy or a presumed pathological macrometastasis based on fine needle aspiration biopsy with cytological examination. Confirmation of clinically detected metastatic disease by fine needle aspiration without excision biopsy is designated with an (f) suffix, e.g. cN3a(f).

^bIsolated tumour cell clusters (ITC) are single tumour cells or small clusters of cells not more than 0.2 mm in greatest extent that can be detected by routine H and E stains or immunohistochemistry (IHC). An additional criterion has been proposed to include a cluster of fewer than 200 cells in a single histological cross section. Nodes containing only ITCs are excluded from the total positive node count for purposes of N classification and should be included in the total number of nodes evaluated.

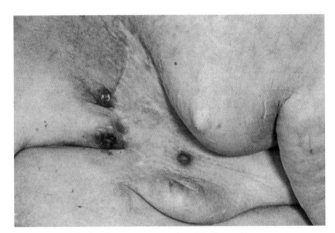

Fig. 26.6 Nodular local recurrence on the skin flaps of a mastectomy scar.

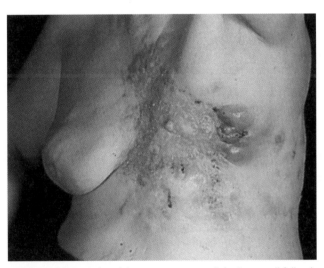

Fig. 26.7 Widespread nodular recurrence over left chest wall following mastectomy, extending to the other breast.

The rationale for mastectomy or whole breast irradiation as treatment for DCIS is related to the potential for multicentric disease and/or the presence of occult invasive cancer. Multifocal disease in the same quadrant is not unusual in patients with DCIS. Following wide excision and negative margins, 24% to 43% of patients will have residual DCIS in the same quadrant. Mastectomy remains the treatment of choice for multicentric DCIS and for large unicentric lesions. Recurrence rates after mastectomy are less than 1%. Regular mammography of the contralateral breast should be carried out because there is an increased rate of contralateral breast cancer of approximately 7 per 1000. If the extent of the lesion is not more than 3 to 4 cm, then an attempt at conservative surgery may be made, aiming to achieve complete excision. The margins of clearance should be at least 1 cm.

ROLE OF POSTOPERATIVE RADIOTHERAPY FOR DUCTAL CARCINOMA IN SITU

The risk of recurrence (both DCIS and invasive) is reduced by postoperative RT for all grades of DCIS by about one-half. However, the absolute benefits in low-grade disease are very small. Four randomised trials have assessed the impact of postoperative RT after breast-conserving surgery for DCIS (NSABP B-17, European Organisation for Research and Treatment of Cancer (EORTC) 10853, UK/ANZ and SweDCIS). All employed 50 Gy in 25 daily fractions over 5 weeks without a boost dose to the site of excision. All show a reduction in DCIS and invasive recurrence. Pooled data from these trials in a Cochrane review showed that RT halved the risk of recurrence after breast-conserving surgery at 10 years. About half the recurrences were DCIS and half invasive. In the Cochrane review, older patients (>50 years) derived more benefit from RT than younger patients. However, none of the trials was prospectively designed for subgroup analysis. International practice varies with all grades of DCIS following breast-conserving surgery and clear margins being treated by postoperative RT in some Western countries. In the United Kingdom, practice tends to be more selective with postoperative RT confined to higher grade tumours. The definition of a truly low-risk group which could be safely treated by breast-conserving surgery alone has proven difficult to determine. Studies suggest that even in apparently low-risk patients, the overall risks of invasive recurrence may be up to 10% to 20% at 15 years.

The role of a boost dose (16 Gy in 8 fractions) after breast-conserving surgery and whole breast irradiation is unclear and is under study in the BIG 3.07 DCIS boost trial. This trial is also comparing standard dose fractionation (50 Gy in 25 daily fractions over 5 weeks) to hypofractionation (42.5 Gy in 16 daily fractions over 3.5 weeks).

There is no indication for axillary dissection or irradiation of the peripheral lymphatics in DCIS because the risk of positive axillary nodes is 4% or less. The overall prognosis of DCIS is excellent with in excess of 97% of patients alive and disease free 10 or more years following diagnosis.

PROGNOSTIC AND PREDICTIVE FACTORS FOR INVASIVE BREAST CANCER

The prognosis for breast cancer in the United Kingdom has substantially improved over the last three decades.

Five-year survival is now around 90% compared with about 50% in the 1970s (Fig. 26.8).

Biomarkers may be prognostic of clinical outcome or predictive of response to treatment or both.

Stage

Prognosis is excellent for stage 1 disease at diagnosis with 98% 5-year survival, falling progressively to 15% for stage IV. The St. Gallen Breast Cancer Consensus has established three well-accepted categories of risk (Table 26.4). These are defined by age, axillary node status, histological and/or nuclear grade, presence or absence of lymphovascular invasion and HER2 status.

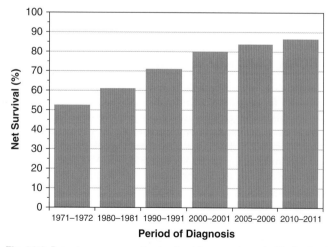

Fig. 26.8 Breast cancer: age standardised 5-year net survival in England and Wales, 1971 to 2011. (From Cancer Research UK, www.cruk.org. With permission.)

Age

Age is an independent prognostic factor. Women aged 35 years or younger have a higher risk of locoregional recurrence and distant relapse. Tumours in women younger than 35 years are more likely to be high grade and ER and PgR negative and HER2 positive. These women are more prone to local recurrence, being diagnosed at an advanced stage and having a lower 5-year survival compared with older premenopausal patients. Encouragingly, the rates of local recurrence in young women with breast cancer are falling. Adjuvant systemic therapy and a radiation boost to the tumour bed after whole breast irradiation reduce the risk of recurrence by 50%. A recent study from The Netherlands of 1000 women with nonmetastatic breast cancer aged younger than 35 years showed that the 5-year risk of local breast recurrence was 3.2% and 3.8% for chest wall recurrence after mastectomy. Comparing 2003 versus 2008 cohorts, the local, regional and distant recurrence rates were as follows: 4.2% and 3.2% (local), 6.1% and 4.4% (regional) and 17.8% and 10% (distant).

Tumour Size

Tumour size is a strong independent prognostic factor for overall and recurrence-free survival. A positive correlation has been found between tumour size and the number of involved axillary lymph nodes. The St. Gallen Consensus panel classify tumours larger than 2 cm as intermediate or high risk, even where there are no other adverse prognostic factors.

Axillary Node Status

Nodal status is the strongest independent prognostic factor in breast cancer. If the axillary nodes are not involved, the 5-year survival rate

TABLE 26.4 St. Gallen Breast Cancer Consensus Risk Categories	
Low risk	Node negative AND all of the following features: Primary tumour (pT) ≤2 cm, AND Grade 1 AND Absence of extensive peritumoral vascular invasionΔ, AND HER2/neu gene neither overexpressed nor amplified◊, AND Age ≥35
Intermediate risk	Node negative AND at least one of the following features: Primary tumour (pT) >2 cm, OR Grade 2–3, OR Presence of extensive peritoumoral vascular invasionΔ, OR Oestrogen receptor (ER) and progesterone receptor (PR) absent HER2/neu gene overexpressed or amplified, OR Age <35 years Node positive (1–3 involved nodes) AND ER and/or PR expressed AND HER2/neu gene neither overexpressed nor amplified
High risk	Node positive (1–3 involved nodes) AND ER and PR absent or HER2/neu gene overexpressed or amplified Node positive (4 or more involved nodes)

Δ, Extensive peritumoral vascular invasion (i.e. neoplastic emboli seen in two or more blocks of the tumour) was a recognized a discriminating feature of increased risk; its presence defined intermediate-risk for node negative disease but did not influence risk category for node positive.
◊, HER2/neu overexpresson or amplification must be determined by quality controlled assays using immunohistochemistry or FISH analysis.

is 98%. If the nodes are involved, 5-year survival rate falls to 84%. There is a direct correlation between number of involved nodes and survival. Nodal micrometastases or isolated tumour cells in lymph nodes should not influence risk allocation.

Tumour grade remains an important prognostic factor with significantly better survival for grade 1 compared with grades 2 and 3. The Gene Expression Grade Index is able to classify grade 2 lesions into two groups at high and low risk of recurrence. There is uncertainty as to the role of grade 2 in defining intermediate-risk prognosis. Unfortunately, 50% of patients fall into the grade 2 category.

HER2/neu Status

HER2 status is both a prognostic and predictive factor in breast cancer. The HER2 gene regulates a protein on the surface of cells that promotes their growth (see later section on HER2-positive breast cancer). In patients with HER2-positive breast cancer, their cancer cells make too many copies of, or overexpress, the HER2 gene. HER2 protein overexpression or gene amplication is an adverse prognostic factor. The incidence of HER2 positivity is 13% to 20%. Testing entails immunohistochemistry (IHC) with more than 10% complete strong membrane staining defining a positive test. Patients with HER2 overexpression are likely to respond to anti-HER2 therapy with trastuzumab.

Lymphovascular Invasion

Lymphovascular invasion is an adverse prognostic factor in axillary node-negative disease. There are conflicting results as to whether or not it is a poor prognostic factor in axillary node-positive disease.

Prognostic Indices

The principal prognostic indices in clinical practice are the Nottingham Prognostic Index (NPI) and Adjuvant! Online (AOL). The NPI is based on three pathological criteria: the size of the lesion (S); the number of involved lymph nodes (N); and the grade of the tumour (G). It is calculated according to the formula: NPI = [.2 × S] + N + G. Fig. 26.9 illustrates the discriminant prognostic value of NPI.

AOL is a web-based decision aid which estimates the impact on risk of relapse and cancer-related mortality of omitting systemic therapy based on prognostic information for the particular patient (age at diagnosis, size of tumour, axillary node status etc.). It predicts the reduction in risks for different therapies. The colour-coded graphical printout helps patients and their clinicians weigh the risks and benefits of different systemic therapies.

Hormonal Receptor Status

Hormone receptor status is both a prognostic and predictive factor in breast cancer. At least 1% of ER-positive cancer is required for hormonal therapy. ER is the only established predictive marker for response to endocrine therapy. However, about one-third of ER-positive and/or PgR-positive patients do not respond to endocrine therapy. ER status is moderately prognostic and highly predictive of response to hormonal therapy. PgR status is strongly prognostic but weakly predictive of response. ER and PgR status have been validated with level 1 evidence.

Ki67

Ki67 represents proliferation status and predicts sensitivity to chemotherapy. However it is not standardised and is not used in standard care. The commonly used cutoff is 20%. Ki67 is moderately prognostic but weakly predictive of response, and there is no level 1 evidence to support its validation.

Molecular Subtype

Immunohistochemical staining for ER, PgR and HER2 is used to approximate breast cancer molecular subtype. Molecular subtype is prognostic of overall survival with the best outcomes for luminal-A and the worst for basal subtype. Luminal-B tumours have an intermediate prognosis.

Gene Profiling

More recently, microarray-based gene profiling has enabled thousands of genes to be studied in one tumour. A microarray consists of known and unknown DNA samples on a solid slide (Fig. 26.10). The probes may be cDNAs or oligonucleotides of varying length. The sequence hybridised to probes on the array can be fluorescently labelled. Expression signatures based on the expression level of large numbers of genes can be determined, reflecting the properties of the cells studied. The microarray in node negative disease may avoid chemotherapy (MINDACT) trial, using MammaPrint 70 gene signature in women with early breast cancer at high clinical risk and low genomic risk for recurrence receiving no chemotherapy based on MammaPrint, resulted in a 5-year survival rate 1.5% lower than the rate with chemotherapy. This implies that 46% of women who are at high clinical risk might not require chemotherapy. However, one limitation is that MammaPrint requires freshly frozen tumour tissue, which makes it more complex to implement. The Oncotype DX signature helps to identify women with intermediate risk stage 1 or 2, axillary node-negative, ER-positive, HER2-negative disease who may or may not benefit from chemotherapy. In the Trial Assigning Individualized Options for Treatment (Rx) (Tailorx trial), patients with a low recurrence Oncotype DX score had a 5-year metastasis-free survival rate with endocrine therapy of 99.3%, and an overall survival of 98%, even without chemotherapy.

Endocrine Therapy

Endocrine therapy is based on blocking the effects of oestrogen which stimulates tumour growth or inhibits its production. Oestrogen passes through the cell membrane and binds the ER. ER alpha, one of the two species of ER binding to ligand, leads to phosphorylation and

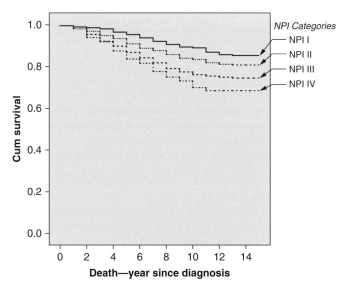

Fig. 26.9 The Nottingham Prognostic Index *(NPI)*: 5- and 10-year data from all-cause survival within a screened population. (From Fong Y et al. The Nottingham Prognostic Index. Five- and ten-year data from all-cause survival with in a screened population. Ann R Coll Surg Eng. 2015;97:37–139. With permission)

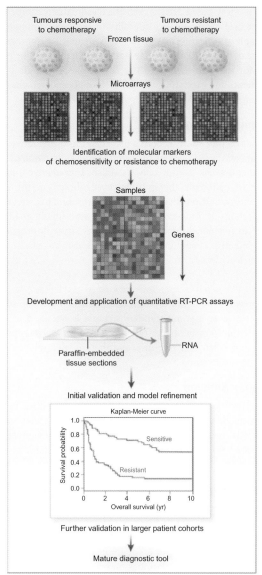

Fig. 26.10 Development of microarray-based diagnostic tests for cancer. Primary or metastatic tumours are resected from patients; DNA microarray profiling is used to obtain gene-expression profiles of the tumours. Next, genome-computational and statistical analyses are used to identify gene-expression markers of responsiveness or resistance to chemotherapy; multiplex quantitative reverse transcriptase-polymerase chain reaction *(RT-PCR)* assays are developed for the best markers, and these assays are applied retrospectively or prospectively to formalin-fixed, paraffin-embedded tissue sections. On the basis of the results, researchers develop diagnostic and predictive models that can be validated in large cohorts of patients, resulting in a mature diagnostic tool. *RNA,* Ribonuclic acid. (From Rawasharmy S. Translating genomics into clinical oncology. N Engl J Med 2004;350:1814–1816. With permission.)

transcription. Most of the oestrogen is sited in the nucleus, but some probably exists in the cell membrane where it may interact with growth factors. Activation of membrane ER by either oestrogen or tamoxifen and the ensuing activation of growth factor signalling may be a cause of tamoxifen resistance in certain patients who overexpress HER2. It is possible that a combination of ER-targeted therapy and growth factor receptor-targeted therapy might reverse tamoxifen resistance. Cross talk between growth factor receptor pathways and ER might elucidate the relationship between PgR expression and response to a variety of hormonal therapies. As a result of an active growth factor kinase cascade, the transcription of the PgR gene may be inhibited. Hence, in some tumours, PgR negativity may be a surrogate for active growth factor signalling. This would suggest that ER-positive, PgR-negative tumours would respond better to aromatase inhibition than to selective ER modulators (SERMs), as in HER2-positive tumours. Indeed, the ATAC trial showed better outcomes in PgR-negative tumours with anastrozole than tamoxifen. There is accumulating data that ER-positive, PgR-negative tumours are a discrete subset with a tendency to higher growth factor receptor activity, relative resistance to SERMs and greater sensitivity to aromatase inhibitors (AIs) such as anastrazole and letrozole.

ER status is predictive for disease-free and overall survival. Irrespective of stage, ER positivity predicts for longer disease-free and overall survival. Higher recurrence and lower survival rates are found in ER-negative patients. About 60% of ER-positive patients will respond to hormonal manipulation. Progesterone receptor status may also help. Oestrogen stimulates PgR production in normal reproductive tissue and in human breast cancer cell lines. The highest response and disease-free survival rate is seen in ER+/PgR+ tumours. Very few tumours are ER-/PgR+, consistent with the production of progesterone receptors being dependent on oestrogen synthesis. Lowest response and disease-free survival rates are seen in ER-/PgR- tumours.

Of the biological markers of prognosis, including p53, cathepsin D, epidermal growth factor receptor and HER2/neu, HER2/neu is the most reproducible. Patients overexpressing HER2/neu have a higher risk of recurrence and a shorter survival rate. There is evidence that tumours that overexpress HER2/neu are relatively resistant to chemotherapy with cyclophosphamide, methotrexate and 5-fluorouracil (5-FU) (CMF) and have greater responsiveness to anthracyclines. In addition, different gene profiles may be found for ER-positive and ER-negative patients.

Mastectomy or Breast Conservation

Breast-conserving surgery is the intended standard of care for most cases of breast cancer. In considering the possibility of breast-conserving surgery, the tumour size, the size of the breast and the mammographic appearance or histology from excision or core biopsy are important. As a general rule, most tumours in excess of 3 cm are unsuitable for breast-conserving therapy unless the breast size is sufficiently large not to result in a marked tissue defect marring cosmesis. Greater flexibility in offering breast conservation is possible with the availability of newer surgical techniques to fill the tissue defect from local excision by a graft. Preoperative systemic therapy with chemotherapy or hormonal therapy, as appropriate, may allow sufficient tumour shrinkage for breast-conserving surgery rather than mastectomy. Tumours of 3 cm or greater at the time of surgery, judged either clinically or radiologically, are generally best treated by mastectomy and axillary node clearance. Patients who have clinical or radiological evidence of multifocal disease or have an extensive intraduct component (EIC) are not suitable for breast conservation. Involved margins after breast-conserving surgery should be re-excised. Mastectomy may be required if it is not possible to clear the margins. Patients should be fully involved in the decision-making process.

There is evidence that local recurrence rates following breast-conserving surgery are higher in younger women. Women under the age of 35 have a higher risk of local recurrence after breast-conserving surgery and RT. This may in part be because of the difficulty of identifying cancers by mammography in younger women who tend to have more radiodense breasts or the more aggressive biology of the disease in younger women.

Lobular Cancer

Some histological forms of breast cancer, typically lobular cancer, are commonly multifocal but poorly imaged by mammography. If a core or excision biopsy of an apparently localised tumour shows lobular carcinoma, an initial wide local excision may be carried out. If the margins are involved with invasive cancer or there is evidence of multifocal disease histologically, then breast conservation is not safe and mastectomy is advised.

Reconstruction After Mastectomy

Mastectomy is a mutilating operation, but much can be achieved in remodeling the breast by use of autologous tissue or implants. Most patients should be offered the possibility of immediate breast construction.

Conservation Therapy (Limited Surgery and Postoperative Radiotherapy)

In patients with T1 and small T2 tumours (≤3 cm), some form of local surgery should be considered. The most popular choice is a wide local excision to obtain clear histological margins. This involves excision of the tumour with a margin of 1 to 2 cm. If the margins are found to be involved, a re-excision to clear the margins is recommended. If re-excision of the margins still shows the tumour at the margin, further re-excision or mastectomy should be considered.

A variety of oncoplastic techniques are available to allow larger resections while maintaining the natural shape of the breast. Reduction mammoplasty is possible in small- and medium-sized breasts. Criteria for breast conservation are summarised in Table 26.5.

Local Recurrence After Breast-Conserving Therapy

The treatment of choice for local recurrence after breast-conserving surgery and postoperative RT is a mastectomy.

Management of the Axilla

Some form of surgical procedure to obtain nodal histology is advised in virtually all women with operable breast cancer. Sentinel node biopsy has become the standard procedure for women with early breast cancer and clinically and ultrasonically negative nodes. Women with palpable nodes should undergo axillary node dissection if they have not received preoperative systemic therapy. Sentinel node biopsy avoids the morbidity of axillary dissection and has become the standard of care in nodal staging of patients without metastases on axillary ultrasound. The sentinel node is the node most likely to drain the primary tumour. It is identified first by the injection of a vital blue dye or a radioactive tracer, or a combination of both. The combination of both techniques is the most accurate. In most patients, the sentinel node is in the axilla but, in a few medially placed tumours, it may be in the internal mammary chain. The axilla is normally explored to identify the sentinel node either by the blue colour of the dye within it or by the high radioactivity scintillation count over it. If the sentinel node biopsy is positive, the surgeon may proceed to a complete axillary dissection or refer the patient for axillary irradiation. In specialist centres, sentinel node biopsy has 97% accuracy.

For patients with clinically involved axillary nodes, a level III axillary clearance up to the level of the medial end of the first rib is recommended. Normally, there should be at least 10 axillary nodes in a level

---

TABLE 26.5 Criteria for Breast-Conserving Therapy

1. Tumours ≥3 cm
2. Satisfactory cosmetic result anticipated
3. Postoperative whole breast radiotherapy technically feasible
4. Medically fit for surgery
5. Clear histological margins at primary excision or re-excision
6. Able to attend regular clinical and mammographic follow-ups

---

III clearance and commonly, there are 20 to 30. The local control in the axilla from a level III clearance is similar to a selective policy of axillary RT in patients with one or more involved nodes on a four-node lower axillary sample. With either policy, the axillary recurrence rate is similar, 5% at 5 years.

REGIONAL NODAL IRRADIATION

Axillary irradiation is an alternative to axillary node clearance. In the EORTC 10891/22023 AMAROS trial 4823 patients with T1-T2,N0 breast cancer were randomised if they had one to two positive sentinel nodes to axillary node clearance or axillary irradiation. At a median follow-up of 6.1 years, the 5-year axillary recurrence rate, the primary endpoint (for which the trial was underpowered), 0.43% (95% confidence interval (CI) 0.00–0.92) after axillary clearance and 1.19% after axillary RT (95% CI 0.31–2.08) were not significantly different. Neither did disease-free or overall survival differ (Fig. 26.11). At 5 years, lymphoedema (arm circumference >10% greater in the ipsilateral upper or lower arm or both) was significantly more frequent after axillary node clearance (13%) compared with 5% for axillary RT. Patients with low volume axillary disease can therefore be spared the morbidity of axillary clearance. For more extensive axillary disease, axillary clearance is still recommended. The Early Breast Cancer Trialists Collaborative Group (EBCTCG) showed that in women treated with or without postmastectomy, irradiation including the supraclavicular fossa, axilla and internal mammary chain, there was an 8% reduction in breast cancer mortality at 20 years in the one to three node-positive group (Fig. 26.17). A Danish internal mammary node trial showed a 3.7% survival benefit with greater gains in N2 disease, and N1 disease with central/medial tumours.

Can we identify particular subgroups that benefit from RNI? The trial populations of MA.20 and the EORTC IMC trial differed. MA.20 studied patients with N1 (85%) and high-risk node negative (10%) disease. The EORTC recruited N0 (44%) and N1 (43%) patients. The larger N0 group in the EORTC is likely to have had a lower risk of internal mammary nodes because the latter are associated with axillary node metastases. It is not clear how much benefit is derived from supraclavicular as opposed to internal mammary nodal irradiation (IMN). Given that RNI only added 3% to 5% improvement in disease-free survival and 1% to 1.6% in overall survival, the absolute benefit from treating any one of these sites is even less. In addition, supraclavicular relapse has a bad prognosis similar to that of de novo supraclavicular node involvement (N3), whereas, clinically involved IMNs have a relatively good prognosis. Both the MA.20 and EORTC trials employed axillary clearance so it is not clear how the results apply to the current practice of sentinel node biopsy. It is possible that IMN irradiation could be an effective salvage therapy for IMN relapse, but there are no data to support this, and it would be difficult to prove. Where the absolute benefits of IMN irradiation are very small, the decision on whether to irradiate the internal mammary nodes or not must be balanced against the risks of radiation pneumonitis (1% absolute increase and 4% lymphoedema in the MA.20 trial). Although neither the MA.20 nor EORTC trial reported any increase in cardiac events, the risk of increased cardiac dosage is higher with left-sided compared with right-sided tumours. It may therefore only be reasonable to treat the internal mammary nodes if anatomy is favourable, minimising doses to heart and lungs. Breath-hold techniques are advised to minimise dose to the heart (Figs 26.12 and 26.13).

Recommendations (based on the statement of the Association of Breast Surgery, 2015) for management of the axilla following sentinel node biopsy after mastectomy or breast-conserving surgery are:

1. If sentinel node shows isolated tumour cells and/or micrometastases, no further treatment.

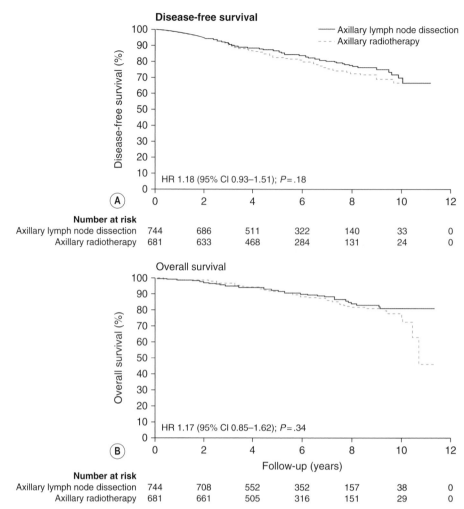

Fig. 26.11 European Organisation for Research and Treatment of Cancer (EORTC) 10891/22023 AMAROS trial; disease-free and overall survival. *CI,* Confidence interval; *HR,* heart rate. (From Donker M et al. Radiotherapy or surgery of the axilla after a positive sentinel node in breast cancer (EORTC 10981-22023 AMAROS: a randomised, multicentre open label, phase 111 non inferiority trial. Lancet Oncol. 2014;15:1303-1310. With permission.)

2. If one to two sentinel node(s) show macrometastases after breast-conserving surgery in patients receiving whole breast irradiation, if postmenopausal TI, grade 1 or 2, ER-positive, HER2-negative, further axillary treatment is no longer mandatory. Patients could be entered into the POsitive Sentinel NOde: Adjuvant Therapy Alone Versus Adjuvant Therapy Plus Clearance or Axillary Radiotherapy (POSNOC) or equivalent trial. If one to two sentinel node(s) show macrometastases after mastectomy or in tumours with one of the following criteria: T3, grade 3, ER-negative or HER2-positive, further axillary treatment should usually be recommended. These patients could also be entered into the POSNOC or equivalent clinical trial. There was no consensus on the management of patients with one or more of the following features: premenopausal status, T2 tumours, lymphovascular invasion or extranodal spread.

3. If three or more sentinel node(s) show macrometastases, patients should usually be recommended to have further axillary treatment.

4. Axillary RT is a valid alternative treatment to axillary lymph node dissection in patients with a low burden of axillary disease.

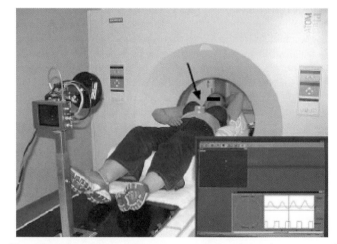

Fig. 26.12 The Varian RPM system displayed in the computed tomography-scanner facility. A passive, infrared light reflecting marker (*arrow*) is placed on the patient's chest wall over the xiphoid process. The vertical motion of the marker is tracked by an infrared-sensitive video camera and the input projected onto a computer screen breathing curve. The insert shows the gating computer screen with the video camera view and the breathing curve.

INDICATIONS FOR INTERNAL MAMMARY IRRADIATION

1. Patients at high risk of locoregional recurrence (i.e. T4 or ≥4 axillary macrometastases).
2. Patients with one to three positive nodes where regional nodal irradiation is advised, taking into account risk factors (e.g. central/medial location of primary in the breast), laterality and likely dose to heart and lungs.

Morbidity of Axillary Treatment

Side effects of an axillary clearance include postoperative seroma and numbness in the upper limb. Lymphoedema occurs in 7% to 8% of cases. If axillary RT is added to the dissection, the risk of lymphoedema is substantially higher (between 30% and 40%).

After conventionally fractionated RT (e.g. 45–50 Gy in 20–25 fractions) to the axilla, the risk of lymphoedema is about 3% to 5%, that is, lower than after axillary dissection. However, there is an increased risk of long-term restriction of shoulder movement and a small risk of brachial plexopathy (≤1%). Brachial plexopathy is a rare but serious complication and is usually irreversible. Very careful attention to RT technique with avoidance of overlap between axillary and breast/chest wall fields or moving the patient between the treatment of these fields is essential.

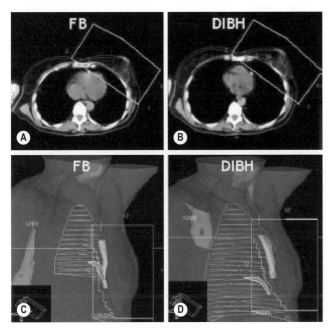

Fig. 26.13 The tangential fields for different respiratory patterns and the volume delineation principles. The transverse view in the same couch position for a sample patient in treatment position during (A) free breathing *(FB)* and (B) deep inspiration breath-hold *(DIBH)* mode are displayed. In addition, beam's eye views of the medial field during (C) FB and (D) DIBH are shown. Note the difference in lung inflation and in cardiac/LACDA *(white encircled)* position. (From Elsevier Ltd. Pedersen AN et al. Breathing adapted radiotherapy of breast cancer: reduction of cardiac and pulmonary doses using voluntary inspiration breath-hold. Radiother Oncol. 2004;72:53-60. With permission.)

Postoperative Radiotherapy

After Breast-Conserving Surgery

In general, postoperative whole breast irradiation should be delivered following wide local excision as part of breast-conserving therapy. The EBCTCG metaanalysis of randomised trials of breast-conserving surgery with or without RT shows a halving of the risk of first recurrence, irrespective of risk category (see Further Reading).

An overall survival benefit was demonstrated by the addition of postoperative RT after breast-conserving surgery (Fig. 26.14).

There is much less randomised data on the role of postoperative RT in older patients, particularly over the age of 65 years, receiving adjuvant endocrine therapy. The most mature data are from the CALGB 9343 trial in which 636 ER-positive patients 70 years of age and older with TI,N0 tumours treated with 5 years of adjuvant tamoxifen were randomised to postoperative whole breast irradiation or no RT. At 10 years, 90% of patients in the tamoxifen group (95% CI, 85%–93%) compared with 98% in the tamoxifen + RT group (95% CI, 96%–99%) were free from locoregional recurrence.

In the PRIME 2 trial in 1386 patients with axillary node-negative T1-2 (<3 cm), pN0, M0 hormone receptor-positive breast cancer

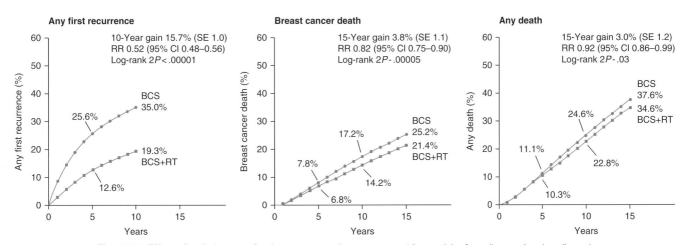

Fig. 26.14 Effect of radiotherapy after breast-conserving surgery on 10-year risk of any (locoregional or distant) first recurrence and on 15-year risks of breast cancer death and death from any cause in 10,801 women (67% with pathologically node-negative disease) in 17 trials. *BCS, RT, RR* (From Early Breast Cancer Trialists Collaborative Group (EBCTCG). Darby S et al. Effect of radiotherapy after breast conserving surgery on 10 year recurrence and 15-year breast cancer death: meta-analysis of individual patient data for 10,801 women in 17 randomised trials. Lancet 2011;378:1707–1716. With permission.)

randomised to whole breast irradiation or no RT following breast-conserving surgery with minimum 1-mm clear margins, the local recurrence rate in the irradiated arm at 5 years of follow-up was significantly lower (1.3% vs 4.1%, 95% CI .0.2–2.3, $P = .0002$), but the absolute difference was very small (2.8%) (see Further Reading). The National Institute for Care and Clinical Excellence (NICE) suggests consideration of omission of RT for invasive cancer in women if margins are clear, there is a low absolute risk of local recurrence ($\geq$65 years, T1,NO, ER positive, grade 1 or 2) and they are willing to take adjuvant endocrine therapy for a minimum of 5 years. Overall survival at 10 years without RT after breast-conserving surgery is the same with or without RT. Current U.K. (PRIME TIME) (postoperative avoidance of radiotherapy:biomarker selection of women at very low risk of recurrence) and North American studies (LUMINA, PRECISION) are evaluating whether biomarkers can assist in identifying a truly low-risk group of older patients from whom postoperative RT can be safely omitted after breast-conserving surgery.

Following Mastectomy

More than half of the locoregional recurrences following mastectomy occur on the chest wall. The mastectomy scar is the commonest site of recurrence (see Figs 26.7 and 26.8). Postmastectomy RT is standard in women with four or more involved axillary nodes and for T3,NI tumours

The role of adjuvant RT following mastectomy in patients with one to three involved nodes remains controversial and both guidelines and practice vary. Before 1997, it was accepted that postmastectomy irradiation improved locoregional control but not survival. However, in 1997, two landmark randomised trials conducted in Denmark and Canada showed a 9% to 10% survival benefit from the addition of locoregional RT following mastectomy to adjuvant CMF chemotherapy. The much larger Danish trial in high-risk premenopausal patients (Fig. 26.15) of over 3000 patients showed that a significant advantage accrued to patients receiving adjuvant irradiation (10-year survival 54% vs 45%). A trial from the same trial group (Fig. 26.16) shows a similar 9% survival (45% vs 36%) benefit in high-risk postmenopausal women receiving locoregional regional irradiation in addition to adjuvant tamoxifen. However, the survival advantage of the benefits of RT only emerged late (i.e. at 10 years). In both the Danish and Canadian trials, all of the peripheral lymphatics (axilla, supraclavicular and internal mammary chain) were irradiated. It is not clear whether irradiation of all of these areas, particularly the internal mammary chain is essential.

The RT technique in the Danish trial differed from the use of a pair of tangential fields in most UK centres to treat the chest wall. A combination of electron beam with limited penetration beyond the chest wall was used to treat the medial part of the chest wall and matched with a photon field to treat the lateral half of the chest wall. Ten-year follow-up data showed no excess of cardiac morbidity or mortality in the RT plus systemic therapy group compared with those receiving systemic therapy alone. The results of the Danish trial emphasise the importance of good RT technique in minimising the dose to the heart.

The most recent Oxford overview of randomised trials of postmastectomy RT (see Further Reading) shows a survival advantage from postmastectomy RT not only in patients with four or more involved nodes but also in those with one to three involved nodes. For 1314 women treated by axillary clearance and one to three positive nodes, RT reduced locoregional recurrence ($P < .0001$), overall recurrence (RR 0.68, 95% CI 0.57–0.82, $P = .00006$) and breast cancer mortality (RR 0.80, 95% CI 0.67–0.95, $P = .01$) (Fig. 26.17). The Oxford overview shows that the higher the baseline risk of recurrence, the higher the survival benefit. This latter observation contrasts with a retrospective analysis of the Danish PMRT trials, which showed a greater survival benefit for patients with low-risk features and luminal subtype. These contradictory findings might be explained by the complex interaction of local control and better systemic therapy. It is not clear whether more aggressive locoregional therapy should be recommended in more aggressive tumours. On the basis of the results of the Oxford overview, some have argued that PMRT should be recommended for all patients with one to three positive nodes. However, the locoregional recurrence in unirradiated patients was 16.5% at 5 years and 20.3% at 10 years, higher levels than seen in the United States and other countries. It is therefore difficult to extrapolate from the EBCTCG analysis to all patients with one to three positive nodes. It remains unclear which subsets benefit.

Consideration has to be given to the serious side effects of nodal irradiation (lymphoedema, pneumonitis, cardiac damage and second malignancy).

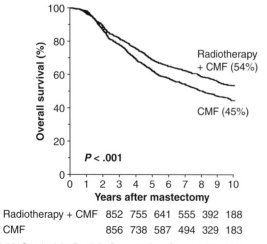

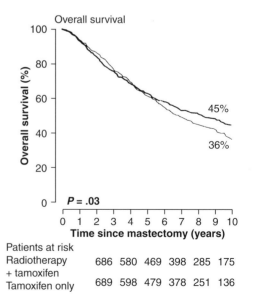

Patients at risk

Radiotherapy + tamoxifen	686	580	469	398	285	175
Tamoxifen only	689	598	479	378	251	136

Radiotherapy + CMF	852	755	641	555	392	188
CMF	856	738	587	494	329	183

Fig. 26.15 Survival in Danish Cooperative Group trials of locoregional radiotherapy after adjuvant cyclophosphamide, methotrexate and 5-fluorouracil (5-FU) *(CMF)* in high-risk premenopausal women. (From Overgaard M et al. Postoperative radiotherapy in high-risk premenopausal women with breast cancer who receive adjuvant chemotherapy. Danish Breast Cancer Cooperative Group 82b trial. N EnglJ Med. 1997; 337:949-955. With permission.)

Fig. 26.16 Survival in Danish Cooperative Group trials of locoregional radiotherapy after adjuvant tamoxifen in high-risk postmenopausal women. (From Elsevier Ltd., Overgaard M. Postoperative radiotherapy in high-risk postmenopausal breast cancer patients given adjuvant tamoxifen: Danish Breast Cancer Cooperative Group 82c randomised trial. from Lancet. 1999;353:1642. With permission.)

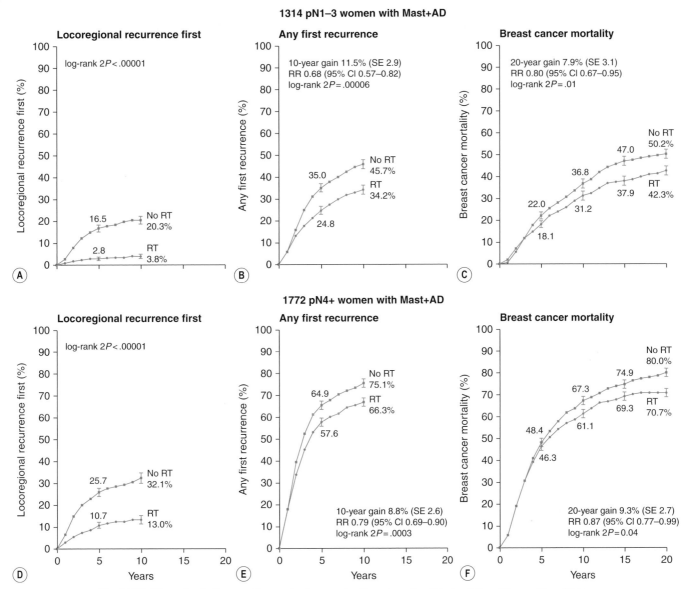

Fig. 26.17 Effect of radiotherapy after mastectomy and axillary dissection (Mast + AD) on 10-year risks of locoregional and overall recurrence and on 20-year risk of breast cancer mortality in 1314 women with one to three pathologically positive nodes (pN1–3) and in 1772 women with four or more pathologically positive nodes (pN4 +). (From Early Breast Cancer Trialists Collaborative Group (EBCTCG). McGale P et al. Effect of radiotherapy after mastectomy and axillary surgery on 10-year recurrence and 20 year breast cancer mortality: meta-analysis of individual data for 8135 women in 22 randomised trials. Lancet. 2014;383:2127-2135. With permission.)

It is known that the risk of local recurrence increases with the cumulative number of risk factors (high tumour grade, nodal involvement and lymphovascular invasion). How these factors should be weighted in the selection of patients for postmastectomy RT is not clear.

The 2017 St. Gallen Consensus statement, taking into account the improvement in disease-free survival in two trials of regional nodal irradiation, the EORTC internal mammary node trial and the MA-17 trial recommended PMRT for patients with one to three positive nodes and adverse biological features (young age (≤40 years), low or negative ER expression, high-grade histology and extensive lymphovascular invasion). However, it is difficult to find a sound basis for selection, particularly subgroups of one to three node-positive for irradiation or not, because none of the trials in the overview had prospectively planned subgroup analyses. Currently in the United Kingdom, the MRC/EORTCSUPREMO trial, now in follow-up phase, is the only prospective trial that is evaluating the role of chest wall irradiation in patients after mastectomy and axillary node clearance with one to three involved nodes or node negative with other risk factors (grade 3 and/or lymphovascular invasion receiving contemporary systemic therapy and, where appropriate, anti-HER2 therapy. It has a biological substudy, TRANS SUPREMO, seeking a molecular signature of radiosensitivity. Hopefully, it may provide the basis for selecting patients for PMRT on the basis of biological as well as clinicopathological factors. In the absence of more definitive evidence, the pros and cons of PMRT in women with one to three positive nodes will have to be discussed in multidisciplinary teams on an individual basis.

Indications for postmastectomy radiotherapy. International consensus supports the routine use of postmastectomy RT for patients who have a 20% or more risk of locoregional recurrence:

1. Tumours greater than 5 cm in diameter.
2. Four or more histologically involved axillary nodes.

Guidelines on postmastectomy RT for patients with one to three involved nodes vary. NICE guidelines (2018) recommend adjuvant RT for all patients with axillary macrometastases.

In addition, RT is indicated for:

1. Close or involved surgical margins.
2. Chest wall recurrence following mastectomy.

TARGET VOLUME AND TECHNIQUES FOR LOCOREGIONAL IRRADIATION

In choosing a technique, guiding principles should be homogeneous irradiation of the target areas, avoidance of overlap of chest wall/breast with fields to the peripheral lymphatics and minimising dosage to critical structures (lung, heart and the brachial plexus).

This is not an easy task because of the variation in shape and thickness of the chest wall and breast in the craniocaudal and transverse planes. In addition, the sternum slopes when the patient is lying flat. The proximity of the lung and heart to the target volume means that some lung is commonly irradiated. Dose inhomogeneity is exacerbated by lung effects because of scatter and lung transmission.

Computed Tomography Simulation

Over the last decade, most UK centres have migrated from two-dimensional to three-dimensional RT planning. Three-dimensional planning is now the standard of care. Radiation planning techniques have expanded to forward planned field-in-field and intensity-modulated RT (IMRT). This range of techniques with better visualisation of target volume (breast, regional nodes and critical structures (heart, brachial plexus)) has allowed treatment to be individualised and risks of morbidity to be diminished. The adoption of three-dimensional planning has enabled a move from field placements based on anatomical landmarks to individualised delineation of target volumes and critical structures and better homogeneity of dose distribution, while minimising dosage to organs at risk. The evidence that postoperative irradiation after mastectomy and breast-conserving therapy improves survival (by mechanisms which remain unclear) and that older RT techniques compromised survival by cardiac damage underpins efforts to optimise maximal antitumour effect with the lowest risk of morbidity.

Full computed tomography (CT) scanning of the breast and/or peripheral lymphatics requires the patient to be planned with the ipsilateral arm abducted behind the head or with both hands holding a bar in front of the patient to fit into the bore of most CT scanners. For treatment of the breast alone, the patient should be scanned in the treatment position from lung apices to the bottom of the lungs and breast and nodal fields from the mastoid to the bottom of the lungs.

Where the internal mammary nodes are to be included as part of regional nodal irradiation, breath hold techniques with wide tangents or rotational techniques to minimise cardiac irradiation are recommended (see Figs 26.12 and 26.13).

INTENSITY MODULATED RADIOTHERAPY

IMRT has become available to provide a more even distribution of radiation dose across the breast/chest wall while reducing unwanted irradiation of critical organs such as the lung and heart. IMRT allows the fluence intensity to be varied across the beam. Virtual simulation, which incorporates a laser positioning system and a CT scanner and treatment planning system, has replaced simulation in many centres. Constraints may be put on doses to critical organs and to the breast and chest wall. It has been shown that IMRT can reduce by 3% to 5% the dose to the top and bottom of the breast where hot spots

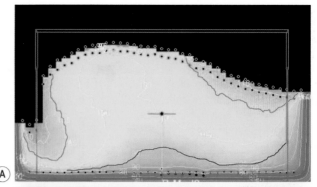

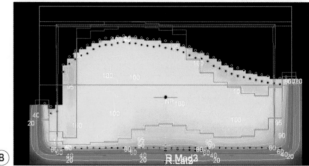

Fig. 26.18 Two beam's eye view images of the same breast with the isodoses displayed as a colourwash. (A) The dose distribution for a standard two-field plan is shown. The high-dose areas equal to or above 107% of the prescribed dose are shown by the deeper orange colour (*outlined in red*). The lower dose areas equal to or below 95% of the prescribed dose are shown by the green colour (*outlined in blue*). (B) The dose distribution is improved by the addition of two additional MLC-shaped fields, which have the effect of decreasing the regions of higher dose and boosting the regions of lower dose. (From Barnett GC et al. A randomised controlled trial of forward-planned radiotherapy (IMRT) for early breast cancer: baseline characteristics and dosimetry results. Radiother Oncol. 2009;92:34-41. With permission.)

commonly occur with conventional wedged fields using two-dimensional planning (Fig. 26.18A, B). The Cambridge IMRT trial comparing forward-planned IMRT to two-dimensional planning showed that IMRT improved the mean volumes receiving more than 107% and less than 95% of the prescribed dose compared with control. Despite the better target coverage and reduced cardiac dosage from three-dimensional planning over two-dimensional planning, the normal tissue complication probability (NTCP) for lung may increase.

Volumetric arc therapy. There is limited experience with volumetric-modulated arc therapy (VMAT). It can provide similar or superior target coverage, better sparing of normal tissues with fewer monitor units and shorter delivery times. It has advantages where bilateral breast irradiation is required with a single isocentre and asymmetric arcs. Simultaneous irradiation boost is also possible.

Respiratory gated radiotherapy. One of the most important principles of adjuvant RT for breast cancer is the minimisation of dose to the heart. The 2005 EBCTCG showed in approximately 40,000 women in 78 randomised trials of adjuvant RT that the beneficial effects of RT were counterbalanced by a 30% increase in cardiac deaths. The deaths were predominantly a result of ischaemic heart disease. Active breathing control is one of the key techniques to reduce cardiac and lung irradiation. It involves computer-controlled temporary suspension of breathing in a reproducible cycle.

Following respiratory training, the patient is positioned in a CT scanner without immobilisation (see Fig. 26.12). Radiotherapy is delivered in maximal deep inspiration when the heart is maximally displaced,

TABLE 26.6 Criteria for Deep Inspiratory Breath-Hold Techniques to Reduce Cardiac Irradiation

1. Breast conservation where tumour bed is lower part of the breast or postmastectomy where cardiac shielding may shield the tumour bed
2. When cardiac doses likely to exceed guidelines of safety
3. Maximum heart depth 1 cm on digital reconstructed radiograph
4. Patients with established cardiac issues or risk factors for cardiac disease

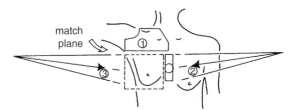

Fig. 26.20 Diagram showing fields to the chest wall/breast, axilla, supraclavicular fossa and internal mammary chain. (From Casebow MP. Matching of adjacent radiation beams for isocentric radiotherapy. Br J Radiol 1984;57:736. With permission.)

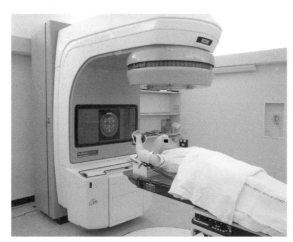

Fig. 26.19 Patient lying on an inclined breast board for adjuvant postoperative radiotherapy planning. (Courtesy Mrs. J Cameron, Edinburgh Cancer Centre.)

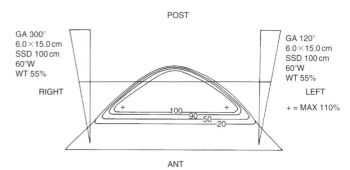

Fig. 26.21 Isodoses of a pair of wedged tangential breast fields shown in Fig. 26.19.

posteriorly away from the treatment beams (see Fig. 26.15). The lung volume irradiated is also reduced. Patients suitable for deep inspiratory breath-holding technique are summarised in Table 26.6. Some form of immobilisation is essential to provide a reproducible treatment set-up. A variety of devices are in use. These may include a breast board (Fig. 26.19) that fits onto the simulator and treatment couch and a custom-made foam mould from the head to the knees. The patient is treated supine with the arm abducted to 90 degrees. The breast board can be inclined to a range of angles to flatten the chest wall/breast.

This technique simplifies matching and avoids the need for rotating the collimator. The disadvantage is that it increases the volume of lung irradiated in the shoulder field. Alternatively, the patient can lie supine with the arm abducted to 90 degrees. Rotation of the collimator is needed to keep the posterior beam edge parallel to the slope of the contour. The disadvantage is difficulty in matching the chest wall to the shoulder field.

For the large or very mobile breast, some additional form of immobilisation (shell or sling) is needed. The very mobile breast tends to fall laterally, moving the posterior beam edge further back than the midaxillary point and increasing the volume of lung irradiated. The immobilising device will bring the breast medially and reduce the volume of lung irradiated. Treating the patient prone is an alternative technique for large-breasted patients.

Separate fields (Fig.26.20) are planned to cover: (1) supraclavicular fossa, axilla and, if desired, the upper internal mammary chain and (2) chest wall/breast. Individualised CT planning is needed to ensure adequate coverage while limiting transmitted dosage to the underlying heart and lungs.

Shoulder Field

A direct anterior megavoltage field (see Fig. 26.20) covers the supraclavicular fossa and axilla. The upper margin should be at the level of the thyrohyoid groove. The lateral margin should encompass the lateral border of the axilla.

The shoulder joint and the part of the larynx within the field should be shielded. Some centres angle the shoulder field 15 degrees to exclude the spinal cord, although this is not essential as long as the dosage and fractionation are within cord tolerance. The lower border of the shoulder field should be nondivergent to avoid overlap with the tangential fields.

The axillary and supraclavicular nodes are commonly at the same depth and, therefore, a single anterior field may suffice. Some centres use a small direct posterior field (posterior axillary boost) to supplement the dose to the axillary nodes. The posterior field is often treated on alternate days unless the mid-axillary separation exceeds 20 cm.

Supraclavicular field. Where the axillary clearance shows four or more nodes to be involved at pathological staging, irradiation of the medial supraclavicular fossa should be given. If the axilla is to be cleared, the surgeon should be asked to place metal clips up to the medial extent of the axillary dissection to ensure that the lateral margin of the supraclavicular field abuts on, but does not overlap, the field of the axillary clearance.

If there are one to three involved nodes and other adverse prognostic factors, for example, grade 3 histology or T3, supraclavicular RT can be considered in fit patients.

Neoadjuvant Therapy

In patients who have undergone neoadjuvant therapy with hormonal therapy or chemotherapy and the axillary nodes are positive cytologically and/or clinically, or radiologically suspicious, and if the nodal status is YpN- after neoadjuvant therapy, irradiation of the supraclavicular fossa should be considered. If the nodal status is positive after neoadjuvant therapy (ypN+), irradiation of the supraclavicular fossa is recommended.

Chest wall and breast. The chest wall or breast is treated isocentrically and can normally be encompassed in a pair of wedged tangential fields (Fig. 26.21), keeping the posterior beam edges parallel to minimise divergence into the lung. This should cover the scar of local excision or of the mastectomy. Before three-dimensional scanning

TABLE 26.7   Locoregional Target Volumes

The Axilla

Level 1: CTVn_L1 (Clinical Target Volume, Nodes)

Identification of axillary level I is influenced by surgical scarring from sentinel node biopsy or axillary node clearance. The medial border abuts on the lateral border of CTVn_L2. Superiorly, the axillary vein should be included with a 5-mm margin. The superolateral border of CTVn_L2 should be delineated 1 cm inferior and medial to the humeral head. More inferiorly, the lateral border is limited by an imaginary line between the lateral border of the pectoralis major and the anterolateral edge of the deltoid muscle. The inferior limit in the midaxillary line is around the level of the 4th–5th ribs. The posterosuperior border of CTVn_L1 is the ventral edge of the subscapular and deltoid muscles, omitting the thoracodorsal artery and vein.

Level 2: CTVn_L2

CTVn_L2 lies posterior to the pectoralis minor muscle. The medial limit is the medial border of pectoralis minor. The superior border includes the axillary artery which lies above the axillary vein, with an extra slice preferably to take account of partial volume effect. The posterior limit extending to a 5-mm margin posterior to the axillary vein into the surrounding fat, normally correspond with the chest wall. The lateral border is the lateral border of the pectoralis minor muscle where artefacts may be seen following axillary node dissection. In the latter case, the inferior border may be adjusted to exclude the surgical bed from the level II volume.

CTVn Interpectoralis

The interpectoral lymph nodes (Rotter's nodes) lie anterior to pectoralis minor and posterior to pectoralis major. The superior, inferior, lateral and medial limits largely reflect the borders of CTVn_L2.

Level 3: CTVn_L3

CTVn_L3 lies medial to pectoral minor and CTVn_L2 and is known at the infraclavicular volume. The medial border is the clavicle and the junction between the subclavian and internal jugular veins. The superior border includes the subclavian artery with an additional slice for partial volume effect and medially follows the superior border of CTVn_L2 and links to the superior limit of CTVn_L4. The superior border is the clavicle. The inferior border is a 5-mm extension into the fat inferior to the subclavian vein. The posterior limit is the 5-mm posterior to the subclavian vessels.

Level 4: CTVn_L4

This is usually known as the supraclavicular volume. The medial limit is the internal jugular vein (without a margin, i.e. excluding the common carotid artery and the thyroid gland). The superior border is the cranial level of the arch of the subclavian artery (i.e. there is a 5-mm margin superior to the subclavian vein. To account for the partial volume effect and computed tomography (CT) scan slice thickness, the superior limit is delineated one slice superior to the subclavian arch. Anterolaterally, the border is the posterior side of the sternocleidomastoid and sternothyroid muscles and the clavicle.

The most lateral part is the connective tissue between the lateral border of the anterior scalene muscle and the clavicle, and links with the medial border of CTVn_L3. The inferior border of CTVn_L4 includes the subclavian vein with a 5-mm margin, so linking to the cranial border of CTVn_IMN. The pleura is the posterior limit.

(at 2- to 3-mm intervals), it is helpful to place temporary radiopaque markers at the margins of the breast/chest wall, while acknowledging that these may not represent the true margins of the clinical target volume (CTV)p_Breast.

Delineation of the target volume. To date, the target volume has been the weakest link in the planning chain. The European Society for Therapeutic Radiology and Oncology (ESTRO) consensus guidelines on target volume definition for breast/chest wall and regional nodes are recommended for early breast cancer (see Further Reading). It should be emphasised that they do not apply to locally advanced disease, for which planning should be individualised. The target volumes for the regional nodes are shown in Table 26.7.

The breast. CTV should be delineated on CT slices sequentially. For the whole breast (CTVp_Breast), the CTV includes the soft tissues of the breast down to the fascia. It is often not possible to identify clearly the borders of the breast. The posterior border of the CTVp_Breast is the ventral side of the pectoralis major muscle, or in its absence, the exterior side of the ribs and intercostal muscles. The ventral border is 5 mm underneath the skin surface with the exception of T4 cancer where full dosage to the skin is advised. The upper border is the inferior edge of the sterno-clavicular joint. The medial border is the ipsilateral edge of the sternum. The lateral thoracic vessels at the lateral border of the breast can be a useful guide to the lateral border of the breast, although it may not be necessary to delineate CTV_Breast that far lateral if glandular tissue is clearly visible.

The CTVp_Breast should include the primary tumour bed and any margin around it.

Typical acceptable dose distributions in the breast and adjacent structures are shown in Figs 26.22 and 26.23.

The chest wall. Radiopaque markers should be placed and the imaginary margins of the breast around along the mastectomy scar.

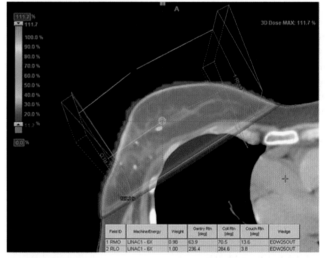

Field ID	Machine/Energy	Weight	Gantry Rtn [deg]	Coll Rtn [deg]	Couch Rtn [deg]	Wedge
1 RMO	LINAC1 - 6X	0.98	63.9	70.5	13.6	EDW25OUT
2 RLO	LINAC1 - 6X	1.00	236.4	284.6	3.8	EDW25OUT

Fig. 26.22 Dose colour wash for a three-dimensional conventional tangential plan through isocentre, off-axis dose maximum, 111.7%. (From Barrett A, Dobbs J, Morris S and Roques T, Practical Radiotherapy Planning, 4th ed. London: Hodder Arnold, 2009. With permission.)

The margins of the CTVp_thoracic wall are similar to the breast. Unless there is invasion of the skin (T4), there is no need to include the pectoral major muscle and ribs in the VCTVp_thoracic wall.

For the planning target volume (PTV), a margin is added to the CTV to take account of patient movement and setup error. The treatment plan should comply with ICRU 50 criteria so that the breast PTV should receive no less than 95% and no more than 107% of the prescribed dose.

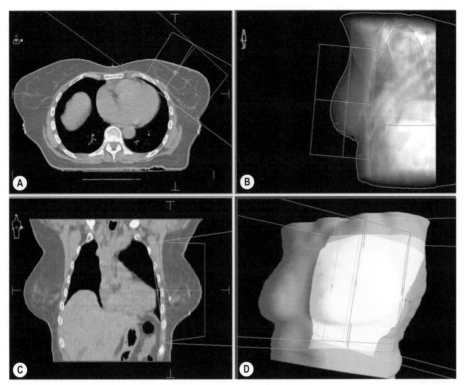

Fig. 26.23 Virtual simulation of breast with clips in tumour bed showing (A) axial scan with adjustment of beam border anteriorly from skin markers to avoid the heart, (B) sagittal, (C) coronal and (D) rendered image of tangential beams. (From Barrett A, Dobbs J, Morris S and Roques T, Practical Radiotherapy Planning, 4th ed, London: Hodder Arnold, 2009. With permission.)

Dose prescription to the breast. Dose prescription to the breast is 40 Gy TAD in 15 daily over 3 weeks (6–10-MV photons).

Dose prescription to the axilla. The dose should be specified both medially at 3-cm depth from the anterior skin surface (point B) and laterally at half patient's thickness in the middle of the posterior-anterior beam (point A). The dose should not vary by 5% or more, and maximally by ±10% across the CTV.

Dose prescription to the axilla or supraclavicular fossa. Dose prescription to the axilla or supraclavicular fossa is 40 Gy in 15 daily fractions over 3 weeks (6–10-MV photons).

Internal mammary nodes: CTVn_IMN. The superior limit is the inferior limit of CTVn_L4 (Table 26.7), delineated 5 mm around the internal thoracic artery. The inferior limit is normally the superior side of the fourth rib but may be extended with one more intercostal space to the fifth rib. The medial border is 5 mm to the internal thoracic vein or the sternum, whichever is the closest. The lateral border is the internal mammary artery and vein with a 5-mm margin. The posterior border is the pleura. The anterior limit is the anterior limit of the vascular area.

Delineation of the heart. The heart is a complex structure for contouring. Atlases have been developed to assist with contouring of the left ventricle and coronary arterial segments on RT CT-planning (see Further Reading). This may assist in research on the relationship between segment doses and cardiac outcomes

Dose prescription to the internal mammary nodes. Dose prescription to the internal mammary nodes is 40 Gy TAD in 15 daily fractions over 3 weeks (6–10-MV photons).

Limiting volume of lung irradiated; I. At the time of simulation, the thickness of lung encompassed in the tangential fields should be measured (the central lung distance perpendicularly from the inner aspect of the chest wall to the posterior beam edge). The central lung distance

should not exceed 3 cm. If it exceeds 3 cm, consideration should be given to bringing the medial and/or lateral margins of the fields inwards, as long as this does not involve skimping on the coverage of the wide excision or mastectomy scars. To avoid divergence into the lung, the posterior beam edges should be kept parallel.

Skin bolus. To overcome the skin-sparing effect of megavoltage, skin bolus (0.5–1 cm depending on the energy of photons) should be applied to the chest wall to ensure full skin dosage in patients where the skin is involved by tumour. Practice varies in the use of bolus for postmastectomy RT when the skin is not involved. Some centres apply bolus to a limited area above and below the scar (where recurrences are commonest) or to the whole of the chest wall, either for the whole or part of the course of RT. It is not clear which approach is optimal.

Field matching. One of the main challenges in breast/chest wall planning is to match the tangential fields to the shoulder field. Immobilisation should minimise movement between the treatment of fields to avoid the risk of overdosage or underdosage at the junction. Fields may be matched using the light beam, and lasers by eye using couch rotation (usually 5–6 degrees) and some collimator rotation. Alternatively, the following can be used:

1. A half beam block (Fig. 26.24A) to counteract beam divergence, allowing the field edges to be abutted. Asymmetric jaws facilitate this. The match plane can be vertical (Fig. 26.24C) or angled (Fig. 26.24D).
2. A vertical hanging block.
3. A single isocentre with blocks, avoiding the need for couch movement between fields.

Dosimetry. Planning is based on multislice CT scanning of the breast and/or peripheral lymphatics. An adequate does for most patients is 6 to 10 MV photons. Wedges are needed to compensate for missing tissue. Lung transmission increases the dose to the posterior breast. A correction factor of 10% may be needed. Variations in depth dose across the breast may be around 20%, particularly in larger breasts. Build-up (the distance over which the dose builds up) to 100% is 5 to 10 mm from the skin surface for 6-MV photons.

Dose, energy and fractionation. Megavoltage irradiation (6-MV photons) is used for the tangential field to the chest wall or breast. For patients with larger breasts, higher energy (10-MV) photons may be needed.

Many of the earlier fractionation regimens were developed empirically. In the United States, 2-Gy fractions were widely adopted under the influence of Professor Gilbert Fletcher of the MD Anderson Hospital in Texas. For much of North America and continental Europe, 50 Gy in 25 fractions over 5 weeks was the international standard for postoperative locoregional RT until evidence emerged from four trials totalling over 7000 patients for the efficacy and safety of shorter hypofractionated dose fractionation schedules. Hypofractionated RT is defined as a dose per fraction in excess of 2 Gy. It was hypothesised that breast cancer may be as sensitive as late-reacting tissues to fraction size. Accordingly, hypofractionation should not be disadvantageous for breast cancer as long as the total dose is appropriately reduced. Indeed hypofractionation may be advantageous in local control by minimising accelerated tumour repopulation. Total dose has to be reduced to compensate for nonlinear increase in normal tissue and anticancer effects, more particularly, for late-reacting normal tissues than for self-renewal tissues. The Canadian and START B trials have been the most influencial in changing this practice. The Canadian trial of axillary node-negative patients treated by breast-conserving surgery and postoperative RT showed at 10 years a nonsignificant difference in cumulative incidence of local recurrence (6.7% in control group and 6.2% in hypofractionated arm). However, hypofractionation was less effective with high-grade tumours (4.7% in control and 15.6% in the hypofractionated group). There was no difference in cosmesis or cardiac events between the two arms. The START trials which included patients treated both by mastectomy and breast-conserving surgery showed no compromise in local control or cosmesis from hypofractionation, some evidence of less late breast toxicity and no increase in cardiotoxicity in the shorter regimen. In the START A trial, the local recurrence rate at 5 years for the 50 Gy/25 fractions, 39 Gy/13 fractions and 41.6 Gy/13 fractions was 7.4%, 8.8% and 6.3%, respectively. For START B, the equivalent figures for the 50 Gy/25 fractions and 40 Gy/15 fractions were 5.5% and 4.3%, respectively. A metaanalysis of START A and B trials showed no adverse effects of fractionation by nodal status or (in contrast to the analysis in the Canadian trial which had less statistical power), by tumour grade. As a result of the START B trial, a dose of 40 Gy in 15 daily fractions has been adopted as the standard dose fractionation regimen recommended by NICE. Shorter fractionation regimens are more convenient for patients and less costly. However, long-term follow-up will be needed to assess the impact of hypofractionated regimens on locoregional control, morbidity and survival.

It is uncertain what the limits of hypofractionation are. The UK FAST trial is investigating two dose fractionation regimens of 27 Gy (5.4 Gy/fraction) and 26 Gy (5.2 Gy/fraction) over a week compared with a standard 3-week schedule.

Boost to the primary tumour volume after whole breast irradiation. Some form of boost of irradiation to the primary tumour is desirable to bring the tumour dose to 60 Gy in women under the age of 50 years. This is most commonly delivered by electrons. Excellent results can also be achieved by implantation with high- or low-dose rate interstitial implantation. The excellent cosmetic results achievable from postoperative whole breast irradiation and interstitial implantation are shown in Fig. 26.25. Either form of boost will give comparable local control. However, interstitial implantation requires significant practical expertise, and its use is in decline in the United Kingdom and United States. Worldwide low-dose rate afterloading systems, sources and iridium wide have been withdrawn. High dose rate (HDR) brachytherapy with

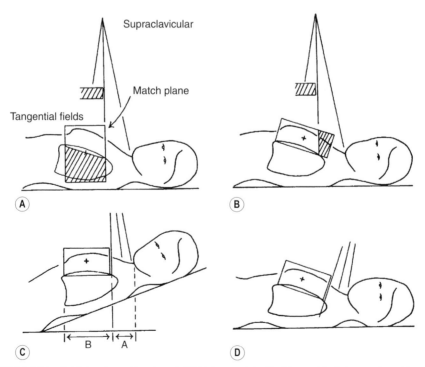

Fig. 26.24 Matching fields in a breast treatment. (A) Using a rotated half-beam block to counteract beam divergence between cervico-axillary and breast fields. (B) Lead block to trim superior edge of the tangential fields to form a vertical match plane. (C) Match plane vertical on an inclined breast board. (D) Match plane angled in supine position. (From Casebow MP. Matching of adjacent radiation beams for isocentric radiotherapy. Br J Radiol. 1984;57:737. With permission.)

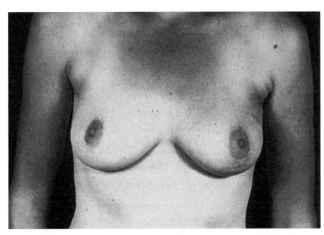

Fig. 26.25 Excellent cosmetic result of postoperative radiotherapy and iridium implant following lumpectomy for early carcinoma of the left breast. (Courtesy Dr. D. Ash, Leeds.)

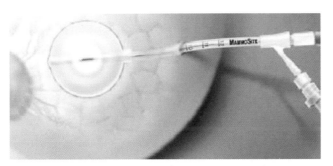

Fig. 26.26 Breast brachytherapy with MammoSite.

iridium-192 using the MammoSite system is practiced in a limited number of centres. The MammoSite HDR system has a catheter comprising a multilumen tube with balloon assembly (Fig. 26.26). The balloon is inflated to fit the size of the excision cavity. An iridium-192 source is inserted into the balloon to deliver the required dose. On completion of therapy, the balloon is deflated and the catheter removed.

A large EORTC trial (Fig. 26.27) of over 5500 patients showed an overall 40% reduction in the risk of local recurrence with the use of the boost. Patients with clear margins after wide local excision were treated with whole breast irradiation (50 Gy in 25 fractions over 5 weeks) and randomised to either a boost (electrons 10 Gy) or implant. Age was an independent risk factor for recurrence. In women under the age of 40 years, the local recurrence with the boost was 10% compared with 20% without the boost.

The absolute reduction in recurrence was smaller in women over the age of 40 years, but still statistically significant up to the age of 50 years. Long-term follow-up of the trial at 20 years showed the cumulative incidence of ipsilateral breast tumour recurrence was 16.4% (99% CI 14.1–18.8) in the no-boost group versus 12.0% (9.8–14.4) in the boost group. The proportional reduction in risk for all risk groups was similar. The absolute reduction in risk was highest in the highest-risk group (i.e. youngest patients). The risk was 36% in the no-boost versus 24.2% in the boost group for women under 40 years; 19.4% (14.7–24.1) versus 13.5% (9.5–17.5) in women 41 to 50 years; 13.2% (9.8–16.7) versus 10.3% (6.3–14.3) in women 51 to 60 years and 12.7% (7.4–18.0) versus 9.7% (5.0–14.4) for women older than 60 years (see Fig. 26.27). At 20 years, the cumulative incidence of severe fibrosis was 1.8% (99% CI 1.1–2.5) in the no-boost group versus 5.2% (99% CI 3.9–6.4) in the boost group ($P < .0001$). On this basis, for patients

with clear excision margins, a boost is recommended for women up to the age of 59 years or with an unfavourable biological profile. For older patients, the risks of a boost probably outweigh the benefits. In patients for whom re-excision of positive margins is not possible, an electron boost would still be indicated.

Indications for breast boost

1. Women up to age of 59 years or with unfavourable features (high grade, node positive, T3, T4).
2. Positive or close excision margins (<1 mm).

Omission of breast boost can be considered in women 60 years (or older) or a favourable biological profile (grade 1–2, node negative, T1-T2)

Breast boost technique. The EORTC 22881-10882 trial used an extra 16 Gy as the boost dose. However, increased rates of moderate to severe fibrosis rose significantly by 15% at 10 years (28.1% vs 13.2%, $P < .001$). Conventionally planning of the boost had been based on a variety of information (mammogram, operation note and position of the scar) and treated with a single electron field. This clinically based approach was often inaccurate compared with using the position of the surgical ligaclips placed at the margins of the tumour bed (Fig. 26.28). There is also evidence that electron-based treatment often underdoses the tumour bed compared with photon-based techniques. Advanced RT techniques (IMRT and image-guided RT, IGRT) enable a simultaneous integrated boost to be delivered within the breast during daily RT sessions compared with the sequential boost.

IMRT provides better dose homogeneity within the boost volume than a single electron field.

This is more convenient to patients and provides cost savings. Studies are in progress to establish whether IMRT and IGRT may have an advantage in reducing boost volumes and the risks of fibrosis. In the UK IMPORT-HIGH trial of patients with early breast cancer: at higher than average risk treated by breast-conserving surgery, IMRT is being assessed: delivering a simultaneous integrated boost: to test whether radiotherapy side effects can be reduced. The control group receive whole breast irradiation (40 Gy in 15 fractions) followed by a sequential photon boost of 16 Gy in 8 fractions with 36 Gy in 15 fractions to the low-risk volume; 40 Gy in 15 fractions to the involved quadrant; and dose escalation to the tumour bed of 48 Gy or 53 Gy in 15 fractions with concomitant boost (Fig. 26.29).

The appropriate electron energy, usually 9 to 12 MeV, is chosen according to the depth of the breast tissue at the site of the tumour-bearing area. This should be accurately measured on the planning CT postoperatively. To avoid transmission of unwanted irradiation to the underlying lung, a Perspex degrader of appropriate thickness can be interposed between the electron applicator and the skin to attenuate the beam. The boosted volume should cover the tumour-bearing area with a margin of 1 to 2 cm (to take account of the inbowing of electron isodoses at depth) judged from clinical, mammographic and perioperative findings. Surgeons place metal clips at the site of the excision, which assist the clinical oncologist in the identification of the tumour bed. Alternatively a field-in-field technique may be used for the breast boost.

Electron boost dose. An electron boost dose is 10 Gy in 5 daily fractions over 1 week or 16 Gy in 8 daily fractions, or a radiobiologically equivalent dose, for example, 12 Gy in 4 daily fractions.

Partial Breast Irradiation

Whole breast irradiation has to date been the standard of care following breast-conserving surgery. The case for partial breast irradiation is based on observations that most ipsilateral local recurrences occur close to the original site of excision (the tumour bed). The tumour bed can be identified by titanium surgical clips. The development of advanced RT techniques has allowed dose to be matched

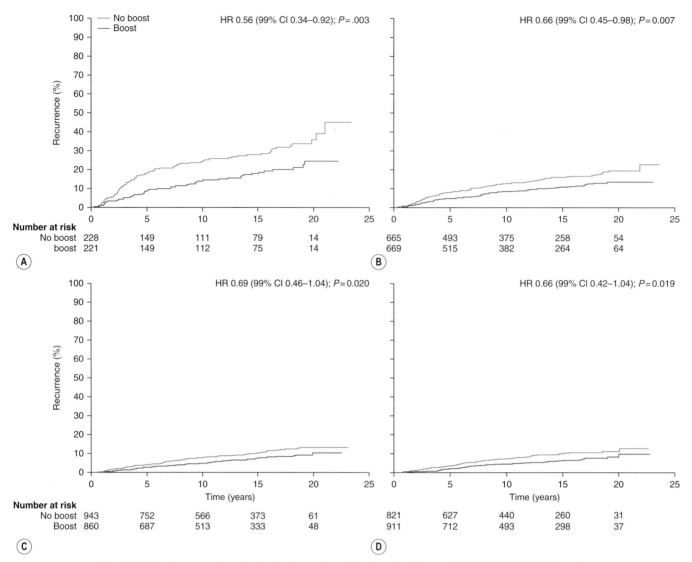

Fig. 26.27 The European Organisation for Research and Treatment of Cancer (EORTC) 22881-10882 Boost vs No-boost trial. Cumulative incidence of ipsilateral breast tumour recurrence by age. For patients aged 40 years or younger, 71 patients in the no-boost group versus 42 in the boost group had recurrence (A); for patients aged 41 to 50 years, 108 versus 74 had recurrence (B) for patients aged 51 to 60 years, 100 versus 64 had recurrence (C); and for patients aged older than 60 years, 75 versus 57 had recurrence (D). *HR,* Hazard ratio. (From Bartelink H et al. Whole breast irradiation with or without a boost for patients treated with breast conserving surgery for early breast cancer: 20 year follow up of a randomised phase 3 trial. Lancet Oncol. 2015;16:47-56. With permission.)

to the spatial variation in risk of local recurrence. There are a variety of partial breast irradiation techniques, including external beam, interstitial brachytherapy and intraoperative. There is mature level 1 evidence for interstitial brachytherapy and for external beam RT. In the GEC ESTRO noninferiority trial, 1184 patients aged 40 years or older, pTis or pT1–2a (lesions of ≤3 cm diameter), pN0/pNmi and M0 breast cancer (stages 0, I and IIA), were treated by breast-conserving surgery and randomised to whole breast irradiation or to accelerated partial breast irradiation (APBI) with multicatheter brachytherapy.

At 5 years of follow-up, the cumulative incidence of local recurrence was noninferior for APBI (1.44% (95% CI .51–2.38) with APBI and .92% with whole breast irradiation). In the larger UK IMPORT-LOW trial of 2018 patients aged 50 years or older with unifocal grade 1–3 breast cancer, 3 cm or less with zero to three positive nodes and minimum 2 mm clear margin were randomised to whole breast irradiation (control), 40 Gy to whole breast or 40 Gy to partial breast, and

36 Gy to whole breast or 40 Gy to partial breast only, in 15 daily fractions. At median follow-up of 72 months, the cumulative incidence of local relapse was 1.1% (95% CI 0.5–2.3) in the control group, .2 (95% CI 0.02–1.2) in the reduced group and .5% (95% CI 0.2–1.4) in the partial breast group. Both reduced group and partial breast group were noninferior. Cosmesis and patient and clinical assessment were similar for all groups.

Intraoperative Radiotherapy

The role of intraoperative RT (IORT) as a method of partial breast irradiation for early breast cancer remains controversial. A number of phase III randomised trials have evaluated IORT. The ELIOT (ELectron InOperative Therapy) trial used a single dose of intraoperative electrons (21 Gy) to the tumour bed following wide local excision. This was an equivalence trial. The 5-year ipsilateral breast tumour recurrence was significantly higher in the IORT group compared with the whole breast irradiation group (4.4% vs .4%, P < .001), although it was within an accepted

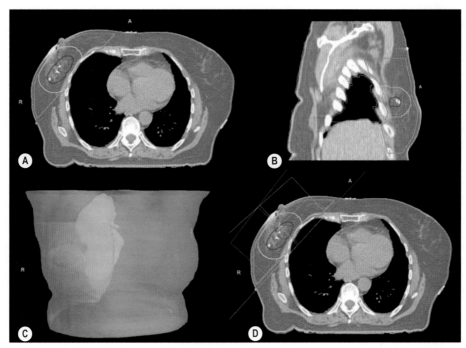

Fig. 26.28 (A) Axial computed tomography (CT) scan with clips in the tumour bed (*dark blue*), boost clinical target volume (CTV) (*cyan*) and whole breast planning target volume (PTV) (*red*). (B) Sagittal view. (C) Three-dimensional image (lung in green). (D) Axial CT scan with beams for whole breast external beam radiotherapy (6 MV, gantry 221 degrees and 47 degrees, 9.5 (W) ×2 0 (L). (From Barrett A, Dobbs J, Morris S and Roques T, Practical Radiotherapy Planning, 4th ed, London: Hodder Arnold, 2009. With permission.)

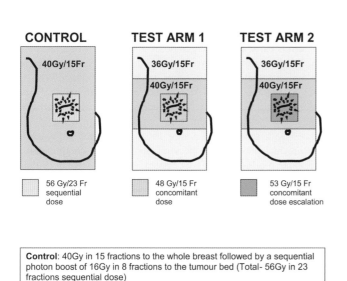

Control: 40Gy in 15 fractions to the whole breast followed by a sequential photon boost of 16Gy in 8 fractions to the tumour bed (Total- 56Gy in 23 fractions sequential dose)

Test Arm 1 and 2: 36Gy in 15 fractions to the low risk volume of the breast, 40Gy in 15 fractions to the index quadrant and dose escalation to the tumour bed with two dose levels of 48Gy and 53Gy in 15 fractions as concomitant boost

Fig. 26.29 Study schema of UK IMPORT HIGH trial. (From Coles CE et al. Breast radiotherapy: less is more?. Clin Oncol. 2013;127-134).

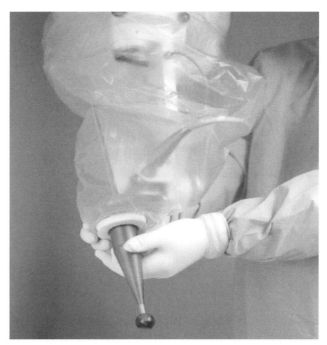

Fig. 26.30 Intrabeam intraoperative radiotherapy.

noninferiority margin of 4.5%. The risk of recurrence was elevated in the index quadrant, the rest of the breast and the regional nodes. There was less breast morbidity with IORT except for fat necrosis. On this basis, intraoperative electron beam therapy is not recommended. The main controversy over IORT relates to the TARGIT-A trial evaluating IORT with a 50-kv device with a range of sizes of spherical applicators

(Fig. 26.30) delivering a single dose of 20 Gy to the tumour bed over 15 to 20 minutes following wide local excision. This was planned as a noninferiority trial with a margin of 2.5% at 5 years. Additional external beam RT was given if there were additional risk factors identified on the pathology excision specimen (15% of IORT arm). At a median follow-up of 29 months, the estimated 5-year local recurrence rate was 3.3% with

IORT and 1.3% with WBI which was not statistically significant ($P =$ .043). There has been criticism of the short follow-up and the statistical design and interpretation of the trial. Further follow-up of the trial will be needed before judging its efficacy.

There are no uniformly agreed-upon criteria for eligibility for partial breast irradiation. Suggested criteria include tumour smaller than 3 cm, unifocal, without an EIC, close or negative margins and zero to three involved nodes.

It should be emphasised that large randomised studies will be needed to assess the clinical and economic effectiveness of partial breast irradiation techniques.

Local Recurrence After Mastectomy

If local recurrence occurs on the chest wall, spot recurrence should be locally excised if feasible. Of patients treated by local excision alone, 60% to 70% will develop a second local recurrence. For multiple spot recurrences (see Figs 26.6 and 26.7), this is unlikely to be practical. Radical RT (40 Gy in 15 daily fractions) to the chest wall and the supraclavicular fossa is recommended. If irradiation of the supraclavicular fossa is omitted, recurrence rates at this site may be as high as 28%.

For an isolated axillary recurrence, a level III clearance should be considered. Axillary irradiation is only considered if there is macroscopic disease remaining after a clearance or a previous clearance has been undertaken. Most of the available evidence does not support the use of axillary irradiation for patients with extracapsular spread who have undergone a level III axillary clearance.

Morbidity of Radical Radiotherapy

The most common toxicities following breast-conserving surgery and postoperative irradiation to the breast and/or regional nodes are acute dermatitis, arm or breast oedema, myositis, breast fibrosis, rib fractures, lung fibrosis and pneumonitis. Less common complications are cardiac damage, brachial plexopathy and second malignancies (see Further Reading).

Acute Dermatitis

Acute radiation dermatitis occurs 0 to 1 day after the start of RT. Acute skin toxicity is a result of impaired repopulation of the epidermis. Features include varying intensities of erythema, itching, hyperpigmentation, and discomfort.

Skin Care During Treatment

The following guidance is based on the recommendations of the Society of Radiographers (https://www.sor.org).

Patients are advised to wear loose fitting natural fibre clothing adjacent to the skin, for example, a cotton T-shirt. The skin should be washed gently with soap and water and gently patted dry. Avoid heat, rubbing, and cooling pads/ice, wax for hair removal and all depilatory creams/products and adhesive tape.

To minimise irritation, a moisturising cream that is free of sodium lauryl sulphate is advised. Topical antibiotics should be avoided, unless there is a microbiologically proven infection. Deodorants can continue to be applied, as long as they do not act as an irritant; deodorants should be stopped if the skin is broken. Direct sun exposure should be avoided and high-factor sun block applied to exposed skin.

If the skin is broken, appropriate dressings/products can be applied to minimise further trauma. Nonadhesive non- or low-paraffin/ petroleum jelly products are recommended. Gentian violet should not be applied.

Monitoring of skin reactions after completion of treatment should be arranged through community nursing services or a general practitioner.

Breast swelling. Swelling of the breast occurs in around 30% of patients following breast-conserving surgery and postoperative RT and settles spontaneously in most cases.

Breast Pain

Acute, sharp, electric-shock–like pains or a dull ache within the irradiated breast commonly occur 0 to 21 days after the start of treatment. Reassurance that it will settle and simple analgesia is often all that is required.

Telangiectasia. Telangiectasia are dilatations of skin capillaries. They have the appearance of spidery red or purple clusters and impair cosmesis. The dilatations develop 2 months to sometimes longer than 6 months progressively after treatment and then stabilise but are permanent. It is important that patients are warned of their development. Telangiectasia are associated with the use of skin bolus or electron breast boosts, particularly using more than 10 MeV compared with low-energy photons or electrons. Forward planned IMRT has a lower risk of inducing telangiectasia than standard RT. No treatment is normally advised.

Chest Wall Pain/Fibrosis

Chest wall pain, skin fibrosis and contracture occur after breast-conserving surgery and postoperative RT, as well as following postmastectomy irradiation. High-energy electrons (>10 MeV) are associated with an increased risk of breast fibrosis. Maximising dose homogeneity within the breast (avoiding the volume of the breast receiving >107%) is important to minimising breast fibrosis.

Lymphoedema

Lymphoedema is one of the serious side effects of adjuvant RT that causes patients distress and can be difficult to manage. Lymphoedema of the arm is particularly likely to occur if the axilla is irradiated after a level 3 axillary clearance. Arm lymphoedema may increase progressively and eventually plateau, often years after its onset. With the decline in axillary node clearance and increase in sentinel node biopsy, the incidence of arm lymphoedema is very much less (1%– 5%) after sentinel lymphadenectomy alone. Lymphoedema may be associated with sensory and motor deficit (associated with damage to the brachial plexus), and pectoral fibrosis. This combination of locoregional morbidities was associated with older RT techniques and when peripheral lymphatic irradiation was combined with axillary node dissection. In extreme cases of severe lymphoedema, the limb may be flail and useless. Patients with lymphoedema are more prone to cellulitis of the arm which should be promptly assessed and treated with antibiotics.

Avoidance of trauma to the skin of the arm (for example, using long-sleeved gloves for gardening), manual lymphatic drainage and compressing bandages or garments are recommended.

Following breast-conserving surgery, the incidence of breast or arm oedema is usually related to axillary node dissection rather than axillary nodal irradiation.

Brachial Plexopathy

Brachial plexopathy is a major complication of regional nodal irradiation. Fortunately it is now rare (1%) but it was more common in the past with older RT techniques employing higher doses per fraction, and when regional nodal irradiation was often combined with level III clearance. The incidence of brachial plexopathy was significantly higher when the total dose to the axilla exceeded 50 Gy. Clinical features include paraesthesia in the affected arm/hand, pain in the shoulder or upper limit, motor weakness and sensory deficit, muscle wasting and loss of tendon reflexes. C7 is particularly affected with lesser involvement of C6 and C8. The median interval between irradiation and onset of brachial neuropathy is typically 1 to 4 years, although onset can sometimes occur as late as 21 years after radiation therapy. Modest hypofractionation (46 Gy in 20 fractions) is not associated with radiation-induced brachial plexopathy. The UK hypofractionation regimen of 40 Gy in 15 daily fractions is considered safe. The important differential diagnosis is malignant infiltration of the brachial plexus. Suspected cases require referral to a neurologist and investigation by MRI and, if appropriate, nerve conduction studies. Clinical symptoms and nerve conduction studies cannot always distinguish between malignant infiltration and radiation-induced brachial plexopathy. Painless upper cervical trunk lesions with lymphoedema usually suggest radiation injury, and painful lower cervical trunk lesions with Horner syndrome usually indicate tumour infiltration. MRI findings characteristic of radiation-induced brachial plexopathy are hyperintensity on T2. A mass is suggestive of malignant brachial infiltration. Metastases show enhancement on gadolinium-enhanced images.

There are no effective treatments for radiation-induced brachial plexopathy. Hyperbaric oxygen was found to be ineffective. Coordinated care between surgeon, oncologist, neurologist, palliative care specialist, physiotherapist, occupational therapist and general practicioner is needed.

Cardiac Damage

Radiation-induced heart disease encompasses coronary artery disease, pericarditis, myocardial dysfunction and valvular heart disease. Radiation-induced pericarditis is a rare acute complication, usually occurring soon after exposure. The majority of other radiation-related cardiac abnormalities are late events, occurring 10 to 15 years after RT. In general, radiation-induced cardiotoxicity occurs at an earlier age than the normal population. A significantly higher risk of cardiac death was seen with a linear dose-response relationship in the Japanese survivors of the atomic bomb.

More recent data among 963 women who had a major coronary event after RT for breast cancer between 1958 and 2011 in Sweden and Denmark compared with 1205 control women who did not have a major coronary event, showed a linear increase in major coronary events with mean dose to the heart by 7.4% per Gy with no apparent threshold. There are higher risks of radiation-induced cardiac events in patients with established risk factors for coronary heart disease. There is limited literature on the effects of specific doses to the heart and specific cardiac substructures.

Myocardial perfusion defects (ischaemic areas of the level ventricle) have been identified in patients irradiated for breast cancer. However, the clinical significance of these abnormalities is not known. The site of these left ventricular perfusion defects is mainly influenced by the borders of the RT fields rather than the distribution of the coronary vessels. This implies that they are caused by damage to the microvasculature of the myocardium rather than coronary artery damage. Damage to the coronary arteries has been demonstrated in breast cancer patients who have undergone adjuvant irradiation and occurs particularly in arterial segments likely to have received high radiation doses.

More data are needed on the combined cardiotoxic effects of anthracycline-based adjuvant chemotherapy. Anti-HER2 therapy with trastuzumab is also cardiotoxic. Little is known of these combined cardiotoxic effects or interaction with other known risk factors (smoking, hypercholesterolaemia, premature menopause). There are wide variations between patients in proneness to radiation-induced toxicity, and some evidence of variation in genetic susceptibility. Appropriate imaging screening procedures and biomarkers of risk of cardiac damage are needed because cardiac events may occur 10 to 15 years or more

after radiation exposure. Answers to these questions will inform prevention strategies for breast cancer survivors in whom cardiac exposure cannot be avoided.

Radiation can cause valvular disease, typically affecting the left-sided valves, with aortic regurgitation being the most common. Rarely, it may result in aortic stenosis, mandating surgical intervention.

Lung

There are two phases of lung toxicity. The first is a subacute inflammatory phase, radiation pneumonitis. The second phase is late radiation fibrosis. Radiation pneumonitis is uncommon. It presents acutely with cough, shortness of breath or fever. On auscultation of the chest, there may be crackles or no added sounds. It is thought cytotoxic damage to the type II pneumocytes and vascular endothelial cells primarily initiates radiation damage. These tissue changes include abnormalities of surfactant-containing lamellar bodies within type II pneumocytes; increases in surfactant production are detected in bronchoalveolar lavage samples within hours of radiation. The immediate phase (within hours or days) is clinically silent. It features an inflammatory response inducing a leucocytic infiltration leading to intraalveolar oedema and vascular congestion. There follows a latent phase (days to weeks) featuring the accumulation of thick secretions from an increase in goblet cells and ciliary malfunction. Subsequently, there is an acute exudative phase (weeks to months) of hyaline membrane formation, type II pneumocyte proliferation, endothelial and epithelial shedding and clinical symptoms of radiation pneumonitis. There follows an intermediate phase (months) mirroring progression of changes noted previously, destruction of hyaline membranes, regeneration of capillaries and fibroblast migration. Finally, there is a fibrotic phase (months to years) of progressive fibrosis with deposition of collagen by fibroblasts distorting alveolar spaces and reducing lung volumes.

The risk of pneumonitis is related to the volume irradiated. With the greater appreciation of lung volumes irradiated on three-dimensional compared with two-dimensional planning, the incidence is likely to fall. The addition of regional nodal irradiation to breast irradiation significantly increases the risk of pneumonitis. A number of cytotoxic agents increase the risk of radiation pneumonitis: taxanes, cyclophosphamide, gemcitabine, doxorubicin, mitomycin C, vincristine and bevacizumab. Chest radiograph and CT scan may show pulmonary infiltrates in the irradiated volume.

Lung function tests may show restrictive ventilatory changes and impaired diffusion capacity that are reversible. Treatment of radiation pneumonitis is with high-dose steroids (prednisone 60 mg per day for 14 days), tailed off by 10 mg per day over 1 to 2 weeks.

Rib fractures. Rib fractures, as a result of ischaemic osteoradionecrosis with or without soft tissue necrosis, can develop around a year after conventionally fractionated breast RT but are rare (.1%–5%). Treatment is normally conservative.

ADJUVANT HORMONAL AND CYTOTOXIC THERAPY

Rationale

It is generally accepted that a substantial number of patients with apparently localised breast cancer harbour systemic micrometastases. These micrometastases are currently beyond the detection of the conventional staging.

All patients should be considered for some form of adjuvant systemic therapy to try to eradicate micrometastases. Selection of therapy is based on the risk of recurrence. Factors to be taken into consideration are tumour size, tumour grade, axillary node status, oestrogen/progesterone receptor and human epidermal growth factor (HER2) status. The addition of information on tumour biology from intrinsic subtypes

TABLE 26.8 Recommendations for Adjuvant Systemic Therapy Based on Prognostic Factors

Low Risk	Intermediate Risk	High Risk
Prognostic Factors		
Premenopausal/ postmenopausal	Premenopausal	Premenopausal or postmenopausal
Tumour size <2 cm	Tumour size >2 cm	Any tumour size
Grade 1 or II	Grade III	Any grade
Axillary node negative	Axillary node negative	
ER positive	Axillary positive (1–3N+)	>4 axillary nodes positive
	ER negative	ER positive or negative
HER2 negative	HER2 positive	HER2 positive/negative
Treatment		
Tamoxifen for 5 years (grade 1)	Anthracycline-containing regimen if node negative	
Tamoxifen for 5 years and OS (goserelin for 2 years or oophorectomy)	Anthracycline-taxane combination if node positive Trastuzumab if HER2 positive postchemotherapy	Anthracycline-taxane combination Trastuzumab if HER2 positive postchemotherapy
	If postmenopausal ER and/ or PgR positive, aromatase inhibitor (AI) (anastrazole or letrozole) for 5 years or AI for 2 years followed by 3 years of tamoxifen	If ER and/or PgR positive and postmenopausal, aromatase inhibitor (anastrazole or letrozole) for 5 years
(if premenopausal and grade II)	If ER and/or PgR positive and premenopausal, tamoxifen for 5 years Consider for further 5 years of tamoxifen	If ER and/or PgR positive and premenopausal, tamoxifen for 5 years Consider for further 5 years of tamoxifen

ER, Oestrogten receptor, *PgR,* progesterone receptor.

TABLE 26.9 Recommendations for Adjuvant Endocrine Therapy for Postmenopausal Patients Based on Prognostic Factors

Risk Category	Endocrine Therapy
Low-risk NPI <3.4 Patients with all of following: • Tumour ≤2 cm • ER and or PgR positive • Grade 1 histology • No lymphovascular invasion • Age ≥35 years • HER2 negative	Tamoxifen for 5 years
Intermediate-risk NPI 3.4–5.4 Node negative and at least one of following: • pT >2 cm • Grade 2 or 3 histology • Lymphovascular invasion • ER and PgR negative • Age <35 years Node positive (1–3 involved nodes) and ER and/or PgR positive and HER2 negative	If ER/PgR positive, AI (anastrazole or letrozole) for 5 years or AI for 2 years followed by 3 years of tamoxifen
High risk NPI >5.4 • Node positive (1–3 involved nodes) And ER and PgR negative • Node positive (4 or more involved nodes) OR HER2 positive (irrespective of NPI)	Anastrazole or letrozole for 5 years

AI, Aromatase inhibitor; *ER,* oestrogen receptor; *NPI,* Nottingham Prognostic Index; *PgR,* progesterone receptor; *pN,* regional lymphnodes; *pT,* primary tumour.

(luminal-A, luminal-B, HER2 enriched and triple negative) may help estimate response to systemic therapy. Luminal-A tumours are more likely to respond to endocrine therapy and less likely to respond to chemotherapy. Luminal-B tumours are more likely to be chemosensitive. HER2-positive tumours are more likely to respond to anti-HER2 therapy. Triple negative tumours (ER, PgR, HER2 negative) are unlikely to respond to endocrine therapy and more likely to be chemosensitive. Recommendations for adjuvant systemic therapy based on prognostic factors are summarised in Table 26.8 (see Further Reading; Table 26.9 reviews endocrine therapy in postmenopausal patients.

Who Benefits?

The EBCTCG has provided a series of 5-yearly metaanalyses of over 75,000 women with early breast cancer. The group's overview shows clearly that both hormonal (tamoxifen or oophorectomy) and cytotoxic therapy (CMF or anthracycline-containing combination chemotherapy) reduce the relative risk of relapse or death by up to 30% at 10 years. The overall survival benefits are more modest, with a 4% to 12% gain in

overall survival. The benefits in overall survival are greater in premenopausal than postmenopausal women. In women over the age of 70years, there are few data on the benefit of adjuvant chemotherapy and some evidence that the degree of benefit falls with increasing age.

Following polychemotherapy, women aged 50 to 59 years gain a 14% reduction in risk of death compared with 8% in women aged 60 to 69 years. Life expectancy is likely to be prolonged on average by 4 years for women under the age of 50 years and by 1 to 3 years in women over the age of 50 years. Adjuvant chemotherapy reduces 10-year breast cancer mortality by 27%. For a woman who has a 50% chance of dying from breast cancer under the age of 50 years, the approximate reduction in risk of death is 13.5%. For a woman with a 10% risk of death at 10 years, the risk of death is about 8%.

There is evidence that anthracycline-containing regimens increase the probability of survival compared with nonanthracycline-containing regimens such as CMF but at the cost of greater toxicity, particularly myelosuppression. For patients at sufficient risk, a combination of a taxane and an anthracycline is recommended.

Adjuvant Endocrine Therapy

British physician, George T. Beatson, first identified the potential role of oestrogen in breast tissue. He observed that rabbits stopped lactating after oophorectomy. Based on these findings, he undertook an oophorectomy in 1895 on a premenopausal patient with inoperable breast cancer. The patient had a complete remission and lived for a further 4 years. Beatson's work set the foundation of modern hormonal therapy in breast cancer.

Adjuvant Tamoxifen

The EBCTCG review of 194 randomised trials showed that 5 years of adjuvant tamoxifen in ER-positive patients reduced breast cancer mortality by 31% and was superior to 1 to 2 years of tamoxifen. In a subsequent EBCTCG metaanalysis, 5 years of adjuvant tamoxifen significantly reduced the risk of recurrence during the first 10 years, and the risk of breast cancer mortality by about one-third during the first 15 years (Fig. 26.31) (see Further Reading). Women with ER-rich tumours have 3 to 10 times the benefits of ER-poor patients. Life expectancy is increased by 2 to 3 years in women on tamoxifen for 2 to 3 years. If tamoxifen is added to chemotherapy in ER-rich tumours, additional benefit accrues, as also happens when chemotherapy is added to tamoxifen. In addition, tamoxifen reduces the risk of contralateral breast cancer.

There is an advantage to extending tamoxifen beyond 5 years. The ATLAS trial compared 12,984 women who had completed 5 years of tamoxifen and were randomised to continue tamoxifen for 10 years or discontinue it at 5 years. In ER-positive women, extended tamoxifen reduced breast cancer recurrence, breast cancer mortality and overall mortality significantly (Fig. 26.32). The standard duration of adjuvant endocrine therapy is usually 5 years. Extending tamoxifen to 10 years may be beneficial but probably not after initial AI.

Aromatase Inhibitors

In postmenopausal women, the ovary no longer produces oestrogen. Instead, it is mainly synthesised from nonglandular tissue (e.g. subcutaneous fat, muscle and liver) through the aromatase enzyme. The first two generations of AIs caused significant side effects because they also inhibited other steroid hormones such as aldosterone and cortisol.

Third-generation AIs have much greater specificity and are classified as either steroidal (type 1) or nonsteroidal (type 2). Steroidal AIs

inhibit the aromatase enzyme irreversibly. Nonsteroidal AIs are reversible competitive inhibitors.

The role of AIs as an alternative to tamoxifen or in combination with it was explored in the ATAC trial. This trial of over 9000 postmenopausal node-negative and predominantly ER-positive patients at a median follow-up of 68 months, showed a significantly longer disease survival in the anastrazole alone group over tamoxifen alone (hazard ratio (HR) 0.86; 95% CI .78–.97, $P = .01$). In addition, there was a highly significant reduction in risk of contralateral breast cancer in the anastrazole alone group. The incidence of endometrial cancer, vaginal bleeding and discharge, venous thromboembolism and cerebrovascular accidents was also reduced in the anastrazole-treated group. However, musculoskeletal symptoms and bone fractures were more common with anastrazole.

In the BIG 1-98 trial, 8028 postmenopausal patients with endocrine-sensitive breast cancer were randomised to 5 years of tamoxifen (20 mg daily), 5 years of letrozole (25 mg daily), 2 years of tamoxifen followed by 3 years of letrozole or 2 years of letrozole followed by 3 years of tamoxifen. Analysis of the comparison of the tamoxifen (5 years) and letrozole (5 years) with a median follow-up of 25.8 months showed a significant advantage survival of letrozole over tamoxifen (84.0% vs 81.4%, respectively). Patients on tamoxifen had significantly more thromboembolic events. Patients on letrozole had significantly more bone fractures (5.7% vs 4%, respectively, $P = .001$) and deaths from cardiac or cerebrovascular causes.

In the TEAM trial, postmenopausal patients were randomised to upfront tamoxifen versus exemestane, tamoxifen followed by exemestane or exemestane alone. At a median follow-up of 30.6 months, disease-free survival was improved by 4.7% with exemestane compared with tamoxifen alone (95% CI 2.8–6.8). However, there was no difference between exemestane alone or when switched to exemestane: from

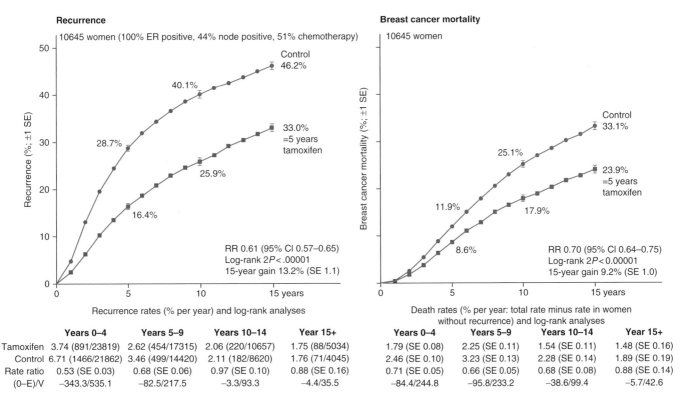

Fig. 26.31 Effects of tamoxifen on 15-year probability of recurrence and breast cancer mortality. *RR* (Reproduced with permission from Davies et al. Early Breast Cancer Trialists Collaborative Group (EBCTCG). Relevance of breast cancer hormone receptors and other factors to the efficacy of adjuvant tamoxifen: patient-level: patient-level meta-analysis of randomised trials. Lancet, 2011;378:771–784.)

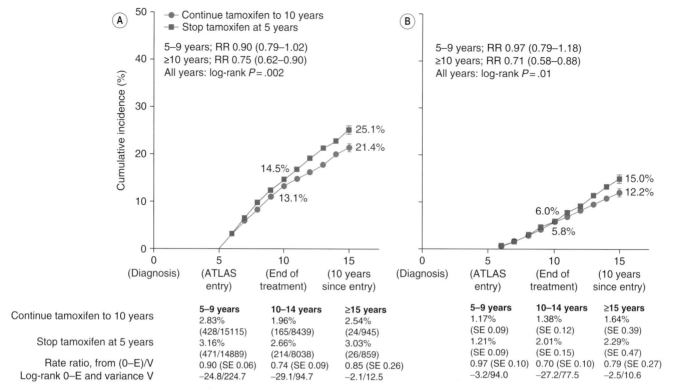

Fig. 26.32 Adjuvant Tamoxifen: Longer Against Shorter (ATLAS trial). Recurrence (A) and breast cancer mortality (B) by treatment allocation for 6846 women with ER-positive disease. Error bars show SE. Recurrence rates are percentage per year (events per patient-years of follow-up). Death rates (overall rate: rate in women without recurrence) are percentage per year (SE). *RR* (Davies C et al. Long-term effects of continuing adjuvant tamoxifen to 10 years versus stopping at 5 years after diagnosis of oestrogen receptor-positive breast cancer. Lancet. 2013;381:805–816).

Tamoxifen. There were significantly fewer contralateral breast cancers in the exemestane group compared with tamoxifen.

The EBCTCG undertook a metaanalysis of 31,920 patients in randomised trials of AIs versus tamoxifen. They compared subgroups (5 years of AI, 5 years of tamoxifen or 2–3 years of tamoxifen followed by AI to complete 5 years of treatment and 2–3 years of an AI followed by tamoxifen). A greater reduction in recurrence was seen in patients taking an AI during any point of the trial.

Switching Trials

Switching to an AI after 2 to 3 years of tamoxifen is an option. The Austrian Breast and Colorectal Cancer Study Group (ABCSG 8) trial undertook a combined analysis with the Arimidex-Nolvadex (ARNO 95) trial which assessed the benefits of switching to anastrazole for 3 years after 2 years of adjuvant tamoxifen. 3224 ER-positive women who had 2 years of adjuvant tamoxifen were then randomised to 1 mg anastrazole, 20 or 30 mg of tamoxifen. At a median follow-up of 28 months, there was a 40% reduction in event rates with anastrazole (67 events) versus tamoxifen (110 events) (HR 0.60; 95% CI .44–.81, $P = .0009$).

In the Intergroup Exemestane Study, patients were randomised after 2 to 3 years of tamoxifen to either a further 2 to 3 years of tamoxifen or the AI, exemestane, 25 mg orally for a further 2 to 3 years. There was an absolute benefit in disease-free survival of 4.7% which was statistically significant and led to early closure of the trial. Overall survival was not significantly different. These trials show that sequential use of AIs and tamoxifen conferred additional benefit. The optimal sequence and duration of treatment however are uncertain.

Adjuvant Hormonal Therapy After 5 Years of Tamoxifen

Breast cancer patients are 60% to 70% ER positive. Despite the efficacy of adjuvant endocrine therapy, 50% of breast cancer recurrences and

66% of deaths occur after the initial 5 years of tamoxifen. This implies that ER-positive breast cancer is a chronic relapsing disease that may remain quiescent for many years. This high rate of late relapse was the basis for investigating extending adjuvant endocrine therapy beyond 5 years. In this extended adjuvant setting, reductions in breast cancer recurrence must be balanced against the cumulative toxicity of longer endocrine therapy.

Recent evidence suggests that extended adjuvant hormonal therapy with the more recent and more potent AIs, such as letrozole and exemestane, may reduce the risk of recurrent breast cancer in patients treated initially with tamoxifen. In the NCI MA17 trial, 1918 patients who had received 4.5 to 6 years of an adjuvant AI were randomised to 2.5 mg of letrozole or placebo for a further 5 years. The 5-year disease-free survival in the extended letrozole group was 96% compared with 91% in the placebo group (HR 0.66; $P = .01$). This benefit was independent of nodal status. However, there was no difference in overall survival between the two groups.

Tamoxifen confers a similar reduction in risk of death in node-positive and node-negative women. However, the absolute reduction in risk is greater in node-positive women. The absolute gain in 10-year survival between 5 years of tamoxifen and no tamoxifen is 6% for node-negative and 11% in node-positive women. It confers benefit in both premenopausal and postmenopausal ER-positive women. Adding tamoxifen to chemotherapy in ER-positive patients confers additional benefit. All patients who are ER positive regardless of their menopausal or nodal status should be considered for adjuvant endocrine therapy for 5 years.

The Dutch IDEAL trial randomised patients who had received 5 years of adjuvant endocrine therapy (tamoxifen alone, AI alone or Tam + AI) to 2.5 or 5 years of letrozole. There was no survival advantage from 5 years of letrozole. Because there are adverse effects and limited absolute benefit in low-risk disease, it may be advisable to reserve extended endocrine therapy for high-risk disease.

Toxicity of Tamoxifen

Postmenopausal symptoms of hot flushes, vaginal dryness and sexual dysfunction are experienced by 20% to 40% of patients. Cognitive deficits also occur (as they do after cytotoxic chemotherapy). These symptoms can significantly interfere with a patient's quality of life. Transient thrombocytopenia occurs in 5% to 10% of patients and vaginal bleeding occurs in 5%. Tamoxifen increases the development of benign endometrial changes, such as hyperplasia. The risk of endometrial cancer, particularly in women who have been on tamoxifen for 5 years or more, is increased three- to fourfold, although the risk remains very small. The risk of endometrial cancer is 0.02%.

Care should be taken to avoid giving tamoxifen concurrently with chemotherapy because it increases the risk of a stroke. Tamoxifen should therefore only be started once chemotherapy has been completed.

Tamoxifen Plus Chemotherapy

Treatment with both tamoxifen and chemotherapy gives added benefit in patients with ER-positive disease in both node-positive and node-negative women. This also applies to postmenopausal ER-positive patients. However, in ER-negative, node-negative women, the NSABP B-23 trial showed no benefit of the addition of tamoxifen to chemotherapy.

Adjuvant Ovarian Suppression

The Oxford overview showed a highly significant increase in recurrence-free survival (25%) in premenopausal women under the age of 50 years treated by oophorectomy (see Further Reading).

For node-positive premenopausal women the gains in recurrence-free and overall survival at 15 years were 10.5% and 13% respectively. Much smaller but still statistically significant benefits in both these parameters were seen in premenopausal node-negative women. Because tamoxifen and chemotherapy became standard adjuvant therapy, the role of ovarian suppression became unclear. A number of prospective trials and a metaanalyses of ovarian suppression using gonatropin releasing hormone (GnRH) showed no gain from addition of ovarian suppression to tamoxifen or chemotherapy.

The Suppression of Ovarian Function trial (SOFT) compared tamoxifen, tamoxifen plus ovarian suppression and the combination of the AI, exemestane, plus ovarian suppression in premenopausal women. Adjuvant therapy was given for 5 years. Options for ovarian suppression were surgical oophorectomy and radiation-induced ovarian suppression of GnRH agonist treatment with triptorelin.

The Tamoxifen and Exemestane Trial (TEXT) compared tamoxifen plus ovarian suppression with the combination of the AI, exemestane and ovarian suppression in 3066 premenopausal patients. At a median follow-up of 67 months, the estimated disease-free survival was 86.6% in the tamoxifen + ovarian suppression group and 84.7% in the tamoxifen group (HR 0.83, 95% CI 0.66–1.04, $P = .10$). There was significant benefit from ovarian suppression in the whole study population. However, for patients at sufficient risk to require chemotherapy and who remained premenopausal, the addition of ovarian suppression improved disease outcomes. In a combined analysis of the SOFT and TEXT trials, at a median follow-up of 68 months, disease-free survival was 91.1% in the exemestane-ovarian suppression group and 87.3% in the tamoxifen-ovarian suppression group.

In the SOFT and TEXT trials, the 5-year breast cancer recurrence rates were significantly lower among premenopausal women who received the AI, exemestane plus ovarian suppression compared with those who received tamoxifen plus ovarian suppression. Adding ovarian suppression to tamoxifen did not result in significantly reduced recurrence rates over those treated with tamoxifen alone.

The American Society of Clinical Oncology (2016) recommends that ovarian suppression in addition to adjuvant endocrine therapy should be considered for premenopausal women with ER-positive breast cancer at higher risk of recurrence based on tumour stage, grade, nodal status or other biological features. If the patient has risk factors to warrant adjuvant chemotherapy, this would also justify ovarian suppression. Ovarian suppression was particularly encouraged in women under the age of 35 years where the SOFT trial showed particular benefits. For low-risk premenopausal patients (stage 1 or node negative with tumour ≤1 cm), ovarian suppression was not recommended.

ADJUVANT/NEOADJUVANT COMBINATION CHEMOTHERAPY (POLYCHEMOTHERAPY)

The use of chemotherapy as adjunct to locoregional therapy dates back to the 1950s. Circulating tumour cells were identified after mastectomy, but assumed to have been detached by surgery. Short-course cyclophosphamide given at the time of surgery reduced the risk of recurrence and mortality. Bernard Fisher, an American surgeon, hypothesised in the 1970s 'that breast cancer is a systemic disease… and that variations in effective local regional treatment are unlikely to affect survival substantially'. A further milestone in the 1970s was the use of combination chemotherapy with CMF by the Italian oncologist, Gianni Bonadonna, and the use of anthracycline-containing regimens in the 1990s and taxanes and anti-HER2 therapy in the early 2000s.

Neoadjuvant Chemotherapy

Neoadjuvant chemotherapy (NACT) has been widely adopted to try to induce a tumour response before surgery. NACT has three principal advantages.

First, it provides information on in vivo chemosensitivity. If there is no response to a particular regimen, it can be discontinued and changed. Second, it allows conversion of mastectomy to breast-conserving surgery if there is sufficient tumour shrinkage. It may allow more time to plan surgery or for genetic testing. Third, it provides prognostic information because a pathological complete response (pCR) in the primary tumour or nodes is a good prognostic sign. If there is no residual disease after NACT, either invasive or noninvasive, this is described as a pCR. Patients who have a higher probability of a pCR are: aged older than 40 years, grade 3, ductal histology, TNBC, ER/PgR negative, HER2 positive receiving transtuzumab and Ki67 greater than 14%. Those with a lower probability of pCR are aged older than 60 years, grade 1, lobular histology, ER/PgR positive and Ki67 less than 14%. About 50% to 60% of patients now achieve a complete pathological response. The pathological assessment after NACT using the TNM classification is preceded by "yp". A complete response in the breast is ypT0/is and in the nodes ypN0. Although the influence of NACT on outcome is clear for invasive disease, the same is not true for DCIS where the significance of residual DCIS is unclear. In terms of disease free and overall survival preoperative (neoadjuvant), chemotherapy is as effective as postoperative chemotherapy. It is particularly suitable for HER2 positive and TNBCs where there is a good correlation between pCR and survival. The 2018 EBCTCG metaanalysis comparing neoadjuvant and adjuvant chemotherapy in 4756 women showed more than two-thirds of patients allocated to NACT achieved a partial or complete response. Patients allocated to NACT were more likely to undergo breast-conserving surgery than patients undergoing adjuvant chemotherapy. NACT was likely to be associated with local recurrence (15-year local recurrence was 21.4% for NACT and 15.9% for adjuvant chemotherapy, an increase

TABLE 26.10 Neoadjuvant Chemotherapy	
Epirubicin 90 mg/m² IV	Day 1
Cyclophosphamide 600 mg/m² IV	Day 1
Repeated every 21 days for 4 cycles	
Docetaxel (Taxotere) 100 mg/m² repeated every 21 days for 4 cycles after 4 cycles of EC	Day 1

EC, Epirubicin and cyclophosphamide; *IV*, intravenously.

of 5.5% (95% CI 2.4–8.6). There were differences in distant recurrence or breast cancer mortality (see Further Reading). Patients with ER-negative high-grade tumours were most likely to achieve a pCR. A number of trials have shown pCR rates up to 83% in HER2-positive disease.

With NACT, a pathological complete response can be achieved in the axilla in 41% to 75% of patients with triple negative or HER2-positive breast cancer. The EBCTCG metanalysis does not provide information on axillary lymph node status before and after NACT. The policies for surgical management have changed with sentinel node biopsy, often replacing axillary node dissection. Sentinel node biopsy after NACT in patients who had a positive axilla before NACT is regarded as accurate if at least three sentinel nodes are removed and examined. Whether axillary dissection or RT should be undertaken when there has been a pCR in the axilla is unknown. A US trial (NSABP B51) is assessing the role of axillary irradiation in patients whose axilla has been converted from node positive to node negative by NACT.

In patients undergoing NACT, the primary and axillary nodes (if involved) should be marked by a metal clip, because these may be difficult to locate if there has been a good response to NACT. Similar regimens can be used for neoadjuvant and postoperative adjuvant chemotherapy. For NACT, a sequential regimen of a combination of epirubicin and cyclophosphamide (EC) followed by docetaxel (Taxotere) is suggested (Table 26.10).

Where there has been a pCR, safe omission of surgery depends on the ability to mark the tumour preoperatively. In most cases where breast-conserving surgery is possible, it is carried out after NACT.

Postoperative Adjuvant Chemotherapy

Postoperative adjuvant chemotherapy should be initiated within the first few weeks after surgery and precede adjuvant RT (if required). Anthracyline- and taxane-containing combination chemotherapy is the standard given concurrently or sequentially over 18 to 24 weeks. Four cycles of an anthracycline-based regimen followed by four cycles of a taxane-based regimen is advised. For node-negative patients, an anthracyline-containing regimen (5-FU, epirubicin, cyclophosphamide (FEC-75)) (Table 26.11C) or a combination of four cycles of epirubicin and four cycles of cyclophoshamide, methotrexate and 5-FU (Epi–CMF) (Table 26.11B) is suggested, and for node-positive patients, an anthracycline-taxane combination is recommended (FEC-100/docetaxel (Table 26.11A)). For patients who do not wish to lose their hair, a combination of CMF (Table 26.12) is suggested, or docetaxel and cyclophosphamide when anthracyclines are contraindicated. For elderly or frail patients, four cycles of epirubicin and cyclophosphamide are recommended. **Physicians should always check evidence based local protocols for chemotherapy regimes.**

Growth factor support may be required because of the high incidence of neutropenia with some anthracycline-containing regimens (e.g. docetaxel, doxorubicin and cyclophosphamide, TAC). The EBCTCG indicated that taxane-containing and anthracycline-containing regimens reduced 10-year breast cancer mortality by approximately one-third (Fig. 26.33) (see Further Reading).

TABLE 26.11   Adjuvant chemotherapy regimes (A) FEC (100)/Taxotere (B) Epirubicin + Cyclophosphamide, Methotrexate and 5-Fluorouracil (C) FEC 75

(A)   FEC-100/Docetaxel
5-FU 500 mg/m² intravenous
Epirubicin 100 mg/m² intravenous
Cyclophosphamide 500 mg/m² intravenous
FEC day 1 and repeated every 21 days for 3 cycles followed by docetaxel
Docetaxel 100 mg/m² intravenously on day one and repeated every 21 days for 3 cycles

(B) Epirubicin + CMF Repeated Every 21 Days for 4 Cycles
Epirubicin intravenous 100 mg/m² on day 1
Followed by 4 cycles of CMF
Cyclophosphamide intravenous 600 mg/m² on day 1 and day 8
Methotrexate intravenous 40 mg/m² on day 1 and day 8
5-FU intravenous 600 mg/m² on day 1 and day 8

(C) FEC-75	
5-FU 600 mg/m² intravenously	Day 1
Epirubicin 75 mg/m² intravenously	Day 1
Cyclophosphamide 600 mg/m²	Day 1
Regimen repeated every 21 days for 6 cycles	

5-FU, 5-Flourouracil; *CMF*, cyclophosphamide, methotrexate and 5-FU; *FEC*, 5-FU, epirubicin, cyclophosphamide.

TABLE 26.12   Adjuvant Cyclophosphamide, Methotrexate and 5-Fluorouracil Regimen

Classical		
Cyclophosphamide	100 mg/m² orally	Days 1–14
Methotrexate	40 mg/m² iv bolus	Days 1 and 8
5-Fluorouracil	600 mg/m² iv bolus	Days 1 and 8
Repeated every 28 days		

HER2 Positive Breast Cancer

Approximately 20% of breast cancers are HER2 positive and are associated with aggressive behaviour and a poor prognosis. HER2 positive tumours are classified as those 3+ on IHC or 2+ on IHC with HER2 gene amplification on in situ hybridisation testing. Trastuzumab is a monoclonal antibody against HER2. It binds to and prevents activation of the receptor, inhibiting downstream signaling for proliferation (Fig. 26.34). Pertuzumab, a more recently developed drug, blocks the dimerisation of HER2 (Fig. 26.35) and works synergistically with trastuzumab, increasing the pathological complete response rate in the neoadjuvant setting.

Four major randomised trials (NSABP B31, Intergroup N9831, BCIRG 006 and the HERA trial) have assessed the role of trastuzumab in the adjuvant setting (Table 26.13). The addition of trastuzumab for one year to a sequence of anthracycline-taxane adjuvant chemotherapy in the NSAPB B31 trial improved overall survival (HR 0.63, 95% CI 0.54–0.73, $P < .001$). Two years of trastuzumab in the HERA trial was no more effective than one year of therapy. Shorter durations of trastuzumab (e.g. FinHER) confer benefit but the PHARE trial shows that 12 months of trastuzumab is superior to 6 months.

Adjuvant trastuzumab is given three weekly intravenously (IV) (Table 26.14) for 12 months after the completion of adjuvant chemotherapy.

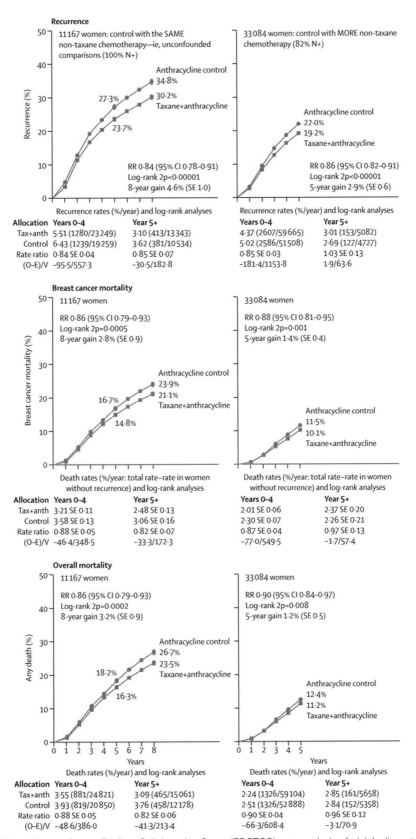

Fig. 26.33 Early Breast Cancer Trialists Collaborative Group (EBCTCG) metaanalysis of trials' adjuvant polychemotherapy. Time to recurrence, breast cancer mortality and overall mortality for taxane-plus-anthracycline-based regimens (Tax + anth) versus control with (*left*) the same or (*right*) more nontaxane chemotherapy trials, versus the same nontaxane chemotherapy (usually 4AC (4 cycles of Anthracyline + cyclophoshamide)). Relative risk (and its 95% confidence interval) = event rate ratio from summed log-rank statistics for all time periods combined. Gain (and its SE (Standard Error)) = absolute difference between ends of graphs. Event rates, % per year, are followed by (first events per woman-years). Error bars show ±1 SE. *RR* (Relative Risk), (From Elsevier Ltd. from Comparison between different polychemotherapy regimens for early breast cancer: meta-analysis of longterm outcome among 100,000 women in 123 randomised trials. Lancet Oncol. 2012; 379:432–444. With permission.)

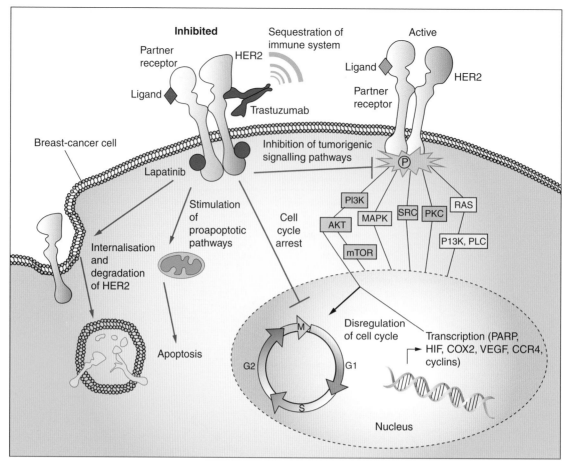

Fig. 26.34 Mechanism of action of current therapies for HER2-expressing breast cancer. Constitutively, active HER2 receptors on the surface of HER2–expressing breast cancer cells dimerize with other HER receptors, activating downstream signalling pathways that mediate tumorigenic cell proliferation, survival and invasion. Trastuzumab prevents constitutive activation of HER2, induces internalisation and degradation of the protein and stimulates the immune system to recognise HER2 overexpressing cells. Lapatinib binds to HER2 and HER1 and inhibits tumorigenic receptor signalling (From Jones KL, Buzdar AU. Evolving novel anti-HER2-strategies. Lancet Oncol. 2009;10:1179-1187. With permission.)

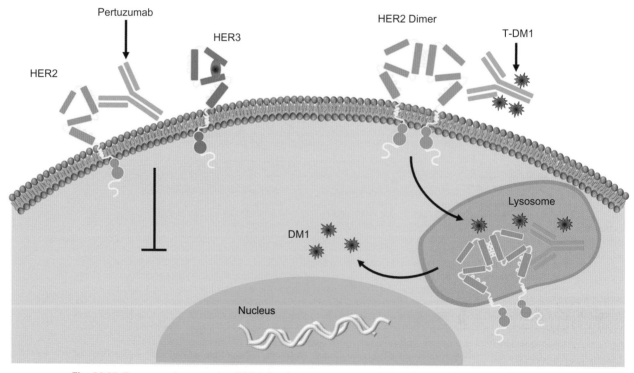

Fig. 26.35 Trastuzumab emtansine *(TDM-1)* and pertuzumab mechanism of action. (From Dixon JM. ABC of Breast Diseases, 4ᵗʰ ed, Oxford: Wiley-Blackwell, 2012.With permission.)

TABLE 26.13 Results from Major Trials Addressing Efficacy of Trastuzumab in Adjuvant Treatment of Breast Cancer

Trial	No. Patients; Years of Observation	Trial Arms	Disease-Free Survival Compared With Experimental Arm	Overall Survival Compared With Experimental Arm
BCIRG006	3222; 5 years	Doxorubicin + cyclophosphamide followed by docetaxel followed by docetaxel + trastuzumab, followed by trastuzumab; docetaxel + carboplatin + trastuzumab followed by trastuzumab	HR .64 (P = -.001)[a], HR 0.75 (P = .04)[b]; 75% vs 84% vs 81%; 257 vs 185 vs 214 events	HR 0.63 (P = .001); HR .77 (P = .04); 87% vs 92% vs 91%; 141 vs 94 vs 113 events
NCCTG N9831 & NSABP B-31	4046; 8.4 years	Doxorubicin + cyclophosphamide followed by paclitaxel; doxorubicin + cyclophosphamide, followed by paclitaxel + trastuzumab, followed by trastuzumab	HR 0.60 (P = .001); 62% vs 74%; 680 vs, 473 events	HR .63 (P < .001); 75% vs 84%; 418 vs 286 events
NCCTG N9831	2184; 6 years DFS analysis at 5 years follow-up	Doxorubicin + cyclophosphamide followed by paclitaxel (A); doxorubicin + cyclophosphamide, followed by paclitaxel, followed by trastuzumab (B); doxorubicin + cyclophosphamide, followed by paclitaxel + trastuzumab (C)	Sequential arm: HR .69 (P < .001); 72% vs 80% (A vs B); 225 vs 165 events Concurrent arm: HR 0.77 (P = .020); 80% vs 84% (B vs C); 174 vs 139 events	Sequential arm: HR 0.88 (P = .343); 88% vs 89% (A vs B); 108 vs 96 events Concurrent arm: HR 0.78 (P = .102); 90% vs 92% (B vs C) 96 vs 76 events
HERA	5099; 8 years	4 cycles of standard chemotherapy; 4 cycles of standard chemotherapy followed by trastuzumab (1 year); 4 cycles of standard chemotherapy followed by trastuzumab (2 years)	HR 0.99 (P = .86); 82% vs 81% (2 years vs 1 year); 367 vs 367 events (2 years vs 1 year; HR .76 (P = .001); 71% vs 65% (1 year vs observation); 471 vs 570 events (1 year vs observation)	HR 1.05 (P = 0. 63); 86% vs 88% (2 years vs 1 year); 196 vs 186 events; HR 0.76 (P ≤ .001); 83% vs 77% (1 year vs observation) 278 vs 350 events (1 year vs observation)
FNCLCC-PACS04	3010; 3 years	FEC or epirubicin + docetaxel followed by trastuzumab	HR 0.86 (P = .41); 78% vs, 81%; 70 vs, 59 events	HR 1.27 (P = NR); 96% vs 95% 18 vs 22 events
FinHER	232; 5.1 years	Docetaxel or vinorelbine, followed by FEC; docetaxel or vinorelbine + trastuzumab followed by FEC	HR 0.65 (P = .12); 73% vs 83%; 31 vs 22 events	HR 0.55 (P = .09); 82% vs 91%; 21 vs 22 events
PHARE	3380; 2 years	Trastuzumab (6 months; trastuzumab (12 months)	HR 1.28 (P = .29); 94% vs 92%;175 vs 219 events	NA
ALLTO	8381; 4.5 years	Lapatinib; trastuzumab; trastuzumab followed by lapatinib; lapatinib + trastuzumab	HR 0.84 P = .048; 88% lapatinib + trastuzumab vs 86% trastuzumab	HR .80 (p = .78); 95% lapatinib + trastuzumab vs 94% trastuzumab
ExteNET	2840; 2–3 years	Docetaxel (12 months); docetaxel (12 months) followed by neratinib	HR 0.67 (P = .009); 92% vs 94%; 109 vs 70 events	NA
TEACH	3147; 4 years	Placebo vs lapatinib	HR 0.83 (P = .053); 83% vs 87%; 264 vs 210 events	HR 0.99 (P = .96); 94% vs 94%; 97 vs 92 events

[a]HR 0.64 (P < .001 for doxorubicin + cyclophoshamide followed by docetaxel vs doxorubicin + cyclophoshamide, followed by docetaxel + trastuzumab, followed by trastuzumab.)
[b]HR 0.75.
FEC, Fluorouracil (5-FU) + epirubicin + cyclophosphamide; HR, hazard ratio; NA, not applicable.
(P = .04 for doxorubicin + cyclophoshamide followed by docetaxel vs docetaxel + carboplatin + trastuzumab, followed by trastuzumab.)
Modified from Loibl S Gianni L. HER2-positive breast cancer. Lancet. 2017;389:2415–2429.

TABLE 26.14 Treatment Schedule for Adjuvant Trastuzumab

8 mg/kg intravenous loading dose
Then 6 mg/kg every 21 days for 1 year

Trastuzumab should not be given concurrently with anthracyclines because of the higher risk of cardiac failure.

Cardiac function should be monitored every 3 months in patients on trastuzumab by left ventricular cardiac ejection fraction. If the latter falls, trastuzumab may have to be temporarily or permanently suspended. Rarely, cardiac failure may occur (around 1%) with sequential anthracycline and trastuzumab but rising to 4% if given concurrently.

Triple Negative Breast Cancer

There is no optimal chemotherapy regimen for TNBC and choice will be influenced by patient preference. For patients who have high-risk disease (e.g. node-positive luminal-B, HER2 positive), an anthracycline is followed by a taxane-containing regimen. For patients with lower risk disease (such as TI, node negative) a nonanthracycline regimen is preferred, although the evidence base is weak. BRCA1-associated breast cancer is commonly triple negative. The pathological complete response rate with platinum-based combination chemotherapy is much higher with BRCAI-associated TNBC (88%) than with sporadic TNBC (34%–40%).

Adjuvant Chemotherapy in Older Patients

Older, fit patients aged 70 years or older should be treated with combination chemotherapy because single agent therapy results in poorer outcomes. Patients' fitness should be carefully assessed, and geriatric assessment is advised. Toxicity should be closely monitored.

MANAGEMENT OF LOCALLY ADVANCED BREAST CANCER

Locally advanced breast cancer (LABC), or stage III breast cancer, refers to tumours larger than 5 cm in diameter (T3) or associated with involvement of the skin or chest wall (T4), inflammatory breast cancer (T4d) or with fixed axillary nodes (N2-3) or ipsilateral supraclavicular nodes (M1). LABC still presents a major challenge in management. With breast screening and greater public awareness, its incidence is falling, accounting for about 4% of European patients presenting with breast cancer. A typical example is shown in Fig. 26.36 These are a very heterogeneous group of tumours with widely differing natural histories. Historically, results with surgery and RT were disappointing with high levels of locoregional and systemic failure. Substantial improvements have been achieved with the addition of systemic therapy. The evidence base is much weaker than for early breast cancer. Much of the published literature is based on case series, with mixed populations of patients, some including patients with inflammatory breast cancer and others not. Often, in studies of systemic therapy, locoregional therapy is not well defined. There are limited internationally agreed-upon guidelines on management (see Further Reading). However, long-term survival remains poor at about 50% and systemic failure remains a major problem.

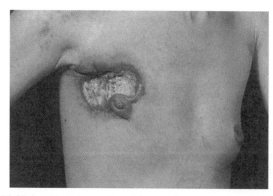

Fig. 26.36 Locally advanced and inoperable carcinoma of the right breast (T4).

Clinical Features

The main features of LABC are skin nodules, peau d'orange (T4b), inflammatory changes (T4d), ulceration and fixity to the chest wall (T4a), fixed axillary nodes (N2) or lymphoedema (N3). Local pain, bleeding, ulceration and infection are common symptomatic problems. The natural history of locally advanced disease varies widely. In some patients, distant metastatic disease will rapidly supervene, in others, the disease remains locoregional and relatively indolent.

Diagnosis

Diagnosis should be confirmed by core biopsy of the primary tumour and suspicious nodes.

Mammography may show the extent of malignant calcification but may not be appropriate for patients with gross bleeding or fungating tumours. Ultrasound may show site and extent. MRI is useful for assessing the extent of axillary/internal mammary node spread and invasion of skin and pectoral fascia.

Principles of Management

Neoadjuvant chemotherapy is the first step in the multimodal management of LABC. All chemotherapy should be given before surgery. Surgery, RT and systemic therapy in different combinations need to be tailored to the clinical features of the patient's cancer to maximise locoregional control and reduce the risk of distant metastases.

For patients with operable T3,N,MO disease, the choice is between breast-conserving surgery with oncoplastic procedures or mastectomy, if negative margins can be obtained, followed by adjuvant systemic therapy and RT or NACT followed by surgery and RT. A radiopaque marker should be placed in the tumour under image guidance to assist in the identification of the primary in case of pCR. NACT shrinks the tumour in 20% to 40% of cases, allowing breast-conserving surgery in some cases where mastectomy would otherwise have been mandated. For patients with inoperable locally advanced disease, systemic therapy, surgery and RT are indicated.

Role of Surgery

Surgery has a limited role in the management of locally advanced disease. It encompasses: (1) initial core biopsy for diagnosis and ER status; (2) mastectomy and axillary clearance in operable patients; (3) mastectomy (ideally with myocutaneous flap reconstruction) for residual masses after chemotherapy and radical RT; and (4) palliative debriding of infected and/or necrotic areas to reduce odour. For inflammatory breast cancer (T4d), only patients with complete clinical resolution of inflammatory changes following chemotherapy should be considered for mastectomy. Mastectomy as the primary procedure or when inflammatory changes persist after neoadjuvant systemic therapy is likely to be followed rapidly by recurrence in the skin flaps.

Trials of adjuvant chemotherapy in patients with stage III disease are rare. The Oxford overview of randomised trials of adjuvant systemic therapy does contain some patients with large operable cancer. The overview showed that all patients gained from adjuvant chemotherapy irrespective of tumour size. On this basis, it is reasonable to extrapolate the results of the overview to patients with operable stage IIIA disease.

Choice of Systemic Therapy

Data on the optimum chemotherapy for LABC are similarly sparse. The recommendations for anthracycline-based chemotherapy for LABC are largely extrapolated from studies of node-positive, metastatic breast cancer. Anthracycline- and taxane-based regimens are the standard NACT regimens. If sufficient tumour debulking has been achieved for surgery, this should be followed by postoperative RT. If there is no response and the tumour remains inoperable, radical RT should follow. Neoadjuvant therapy with anthracycline-containing chemotherapy downstages involved axillary nodes in 30% of cases and the anthracycline-taxane combination downstages in 40%. Even higher rates are achievable in HER2-positive patients treated with trastuzumab.

Hormonal Therapy

Patients with LABC who are ER and/or PgR positive should receive an AI at the end of chemotherapy for 5 years. For patients who are not suitable for chemotherapy and are hormone-receptor positive, primary treatment with an AI such as letrozole (2.5 mg daily) is recommended. Responses to hormonal therapy may take 6 to 8 weeks to occur. Patients who are premenopausal and hormone-receptor positive and are not suitable for chemotherapy should receive a luteinising hormone releasing hormone (LHRH) agonist (goserelin, 3.6 mg subcutaneously monthly).

Locoregional Therapy

If erythema of inflammatory changes or peau d'orange resolve with NACT, mastectomy and axillary clearance should follow. Postoperative RT is given to the chest wall and, if there are four or more involved axillary nodes, given to the medial supraclavicular fossa. There is no good evidence to determine whether or not the internal mammary nodes should be irradiated. Breast-conserving therapy for LABC is not standard therapy. However, there are some patients in whom the degree of debulking achieved by chemotherapy does make breast-conserving therapy possible. In addition, there are select patients with very small tumours which involve the skin early because of their proximity to the inframammary fold where the amount of breast tissue is small.

Target Volume

The target volume should include the chest wall or breast (in the case of conservative surgery) and, if the axilla has not been cleared, the peripheral lymphatics.

Technique

The principles of radical RT for early breast cancer apply also to locally advanced disease, both for the intact breast or following mastectomy. The only difference is that 0.5 to 1 cm of skin bolus should be applied to the breast or chest wall to ensure that the skin receives a full dose (to overcome the skin-sparing effect of megavoltage RT). Axillary surgery is not normally carried out at staging and, therefore, the peripheral lymphatics will normally be irradiated. If mastectomy and a level III axillary clearance have been carried out, the axilla should not be irradiated. Where there is macroscopic disease which would cross the conventional breast/shoulder field junction, it is best to use an en bloc technique, treating both the breast and the peripheral lymphatics in a Perspex jig.

Dosage and Fractionation (Radical)

Dosage and fractionation for LABC is 40 Gy in 15 daily fractions over 3 weeks (6–10 MV photons).

A boost of 10 Gy in 5 daily fractions (if primary tumour is sufficiently small) is to be encompassed within the boost volume.

Locoregional Palliative Radiotherapy

In some patients, radical RT is not advised, because of poor medical condition, advanced age or evidence of metastatic disease elsewhere. Locoregional recurrence occurs in approximately 5% to 15% of patients in trials treated by locoregional RT after breast-conserving surgery or mastectomy. Palliative RT can be very effective with minimal toxicity for symptomatic relief of local bleeding, ulceration from localised advanced disease, pain or discharge from skin metastases or flap recurrence after mastectomy, or axillary involvement with or without upper limb lymphoedema. Palliative RT to limited volumes is often possible in areas treated with radical locoregional RT. Responses are usually only partial but may be sufficient for symptomatic relief and may be prolonged. Dry or moist desquamation usually settles within 2 to 3 weeks.

Technique

The technique should be simple, either with parallel-opposed or tangential fields at megavoltage confined to the macroscopic area of tumour with 1- to 2-cm margins with bolus or a single electron field using a Perspex degrader to bring up the skin to full dose.

Dose

Dosing consists of 20 Gy in 5 daily fractions over 1 week (electrons of appropriate energy or 4–6 MV photons),or 36 Gy in 6 fractions of 6 Gy given once or twice weekly over 6 weeks, particularly in frail patients.

BONE METASTASES: PREVENTION AND TREATMENT

Approximately 20% to 30% of patients present with bone metastases as the first site of metastatic disease. They are associated with more aggressive tumours, particularly in younger women with large tumours, higher grade or several involved axillary lymph nodes. Bone metastases will develop in 60% to 70% of patients at some stage in the course of their disease. Life expectancy of patients with bone metastases is about 2 to 3 years, and less than a year if visceral metastases are present. Bone metastases cause significant morbidity because of pain, pathological fractures, hypercalcaemia or spinal cord compression. Patients with bony metastases should be considered for up to 2 years of bisphosphonate therapy.

Adjuvant bisphosphonates (zoledronic acid or sodium clodronate) are recommended for postmenopausal women with node-positive invasive breast cancer or those at high risk of recurrence. A baseline bone mineral density (DEXA) scan should be arranged at baseline.

Side effects of bisphosphonates include osteoradionecrosis of the jaw, atypical femoral fractures and osteonecrosis of the external auditory canal.

The optimum duration for bisphosphonate therapy is uncertain. There is evidence that benefit diminishes after 2 years of therapy so that 2 years of therapy seems reasonable. It is thought that the antimetastatic effect of bisphosphonates might be because of a fall in disseminated tumour cells in the bone marrow in women undergoing NACT for breast cancer.

A Cochrane systematic review of 44 randomised trials in 37,302 women with early or advanced breast cancer showed that bisphosphonates reduced the risk of bone metastases in early breast cancer compared with placebo/no bisphosphonate (RR 0.86, 95% CI 0.75–0.99, $P = .03$. There was a survival benefit in postmenopausal women (HR 0.77, 95% CI 0.66–0.90, $P = .001$) but not in premenopausal women. In advanced breast cancer without clinically evident bone metastases there was no evidence of an effect on bone metastases or overall survival. In patients with bone metastases, oral or IV bisphosphonates reduced the risk of a skeletally related event by 14% (RR 0.86, 95% CI 0.78–0.95, $P = .003$) compared with placebo. Bisphosphonates reduced pain but had no impact on survival. Toxicities were generally mild. The incidence of osteonecrosis of the jaw was rare (<5%) in the adjuvant setting.

Approved agents for patients with bone metastases include denosumab (120 mg subcutaneously every 4 weeks, IV pamidronate 90 mg over ≥2 hours, and zoledronic acid (4 mg given IV over

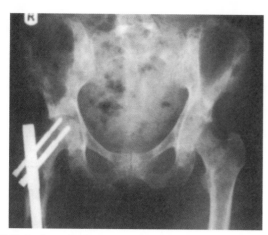

Fig. 26.37 Radiograph of pelvis showing pinning of pathological fracture of right hip as a result of extensive mixed and sclerotic disease from breast cancer.

≥15 minutes every 3–4 weeks)). Dosage must be adjusted according to renal function because bisphosphonates are renally excreted and potentially nephrotoxic.

Oral clodronate (1600 mg day) is an alternative but its bioavailability is limited and GI intolerance is common. Patients at risk of pathological fracture should be referred to an orthopaedic surgeon for consideration of mechanical stabilisation (Fig. 26.37) followed by postoperative palliative RT.

Palliative Radiotherapy for Bone Metastases

Technique
Single or parallel-opposed fields are used in palliative RT. Single fields suffice for the thoracic, lumbar spine and sacroiliac joints. The cervical spine can be treated by a single posterior field, but this will cause a sore throat because of the exit dose through the mouth. Lateral opposed fields reduce the dose to the mouth and resulting mucositis.

Dose
Single fractions of 8 Gy are recommended at megavoltage. Following surgical stabilisation, fractionated RT is given: 20 Gy in 5 fractions over 1 week at megavoltage.

Palliative Surgery

Where there is extensive ulceration and secondary infection causing distressing and offensive odour, surgical debridement of the affected area is often helpful in improving these symptoms. This can be repeated if necessary.

Principles of Management

Multidisciplinary management is essential in view of the complexities of advanced disease and must be adapted to the differing requirement of individual patients. Psychosocial support is needed from the time of diagnosis from specialised oncology nurses. Patients should be told that metastatic breast cancer is incurable but amenable to treatment. Given that treatment is palliative, a careful and difficult balance has to be struck between toxicity and its adverse effects on quality of life and disease control.

The minimum of staging is history, physical examination, full blood count, liver function tests, CT scan of chest and abdomen and bone scan. The brain should not be imaged in asymptomatic patients.

The choice of treatment must consider the age, general medical condition, comorbidities (including organ dysfunction) and performance of the patient, menopausal status, ER status, previous therapies and toxicities, number and sites of metastatic involvement, the tempo of the disease and expression of HER2. An elevated serum level of HER2 in ER-positive women with metastatic disease correlates with an inferior and shorter response to endocrine therapy. There are two general forms of systemic therapy: hormonal and cytotoxic. Concomitant endocrine and chemotherapy should not be administered outside a trial setting. In addition, patients whose tumour overexpresses HER2 (defined as a score of 3+ on IHC or 2+ on IHC with a positive fluorescent in situ hybridisation (FISH) test) may benefit from trastuzumab as a single agent or in combination with chemotherapy. In selected patients with HER2-positive, ER-positive breast cancer in whom endocrine therapy is preferred to chemotherapy, hormonal therapy can be combined with anti-HER2 therapy. In general, hormonal therapy is better tolerated than cytotoxic therapy and, in the absence of immediately life-threatening aggressive disease, is the preferred first line of treatment in ER-positive disease. For ER-negative disease and disease progressing on endocrine therapy, aggressive disease or rapidly evolving visceral disease, chemotherapy is the treatment of choice in fit patients. Types and durations of chemotherapy regimens should be individualised and take account of patients' preference. Response to endocrine therapy should be assessed every 2 to 4 months and after two to four cycles of chemotherapy. To date, there is no multigene technology to support choice of treatment in advanced breast cancer. The general schema of systemic therapy for metastatic cancer is summarised in Fig. 26.38.

Medical Management of Advanced and Metastatic Disease

Less than 10% of patients present with advanced or metastatic disease. About 50% of patients with involved nodes and 10% of those who are node negative will relapse within 5 years. There is no curative treatment for metastatic disease. Prognosis is poor with a median survival of 2 to 4 years and a 5-year survival rate of about 25%, although control of metastatic disease with anti-HER2 therapy now commonly exceeds 2 to 3 years. Nonetheless, durable and clinically useful disease control can be obtained by hormonal and/or cytotoxic therapy. In addition, therapy with bisphosphonates can be useful in reducing the risk of complications of bony metastases. Therapeutic intent is palliative. Aims of treatment are principally relief of cancer-related symptoms, improvement in quality of life and prolongation of life. Prognosis is governed by a complex interaction of factors, including number and site of metastases, disease-free interval, hormonal sensitivity and expression of the epidermal growth factor, HER2. Early introduction of aggressive chemotherapy increases the likelihood of treatment-resistant disease. Better prognosis is associated with hormone sensitive, HER2-negative tumours, a long disease-free interval (>1 year), absence of visceral involvement and a limited number of sites of metastases. The level of the evidence base for most recommendations is low (see ESO-ESMO guidelines for advanced breast cancer in Further Reading). Our understanding of the biology of advanced breast cancer and the mechanisms of treatment resistance is limited.

Menopausal Status and Hormone Receptor Status

In general, more postmenopausal than premenopausal patients are ER positive. Premenopausal patients tend to have more aggressive disease and are more commonly ER negative, especially under the age of 40. Patients with aggressive and/or ER-negative disease require chemotherapy.

ER and PgR status is a useful guide to clinical response. ER+/PgR+ tumours have a response rate of 77%: ER+/PgR- 27%; ER-/PgR+ 46%; and ER-/PgR- 11%. In premenopausal ER-positive patients, options include ovarian suppression by medical means (goserelin 3.6 mg

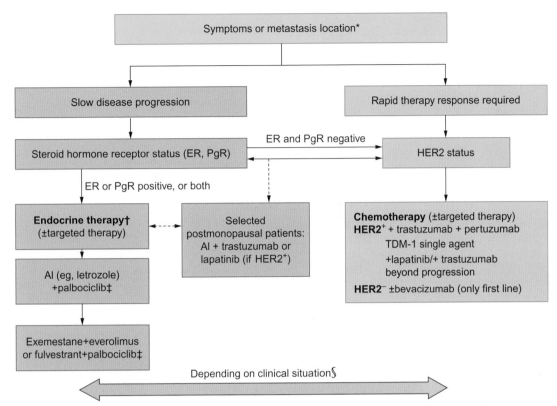

Fig. 26.38 Principles of systemic therapy for metastatic breast cancer. (From Harbeck N, Gnant M. Breast cancer. Lancet. 2017;389:1134–1150. With permission. * if bone metastases: bisphoshonates or denosumab, § only applicable if ER or PgR positive or both.)

monthly subcutaneously) or oophorectomy combined with tamoxifen. There is evidence in advanced disease that goserelin and tamoxifen have synergistic effects with a higher response rate (but no additional survival benefit) and are best prescribed together.

The advantage of goserelin is that it is reversible once withdrawn. This has particular advantages in women who tolerate poorly the menopausal symptoms that it induces and wish to stop the treatment and continue tamoxifen alone. Oophorectomy is usually performed as a laparoscopic procedure.

In general, response to one hormonal agent predicts response to subsequent hormonal therapy. Overall, 50% to 60% of ER-positive patients will respond. The duration of disease control by first-line hormonal therapy is usually about 18 months. About 25% of patients who respond to first-line hormonal agent will respond to second-line hormonal therapy. However, only 15% of patients who fail to respond to first-line therapy will respond to second-line hormone therapy.

For first-line therapy in premenopausal ER-positive women in the absence of visceral life-threatening disease, a combination of tamoxifen (20 mg orally daily) and ovarian suppression with goserelin (3.6 mg subcutaneously monthly) is suggested; for second-line therapy, anastrazole, an AI, can be substituted for tamoxifen while continuing ovarian suppression with goserelin. If second-line hormonal therapy fails, cytotoxic chemotherapy should be considered.

For first-line therapy for recurrent disease in postmenopausal women, even in the presence of visceral disease (unless there is visceral crisis), the choice is between tamoxifen (20 mg per day), an AI, anastrazole (1 mg orally daily) or letrozole (2.5 mg orally daily); for second-line therapy, an AI, exemestane (25 mg orally daily) or fulvestrant, a selective ER downregulator (SERD) (500 mg monthly with initial loading dose), is recommended. Anastrazole commonly causes joint stiffness because of its musculoskeletal effects. Everolimus can be added

to an AI if there has been progression on a nonsteroidal AI. More recently, the addition of a CDK4/6 inhibitor, palbociclib, to an AI as first-line therapy for postmenopausal patients (with the exception of those relapsing less than a year after from the end of adjuvant AI) is also an option. The main toxicity of palbociclib is neutropenia. The optimum sequence of endocrine therapy after first-line therapy is unclear. Options include tamoxifen, fulvestrant combined with palbociclib, AI plus everolimus and megestrol acetate and fulvestrant.

Patients who are most likely to benefit from hormonal therapy for relapsed disease have one or more of the following characteristics:

- Disease-free survival over 2 years
- Soft tissue or bone disease
- Older postmenopausal

Sites of Metastases and Impact on Management

Visceral metastases (e.g. liver disease) tends to respond less well to hormonal therapy and better to cytotoxic therapy. However, durable responses to hormonal therapy are occasionally seen with ER-positive liver metastases.

Cytotoxic Therapy

Breast cancer is moderately sensitive to chemotherapy. In general, combination chemotherapy has a higher overall response rate and a slight advantage in survival over monotherapy. Commonly used agents are doxorubicin, taxanes (doxetacel and pacilitaxel), epirubicin, methotrexate and 5-FU, trastuzumab (Herceptin) and capecitabine. New additions are eribulin, lapatinib and pertuzumab, T-DM1 and palbociclib. The schema for chemotherapy for metastatic breast cancer is summarised in Fig. 26.39. The sequence of systemic therapy in HER2 positive metastatic breast cancer is summarised in Fig. 26.40. For patients who have already received anthracyclines and taxanes,

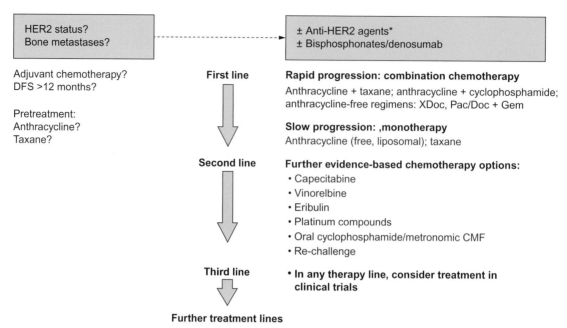

Fig. 26.39 Chemotherapy for metastatic breast cancer. Approved targeted drugs for addition to chemotherapy: trastuzumab, pertuzumab or lapatinib for HER2-positive tumours; bevacizumab (first-line therapy) for HER2-negative tumours. *CMF*, Cyclophosphamide, methotrexate and 5-fluorouracil; *DFS*, disease-free survival; *Gem*, gemcitabine; *Pac*, paclitaxel; *XDoc*, capecitabine and docetaxel. (From Harbeck N, Gnant M. Breast cancer. Lancet. 2017;389:1134–1150. With permission.)

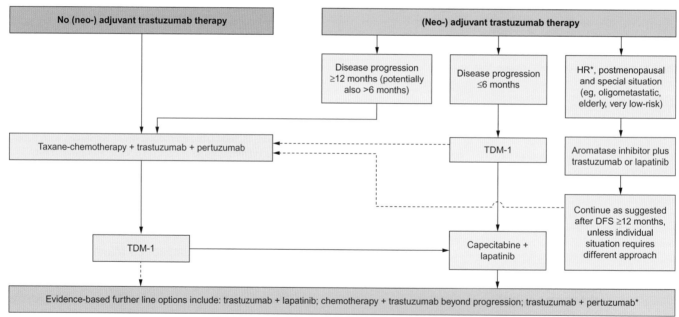

Fig. 26.40 Evidence-based sequence of systemic therapy in HER2 positive metastatic breast cancer. Please note the currently available evidence does not cover all situations because of individual differences in pretreatment. Thus, extrapolations from available evidence were applied when needed. Solid lines represent evidence-based and dotted lines are reasonable options without evidence. *DFS*, Disease-free survival; *HR +*, hormone receptor positivie (ER or PgR positive, or both); *TDM-1*, trasutuzumab emtansine. * If no previous pertuzumab. (From Harbeck N, Gnant M. Breast cancer. Lancet. 2017;389:1134–1150. With permission.)

capecitabine, vinorelbine and eribulin are the preferred agents based on efficacy and toxicity. Rechallenge with anthracyclines is possible if there has been at least a 12-month period disease free. Eribulin is a microtubule inhibitor usually used in third or subsequent lines of chemotherapy. Lapatinib is a small-molecule, reversible inhibitor of both

epidermal growth factor receptor and (HER2 tyrosine kinases. Its mechanism of action is shown in Fig. 26.34.

Pertuzumab has a complementary mechanism of action (see Fig. 26.35) to that of trastuzumab, binding the extracellular domain 11 of HER2 and inhibiting ligand-dependent dimerisaton of

TABLE 26.15 Palliative Schedule of Trastuzumab

Loading dose 4 mg/kg intravenous by infusion over 90 minutes
If loading dose is tolerated, subsequent weekly doses of 2 mg/kg intravenous by infusion over 30 minutes

TABLE 26.16 Palliative Doxorubicin/Epirubicin and Cyclophosphamide

Doxorubicin intravenous 60 mg/m^2 or epirubicin 75 mg/m^2
Cyclophosphamide intravenous 600 mg/m^2
Given every 3 weeks

TABLE 26.17 Palliative Regimen With Docetaxel

Docetaxel 75 or 100 mg/m^2
Repeated every 21 days for up to 6 courses
Dose reduction to 75 mg/m^2 if liver function disturbed or toxicity Prophylaxis with growth colony stimulating factor if using docetaxel 100 m/m^2

TABLE 26.18 Palliative Capecitabine

1250 mg/m^2 twice daily (bd) orally days 1–14 every 21 days
Consider starting frailer patients at 1000 mg/m^2

TABLE 26.19 Palliative Capecitabine and Lapatinib

Capecitabine 1000 mg/m^2 twice daily (bd) orally on days 1–14 every 21 days
Lapatinib 1250 mg orally once daily until disease progression

HER2-HER3 and diminishing signalling via intracellular pathways (e.g. phosphatidylinositol 3-kinase (PI3K/AKT)). Trastuzumab emtansine (TDM-1) is an antibody–drug conjugate made up of trastuzumab, stably linked to a very potent chemotherapy drug (DM-1) derived from maytansine. The mechanism of action of TDM-1 is shown in Fig. 26.35.

HER2-positive patients who receive anti-HER therapy in the adjuvant setting and relapse should be considered for further anti-HER2 therapy (unless there are specific contraindications to its reintroduction). The palliative dose schedule for trastuzumab is shown in Table 26.15.

For patients who have received anti-HER2 therapy in the (neo) adjuvant setting, chemotherapy combined with dual blockage with trastuzumab and pertuzumab should be considered. However, there is no evidence to support continuing dual blockade beyond progression. TDM-1 should be considered after first-line trastuzumab-based therapy as it provides a benefit in overall survival.

The optimum period of anti-HER2 therapy is uncertain. Nor is it known in patients who obtain a complete response to anti-HER2 therapy, how long it should be continued. Stopping it may be an option after several years of durable response, keeping open the possibility of reintroduction if there is recrudescence of disease. Lapatinib plus trastuzumab without chemotherapy is a useful option for some patients after progression on chemotherapy plus trastuzumab.

For first-line therapy when trastuzumab is used as the only anti-HER2 therapy, the preferred chemotherapeutic agents are a taxane or vinorelbine. For second and subsequent lines of chemotherapy, trastuzumab can be combined with nearly all chemotherapeutic agents including vinorelbine, taxanes, capecitabine, eribulin, anthracyclines, platinum or gemcitabine.

For advanced (TNBC) chemotherapy is indicated. The TNT study, which compared standard docetaxel to carboplatin in TNBC, demonstrated the superiority of carboplatin in BRCA-positive patients alone, but similar efficacy for both agents in unselected TNBC patients.

Capecitabine is an oral fluoropyrimidine with a slow release of 5-FU. The usual dose is 1250 mg/m^2 bd for 14 days. Gastrointestinal or renal toxicity may be dose limiting. The combination of capecitabine and docetaxel improves time to progression, overall survival and response rates in women whose disease has progressed on or after anthracycline therapy.

Combination Chemotherapy and Anti-HER2 Therapy

Median time to response varies from 6 to 14 weeks. Median duration of response is 6 to 12 months. Response rates to second-line combination chemotherapy are generally much lower (about 20%), and to third-line therapy, 5% or less. In only about 15% to 20% of patients is a complete response obtained. There are wide variations in the combinations of chemotherapy used in metastatic breast cancer. For fitter patients, particularly in patients with visceral disease, an anthracycline (adriamycin) combined with cyclophosphamide is an appropriate first-line combination (Table 26.16). For patients whose disease has progressed on an anthracycline-containing regimen, a taxane (Table 26.17) (combined with herceptin in HER2-positive patients) is recommended. The optimal duration of chemotherapy is unclear. For most agents, administration of two initial courses to test responsiveness of the tumour followed by up to four additional courses if there is continuing response with acceptable toxicity is common practice. Decisions about the continuation or cessation of treatment should be taken by patient and doctor, taking account of symptoms, signs, toxicity, quality of life and patient preference.

If patients are unfit for anthracylines, then CMF is recommended (as per adjuvant therapy) (see Table 26.12). The response rate to CMF is 40% to 50%.

Capecitabine is an orally active prodrug of 5-FU with an objective response rate of 36% (Table 26.18). Response rates are similar to taxanes in patients previously treated by anthracyclines. Hand-foot syndrome and GI toxicity are common and commonly require reductions in dose (e.g. to 2000 mg/m^2) or occasionally, cessation of therapy. It may be combined with lapatinib (Table 26.19) in HER2-positive metastatic patients who have had previous treatment with an anthracycline, taxane and trastuzumab with normal cardiac function. There is a synergistic cytotoxic effect if capecitabine is combined with docetaxel. The combination of docetaxel with capecitabine has a higher response rate (42% vs 30%) when compared with docetaxel alone. Median survival with the combination was 14 months compared with 11 months with docetaxel alone. Gemcitabine has a first-line response rate of between 23% and 37% (Table 26.20). There are synergistic effects when it is combined with either cisplatin or paclitaxel.

Other options are eribulin (Table 26.21), vinorelbine (Table 26.22) or gemcitabine combined with paclitaxel (Table 26.23).

Physicians should always check evidence based local protocols for chemotherapy regimes.

TABLE 26.20   Single Agent Chemotherapy First-Line Responses Rates in Metastatic Breast Cancer

Paclitaxel/docetaxel	36%–68%
Doxorubicin and epirubicin	40%
Cyclophosphamide	36%
Mitoxantrone (mitozantrone)	27%
Methotrexate	26%
5-Fluorouracil	28%
Vinorelbine	40%–52%
Gemcitabine	23%–37%
Eribulin	29%

TABLE 26.21   Palliative Eribulin

1.23 mg/m^2 (1.4 mg/m^2 eribulin mesylate) iv over 2–5 minutes, day 1 and day 8, every 21 days until disease progression

TABLE 26.22   Palliative Vinorelbine

25–30 mg/2× weekly (or days 1 and 8 every 21 days if used in combination schedules)

60 mg/m^2 orally weekly for cycles 1–3, then increasing to 80 mg/m^2 except if neutrophil count falls to <500/mm^3 more than once during first three cycles between 500 and 1000/mm^3

TABLE 26.23   Palliative Gemcitabine and Paclitaxel

Gemcitabine intravenous 1250 mg/m^2 days 1 and 8	
Paclitaxel 175 mg/m^2 iv day 1 every 21 days	

Morbidity of Chemotherapy (Adjuvant and for Metastatic Disease)

The morbidity of adjuvant cytotoxic therapy may be both physical and psychological. For CMF chemotherapy, acute toxicity includes nausea and vomiting, temporary alopecia, lassitude, and soreness of the eyes (the latter because of secretion of methotrexate into the tears). Neutropenia-related infection is less common with CMF than with more intensive anthracycline-based chemotherapy. The anthracyclines (doxorubicin and epirubicin) cause complete, although reversible, alopecia. They are also potentially cardiotoxic, and cardiac function, judged clinically and by electrocardiogram and cardiac ejection fraction, should be adequate before use. The risk of symptomatic cardiac dysfunction, for example, using a combination 5-FU, epirubicin (at a dose of 100 mg/m^2) and cyclophosphamide (FEC-100) is 2% at 8 years. The risk of cardiac death is less than 1% if guidelines on maximum cumulative dose are respected. There appears to be no added risk of cardiotoxicity from combining taxanes with anthracyclines. With cumulative doses of anthracyclines, the long-term risk of inducing leukaemia increases. However, if a total dose of 720 mg of epirubicin is not exceeded, there is no increased risk of leukaemogenesis. More recently, cognitive dysfunction has been recognised as a complication of chemotherapy caused by damage to the frontal cortex. The risk factors for this

TABLE 26.24   Side Effects of Chemotherapy and Route of Administration

Capecitabine Oral
Severe nausea or vomiting
Diarrhoea
Stomach pains
Loss of appetite
Constipation
Fatigue/weakness
Back/joint/muscle pain
Headache
Hand-Foot syndrome

Carboplatin (Usually Given Intravenously)
Reduced blood count
Nausea, vomiting and/or diarrhoea
Hair loss (reversible)
Confusion

Cisplatin (Usually Given Intravenously)
Reduced blood count
Allergic reactions
Nausea and vomiting
Tinnitus and hearing loss
Renal damage

Cyclophosphamide (Given Intravenously or Orally)
Reduced blood count
Nausea, vomiting
Abdominal pain
Anorexia
Hair loss (reversible)
Impaired fertility
Bladder damage
Pulmonary or cardiac toxicity (at high dose)

Docetaxel (Taxotere) (Given Intravenously)
Reduced blood count
Allergic reactions
Fluid retention with weight gain; ankle or abdominal swelling
Peripheral neuropathy
Nausea
Diarrhoea
Mouth ulcers
Hair loss
Fatigue and weakness

Doxorubicin (Given Intravenously)
Reduced blood count
Mouth ulcers
Nausea and vomiting
Hair loss (reversible)
Cardiac damage

Continued

are unknown. The taxanes are associated with fluid retention, peripheral neuropathy and allergic reactions. The common toxicities of a selection of anticancer agents used in treating breast cancer are summarised in Table 26.24. Nausea and vomiting can be reduced by the use of steroids and anti-5HT3 antagonists.

Bone Marrow Involvement

Bone marrow involvement complicates the delivery of cytotoxic therapy because the associated leukopenia and thrombocytopaenia of

TABLE 26.24 Side Effects of Chemotherapy and Route of Administration—cont'd
Eribulin (Given Intravenously)
Reduced blood count
Fatigue/weaknes
Hair loss
Nausea
Peripheral neuropathy
Etoposide (Given Intravenously)
Reduced blood count
Nausea and vomiting
Mouth ulcers
Allergic reactions
Hypotension (during administration)
Anorexia
Diarrhoea and abdominal pain
Flu-like symptoms
Brochospasm
5-Fluorouracil (Given Intravenously)
Reduced blood count
Mouth ulcers
Diarrhoea
Dry skin
Photosensitivity
Gemcitabine (Given Intravenously)
Reduced blood count
Nausea and vomiting
Fever and flu-like symtptoms
Rash
Methotrexate (Given Intravenously, Intrathecally or Orally)
Reduced blood count
Mouth ulcers
Skin rashes and photosensitivity
Hair loss (reversible)
Liver damage
Kidney damage (at high dose)
Seizures
Paclitaxel (Taxol) (Given Intravenously)
Reduced blood count
Allergic reactions
Mouth ulcers
Peripheral neuropathy
Nausea and vomiting
Diarrhoea
Anorexia
Altered taste
Hair loss
Joint pains
Vinorelbine (Given Intravenously or Orally)
Low blood count
Nausea
Vomiting
Fatigue/weakness
Constipation
Diarrhoea
Dizziness

impaired marrow function may compromise the delivery of full-dose chemotherapy. Doses of chemotherapy have to be reduced to 50% or less of standard dosage. Weekly low-dose IV epirubicin (20 mg/m^2) is generally well tolerated. If chemotherapy is successful, haemoglobin, white count and platelet levels should eventually rise. Bone marrow involvement is not an absolute indication for cytotoxic therapy because responses are seen in ER-positive patients. However, rapidly evolving bone marrow infiltration will require chemotherapy.

Growth Factor Support

For patients who are experiencing treatment delays because of febrile leucopenia, treatment with granulocyte colony-stimulating factor (GCSF) is recommended. GCSF is given daily by subcutaneous injection, starting not less than 24 hours after chemotherapy and continuing until the predicated neutrophil nadir has passed and recovered into the normal range. Duration of treatment is normally up to 14 days depending on the drug regimen, dosage and scheduling. Common side effects include pain and redness at the injection site and bone pain.

CLINICAL OUTCOMES IN EARLY AND ADVANCED METASTATIC BREAST CANCER

Clinical outcomes have improved steadily after the last three decades due to a combination of factors: breast screening and better surgery, RT and systemic therapy. Local relapses after breast-conserving surgery have fallen from around 5% at 5 years 2 decades ago to around 2% to 3% currently. The Edinburgh Breast Conservation series of over 1812 patients typifies these improvements. It includes patients presenting through the breast screening programme or symptomatically, and treated between 1990 and 1998. The actuarial overall survival (deaths from all causes) is 88.5% at 5 years, 77.2% at 10 years, 65.9% at 15 years and 55.8% at 20 years. At 10 years, the cumulative risk of ipsilateral breast relapse was 8.4% (.84% per annum). The time to ipsilateral breast tumour recurrence is shown in Fig. 26.41.

Life expectancy from the time of diagnosis of advanced and metastatic disease has improved about 2 to 3 years with a few long-term survivors over 5 years with HER2-positive breast cancer controlled by trastuzumab.

FOLLOW-UP

The main goals of follow-up are:
1. Detection of locoregional or metastatic recurrence, second primary tumour and contralateral breast cancer.
2. Assessment and treatment of complications of treatment.
3. Encouragement of compliance with therapy.
4. Psychosocial support.
5. Maintenance and monitoring of response to treatment and treatment-induced morbidity and to facilitate rehabilitation.

Clinical trials have failed to show an improvement in patient outcomes from more intensive versus less intensive follow-up for systemic recurrence. There is no evidence that the early detection of asymptomatic disease at distant sites improves survival or quality of life. Routine imaging apart from mammography is not recommended as part of follow-up care.

From the patient's perspective, reassurance that there is no evidence of recurrence or of progressive disease is probably the most important. Most of the evidence suggests that, at least for women treated for operable breast cancer, most recurrences, whether after breast conservation or mastectomy, present symptomatically. It is probable that a policy of annual mammography to detect local recurrence in the conserved or

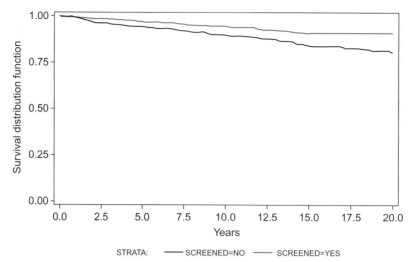

Fig. 26.41 Time to ipsilateral breast tumour recurrence by screened or symptomatic presentation. (From Kunkler IH, Kerr GR, Thomas JR, et al. Impact of screening and risk factors for local recurrence and survival after conservative surgery and radiotherapy for early breast cancer: results from a large series with long-term follow-up. Int J Radiat Oncol Biol Phys. 2012;83:829–838. With permission.)

contralateral breast and rapid access to the breast/oncology clinic for women with new symptoms would be much more cost effective.

Follow-Up After Breast-Conserving Therapy

For patients managed by breast-conserving therapy, the priorities are the detection of local recurrence which can be treated by mastectomy and of contralateral breast cancer. The risk of contralateral breast cancer is three to five times that of the normal population. Guidelines on optimal duration of follow-up vary considerably. NICE recommends annual mammography for 5 years.

Although distant relapses peak in the first 5 years of follow-up, recurrence rates within the treated breast remain constant at 1% to 1.5% per year for at least 10 years. This argues that the frequency of follow-up does not need to be any more frequent in the early years after completion of treatment than in later years. Most studies of follow-up show that multiple clinical visits are of little value in detecting recurrence. In a study from Edinburgh of 1312 women followed up for 10 years after breast-conserving surgery and postoperative RT treated between 1991 and 1998, only 15 relapses were detected clinically (see Further Reading). Discharge from clinical follow-up at 3 years while maintaining annual mammography up to 10 years seems reasonable. At this point, women who still lie within the UK screening age group (i.e. aged <69 years) should be returned to the 3-yearly breast-screening programme. For women over the age of 70 years, further follow-up should be decided on an individual basis between the patient and their surgeon/oncologist.

Follow-Up After Mastectomy

Local recurrences on the chest wall are commonest in the first 2 years after mastectomy and 80% of chest wall and axillary recurrences occur within the first 5 years. The evidence-based guidelines of the American Society of Clinical Oncology recommend a careful history and clinical examination every 3 to 6 months for 3 years, then visits every 6 to 12 months for 2 years, and then annually thereafter. Optimum duration of follow-up is uncertain. NICE recommends annual mammography for 5 years.

BREAST CANCER IN PREGNANCY

The diagnosis of breast cancer in pregnancy is uncommon but presents difficult decisions for patient, oncologist and obstetrician. Close liaison between oncologist and obstetrician is essential. The interests of both mother and child need to be taken into account. In women aged 30 years or younger, 10% – 20% of cases may be associated with pregnancy or within 1 year postpartum.

Histology is similar to age and stage-matched nonpregnant controls. Most tumours are high grade and lymphovascular invasion is common. Lymph node involvement is reported to be as high as 79%. Most tumours (>70%) are ER-negative.

Management will be influenced by the stage of pregnancy, the preference of the patient and the stage of the disease. There is no level 1 evidence on pregnancy and breast cancer. There are guidelines (e.g. Royal College of Obstetrics and Gynaecology (see Further Reading)). However, it should follow as far as possible the protocol for nonpregnant patients. A subsequent pregnancy after the diagnosis of breast cancer does not adversely affect prognosis. Indeed, there is some evidence that it may have a favourable effect on survival.

Ultrasound is used initially to image a breast lump. A tissue diagnosis should be obtained by ultrasound guided biopsy. With adequate fetal shielding, mammography should not be harmful. However, the increased density of the breast during pregnancy may obscure the radiological signs of malignancy. Staging for metastases should only be undertaken if there is a high level of clinical suspicion and should be restricted to chest radiograph and liver ultrasound.

Continuing the pregnancy should take account of prognosis, treatment and future fertility between patient, partner and the multidisciplinary team. In the first trimester, termination is normally advised and followed by standard treatment.

Surgery can usually be safely performed during all trimesters. In general, this is delayed until at least the 12th week of gestation because, before this point, the risk of spontaneous abortion is highest. Breast-conserving surgery or mastectomy is carried out, depending on tumour features and breast size. Sentinel node biopsy is recommended if preoperative axillary ultrasound and needle biopsy are negative. Radioisotope scintigraphy is allowable because it does not cause significant uterine irradiation. However, blue dye should be avoided because its effects on the fetus are unknown. If the axilla is positive, axillary lymph node dissection should be performed. Reconstruction should be delayed to avoid prolonged anaesthesia. In the first trimester, adjuvant chemotherapy is contraindicated because there is a high risk of fetal abnormality. However, in the second trimester, it is safe. Anthracyclines may be safely administered. The combination of 5-FU epirubicin and cyclophosphamide can be delivered without adverse effect on the infant. There are few data on taxanes, which should therefore be reserved for high-risk node positive or metastatic disease. A standard 5HT3 antagonist and dexamethasone are used as antiemetics. Growth factors are also permitted during pregnancy. Tamoxifen and trastuzumab are contraindicated in pregnancy but may be used after delivery. No adjuvant RT is given until after the delivery of the baby.

Most patients can proceed to term with natural or induced delivery followed, if indicated, by postoperative RT (with same criteria as in the nonpregnant patient). Radiotherapy can be safely delayed up to 6 months after surgery.

Hormonal therapy, if indicated, should be started after delivery, and after chemotherapy has been completed.

Pregnancy per se does not appear to impair the prognosis of breast cancer for women diagnosed in pregnancy when compared with nonpregnant controls matched for age and stage. However, because pregnancy-associated breast cancer occurs in younger women with many adverse risk factors conferring a higher risk of metastasis (high grade, ER negative), such women may be expected to have a poorer prognosis.

BREAST CANCER IN MALES

Breast cancer in men is rare, only representing 1% of breast cancer. Most cases occur in an older age group than in women, typically occurring over the age of 60 years. It has its own biological and clinical features, distinct from female breast cancer. In the largest series to date, the EORTC 100085/TBCRC/BIG/NABCG international male breast cancer programme of 1822 patients, the median age was 68.4 years. Of these, 56% were node negative and 48% TI. Nearly 85% were invasive ductal carcinomas, just over half were grade 2, 99% were ER positive, 81% PgR positive and over 96% androgen-receptor (AR) positive; 41% were luminal-A–like, 48% Luminal-B-like, HER2 negative, 8% Luminal B-like, Her2-positive and <3% triple negative basal. Like female breast cancer, histological grade was not associated with clinical outcome. In men under the age of 50 years, breast cancer-specific mortality was higher. Overall and recurrence survival were superior in strongly ER-, PgR- or AR-positive patients.

In some cases, there is a genetic predisposition. A variable proportion of cases (3% to 20%) carry a mutation of the BRCA2 gene. A family history of male breast cancer is a major predisposing factor to female breast cancer. In addition, BRCA2 mutations are associated with an increased risk of other cancers such lymphomas, laryngeal and kidney cancer.

Presentation is typically with locally advanced disease, often affecting the nipple. Fixation to the chest wall is common. The advanced state of the local disease is in part, probably as a result of the limited amount of breast tissue that the tumour has to invade and the lack of awareness among men that they can develop breast cancer.

The rarity of the tumour means that there are no trials of adjuvant therapy. The specific metabolic and endocrine context of male breast cancer suggest that treatment should not be directly extrapolated from that of female breast cancer. In men, 80% of circulating oestrogen is generated from peripheral aromatisation of androgens. The testes account for the other 20%. If aromatisation alone is inhibited, a feedback loop of luteinising hormone (LH) and follicle-stimulating hormone (FSH) production may develop, resulting in increased hormonal testicular production. As a result, it is recommended that AIs are only used in combination with LHRH agonists or orchidectomy. If the disease is operable, simple mastectomy (because there is little breast tissue) and sentinel node biopsy is preferred, proceeding to axillary node clearance if node positive. The principles of postoperative RT and chemotherapy apply as per female breast cancer. For ER-positive patients, tamoxifen is safe, both in the adjuvant and metastatic setting. For ER-negative disease, chemotherapy is recommended. The outcome of the disease is usually poor with a 5-year survival rate of about 65%, reflecting the commonly advanced nature of the disease at presentation.

FURTHER READING

Poortmans P, Collette S, Kirkove S, et al. Internal and medial supraclavicular irradiation in breast cancer. N Engl J Med 2015;373:317–27.

Early Breast Cancer Trialists' Collaborative Group (EBCTCG). Effect of radiotherapy after breast-conserving surgery on 10-year recurrence and 15-year breast cancer death: meta-analysis of individual patient data for 10 801 women in 17 randomised trials. Lancet 2011;378:1707–16.

Kunkler IH, Williams LJ, Jack W, et al. Breast-conserving surgery with or without irradiation in women aged 65 years or older with early breast cancer (PRIME II): a randomised controlled trial. Lancet Oncol 2015;16:266–73.

McGale P, Taylor C, Correa C, et al. Effect of radiotherapy after mastectomy and axillary surgery on 10-year recurrence and 20-year breast cancer mortality: meta-analysis of individual patient data for 8135 women in 22 randomised trials. Lancet 2014;383:2127–35.

Offersen B, Boersma JL, Kirkove C, et al. ESTRO breast cancer consensus guideline on target volume delineation for elective radiation therapy of early breast cancer. Radiother Oncol 2015;114:3–10.

Boggs DH, De Los Santos J. Radiation therapy effects in breast cancer. In: Koonitz BF, editor. Radiation therapy effects. An evidence based guide to manging toxicity. New York: Demos; 2018. p. 79–99.

Harbeck N, Gnant M. Breast cancer. Lancet 2017;389:1134–50.

Early Breast Cancer Trialists' Collaborative Group (EBCTCG). Comparisons between different polychemotherapy regimes for early breast cancer meta-analyses of long-term outcome among 100,000 women in 123 randomised trials. Lancet 2012;379:432–44.

Cardoso F, Costa A, Senkus E, et al. 3rd ESO-ESMO international consensus guidelines for advanced breast cancer. Annals Oncol 2017;28:16–33.

Montgomery DA, Krupa K, Jack WJL, et al. Changing pattern of detection of loco-regional relapse in breast cancer: the Edinburgh experience. Br J Cancer 2007;96:1802–7.

27

Gynaecological Cancer

Christopher Kent, Paul Symonds

CHAPTER OUTLINE

ANATOMY

The female reproductive organs lie within the pelvis and are the vulva, vagina, uterus, fallopian tubes and ovaries. These are represented in Figs 27.1 and 27.2.

INCIDENCE OF GYNAECOLOGICAL CANCER

The incidence of gynaecological cancer in England in 2014 is shown in Table 27.1. The incidence of cervical cancer has declined markedly since 1978. This falling trend has been accelerated by the success of the cervical screening programme (Fig. 27.3). However, cervical cancer is the most important female cancer in much of the developing world including South Asia, sub-Saharan Africa and South America. In the last 20 years, the incidence of carcinoma of the body of the uterus has almost doubled in the United Kingdom and the United States. This may be associated with the epidemic of obesity in both the United Kingdom and North America.

CARCINOMA OF CERVIX

Causes of Cervical Neoplasia

In virtually all cases of cancer of cervix, there is evidence that the tumour is associated with infection with the human papilloma virus (HPV), particularly types 16 and 18. The human papilloma virus produces proteins that bind to the products of two important tumour suppressor genes, p53 and Rb1.

Risk factors associated with cervical cancer are those that promote sexually transmitted disease. These are in particular, the age of first intercourse and the number of sexual partners. There is a lower incidence of cervical carcinoma in women using barrier methods of contraception. Male behaviour is also important. Partners of men in certain occupations, such as seamen, deep-sea fishermen and long-distance lorry drivers, have a higher incidence of cervical cancer. So do those partners of men whose previous partners have developed cervix cancer. Smoking and immunosuppression are also associated with cervical cancer. Cervical neoplasia is more common in women who are HIV positive. Currently, girls aged 12 to 14 in the United Kingdom are offered vaccination against HPV. In time, this will reduce the incidence of cervical cancer and also HPV-associated head and neck cancer.

Pathology of Cervical Cancer

Viral infection of the cervix may lead to premalignant change which is called dysplasia (dyskaryosis). This can be detected in exfoliated cells removed during a cervical smear. Cervical dysplasia (dyskaryosis) is graded mild, moderate or severe. The terms CIN1, CIN2 and CIN3 are histological terms used to describe increasing degrees of dysplasia, mild, moderate and severe, in biopsy material. In some women, there is a progression from mild to severe dysplasia and then invasive cancer. This often takes many years to develop and can be detected during cervical screening. Treatment of premalignant disease is highly effective. Patients with moderate or severe dysplasia are offered ablative treatment using large loop excision, laser vaporisation or cryotherapy. However, in most cases, dysplasia is self-limiting. Even the most severe form of dysplasia, CIN3 (previously called carcinoma in situ), will only

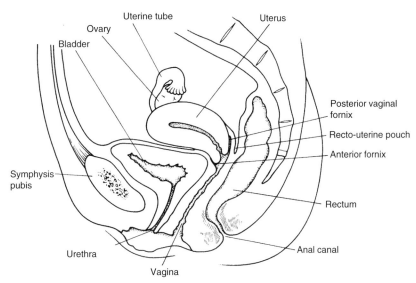

Fig. 27.1 Sagittal section of the uterus and its relations. (Modified from Ellis. Clinical anatomy. 5th ed. Oxford: Blackwell; 1975.)

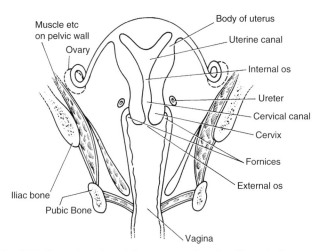

Fig. 27.2 Coronal section of the uterus and vagina. Note the important relationship of the ureter to the cervix.

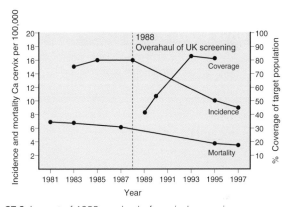

Fig. 27.3 Impact of 1988 overhaul of cervical screening programme on incidence and mortality of cervical cancer in the United Kingdom.

TABLE 27.1 **Incidence of Gynaecological Cancer in the United Kingdom in 2014**		
Site	**Number of Cases per Annum**	**Incidence per 100,000 Women**
Vulva	1289	4.2
Cervix	3224	10.3
Body of uterus	9324	28.4
Ovary	7378	22.5

progress to invasive cancer in between 20% and 40% of women if left untreated. Between 85% and 95% of cases of invasive cancer of cervix are squamous carcinomas. The remainder are adenocarcinoma or adenosquamous tumours. There is some evidence that the incidence of adenocarcinoma is increasing among younger women. Some authorities, but not all, have found adenocarcinoma of the cervix has a worse prognosis than squamous cancer when treated by radiotherapy (RT).

Carcinoma of the cervix spreads predominantly by direct invasion and through the lymphatic system. Initially, the tumour spreads into the uterus or vagina and parametrium (the tissues around the uterus). Later, it can infiltrate the bladder or rectum. The tumour spreads to the iliac and then paraaortic lymph nodes (Fig. 27.4). Bloodborne spread is less common and this may lead to liver, lung and bone metastases.

Symptoms and Investigations of Cervical Cancer

Premalignant changes are usually asymptomatic. The cardinal symptom of invasive cervix cancer is irregular vaginal bleeding. This may be bleeding after intercourse or bleeding in between periods. Sometimes, the presenting symptom is a brown vaginal discharge. Pain is usually a symptom of advanced disease and suggests spread to adjacent organs around the cervix. Backache may be associated with para-aortic lymph node spread.

Patients with cervical cancer are staged clinically according to the International Federation of Gynaecology and Obstetrics (FIGO) staging system (Table 27.2). Accurate staging of cervical cancer is essential so that appropriate treatment can be planned. The cornerstone to staging is an examination under anaesthesia (EUA). The cervix and vagina are inspected and palpated for evidence of tumour. Rectal examination is essential to assess the degree of parametrial spread and to find if the

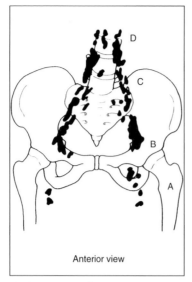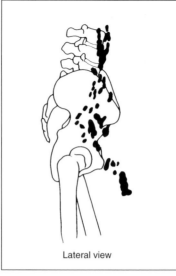

Anterior view   Lateral view

Fig. 27.4 Lymphatic drainage of the cervix: (A) obturator; (B) internal, external and common iliac; (C) lateral sacral; and (D) para-aortic. (From Souhami, Tobias. Cancer and its management. Oxford: Blackwell; 1986.)

TABLE 27.2   International Federation of Gynaecology and Obstetrics 2009 Staging: Carcinoma of the Cervix Uteri

Stage I	The carcinoma is strictly confined to the cervix (extension to the corpus would be disregarded)	
	Ia	Invasive carcinoma, which can be diagnosed only by microscopy. All macroscopically visible lesions, even with superficial invasion, are allotted to Stage Ib carcinomas. Invasion is limited to a measured stromal invasion with a maximal depth of 5.0 mm and a horizontal extension of not >7.0 mm. Depth of invasion should not be >5.0 mm taken from the base of the epithelium of the original tissue, superficial or glandular. The involvement of vascular spaces, venous or lymphatic, should not change the stage allotment
	Ia1	Measured stromal invasion of not >3.0 mm in depth and extension of not >7.0 mm
	Ia2	Measured stromal invasion of >3.0 mm and not >5.0 mm with an extension of not >7.0 mm
	Ib	Clinically visible lesions limited to the cervix uteri or preclinical cancers greater than stage 1a
	Ib1	Clinically visible lesions not >4.0 cm
	Ib2 (see Figs 27.9 and 27.10)	Clinically visible lesions >4.0 cm
Stage II	Cervical carcinoma invades beyond the uterus, but not to the pelvic wall or to the lower third of the vagina	
	IIa	No obvious parametrial involvement
	IIa1	Clinically visible lesion ≤4.0 cm in greatest dimension
	IIa2	Clinically visible lesion >4 cm in greatest dimension
	IIb (see Figs 27.5 and 27.6)	Obvious parametrial involvement
Stage III	The carcinoma has extended to the pelvic wall. On rectal examination, there is no cancer-free space between the tumour and the pelvic wall. The tumour involves the lower third of the vagina. All cases with hydronephrosis or nonfunctioning kidney are included, unless they are known to be because of other causes	
	IIIa	Tumour involves lower third of the vagina, with no extension to the pelvic wall

Continued

TABLE 27.2   International Federation of Gynaecology and Obstetrics 2009 Staging: Carcinoma of the Cervix Uteri—cont'd

	IIIb (see Figs 27.18 and 27.19)	Extension to the pelvic wall and/or hydronephrosis or nonfunctioning kidney
Stage IV	The carcinoma has extended beyond the true pelvis, or has involved (biopsy-proven) the mucosa of the bladder or rectum. A bullous oedema, as such, does not permit a case to be allotted to stage IV	
	IVa (see Figs 27.12–27.14)	Spread of the growth to adjacent organs
	IVb (see Figs 27.20–27.22)	Spread to distant organs

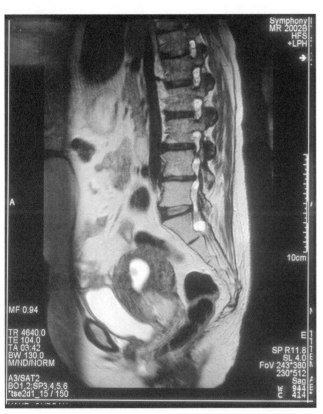

Fig. 27.5 Large cervical tumour in endocervical canal.

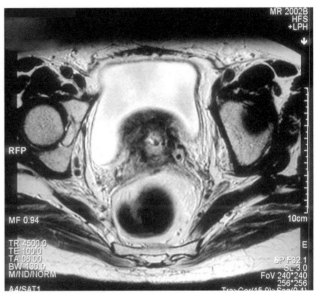

Fig. 27.6 Cervical tumour extending into R parametrium.

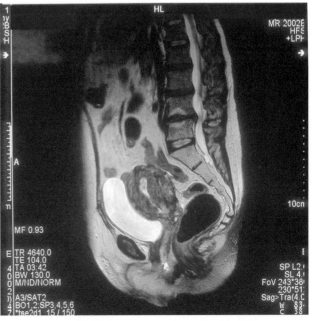

Fig. 27.7 Residual tumour in endocervical canal.

tumour is fixed to the pelvic sidewall. This is usually accompanied by a cystoscopy and, if necessary, a proctoscopy and sigmoidoscopy. Patients usually have a computed tomography (CT) or magnetic resonance imaging (MRI) scan of the abdomen and pelvis looking for nodal spread and urinary obstruction. MRI scanning is a more effective method for imaging the primary tumour (Figs 27.5, 27.6 and 27.7). Although spiral CT scanning and MRI are probably equally effective in the evaluation of lymph node metastasis, increasingly positron emission tomography (PET) scanning is used to detect occult metastatic disease (Fig. 27.8). To fulfill FIGO staging rules, because cervix cancer is particularly common in the developing world where imaging facilities are limited, staging should be based on the results of the EUA, cystoscopy, chest radiograph and abdominal ultrasound only. Patients may be assigned a FIGO clinical stage and a stage following sophisticated radiology.

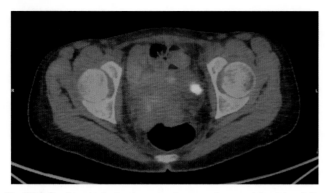

Fig. 27.8 Positron emission tomography scan shows avid uptake of flurodeoxyglucose (FDG) in left pelvic lymph node containing metastatic cervical cancer.

TABLE 27.3 Carcinoma of the Cervix: Cancer-Specific 5-Year Survival	
Stage	**Overall 5-Year Survival (%)**
Ia1	97–100
Ib2	95–97
Ib	80–90
IIa	70–75
IIb	65–75
IIIa	40–50
IIIb	45–50
IVa	15–25
IVb	5–10

Treatment

Stage is the most important factor related to outcome. However, tumour size is also an important prognostic feature. Typical survival figures are listed in Table 27.3. The prognosis for locally advanced disease has improved following the widespread use of combined chemotherapy and radiation treatment (Figs 27.9 and 27.10). The results may well improve further over the next few years with the increasing use of intensity-modulated RT (IMRT) or volumetric arc therapy (VMAT) and image-guided adaptive brachytherapy (IGABT).

Treatment of Stage I Disease

Stage I tumours are subdivided into stage Ia and stage Ib. They are further subdivided according to tumour size. Stage Ia cases are those that are treated by less than radical means. The prognosis is excellent for stage Ia1 patients and the problem is to avoid overtreatment. A cone biopsy or simple hysterectomy offers many of these patients a virtual 100% chance of cure. The outlook is almost as good for stage Ia2 patients. The optimum management of this group has not been clearly defined. The management options vary from cone biopsy to simple or modified radical hysterectomy.

Stage Ib is divided into patients with tumours confined to the cervix and uterus up to 4 cm in size (stage Ib1) or greater than 4 cm (stage Ib2). Patients with stage Ib1 tumour may be treated by radical hysterectomy. Usually, such patients are relatively slim, fit and often premenopausal. In a radical hysterectomy (a Wertheim's hysterectomy), the ureter is mobilised to allow wide excision of the uterus and cervix with removal of the cardinal ligaments and a wide cuff of vagina. The pelvic lymph nodes are also usually removed. Radiotherapy is an alternative for those unwilling to undergo surgery or unfit for a radical operation.

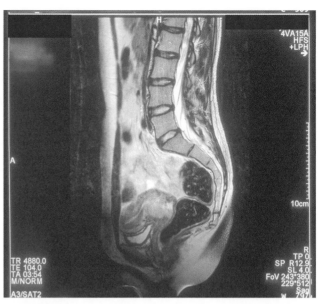

Fig. 27.9 Large stage Ib2 cervical tumour before treatment.

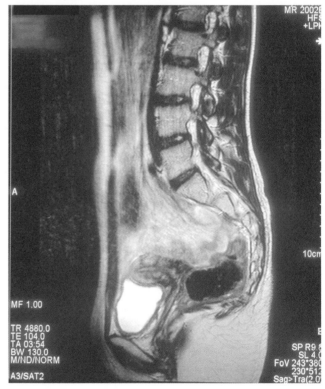

Fig. 27.10 Complete regression after chemoradiotherapy of tumour shown in Figs. 27.9.

Stage Ib2 patients are usually treated by RT as these tumours have often spread to pelvic lymph nodes. If treated by surgery, such patients usually require postoperative RT.

The only large randomised trial (Landoni et al., 1997) of RT and surgery in operable cervical cancer showed equally good results for both modalities (Fig. 27.11). The number of serious complications was higher in the surgical arm. However, complications of surgery are usually easier to rectify than the complications of RT.

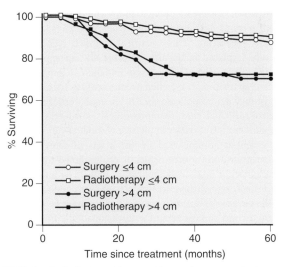

Fig. 27.11 Survival of stage 1b operable carcinoma cervix in a randomised trial of 343 patients treated by surgery or radiotherapy.

Postoperative Radiotherapy

RT is given after surgery if there is an increased risk of local recurrence. RT is mandatory if a stage Ib tumour is inadvertently treated by simple hysterectomy, because retrospective studies have shown 5-year survival figures of only 50% in this situation without RT. Indications after radical surgery include positive surgical excision margins and lymph nodes involved by tumour. Treatment may be external beam RT with or without brachytherapy (intracavitary treatment) to the upper one-third of vagina. Concomitant chemotherapy has been shown to improve long-term survival in clinical trials.

Treatment of Stage II–IVa

A few patients with stage IIa disease with early involvement of the vaginal vault are suitable for treatment by radical hysterectomy. Most are treated by RT, which remains the mainstay of treatment of patients with stages IIb–IVa (Figs 27.12, 27.13 and 27.14). There are three components to a radical RT treatment: external beam irradiation, brachytherapy and concomitant chemotherapy.

External Beam Radiotherapy

Most UK and European centres have moved away from planning treatment volumes based on bony landmarks. The gross tumour volume (GTV) at diagnosis is the cervical tumour plus any extra cervical spread as assessed by MRI T2 weighted scans plus clinical examination. The GTV is included in the clinical target volume (CTV), which encompasses the whole of both parametria and the uterus and at least 20 mm of uninvolved vagina below any palpable tumour. Allowance is made for organ movement during the course of treatment in the internal target volume (ITV) and a further margin is added to make up the planned target volume (PTV). Lymph nodes (plus a 5-mm margin), which may contain metastatic cancer, are included in the PTV. The volume of nodes irradiated depends on the primary tumour size and the presence or absence of lymph nodes bigger than 1 cm on imaging or PET scan being positive. Briefly, patients with small tumours and lymph node negative on scanning will have nodal irradiation to the iliac artery bifurcation. The treated volume is extended to 15 mm above the aortic bifurcation in patients with larger tumours or suspicious looking lymph nodes below the iliac bifurcation. If the common iliac nodes are enlarged, treatment is extended into the para-aortic chain up to the renal vein. In the case of stage 3a patients with involvement of the lower

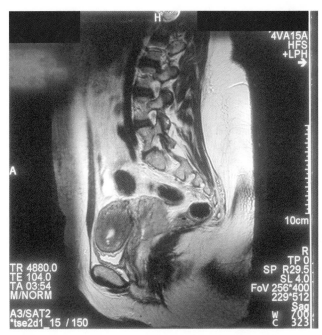

Fig. 27.12 Saggital view of large cervical tumour involving rectum, stage IVa before treatment.

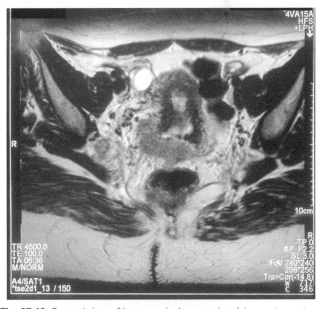

Fig. 27.13 Coronal view of large cervical tumour involving rectum, stage IVa before treatment.

third of the vagina, the inguinal nodes may be included in the treatment volume. IMRT or VMAT (VMAT is quicker) markedly reduces the volume of bladder and bowel, which is irradiated, and consequently the risk of late damage (Figs 27.15 and 27.16). A commonly used dose is 45 gray (Gy) in 25 fractions using 6-MV x-rays. Dose escalation studies using a concomitant boost to either parametrial tumour or lymphoid masses are ongoing, including the National cancer research Network-UK (NCRN)-DEPICT trial study. Results so far show that a boost of 54 Gy and possibly 58 Gy can be given safely.

During treatment, patients are supine with head, knee and ankle immobilisation. Treatment set-up is aided by the use of room lasers and skin marks. In our centre in Leicester, patients have a daily on treatment CT scan using the cone beam CT scanner incorporated into the treating linear accelerator with adjustments made for organ movement to the PTV.

Brachytherapy

Brachytherapy (short-distance treatment) is high-dose treatment from applicators placed either against the tumour or into the cervix. It allows very high doses to be given to the cancer with sparing of the surrounding organs at risk, particularly the bladder, rectum and sigmoid colon. Rather than prescribing treatment to an arbitrary point such as Manchester point A, modern practice is an individual approach. The prescribed radiation dose is adjusted to incorporate the residual tumour demonstrated after external beam radiation and chemotherapy on an

MRI scan taken just before brachytherapy (the D90 isodose line) and takes into account the dose received by nearby organs at risk, such as the bladder or rectum. This treatment is called IGRT. Typically a central tube is placed in the uterine canal and an applicator placed against the cervix (Fig. 27.17). A combination of intracavitary (IC) and interstitial treatment (IS) when needles are inserted into the tumour usually through a ring applicator (IC/IS brachytherapy) has been shown in the retroEMBRACE study to improve local control compared with the use of a standard intracavitary applicator without any increase in toxicity. Treatment is administered in just a few minutes using a very high-intensity iridium source, which is programmed to enter each of the intracavitary or interstitial applicators, in turn, for a variable period of time. Usually two or three treatments are given up to a week apart.

For the purpose of dosimetry, the external dosage is combined with the brachytherapy dosage using the linear quadratic formula as 2-Gy equivalents (EQD2). Maximum doses to the organs at risk are calculated over an area of 2 cm^2 (D2cc). Typical given doses are an EQD2 of 85 to 95 Gy to 90% isodose line enclosing the residual tumour (D90), a D2cc less than 80 Gy to the bladder and less than 65 Gy to

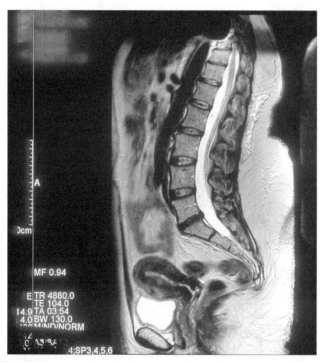

Fig. 27.14 Complete response after treatment without a recto-vaginal fistula.

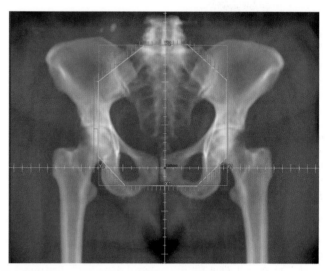

Fig. 27.16 Traditional nonintensity-modulated radiotherapy anterior pelvic field with large amounts of bowel in the treated volume.

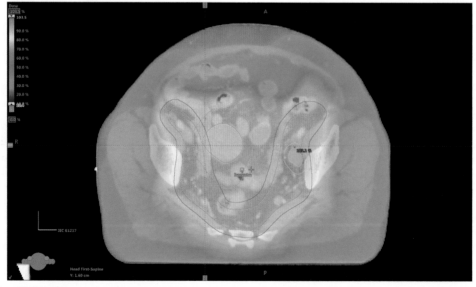

Fig. 27.15 U-shaped intensity-modulated dose distribution to treat pelvic lymph nodes, avoiding the small bowel.

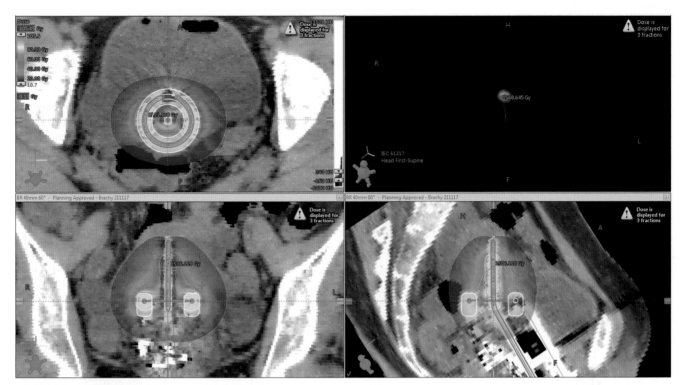

Fig. 27.17 Computed tomography scan showing a central tube in the uterus and a ring applicator placed against the cervix.

rectum and sigmoid colon. Further information is available in the International Commission for Radiation Units and Measurement (ICRU) report 89. Ideally, both external beam and brachytherapy should be completed in 42 to 48 days because cervical tumours can repopulate (regrow) during gaps in treatment.

Concomitant Chemotherapy

The addition of chemotherapy to RT in the treatment of carcinoma of cervix improves prognosis. The latest Cochrane metaanalysis of individual trial patient data (2010) shows concomitant chemotherapy reduces the odds of death by 31% (hazard ratio .69) with an absolute all-stage improvement in survival by 10% (Figs 27.18 and 27.19). Cisplatin given weekly (40 mg/m^2) is the current regimen of choice. The results are as good as more toxic regimens.

Complications of Treatment

During RT, the majority of patients develop diarrhoea, which can be reduced by agents such as loperamide. Nausea and vomiting are uncommon but respond to antiemetics such as ondansetron. Radiotherapy for cervical cancer gives some of the highest late complications of treatment. Patients may develop bladder or rectal fistulae. Endarteritis of small blood vessels and fibrosis may result in stenosis of the small or large bowel leading to intestinal obstruction. These severe late effects may develop up to 4 years after treatment. The incidence of severe damage (grade 3) after radical chemoradiotherapy recorded in the Royal College of Radiologists audit was 3% rectum, 1.5% colon, 2% small bowel and 2% bladder. Some patients had more than one site involved by complications. The site with the highest incidence of grade 3 damage is the vagina (5%). In part, this is because if the vagina is extensively involved by tumour, it will heal with fibrosis leading to stenosis. The use of vaginal dilators can reduce the incidence of vaginal stenosis. There is no evidence currently that giving chemotherapy along with RT increases the frequency of late effects.

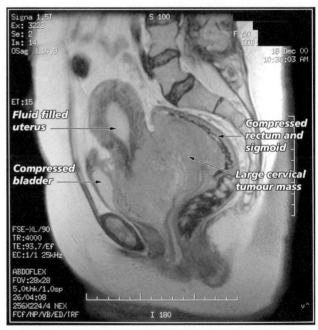

Fig. 27.18 Large stage III cervical tumour fixed to both pelvic sidewalls and involving the vagina. The tumour is compressing on both bladder and rectum.

Future Trends

Current clinical trials aim to increase local control and ultimate survival in patients with locally advanced cervical cancer without increasing complications. These include the UK NCRN Interlace trial where patients are randomised to receive either standard chemoradiotherapy

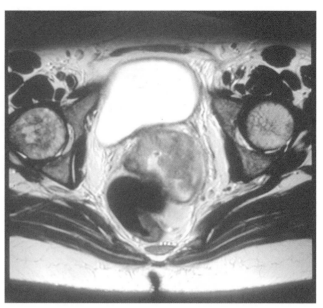

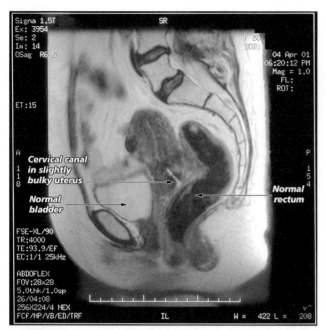

Fig. 27.19 Large stage III tumour 3 months after chemoradiotherapy. Complete response. This patient was discharged from the clinic in 2007, 7 years after treatment.

Fig. 27.21 Same tumour as Fig. 27.20 extending around rectum.

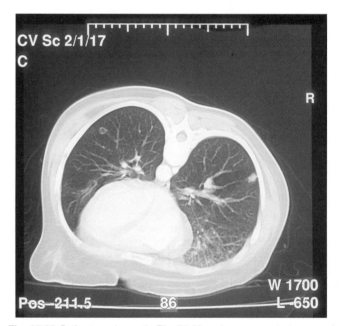

Fig. 27.22 Patient as shown in Fig. 27.20: pulmonary metastases and lymphangitis.

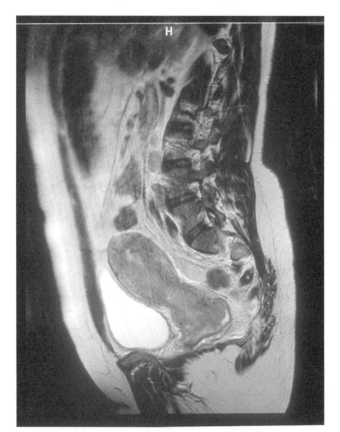

Fig. 27.20 Stage IVb cervical tumour involving virtually the whole of the uterus plus upper vagina with para-aortic node metastases.

with weekly cisplatin or, in addition, 6 weekly treatments with carboplatin and paclitaxel before the start of standard therapy. The European EMBRACE study is exploring radiation dose escalation using both IMRT and IGRT.

CARCINOMA OF ENDOMETRIUM

The causes of endometrial cancer are unknown. Physiological conditions and diseases that expose the endometrium to high levels of oestrogen are important in the development of this condition. These include early menarche, late menopause, nulliparity, polycystic ovarian disease and, rarely, oestrogen-producing ovarian tumours. Patients who are obese have a greater risk of endometrial cancer as adrenal steroids are metabolised to oestrone and oestrogen in adipose tissue. Both oestrogen-only hormone replacement therapy (HRT) and tamoxifen (used in the treatment of breast cancer) can lead to endometrial hyperplasia and endometrial cancer. Recently, it has been shown that up to

25% of endometrial cancers in patients aged under 60 years may be caused by a hereditary defect in DNA mismatch repair genes (Lynch syndrome).

Pathology

The majority of tumours are adenocarcinoma of endometrioid type. Atypical types, such as clear cell or serous papillary tumours, carry a worse prognosis. Tumour grade and spread into the myometrium are useful predictors of pelvic node spread. Patients with poorly differentiated tumours are at higher risk of developing both vaginal vault recurrence and spread to pelvic lymph nodes than patients with well-differentiated tumours. Survival tends to fall with increasing depth of myometrial invasion as the extent of myometrium invasion correlates with involvement of pelvic and paraaortic lymph nodes by tumour. This is especially true of poorly differentiated tumours.

Routes of Spread

Tumour may extend beyond the endometrial cavity to involve the cervix or vagina. Parametrial spread is extremely uncommon. Distant spread is first to iliac lymph nodes or occasionally directly to para-aortic nodes without iliac involvement. Blood stream spread is unusual. Staging takes into account pathological features and the pattern of spread. The current FIGO staging is shown in Table 27.4. Over 80% of patients have stage I tumours.

Treatment

The mainstay of treatment is simple hysterectomy. There is no evidence from randomised clinical trials (confirmed by a 2017 Cochrane metaanalysis) that lymphadenectomy improves survival. Clinically enlarged nodes though, should be removed at the time of hysterectomy. Patients with moderate to well-differentiated tumours confined to the inner half of the myometrium require no further treatment.

Radiotherapy

RT may be given as an alternative to surgery, as postoperative adjuvant treatment or to treat pelvic or vault recurrence. Patients who are treated primarily by local RT are often extremely obese or have serious intercurrent disease, which are both contraindications for surgery. Five-year survival of 72% has been reported in Manchester patients treated by two intrauterine caesium insertions. Patients who require external beam RT before an intrauterine insertion can be selected by MRI scanning, which is good at showing myometrial invasion by tumour. Doses used are similar to those used to treat carcinoma of cervix.

Postoperative Radiotherapy

Both The Netherlands' PORTEC trial and the Medical Research Council (MRC) ASTEC trials showed no survival advantage for routine postoperative RT for patients with immediate risk (grade I FIGO Ib, G2 Ib, G3 Ia) tumours. There was a statistically significant decrease in pelvic recurrence compared with observation alone after surgery, but no overall survival benefit.

Patients with more aggressive tumours may benefit from postoperative RT. A metaanalysis and systematic review by Johnson and Cornes showed postoperative RT increased survival by 10% for patients with poorly differentiated tumour penetrating more than halfway through the myometrium (stage Ib G3). When planning RT, the target volume should include the internal and external iliac lymph nodes plus the upper two-thirds of the vagina. Field arrangements and volume irradiated are very similar to those used in the treatment of cervical cancer. Doses of 40 to 45 Gy are given in 1.8- or 2-Gy fractions.

Radiotherapy can be used with curative intent if previously unirradiated patients develop an isolated pelvic recurrence. Five-year survival rates of 50% to 80% have been reported in patients with isolated vaginal vault recurrence, although this falls to about 20% in patients with pelvic side-wall disease.

Brachytherapy

Brachytherapy in addition to external beam RT reduces the risk of vaginal recurrence and improves survival in patients with stage II (involvement of cervix) tumours.

The major use for vaginal brachytherapy is to treat patients with intermediate-risk tumours rather than external beam RT. The Netherlands' PORTEC-2 study showed an identical survival and very similar local recurrence rates at 3 years after treatment, but brachytherapy patients had fewer radiation-induced side effects and a better quality of life. Brachytherapy is easy to administer via a vaginal cylinder that can be inserted without an anaesthetic.

Combined Chemoradiotherapy

Unlike the situation in cervix cancer unpublished and published results from the PORTEC3, Gynaecology Oncology Group GOG249 and GOG258 randomised trials showed there is no role for combined radiation and chemotherapy as postoperative treatment in high-risk stage 1 and stage 2 patients. RT alone is the standard of care for these patients. There may be a case for combined treatment for stage 3 (node positive) patients as a provisional analysis in the PORTEC-3 trial found the 5-year survival in the chemoradiotherapy group was 69% compared with 58% in the radiation-only group. Serous or carcinosarcoma histology may also be an indication for combined treatment. Carcinosarcomas are not true sarcomas but a particularly aggressive form of endometrial cancer.

Other Treatment Modalities

Some endometrial cancers exhibit progesterone and/or oestrogen receptors. About one-third of patients with endometrial cancer will show an objective response to progesterogenic hormones such as

TABLE 27.4 International Federation of Gynaecology and Obstetrics 2009 Staging: Carcinoma of the Endometrium	
Stage I	Tumour confined to the corpus uteri
Ia	No or less than half myometrial invasion
Ib	Invasion equal to or more than half of the myometrium
Stage II	Tumour invades cervical stroma, but does not extend beyond the uterus
Stage III	Local and/or regional spread of the tumour
IIIa	Tumour invades the serosa of the corpus uteri and/or adnexa
IIIb	Vaginal and/or parametrial involvement
IIIc	Metastases to pelvic and/or para-aortic lymph nodes
IIIc1	Positive pelvic nodes
IIIc2	Positive para-aortic lymph nodes with or without positive pelvic lymph nodes
Stage IV	Tumour invades bladder and/or bowel mucosa, and/or distant metastases
IVa	Tumour invasion of bladder and/or bowel mucosa
IVb	Distant metastases, including intra-abdominal metastases and/or inguinal lymph nodes

megestrol acetate (160 mg daily). Response rates tend to be higher in patients with well-differentiated tumours, especially those who are progesterone receptor positive. Chemotherapy is of limited value in the treatment of endometrial cancer. Doxorubicin is the best single agent with a 20% to 40% response rate. Response rates greater than 50% have been reported with doxorubicin and cisplatin combinations. Recently, paclitaxel has also been used in combination with carboplatin with response rates of up to 70%. However, there is little evidence of improved survival for combination chemotherapy compared with single agent doxorubicin. Responses tend to be of short duration and survival tends to be about 9 months in patients with metastatic disease. The response rate to carboplatin is between 25% and 35% and may be the drug of choice for elderly unfit patients.

Results of Treatment

The majority of patients suffer from stage I cancers. Five-year survival for patients with stage Ia grade1-well differentiated (G1)/grade2 moderately differentiated (G2) disease is over 90%. This falls to about 70% for patients with stage IB Grade3-poorly differentiated (G3) disease. Reported 5-year survival for patients with stage II disease is between 85% and 60%, and stage III disease is between 75% and 40%, depending on the treatment modality and the degree of histological differentiation of the tumour.

Future Trends

Patients with endometrial cancer tend to be older and less fit than patients with cervical cancer and tolerate chemotherapy less well. Research is centered around less toxic forms of chemotherapy and molecular targeted agents for use in the small group of high-risk cases requiring additional treatment after surgery.

SARCOMAS OF THE UTERUS

The most common true sarcoma of the uterus is a leiomyosarcoma, which is a rare tumour arising from the smooth muscle of the uterus. Metastatic spread through is the bloodstream especially to the lungs is common. Primary treatment is by hysterectomy. Unlike soft tissue sarcomas at other sites where postoperative RT is of proven value, an European Organisation for the Research and Treatment of Cancer (EORTC) randomised trial failed to show either a survival advantage or an improvement in local control following postoperative RT. In common with other soft tissue sarcomas, adjuvant chemotherapy delays, but does not prevent, the development of distant metastases. The overall 5-year survival is 30% to 40%.

CANCER OF THE OVARY

Aetiology

In the majority of cases, the cause of ovarian cancer is unknown. However, epithelial ovarian cancer is more common in women who have never been pregnant or had an early menarche or late menopause. Conversely, the incidence of ovarian cancer is reduced in women who have had multiple births, and there is good evidence that oral contraceptives reduce the incidence of this disease. The protective effect of birth parity and oral contraceptives is probably through suppression of ovulation. About 5% of ovarian cancers are familial. The most important hereditary syndromes are associated with carriage mutations of the BRCA1 complex on chromosome 17 and the BRCA2 complex on chromosome 13. The BRCA1 and 2 genes are also associated with breast cancer and sometimes colon and endometrial cancers. Familial tumours tend to develop at a younger age than sporadic cancers. Women with two or more first-degree relatives who have developed ovarian cancer or one who has developed breast cancer and one other relative who has developed ovarian cancer before the age of 50 may be offered genetic counselling and testing for mutations in the BRCA1 and 2 genes. These patients also may be offered screening for ovarian and breast cancer. Prophylactic oophorectomy including removal of the fallopian tubes also may be recommended in certain cases.

Pathology

Benign or malignant ovarian tumours may be solid or cystic. Some benign ovarian cysts may exceed 30 cm in diameter and weigh many kilograms. About 10% of ovarian tumours may be classified as borderline. These are tumours that have some histological features of malignancy but lack stromal invasion.

Malignant ovarian tumours are subdivided into epithelial, germ cell and sex cord. Some 85% of ovarian tumours are classified as of epithelial origin. The most common type of ovarian cancer is high-grade serous, which accounts for about 70% of all cases. Mainly by studying the ovaries and fallopian tubes from patients with BRCA1/2 mutations undergoing prophylactic oophorectomy, a considerable amount has been learnt about the origin of these tumours. In fact, they originate from malignant transformation of cells in the fimbria of the end of the fallopian tubes. Malignant cells then implant into the surface of the ovary and into the peritoneal cavity. This explains why many ovarian cancers are at an advanced stage by diagnosis. Unlike high-grade serous tumours, clear cell and mucinous malignant tumours do not usually present at stage 1.

Method of Spread

Ovarian cancer tends to be a disease of the abdominal cavity and rapidly spreads across the peritoneal cavity to involve the omentum, a fatty apron close to the spleen and left kidney. There may also be multiple peritoneal deposits, particularly in the subdiaphragmatic areas. These peritoneal deposits may produce large volumes of ascitic fluid. A potentially fatal consequence of peritoneal disease is intestinal obstruction. The cancer may also spread to pelvic and para-aortic lymph nodes, the liver and pleural cavity of the chest by direct spread across the peritoneum or via the blood stream. Involvement of lung parenchyma is less common. Metastasis to other sites, particularly bone and brain, is rare.

Clinical Features

Late-stage diagnosis is the rule rather than the exception and, justifiably, ovarian cancer has the nickname the silent killer. There are no typical symptoms. Women may complain of abdominal bloating or nonspecific gastrointestinal symptoms. One of the first signs may be the discovery of a large pelvic mass or ascites.

Investigations and Staging

Investigations in most cases are for a pelvic mass with or without ascites. The tumour marker CA125 is elevated (>35 international units per litre (IU/L)) in about 50% of patients with early stage, and 80% of patients with more advanced stage disease. CT scanning of the abdomen is excellent for demonstrating primary tumour with significant peritoneal spread and involvement of the omentum. CT scanning can also show the degree of spread to adjacent organs and is useful for predicting operability. Between 60% and 70% of patients have spread beyond the pelvis at diagnosis and are placed in stages III or IV. FIGO staging of this disease is listed in Table 27.5.

Needle biopsy under CT control from the primary tumour or omental metastases can confirm the diagnosis in inoperable cases. Ascites

TABLE 27.5 International Federation of Gynaecology and Obstetrics 2009 Staging: Carcinoma of the Ovary

Stage I	Growth limited to the ovaries	
	Ia	Growth limited to one ovary; no ascites present containing malignant cells. No tumour on the external surface; capsule intact
	Ib	Growth limited to both ovaries; no ascites present containing malignant cells. No tumour on the external surfaces; capsules intact
	Ic	Tumour either stage Ia or Ib, but with tumour on surface of one or both ovaries, or with capsule ruptured, or with ascites present containing malignant cells, or with positive peritoneal washings
Stage II	Growth involving one or both ovaries with pelvic extension	
	IIa	Extension and/or metastases to the uterus and/or tubes
	IIb	Extension to other pelvic tissues
	IIc	Tumour either stage IIa or IIb, but with tumour on surface of one or both ovaries; or with capsule(s) ruptured; or with ascites present containing malignant cells or with positive peritoneal washings
Stage III	Tumour involving one or both ovaries with histologically confirmed peritoneal implants outside the pelvis and/or positive retroperitoneal or inguinal nodes. Superficial liver metastasis equals stage III. Tumour is limited to the true pelvis, but with histologically proven malignant extension to the small bowel or omentum	
	IIIa	Tumour grossly limited to the true pelvis, with negative nodes, but with histologically confirmed microscopic seeding of abdominal peritoneal surface, or histologically proven extension to small bowel or mesentery
	IIIb	Tumour of one or both ovaries with histologically confirmed implants; peritoneal metastasis of abdominal peritoneal surfaces, none exceeding 2 cm in diameter; nodes are negative
	IIIc	Peritoneal metastasis beyond the pelvis >2 cm in diameter and/or positive retroperitoneal or inguinal nodes
Stage IV	Growth involving one or both ovaries with distant metastases. If pleural effusion is present, there must be positive cytology to allot a case to stage IV. Parenchymal liver metastasis equals stage IV	

may have to be drained to relieve discomfort and shortness of breath. Ascitic fluid should always be examined cytologically for the presence of malignant cells.

Treatment

Surgery

The role of surgery is both diagnostic and therapeutic. At laparotomy, the full extent of peritoneal spread must be assessed, particularly the subdiaphragmatic areas and the paracolic gutters (the areas adjacent to the large bowel). The aim of surgery is to remove as much tumour as possible. If possible, both ovaries and the uterus should be removed along with the omentum. All macroscopic disease should be removed if possible. If not, residual peritoneal disease should be debulked to leave individual residual tumours of less than 1 cm. There are numerous nonrandomised studies that indicate that optimal debulking improves prognosis but there have been no randomised controlled trials comparing aggressive debulking against more conservative surgery.

Chemotherapy

Following surgery, the mainstay of treatment is chemotherapy. Primary debulking surgery is only possible in 40% to 50% of women. A large number of patients have bulk residual disease after surgery. Patients with stage III or IV disease even after optimal surgery will rapidly

relapse without further treatment but, fortunately, epithelial ovarian cancer is fairly chemosensitive. For the last 20 years, a combination of paclitaxel and carboplatin has been standard chemotherapy. Although 60% to 80% of patients with advanced disease have significant tumour shrinkage after this chemotherapy, the median progression-free survival is only 16 to 18 months, and by 2 years, three-quarters of all patients have relapsed. Recent research has concentrated on the addition of biological agents to standard chemotherapy. Bevacizumab (Avastin) is a monoclonal antibody, which is an antagonist of the tumour growth factor, vascular endothelial growth factor (VEGF). In the NCRN ICON7 trial (2015), the addition of bevacizumab to standard chemotherapy increased progression-free survival in the short term but not ultimate 5-year survival. The oral anti-VEGF drug, cediranib, may be more effective. In the ICON6 trial (2016), which compared the treatment of platinum-based chemotherapy in relapsed disease when patients were given cediranib or a placebo, early results show a sustained 3-month improvement in progression-free survival at 2 years in the cediranib group.

Radiotherapy

The major role of RT is largely palliative and is used to shrink symptomatic ovarian masses, especially tumours causing pain or vaginal bleeding. Doses of 20 to 30 Gy in 5 to 10 fractions are usually given using parallel-opposed fields. Clear cell carcinoma is less chemosensitive than the commoner serous subtype. Studies have shown an improved survival by the addition of RT to adjuvant chemotherapy in stages 1c and 2 clear cell patients.

Results of Treatment of Epithelial Tumours

In the past, the 5-year survival associated with stage I disease was about 65%. This may have reflected rather poor staging. Recently, trials of adjuvant chemotherapy have demonstrated 5-year survivals of up to 90% in this group of women. The 5-year survival for stage II disease is 40% to 60%. True stage II cases are relatively uncommon. The majority of women have stage III disease, which carries a 30% to 40% 5-year survival. The 5-year survival for stage IV disease is about 5% to 10%.

Future Trends

Trials investigating the addition of biological agents to standard chemotherapy are ongoing. Poly ADP-ribose polymerase (PARP) inhibitors show promise in patients with BRCA1/2 mutations either in the germline or within the tumour itself. Further investigations of the role of RT in clear cell tumours seem warranted.

RARE TUMOURS OF THE OVARY

Sex-Cord Tumours

The most common of the sex-cord tumours are granulosa cell tumours. These display a spectrum of aggressiveness. Some may behave in benign fashion and others are extremely aggressive. They are found predominantly in postmenopausal women but can occur at any age, including before puberty. These tumours often produce steroid hormones, particularly oestrogens, which can cause postmenopausal bleeding in older women and precocious puberty in young girls. Over 80% of patients present with stage I disease. Treatment is predominantly by surgery. Bilateral ovarian disease occurs in up to 25% of patients. Usually, both ovaries are removed along with the uterus. A single ovary may be removed in young women with stage I disease preserving fertility. Granulosa cell tumours can recur up to 30 years after initial surgery. The site of recurrence is usually within the abdominal cavity or the liver. Metastases from granulosa cell tumour can be hemorrhagic leading to internal bleeding. Because of the rarity of this tumour, there have been few comparative studies of chemotherapy in this disease but cisplatin-based regimens, such as the BEP regimen (bleomycin, etoposide and cisplatin) or CAP (cyclophosphamide, adriamycin, cisplatin), can offer very useful palliation.

Most of the RT literature comes from the 1970s, but this tumour is more radiosensitive than the more common epithelial cancers. Pelvic RT is sometimes used as an adjuvant after surgery or in the palliation of advanced disease. Pelvic fields are treated with doses of 45 to 50 Gy in 20 to 25 fractions depending on the size of treated volume. Overall, the prognosis is good in the short term with a 5-year survival of over 80%.

Leydig-Sertoli cell tumours are rare. More than half of these tumours produce male hormones that can cause virilisation. The majority of these tumours behave in a benign fashion and present with stage I disease. Malignant lesions are exceedingly rare.

Germ-Cell Tumours

Dysgerminomas account for 2% to 5% of all ovarian tumours and usually occur in women under 30 years old. Histologically, they are similar to seminoma of the testes in men and tend to spread in a similar way via the pelvic and para-aortic lymph nodes. The majority of tumours present with stage I disease, although up to 15% of tumours can be present in both ovaries. Surgery is usually aimed at conservation of fertility with removal of only one ovary, but such patients need very close

follow-up owing to the risks of developing a further tumour in the remaining ovary.

This tumour is extremely chemosensitive. The BEP regimen is effective if patients relapse after surgery with a 5-year survival of about 85%. The tumour is quite radiosensitive and, in the past, patients have been treated with wide-field RT with doses between 20 and 40 Gy in 2 to 4 weeks. Good long-term survival has been reported following wide-field RT. However, our experience is that chemotherapy gives better results than RT. An added advantage is that fertility is more likely to be preserved following chemotherapy than RT.

More than 98% of ovarian teratomas are benign, most commonly cystic teratomas or dermoid cysts. Malignant teratomas are rare and have a similar histological appearance to those arising in the testes. The same chemotherapy regimens used to treat the more common testicular teratomas in males are also used in ovarian disease, particularly the BEP regimen. The outlook for such patients is not as good as male testicular teratoma patients with a 5-year survival of about 50%.

TUMOURS OF THE VAGINA AND VULVA

There were only 254 new cases of vaginal cancer in the United Kingdom in 2014. This may be because the FIGO rules state that if the cervix or the vulva is involved, the tumour should be assigned to either site. The staging of vaginal cancer is listed in Table 27.6.

The majority of tumours are squamous and tend to occur in women over 60 years of age. Surgery as a primary treatment has a limited role and the majority of patients are treated in a similar fashion to cervical cancer. Usually, such patients receive pelvic RT, the target volume being the whole vagina and the pelvic lymph nodes. If the patient is fit enough, cisplatin should be given along with external beam RT. This would be followed by an intracavity insertion for tumours in the upper half of the vagina, or an external beam boost treatment for tumour in the lower half of this structure. Results of treatment tend to be somewhat worse than in cervical cancer with about a 75% 5-year survival for stage I, 60% for stage II, 30% for stage II and 15% for stage IV.

Vulval cancer tends to be a disease in elderly women with a mean age of diagnosis of approximately 70 years. Of vulval cancer, 75% are squamous carcinoma and they predominantly metastasise via the lymphatic system to the groin. Staging takes into account the tumour size and whether lymph node metastases are present (Table 27.7). The primary treatment of vulval carcinoma is surgery using the triple incision technique, a bilateral groin node dissection and radical vulvectomy. Because many of the women with this disease are elderly and have intercurrent disease, some are not suitable for this treatment. However,

TABLE 27.6	International Federation of Gynaecology and Obstetrics 2009 Staging: Carcinoma of the Vagina	
Stage 0	Carcinoma in situ, intraepithelial neoplasia grade III
Stage I	The carcinoma is limited to the vaginal wall
Stage II	The carcinoma has involved the subvaginal tissue but has not extended to the pelvic wall
Stage III	The carcinoma has extended to the pelvic wall
Stage IV	The carcinoma has extended beyond the true pelvis or has involved the mucosa of the bladder or rectum; bullous oedema as such does not permit a case to be allotted to stage IV
IVa	Tumour invades bladder and/or rectal mucosa and/or direct extension beyond the true pelvis
IVb	Spread to distant organs

TABLE 27.7 International Federation of Gynaecology and Obstetrics 2009 Staging: Carcinoma of the Vulva

Stage I	Tumour confined to the vulva
Ia	Lesions ≤2 cm in size, confined to the vulva or perineum and with stromal invasion ≤1.0 mm, no nodal metastasis
Ib	Lesions >2 cm in size or with stromal invasion >1.0 mm, confined to the vulva or perineum with negative nodes
Stage II	Tumour of any size with extension to adjacent perineal structures (1/3 lower urethra, 1/3 lower vagina, anus) with negative nodes
Stage III	Tumour of any size with or without extension to adjacent perineal structures (1/3 lower urethra, 1/3 lower vagina, anus) with positive inguino-femoral lymph nodes
IIIa	1. With 1 lymph node metastasis (≥5 mm) or 2. 1–2 lymph node metastasis(es) (<5 mm)
IIIb	1. With 2 or more lymph node metastases (≥5 mm) or 2. 3 or more lymph node metastases (<5 mm)
IIIc	With positive nodes with extracapsular spread
Stage IV	Tumour invades other regional (2/3 upper urethra, 2/3 upper vagina) or distant structures
IVa	Tumour invades any of the following: 1. Upper urethral and/or vaginal mucosa, bladder mucosa, rectal mucosa or fixed to pelvic bone or 2. Fixed or ulcerated inguinofemoral lymph nodes
IVb	Any distant metastasis including pelvic lymph nodes

there is difficulty in administering RT to this region. The folds of the groin and vulva lead to loss of skin sparing when megavoltage RT is administered to this region and patients develop a risk of radiation reactions with moist desquamation after relatively modest doses of RT such as 45 Gy in 25 fractions. This limits the scope of RT in this disease. Radiotherapy has been shown to reduce pelvic and groin recurrences when given postoperatively in patients with one or more positive lymph nodes. There is also an improvement in 5-year survival.

Chemoradiotherapy is being used increasingly in patients who have initially inoperable disease. Drugs such as cisplatin, 5-fluorouracil (5-FU) and mitomycin have been given along with radiation therapy.

A review of published data has shown that the complete response rate is 60% following chemoradiotherapy but the complication rate for this treatment can be high with up to a 10% death rate, particularly secondary to neutropenic sepsis. Owing to the toxicity of combination regimens, single-agent cisplatin is the preferred treatment. Chemoradiotherapy can shrink inoperable tumours and make such lesions operable. However, wound healing may be impaired.

The most important factor in vulval cancer is the presence of inguinal nodal metastases. Patients without nodal involvement have a 70% to 80% 5-year survival. Survival falls to 50–30% for those with involved inguinal lymph nodes (one to more than four positive lymph nodes).

FURTHER READING

Pecorelli S. Revised FIGO staging for carcinoma of the vulva, cervix and endometrium. Int J Gynaecol Obstet 2009;105:103–4.

Landoni F, Maneo A, Columbo A, et al. Randomised study of radical surgery versus radiotherapy for stage Ib–IIa cervical cancer. Lancet 1997;350:28–33.

Vale CL, Tierney JF, Davidson SE, Drinkwater KJ, Symonds P. Substantial improvements in UK cervical cancer survival with chemoradiotherapy: results of a Royal College of Radiologists Audit. Clin Oncol 2010;22:590–601.

Mazeron R, Fokal LU, Kirchheiner K, et al. Dose-volume effect relationships for late rectal morbidity in patients treated with chemoradiation and MRI-guided adaptive brachytherapy for locally advanced cervical cancer: results from the prospective multicenter EMBRACE study. Radiother Oncol 2016;120:412–9.

Fokdal L, Sturdza A, Mazeron R, et al. Image guided adaptive brachytherapy with combined intracavitary and interstitial technique improves the therapeutic ratio in locally advanced cervical cancer: analysis from the retroEMBRACE study. Radiother Oncol 2016;120:434–40.

International Commission for Radiation Units and Measurement. Prescribing, recording and reporting brachytherapy for cancer of the cervix. ICRU report 89. Oxford: Oxford University Press; 2016.

Faust G, Davies Q, Symonds P. Changes in the treatment of endometrial cancer. Br J Obstet Gynaecol 2010;117:1043–6.

de Boer SM, Powell ME, Mileshkin L, et al. Toxicity and quality of life after adjuvant chemoradiotherapy versus radiotherapy alone for women with high risk endometrial cancer (PORTEC-3): an open-label multicenter randomised phase 3 trial. Lancet Oncol 2016;17:1114–26.

Ledermann JA, Embleton AC, Raja F, et al. Cediranib in patients with relapsed platinum-sensitive ovarian cancer (ICON6): a randomized, double-blind, placebo-controlled phase 3 trial. Lancet 2016;387:1066–74.

Oza AM, Cook AD, Pfisterer J, et al. Standard chemotherapy with or without bevacizumab for women with newly diagnosed ovarian cancer (ICON7): overall survival results of a phase 3 randomised trial. Lancet Oncol 2015;16:928–36.

Ledermann JA, El- Khouly F. PARP inhibitors in ovarian cancer: clinical evidence for informed treatment decisions. Br J Cancer 2015;113:S10–6.

Koh W-J, Greer BE, Abu-Rustum NR, et al. NCCN clinical practice guidelines in oncology: vulval cancer version 1.2017. JNCCN 2017;15:92–120.

28

Cancer of Kidney, Bladder, Prostate, Testis, Urethra and Penis

Aravindhan Sundaramurthy, Duncan B. McLaren

CHAPTER OUTLINE

KIDNEY

Anatomy

The kidneys lie retroperitoneally on the posterior abdominal wall. They are approximately 11 cm long and 6 cm wide in adults. The left kidney is 1 cm higher than the right. The right kidney is related in front to the liver, the second part of the duodenum and the ascending colon. In front of the left kidney are the stomach, pancreas, descending colon and spleen. On the top of each kidney lies an adrenal gland. Behind the kidneys lie the diaphragm and the 12th rib. On the medial side of the kidney there is an opening, the hilum, through which pass the renal artery and vein, and the ureter. The renal vein drains into the inferior vena cava. The lymphatic drainage is to the paraaortic nodes. The anatomical relationships are shown in Fig. 28.1.

Pathology

The three principal malignant tumours of the kidney are Wilms tumour (nephroblastoma) in children (described in Chapter 33), renal cell carcinoma (RCC) and transitional cell carcinoma (TCC) of the renal pelvis. RCC is the most common adult renal epithelial cancer accounting for more than 90% of all renal malignancies. The most frequent histological subtype of RCC includes clear cell (75%), papillary (10%) and chromophobe (5%). Other rare subtypes are cystic-solid, collecting duct, medullary, mucinous and Xp11 translocation tumours. Macroscopically, the clear cell RCC appears as a yellowish vascular mass. Microscopically, the tumour cells are large with a foamy or clear appearance to the cytoplasm. The nucleus is small, central and densely staining.

Renal cancer is uncommon, accounting for 3% of all cancers and 1.5% of cancer deaths. Over the last 10 years, the incidence has risen by 23% in men and 29% in women within the United Kingdom, a pattern reflected throughout the world. Overall there is a 2:1 male to female ratio in incidence and the disease occurs mainly in the 5th to 7th decades of life. The aetiology of renal cell carcinoma is unknown, although smoking and obesity are risk factors. Some 30% of patients present with metastatic disease.

Spread

There is direct spread through the renal substance and into the perinephric fat of the renal bed. The characteristic mode of spread is

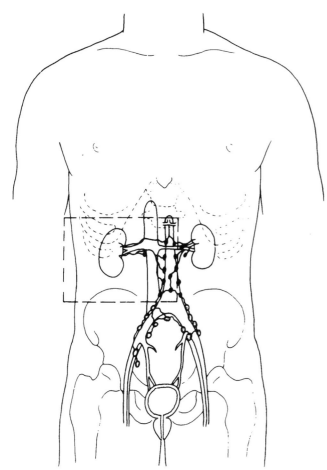

Fig. 28.1 Anatomical relationships of the kidney with lymphatic drainage pathways and typical treatment volume when irradiating the renal bed. (From Souhami, Tobias. Cancer and its management. Oxford: Blackwell; 1986. With permission.)

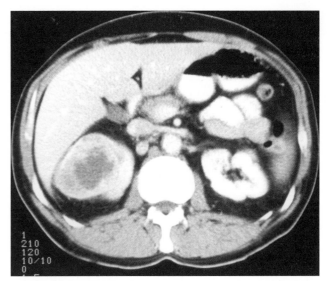

Fig. 28.2 Computed tomography scan showing a typical renal cell carcinoma in the right kidney.

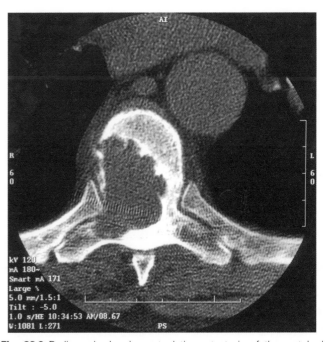

Fig. 28.3 Radiograph showing osteolytic metastasis of the vertebral body from renal cell carcinoma.

permeation along the renal vein and into the inferior vena cava. Tumours may rarely extend up to the right side of the heart, completely blocking the inferior vena cava. Lymphatic spread to local renal hilar and paraaortic lymph nodes and hematogenous metastatic spread to lung, bone and brain are common. The tempo of metastatic disease may be unpredictable; however, less than 10% of patients remain alive 5 years from diagnosis. Rarely, spontaneous regression of metastases may occur following nephrectomy.

Clinical Features

Presentation is usually with local symptoms. Painless hematuria is the most common, or colicky pain secondary to clots of blood. Other symptoms are aching or a mass in the loin, which may be noticed by the patient. A coincidental finding following radiological imaging of the abdomen is an increasingly common presentation. Distant metastasis may be the first presentation, such as pathological bone fracture, haemoptysis from pulmonary metastases or symptoms of raised intracranial pressure from cerebral deposits. Systemic features such as anaemia, loss of weight and unexplained fever may occur. The kidney may be palpably enlarged.

Investigation and Staging

The urine may contain frank or microscopic evidence of blood. Urine cytology may show malignant cells. Ultrasound and computed tomography (CT) scanning (Fig. 28.2) are helpful in distinguishing between solid and cystic renal masses. Ultrasound may show extension of tumour into the renal vein or inferior vena cava. CT scanning of the chest, abdomen and pelvis may show direct tumour spread, venous and lymph node involvement and soft tissue metastases in liver and lung. Angiography is an invasive procedure and its use is diminishing. It still has a role in demonstrating the renal artery and new vessel formation when the kidney is to be embolised (i.e. material introduced into the renal arterial to cut off its blood supply and cause death of part of or the whole of the kidney). Bone metastases are typically osteolytic (Fig 28.3).

The Union for International Cancer Control (UICC) TNM 8 staging system is shown in Table 28.1.

TABLE 28.1 Union for International Cancer Control TNM 8 Staging of Primary Renal Tumours

Stage	Clinical Findings
Tumour	
Tx	Primary tumour cannot be assessed
T0	No evidence of primary tumour
T1	Tumour ≤7.0 cm in greatest dimension, limited to the kidney
	T1a tumour ≤14.0 cm
	T1b tumour >4.0 cm but ≤7.0 cm
T2	Tumour >7.0 cm in greatest dimension, limited to the kidney
	T2a tumour >7.0 cm but ≤10.0 cm
	T1b tumour >10.0 cm but limited to the kidney
T3	Tumour extends into major veins or perinephric tissues but not into the ipsilateral adrenal gland and not beyond Gerota fascia
T3a	Tumour extends into the renal vein or its segmental branches, or tumour invades the pelvicalyceal system, or tumour invades perirenal and/or renal sinus fat (peripelvic) fat but not beyond Gerota fascia
T3b	Tumour extends into the vena cava below diaphragm
T3c	Tumour extends into vena cava above the diaphragm or invades the wall of the vena cava
T4	Tumour invades beyond Gerota fascia (including contiguous extension into the ipsilateral adrenal gland)
Nodes	
Nx	Regional lymph nodes cannot be assessed
N0	No regional lymph node metastasis
N1	Metastasis in regional lymph nodes
Metastases	
Mx	Distant metastases cannot be assessed
M0	No distant metastases
M1	Distant metastases
Histological Grading	
Gx	Grade of differentiation cannot be assessed
G1	Well differentiated
G2	Moderately differentiated
G3–4	Poorly differentiated/undifferentiated

Treatment

Surgery is the main treatment for localised renal cell cancer. Radiotherapy (RT) and embolisation have more limited roles. Chemotherapy is of unproven value. Oral tyrosine kinase inhibitors (TKIs) are the first-line therapy for metastatic disease. There is now a renewed interest in immunotherapy both in the adjuvant as well as the palliative setting.

Surgery

Nephrectomy is indicated for tumours confined to the kidney and/or regional nodes. Extension into the inferior vena cava is not necessarily a contraindication to surgery. T1 tumours (≤7 cm) could be treated with a nephron-sparing surgery or partial nephrectomy if feasible. There are no randomised controlled trials (RCTs) assessing oncological outcomes of laparoscopic versus open radical nephrectomy; however laparoscopic surgery is associated with less blood loss, less analgesic requirement and a shorter length of stay. Tumours up to T3a could be treated with a laparoscopic approach, and open nephrectomy

reserved for stage T3b and higher. Currently, in the era of TKIs, there is debate as to the role of cytoreductive nephrectomy in the presence of metastatic disease. Bulky, symptomatic tumours with small volume metastases may still be considered for cytoreductive nephrectomy before starting TKIs at subsequent radiological progression. In selected patients, aggressive surgical removal of the primary tumour together with solitary metastases, particularly in lung and bone, may be followed by up to 35% 5-year survival. Palliative removal of the kidney may be required to control pain or haemorrhage, or if a painful syndrome following embolisation occurs.

Embolisation

Embolisation of the kidney via a catheter inserted into the renal artery may be useful in both operable and inoperable cases. In operable cases, embolisation is indicated where there is concern about blood loss at nephrectomy, for example, in patients who refuse blood transfusion on religious grounds. In inoperable cases, it is effective in controlling renal pain and haematuria. A postembolisation syndrome with pain, ileus, and infection may complicate embolisation.

Radiotherapy

Renal cell carcinoma is relatively resistant to radiation. Pre- or postoperative RT does not reduce local recurrence where the tumour has spread locally outside the kidney. Its role is palliative to relieve symptoms from the primary tumour or from distant metastases.

Kidney

Target volume. The whole of the kidney and the regional nodes should be included (see Fig. 28.1).

Technique. A parallel-opposed anterior and posterior pair of fields is used.

Dose and energy. Dose and energy are comprised of 30 gray (Gy) in 10 daily fractions over 2 weeks (6–15 MV photons) or a single 8 to 10 Gy for haematuria.

Distant metastases. Palliative radiotherapy can be offered for symptomatic bone or nodal metastasis.

Technique. Parallel-opposed field or single direct field.

Dose and energy. Single 8–10 Gy to 30 Gy in 10 daily fractions using 6–15 MV photons.

Brain metastasis. Can be treated depending upon fitness using 20 Gy in 5 daily fractions to 30 Gy in 10 daily fractions using 6 MV photons using a parallel-opposed field.

Chemotherapy

Chemotherapy has little value in renal cancer. Single-agent vinblastine has a less than 10% response rate. Oral progestogens such as Provera have been claimed to benefit 20% of patients; however, in randomised clinical trials, the benefit has fallen below 10%. Their major use is in the palliation of systemic symptoms such as anorexia.

Tyrosine Kinase Inhibitors

Systemic therapy in metastatic renal cancers has progressed in the last decade with the development of various oral TKIs. Sunitinib and pazopanib are now used as first-line therapy. TKIs inhibit a number of tumour-cell proliferations and angiogenesis pathways, particularly vascular endothelial growth factor receptor (VEGFR), platelet-derived growth factor receptor (PDGFR) and the stem cell receptor, c-kit. Sunitinib has been shown to give a longer median progression-free survival (11.9 months vs 5 months) than alpha-interferon in a large randomised trial of previously untreated patients with metastatic renal cancer along with a higher objective response rate (31% vs 6%). Diarrhoea, skin marks (hand–foot syndrome) and hypertension are the most common adverse effects. At progression, second-line treatments such as other

TKIs (axitinib, cabozantinib), mTOR inhibitors (everolimus) or programmed death (PD-1) receptor blockers (nivolumab) appear to offer potential further survival benefit.

Immunotherapy

There is now a renewed interest in immunotherapy in renal cancers. Earlier studies using interferon-alpha and interleukin-2 (IL-2) to stimulate the body's immunological attack on tumours were associated with marked toxicities such as profound flu-like illness with fever, rigors, anorexia, weight loss, myalgia and fatigue. The CheckMate 025 study (study using immune check point inhibitor, Nivolumab) showed that compared with everolimus, an improved median survival of 25 months versus 19.6 months was achieved with nivolumab. Nivolumab is a human monoclonal antibody that binds to PD-1 receptor, thereby potentiating T-cell response, including antitumour response. This is currently approved for patients progressing after prior TKI therapy. There are currently other immunotherapy agents, such as monoclonal antibody checkpoint inhibitors (atezolizumab and pembrolizumab) being tested in various studies.

Results of Treatment

The outlook of treatment depends on the stage at diagnosis. For tumours confined to the kidney, 5-year survival varies from 50% to 80%. Extrarenal or renal vein invasion, lymph node and bloodborne metastases all confer a poor prognosis. Patients with metastatic disease at presentation have a median survival of only 12 months, with 20% remaining alive 2 years from diagnosis.

BLADDER

Anatomy

The bladder is related anteriorly to the pubic symphysis; superiorly to the small intestine and sigmoid colon; laterally to the levator ani muscle; inferiorly to the prostate gland; and posteriorly to the rectum, vas deferens and seminal vesicles (see Fig. 28.7) in the male, and to the vagina and cervix in the female. At cystoscopy, the bladder mucosa and ureteric orifices can be inspected. Lymphatic drainage is to the iliac and paraaortic nodes.

Pathology

The bladder, ureters and renal pelvis are lined by transitional cell epithelium (urothelium). The same type of tumours may arise anywhere along the urinary tract but cancers in the renal pelvis and ureter are rare compared with those in the bladder. Prostatic adenocarcinoma and other pelvic tumours are also sometimes secondarily involved with the bladder.

Aetiology

In the majority of cases of bladder cancer, the aetiology is unknown. However, as discussed in Chapter 15, occupational exposure to certain carcinogens has accounted for some cases. The production of aniline dyes and the processing of rubber are associated with 2-naphthylamine, which is now recognised as a procarcinogen. Workers in these industries are now offered regular cytological examination of urine to detect abnormalities or tumours at an early stage.

Smoking is perhaps the most common factor that predisposes to bladder cancer. Bladder cancer is up to six times more common in smokers than nonsmokers and increases in frequency with the number of cigarettes smoked. Phenacetin, formerly used as an analgesic drug, and the cytotoxic alkylating agent, cyclophosphamide, may give rise to urothelial tumours. Squamous carcinoma tends to be associated with chronic irritation of the bladder, including a parasitic disease, schistosomiasis (formerly known as bilharziasis), which is common in Egypt and Central Africa. Adenocarcinoma occurs on the dome of the bladder in relation to embryological remnants of the urachus, and from the trigone at the bladder base.

Genetic alterations in bladder cancer are common. Deletion of markers on chromosome 9 is an early event. Subsequent mutation in *p53* allows cells with DNA damage to proceed through the cell cycle, replicating genetic errors. Loss of the pRb (retinoblastoma) gene product disrupts cell cycling and increases the mitotic index. Patients with both mutations have higher-grade more advanced disease and a poor response to treatment.

Epidemiology

Bladder cancer is common and accounts for 3% of all new cancers (2015) and 3% of cancer deaths (2014) in the United Kingdom. The male to female ratio is 2.5:1 and it has a peak incidence at the age of 75 years. The impact of smoking in women has seen a greater rise in incidence in this group over the last 10 years compared with men. It is twice as common in Caucasians as in those of African descent. Over 90% are TCCs.

Macroscopic Appearance

The chief types on inspection of the bladder are (1) papillary and (2) solid. Multiple growths are common.

Papillary carcinoma has a base with surface fronds. The tumours tend to be multiple and to appear in crops. Confined at first to the mucosa and submucosa, they eventually invade the submucosa, muscle coat and then outside the bladder.

Solid carcinoma is nodular, often ulcerated, grows more rapidly and infiltrates early.

From the point of prognosis, a division can be made between superficial (papillary) and invasive (solid) bladder cancer. Superficial bladder tumours are the most common (80%) and become invasive in 10% to 20% of cases. By contrast, invasive cancer, untreated, carries a very poor prognosis with less than 10% of patients alive after 2 years. The degree of invasion correlates with the risk of metastatic disease. Invasion of the lamina propria (the layer of tissue between the epithelium and the muscle layer of the bladder), and superficial and deep muscle is associated with 20%, 30% and 60% incidence of lymphatic invasion.

Microscopic Appearance

Benign tumours of the bladder are very uncommon. However, low-grade transitional cell malignant tumours are often erroneously referred to as papillomas.

Malignant tumours of the bladder include:
- TCC; papillary and solid variants
- Small cell carcinoma (<1% in the United Kingdom)
- Adenocarcinoma (uncommon)
- Squamous carcinoma (≈5% in the United Kingdom)
- Sarcomas (very rare)

Transitional carcinoma accounts for 90% of bladder cancer and is classified histologically into grades 1 to 3 corresponding to well-, moderately and poorly differentiated tumours. The degree of differentiation is important. Patients with high-grade tumors have a significant risk of dying of their cancer even if it is not muscle-invasive and therefore require aggressive management.

After muscle has been invaded, lymphatic spread is to the pelvic and then paraaortic nodes. Bloodborne metastases are common to lung, liver and bone. Small cell carcinoma of the bladder is rare and has a poor prognosis. Therefore, any amount of small cell histology, even when present with predominantly urothelial elements, is classified as primary small cell bladder cancer, rather than urothelial carcinoma with small cell differentiation.

Clinical Features

The presenting symptom is usually painless frank haematuria. Occasionally, clots of blood are passed and are even more suggestive of the diagnosis. Carcinoma in situ is often associated with dysuria, nocturia and urinary frequency. Papillomatous types grow slowly and may cause no other symptoms for a long time. When aggressive carcinomas invade muscle, there may be urinary frequency, dysuria and pain, especially when there is extravesical (i.e. outside the bladder) spread into the pelvic soft tissues. Bacterial cystitis may be associated with the tumour and may aggravate symptoms.

Obstruction of one or both ureters can occur at any time, with no symptoms at first. Later, there may be upper urinary tract infection, pain in the flank(s) and eventual renal failure from backpressure. In localised bladder disease, clinical examination is usually unremarkable.

Investigation and Staging

Urine

The urine should be examined for red cells, pus cells and bacteria as well as undergoing cytology for malignant cells. Urine cytology is a valuable screening method for industrial workers at risk. Malignant cells are present in the urine of 60% of cases of bladder cancer, particularly the higher grade tumours. However, negative cytology does not exclude malignancy.

Biochemistry

Serum urea, creatinine and electrolytes are measured for evidence of renal impairment.

Radiology

Radiology is important in the diagnosis and staging of bladder cancer. A CT urogram will determine the site of the tumour in the bladder and exclude a lesion higher up in the renal tract. Obstruction at the lower end of the ureter(s) will be shown by dilatation of the ureter and renal pelvis (hydroureter and hydronephrosis). A CT scan of the chest and abdomen is required to complete radiological staging. MRI scanning is the more effective modality to demonstrate deep muscle invasion and spread to pelvic lymph nodes.

Cystourethroscopy

Cystourethroscopy is the most important investigation of all. Under general anaesthesia, the urethra and the whole of the bladder are inspected. The number, site, size and character of the tumours are noted and a biopsy is taken. While the patient is relaxed under the anaesthetic, a bimanual examination of the pelvis is made, with a finger in the rectum and the other hand on the lower abdomen. In this way, the tumour may be palpated and any extravesical spread assessed.

Clinical staging of bladder cancer is according to the UICC TNM 8 classification (Fig. 28.4 and Table 28.2).

Treatment

Treatment will depend on the stage, histology, size and multiplicity of tumours and the age and general medical condition of the patient.

Superficial Tumours Ta, Tis and T1

Superficial tumours are biopsied and removed by transurethral resection (TUR) or diathermy at the time of cystoscopy. Random biopsies of the bladder are carried out to exclude carcinoma in situ. In the majority

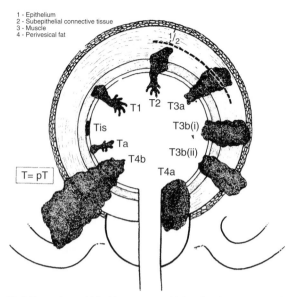

1 - Epithelium
2 - Subepithelial connective tissue
3 - Muscle
4 - Perivesical fat

Fig. 28.4 T staging of bladder cancer—Union for International Cancer Control classification. (From Hermanek P, Hutter RVP, Sobin LH, editors. International Union Against Cancer TNM Atlas. Illustrated guide to the TNM classification of malignant tumours. 4th ed. London: Springer-Verlag; 1997. With permission.)

TABLE 28.2 Union for International Cancer Control TNM 8 Staging of Bladder Cancer

Stage	Clinical Findings
Tumour	
Tis	Carcinoma in situ
Ta	Papillary noninvasive carcinoma
T1	Invasion into submucosa but not beyond the lamina propria
T2a	Tumour invades superficial muscularis propria (inner half)
T2b	Tumour invades deep muscularis propria (outer half)
T3a	Invasion into perivesicular tissues microscopically
T3b	Invasion into perivesicular tissues macroscopically (extravesical mass)
T4a	Tumour invades prostate stroma, seminal vesicles, uterus or vagina
T4b	Tumour invades pelvic wall or abdominal wall
Nodes	Regional lymph nodes include both primary and secondary drainage regions. All other nodes above the aortic bifurcation are considered distant lymph nodes
N0	No evidence of nodal involvement
N1	Single regional lymph node metastasis in the true pelvis (hypogastric, obturator, external iliac, or presacral lymph node)
N2	Multiple regional lymph node metastasis in the true pelvis (hypogastric, obturator, external iliac, or presacral lymph node metastasis)
N3	Lymph node metastasis to the common iliac lymph nodes
Metastases	
M0	No metastases
M1a	Nonregional lymph nodes
M1b	Other distant metastases

of patients, these tumours tend to recur rather than invade (≤60% recurrence rate). For this reason, cystoscopic follow-up needs to be lifelong.

In cases of high-grade disease or carcinoma in situ, intravesical BCG should be used to reduce the recurrence rate to 40% and may also delay the rates of progression. Cystectomy is indicated if these measures fail.

Superficial tumours do respond completely to radical RT in over 75% of cases, but there is recurrence in more than 50%. For this reason, radical RT is rarely used in T1 lesions.

Invasive Bladder Cancer (T2 and T3)

Surgery or RT is the standard treatment for invasive bladder cancer.

T2 tumours. Endoscopic resection (TURBT) alone is inadequate to control T2 tumours. Additional radical treatment with either cystoprostourethrectomy (removal of the bladder and prostate with diversion of the ureters onto the abdominal wall) or radical RT is required. Local practice will determine treatment. Europe and the United States have favored cystoprostourethrectomy as the treatment of choice. In the United Kingdom, radical RT with salvage cystectomy for those patients with persistent or recurrent tumour remains a valid option. This policy has the advantage that the patient has a better chance of tumour control with the bladder intact. If RT fails, there is a 30% chance of successful salvage by cystectomy. By contrast, if primary cystectomy fails, radical RT is rarely successful for recurrent disease. Each policy carries a similar 5-year survival of about 50% to 60%.

T3 tumours. If bimanual palpation and/or radiological imaging have demonstrated macroscopic extension of disease outside the bladder, cure rates fall to around 40% at 5 years. Such patients are more commonly treated with radical RT than with surgery. Combined modality treatment with concurrent chemotherapy (5-fluorouracil (5-FU) and mitomycin C) and RT appears to improve local control at 2 years in comparison to standard conformal RT alone in patients with T2-T3 disease.

T4 tumours. A distinction must be made between T4a and T4b tumours. T4a means tumour penetration into the prostate or vagina. T4a includes both aggressive deeply invasive tumours infiltrating the prostate and less aggressive superficial tumours extending into the prostatic urethra and/or ducts. The latter has a much better prognosis than the former. T4a tumours should be treated radically. T4b tumours are fixed to neighboring structures, are inoperable and should be treated with palliative RT.

Adenocarcinoma and Squamous Carcinoma of the Bladder

Neither adenocarcinoma nor squamous carcinoma of the bladder is very radiosensitive and they are better treated by cystectomy.

Small Cell Carcinoma of the Bladder

Small cell tumours often present with metastatic disease. Platinum and etoposide combination chemotherapy is the cornerstone in the management of small cell carcinoma. This may be followed by RT to consolidate the response in cases of localised disease. However, the prognosis still remains poor with 5-year overall survival for all stages combined of approximately 20%.

Neoadjuvant or Adjuvant Chemotherapy

Combination cisplatin-based chemotherapy for two to four cycles before radical therapy improves survival for muscle-invasive TCC by 5% at 5 years. A complete response at cystoscopic re-evaluation predicts for better survival, and organ preservation should be considered. Cystectomy and pelvic nodal clearance is indicated for a poor response. Concerns over delaying definitive treatment and chemotherapy-related toxicity exist. Appropriate patient selection for neoadjuvant chemotherapy is important.

To date, all adjuvant chemotherapy studies have failed to recruit adequate patient numbers. The European Organisation for Research and Treatment of Cancer (EORTC) 30994 study is the largest study that managed to recruit 284 patients of the planned 660 and showed only a trend towards better overall survival, but a significant improvement in time to treatment failure. A metaanalysis of nine RCTs with 945 patients showed a 22% relative decrease in risk of death with adjuvant chemotherapy. Therefore four cycles of adjuvant cisplatin-based chemotherapy may be considered in patients with poor prognostic features, such as pT3 or pT4 or node-positive disease, who could not get neoadjuvant chemotherapy.

Radical Radiotherapy

The following are criteria for accepting patients for radical RT:

- Age younger than 80 years (unless particularly fit)
- Adequate general medical condition
- No inflammatory bowel disease or symptomatic adhesions
- Good bladder function
- Minimal or no carcinoma-in-situ
- TCC
- Single tumour smaller than 7 cm maximum diameter
- Recurrent T1G3, T2–T4a
- No metastases

Target volume. Target volume includes the whole bladder with a 1 to 2 cm margin. The bladder is emptied before CT simulation and before each treatment.

Radiation planning technique. The patient is simulated supine with feet in foot stocks and hands elevated onto the chest. The clinical target volume (CTV) includes the whole bladder and the planning target volume (PTV) is obtained by a 1 to 2 cm expansion. It is common practice to cover the prostatic urethra in the PTV in view of the risk of local recurrence. The organs at risk, the rectum and the femoral heads, are contoured on the planning CT scan. An open anterior and two lateral wedged or posterior oblique wedged fields are used, treating isocentrically, however, a four-field technique is employed in occasional cases (Figs 28.5 and 28.6). A direct lateral field is preferred at our institution, the Edinburgh cancer centre to reduce rectal doses in view of the sharp fall-off of the field. With high-energy photon beams such as 15 MV, femoral-head doses are kept below 50% of the tumour dose. The use of conformal therapy techniques is routine and improves treatment-related morbidity in addition to possible dose escalation in the future. In addition, intensity-modulated RT (IMRT) is increasingly being used to treat patients at risk of pelvic lymph-node involvement (Fig. 28.7); whether this improves survival, however, is unproven. The use of megavoltage cone beam CT to aid soft tissue matching has allowed development of different adaptive RT strategies such as 'plan of the day' where pretreatment images are used to select the best fit plan from a library of predesigned treatment plans. The RAIDER study (**R**andomised phase II trial of **A**daptive **I**mage guided standard or **D**ose **E**scalated tumour boost **R**adiotherapy) explores the feasibility of adaptive and dose escalated tumour boost using fiducial markers (Lipoidol) injected around the tumour to aid image guidance.

Dose and energy. Radical treatment doses are either 55 Gy in 20 daily fractions over 4 weeks (10–15 MV photons) or 64 Gy in 32 daily fractions over 6.5 weeks (10–15 MV photons).

Concurrent Chemotherapy and Radiotherapy

Concurrent chemotherapy with radiation (chemo-rt) should be considered for all patients fit enough to receive it, and can be given safely after neoadjuvant chemotherapy or on its own. The BC 2001 study (Bladder cancer 2001) reported improved local control at 2 years to 71% after concurrent chemo-rt with 5-FU and mitomycin-C over RT alone. Similarly, in an attempt to overcome tumour hypoxia in the bladder, nicotinamide and carbogen in combination with RT within the phase II

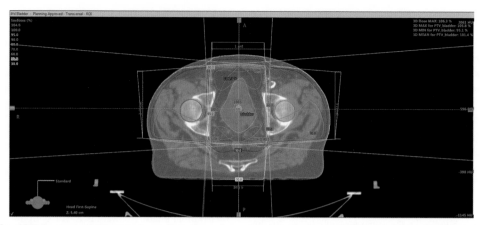

Fig. 28.5 Isodose distribution for radical three-dimensional conformal radiotherapy of the bladder using four fields.

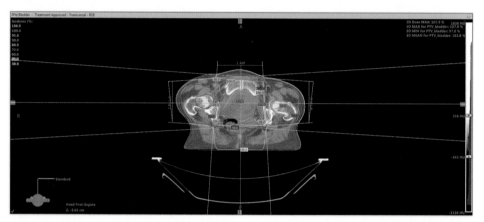

Fig. 28.6 Isodose distribution for radical three-dimensional conformal radiotherapy of the bladder using the anterior and two lateral fields.

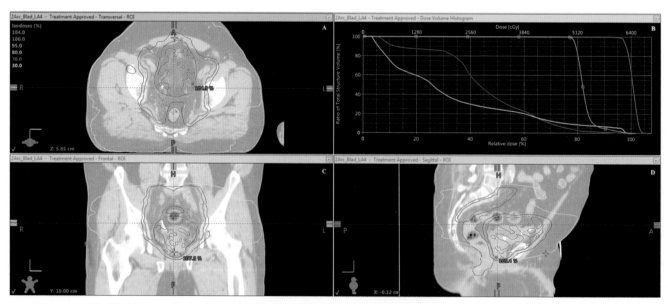

Fig. 28.7 Isodose distribution of a bladder and pelvic nodes radical radiotherapy treatment plan using volumetric arc therapy. Axial view (A), DVH with planning target volume (PTV) bladder in red, PTV lymph nodes in green, rectum in brown and bowels in yellow (B), coronal view (C) and sagittal view (D).

BCON study has improved local control and survival in comparison with RT alone. In the United Kingdom, a 5-FU and mitomycin C combination is the most common agent used in chemo-rt.

Radiation reaction. Before radiation begins, attention is paid to the patient's general condition and nutrition. The patient's hemoglobin level should be maintained over 12 g/dL, by blood transfusion if necessary, because anaemia will reduce the amount of oxygen available to the tumour. It is known that reduced oxygenation in parts of the tumour contributes to resistance to radiation. Urinary infection should be treated with antibiotics. The urine should be made sterile if possible before radiation begins because inflammation has adverse effects on radiation response. However, with an ulcerated mass this may not be possible until the tumour has shrunk in response to radiation.

Acute reactions.

1. Frequency and urgency, from radiation cystitis during and after the course, are common but not usually serious unless bacterial infection is gross. Painful spasm may require an antispasmodic drug such as oxybutynin or solifenacin. Fluid intake must be strongly encouraged. The patient should be warned that he or she might pass fragments in the urine (blood clot and tumour) and a little fresh blood.
2. Bowel reactions are also to be expected in almost every case – usually mild diarrhea and tenesmus. If they are severe, treatment may have to be suspended or dosage reduced.

Late reactions.

1. Fibrosis of the bladder. The bladder wall may be so contracted by fibrosis and the bladder volume so reduced that uncontrollable frequency may make life intolerable. Ureteric diversion may be required.
2. Telangiectasia on the bladder lining may develop, with repeated bleeding. It may be possible to seal them off with the diathermy point at cystoscopy. If they are uncontrolled by this means, cystectomy may be required.
3. Late bowel reactions are similar to those after the irradiation of cancer of the cervix (p. 451), although less common (<5%). Loops of bowel trapped in the pelvis by adhesions after previous surgery or inflammatory disease are especially at risk. There may be bleeding from telangiectasia on the bowel mucosa, ulceration, and even necrosis and perforation. If conservative measures fail (e.g. steroid enemas), a defunctioning colostomy may be required.

Palliative Radiotherapy

Palliative RT should be considered in the following circumstances: age (>80 years) or poor general condition with either significant local symptoms (e.g. haematuria) or symptomatic metastases, for example, bone and skin.

Technique. The patient is simulated supine with feet in foot stocks and hands by the side. A parallel-opposed anterior and posterior pair of fields is used. The treatment volume includes the bladder with a 2-cm margin or bladder and pelvic nodes if involved.

Dose and energy. Depending upon the intent of palliation and fitness of the patient, different dose schedules can be considered.

30 Gy in 10 daily fractions over 2 weeks (10 – 15 MV photons) or 21 Gy in 3 fractions over 1 week (10 – 15 MV photons) or 20 Gy in 5 daily fractions (10 – 15 MV photons).

For symptoms such as hematuria, a single fraction of 8 – 10 Gy using 10 – 15 MV photons should be considered.

Palliative Chemotherapy and Immunotherapy

Response rates of greater than 50% have been reported using cisplatin-based regimens, such as cisplatin, methotrexate and vinblastine (CMV), methotrexate, vinblastine, doxorubicin and cisplatin (MVAC)

or gemcitabine and cisplatin (GC) for metastatic disease. Median survival following chemotherapy depends on sites of disease. Nodal disease carries a relatively good prognosis with a median survival of 24 months; in comparison, median survival for disease in organs such as the liver, remains disappointing at less than 12 months. Immunotherapy agents targeting the checkpoint pathway are trialed in various studies. Currently, Pembrolizumab is approved as a second-line agent in patients with metastatic bladder cancer who have progressed after a prior platinum-containing chemotherapy.

Results of Treatment

The 5-year survival for radical RT is 80% for T1, 55% to 60% for T2, 40% to 45% for T3 and 25% to 30% T4 tumours.

PROSTATE

Anatomy

The prostate gland lies just below the base of the bladder and in front of the rectum (Fig. 28.8). It resembles a chestnut in size and shape. Through it passes the prostatic urethra. Into the urethra empty the ejaculatory ducts. These carry sperm from the seminal vesicles, which lie behind and to each side of the prostate gland. The prostate is divided into two lobes by a median groove. From a functional point of view, it is divided into a peripheral zone, central zone and transitional zone. It is surrounded by a thin layer of fibrous tissue (true capsule) and a layer of fascia continuous with that surrounding the bladder (false capsule). Between these two layers lies the prostatic venous plexus. Part of the venous drainage is to a plexus of veins lying in front of the vertebral bodies. This may account for the tendency of prostate cancer to spread to the vertebrae.

Pathology

Cancer of the prostate gland is the second most common malignancy in men in the United Kingdom. In total, 47,200 new cases and 11,300 deaths were recorded in 2014 to 2015. There has been a significant rise in the incidence of prostate cancer in the last 20 years as a result of a combination of increased awareness, prostate-specific antigen (PSA) testing and an ageing population with the opportunity to develop the disease.

The exact aetiology of prostatic cancer is unknown. It is most common in the 7th and 8th decades and is rare under the age of 40 years. Marked worldwide variations in incidence exist. In particular, Japan has rates considerably lower than in the United States. A correlation with diet and, in particular, high-fat consumption is directly implicated. Genetic factors have a role; siblings are at increased risk with a positive

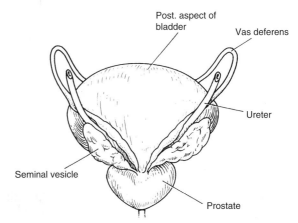

Fig. 28.8 Prostate, seminal vesicles and vas deferens in a posterior view of the bladder. (Modified from Ellis. Clinical anatomy, 5th ed. Oxford: Blackwell; 1975.)

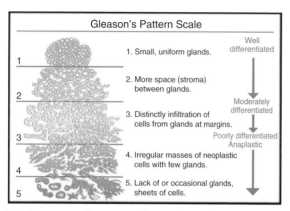

Fig. 28.9 Gleason grading system for carcinoma of the prostate. (From Kirby RS, Brawer MK, Denis LJ, editors. 2001. Prostate cancer fast facts. 3rd ed. Abington: Health Press. With permission.)

family history and African Americans have higher levels of disease compared with Americans of European descent. Mutations in the BRCA gene are a risk for developing prostate cancer. Men with BRCA1 mutation are 3.4 times more likely to develop prostate cancer by age 65 years and this risk is 8.6-fold higher in men with mutation in the BRCA2 gene. Environmental factors include exposure to radiation, heavy metals and chemical fertilisers, although no definitive link has been determined.

Over 95% are adenocarcinomas, 70% arising from the peripheral part of the gland. Other rare histological subtypes include small cell carcinoma, carcinosarcoma, mucinous adenocarcinoma and ductal carcinoma. The ductal and mucinous carcinomas tend to behave similar to conventional prostatic adenocarcinoma, whereas the small cell carcinoma and carcinosarcoma tend to present with metastatic disease frequently and follows an aggressive course. The differentiation of prostate cancer is graded according to the Gleason grading system. It is based on the extent to which the tumour cells are arranged into recognisable glandular structures, grade 1 tumours forming almost normal glands, whereas grade 5 tumours consist of sheets of cells (Fig. 28.9). Because of the heterogeneity in prostate cancer, the two most common grades seen are added together to give a Gleason score.

Before the advent of PSA testing, in 75% of cases, the tumour had spread beyond the gland at the time of presentation, and 50% had distant metastases. However, the introduction of PSA screening in countries such as the United States has dramatically reduced the number of patients presenting with advanced disease.

Prostate cancer may spread directly to the bladder, seminal vesicles and rectum. Lymphatic spread is to the obturator and to the presacral, internal and external iliac nodes. Further spread is to the common iliac and paraaortic nodes. It readily invades the pelvic veins and thence the pelvic bones and vertebrae. Bone secondaries are typically of sclerotic type, showing as an increased density on the radiograph because they induce new bone formation.

The natural history of the disease is quite variable. It may be indolent in the elderly patient with a well-differentiated tumour and an incidental finding at postmortem. The disease tends to run a more aggressive course in younger men, particularly with poorly differentiated tumours. Prostate cancer in men with germline BRCA mutation is associated with higher risk of nodal involvement, distant metastasis and poor survival outcomes. Preliminary results from the IMPACT study, **I**dentification of **M**en with genetic predisposition to **P**rost**A**te **C**ancer: **T**argeted screening in BRCA 1/2 mutation carriers and controls suggest a high positive predictive value of PSA screening, and final results of the study are awaited.

Hormonal Sensitivity

The prostate has analogies with the breast and is under hormonal control. Removal of male hormones by orchidectomy, or administration of female hormones (oestrogens), causes shrinkage of the normal gland, and of 80% of tumours.

Prostate-Specific Antigen and Screening

PSA is a glycoprotein that liquefies semen. Approximately 20% of men with PSA levels above the normal range of 4 ng/mL have prostate cancer, and this risk increases to more than 60% in men with a PSA level above 10 ng/mL. PSA levels increase in proportion to the volume of disease and can be used to monitor the response to treatment and development of metastatic disease. PSA has largely superseded the use of an enzyme, acid phosphatase, secreted by normal and malignant prostate tissue, in the diagnosis and assessment of response to treatment.

The benefits of screening for prostate cancer are as yet unproven. The results of two large screening RCTs were conflicting. The European Randomised Study of Screening for Prostate Cancer (ERSPC) improved prostate cancer survival by 20% but at the expense of significant overtreatment. After 13 years of follow-up, 27 men required a prostatectomy to save the life of one additional man. The US-based Prostate, Lung, Colorectal, and Ovarian (PLCO) cancer screening trial did not show a survival advantage; however, many men in the control arm had PSA screening performed outside of the study and so reduced any potential benefit to the screening arm. A single PSA screening intervention in the cluster randomisation trial of PSA testing in prostate cancer (CAP trial) did not show a significant difference in prostate cancer mortality after a median follow-up of 10 years compared with standard practice without screening. However, more prostate cancers with a lower grade were detected. The ERSPC study with a mean of 2.1 PSA test per intervention group participant showed a higher cumulative risk of prostate cancer with 3.4 more diagnoses per 1000 person-years over the 13 years of follow-up. In 2017, the U.S. Preventive Services Task Force (USPSTF) revised their earlier recommendation against screening and currently recommends shared decision making for screening healthy men 55 to 69 years of age. At present there are no plans to introduce a U.K. mass prostate-screening program; however, there is an informed-choice program where men aged 50 years and over can discuss with their doctor and request that their PSA levels be tested.

Clinical Features

The prostate often undergoes benign enlargement, and the early symptoms of cancer may be similar, that is, increased frequency and difficulty of micturition. Haematuria and urinary obstruction can occur. Bone pain or pathological fracture may be the first presenting symptom. Back pressure on the kidneys may cause renal impairment. Sacral, sciatic or perineal pain may occur from infiltration of nerves in the pelvis. Clinical evidence of disease is rare under the age of 45 years.

Diagnosis and Staging

The presence of a hard irregular gland on rectal examination suggests the diagnosis. This should be confirmed by a biopsy of the prostate. Usually, 10 to 12 biopsies of the prostate (5 or 6 from each lobe) are conducted under transrectal ultrasound guidance. Transperineal biopsies could be considered in patients with an anterior gland tumour. Prostatic carcinoma is staged using the TNM classification (Table 28.3). The local stage of the disease is mainly based on digital rectal examination and may be supplemented by ultrasound, CT or MRI scanning. Multiparametric MRI of the prostate is increasingly used both as an initial screening tool

TABLE 28.3 Union for International Cancer Control TNM 8 Staging of Prostate Cancer

Stage	Clinical Findings
Tumour	
T1	Clinically inapparent tumour not palpable or visible by imaging
T1a	Tumour incidental finding in ≤5% of tissue resected
T1b	Tumour incidental finding in >5% of tissue resected
T1c	Tumour identified by needle biopsy (e.g. because of elevated PSA)
T2	Palpable tumour confined to the gland
T2a	Tumour involves half a lobe or less
T2b	Tumour involves more than half a lobe
T2c	Tumour involves both lobes
T3	Tumour extending through the capsule
T3a	Extraprostatic extension (unilateral or bilateral) including microscopic bladder neck involvement
T3b	Tumour invades seminal vesicle(s)
T4	Tumour fixed or invading adjacent structures
Nodes	
N0	No nodes involved
N1	Regional lymph nodes involved
Metastases	
M0	No distant metastases
M1a	Nonregional lymph node(s)
M1b	Bone(s)
M1c	Other sites

PSA, Prostate-specific antigen.

TABLE 28.4 Prostate Cancer Risk Stratification

Risk category	
Low risk	T1-T2a and Gleason <7 and PSA <10
Intermediate risk	T2b-T2c or Gleason 7 or PSA 10–20 with no high-risk features
High risk	≥T3 or Gleason 8–10 or PSA >20

PSA, Prostate-specific antigen.

- External beam RT
- Prostate brachytherapy
- External beam RT with brachytherapy boost
- Radical prostatectomy

Men with localised disease could be considered for any of the above-mentioned treatment options depending upon their fitness, personal preferences and symptoms.

Active surveillance. The Prostate Testing for Cancer and Treatment study (ProtecT) is the first RCT to determine the optimum treatment for early prostate cancer. The study randomised patients to active monitoring, radical prostatectomy or radical RT. Although the incidence of distant metastasis in the active surveillance arm was approximately double the radical treatment arm, there was no difference in overall survival or prostate cancer-specific survival after a median follow-up of 10 years. The study idea was conceived almost 2 decades ago and therefore the active surveillance protocol in the study reflects the practice in the late 1990s. Currently, the selection of patients suitable for active surveillance has improved with the advent of multiparametric MRI and transperineal prostate biopsies, and this can potentially improve distant metastasis-free survival. Younger, fitter men with low-risk prostate cancer may be treated with active monitoring initially, with radical treatment offered on progression of disease based on an increase in Gleason grade on repeat biopsy or significant rise in PSA. The philosophy behind this approach is to spare treatment-related toxicity in men who may have indolent disease.

Watchful waiting. Elderly, medically unfit men with less aggressive histological features may be managed by watchful waiting (with deferred hormonal therapy and/or palliative RT for symptomatic progression).

External beam radiotherapy. External beam RT in prostate cancer is a noninvasive treatment that has been through significant changes over the past two decades. The Medical Research Council UK Prostate 07 study (PR07) showed an overall survival benefit with the addition of RT to hormones alone in locally advanced prostate cancer. The chance of local control with RT decreases with increasing PSA, grade and stage of disease. Neoadjuvant hormonal therapy for 3 months before RT has demonstrated improved local control in low- and intermediate-risk prostate cancers over RT alone. The hormonal treatment reduces the size of the prostate by 30% and hence, the treatment volume. It also reduces the number of tumour cells to irradiate, possibly through synergistic apoptotic mechanisms.

Dose escalation and intensity-modulated radiotherapy. Many randomised trials and single institution series suggest that dose-escalated RT improves local control and PSA relapse-free survival (a surrogate for actual survival). The Medical research council radiotherapy study (RT01) has demonstrated the safety and efficacy of increasing dose from 64 Gy to 74 Gy in U.K. institutions. At 10 years, the biochemical progression-free survival was significantly improved to 55% versus 43% in favor of 74 Gy using three-field conformal RT. A study in The Netherlands comparing 68 Gy versus 78 Gy has also shown better progression-free survival at 5 years (64% vs 54%) but no difference

as well as part of the staging process. The recent Prostate Magnetic Resonance Imaging Study (PROMIS) has shown that a multiparametric MRI can decrease at least one-quarter of men with raised PSA up to 15 ng/mL from getting a biopsy.

A multiparametric MRI scan, in particular is helpful in showing the intraprostatic tumour and is a useful tool to assess extracapsular spread, enlarged pelvic nodes and local invasion of the bladder, seminal vesicles and rectal wall. Surgical dissection of the pelvic nodes to assess pelvic node involvement has not gained wide acceptance in the United Kingdom because it does not improve survival. A bone scan is recommended in view of the high incidence of bone metastases if the PSA is greater than 10 or the Gleason score is 7 or above. Prostate-specific membrane antigen (PSMA) is a promising and specific target for prostate cancer imaging. Positron emission tomography (PET) using novel PSMA agents with CT or MRI scans has gained increasing interest and shows great promise for improving prostate cancer staging, both systemic and local.

Treatment

Localised Prostate Cancer

The overarching goal in the management of prostate cancer is cure with minimal impairment of quality of life. Aggressive treatment of indolent disease exposes patients to the toxicity of treatment, whereas under-treatment may lead to potentially curable disease-causing significant morbidity or cancer-related death. Balancing these issues requires time and experience. Risk classification systems based on PSA, Gleason score and T stage may guide management (Table 28.4).

Treatment options include:

- Active surveillance (radical treatment still offered at progression)
- Watchful waiting (noncurative hormonal therapy offered at progression)

in overall survival. The low alpha/beta ratio of prostate cancer suggests that prolonged fractionated schedules may not be radiobiologically as efficient as hypofractionation. Two studies using moderate hypofractionation, the CHHiP study (Conventional versus hypofractionated high-dose intensity-modulated radiotherapy for prostate cancer) and the PROFIT study (Prostate Fractionated Irradiation Trial), showed that 60 Gy in 20 fractions is not inferior to dose-escalated RT, 74 Gy or 78 Gy, respectively. This has now been adopted in most U.K. institutions, offering a moderate hypofractionated regime of 60 Gy in 20 fractions for patients with low- and intermediate-risk prostate cancer. Hypofractionation in high-risk patients is still debatable, because this subgroup constituted only 12% in the CHHiP study. In the era of dose escalation, either using standard 2 Gy per fractionation or moderate hypofractionation, it is unclear whether there is any extra benefit with addition of neoadjuvant hormonal therapy versus radiation alone in the low- and intermediate- risk cases.

The ability of IMRT to tightly sculpt dose to the prostate, particularly at the prostate–rectal interface is of particular value. Doses in excess of 80 Gy have already safely been administered with excellent PSA relapse-free survival without additional neoadjuvant hormonal therapy.

For these radiation doses to be delivered, tight treatment margins are required, which in turn requires accurate tumour localisation. Using online portal imaging to localise bony anatomy ensures accurate field set-up only. The prostate is a mobile organ, the position of which is influenced by changes in rectal and bladder filling. The two most popular methods of image- guided RT (IGRT) to ensure accurate treatment delivery are daily megavoltage imaging or kilovoltage imaging of fiducial markers placed within the prostate via transrectal ultrasound or the use of weekly cone beam CT.

Stereotactic ablative body radiotherapy. With growing evidence on the response of prostate cancer to hypofractionation, other ultrahypofractionated RT schedules, such as stereotactic ablative body radiotherapy (SABR), are currently being tested in multiple ongoing trials. In the United Kingdom, the PACE study (Prostate Advances in Comparative Evidence) is currently evaluating a dose of 36.25 Gy in five fractions in low- and intermediate-risk prostate cancers.

Prostate brachytherapy – low-dose rate seeds. Prostate brachytherapy is now an accepted treatment modality for early prostate cancer. In the traditional preplan technique, the treatment is delivered in two phases. In the first phase, a volume study is performed with the patient in an extended dorsal lithotomy position, usually under a general anaesthetic. A transrectal ultrasound probe mounted on a stepping unit scans the prostate from base to apex in 5-mm slices. On each slice, the prostate is outlined and the volume calculated. Prostate volumes above 50 mL may lead to pubic arch interference at the time of implantation. In these cases, a volume of up to 70 mL may be reduced by 30% and so be suitable for subsequent implantation after 3 months of androgen-deprivation therapy.

Once the volume study has been performed, the images are transferred to the planning computer. The exact seed location and number of needles required to deliver the implant is then determined using three-dimensional planning. The x and y coordinates are provided by the template grid against the perineum, and the z coordinate is set by the transrectal probe position in relation to the base of the prostate. Dose constraints to the rectum and urethra are built into the plan.

The second phase of the procedure is the implant itself. The patient is repositioned as for the volume study and the prostate position is checked. The brachytherapist guides the implant needles directly into the prostate through a closed transperineal approach (Fig. 28.10). Each needle is loaded with either iodine-125 or palladium-103 seeds. It has been suggested that palladium should be used for higher-grade tumours

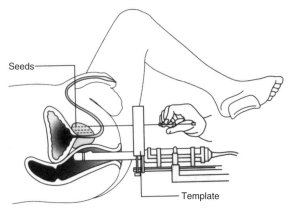

Fig. 28.10 Brachytherapy for early prostate cancer. (From Kirby RS, Brawer MK, Denis LJ, editors. 2001. Prostate cancer fast facts. 3rd ed. Abington: Health Press. With permission.)

owing to its greater dose rate. In practice, however, there are no data to demonstrate any difference in PSA relapse-free survival using either isotope. In the United Kingdom, the majority of centres use iodine-125. A dose of 145 Gy to a PTV of the prostate capsule plus 3 mm is delivered. The inverse square law determines that the dose to the rectum, bladder and neurovascular bundles is very low, with resultant decreased toxicity in comparison to external beam and surgery. The procedure takes approximately 1 hour and the patient is usually discharged the same day with rapid resumption of normal activity.

An alternative and increasingly popular approach to the two-phase technique is intraoperative planning. With this technique, the whole treatment is delivered in a single visit. The patient is positioned in theatre as before. The brachytherapist places the needles under transrectal ultrasound control into the prostate, usually adopting a modified peripheral loading pattern. A plan is produced based around the needle position. Optimisation of the plan via adjustment of the needle position is performed before loading as an afterloading technique. Whichever technique is adopted, the aim is to deliver a dose of 145 Gy to at least 90% of the prostate (D90) on posttreatment dosimetry.

The appropriate selection criteria are listed here:
- Life expectancy of 10 years.
- Organ-confined disease (T1–T2b) on MRI.
- PSA less than 20.
- Gleason score of 7 or less.
International Prostate Symptom Score (IPSS) less than 20 (a high score indicates marked irritative or obstructive symptoms and predicts for posttreatment urinary retention and significant urinary toxicity).
- Maximum flow rate (Qmax) greater than 10 mL/s (if below 10 mL/s then greater risk of posttreatment urinary retention)
- No previous trans-uretheral resection of prostate (TURP) (seeds fall into cavity and affect dosimetry)
- Prostate volume 50 mL or less (above this, the risk of pubic arch interference increases)

The major toxicity is radiation-induced urethritis that may last some months. Frequency, dysuria and mild obstructive symptoms are common. Urinary retention and proctitis may be seen in 5% of patients. Patients are routinely placed on an alpha blocker for 3 to 6 months and encouraged to have a high fluid intake. Proctitis is treated as for external beam RT. In carefully selected patients, outcomes appear very good, with PSA relapse-free survival of greater than 90% at 10 years of follow-up in good-prognosis patients. Clinical trials comparing radical prostatectomy with prostate brachytherapy have so far not been undertaken.

External beam radiotherapy with brachytherapy boost. High-dose rate brachytherapy is increasingly being adopted as a treatment for men with unfavorable intermediate- and high-risk prostate cancer in combination with external beam RT. A high-dose rate (HDR) implant can deliver very high biologically effective radiation doses in a shortened overall treatment time to the tumour whereas the rapid falloff in dose limits surrounding normal tissue toxicity. HDR brachytherapy as a monotherapy is currently evaluated in trials either as a whole gland approach or a focal approach treating the intraprostatic gross tumour volume (GTV) in the low and favorable intermediate-risk group.

A single high-dose 15 Gy HDR boost followed by either 37.5 Gy in 15 fractions of external beam to the prostate in unfavorable intermediate-risk prostate cancer or 46 Gy in 23 fractions to prostate and pelvic lymph nodes in high-risk prostate cancer has been commonly used.

Low-dose rate (LDR) brachytherapy boost to external beam RT is gaining increased acceptance among oncologists since publication of the ASCENDE-RT study (**A**ndrogen **S**uppression **C**ombined with **E**lective **N**odal and **D**ose **E**scalated **R**adiation **T**herapy). The study compared dose-escalated external beam RT, 78 Gy versus external beam RT, 46 Gy to the prostate and pelvic nodes and LDR brachytherapy boost to prostate, 110 to 115 Gy. The brachytherapy boost arm had a superior biochemical control at the cost of late urinary toxicity; prevalence of G3 urinary toxicity at 5 years was 8%. Men with high-risk features but cancer confined to the prostate gland alone are suitable for this approach. It is not feasible to implant LDR seeds into the involved seminal vesicles (SV), but if the involvement is confined to the SV base alone, then an LDR implant could be considered.

Radical prostatectomy. Patients who are medically fit with organ-confined disease are suitable for surgery. A nerve-sparing radical prostatectomy has improved potency rates postprocedure. Severe incontinence is noted in less than 5% of cases, but a higher proportion may have mild stress incontinence. Positive surgical margins in at least 30% of carefully staged patients are common. Laparoscopic prostatectomy is gaining popularity because of improved surgical visualisation of the urethral anastomosis and neurovascular bundles, and potentially shorter inpatient postoperative stay. The use of robotic-assisted laparoscopic prostatectomy can shorten the surgical learning curve and is now available in a number of U.K. urology centers.

External beam radiotherapy planning

Target volume. When planning external beam RT (EBRT), if the tumour staging demonstrates that the tumour is confined to the prostate and there is no obvious involvement of the pelvic nodes, the target volume is confined to the tumour and any local extension (e.g. seminal vesicles), with a 1-cm margin of normal tissue around it. At the rectal–prostate interface, a margin of 0.5 cm is satisfactory if using IGRT. The role of additional pelvic RT is unclear; however, an increasing number of protocols treat the pelvis if there is a risk of nodal involvement of at least 15%.

Technique. A three-field technique, with one anterior and two posterior oblique fields at 120 degrees to each other, or one anterior and two wedged lateral fields, are still used in some institutions. Most U.K. centers offer IMRT using either a multifield-based technique or volumetric arc therapy (VMAT). The patient lies supine with the feet in foot stocks. Localisation is done with a CT planning scan. The bladder should be full to displace the dome of the bladder and small bowel out of the field. CT cuts of 3 to 5 mm are taken through the pelvis. The CTV of prostate ± seminal vesicles is outlined. Difficulty in localisation of the prostatic apex and extension into the bladder are common areas of fault.

In our institution, based on the CHHiP study experience, we treat localised prostate cancer to 60 Gy in 20 fractions.

Technique and dose fractionation. A simultaneous integrated boost technique is used to plan and treat two volumes, namely PTV 57 Gy and PTV 60Gy in 20 daily treat two volumes, namely PTV 57Gy and PTV 60Gy in 20 daily fractions. It is appropriate to change these two volumes to PTV 71 Gy and PTV 74 Gy respectively, when a total dose of 74 Gy in 37 daily fractions is considered.

The Roach formula (PSA + [(GS−6) × 10)]) is used to decide on the extent of seminal vesicle to be included in the clinical target volume 57 Gy (CTV 57 Gy). If the risk of seminal vesicle invasion is ≥15% as per Roach formula, the base of the seminal vesicle should be included in the CTV 57 Gy. In cases where there is T3b disease (involvement of seminal vesicle), the whole seminal vesicle should be included in the CTV 57 Gy.

The CTV 60 Gy is made of prostate alone or the prostate with involved seminal vesicle (in T3b disease).

In general a margin of 0.5 – 1 cm is applied to obtain the PTV.

At the Edinburgh cancer centre, we use PTV 57 Gy = CTV 57 + 1 cm all round except 0.5 cm posteriorly PTV 60 Gy = CTV 60 + 0.5 cm all round except 0.3 cm posteriorly

Organs at risk to be contoured are: Rectum (Inferior limit – level of ischial tuberosities; superior limit – sigmoid flexure), Bladder (whole) & Femoral heads.

With IMRT, the volume is shaped to follow the prostate and, in so doing, as much of the normal tissues such as the rectum are avoided. A typical isodose distribution is shown in Fig. 28.11A, B.

Typical OAR dose constraints used for planning are outlined in Table 28.5.

Dose and energy. Dose administrated are 60 Gy in 20 daily fractions over 4 weeks or 74 Gy in 37 daily fractions over 7.5 weeks.

Acute reactions. About half way through a radical course, urinary frequency and, occasionally, dysuria occur. These can often be relieved with an antiinflammatory agent, such as Froben, 50 mg, 3 × daily (tds) and normally settle within 4 weeks of the end of treatment. Diarrhoea and tenesmus from acute proctitis have a similar time course and are treated with a low-residue diet, Fybogel and, on occasion, steroid suppositories.

Late reactions. Significant late reactions may occur in 3% to 5% of patients. The main late urinary effects are chronic cystitis, urethral stricture or incontinence. Loss of sexual potency also occurs. At 2 years from completion of combined neoadjuvant hormonal therapy and radical RT, 50% of previously potent men will be impotent. Bowel morbidity includes rectal ulceration or stricture and small bowel obstruction. Symptoms are tenesmus, rectal bleeding or incontinence. Proctitis may respond to steroid (Predsol) enemas but, ultimately, a defunctioning colostomy is required in exceptional circumstances.

Results of radical radiotherapy. The 5-year PSA relapse-free survival for low-, intermediate- and high-risk prostate cancers are 95%, 85% and 60%, respectively.

Pelvic Lymph Node Irradiation

The treatment of pelvic lymph nodes remains controversial but is increasingly being adopted for high-risk patients within the United Kingdom. A Radiation Therapy Oncology Group (RTOG) trial has shown better progression-free survival when pelvic irradiation (45 Gy in 25 fractions) is combined with definitive irradiation to the prostate (72.2 Gy). Many centres offer whole pelvic RT if the risk of nodal metastases exceeds 15%. The risk of pelvic lymph node involvement is calculated by the following formula:

$$2/3\,PSA + (Gleason\ score - 6 \times 10)$$
$$= percentage\ risk\ of\ nodal\ spread$$

Ideally, the pelvic nodes and the prostate should be treated using an IMRT technique.

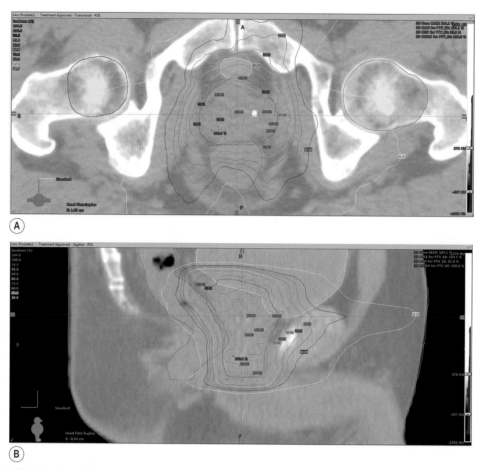

Fig. 28.11 Isodose distribution of a prostate radical radiotherapy treatment plan using volumetric arc therapy. Axial view (A) and sagittal view (B).

TABLE 28.5 Prostate External Beam Radiotherapy Planning Organs at Risk Dose Constraints

Rectum	Dose	Target Volume %
•	V100%	3
•	V95%	25
•	V90%	30
•	V75%	50
•	It is recommended that the 60% isodose should not cross the posterior rectal wall.	
Bladder	V100%	25
•	V90%	50
Femoral heads: ≥ 2 cm^3 to receive <70% of dose to isocentre.		

TABLE 28.6 Guide to Prostate Cancer Treatment Based on Risk Stratification

Risk Category	Radical treatment options to consider depending upon patient preference and other individual risks
Low risk	Active surveillance, prostatectomy, EBRT to prostate, LDR monotherapy
Intermediate risk	Prostatectomy, EBRT to prostate, LDR monotherapy, EBRT with seed boost in select patients with unfavourable features such as Gleason 4 + 3
High risk	Prostatectomy in selected patients, EBRT to prostate, EBRT to prostate and pelvic nodes, EBRT to prostate and pelvic nodes with brachytherapy boost
Locally advanced ± nodes	EBRT to prostate, EBRT to prostate and pelvic nodes

EBRT, External beam radiotherapy; *LDR*, low-dose rate.

Treatment guide in prostate cancer. Treatment based on risk stratification as in Table 28.6 could guide treatment decisions.

Androgen-deprivation therapy in high-risk prostate cancer. It is now accepted that for men with locally advanced prostate cancer (T3/4 Gleason Score 8–10), longer-term hormonal therapy of at least 2 years improves survival over a shorter 6-month therapy. It is important that hormonal therapy is given concurrently with the RT. In our institution, we offer 3 months of neoadjuvant and concurrent hormonal therapy before stopping the adjuvant hormonal therapy after 2 years if the

PSA is 0.1 or less. The definition of treatment failure following radical RT is the nadir PSA value posttreatment + 2 ng/mL as per the Phoenix consensus conference definition.

Salvage Radiotherapy

Following surgery, biochemical failure is defined as two consecutive rising PSA levels and a PSA of greater than 0.2 ng/mL. Aim to institute treatment before PSA rises above 0.5 ng/mL. The RTOG 96–01 study shows a 5% improvement in survival at 12 years with the addition of

2 years of bicalutamide, 150 mg. This benefit was more pronounced in patients with PSA >0.7.

Technique and dose/fractionation schedule. Technique and dose/fractionation schedule should be as follows:

For prostate bed: 3-field, CT-planned conformal RT using 15 MV photons; 52.5 Gy in 20 daily fractions over 4 weeks (or equivalent) to isocentre for microscopic disease (55 Gy in 20 daily fractions to be considered in cases with macroscopic disease).

For prostate bed and pelvic lymph nodes: 66 Gy in 33 daily fractions using VMAT.

For PTV prostate bed: CTV with 1 cm margin except 0.6 cm posteriorly; 64 Gy in 32 daily fractions.

For PTV Pelvic Lymph nodes: CTV Lymph nodes + 0.5 cm isotropic margin; 52 – 54 Gy in 33 daily fractions.

Metastatic Disease

Androgen-deprivation therapy. Most prostatic tumours contain elements sensitive to the androgenic hormone testosterone. Hormonal treatment is designed to reduce levels of testosterone circulating in the blood. This may be achieved in a number of different ways:

1. Removal of the testes, which secrete testosterone (orchidectomy).
2. Chemical compounds, similar to luteinising hormone-releasing hormone (LHRH analogues), which diminish the pituitary production of luteinising hormone (LH) and thus reduce testosterone production; these are administered by a monthly or 3-monthly depot injection.
3. Oral agents, which block the cellular action of androgens (e.g. cyproterone acetate, biclutamide).
4. Oral oestrogens, for example, diethylstilbestrol (out of fashion because of higher cardiovascular risks and development of newer agents).

About 80% of patients will respond to hormonal therapy. The median duration of response is 18 to 24 months. Early intervention with hormonal therapy reduces complications of the disease, such as pathological fractures; however, it does not appear to improve survival. In general, androgen deprivation is achieved today using either an LHRH analogue or an LHRH antagonist. Antiandrogen monotherapy (bicalutamide 150 mg alone) has shown inferior biochemical outcomes compared with an LHRH agent. Patients who progress on androgen-deprivation therapy (ADT) could be considered for maximum androgen blockade (MAB) with addition of an antiandrogen such as bicalutamide, 50 mg once daily. The median duration of response for patients on MAB is approximately 10 months. Patients with poor fitness, who progress on MAB may be considered for low-dose dexamethasone, 0.5 mg instead of the antiandrogen. Fitter patients who progress on an LHRH agent alone or MAB, should be offered systemic therapy, such as docetaxel or abiraterone or enzalutamide.

Up-front docetaxel or abiraterone. Recent evidence from the STAMPEDE study (**S**ystemic **T**herapy in **A**dvancing or **M**etastatic **P**rostate cancer: **E**valuation of **D**rug **E**fficacy) shows that adding a stronger anticancer agent earlier in the treatment, within 12 weeks of ADT has improved overall survival in men with metastatic prostate cancer. Consider chemotherapy, six cycles of docetaxel or the CYP17 blocker, abiraterone, for hormone-naïve new presentation of metastatic prostate cancer.

Agents in management of metastatic castrate-resistant prostate cancer. There are now multiple agents that could be considered for metastatic castrate-resistant prostate cancer (CRPCa). Docetaxel, 75 mg/m^2 once every 21 days with prednisolone, 5 mg twice daily (bd), continuously over 6 to 10 cycles have demonstrated a 3-month survival advantage over mitoxantrone in the TAX 327 (Taxane 327) study. Both abiraterone (CYP17 blocker) and enzalutamide

(a novel antiandrogen) have been approved for use either pre- or post-docetaxel in the United Kingdom. Ra-223 is a bone-seeking isotope of radium that has shown to improve survival and pain in symptomatic, bone-only metastatic CRPCa. The dosage for cabazitaxel is 20 to 25 mg/m^2 once every 21 days; up to 10 cycles are approved post-docetaxel in patients with metastatic CRPCa.

Palliative radiotherapy. RT has a useful role in relieving pain from bone metastases. It can also shrink advanced local disease causing symptoms of outflow obstruction and pelvic nodes causing lymph-edema and nerve compression.

Technique. Parallel-opposed field or single fields to be considered depending upon the location of the metastasis.

Dose and energy.

1. Prostate: 30 Gy in 10 daily fractions over 2 weeks (10 – 15 MV photons) using a parallel-opposed field.
2. Bone metastases confined to a limited area, for example, lumbar spine: single fraction of 8 Gy or 20 Gy in 5 daily fractions (6 – 15 MV photons).

Widespread hemibody irradiation. Where there are widespread painful bony metastases, hemibody irradiation may be considered to encompass all the painful areas. Improvement in pain control tends to be prompt and may last the few months until death. Treatment of the lower half of the body is better tolerated because the side effects are minimal.

Preparation. The patient is given intravenous fluids and fasted before treatment. Regular antiemetics are given before and after treatment.

Treatment volume. For the lower half, the field usually extends from the umbilicus to the knees and for the upper half, from the top of the head to the umbilicus. Overlap with the lower field is avoided.

Acute reaction. Nausea and vomiting occur at the end of treatment and last for up to 6 hours. Lethargy is common. If the upper half is treated, hair loss starts at about 10 days. The mouth becomes dry and taste sensation is altered. The blood count reaches its low point between 10 and 14 days. Hemoglobin, white blood cell and platelet counts are all reduced (pancytopenia) and remain so for up to 8 weeks. Cough and shortness of breath occurring at 6 weeks are usually indicative of radiation pneumonitis. If both halves of the body are treated, an interval of at least 6 weeks is left after the first hemibody irradiation to allow the systemic effects to settle and the blood count to recover.

Technique. The patient is treated supine. Parallel-opposed anterior and posterior fields are used at extended focus skin distance (FSD) (140 cm).

Dose and Energy. For lower half of body, use 8-Gy midplane dose in a single fraction (9–10 MV photons).

For upper half of body, use 6-Gy midplane dose in a single fraction (9–10 MV photons).

TESTIS

Anatomy

Each testis (the diminutive form *testicle* is also in common use, with its adjective *testicular*) lies within a fibrous capsule (tunica albuginea) inside the scrotum (Fig 28.12). In the embryo, the testes arise on the posterior abdominal wall and migrate downwards through the inguinal canal to the scrotum.

The testis is divided into 200 to 300 lobules. Each of these contains one to three seminiferous tubules. These drain into the epididymis, which lies on the posterior border of the testis. The lymphatic drainage of the testis is to the paraaortic nodes. Note that the skin of the scrotum drains to the inguinal nodes. To avoid surgical contamination of the scrotal skin, the testis is surgically removed through an inguinal incision.

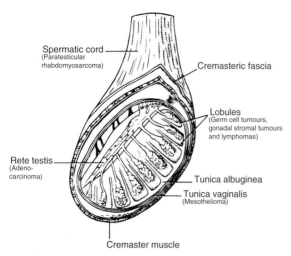

Fig. 28.12 Diagram of testis and spermatic cord indicating sites of tumour origin. Paratesticular rhabdomyosarcoma may arise from connective tissue of the cord or of adjacent structures. (From, Williams CJ, Krikorian JG, Green MR. Textbook of uncommon cancers. Wiley & Sons Limited, 1988. With permission.)

Pathology

Aetiology

The main factor predisposing to the development of germ cell tumours of the testis is an undescended testis. This accounts for 10% of cases. The risk is increased fivefold if one testis is maldescended and 12-fold if both are maldescended. However, even if one testis is maldescended, there is an increased risk of testicular cancer in the normally descended testis on the other side. Intratubular germ cell neoplasia or carcinoma in situ is a premalignant condition, which gives rise to malignancy in 50% of patients within 5 years.

Testicular cancer is the most common form of malignancy in men between the ages of 20 and 40 years. The incidence is rising, possibly through increased exposure to environmental oestrogens. Currently, there are about 2300 new cases per year in the United Kingdom (year 2015 figures). Testicular cancer accounts for 0.1% of deaths from cancer. The types of common (germ cell tumours) and rarer tumours and their sites of origin in the testis are illustrated in Fig. 28.12.

Germ cell tumours. There are two main tumour types that arise from the germ cells: seminoma and teratoma. Teratoma occurs mainly between the ages of 20 and 35 years, and seminoma between ages 25 and 40 years. Over the age of 50 years, tumours are more likely to be nongerm-cell tumours. These are non-Hodgkin lymphomas and tumours arising from other structures of the testis (Sertoli and Leydig cell tumours). Paratesticular rhabdomyosarcoma (see Fig. 28.12) occurs in infancy and in young adult life.

Seminoma. Seminoma is the most common type of germ cell tumour (60%). It arises from the cells of the seminiferous tubules. Seminoma is solid with a pale cut surface like a potato. There are two principal types: classical and spermatocytic. The characteristic histological feature of classical seminoma is its uniform appearance. The cells are rounded with a central nucleus and clear cytoplasm. The tumour is divided into lobules by a fibrous stroma, associated with a variable infiltration of lymphocytes.

Spread of seminoma may be local to the epididymis and to the spermatic cord, but lymphatic spread is more important. The first group of nodes to be invaded is the upper paraaortic, at the level of the renal hilum. Further lymphatic spread may be upward to the mediastinum and even to the supraclavicular nodes through the thoracic duct, or downward to the lower paraaortic and pelvic nodes. If extratesticular

tissues of the scrotum are invaded, including the scrotal skin, their draining inguinal lymph nodes may be invaded. Bloodborne spread is much less common.

Spermatocytic seminoma is uncommon and generally seen in older men. The tumour cells show differentiation to spermatocytes, and their behavior is benign. Metastases are extremely rare.

Teratoma. Teratoma accounts for the remainder of germ cell tumours. Strictly speaking, a teratoma shows differentiation towards all three embryological germ cell layers of ectoderm (e.g. skin, neural tissue), endoderm (e.g. gut, bronchi) and mesoderm (e.g. fat, cartilage). In practice, the British classification applies the term more widely (although American terminology refers to this group as nonseminomatous germ cell tumours). Teratomas are subtyped according to their cell constituents as:

- Teratoma differentiated
- Malignant teratoma intermediate
- Malignant teratoma undifferentiated
- Malignant teratoma trophoblastic

Teratoma differentiated (TD) shows cysts lined by various mature-looking epithelium surrounded by smooth muscle, with islands of cartilage and neural tissue. In infants, its behavior is benign but, in adults, it is rare and can give rise to metastases. Malignant teratoma undifferentiated (MTU), by contrast, has no recognisable differentiated structures, but has undifferentiated rather than carcinomatous tissue. It often has tissue resembling yolk sac (YST), and there are frequently syncytiotrophoblast giant cells. These account for secretion of alpha-fetoprotein (AFP) and human chorionic gonadotrophin (HCG), respectively, which can be measured in the blood and are invaluable as markers of tumour load. MTU has an aggressive clinical behavior with early metastasis via lymphatics to paraaortic lymph nodes, and bloodborne spread to the lungs. Malignant teratoma intermediate (MTI) has a mixture of differentiated and undifferentiated tissues. Malignant teratoma trophoblastic (MTT) has tissue resembling gestational choriocarcinoma (i.e. syncytiotrophoblast and cytotrophoblast), either throughout or in combination with features of other teratomas. Large amounts of HCG are secreted and the clinical course is very aggressive with widespread bloodborne metastases.

Tumour Markers

The two tumour markers, AFP and HCG are helpful in the diagnosis, staging and monitoring of response to treatment (Fig. 28.13). AFP has a half-life of about 5 days. It is produced by yolk sac elements but is not specific to teratoma. Elevated levels occur in the presence of liver damage. HCG is mainly a marker of trophoblastic neoplasms; it can, however, occur in seminoma. The half-life of HCG is 24 hours and of the beta subunit, 45 minutes. Markers for the presence of seminoma are much less reliable. Serum placental alkaline phosphatase (PLAP) is often raised in the presence of seminoma, particularly if there is bulky disease. However, false-positive and false-negative results for PLAP are common. Lactate dehydrogenase (LDH) is an important nonspecific marker of disease volume and has been incorporated into the International Germ Cell Consensus Classification (Table 28.7).

Clinical Features

Testicular germ cell neoplasia usually present as a gradually enlarging painless testicular swelling, although atrophy of a testis may occur. The tumour feels hard. Around 30% of patients describe pain in the testis, and an equal number of patients present with a dragging sensation. A small number of patients give a history of trauma. The first symptoms and signs may be of metastatic spread (hemoptysis from lung metastases, back pain from paraaortic metastases, loin pain from ureteric obstruction or neck lymphadenopathy). Malignant

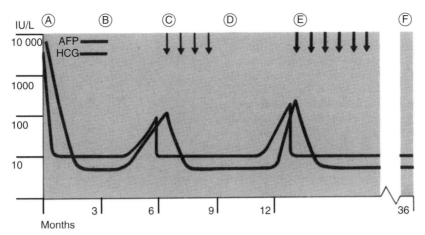

Fig. 28.13 Tumour markers in the management of testicular cancer. (A) Both human chorionic gonadotrophin *(HCG)* and alpha-fetoprotein *(AFP)* are elevated before orchidectomy but fall following operation (HCG more rapidly because of its short half-life). (B) No evidence of recurrence, followed by a rise in marker levels. (C) Combination chemotherapy for recurrence is followed by a fall in levels to normal (D). (E) A further rise in marker levels is treated more intensively and the patient is disease free at 3 years (F). (From Souhami, Moxham. Textbook of medicine. London: Churchill Livingstone; 1990. With permission.)

TABLE 28.7 The International Germ Cell Consensus Classification (IGCCC) Prognostic Grouping

Teratoma	Seminoma
Good prognosis with all of:	
Testis/retroperitoneal primary	Any primary site
No nonpulmonary visceral metastases	No nonpulmonary visceral metastases
AFP <1000 ng/mL	Normal AFP
HCG <5000 IU/L	Any HCG
LDH <1.5 upper limit of normal	Any LDH
56% of teratomas	90% of seminomas
5-year survival, 92%	5-year survival, 86%
Intermediate prognosis with all of:	
Testis/retroperitoneal primary	Any primary site
No nonpulmonary visceral metastases	Nonpulmonary visceral metastases
AFP ≥1000 and ≤10,000 ng/mL or	Normal AFP
HCG ≥5000 and ≤50,000 IU/L or	Any HCG
LDH ≥1.5 normal and ≤10 normal	Any LDH
28% of teratomas	10% of seminomas
5-year survival, 80%	5-year survival, 73%
Poor prognosis with any of:	
Mediastinal primary or nonpulmonary visceral metastases	No patients classified as poor prognosis
AFP >10,000 ng/mL or	
HCG >50,000 IU/L or	
LDH >10 normal	
16% of teratomas	
5-year survival, 48%	

AFP, Alpha-Fetoprotein; *HCG*, human chorionic gonadotrophin; *IU*, International Units; *LDH*, lactate dehydrogenase.

teratoma trophoblastic (choriocarcinoma) may produce gynaecomastia (breast enlargement).

Diagnosis and Staging

The diagnosis of testicular germ cell neoplasia is made by surgical removal of the testis through an inguinal incision (inguinal orchidectomy) and histological examination. Immunocytochemical stains of the tumour for the presence of AFP and HCG may be positive. Blood levels of AFP and HCG are measured pre- and postoperatively. A chest radiograph is required (for overt lung metastases), together with a CT scan of the thorax (for small-volume lung and mediastinal metastases) and of the abdomen (abdominal nodal and liver metastases).

The Royal Marsden staging classification (Table 28.8), based on the extent of spread and bulk of disease, has been widely used for determining management. Although still useful for seminoma stage II nodal size subgrouping, it has been largely superseded by the International Germ Cell Consensus Classification (IGCCC) prognostic grouping.

TABLE 28.8 The Royal Marsden Hospital Staging Classification of Testicular Tumours

Stage	Clinical Findings
Mk+	Rising serum markers with no other evidence of metastases
I	No evidence of metastases
II	Abdominal node involvement
a	<2 cm diameter
b	2–5 cm diameter
c	>5 cm diameter
III	Nodal involvement above the diaphragm
IV	Extralymphatic metastases
L1	Lung metastases ≤3 in number
L2	Lung metastases >3 in number (all ≤2 cm or less in diameter)
L3	Lung metastases >3 in number (>2 cm in diameter)

Treatment

Seminoma

Stage I. The majority (70%) present as stage I disease. Approximately 15% to 20%, however, will relapse; 90% of which will be in the paraaortic nodes. There is a slight increased chance of relapse with tumours larger than 4 cm or rete testis invasion. Options include surveillance, prophylactic irradiation or adjuvant chemotherapy.

Surveillance. This is the preferred option for stage I disease for many patients and the importance of attendance for clinic and follow-up scans should be discussed with the patient. Active surveillance for patients with stage I seminoma results in a relapse rate of 17% and a cause-specific survival of 99.7%. Approximately 2% of stage I seminoma patients on active surveillance will relapse after 2 years, accounting for 9% of all relapses.

Adjuvant radiotherapy. Depending upon patient preference or if there is concern about subsequent fitness for curative chemotherapy in the event of relapse, adjuvant RT should be strongly considered. Prophylactic irradiation of the paraaortic and if indicated, the ipsilateral pelvic nodes reduces the relapse rate to 2% to 3%. The medical research council testicular cancer study 18 (MRC TE18), has shown that 20 Gy in 10 daily fractions to the para-aortic strip can safely replace the previous standard of 30 Gy in 15 daily fractions.

Adjuvant chemotherapy. The Medical research council testicular cancer study 19 (MRC TE19) showed that Carboplatin prescribed to a dose of area-under-curve (AUC) 7 (based on glomerular filtration rate calculated using ethylenediamine tetraacetic acid (EDTA) clearance) reduces the relapse rate to about the same as RT; however, the duration of follow-up in the TE 19 study is shorter. The site of relapse is often the paraaortic nodes. Hence, follow-up must include CT or MRI scanning of abdomen.

Spermatocytic seminoma is a different pathological entity to classical seminoma and no further treatment is indicated following orchidectomy.

Stage IIa. Stage IIa disease (nodes ≤2 cm) can be treated with either postoperative dog-leg RT (30 Gy in 15 fractions) or chemotherapy.

Stage IIb. Based on the Royal Marsden hospital experience, for stage IIb (nodes 2–5 cm), a single cycle of carboplatin at AUC7 followed by paraaortic RT (30 Gy in 15 fractions) has shown to reduce the relapse rate by less than 10% at 5 years, which is similar to good-prognosis seminomas treated with three cycles of bleomycin, etoposide and cisplatin (BEP) or four cycles of cisplatin and etoposide.

Radiotherapy target volume. The upper margin of the paraaortic field is at the level of the junction of the 10th and 11th thoracic vertebrae. The lower limit is the junction of the 5th lumbar vertebra and the first sacral vertebra. Where there has been previous inguinoscrotal surgery, such as hernia repair, the field is extended to cover the ipsilateral pelvic and inguinal nodes (Fig. 28.14). This 'dog-leg'-shaped field is vertical in the paraaortic region and diverges at the level of the junction of the fourth and fifth lumbar vertebrae. The lower limit of the field is the bottom of the obturator foramina and should include the inguinal scar. In addition, previous orchidopexy, removal of the testis through the scrotum or extension of tumour to the tunica vaginalis, requires the ipsilateral scrotum to be irradiated.

Technique. The patient is simulated supine with feet in foot stocks and hands by the side. CT-based simulation and planning allows better visualisation and efficient use of multileaf collimators (MLCs) to shield as much of the normal tissue as possible.

Paraaortic strip radiotherapy: Used for adjuvant radiotherapy in Stage I seminoma when there is no previous inguinoscrotal surgery. An anterior and posterior pair of fields is used. The patient is simulated supine at normal FSD. The width of the paraaortic field is normally 8 to 10 cm. The field is offset to include the renal hilar nodes on the side of

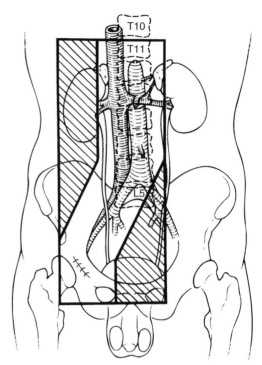

Fig. 28.14 Treatment volume for ipsilateral pelvic and paraaortic (dog-leg) irradiation for testicular seminoma.

the orchidectomy. The contralateral border is the lateral extent of the pedicle of the vertebral body. Care should be taken not to include more than one-third of the renal substance within the paraaortic fields on either side.

Dog-leg radiotherapy: Used for adjuvant radiotherapy in Stage I seminoma where patients had previous inguinoscrotal surgery or in stage IIa disease. An anterior and posterior pair of fields is used. The patient is simulated supine throughout, if treatment under couch at an extended FSD (about 140 cm) can be achieved. MLCs protect tissue outside the treatment volume. Care should be taken not to include more than one-third of the renal substance within the paraaortic fields on either side. If there is involvement of the lower paraaortic nodes and risk of retrograde spread to the pelvic lymph nodes, then an 'inverted Y'-shaped field should be used to treat the paraaortic and pelvic nodes. If the hemiscrotum is to be treated, a direct electron field of appropriate energy, or 300 kV x-rays may be used with shielding of the contralateral testis.

Dose and energy. Seminoma is one of the most radiosensitive of all cancers and can be cured with relatively modest doses. The present standard dose is:

Stage I: 20 Gy in 10 daily fractions over 2 weeks (9–16 MV photons) to the PA strip and consider dog-leg field in cases of scrotal contamination.

Stage IIa: 30 Gy in 15 fractions over 3 weeks (9–16 MV photons) using dog-leg field.

Stage IIb: 30 Gy in 15 fractions over 3 weeks (9–16 MV photons) to the PA strip 4 to 6 weeks after carboplatin at AUC7.

Acute reaction. About 50% of patients will experience nausea lasting for 2 to 3 hours following treatment. Regular use of a 5-HT$_3$ antagonist is recommended.

Late reactions. Late side effects are rare. Dyspepsia occurs in 5%, occasionally with evidence of peptic ulceration. Using the radiation technique and dosage described, the dose to the contralateral testis is very low (less than 0.5 Gy). Nonetheless, this dose is sufficient to cause a moderate reduction in sperm count for 2 to 3 years, but it is not associated with permanent infertility. There are some concerns about the

TABLE 28.9 Bleomycin, Etoposide and Cisplatin Chemotherapy Regimen

Bleomycin	30,000 units IV infusion	Days 1, 8, 15
Etoposide	100 mg/m^2 IV infusion	Days 1–5
Cisplatin	20 mg/m^2 IV infusion	Days 1–5
Repeated every 21 days		

IV, Intravenous.

long-term complications of adjuvant RT, such as second malignancy and hypertension.

Stage IIc, III and IV. Four cycles of combination chemotherapy with BEP (Table 28.9) are recommended for these stages. In good-prognosis seminoma in men aged over 40 years or in those with previous chest irradiation, etoposide and cisplatin (EP) may be used to decrease the risks of bleomycin lung.

Results of Treatment. The results of treatment in early-stage seminoma are excellent, reflecting its radiosensitivity: 5-year survival rates by stage are 95% for stage I and 90% for stages IIa and IIb. For more advanced stages, cure rates have improved with the availability of effective combination chemotherapy: 5-year survival for stages IIc and III is 75% and for stage IV, 65%.

Teratoma

Stage I. Teratoma has a higher incidence of extralymphatic spread. In the presence of extralymphatic metastases, irradiating the paraaortic nodes prophylactically may compromise the ability to deliver subsequent combination chemotherapy at desired dosage and frequency. About 30% of patients with stage I disease following orchidectomy will have subclinical metastases and will relapse (80% of whom will relapse in the first 12 months). To avoid overtreatment of the majority of patients, a policy of close surveillance with treatment at relapse is recommended. Patients with lymphatic or vascular invasion are at greater risk of relapse (40%) and are not suitable for surveillance. Such patients are best treated by two cycles of adjuvant combination chemotherapy.

Surveillance. In patients for whom a surveillance policy is adopted, tumour markers, chest x-ray (CXR) and clinical examination are performed monthly in the first year with 3-monthly CT scans of chest and abdomen. In the second year, follow-up should be 2-monthly with CT scans at 18 and 24 months. Subsequent follow-up should be 3-monthly for the third year, 6-monthly to the fifth year and annually thereafter to 10 years.

Stages II–IV. These stages should be managed by combination chemotherapy (see later).

Cytotoxic chemotherapy. The development of curative combination chemotherapy for advanced testicular cancer in the 1980s has been one of the most important advances in oncology.

The combinations of drugs used for treating seminoma are the same for teratoma. The most effective regimens contain cisplatin. Cisplatin was successfully combined with vinblastine and bleomycin (PVB). Now, vinblastine is replaced by etoposide, which is less myelotoxic, without loss of efficacy. This regime is known as BEP (see Table 28.9). An attempt to reduce toxicity by replacing cisplatin with carboplatin has proved to be less effective. Before each course of chemotherapy, a number of investigations are carried out to assess fitness to treat, and to modify dosage if necessary, because of the toxicity of the agents. A full blood count is required because of the myelotoxicity of etoposide.

Cisplatin is toxic to the kidney and to hearing. Renal function tests (serum urea, electrolytes and creatinine, 24-hour urine creatinine clearance or formal EDTA GFR) and hearing (audiometry) should be measured before, during and after treatment.

Bleomycin can be toxic to the lung (see below). Full lung function tests (including gas transfer factor) are carried out before treatment and repeated if toxicity is suspected.

Sperm storage, if available, is desirable for men wishing to father children following chemotherapy because sterility is commonly induced. Normally, an initial sample is examined to count the number and motility of the sperm. If satisfactory, two additional samples are taken for sperm banking. However, chemotherapy, if urgently required, should not be delayed to await this procedure.

Dosage and scheduling. Normally, four courses of BEP are given at 3-weekly intervals. Patients with good-risk disease can be cured with just three cycles as demonstrated in the MRC TE 20 trial without compromising the 90% overall survival. For those patients in the intermediate- or poor-risk IGCCC groups, survival is 40% to 70%. Efforts to increase the efficacy of chemotherapy schedules through dose intensification and new combinations are ongoing. As yet, there has been no improvement over standard BEP.

Monitoring response to treatment. Clinical examination, chest radiograph, tumour markers, full blood count and renal function tests are repeated before each cycle of treatment to monitor the response to and toxicity of treatment.

Following surgery, a fall in tumour marker levels in line with their half-lives usually indicates that there is no residual disease. A slower fall or rising levels suggest residual disease.

It may be necessary to delay the next cycle of chemotherapy or modify its dosage if blood count, renal function or hearing deteriorate below certain thresholds. Every effort should be made to deliver the chemotherapy on schedule and granulocyte colony-stimulating factor (GCSF) support may be required. Chemotherapy should not be given if the neutrophil count is below 1.0×10^9/L. CT scan of chest and abdomen is repeated after three cycles to confirm that the disease is responding. Rapid resolution of disease is usual after the first course. Residual 2 to 4 cm masses may, however, persist for several years.

Management of residual abdominal masses. Resection of residual abdominal masses following chemotherapy is indicated for teratoma. Seminoma resection is difficult and usually not indicated because of a lack of tissue planes and tumour infiltration beyond resection margins. A policy of observation is usually recommended. Resection of residual masses after treatment for teratoma shows that most of them (44%) are the result of differentiated (mature) teratoma or to fibrosis and necrosis (34%). Residual tumour is found in 22% of cases. If recurrence occurs, as it does in 10% to 20% of patients, it is most likely to develop at a site of initial involvement. If surgical expertise is available, resection of residual masses is desirable. It serves both as a diagnostic and therapeutic procedure. Further chemotherapy is indicated if residual disease is found, but the outlook is poor, with less than 50% of such patients remaining free of disease.

Toxicity. In addition to renal damage and ototoxicity (impaired hearing), cisplatin causes severe nausea and vomiting, and peripheral neuropathy. The 5-HT antagonists (ondansetron and granisetron) can reduce nausea and vomiting. Intravenous hydration is required 24 hours before cisplatin is given and for 24 hours afterwards to reduce the risk of renal damage. Nonetheless, the majority of patients will experience temporary renal damage. A 20% to 25% reduction in glomerular filtration rate is usual.

Etoposide causes alopecia and myelosuppression. The incidence of septicemia with etoposide is less than with vinblastine because it is less myelosuppressive.

Bleomycin may cause pneumonitis. Presentation is with progressive dyspnea. This complication may occur after relatively modest doses (e.g. 200 mg). It can be progressive, is irreversible and carries a 1%

mortality. Other side effects are fever, skin rashes, pigmentation and Raynaud's phenomenon.

Results of treatment. Some 90% of patients with small-volume disease are cured following chemotherapy. For large-volume disease in extralymphatic sites, the probability of survival is reduced to 50% to 70%.

The 5-year survival is 90% for stages I and IIa, 70% for stages IIb and III, and 50% to 60% for stage IV.

TESTICULAR LYMPHOMA

Testicular lymphomas are rare (4% of testicular tumours). They are mainly non-Hodgkin lymphomas. Most patients present at an early stage with a unilateral testicular mass; however, bilateral testicular involvement occurs in about 10% of the cases. Clinical features that help to differentiate them from germ cell tumours are an older age group (age >50 years), different pattern of metastases, absence of maldescent and of gynaecomastia. They are usually of high grade (diffuse large B cell) and contralateral testis and brain are sanctuary sites. Patients initially undergo orchidectomy. The recommended treatment for stages IAE and IIAE are a combination of six cycles of combination chemotherapy using rituximab, cyclophosphamide, doxorubicin, vincristine and prednisolone, commonly called as R-CHOP regime and RT to the scrotum (IA) and involved nodes (IIA) and central nervous system (CNS)-directed therapy with either intrathecal methotrexate or high dose intravenous methotrexate. Treatment of stages III and IV disease is not different from early-stage disease with chemotherapy, CNS prophylaxis and scrotal irradiation.

Dose and Energy

Stage IA: Prophylactic radiotherapy to the scrotum including remaining testicle to a dose of 30 Gy in 15 fractions over 3 weeks using 6 MV photons or electrons of appropriate energy.

Stage IIA: In addition to scrotal radiotherapy, the involved nodal basin should be treated to 30 Gy in 15 daily fractions over 3 weeks (6 – 15 MV photons) using a parallel opposed field or 3-D conformal technique.

Results of Treatment

With aggressive treatment approaches, the outcome of primary testicular lymphoma is improving. Prognosis is based on a 5-point scoring system, international prognostic index (IPI): 1 point each for stage III/IV disease, raised LDH, performance status 2 or more, age older than 60 years and more than 1 extra nodal site. Depending upon the IPI score, the 5-year overall survival ranges from 25% to 75%.

URETHRA

Tumours of the urethra are rare and are usually transitional carcinomas. Predisposing factors are as for bladder cancer. Presenting symptoms and signs are pain and hematuria.

Female Urethra

The tumour is twice as common in women as in men. In the proximal third, transitional carcinoma predominates and, in the distal two-thirds, squamous carcinoma predominates. The distal urethra drains to the inguinal nodes and the proximal urethra to the iliac nodes. Presenting features are offensive discharge, bleeding or a mass.

Treatment

Surgery in the form of a cystourethrectomy is perhaps the treatment of choice. In those who are unsuitable, then attempts at organ preservation can be considered. For superficial squamous carcinoma of the urethral orifice, three iridium hairpins are an alternative treatment. A dose of 60 to 65 Gy is given in 6 to 7 days. For more proximal lesions, radical external beam irradiation using an anterior and two lateral wedged fields is used. A dose of 55 Gy is given in 20 daily fractions over 4 weeks using megavoltage.

Results of Treatment

The cure rates with surgery and RT are similar, at about 50%.

PENIS

Cancer of the penis is a rare tumour in the United Kingdom with an age-standardised incidence rate of 2.3 and mortality of 0.5 per 100,000 men. The incidence increases with age and is common during the sixth decade of life, although it does occur in younger men. The disease is more common in Southeast Asia, China and Africa. In Uganda, penile carcinoma is currently the most commonly diagnosed male cancer.

Pathology
Aetiology

Human papilloma virus (HPV) is an important risk factor for penile cancer, however, it remains unclear if an HPV-related penile cancer has a different prognosis compared with non-HPV-related penile cancer. It is less prevalent in communities practicing neonatal circumcision, as this removes approximately half the tissue that can develop into penile cancer. Phimosis is present in up to 50% of cases. Poor penile hygiene is thought to be an important predisposing factor. Other risk factors include smoking, chronic penile inflammation and premalignant conditions such as giant condylomata, erythroplasia of Queyrat, Bowen disease and Paget disease. Squamous cell carcinoma accounts for the majority of the penile cancers, and other rare pathologies include sarcomatoid carcinoma, adenosquamous carcinoma and mucoepidermoid carcinoma.

Clinical Features

These tumours occur as warty growths or, more commonly, as indurated ulcers on the glans or the sulcus at the base of the glans. Symptoms have often been present for a year or more before presentation. The first sign may be an infected or bloody discharge from beneath the prepuce. Growth is superficial at first, then by invasion of the penile shaft. If the lesion is visible, the diagnosis is usually obvious. If phimosis hides it, the glans must be exposed by incising and peeling back the prepuce (dorsal slit) or by complete circumcision, under anaesthesia. A biopsy is taken at the same time.

Inguinal and pelvic nodes are the regional drainage basin for the penis. Lymphatic spread first occurs to the inguinal nodes (superficial and deep) and then to the ipsilateral pelvic nodes. Bloodborne metastases are rare and late.

Staging

Both the UICC TNM 8 and Jackson staging systems are in use (Table 28.10). Physical examination is an important part of the diagnostic process and an MRI can provide valuable information to assess local invasion to aid surgical planning. Conventional cross-sectional imaging such as CT or MRI can be used to assess regional nodes and distant metastatic disease. However, the risk of micrometastatic disease to the draining lymph nodes is 25% even in the absence of clinically palpable disease, and these imaging modalities are often unreliable to detect micrometastatic disease. There are no established tumour markers in penile cancers.

TABLE 28.10 Union for International Cancer Control TNM 8 and Jackson Staging Systems for Penile Cancer

Stage	Clinical Findings
Tumour	
Tis	Carcinoma in situ (penile intraepithelial neoplasia, PeIN)
Ta	Noninvasive localised squamous cell carcinoma
T1	Tumour invades subepithelial connective tissue
T1a	Tumour invades subepithelial connective tissue without lymphovascular invasion or perineural invasion and is not poorly differentiated
T1b	Tumour invades subepithelial connective tissue with lymphovascular invasion or perineural invasion or is poorly differentiated
T2	Tumour invades corpus spongiosum with or without invasion of the urethra
T3	Tumour invades corpora cavernosum
T4	Tumour invades other adjacent structures
Nodes	
N0	No palpable or visibly enlarged inguinal lymph nodes
N1	Palpable mobile unilateral inguinal lymph node
N2	Palpable mobile multiple or bilateral lymph nodes
N3	Palpable fixed inguinal nodal mass or pelvic lymphadenopathy, unilateral or bilateral
Metastases	
M0	No distant metastases
M1	Distant metastasis – includes lymph node metastasis outside of the true pelvis in addition to visceral or bone sites
Jackson classification	
I	Tumour confined to the glans or prepuce
II	Tumour extending on to the shaft of the penis
III	Tumour with operable inguinal nodes
IV	Tumour with inoperable metastases

Treatment

Superficial noninvasive disease could be treated with topical chemotherapy such as imiquimod or 5-FU, laser treatment, photodynamic therapy and total or partial glans resurfacing. Surgery and RT are the main treatments for invasive penile cancer. Factors that influence the choice of treatment, are the age and general condition of the patient, the extent of the disease, the desire to retain sexual function and the capacity to pass urine in the standing position for young males. In patients with locally advanced disease, cisplatin-based neoadjuvant chemotherapy followed by surgery may be considered for responders.

Surgery

Specialised surgical techniques are now available, which can excise early invasive tumours and reconstruct the penis with a split skin graft for an excellent cosmetic and functional result. More advanced tumours involving the deeper corpora and urethra require amputation of part or the whole of the penis. Although curative if the inguinal nodes are not involved, the procedure is associated with considerable psychological morbidity, especially for young males.

Radiotherapy

Radical RT is still an effective treatment for early penile cancer because it permits the organ to be conserved. However, if there is deep invasion of the shaft, the chances of control by radiation are poor and surgery is preferable. Invasion of the urethra also favors surgery because postradiation fibrotic stricture is very liable to occur. Circumcision should be considered in appropriate patients if planned for RT because this allows better inspection and staging of the lesion.

Treatment techniques and dosage. The choice of technique and energy will depend on the extent and site of the disease. For tumours confined to the glans or the prepuce, superficial, orthovoltage, electron beam or implants are possibilities. For infiltrating tumours or where the inguinal nodes are involved, megavoltage irradiation is required. In general, a total dose less than 60 Gy (2 Gy/fraction) to the primary tumour is associated with higher risk of local recurrence.

Implantation. Brachytherapy for penile cancers is rarely done in the United Kingdom. Tumours greater than 4 cm in any dimension or invading the corpora cavernosa should not be implanted. A recent French study on long-term outcomes with penile brachytherapy suggests a good local control with a local relapse rate of 18.9%, with surgery reserved for local failures. Penile brachytherapy can be done using either an LDR or an HDR implant. In LDR brachytherapy, a two- to three-plane implant should cover the tumour with at least a 1-cm margin. The Paris system of dosimetry is used to guide needle placement at appropriate spacing to cover the lesion with a margin. In general, 12 to 18 mm spacing is acceptable for LDR brachytherapy. LDR brachytherapy is largely superseded by HDR brachytherapy because of advantages of remote afterloading and radioprotection. In an HDR implant, adequate dose coverage could be achieved by dwell position and time adjustment; however, a closer spacing is recommended, generally 10 to 12 mm.

Dose. LDR brachytherapy should be treated with 60 to 65 Gy at 0.5 to 0.6 Gy/h with treatment completed in 5 to 6 days. HDR brachytherapy should be treated with 3.2 Gy twice daily to a total of 38.4 Gy in 6 days.

Superficial or orthovoltage therapy. For very small (T1) superficial tumours, 100- or 250-kV x-ray therapy may suffice. A 0.5 cm margin of normal surrounding tissue is included in the treated volume. A dose of 50 Gy is given in 15 fractions over 3 weeks. Alternatively, low-energy (6 MeV) electrons can be used, using an appropriate thickness of Perspex over the lesion to bring up the surface dose to 100%.

Megavoltage.

Treatment volume. If there is evidence of spread on to the shaft of the penis, the whole of the penis should be treated.

Technique. A rectangular wax block with a central cylindrical cavity is made to encompass the penis and ensure homogeneous irradiation of the whole volume. The penis is treated en bloc by a parallel-opposed pair of lateral fields.

Dose and energy. Doses should be given as 50 to 55 Gy in 20 daily fractions over 4 weeks using megavoltage (4–6 MV) photons or 60 to 66 Gy in 30 to 33 daily fractions over 6 to 7 weeks using megavoltage (4–6 MV) photons.

Acute reactions. Acute reactions are like skin reactions elsewhere but more marked, and moist desquamation is commoner. The urethral reaction causes discomfort and dysuria. If very severe, the reaction may result in acute retention requiring catheterisation.

Late reactions. Late reactions include telangiectasia, skin atrophy, urethral stricture and necrosis. Urethral dilatation is required for stricture. Necrosis occurs in less than 10% of cases.

Management of regional nodes. The management of lymph nodes in clinically node-negative (cN0) patients depends upon stage, grade and presence or absence of lymphovascular invasion. In patients with no palpable nodes, dynamic sentinel node biopsy (DNSB) is promising with a false negative rate of 7%. Early lymphadenectomy in clinically node-negative patients improves overall survival compared with delayed lymph node dissection (at the point of recurrence). Uni- or bilateral palpable lymphadenopathy is very likely disease related and a block dissection of the groin should be carried out. The use of antibiotics to exclude node enlargement because of infection is discouraged. Following management of the lymphatics, the primary tumour can be addressed with radical RT. There is no value in giving prophylactic groin node irradiation. The only role for RT in the treatment of groin nodes is for palliation. For fixed inoperable nodes, neoadjuvant chemotherapy for downstaging before lymphadenectomy for locally advanced patients, can be considered.

Palliative radiotherapy

Technique. Palliative therapy is comprised of a simple parallel-opposed pair of fields to the affected groin.

Dose and energy. Doses should be given as 30 Gy in 10 daily fractions over 2 weeks using 10 – 15 MV photons.

Palliative Chemotherapy

Cisplatin-based chemotherapy can be considered for fit patients. Response rates of 30% to 40% have been reported.

Results of Treatment

Early superficial tumours have a high cure rate: 5-year survival for stage I disease is about 90%. This falls to 60% in stage II and 30% to 40% in stage III.

FURTHER READING

Motzer RJ, Hutson TE, Cella D, et al. Pazopanib versus sunitinib in metastatic renal-cell carcinoma. N Engl J Med 2013;369(8):722–31.

Escudier B, Eisen T, Stadler WM, et al. Sorafenib in advanced clear-cell renal-cell carcinoma. N Engl J Med 2007;356(2):125–34.

Motzer RJ, Escudier B, DF McDermott, George S, Hammers HJ, Srinivas S, et al. Nivolumab versus everolimus in advanced renal-cell carcinoma. N Engl J Med 2015;373(19):1803–13.

Choueiri TK, Escudier B, Powles T, et al. Cabozantinib versus everolimus in advanced renal-cell carcinoma. N Engl J Med 2015;373(19):1814–23.

Vale C. Neoadjuvant chemotherapy in invasive bladder cancer: a systematic review and meta-analysis. Lancet 2003 Jun 7;361(9373):1927–34.

James ND, Hussain SA, Hall E, et al. Radiotherapy with or without chemotherapy in muscle-invasive bladder cancer. N Engl J Med 2012;366(16):1477–88.

Schröder FH, Hugosson J, Roobol MJ, et al. Screening and prostate cancer mortality: results of the European Randomised Study of Screening for Prostate Cancer (ERSPC) at 13 years of follow-up. Lancet 2014;384(9959):2027–35.

Hamdy FC, Donovan JL, Lane JA, et al. 10-Year Outcomes after Monitoring, Surgery, or Radiotherapy for Localized Prostate Cancer. The New England journal of medicine 2016;375(15):1415–24. https://doi.org/10.1056/NEJMoa1606220.

Warde P, Mason M, Ding K, et al. Combined androgen deprivation therapy and radiation therapy for locally advanced prostate cancer: a randomised, phase 3 trial. Lancet 2011;378(9809):2104–11.

Bolla M, Van Tienhoven G, Warde P, et al. External irradiation with or without long-term androgen suppression for prostate cancer with a high metastatic risk: 10-year results of an EORTC randomized study. Lancet Oncol 2010;11(11):1066–73.

Bolla M, De Reijke TM, Van Tienhoven G, et al. Duration of androgen suppression in the treatment of prostate cancer. N Engl J Med 2009;360(24):2516–27.

Dearnaley D, Syndikus I, Mossop H, et al. Conventional versus hypofractionated high-dose intensity-modulated radiotherapy for prostate cancer: 5-year outcomes of the randomised, non-inferiority, phase 3 CHHiP trial. Lancet Oncol 2016;17(8):1047–60.

James ND, Sydes MR, Clarke NW, et al. Addition of docetaxel, zoledronic acid, or both to first-line long-term hormone therapy in prostate cancer (STAMPEDE): survival results from an adaptive, multiarm, multistage, platform randomised controlled trial. Lancet 2016;387:1163–77.

James ND, de Bono JS, Spears MR, et al. Abiraterone for prostate cancer not previously treated with hormone therapy. N Engl J Med 2017;377(4):338–51.

Morris WJ, Tyldesley S, Rodda S, et al. androgen suppression combined with elective nodal and dose escalated radiation therapy (the ASCENDE-RT Trial): an analysis of survival endpoints for a randomized trial comparing a low-dose-rate brachytherapy boost to adose-escalated external beam boost for high- and intermediate-risk prostate cancer. Int J Radiat Oncol 2017;98(2):275–85.

Jones WG, Fossa SD, Mead GM, et al. Randomized trial of 30 versus 20 Gy in the adjuvant treatment of stage I testicular seminoma: a report on Medical Research Council Trial TE18, European Organisation for the Research and Treatment of Cancer Trial 30942 (ISRCTN18525328). J Clin Oncol 2005;23(6):1200–8.

Mosconi AM, Roila F, Gatta G, Theodore C. Cancer of the penis. Crit Rev Oncol Hematol 2005;53:165–77.

Oliver RTD, Mead GM, Rustin GJS, et al. Randomized trial of carboplatin versus radiotherapy for stage I seminoma: mature results on relapse and contralateral testis cancer rates in MRC TE19/EORTC 30982 Study (ISRCTN27163214). J Clin Oncol 2011;29(8):957–62.

De Wit R, Roberts JT, Wilkinson PM, et al. Equivalence of three or four cycles of bleomycin, etoposide and cisplatin chemotherapy and of a 3- or 5-day schedule in good prognosis germ cell cancer; a randomized study of the EORTC and treatment of genitourinary tract cancer group and the MRC. J Clin Oncol 2001;19(6):1629–40.

29

Lymphoma and Disease of Bone Marrow

Matthew Ahearne, Lesley Speed

CHAPTER OUTLINE

INTRODUCTION

Lymphomas present as solid masses arising in lymph nodes or at extranodal sites anywhere in the body, whereas leukaemias and multiple myeloma are diseases primarily of the bone marrow. They are chemo- and radiosensitive and, in contrast to the common solid tumours, many are curable despite being widespread. Treatments range from simple oral chemotherapy and low-dose radiotherapy (RT) to high dose chemotherapy, total body irradiation (TBI) and haemopoietic stem cell transplantation (HSCT). Small molecule inhibitors, monoclonal antibodies, and immunotherapy are also making their way into the clinic.

Lymphomas derive from malignant lymphocytes, with 90% of B cell and 10% of T cell origin. Lymphomas are conventionally divided into Hodgkin's (HL) and non-Hodgkin's (NHL) types. The former, named after Thomas Hodgkin who described it in 1832, is highly curable, whereas NHL is a diverse group of conditions.

Aetiology and Epidemiology

HL accounts for 0.7% of all cancers and 0.4% of cancer deaths. In the United Kingdom, the incidence is 3 per 100,000 population per year in men, and 1.8 in women. There are two age peaks, from 15 to 35 years, and a smaller old-age peak. There is an association with the Epstein-Barr virus (EBV) and with higher social class.

NHL occurs in 11 per 100,000 people and the median age is 55 to 60 years. Childhood incidence is very low, but higher (particularly Burkitt lymphoma) in developing countries. Overall, the male to female ratio is 1.5:1, although this varies between subtypes.

The causes of most NHL are unknown, but the risk is increased in immunodeficiency syndromes, immunosuppression following organ transplantation, acquired immunodeficiency syndrome (AIDS), autoimmune disorders, coeliac disease and following certain infections or exposure to ionising radiation and carcinogenic chemicals. Characteristic acquired chromosomal defects include the following translocations, involving the immunoglobulin (Ig) genes on chromosome 14q32:

- t(14;18)(q32;q21) in about 80% of follicular lymphoma, involving the *BCL2* gene on chromosome 18q21
- t(11;14)(q13;q32) in all cases of mantle-cell lymphoma, involving the *Cyclin D1* gene on chromosome 11q13
- t(8;14)(q24;q32) in Burkitt lymphoma, involving the *MYC* gene on chromosome 8q24

NHL can result from chronic antigenic stimulation of lymphocytes, as in marginal zone lymphoma of mucosa-associated lymphoid tissue (MALT) following *Helicobacter pylori* infection, usually in the stomach or, rarely, following *Chlamydia psittaci* infection. Burkitt lymphoma, originally described in East African children and classically in the jaw, is associated with the EBV. A rare but very aggressive type of

T-cell NHL is caused by infection with the human T-cell leukaemia virus type 1 (HTLV-1).

Pathological Characteristics

Prognosis and therapy depend on the maturity and subtype of the cell of origin. This is defined by:

1. Morphology: appearance and arrangement of cells
2. Immunophenotyping: cellular differentiation (CD) cell surface antigens identified by a panel of antibodies
3. Cytogenetics: chromosome translocations
4. Molecular biology: gene expression and genetic mutations

The World Health Organisation (WHO) classification includes HL and NHL (Table 29.1). A specialist haematopathologist is essential for accurate categorisation. Morphologically, aggressive NHL can resemble poorly differentiated carcinoma and indolent NHL may be confused with benign lymphadenopathy.

TABLE 29.1 Simplified World Health Organisation Classification of Tumours of Haematopoietic and Lymphoid Tissues

Chronic myeloproliferative diseases
Chronic myeloid leukaemia
PRV
Myelofibrosis
Thrombocythaemia
Myelodysplastic/myeloproliferative diseases and syndromes
Acute myeloid leukaemias
Acute myeloid leukaemia with cytogenetic abnormalities or with prior dysplasia/therapy
Precursor B-cell neoplasm
Precursor B lymphoblastic leukaemia/lymphoma
Mature B-cell neoplasms
Chronic lymphocytic leukaemia/small lymphocytic lymphoma
Marginal zone lymphoma: splenic/nodal/mucosa-associated lymphoid tissue
Myeloma and plasmacytoma
Follicular lymphoma
Mantle cell lymphoma
Diffuse large B-cell lymphoma
Mediastinal large B-cell lymphoma
Burkitt lymphoma
B-cell proliferations of uncertain malignant potential
Posttransplant lymphoproliferative disorder
Precursor T-cell neoplasms
Precursor T-lymphoblastic leukaemia/lymphoma
Mature T-cell and natural killer-cell neoplasms
T-cell and natural killer-cell leukaemias
Natural killer/T-cell lymphoma
Peripheral T-cell lymphoma
Anaplastic large-cell lymphoma and cutaneous anaplastic large-cell lymphoma
Mycosis fungoides and Sézary syndrome
Angioimmunoblastic T-cell lymphoma
Enteropathy-type T-cell lymphoma
Hodgkin's lymphoma
Nodular lymphocyte-predominant Hodgkin's lymphoma
Classic Hodgkin's lymphoma
Nodular sclerosis
Lymphocyte-rich
Mixed cellularity
Lymphocyte-depleted

Hodgkin's Lymphoma

Hodgkin's lymphoma is characterised by Reed-Sternberg (RS) cells, although these are only 2% to 4% of the cells present: the bulk of the tumour consists of normal, reactive lymphocytes, histiocytes, plasma cells, granulocytes and fibroblasts. RS cells are large and multinucleate with prominent eosinophilic nucleoli and express CD30 and CD15. Overall survival is excellent, around 85% at 5 years.

There are four histological subtypes termed classical HL (cHL), lymphocyte rich, nodular sclerosing grades 1 and 2, mixed cellularity and lymphocyte depleted, which is very rare but carries a poor 5-year survival of 20%. The most common is nodular sclerosing, with nodules of cells within sclerosing fibrous bands, which often persist as a residual inactive mass after treatment. The fifth category of HL, lymphocyte predominant, differs histologically and clinically. It has an extremely long natural history with distant relapses, more like indolent NHL.

Non-Hodgkin's Lymphoma

Follicular lymphoma and diffuse large B-cell lymphoma (DLBCL) together make up 80% of all NHL seen in the West. They may be described as indolent and aggressive respectively, and grouped with other NHL subtypes although each is quite distinct.

Aggressive non-Hodgkin's lymphoma. DLBCL behaves aggressively but is curable in up to 60% of patients. Bone marrow is involved in 10% to 15% of cases. It forms sheets of large cells, often multinucleate with prominent nucleoli. Adverse prognostic markers include expression of p53 and BCL2 proteins and MIB-1 (Ki67). High proliferation rates (100% MIB-1 staining) are associated with programmed cell death (apoptosis) as in Burkitt lymphoma. Pale apoptotic cells in a uniform background of dark blue malignant lymphocytes appear as a starry sky. Thus at the aggressive end of the spectrum of DLBCL, it may appear and behave like Burkitt or lymphoblastic lymphoma, which are the truly high-grade types that grow and spread most rapidly but are curable with aggressive treatment. Gene expression profiling of DLBCL cases have identified two major subtypes based on unique gene signatures: germinal centre B-cell like (GCB-DLBCL) and activated B-cell like (ABC-DLBCL). The latter is associated with greater resistance to conventional chemotherapy and worse clinical outcomes.

Mantle cell lymphoma, characterised by cyclin-D1 and CD5 expression, progresses slowly but has a poor prognosis (median survival 3–4 years) because of chemoresistance. Peripheral T-cell lymphoma is a heterogenous group of diseases that typically behave aggressively with poor clinical outcomes.

Indolent non-Hodgkin's lymphoma. In follicular lymphoma, cells arise from lymph node germinal centres and form structures resembling normal follicles. The number of large follicular lymphoma cells seen under the microscope determines the grade. Grade 3b behaves as DLBCL and grades 1, 2 and 3a behave in a low grade indolent way (median survival 7–9 years). It inevitably recurs, unless truly localised at diagnosis (15%). It can transform into DLBCL with a poor prognosis. Bone marrow involvement is common (>60%). Marginal zone lymphomas, presumed to arise from the small B cells of nodal or splenic marginal zones, also behave indolently.

Extranodal non-Hodgkin's lymphoma. DLBCL is the usual type of NHL presenting in the head and neck (Waldeyer's ring, nasal sinuses, thyroid), bone, testis, breast and brain. In the stomach, orbit, salivary glands, lung and spleen, the marginal zone lymphoma predominates, whereas intestinal lymphoma is commonly of T-cell origin and associated with coeliac disease. NHL may arise in the skin from either B or T cells. Histological diagnosis is often difficult and clonality studies using *IG* or *TCR* rearrangements are needed to distinguish reactive conditions. Mycosis fungoides is a very slowly progressive epidermal tumour of T-cell origin which may develop a leukaemic form (Sézary syndrome). Anaplastic large-cell lymphoma (ALCL) also of T-cell origin, may arise in skin or elsewhere, and has a good prognosis if CD30 and ALK antigens are expressed. Cutaneous B-cell NHL includes follicular, marginal zone and DLBCL.

Clinical Features

All lymphomatous nodes may spontaneously wax and wane. They have a rubbery consistency and tend to be smooth, multiple, discrete, mobile and painless. These nodes can enlarge to 10 cm or more without fixation or skin involvement, in contrast to carcinomatous nodes which invade surrounding structures early. However, patients with aggressive lymphoma can deteriorate rapidly with dehydration, hypercalcaemia, anaemia, infection and damage to critical organs.

HL usually presents with enlarged nodes in the neck (60%), mediastinal mass, axilla (20%) or groin (15%). The spleen (10%) or, rarely, liver may be enlarged. Mesenteric nodes, bone marrow and extranodal sites are rarely involved in HL but commonly in NHL. Spread of HL is contiguous, from one lymph node group to the next; in NHL it may not be, and only 10% are localised at presentation.

Three characteristic B symptoms are associated with lymphoma and a worse prognosis: drenching night sweats, weight loss (>10% of body weight in previous 6 months) and fever (>38°C) which may be of a specific periodicity (Pel–Ebstein fever). The disease is staged as A (none of these) or B (any of these). Itching (pruritus) occurs in 12%, but is not classed as a B symptom. Pain felt in involved lymph nodes after drinking alcohol is a symptom peculiar to cHL.

In NHL, 20% have involvement of extranodal sites. In the head and neck there is swelling, proptosis or nasal blockage. Thyroid lymphoma presents as a mass with stridor from tracheal compression, and sometimes a history of Hashimoto thyroiditis. Primary NHL of bone mainly affects proximal long bones, with pain, swelling and pathological fracture. Testicular NHL presents at ages 60 to 80 years with a painless smooth swelling. Bilateral involvement occurs in 20% of patients. NHL of the breast presents with a mass often indistinguishable from carcinoma. Gastrointestinal lymphoma can present with pain, anaemia or bowel obstruction. Primary cerebral lymphoma presents with raised intracranial pressure or focal neurological deficits, including seizures. In the skin, mycosis fungoides starts as erythematous, flat, slightly scaly itchy lesions on the buttocks, upper thighs or breasts. These develop into thicker plaques, and then to fungating tumours with nodal and visceral involvement. The whole skin may become involved, resulting in generalised erythroderma or l'homme rouge. B cell cutaneous lymphoma is more likely to present as a discrete fleshy nodular lump with a tendency to ulcerate. Cutaneous ALCL occasionally undergoes spontaneous remission.

Diagnosis and Staging

A formal excision biopsy is preferred and should ideally be sent fresh to the laboratory. Increasingly, core biopsies are obtained because of logistical ease but may risk inconclusive results requiring the need for further biopsies. Fine needle aspiration is inadequate for accurate diagnosis of lymphoma. There is usually no need to debulk the tumour surgically except when large mediastinal masses compromise the major airways.

Staging establishes the extent of the disease, using the Ann Arbor classification (Table 29.2), clinical assessment and essential investigations:

1. Blood tests: full blood count, plasma viscosity, serum urea and electrolytes, calcium, liver function tests, lactate dehydrogenase (LDH), β2-microglobulin and serum Igs.
2. Computed tomography (CT) scan of chest, abdomen and pelvis with intravenous and oral contrast.

TABLE 29.2 Ann Arbor Staging Classification of Lymphoma

I. Involvement of a single lymph node region (I) or single extralymphatic organ or site (IE)

II. Involvement of two or more lymph node regions on the same side of the diaphragm (II) or localised involvement of an extralymphatic organ or site and one or more lymph node regions on the same side of the diaphragm (IIE)

III. Involvement of lymph node regions on both sides of the diaphragm (III) which may be accompanied by localised involvement of an extralymphatic organ or site (IIIE) or by involvement of the spleen (IIIS) or both (IIISE)

IV. Disseminated involvement of one or more extralymphatic organs or tissues with or without associated lymph node involvement

3. Positron emission tomography (PET) shows uptake of fluorodeoxyglucose (FDG) into areas actively metabolising glucose. The majority of lymphomas are metabolically very active and so show up clearly.
4. A bone marrow aspirate and a small core of bone (trephine) are taken from the posterior iliac crest. This is however, no longer required in HL where absence of PET uptake in bone has been shown to adequately exclude bone marrow involvement.
5. Lumbar puncture for high-risk groups (see below). At the time of the procedure, it is usual to inject methotrexate 12.5 mg.

Clinical Prognostic Factors

Early HL is very favorable if stage 1A, NS or LP type, aged younger than 40 years and female, and unfavorable if aged over 50 years, four or more sites involved, raised erythrocyte sedimentation rate (ESR) and a large mediastinal mass.

Advanced HL is unfavorable if stage 4, age over 50 years, low lymphocyte count, eosinophilia, low hemoglobin, low serum albumin and male.

In DLBCL, the international prognostic index (IPI), validated in the pre-Rituximab era, remains a widely accepted prognostic score from 0 to 5, with one point for each of the following features:

1. Age 60 years or older
2. More than one extranodal site
3. Stage III or IV disease
4. High LDH
5. WHO performance status 2 to 4

The National Comprehensive Cancer Network (NCCN)-IPI score has been validated in the rituximab era and appears to better discriminate good- and poor-risk DLBCL. There is an increased risk of central nervous system (CNS) relapse in DLBCL involving the testis, breast, and epidural space and in those with raised LDH and more than one extranodal site. Burkitt and lymphoblastic lymphomas carry a significant risk of CNS disease with treatment protocols including CNS-directed therapy.

Treatment
Initial Management

It is important to avoid treatment before any biopsy. If awaiting results, then steroids may be given (e.g. prednisolone 100 mg daily) to arrest clinical deterioration. In an emergency, such as airway obstruction, treatment may have to be given with RT. Urgent chemotherapy can rescue very ill patients despite toxicity. Rapid tumour breakdown can cause a tumour lysis syndrome because of release of cytokines and intracellular products causing raised serum urate, phosphate and potassium, reduced calcium and impaired renal and, rarely, lung function.

To prevent this, patients should start allopurinol (300 mg daily), ideally at least 24 hours before chemotherapy, and be very well hydrated. Individuals deemed at very high risk of tumour lysis (very high tumour burden as in Burkitt lymphoma) may receive rasburicase, a synthetic enzyme that breaks down the damaging urate.

Men should be offered sperm storage before chemotherapy. Fertility preservation in females requires ovarian stimulation before egg or embryo storage, which may not be feasible if there is a need to initiate chemotherapy urgently. Preservation of ovarian tissue is under study.

Hodgkin's Lymphoma

RT was the first curative treatment for stage I–III HL. Total nodal irradiation (TNI) was given using extended fields—a mantle field covered all supradiaphragmatic nodes and an inverted Y field covered the infradiaphragmatic nodes and spleen or splenic pedicle.

Chemotherapy was first used in HL for disease incurable with RT. Although side effects were severe with initial regimens such as mustine, vincristine, procarbazine and prednisolone (MOPP), additional cures were achieved, and six to eight cycles of chemotherapy plus extended field radiotherapy became routine. Unfortunately, the intense treatment resulted in up to 10% of patients developing secondary acute myeloid leukaemia (AML) and subsequently other secondary malignancies, particularly in irradiated areas. Heart disease was also increased. After 10 to 15 years, the risk of death from these causes was greater than from relapse of HL, with many patients rendered infertile. The most common second tumour is lung cancer, with an enhanced risk in smokers. In young women treated with mantle fields, the risk of breast cancer increases with age from 8 years after treatment up to as high as 50% in middle age for those treated in their early teens, or up to 25% if treated at ages 20 to 29 years, and early screening is now offered. Thyroid cancer, colon cancer and sarcomas are also seen.

Cure rates have been maintained using less toxic chemotherapy and smaller radiation fields with lower doses to minimise second malignancies and cardiotoxicity. Chemotherapy is used in young patients for all stages. Doxorubicin, bleomycin, vinblastine and dacarbazine (ABVD) has become standard, although it causes acute myelotoxicity, a small risk of cardiomyopathy and a 1% risk of fatal bleomycin lung toxicity. Two to four cycles plus RT is used in stage 1A and 2A and six to eight cycles ± RT for others. PET scanning helps to define complete response and can influence the need for RT. Recent trials, such as the U.K. National Cancer Research Institute (NCRI) (RAPID) and European Organisation for Research and Treatment of Cancer (EORTC) HD10 have shown that the omission of RT in early PET-negative patients reduces progression-free survival but there is no difference in overall survival (in current limited length of follow-up). Decisions are now being made on a more patient-specific basis because of factors such as age, sex, site of disease and size of RT field to determine if patients should receive combined modality treatment or chemotherapy alone. PET-positive patients are escalated to more intensive regimens, such as bleomycin, etoposide, doxorubicin, cyclophosphamide, vincristine, procarbazine, and prednisone (BEACOPP), whereas those with stages III and IV disease may be de-escalated for example by omitting bleomycin as done in the RATHL study.

Extended field RT is used after a partial response to chemotherapy with disease at several sites or where chemotherapy has had to be curtailed, especially in patients who would be unsuitable for HSCT. For elderly and unfit patients with early disease, RT alone may be the treatment of choice.

The overall 5-year survival rate is 85%.

Relapsed cHL may be cured with HSCT or sometimes further conventional chemotherapy or RT. Anti-CD30 antibodies such as brentuximab vedotin and checkpoint inhibitors (immunotherapy), such as nivolumab, offer relapsed patients further options.

Non-Hodgkin's Lymphoma

Aggressive non-Hodgkin's lymphoma. For more than 20 years, six to eight cycles of cyclophosphamide, hydroxydaunorubicin, Oncovin (vincristine) and prednisolone once every 3 weeks (CHOP-21) was the best treatment for DLBCL despite many trials of more intensive regimens. The recent addition of an anti-CD20 human/mouse monoclonal antibody (rituximab) to each cycle (R-CHOP) has increased complete response rates from 63% to 76% and overall survival at 3 years from 51% to 62% with minimal toxicity, and so is the new gold standard. Newer generation anti-CD20 monoclonal antibodies have been tested but to date have not proven superior to rituximab combinations.

In high-risk groups, prophylactic CNS treatment is given concurrently as intrathecal or high-dose intravenous methotrexate. RT to sites of bulk is conventional, but whether PET imaging can identify those in whom RT can be safely omitted is currently under investigation.

For stage IA or IIA DLBCL, including extranodal sites, RT alone is curative in about 50%, but adding three cycles of chemotherapy increases the cure rate to 80% in chemosensitive patients. Eight cycles of CHOP seemed as effective as CHOP × 3 plus RT in one prerituximab trial, but others show an advantage for RT and the combination is preferred. Full-course chemotherapy should be given if there is bulky disease or B symptoms or a high IPI score, usually with RT afterwards. Only 40% of DLBCL cases are truly localised. In testicular DLBCL, the contralateral testis should be irradiated to reduce the risk of recurrence.

At relapse after full-course chemotherapy, HSCT can be curative if chemosensitivity can be shown with salvage regimens (Ifosfamide Etoposide Epirubicin (IVE), Ifosfamide Carboplatin Etoposide (ICE), Etoposide Methylprednisolone Cytarabine Cisplastin (ESHAP), Dexamethasone Cytarabine Cisplatin (DHAP)). Time to relapse is the most important predictive factor with rituximab refractory disease showing the worst outcome. Current clinical trials are exploring the role of immunotherapy

Burkitt lymphomas are treated with mores intensive regimens, such as the Cyclophosphamide, Vincristine, Doxorubicin, Methotrexate, Ifosfamide, Etoposide, Cytarabine (CODOX-M/IVAC) regimen, now combined with rituximab, and can cure around 50% of patients.

In primary cerebral lymphoma, standard chemotherapy can cross the blood–brain barrier initially while there is oedema around the tumour. CNS-penetrating drugs (high-dose methotrexate, cytarabine) are also used. Steroids are effective. RT may prolong remission but causes lethargy and also significant cognitive impairment. Optimal chemotherapy, and the role of RT, are under investigation; prognosis is poor.

For mantle cell lymphoma (MCL), fitter younger patients often receive intensive chemotherapy followed by autologous stem cell transplantation. Bruton's tyrosine kinase (BTK) inhibitor ibrutinib is particularly active in MCL and has recently become available for some patients in the United Kingdom. Rare patients with localised disease may be considered for radical RT. Newer agents currently being tested alone and in combination with chemotherapy include lenalidomide, bortezemib and temsirolimus.

Optimal treatment for peripheral T-cell lymphoma remains unclear with the majority of patients treated with combination chemotherapy (CHOP, Cyclophosphamide Doxyrubicin Vincristine Etoposide Prednisolone (CHOEP), Gemcitabine Methylprednisolone Cisplatin (Gem-P))

Indolent non-Hodgkin's lymphoma. Truly localised (15%) follicular NHL may be cured with RT alone. For palliation, low doses can achieve lasting control.

In widespread disease, a watch and wait approach is acceptable for asymptomatic patients. Immediate treatment with rituximab has not been shown to alter survival but may reduce patient anxiety. On symptomatic progression, treatment options include rituximab/benda-musting, Rituximab Cyclophosphamide Vincristine Prednisolone (RCVP) or, for bulky higher risk disease, Rituximab Cyclophospha-mide Doxyrubicin Vincristine Prednisolone (RCHOP). Oral chloram-bucil may be an option for elderly, less fit patients.

There is now increasing evidence that following induction and second-line chemotherapy, maintenance rituximab (375 mg/m^2 every 2–3 months for up to 2 years) significantly improves progression-free survival. However, to date, survival benefits have not been shown and there is increasing awareness of infective toxicity.

At relapse, rebiopsy is advisable to detect high-grade transforma-tion. Selection and timing of treatment depends on the disease-free interval, extent of relapse, age and general condition, and includes HSCT. Rituximab alone (375 mg/m^2 weekly for 4 weeks) gives a 50% response rate with 13 to 17 months median time to progression in heavily pretreated patients and can be repeated with equal effect.

Marginal zone NHL is described as three types: splenic, nodal and those of mucosa-associated lymphoid tissue (MALT) origin. Sple-nectomy is appropriate for the first, and the others respond to the same agents and general approach as follicular NHL. Although the pattern of disease is different with more extranodal sites, RT can still be curative for disease truly localised to, for example, the stom-ach or parotid. Antihelicobacter therapy is potentially curative in gastric MALT NHL. Gastric MALT can be monitored by regular endoscopies.

Mycosis fungoides has a median survival of 10 years. In the early stages, topical steroids can be used, then often photochemotherapy, using long-wave ultraviolet light with oral psoralens (PUVA). RT can be local or to the whole skin surface using low-energy electrons. Systemic treatments include Alemtuzumab (anti-CD52 antibody) which targets T cells. Combination chemotherapy with a CHOP-type regimen is used in visceral disease, but complete response rates are low (20%–25%).

Special Situations

Lymphoma in children. RT in children causes growth retardation in the treated area, and they are particularly susceptible to second malig-nancies, so chemotherapy is used alone whenever possible. Lower radi-ation doses have been shown to be adequate in paediatric Hodgkin and extranodal presentations are rarer: lymphadenopathy is the presenting feature in 90% of cases.

Lymphoma in pregnancy. HL is the most common diagnosis. Stag-ing should avoid exposure to ionising radiation, using magnetic reso-nance imaging (MRI) or ultrasound in preference to CT. RT is potentially teratogenic during the first trimester. Above a dose of 0.1 gray (Gy) to the fetus, there is a risk of inducing an abnormality. Chemotherapy has an unquantified risk of teratogenesis or carcinogen-esis to the fetus.

Termination should be considered if treatment is essential before the early second trimester, if the fetal dose would exceed 0.1 Gy or if chemotherapy is indicated. If the diagnosis is made late in the second or in the third trimester, it may be possible to postpone treatment until delivery is induced at 32 to 34 weeks. Localised RT above the diaphragm can be safely given, and single-agent chemotherapy may control symp-toms in HL for a few weeks but, if the disease is life threatening, then combination chemotherapy is best. With ABVD, the risk of carcino-genesis or infertility in the child should be low.

Patients who have been successfully treated for HD should be advised to avoid pregnancy for 2 years after the end of treatment because after this, the risk of relapse falls markedly. Subsequent preg-nancy does not increase the risk of relapse.

Lymphoma in human immunodeficiency virus and posttransplant. Human immunodeficiency virus (HIV)-associated lymphoma is usually aggressive, presenting with high IPI scores and often CNS dis-ease. Patients are more prone to succumb to infective complications of treatment. NHL is an AIDS-defining illness, but HL is not. Historical survival outcomes were poor but have significantly improved with RCHOP and the use of highly active antiretroviral therapy (HAART) and are now similar to non-HIV lymphoma.

Posttransplant lymphoproliferative disease (PTLD) is an often loca-lised NHL presenting after organ transplantation. It usually remits on gradual withdrawal of immunosuppressive therapy but, if not, then options include infusion of HLA-matched cytotoxic T lymphocytes.

MULTIPLE MYELOMA

Multiple myeloma accounts for 0.9% of all cancers and 1.3% of cancer deaths. Its incidence is 3 per 100,000 per year with about 3000 new cases annually in the United Kingdom. The median age at diagnosis is 62 years and the male to female ratio is 1.5:1. The aetiology is unknown. Median survival is 3 to 4 years from diagnosis with wide variations.

Pathology

Myeloma is a tumour of plasma cells, which are Ig-producing B lym-phocytes. Their bone marrow microenvironment is increasingly well understood and there are new molecular targets for treatment identi-fied as a result. Myeloma cells potentiate osteoclast activity and inhibit differentiation of osteoblast precursors, uncoupling bone formation from resorption so multiple lytic bone lesions are characteristic. They also produce a specific Ig or paraprotein, detectable by immunoelectro-phoresis and useful for diagnosis and treatment monitoring. Although an intact Ig molecule is too large to enter the renal tubules, free light chains (Bence Jones protein) may be produced and are found in the urine. Serum-free light chains can also be quantified in the blood. Nor-mal Igs are reduced, resulting in recurrent infections (immune paresis). In 5%, there is no secreted protein and the disease is termed nonsecre-tory. Bence Jones only is found in 20%, whereas Ig subtypes are found with frequencies reflecting normal levels, that is, IgG in 50% to 60%, IgA in 20% to 25%, IgD in 2%, IgE and IgM in less than 1%. Parap-roteinemia is also found in lymphoma. IgM is associated with Walden-strom macroglobulinemia or marginal zone lymphoma. In the normal population, paraproteinemia is found in 1% aged over 25 years, 3% over 70 years and 25% over 90 years old. This is monoclonal gam-mopathy of uncertain significance (MGUS) and carries an annual risk of 1% of progression to multiple myeloma. Asymptomatic early mye-loma is termed *smoldering*.

Clinical Features

The most common presenting feature is bone pain (70%) from a rib or vertebra. The destruction of cortical bone leads to pathological fractures in about 25% and hypercalcemia in 30%. Alkaline phospha-tase is normal, and bone lesions lytic. Spinal cord compression is occa-sionally the presenting feature and is an emergency. Humoral and cell-mediated immunity are impaired and recurrent infections are com-mon. Most patients have a cytokine-mediated anaemia; pancytopenia as a result of marrow replacement is uncommon at presentation. A third have reduced white cell count and/or platelets. ESR is raised. Renal failure occurs because of deposition of Bence Jones protein in the renal tubules, dehydration, infection and nonsteroidal anti-inflammatory drugs.

If the paraprotein level is high enough, a hyperviscosity syndrome develops, characterised by visual impairment, lethargy and coma. This is most commonly associated with IgM subtype as these form larger structures in the blood. Amyloidosis, a deposition of abnormal protein in the kidneys, heart, nerves or other sites, is seen in about 10% of mye-loma patients.

A plasmacytoma is a solitary plasma cell mass, usually arising in a rib or vertebra but also other bones and soft tissues, with or without a paraprotein. Progression to multiple myeloma is probable, but not inevitable.

Diagnosis

There are three requirements:

1. Serum or urine paraprotein
2. Plasma cell numbers increased in the bone marrow (>10%) or biopsy of a mass
3. End-organ damage: hypercalcaemia, renal impairment, anaemia or bone lesions (CRAB).

   Investigations

1. Full blood count
2. Serum urea, creatinine and electrolytes
3. Serum calcium
4. Serum electrophoresis
5. Urine electrophoresis (increasingly replaced by serum-free light chain quantitation)
6. Bone marrow examination
7. Skeletal survey (plain x-ray of whole skeleton to show lytic lesions, especially skull, ribs and vertebrae, or diffuse osteoporosis). Bone scans using technetium-labelled colloid are not helpful in myeloma as lytic lesions are not usually shown
8. MRI imaging of the spine if cord compression is suspected
9. PET scanning increasingly used to establish total tumour burden

Prognostic Factors

Poor prognosis is associated with:

1. Increase in plasma-cell labelling index
2. Increase in B2-microglobulin level
3. Low serum albumin
4. Plasmablastic features in the bone marrow
5. Circulating plasma cells
6. 17p and chromosome 13 deletions
7. t(4;14) or t(14;16) translocation
8. Increased density of bone marrow microvessels

Treatment

Prophylactic bisphosphonate therapy is standard for all patients to inhibit bone resorption. Severe hyperviscosity is treated by plasmapheresis, in which some of the patient's plasma is replaced by an appropriate colloid solution (usually albumin) to reduce the level of paraprotein. Nephrotoxic agents should be avoided if possible. Dialysis may be required for renal failure. Control of pain and infection is important.

Chemotherapy is aimed at response defined by a reduction in paraprotein level to 50% or less, healing of radiological lesions and more than 50% reduction in size of a plasmacytoma. Complete response is defined as the absence of detectable paraprotein or urinary light chains and normalisation of the bone marrow with less than 5% plasma cells. Usually a plateau phase is reached where the disease is measurable but stable. It should be considered at an early stage whether each patient is a candidate for high-dose therapy with HSCT. Survival is prolonged by using melphalan at 200 mg/m^2 followed by autologous transplantation. The oral regimen of cyclophosphamide, thalidomide, dexamethasone (CTD) is now the most widely used induction regimen. Thalidomide exerts an antiangiogenic and anti-inflammatory effect. Patients with a durable remission following first autograft often benefit from a repeat autograft. A mini-allograft (see HSCT under the heading Leukaemia) may be superior to a second autograft for a high-risk young patient with a sibling donor, but carries significant transplant-related morbidity and mortality and therefore remains controversial.

For elderly patients and those not fit for HSCT, thalidomide-containing regimens remain the first choice—an attenuated dose of CTD can be used, or thalidomide combined with melphalan and steroid. Bortezumib, a proteosome inhibitor, and lenalidomide, a novel analogue of thalidomide, are often used in combination with dexamethasone in relapsed disease. Combinations of these two drugs with more established chemotherapy agents continue to be investigated for first-line treatment in high-risk patients.

Radiotherapy in Myeloma

Solitary plasmacytoma are treated radically with surgery and RT.

In diffuse disease, palliative RT relieves bone pain and is often used concomitantly with chemotherapy. Single fractions are commonly used but higher doses, for example, may be needed if there is soft tissue associated with the bony abnormality or fracture risk. Hemibody treatments are effective for generalised pain in advanced disease, although as a result of better systemic and bone-directed therapies, these are less frequently undertaken.

Spinal cord or cauda equina compression may occur at presentation or at any stage of the disease, and may be as a result of extradural disease or a collapsed vertebra. In diffuse disease, urgent RT (usually fractionated) is often preferable to surgery, but decompression and stabilisation followed by RT is sometimes more appropriate so surgical consultation should be considered.

TBI is sometimes used as part of HSCT.

LEUKAEMIA

Bone marrow (haemopoietic) stem cells develop into lymphocytes (lymphoid cell line) or red blood cells, platelets or granulocytes (myeloid cell line). Cells of all lineages at virtually any stage of differentiation may become malignant.

In acute leukaemia, the marrow fills with immature lymphoid or myeloid leukaemic cells which displace normal cells and enter the peripheral blood. Untreated, death rapidly results from anaemia, bleeding and immunosuppression.

In chronic leukaemias, which arise from more mature cells, the disease can be stable with few symptoms for many years.

Leukaemia accounts for 2.1% of all cancers and 2.6% of cancer deaths and is more common in males. Described here are:

1. Acute leukaemia
   a. Lymphoblastic (ALL)
   b. Myeloid (AML)
2. Chronic leukaemia
   a. Lymphocytic (chronic lymphocytic leukaemia, CLL)
   b. Myeloid (granulocytic) (chronic myeloid leukaemia, CML)
3. Other myeloproliferative disorders

Acute Leukaemia

Acute lymphoblastic leukaemia (ALL) constitutes 80% of paediatric cases and AML constitutes 80% of adult cases.

AML increases with age (median 65 years). It may arise from myelodysplastic syndrome (MDS), a group of clonal stem cell disorders characterised by dysplasia in one or more lineages, ring sideroblasts and bone marrow blasts (if >20% this becomes AML). Radiation can cause AML evidenced by survivors of atomic bombs (20:1) and whole-spine irradiation for ankylosing spondylitis (10:1). The risk rises from about 3 years after exposure and peaks at 7 to 8 years.

Some cytotoxic drugs (alkylating agents, etoposide) can induce leukaemia. The risk after MOPP chemotherapy is 3%, and, if given with wide-field irradiation for HL, the relative risk is about 6:1. Industrial chemicals, mainly benzene, can also induce AML.

An inherited predisposition is evident in Down syndrome (20:1). Ataxia telangiectasia and other DNA repair defect syndromes, such as Bloom syndrome and Fanconi anaemia, all predispose to either acute lymphoblastic leukemia (ALL) or acute myeloid leukemia (AML), but these are very rare. Infection is not the cause of leukaemia except in the rare adult T-cell leukaemia/lymphoma syndrome (HTLV1 virus).

Chromosomal abnormalities and translocations are numerous and useful in defining prognostic groups; their absence after treatment verifies remission.

Clinical Features

The clinical features of ALL and AML are similar and are described elsewhere along with the treatment of ALL.

Treatment of Acute Myeloid Leukaemia

Intensive combination chemotherapy is used to induce remission. Standard regimens involve cytarabine and daunorubicin, plus etoposide if younger, which can achieve results of about 80% remission in patients under 60 years but, in older patients, remission is only about 40%. Relapse is usual without further treatment, if possible with HSCT to obtain long-term remission/cure. There is a favorable good-risk subgroup of whom two-thirds may be cured and where transplantation may be reserved for relapse, including those with promyelocytic disease where all-trans retinoic acid (ATRA) can induce blast cells to differentiate. New agents include antibody to CD33, found on the leukaemic cell surface, which has been linked with a novel cytotoxic agent (gemtuzumab-ozogamicin, Mylotarg) and is currently being investigated in a large national U.K. trial. Such agents may improve complete response (CR) rates and it is therefore important that younger, fitter patients are entered into national trials.

Long-term cure is possible in 30% of younger patients with HSCT, but cure is very unlikely in older patients or following relapse. Clofarabine, a purine analogue similar to fludarabine, is being trialled in older patients with AML to assess for improved response rates. In patients unfit for intensive chemotherapy, low-dose cytarabine or hydroxyurea is used to obtain some disease control. The prognosis is poor if AML has been preceded by MDS.

Chronic Myeloid Leukaemia

CML is a rare disease that occurs mainly in the fifth and sixth decades. The incidence in the United Kingdom is 1 in 100,000. There is a slight male predominance (1.4:1). In over 90% of cases, the *Philadelphia chromosome* is present, the result of a translocation from chromosome 22 to chromosome 9, resulting in a fusion *BCR-ABL* gene whose protein product ($p210^{BCR-ABL}$) is a tyrosine kinase enzyme essential for malignant transformation. Tyrosine kinase inhibitors, such as imatinib (Gleevac), are a class of drug designed to inhibit these enzymes.

Clinical Features

Presentation is with tiredness because of anaemia, or with splenomegaly which may be massive. The total white cell count is typically between 100 and 500 × 10^9/L, a mixture of myeloid cells at varying stages of differentiation and less than 5% blasts, with this picture reflected in the marrow. The platelet count is normal or raised.

The natural history is of a chronic stable phase of 4 to 6 years, although this can be 1 to 20 years. A 6-month accelerated phase precedes the terminal blastic phase.

Treatment

Tyrosine kinase inhibitors are highly effective at inducing both clinical and cytogenetic complete remission in chronic phase in the majority of patients. Patients who fail to respond to a specific tyrosine kinase inhibitor can be switched to an alternative drug within the same class. Allogeneic HSCT is now only reserved for a minority of high-risk patients. Hydroxyurea is useful to control high white cell counts during end-stage disease.

Chronic Lymphocytic Leukaemia

CLL is the most common form of leukaemia in the Western world. Its incidence in the United Kingdom is 5 per 100,000. The male to female ratio is 2:1. CLL is usually seen in middle age, with the incidence increasing with age. About 5% of cases exhibit some family history of B-cell lymphoproliferative disease, but the nature of the involved gene(s) remains unknown. It is not linked to radiation or chemical exposure or chemotherapy.

Clinical Features

Symptoms of CLL are mainly because of anaemia or infection, although diagnosis is often made incidentally on a full blood count. The white cell count is usually between 30 and 300 × 10^9/L and composed of small mature lymphocytes with condensed nuclei and scant cytoplasm. The bone marrow is hypercellular with an infiltrate composed of mature lymphocytes. Biopsy of enlarged nodes shows monotonous sheets of cells with characteristic proliferation centres.

Enlargement of lymph nodes of the neck and other peripheral sites, spleen and liver is common; staging systems are currently based on the number of enlarged lymph nodes and on normal and abnormal cell counts into stages A, B and C (Binet staging). Adverse prognostic factors include stage B or C, male gender, age older than 60 years, lymphocyte doubling time less than 12 months, diffuse marrow infiltration and more than 10% circulating prolymphocytes. Molecular markers of prognosis are p53 abnormalities, 11q23 deletions, high CD38/ZAP-70 expression and having an unmutated IgVH gene.

CLL is slowly progressive, although occasionally, notably with mutations of the p53 gene, resistant to all conventional therapy. In some patients, the disease is stable for over 20 years.

Treatment

Treatment is indicated for symptoms or if critical organs are threatened. Oral chlorambucil has historically been given first line at doses of, for example, 10 mg daily for 2 weeks out of 4. Rituximab, fludarabine, cyclophosphamide (FCR) or rituximab/bendamustine is used for the majority of patients. Patients who cannot tolerate these drugs, carry a specific cytogenetic deletion of the gene TP53, or who relapse after these therapies, are typically treated with the BTK inhibitor ibrutinib. Venetoclax is an oral drug that inhibits a pathway that promotes CLL cell survival. Sometimes, CLL can transform into a high-grade lymphoma (Richter transformation) and is treated as for DLBCL.

MYELOPROLIFERATIVE DISORDERS

This is a related group of disorders including CML (described earlier), polycythemia vera (PV), essential thrombocythemia (ET) and idiopathic myelofibrosis (IMF). They are slowly progressive with median survival of about 10 years. PV (excess red cells) and ET (excess platelets) can lead to myelofibrosis and to AML.

PV causes pruritus, splenomegaly and gout because of hyperuricemia, and PV and ET cause thromboses, particularly arterial, and less often, haemorrhages.

Treatment is with antiplatelet drugs and hydroxyurea (a cytotoxic drug). Interferon is used less often but has a role in selected patients unable to take hydroxyurea. Anagrelide is useful in ET because it prevents the maturation of platelets. Busulfan and radioactive phosphorus (P32) injections are effective but rarely used now because of the increased risk of leukaemia. Repeated venesection is used in PV to prevent the haematocrit rising to dangerous levels.

In IMF, there is bone marrow fibrosis and failure with associated splenomegaly. It may be as a result of stimulation of fibroblasts by abnormal megakaryocytes. Irradiation is effective at very low doses in shrinking the spleen.

It has recently been discovered that a mutation in another tyrosine kinase, JAK2, can be found in 90% of patients with PV and around 50% of ET and IMF. JAK2 inhibitors are now well developed and can be used for certain patients fulfilling criteria.

HAEMOPOIETIC STEM CELL TRANSPLANTATION

The term haemopoietic stem cell transplantation (HSCT) is used to describe the collection and transplantation of HSC from bone marrow, peripheral blood or umbilical cord blood. It is essential to the delivery of high-dose treatments used increasingly in haematological malignancies and will be referred to throughout this chapter.

Stem cells from the patient's own marrow are autologous and, if donated by another, HLA-matched person, allogeneic. Cells are transplanted by infusion through a central venous Hickman line and are then described as the *graft*.

Autografting has a 1% to 2% mortality. Stem cells are harvested from the peripheral blood after stimulating them to proliferate by giving conventional chemotherapy and granulocyte-colony stimulating growth factors (GCSF), and they are reinfused after high-dose therapy which would otherwise be fatally myelosuppressive. It may not be possible to harvest cells following prior chemotherapy, especially with alkylating agents and fludarabine, and this problem has altered first-line treatments. Plerifixor inhibits a molecule in the bone marrow releasing stem cells into the peripheral blood and has shown to increase the success of harvesting procedures.

Allografting has about a 30% mortality, lower with a sibling than with a matched unrelated donor (MUD) but is the only curative option when there is residual disease in the marrow or when autografting has failed. High-dose conditioning therapy is given to eradicate the underlying disease and to immunosuppress the patient enough to prevent rejection of the transplant, for example, cyclophosphamide (Cy) 100 mg/kg over 2 days and TBI (Cy/TBI). Chemotherapy may be used alone, for example, cyclophosphamide and busulfan (Bu/Cy). Donor harvesting may be from peripheral blood or directly from bone (multiple punctures under general anaesthesia) which gives a better yield of cells. Allografting has the beneficial effect of donor T lymphocytes recognising residual malignant cells as foreign and destroying them.

Following chemoradiotherapy, the white cell and platelet counts drop within 10 days and recover after 3 to 6 weeks of intensive support with antibiotics, and red cell and platelet transfusions. Graft-versus-host disease (GvHD) occurs when T cells from the donor react with antigenic targets on host cells. It may be acute (jaundice, skin rashes, diarrhoea and weight loss) or chronic (arthritis, liver disease, malabsorption, oral mucositis and sicca syndrome, lung disease, pericardial and pleural effusions, scleroderma, skin rashes) and has a high mortality. The incidence is reduced by immunosuppression with cyclosporin A or tacrolimus, and by depleting the donor T cells using monoclonal antibodies such as alemtuzumab (CAMPATH) and antithymocyte globulin (ATG). Blood products are irradiated to kill any T lymphocytes which may precipitate GvHD.

New treatments for GvHD include antibodies to tumour necrosis factor and interleukin-2, and extracorporeal photopheresis.

Immunodeficiency as a result of defects of T-cell and B-cell functions occurs during the first 6 months and for longer in the presence of GvHD. Viral, bacterial and fungal infections may be fatal.

In the event of relapse after transplantation, donor T lymphocytes can be used therapeutically for their graft-versus-disease effect. This is exploited in mini-allografting in patients unfit to undergo a myeloablative transplant: after reduced-intensity conditioning (no TBI), the host normal marrow survives and coexists with the donor marrow, and the donor T cells control the leukaemia.

RADIOTHERAPY DOSES, TECHNIQUES AND TOXICITIES

Various techniques and doses can be employed in the management of lymphomas with radiation. These are dependent on tumour site and volume, intent of treatment, available imaging and patient characteristics.

Involved-node radiotherapy (INRT): planned volume with the clinical target volume (CTV) = involved node/s with margin which follows node chains.

Involved-site radiotherapy (ISRT): planned volume with the CTV = the involved site (may be nodal as above) with defined margins.

Involved-field radiotherapy (IFRT): parallel-opposed beams covering the classical defined involved field, encompassing a node region.

Extended-field radiotherapy (EFRT): extended field encompassing all node regions on one side of the diaphragm: mantle (nodes above) and inverted Y (nodes below).

Megavoltage is used (4–10 MV photons bolus may be needed to ensure an adequate dose to superficial nodes or any skin involvement. Reference to prechemo PET-CT and contrast-enhanced CT is essential.

Hodgkin's Lymphoma

Following chemotherapy: the standard is 30 Gy in 15 fractions to involved node/site.

Early favourable-stage patients can receive 20 Gy in 10 fractions (following 2 cycles of ABVD).

Patients with early or advanced disease may have RT decisions made based on functional imaging results such as PET-CT after 3 cycles of ABVD but generally omission of RT is not advised if there is bulky disease.

RT alone: 30 to 34 Gy in 15 to 20 fractions to extended, or at least to the involved field.

Palliative treatment: options of 8-Gy single fraction, 20 Gy in 5 fractions or 30 Gy in 10 fractions, dependent on clinical situation.

Non-Hodgkin's Lymphoma
Diffuse Large B Cell Lymphoma

Radical: postchemotherapy: 30 Gy in 15 daily fractions over 3 weeks to involved node/site.

RT alone: 30 Gy in 15 fractions to extended field. Palliative: 20 to 30 Gy in 5 to 10 fractions to involved field is usual. Large single fractions, for example, 8 Gy, may be appropriate for bone.

Indolent Lymphoma: Follicular and Marginal Zone

Radical: generally RT alone: 24 Gy in 12 fractions is usually adequate to involved field or modified involved site. If chemotherapy has been given, treat involved site/nodes. If bulky or at a site at risk of organ impairment, consider 30 Gy.

Palliative Treatment: 4 Gy in two fractions can give prolonged remission.

Treatment Techniques

Mantle. Mantle field radiotherapy is less frequently used because of known toxicities of large volumes, but may be useful for salvage/treatment of recurrence in patients not fit for high dose chemotherapy. Target volume: all supradiaphragmatic nodes.

Position: supine with neck extended. Arms abducted and supported with hands on hips.

Field borders

Superior: mastoid process.

Inferior: junction of 10th and 11th thoracic vertebrae.

Lateral: lateral to the humeral head to include the whole axilla.

Nodal volumes can be outlined for more accurate definition.

Shielding

Lungs do not need to be treated, nor does the cervical spine or larynx. Thoracic spine doses will depend on the extent of mediastinum required to be treated.

Tattoos are placed to avoid rotation of the thorax.

It can be challenging to get an even dose distribution because of the contour of the body (Fig. 29.1).

Inverted Y

As with mantle fields, inverted Y fields are less commonly treated. Target volume: all infradiaphragmatic nodes: paraaortic, pelvic, iliac and femoral. This can be extended to also cover the spleen.

Field borders

Superior: junction of the 10th and 11th thoracic vertebrae or if matching to a mantle field, a gap (about 2 cm on skin) is calculated to have the 50% isodoses meet just posterior to the vertebral bodies on a lateral x-ray.

Inferior: the inferior margin of the obturator foramen, or covering involved nodes plus 5 cm.

Lateral: the greater trochanters of the femora.

Shielding. The paraaortic nodes should be treated but abdominal cavity lateral to this area can be shielded. In the pelvis, the bladder and genitalia should be avoided where possible.

Involved fields. Target volume: All pretreatment macroscopic and PET-positive disease and at least one anatomical node group such as the axilla or inguinal area, in an area in which a node mass with a well-defined edge has shrunk with chemotherapy away from an adjacent dose-limiting structure, such as lung, spinal cord or kidney, CTV can be modified to avoid the organ. There should be at least a 5-cm margin along the lymph node chain above and below the pre-chemotherapy disease, which may mean inclusion of part of the adjacent region, for example, where the superior mediastinum

was involved; it is usual to treat both supraclavicular fossae (Figs. 29.4 and 29.6).

Involved sites. ISRT if nodal, may be referred to as INRT. It is much more common now to use involved site volumes rather than involved fields to reduce toxicity. Volumes are irregular in shape and a good knowledge of anatomy is required to define them, with reference to standard atlases, radiological opinion, prechemotherapy PET scans and contrast-enhanced CT scans for planning (Fig. 29.2).

A CTV is defined on the CT planning system. Where there is a residual node mass adjacent to another tissue, such as lung, the CTV may be at the edge of this mass in the axial plane, and does not need to encompass the original size. However, in the direction of the lymph node chain, the CTV is the pretreatment extent of abnormal nodes on PET-CT plus a 1.5-cm margin. This direction may not be directly superior-inferior, for instance, at the junction between node regions in the mediastinum/neck or abdomen/pelvis. Given this anatomical issue, the CTV should ideally be hand drawn and the use of automated planning software margins should be avoided.

Where there is no residual mass, the volume describes the lymph node chain in the space bounded by other structures, such as muscle, large vessels, lung and bone.

A margin is added to the CTV to give the required PTV according to the site, set-up error, likely movement, and local departmental practice, and might vary from 3 to 4 mm to 1.5 cm (Fig. 29.7).

Extra-Nodal Sites

ISRT for extranodal sites following chemotherapy is CT-planned in a similar way to involved nodes. The CTV may define the whole organ, for example, stomach, spleen or thyroid, where there were no adjacent nodes involved, or part of a node chain may need to be outlined in addition.

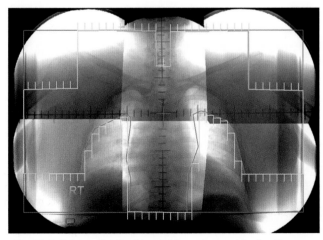

Fig. 29.1 "Mantle field" with shielding using multileaf collimators.

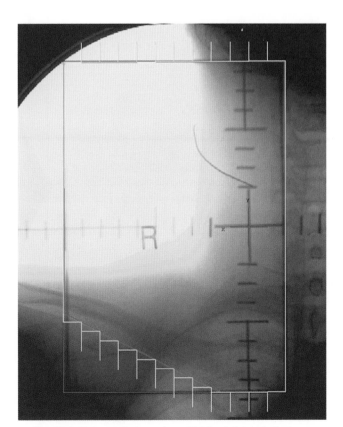

Fig. 29.2 Submandibular nodes: shielding infraclavicular lung.

Head and neck. The patient is immobilised in a supine shell, and CT planning is used (Figs. 29.3, 29.5 and 29.8).

Waldeyer's ring. Although Waldeyer's ring can be thought of as one site for staging purposes, the entire volume does not need to be treated if localised disease, for example, unilateral tonsillar involvement is present. The single structure can be outlined with appropriate margins based on prechemotherapy volumes. For extensive involvement and/or partial response to chemotherapy, larger fields may be considered but can lead to considerable toxicity.

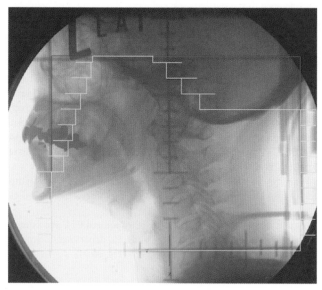

Fig. 29.3 Waldeyer's ring and whole neck: lateral fields.

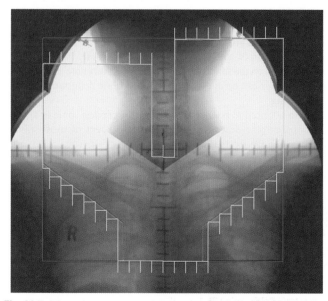

Fig. 29.5 Bilateral neck with sparing of salivary glands on right where only supraclavicular nodes were involved.

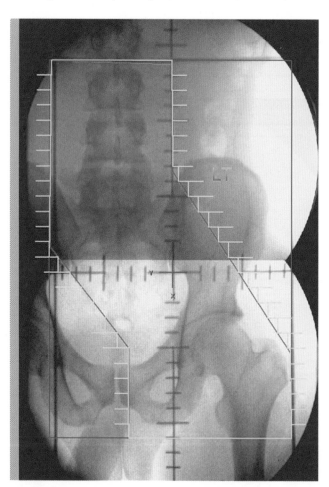

Fig. 29.4 Lower paraaortic, iliac and inguinal nodes: dog-leg–shaped field.

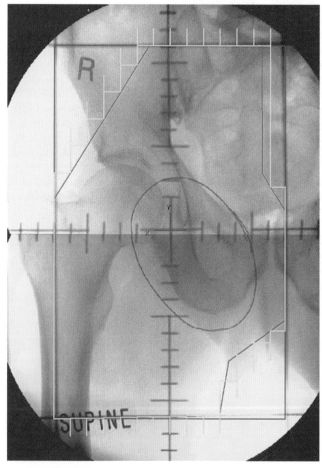

Fig. 29.6 Right pelvic and inguinofemoral nodes.

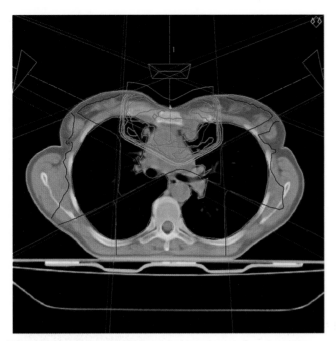

Fig. 29.7 Anterior mediastinal residual lymphoma after chemotherapy: anterior-wedged pair of angled beams.

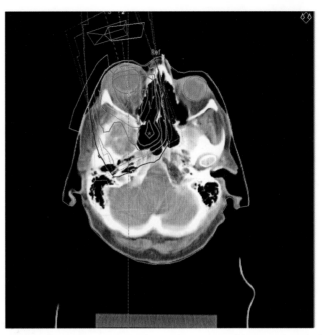

Fig. 29.9 Orbital lymphoma with anterior mass: axial view of sagittal beams and bolus.

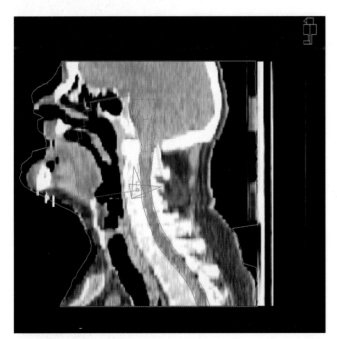

Fig. 29.8 Nasopharyngeal lymphoma: lateral fields covering Waldeyer's ring.

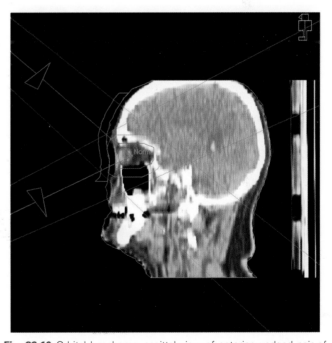

Fig. 29.10 Orbital lymphoma: sagittal view of anterior-wedged pair of angled beams.

Thyroid. The thyroid gland, with or without cervical lymph node chains on both sides, are included. Immobilisation, as for a head and neck tumour, and CT planning are adopted.

Orbit. The whole orbit is treated using CT planning. For small lateral and conjunctival indolent NHL, a single beam may suffice. Beams are angled to avoid the other eye (Figs. 29.9, 29.10 and 29.11).

Nasal sinuses. Planning is the same as for carcinoma (Figs. 29.12 and 29.13).

Brain. The whole brain is treated with a parallel pair of lateral beams. As meningeal involvement is likely, the fields are extended down the neck to C2/3 and to cover the posterior orbit and facial nerve root as for ALL (Figs. 29.14 and 29.15).

Gastrointestinal lymphoma. For gastric NHL, plan on using oral contrast and treat the stomach empty. CT planning can help spare the kidneys or spinal cord, especially for large postchemotherapy residual abdominal masses. Rectal lymphoma is planned as for carcinoma.

Bone. The whole of the affected bone should be included in the volume. A parallel-opposed pair of fields may be adequate, shielding soft tissues with a 2-cm margin.

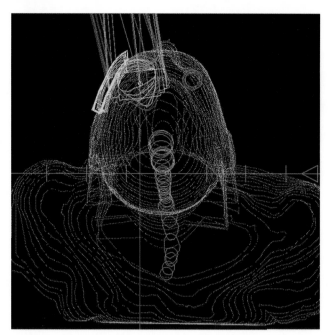

Fig. 29.11 Orbital lymphoma: outline view of volume and beam arrangement.

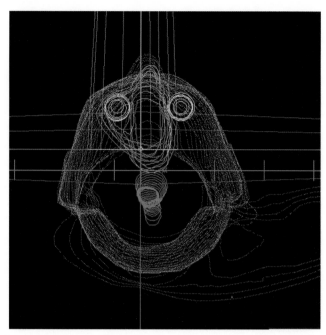

Fig. 29.13 Nasal natural killer/T cell lymphoma: volume and critical structures — contralateral eye and brainstem.

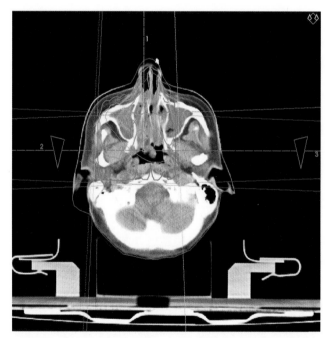

Fig. 29.12 Nasal natural killer/T cell lymphoma: three-field plan.

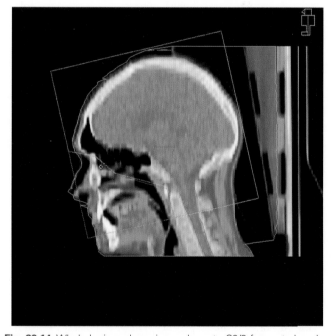

Fig. 29.14 Whole brain and meninges down to C2/3 for acute lymphoblastic leukemia.

Breast. The whole breast is included as CTV. Uninvolved lymph nodes do not need to be treated. This is planned with tangents as per breast carcinoma irradiation.

Spleen. The CTV is the edge of the spleen. CT planning may help minimise the dose to the kidney. Palliative splenic RT is described later under the heading Leukaemia.

Toxicity

Acute side effects. All treatments cause tiredness and temporary hair loss and mucositis in the treated area, from 2 weeks into treatment and for several weeks afterwards. Dry mouth and altered taste are usual where salivary tissue has to be treated, and may be lasting after bilateral high-neck fields, with an increased risk of dental problems. There is a small chance of lymphoedema in the leg or arm, especially if there has been previous surgery in the axilla or inguinal region.

Late effects. The organs most subject to late effects are the thyroid, lung, heart and spinal cord. There is an increased risk of solid tumours in irradiated areas.

Thyroid. Up to 30% develop clinical or biochemical hypothyroidism several years after bilateral neck treatment, requiring thyroxine replacement therapy.

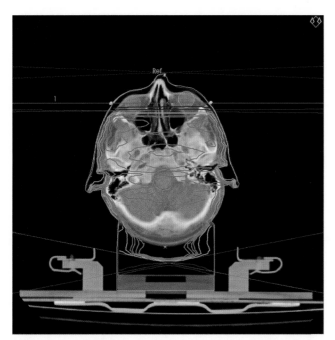

Fig. 29.15 Computed tomography plan for acute lymphoblastic leukemia.

Lung. Lung function is minimally impaired in about one third of patients undergoing mantle therapy. Symptoms, if any, are seen after about 6 weeks: dry cough and dysponea, which usually settle with steroids (prednisolone 40–60 mg/day).

Cardiac. Radiation-induced cardiac disease occurs in less than 5% of patients after mantle treatment and less with involved fields, although data are scarce. It can rarely present as transient pericarditis within a few months of treatment or much later as cardiomyopathy or premature coronary artery disease.

Neurological. Lhermitte syndrome is a transient numbness, tingling (paresthesia) or an electric shock-like sensation in the arms or legs following mantle or neck irradiation from 2 to 4 months afterwards. It may be as a result of transient demyelination of the spinal cord because of damage to oligodendrocytes

Bone. Avascular necrosis of the femoral head occurs in 2% of Hodgkin patients, particularly following chemotherapy and steroid treatment, but RT including the hip is a contributory factor. Symptoms of hip pain develop on average about 2 years following the start of chemotherapy. Total hip replacement may be necessary. The humeral head may also be affected if it could not be shielded.

Fertility. Pelvic RT with lymphoma doses will cause infertility in most young people: for males sperm banking is effective, but for women surgical oophoropexy and, if possible, cryopreservation of ovarian tissue are advised. Hormone replacement therapy (HRT) should be prescribed for premature menopause.

Growth. Growth retardation in children after RT includes limited height, but also, for instance, thinning of the neck muscles and shortening of the clavicles from neck treatment.

Leukaemia

Cranial irradiation may be given as described elsewhere for ALL.

Total Body Irradiation

A 14.4 Gy midplane dose in 8 twice-daily fractions over 4 days (6-MV photons) or 12 Gy in 6 fractions over 3 days. Doses and schedules are generally determined by current trials.

Technique. Techniques vary in detail from centre to centre, and some have machines dedicated to extended field treatment for TBI.

Using a linear accelerator at extended focus to skin distance (FSD) (about 4 metres), a lateral beam can treat the whole patient, who is then turned 180 degrees for the other side.

Thermoluminescent dosimeters (TLDs) are positioned at regular intervals along each side of the body and tissue compensators can be conveniently attached to a rectangular Perspex screen placed alongside the patient. Typically, 1-mm, 8-mm and 6-mm brass compensators are placed over the head, neck and thorax, respectively. Doses are measured at each fraction so as to adjust arm position and compensators, if necessary, to ensure dose homogeneity within around 5%.

Side effects. Side effects are more common with single-fraction than with fractionated TBI.

1. Pneumonitis. Lungs are the dose-limiting organs. Because pneumonitis commonly occurs following bone marrow transplantation in the absence of radiation, the role of TBI in its causation is difficult to assess.
2. Cataract. The incidence of cataract is about 20% between 3 and 6 years.
3. Hepatic venooclusive disease. This is seen in up to 25% of patients but is usually mild. However, the mortality of established disease is high (30%).
4. Fertility. In females under 25 years, periods may return, but in others permanent sterility is to be expected. Men are rendered azoospermic and should have sperm frozen.
5. Hypothyroidism. Hypothyroidism occurs in up to 30%.
6. Growth delay. Growth hormone secretion may be impaired, especially if previous cranial irradiation has been given.
7. Second malignancy.

Splenic Radiotherapy

Splenic RT is used in myeloproliferative disorders, mainly CML and myelofibrosis, to shrink an uncomfortably large spleen and/or to improve blood counts by reducing splenic consumption; this is a delicate balance as counts will initially drop.

Dose. The dose is 0.25 to 0.5 Gy/day up to a total dose of 1 to 10 Gy with 4 to 6 MV photons if there is extramedullary haematopoiesis. Higher dose per fraction, 1 to 1.5 Gy, can be used for other causes of splenomegaly.

Target volume. Irradiation of the whole of the spleen is not necessary to achieve shrinkage and symptomatic benefit. The kidney is dose-limiting but can tolerate 20 Gy so treatment can be repeated.

The spleen is outlined on the CT planning scan and a parallel pair is often adequate.

Myeloma

Radical treatment of solitary plasmacytoma: 40 to 50 Gy in 20 to 25 fractions (Fig. 29.18).

Palliative Treatment of Multiple Myeloma

Spinal deposits. 8 Gy single fraction with a posterior beam to cover abnormal bone(s) plus one vertebra on either side, about 8 cm width to include the transverse processes of the vertebrae, wider to include any paravertebral mass.

Soft tissue mass/spinal cord compression/pathological fracture/ severe pain. 20 Gy in 5 fractions. Consider 30 Gy in 10 fractions for example soft tissue with extensive bone destruction when disease is mainly in one area.

Rib deposits. 8 Gy single fraction

Orthovoltage or electron treatment can be used to the painful area plus a margin of a few centimeters along the rib.

Hemibody radiotherapy for widespread deposits. This is now rarely used because systemic treatment options have increased.

If treating both in sequence, a gap of 6 weeks is necessary for recovery of blood counts.

Position. Supine with arms folded across the chest, hands on shoulders.

Upper half: 6 Gy single fraction—chin to umbilicus, wide enough to cover shoulders.

Lower half: 8 Gy single fraction—umbilicus to maximum field size inferiorly and width to cover iliac bones.

Technique. Extended FSD (140 cm), and anteroposterior parallel beams.

Acute side effects. Nausea and vomiting, prevented with, for example, ondansetron 1 hour before RT, dexamethasone 4 mg twice daily (bd), plus metoclopramide 10 mg as needed (prn). Pneumonitis is rare at 6 Gy, but has an increasing incidence above this dose to the whole lungs.

Diarrhoea occurs in one-third of patients 3 to 5 days after lower hemibody treatment, controllable with codeine or loperamide.

Pancytopenia is common and contributes to lethargy. Blood and platelet transfusions may be required.

Mycosis Fungoides
Local
Use 10 Gy in 5 daily fractions, 8 Gy single fraction to small lesions, higher doses may be needed for tumour stage.

Use 80 to 120 kV for superficial lesions and 220 to 300 kV, or electrons of appropriate energy, for plaque or tumour stage.

Total Body Electron Therapy
Total body electron therapy (TSEBT) is a specialised treatment offered in regional centres, and techniques vary.

Doses can vary but typically are 12 Gy in 8 fractions over 2 weeks with an 8-Gy boost in 2 fractions over 2 days or the more conventional 30 Gy in 20 fractions over 5 weeks.

Four fields can cover the whole body at extended source to surface distance (SSD) (120 cm) with the patient supine. Lead shielding is applied to protect the eyes and the finger nails. If the eyelids are involved, a lead internal eye shield is used. If 5 or 8 MeV electrons are used, Perspex is used to reduce the depth of penetration. Skin in folds (e.g. axilla and groin) is spared with this technique and may be marked for separate treatment when skin erythema develops. This can be minimised by positioning patients carefully.

Temporary alopecia and loss of nails are followed by permanent skin atrophy, oedema and radiodermatitis (Figs. 29.16 and 29.17).

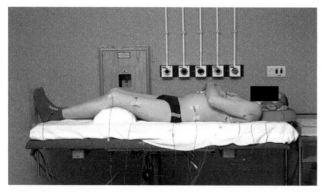

Fig. 29.16 Patient with dosimeters placed ready for treatment.

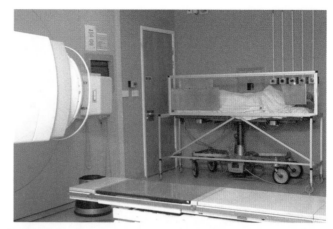

Fig. 29.17 Machine head and patient showing extended focus to skin distance (FSD).

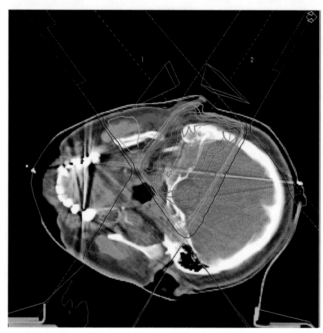

Fig. 29.18 Plasmacytoma of petrous bone: lateral-wedged pair of angled beams.

CHEMOTHERAPY REGIMENS AND TOXICITIES

The majority of chemotherapy regimens cause myelosuppression and the risk of life-threatening neutropaenic sepsis. Chemotherapy typically causes alopecia. There is also the risk of infertility, particularly in men, although this is more commonly encountered with intensive regiments. The problems of nausea and vomiting (particularly because of anthracyclines, dacarbazine and mustine) have been transformed by new antiemetics in the HT3 blocker class (ondansetron, granisetron). Anthracyclines cause cardiomyopathy if a high cumulative dose has to be given, but this is rarely a problem with first-line treatment. The vinca alkaloids (vincristine, vinblastine) cause peripheral neuropathy and constipation. Bleomycin may rarely cause pulmonary fibrosis, which can be fatal. Oral chlorambucil alone is the least acutely toxic treatment used; it does not cause alopecia or much nausea but, like other alkylating agents (cyclophosphamide, melphalan, mustine), causes some irreversible toxicity to bone marrow and gonads.

Hodgkin's Lymphoma
Doxorubicin, Bleomycin, Vinblastine and Dacarbazine
The ABVD drug regimen is shown here.

Doxorubicin (adriamycin) 25 mg/m^2 intravenously (IV)	Days 1 and 15
Bleomycin 10,000 units/m^2 IV	Days 1 and 15
Vinblastine 6 mg/m^2 IV	Days 1 and 15
Dacarbazine 375 mg/m^2 IV	Days 1 and 15
Repeated every 28 days	

Acute toxicity is marked (alopecia is usual, nausea, myelosuppression, constipation, painful veins, pulmonary fibrosis from bleomycin which is fatal in 1% to 30%, and highest in elderly patients, but there is minimal risk of infertility or leukaemia with ABVD, so this is standard treatment.

Ch1VPP
The ChlVPP regimen is shown here.

Chlorambucil 6 mg/m^2 (max. 10 mg) orally	Days 1–14
Vinblastine 6 mg/m^2 (max. 10 mg) intravenously	Days 1 and 8
Procarbazine 100 mg/m^2 orally	Days 1–14
Prednisolone 40 mg orally	Days 1–14
Repeated every 28 days	

This regimen is well tolerated but with a 3% risk of later leukemogenesis; infertility is induced in men, but less likely in women. Only the vinblastine is intravenous and hair loss is unusual. Ch1VPP is used less commonly, but may be considered if ABVD is deemed unsuitable.

Stanford V
The Stanford V is a multiple-drug, 12-week regimen with high control rates, but RT to all masses greater than 5 cm is mandatory.

BEACOPP
BEACOPP is an intensive first-line treatment, suitable for high-risk patients.
Bleomycin
Etoposide
Adriamycin
Cyclophosphamide
Vincristine (Oncovin)
Procarbazine
Prednisolone

Non-Hodgkin's Lymphoma
Follicular grade 1 and 2 and marginal zone:
Oral chlorambucil: 10 mg daily for 14 days every 28 days × 6.
Well-tolerated with rare reports of serious toxicity, but myelotoxic.
　R-COP (also known as R-CVP). R-COP follows the same drug regimen as R-CHOP (see later) but without doxorubicin.

Mantle Cell
FC
Fludarabine
Cyclophosphamide
Repeated every 28 days
　FC is myelotoxic, but a well-tolerated oral regimen without alopecia.

Diffuse Large B Cell, T-Cell-Rich, B Cell, Follicular Grade 3b (and for T-Cell Lymphomas)
Use CHOP alone without rituximab for T-cell lymphoma.
　R-CHOP. Side effects include alopecia, nausea, myelosuppression, peripheral neuropathy, antibody reaction, steroid effects and cardiomyopathy.

Rituximab 375 mg/m^2	Day 1
Cyclophosphamide 750 mg/m^2 intravenously (IV)	Day 1
Doxorubicin 50 mg/m^2 IV	Day 1
Vincristine 1.4 mg/m^2 (max. 2 mg) IV	Day 1
Prednisolone 50 mg/m^2 orally	Days 1–5
Repeated every 21 days (minimum six courses)	

In those assessed to be at high risk of CNS disease prophylaxis by intrathecal or systemic intravenous methotrexate can be given with 3–4 cycles.
　R-PMitCEBO. R-PMitCEBO provides an equivalent outcome but on a weekly regimen; may be easier to tolerate for some patients.

Mitoxantrone	Day 1
Cyclophosphamide	Day 1
Etoposide	Day 1
Bleomycin	Day 8
Vincristine	Day 8
Rituximab 375 mg/m^2	Days 1, 21, 42, 63
Continued weekly, alternating days 1 and 8 for 12–16 weeks	

CNS Prophylaxis
Methotrexate ×4 doses
1 g/m^2 IV on day 14
or 12.5 mg IV on day 1 or 2
with each of 1st 4 cycles

Burkitt Type, Lymphoblastic (Some DLBCL if 100% MIB-1 Staining)
　CODOX-M/IVAC. This is an intensive myelosuppressive regimen with CNS treatment

Relapsed Non-Hodgkin's Lymphoma
　(R)IVE, (R)ICE
Rituximab
Ifosfamide
Etoposide (Vepesid) in IVE or carboplatin in ICE
Epirubicin in IVE or carboplatin in ICE
Reinduction regimens to minimise bulk and mobilise stem cells for harvesting.
　BEAM
Busulfan
Etoposide
Cytosine arabinoside (Ara-C)
Melphalan
　Myeloablative regimen. Oral etoposide: 50 mg bd per os daily for 10 days, q 3 to 4 weeks: palliative single agent.

Myeloma
CTD
Cyclophosphamide
Thalidomide
Dexamethasone

CTD is a generally well-tolerated oral regimen. Specific side effects include pulmonary fibrosis (cyclophosphamide), neuropathy, thrombosis, teratogenesis and thyroid dysfunction (thalidomide).

Bortezomib

Bortezomib is a proteosome inhibitor with various sites of action. Main side effects include neuropathy and thrombocytopenia.

Lenalidomide

Lenalidomide is a novel analogue of thalidomide with similar side effects but neuropathy less likely.

Acute Myeloid Leukaemia
DA

Daunorubicin

Cytarabine (Ara-C)

DA is significantly myelosuppressive. It commonly causes mucositis (oral ulcers, diarrhoea) and, more rarely, conjunctivitis and cardiomyopathy.

FURTHER READING

Kyle RA, Rajkumar SV. Treatment of multiple myeloma: a comprehensive review. Clin Lymphoma Myeloma 2009;9:278–88.

Yahalom J. Radiation therapy after R-CHOP for diffuse large B cell lymphoma: the gain remains. J Clin Oncol 2010;28:4105–7.

Herbst C, Rehan FA, Brillant C, et al. Combined modality treatment improves tumour control and overall survival in patients with early stage Hodgkin's lymphoma: a systematic review. Haematologia (Budap) 2010;95:494–500.

Girinsky T, van der Maazen R, Specht L, et al. Involved-node radiotherapy (INRT) in patients with early Hodgkin lymphoma: concepts and guidelines. Radiother Oncol 2006;79:270–7.

Yahalom J, Mauch P. The involved field is back: issues in delineating the radiation field in Hodgkin's disease. Ann Oncol 2002;13(Suppl.1):79–83.

Press OW. Radioimmunotherapy for non-Hodgkin's lymphomas: a historical perspective. Semin Oncol 2003;30(Suppl. 4):10–21.

Gustavsson A, Osterman B, Cavallin-Stahl E. A systematic overview of radiation therapy effects in Hodgkin's lymphoma. Acta Oncol 2003;42:589–604.

Kheng-Wei Y, Mikhaeel NG. Role of radiotherapy in modern treatment of Hodgkin's lymphoma. Adv Hematol 2011. Article ID 258797.

Ganem G, Cartron G, Girinsky T, et al. Localised low-dose radiotherapy for follicular lymphoma: history, clinical results, mechanisms of action, and future outlooks. Int J Radiat Oncol Biol Phys 2010;78:975–82.

Hoppe RT. The indolent extranodal lymphomas: what is the role of radiation therapy? Haematol Meet Rep 2009;3:10–4.

Strauchen JA. Immunophenotypic and molecular studies in the diagnosis and classification of malignant lymphoma. Cancer Invest 2004;22:138–48.

Coiffier B, et al. CHOP chemotherapy plus rituximab compared with CHOP alone in elderly patients with diffuse large B-cell lymphoma. N Engl J Med 2002;346:235–42.

Salles G, Seymour JF, Offner F, et al. Rituximab maintenance for 2 years in patients with high tumour burden follicular lymphoma responding to rituximab plus chemotherapy (PRIMA): a phase 3, randomised controlled trial. Lancet 2010;377:42–51.

Hallek M, Fischer K, Fingerle-Rowson G, et al. Addition of rituximab to fludarabine and cyclophosphamide in patients with chronic lymphocytic leukaemia: a randomised, open-label, phase 3 trial. Lancet 2010;376:1164–74.

The diagnosis and management of multiple myeloma, British Committee of Standards in Haematology, Available online: http://www.bcshguidelines.com/; 2010.

Armitage JO. Early stage Hodgkin's lymphoma. N Engl J Med 2010;363:653. 562.

Barrett AJ, Savan BN. Stem cell transplantation with reduced-intensity conditioning regimens: a review of ten years experience with new transplant concepts and new therapeutic agents. Leukaemia 2006;20:1661–72.

Bruker B. Translation of the Philadelphia chromosome into therapy for CML. Blood 2008;112:4808–17.

Younes, et al. Brentuximab vedotin (SGN-35) for relapsed CD30-positive lymphomas. N Engl J Med 2010;363:1812–18221.

Burger JA. Inhibiting B-cell receptor signaling pathways in chronic lymphocytic leukaemia. Curr Hematol Malig Rep 2012;7(1):26–33.

30

Tumours of the Central Nervous System

Pinelopi Gkogkou, Sarah J. Jefferies, Neil G. Burnet

CHAPTER OUTLINE

INTRODUCTION

Primary tumours of the central nervous system (CNS) are relatively uncommon: the overall annual incidence of primary CNS tumours is around 14 per 100,000 population, with approximately 5300 newly diagnosed patients in the United Kingdom each year. Although accounting for only 2.6% of cancer deaths, brain tumours lead, on average, to a greater loss of life per patient than any other adult tumour and the effect on the individual with a primary CNS tumour is frequently devastating. Primary CNS tumours affect patients of all ages, from childhood to old age, with a rising incidence from middle age onwards. In childhood, they are the most common solid tumours (as opposed to leukaemias).

There is a huge range in outcome for patients with primary CNS tumours, from almost guaranteed cure in some conditions (e.g. germinoma) to almost guaranteed fatality in others (e.g. glioblastoma [GBM]). For patients with CNS tumours, a holistic approach is always required and, for many, involvement of palliative care services is highly desirable. For many patients, driving is forbidden after the diagnosis of brain tumour (see later).

TUMOUR TYPES

Overall, about 80% of CNS tumours are primary and 20% secondary. However, the proportions depend exactly on how the patient population is gathered. Patients presenting with cerebral metastases are generally seen and looked after by the site-specific specialist teams, based on the tissue of origin.

The major types of primary tumour are given in Table 30.1. The majority of primary tumours are gliomas. Of the gliomas, two-thirds are GBMs (Fig 30.1), making this the most common type of primary CNS tumour in adults. Gliomas in general, and GBMs in particular, are devastating tumours, and therefore consume much of the energy and resources of the neurooncology unit. Although gliomas represent the major diagnosis of primary brain tumours, over one-third of new referrals are for other tumour types, so appropriate attention also needs to be directed towards those.

Gliomas are graded according to the World Health Organization (WHO) classification, significantly updated in 2016 on a scale of I to IV, where IV is the most malignant. Grade I and grade II gliomas together are termed low grade. Grade I tumours are more typical of childhood, but occasionally occur in adults. Grade III and grade IV tumours together constitute high-grade gliomas (HGGs). Grade III tumours may also be called *anaplastic* and grade IV gliomas are known as *glioblastomas*.

Gliomas arise from astrocytes and oligodendrocytes, cells which nourish and support neurons. Primary tumours of neurons alone are extremely uncommon, though they do exist (e.g. neurocytoma). There is a surprisingly large range of very rare tumours within the brain, but apart from those mentioned explicitly in Table 30.1 and described later, their overall management and outcome can generally be inferred from the grade and molecular biology of the tumour.

Gliomas have a slight male predominance, with 55% occurring in men. Meningiomas are more common in females than males, in the ratio of 2:1, which is unusual in oncology. There are only two definite etiological factors for the development of brain tumours: exposure to ionising radiation and genetic predisposition. Genetic syndromes include Li-Fraumeni syndrome, neurofibromatosis types 1 and 2, Gorlin syndrome, tuberous sclerosis, Cowden disease, Turcot syndrome and von Hippel-Lindau, which are proposed as predisposing factors. Rare cases are familial, defined as two or more gliomas diagnosed in first- or second-degree relatives. However, the majority of CNS tumours are sporadic.

TABLE 30.1   A Simplified Classification of the Major Categories of Brain Tumour

Intrinsic Tumours (i.e. Those Arising Within the Brain Substance)

Glial tumours
    astrocytoma
    oligodendroglioma
    glioblastoma (GBM)
    pendymoma medulloblastoma
Germinoma/teratoma
Primary central nervous system lymphoma

Extrinsic Tumours of the Brain Covering

Meningioma

Other Tumours

Pituitary adenoma and craniopharyngioma
Vestibular schwannoma
Skull base chordoma and chondrosarcoma

Cerebral Metastases

Notes

1. GBM used to be known as *glioblastoma multiforme*.
2. The glial tumours are divided into four grades: grades I and II together constitute low-grade gliomas, whereas grades III and IV tumours together are the high-grade gliomas. The term *anaplastic* is equivalent to a grade of III. A grade IV glioma is a GBM.
3. Grade I tumours are rare in adults, although they do occur. They also appear in adult practice in patients treated as children who have outgrown the paediatric services.
4. A large number of other uncommon tumours also occur.
5. Medulloblastoma is predominantly a disease of childhood, but does occasionally occur in adults (i.e. patients over 16).

Secondary CNS metastases may arise from primary tumours at almost any site. However, certain cancers have a propensity to metastasise to the brain. Lung cancer accounts for 60% of metastases, followed by breast (15%), melanoma (6%–11%) and renal cancer (1%–4%). Other tumours causing metastases include colon, pancreas and ovary. Metastases are usually multiple but occasionally can be solitary.

ANATOMY OF THE CENTRAL NERVOUS SYSTEM

Anatomy is the key to understanding the presentation of neurological tumours, their spread and concepts about treatment, particularly with radiotherapy (RT) and surgery.

Anatomy of the Brain

Tissues of the Brain

Within the brain substance itself, tissue is divided into gray and white matter. Gray matter covers the surface folds of the brain (gyri), and broadly is the location of active neurons. White matter lies below the gray matter and contains fibres which communicate with other parts of the brain and body, equivalent to electrical cabling. At a cellular level, the brain is composed of both neurons and cells designed to support the structure and function of those neurons, the glial supporting cells. In right-handed patients, the left hemisphere is almost invariably dominant.

The frontal lobe is very large, extending back to the central sulcus, which divides it from the parietal lobe. The motor cortex sits

Percentage diagnoses for 1000 neuro-oncology referrals

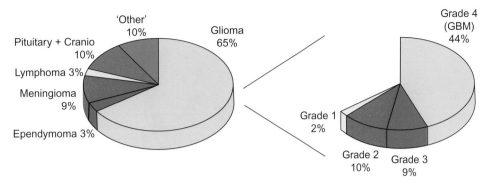

Fig. 30.1 Frequency of the main tumour types. Percentages of different grades of glioma. Grade IV glioma is glioblastoma) (Courtesy Professor NG Burnet.)

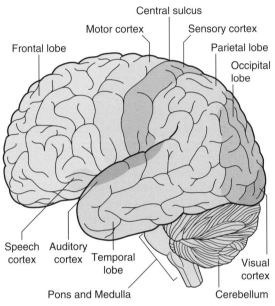

Fig. 30.2 The major anatomical divisions of the brain.

immediately in front of the central sulcus. More anteriorly, the frontal lobe is responsible for intellect, motivation and emotional response. Damage to the frontal lobes can affect intellectual performance, including reasoning, memory, the initiation of activity and insight. The medial frontal lobe is particularly important for these activities and damage to both medial frontal lobes is extremely destructive to the intellect. The motor speech centre (Broca's area) lies in the dominant frontal lobe (Fig. 30.2).

The parietal lobe extends from the central sulcus posteriorly onto the occipital lobe and is also large. The parietal lobe has large areas which are silent, with no obvious functional activity. Immediately behind the central sulcus is the sensorimotor cortex, which deals predominantly with reception of sensory information. In reality, there are other areas adjacent to both motor and sensory cortices which support those functions. At the most posterior part of the cerebral hemisphere is the occipital cortex, which deals with central processing of visual information. The optic radiation connects the optic tracts to the occipital cortex, and runs through the temporal and parietal lobes to arrive at its destination. Tumours lying along that pathway can therefore affect vision.

Inferiorly and laterally, with its tip in the middle cranial fossa, lies the temporal lobe. The medial part is involved in short-term memory. In the dominant hemisphere, the temporal lobe is the location for one of the speech centres, the auditory cortex.

The pons and medulla together form the brainstem. These have processing functions, important functional centres such as the respiratory centre, and also carry all motor and sensory information between the cerebral cortex and spinal cord (Figs 30.2 and 30.3). Even small lesions within the brainstem have very severe neurological effects. The function of the cerebellum is the subconscious control of movement. Damage to the cerebellum therefore leads to ataxia and other difficulties with coordinated movement.

The lobes of the brain communicate by extensive pathways made up of white matter. These run from front to back, side to side, and up and down through the brain. Tumours which spread through white matter tracts (especially the gliomas) therefore have access to pathways which can allow them to spread extensively. The corpus callosum (Fig. 30.3) is the major route of side-to-side communication between the two cerebral hemispheres. HGGs lying medially in the hemisphere often involve this structure, which allows spread into the opposite hemisphere.

Functional imaging, especially using magnetic resonance imaging (MRI), has demonstrated that damage to particular areas of the brain, for example the motor cortex, can lead to some function being taken over by other areas, provided that the rate of damage is slow. In the adult, this can occur in only a modest way, but can explain why, in some circumstances, patients do not lose all the neurological function that might be expected.

Anatomy of the Cerebrospinal Fluid Pathways and Hydrocephalus

The major cerebrospinal fluid (CSF) structures are shown in Fig. 30.4. CSF is produced by the choroid plexus within the two lateral ventricles, and flows into the third ventricle anteriorly through the foramen of Munro (see Fig. 30.4). CSF exits the third ventricle posteriorly through the aqueduct and flows into the fourth ventricle. From there, CSF leaves the fourth ventricle through three foramina (the foramina of Luschka laterally and the foramen of Magendie in the midline) to surround the outside of the brain. A small amount also passes down the central canal in the spinal cord. CSF is actively absorbed by the arachnoid granulations which protrude into the major venous sinuses, especially the superior sagittal sinus at the vertex of the skull. The CSF canals are lined by ependymal cells, from which ependymomas arise. These tumours are therefore related in space to the ventricular system.

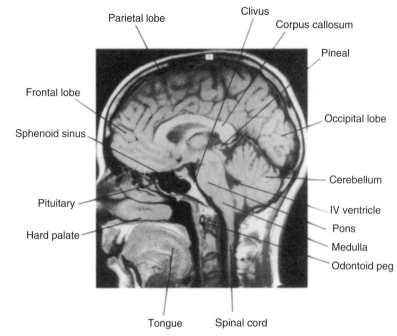

Fig. 30.3 Normal anatomy of the central nervous system. Magnetic resonance midline sagittal section. (Courtesy Dr. L Turnbull, MRI Unit, Sheffield.)

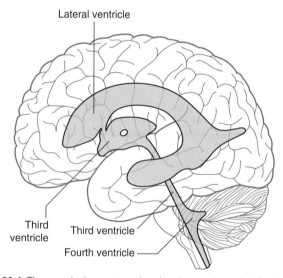

Fig. 30.4 The ventricular system showing the cerebrospinal fluid pathways. (See text for further details.)

Disturbance in the flow or absorption of CSF causes hydrocephalus. Obstruction of the flow before the exit foramina in the fourth ventricle leads to obstructive hydrocephalus. Obstruction of the arachnoid granulations leads to communicating hydrocephalus.

In neurooncology, tumours most commonly cause obstructive hydrocephalus. This is normally the result of obstruction in the fourth ventricle, by tumours growing in or around the ventricle (e.g. medulloblastoma or ependymoma), or within the cerebellum (most commonly metastases). The next most common location for obstruction is the aqueduct, from compression by tumour in adjacent brain or the pineal gland. More proximal obstruction can also occur at the foramen of Munro, usually from infiltrative HGG, causing hydrocephalus in one or both lateral ventricles.

Communicating hydrocephalus can be caused directly by tumour, when extensive meningeal involvement occurs. This is almost always metastatic (most commonly from breast cancer), and it is rare. A more common cause of communicating hydrocephalus in neurooncology practice is blood in the CSF, resulting from surgery or a spontaneous bleed directly from a tumour. Blood can occlude the pores in the arachnoid granulations. Often this resolves spontaneously but, occasionally, a CSF shunt (such as a ventriculoperitoneal (VP) shunt) must be inserted. Infection is also a cause through the same mechanism.

Anatomy of the Skull and Meninges

The skull itself is divided into three fossae. The frontal fossa contains the frontal lobe; the middle cranial fossa contains the temporal lobe; the posterior cranial fossa contains the cerebellum. The cerebellum is divided from the cranial contents by the tentorium cerebelli ("tent"), except for an aperture through which the brainstem passes. The cerebral hemispheres are divided by the falx cerebri. These two structures are composed of layers of tough meninges, and are designed to damp movements of the brain which might otherwise be damaging to the delicate brain substance. They are relatively rigid. The falx and tentorium cannot be infiltrated by gliomas, and so present efficient barriers to their spread. Meningiomas, on the other hand, can spread along their surface, and their potential direction of spread can be appreciated by understanding this anatomy.

The meninges consist of three layers. The outer dura mater (usually known simply as dura) is a tough membrane, which acts like a periosteum; it is the part visible on imaging and forms the falx and tent. Below and closely applied to the dura is the arachnoid mater. Below this lies the pia mater, a thin delicate layer which covers every surface and fold of the brain substance. In some places, there is a space (the subarachnoid space) between the arachnoid and pia, crossed by thin strands with a cobweb-like appearance (hence the origin of the name arachnoid). The dura lines the whole cranial cavity, including the skull base. In some areas, the dura splits to form venous channels, such as the superior sagittal sinus, and the cavernous sinuses. It also forms the two important folds, the tentorium cerebelli and the falx cerebri, which are continuous with the dura covering the skull vault and skull base.

CLINICAL FEATURES—PRESENTATION OF BRAIN TUMOURS

Presenting symptoms and signs of CNS tumours are characteristic; patients may present with one or more classes of symptoms, as follows.

Specific Focal Neurological Deficit

CNS tumours may make their presence known by local damage, leading to specific deficits dependent on the location of the tumour. For example, a meningioma affecting the motor cortex will produce weakness and stiffness typically in a limb, specifically depending on which part of the motor cortex is affected. A GBM affecting the frontal lobe produces intellectual, motivational and memory problems. In this way, symptoms and signs indicate the site of the tumour, which can be confirmed with imaging. Tumours arising in eloquent areas typically present earlier than those in silent areas of the brain, simply because they produce symptoms when they are smaller. Tumours which grow slowly, for example meningioma, produce an insidious onset, with relatively mild symptoms and signs, despite often being surprisingly large when detected. Tumours which grow rapidly, and destructively, such as GBM, produce symptoms and signs that often appear to commence abruptly.

Symptoms and signs relating to specific parts of the brain are as follows:
- Frontal lobe: intellectual impairment and personality change.
- Parietal lobe: sensory or visual inattention.
- Fronto-temporo-parietal: speech disturbance, especially dysphasia.
- Occipital lobe: visual field defects.
- Brainstem: cranial nerve defects, sensory or motor disturbance.
- Cerebellum: loss of coordination of movement.

Epileptic Seizure

Almost all CNS tumours can potentially cause epileptic seizures (as can craniotomy to treat them). These can take a number of forms, including generalised grand mal seizures, Jacksonian motor seizures, sensory seizures and petit mal absence attacks. Seizures are typically associated with slow-growing, low-grade gliomas (LGGs), especially oligodendrogliomas. Seizures will often bring a tumour to light before other symptoms and signs and, for that reason, the presence of seizure is associated with a slightly improved survival in patients with HGG. However, a recurrence or worsening of a seizure following first-line treatment usually indicates disease progression. The efficacy of anticonvulsant medication depends on age, sex, organ dysfunction, comorbidity and cotherapies. Most patients are controlled with simple antiepileptic medication, but where this is problematic, the advice of a neurologist should be sought. Seizure control can be improved by surgical resection, RT and chemotherapy.

Raised Intracranial Pressure

Raised intracranial pressure (ICP) typically produces a triad of symptoms and signs: headaches, which are typically worse in the morning; nausea and vomiting; and papilloedema (oedema of the optic disk). Raised ICP most commonly arises as the result of obstructive hydrocephalus, and is therefore, particularly associated with tumours in the posterior fossa. It can also be associated with drowsiness, mild confusion and sometimes with personality changes. In severe cases, it can be followed by stupor and coma, hemiparesis or quadriparesis, respiratory abnormalities and eventually cardiopulmonary arrest. Management of elevated ICP depends on the patient's physical condition. CSF drainage should be attempted as appropriate, along with surgical removal of the lesion. Occasionally, other medical options (e.g. mannitol) need to be explored. Osmotic diuretics (mannitol) can be used in the acute situation to relieve pressure before commencing on a more definitive treatment. The first-line management in reducing intracranial pressure and symptomatic relief of symptoms is corticosteroids (e.g. dexamethasone).

Nonspecific Symptoms

Nonspecific symptoms are common and typical of CNS tumours. Such symptoms may be very difficult to identify as significant in the early phase of the illness. Headache, which may be local or generalised, but not related to raised ICP, occurs in some patients. The other characteristic symptom, particularly of HGG, is tiredness. Early symptoms may be frustratingly nonspecific, and a patient who complains of vague headache, tiredness and feeling off color is not likely to be investigated for a primary CNS tumour.

PRINCIPLES OF MANAGEMENT

Although most patients come to oncology with a definitive diagnosis, it is important for oncologists to contribute to the multidisciplinary management of CNS patients.

Diagnosis—A Combination of History, Imaging and Pathology

In neurooncology, perhaps more than any other area, it is helpful to combine information from the patient's history and examination findings, as well as imaging results and histology in determining the definitive diagnosis. The history and physical signs, especially the duration and any family history, may indicate a likely diagnosis or help to indicate whether the condition is a high-grade malignancy rather than a low-grade or benign tumour.

Typically, the diagnosis is suggested by computed tomography (CT) or MRI. In some tumour types, such as vestibular schwannoma (acoustic neuroma), imaging is definitive; in other cases, imaging offers only a differential diagnosis. Classical difficulties arise in distinguishing glioma from primary cerebral lymphoma and solitary metastasis from abscess or small glioma. Benign lesions can also have imaging appearances suggestive of malignancy. Therefore biopsy is crucial for obtaining a definitive diagnosis.

Some CNS tumours, especially gliomas, are rather heterogeneous, and it is understood that biopsy material may not necessarily be representative of the whole tumour. Occasionally, it may contain necrotic material only. Thus, clinical history and imaging appearances must also be considered in defining the exact diagnosis.

Performance Status in the Treatment Decision

Performance status (PS) is an important predictor of outcome, including survival, particularly for patients with glioma (Table 30.2). It also indicates how well the patient is likely to tolerate treatment. This is an important factor when recommending a treatment program. The choice can be between radical, palliative or active supportive care. For patients with disabling neurology, especially those with GBM, supportive care may be the most appropriate option.

Principles of Neurosurgery

The acquisition of histological material to define the diagnosis is extremely important. However, in many cases, there is also a role for a more extended procedure to debulk or remove the tumour and relieve

TABLE 30.2 WHO performance status, Glasgow coma scale (GCS) and Karnofsky Performance Status

The WHO performance status is useful in assessing patient capabilities, especially with respect to activities of daily living. The GCS is a measure of conscious level.

WHO PERFORMANCE STATUS

0. Able to carry out all normal activity without restriction.
1. Restricted in physically strenuous activity but ambulatory and able to carry out light work.
2. Ambulatory and capable of all self-care but unable to carry out any work; up and about >50% of waking hours.
3. Capable of only limited self-care; confined to bed or chair >50% of waking hours.
4. Completely disabled. Cannot carry out any self-care; totally confined to bed or chair.

Glasgow Coma Scale (GCS)

Eyes open	Spontaneously	4
	To speech	3
	To stimulus	2
	None	1
Best verbal response	Oriented	5
	Confused	4
	Inappropriate words	3
	Incomprehensible	2
	None	1
Best motor response	Obeys commands	6
	Localised stimulus	5
	Flexion–withdrawal	4
	Flexion–abnormal	3
	Extension	2
	No response	1

Best score 15
Worst 3

Karnofsky Status

Normal, no complaints	100
Able to carry on normal activities. Minor signs or symptoms of disease	90
Normal activity with effort	80
Care for self. Unable to carry on normal activity or to do active work	70
Requires occasional assistance, but able to care for most of his needs	60
Requires considerable assistance and frequent medical care	50
Disabled. Requires special care and assistance	40
Severly disabled. Hospitalisation indicated thought death nonimminent	30
Very sick. Hospitalisation necessary. Active supportive treatment necessary	20
Moribund	10
Dead	0

GCS, Glasgow Coma Scale; *WHO*, World Health Organization.

pressure effects (see sections on individual tumours). Surgical decompression improves symptoms quickly, allows reduced steroid doses, and facilitates RT, especially in patients with HGGs. Although maximum debulking of the tumour is a positive prognostic factor, gliomas are not cured by excision due to infiltration of tumour cells far beyond the visible lesion. Resection of lesions located in eloquent areas of white matter is not always the best treatment option as it can cause permanent neurological deficits and reduce the quality of life (QoL). Use of techniques such as fluorescent 5-aminolevulinic acid hydrochloride

(5-ALA) which permits intraoperative identification of anaplastic foci and awake craniotomy with accompanying functional monitoring have improved the safety of tumour resections. Occasional HGGs grow with a cystic component to the tumour. If fluid reaccumulates, then a small catheter can be placed into the cyst and attached to a subcutaneous (Ommaya) reservoir. By inserting a needle through the skin, fluid can be aspirated without the need for a further surgical procedure. Patients who present with, or develop, hydrocephalus may need a shunting procedure to redirect the flow of CSF. In adults, this is usually done with a VP shunt. Some patients with obstructive hydrocephalus can be successfully treated by a third ventriculostomy, avoiding the need for a shunt. In this procedure, a perforation is made in the floor of the third ventricle, allowing CSF to escape, and circumventing the obstruction.

Principles of Radiotherapy Planning for Central Nervous System Tumours

The fundamental principles of RT planning and treatment delivery apply to CNS tumours. These include accurate and reproducible immobilisation and high-quality imaging to localise the tumour and critical normal structures, using either three-dimensional conformal RT or preferably, intensity-modulated RT (IMRT), typically with rotational techniques, including TomoTherapy and volumetric arc therapy (VMAT). Brain tumours are characterised by irregular shapes which change in three dimensions. IMRT combined with image guidance has facilitated optimal RT especially for tumours considered difficult to treat because of their location (e.g. meningiomas of the skull base, gliomas located near the orbit and the brainstem). However, more recently, proton treatment is used generating highly conformal and complex dose distributions in these anatomic locations, allowing for dose escalation, especially in the management of radioresistant tumours (see Proton chapter 36). The other key clinical consideration in CNS tumour treatments is reduction of RT toxicity, especially to serial structures such as brainstem and optic pathway. Lower doses to the whole brain can also be achieved. IMRT does not increase the integral dose to the healthy brain, thus, can lead to reduced acute and late neurotoxicity, especially relevant with the addition of chemotherapy for some tumours in patients with increased overall survival. However, concerns have been raised about the long-term side effects of IMRT due to low-dose bath to the normal brain, particularly when irradiating benign tumours. The benefits of IMRT can be achieved with the addition of image-guided RT (IGRT) which can result in reduced margins and lead to further reduction of the total cumulative dose to normal untreated tissues (integral dose-total energy). IGRT allows for correction of both systematic (treatment preparation) and random (treatment delivery) errors.

Immobilisation devices include thermoplastic shells, Orfit shell or a relocatable stereotactic head frame. The optimal treatment position depends on the location of the tumour and on the immobilisation devices available. A supine position is more comfortable for the patient. Using couch extensions, such as an "S" frame or a relocatable stereotactic radiotherapy (SRT) head frame, allows treatment of posterior lesions with the patient supine.

For cranial spinal irradiation (CSI) IMRT-IGRT should be considered as the standard of care, achieving reduced dose to organs at risk (OARs) and better target dose homogeneity than older techniques.

Most planning is based on CT because this delivers exact patient geometry and position without distortion and because CT density is required for accurate dosimetry calculation. Preferably, intravenous (IV) contrast should be used because it enhances discrimination of the target. Although this changes the CT numbers slightly, dosimetry is affected by less than 1%. In most circumstances, tumours are less well demonstrated on CT than on MRI, and MRI should be considered an essential modality for planning. All efforts should be made to perform the MRI in the treatment position. The MR images are then coregistered with those of the CT scan.

The correct choice of MRI sequence must be made to optimise definition of the tumour. T1-weighted MRI (T1W) with contrast enhancement provides information on tumour extent; however, the appearances can be influenced by areas of blood-brain barrier (BBB) breakdown. T2-weighted (T2W) and fluid-attenuated inversion recovery (FLAIR) images can help identify a nonenhancing component of the tumour. The FLAIR sequence is helpful in low-grade gliomas, as well as in demonstrating progression of the tumour in secondary GBMs.

CT and MRI are complementary. Although MRI is in general the better modality for showing tumour, CT is extremely useful to determine the exact position of the bone, extent of bone involvement, or the barriers to spread of a noninvasive tumour which is limited by bone. MRI sequences (such as diffusion weighted and diffusion tensor imaging) can be used to help distinguish the tumour cell density and the fractional anisotropy at resection margins in low-grade gliomas. MR perfusion measures cerebral blood volume in tumours and can be used to identify the best area to obtain a biopsy, as it can help in distinguishing malignant activity from tumour necrosis. MR spectroscopy and positron emission tomography (PET) imaging can provide information on the metabolic activity of the tumour. They can also be helpful in tumour grading and differentiating between response to treatment and necrosis. In some meningiomas that have been completely resected, coregistration with the preoperative MRI may be helpful in determining the location of the tumour and possible spread. PET scanning can be useful for planning in some circumstances, using methionine (an amino acid) or DOTATOC (1,4,7,10-tetraazacyclododecane-$N^I,N^{II},N^{III},N^{IIII}$-tetraacetic acid (D)-Phe^1-thy^3-octreotide).

Planning Volumes

The International Commission on Radiation Units (ICRU) report 83 sets guidelines on planning IMRT and offers useful recommendations for planning volumes. The definitions of gross tumour volume (GTV), clinical target volume (CTV) and planning target volume (PTV) as outlined in ICRU 83 should be used for planning purposes. Imaging shows the extent of the GTV. For GBMs, early recurrence after the operation is common and can even be visible in the MRI RT planning scan. New imaging approaches mentioned above could be used for the gliomas and meningiomas to improve the target volume definition and add to the individualisation of the treatment. Historical data are used to define a CTV margin around it, which is typically the same in all patients with the same condition. Following an isotopic growth from GTV, the CTV is edited to account for anatomical barriers of tumour spread (e.g. bone). The PTV margin is designed to account for uncertainties in planning and treatment and has systematic (i.e. treatment preparation) and random (i.e. treatment delivery) elements. The margin should be added based on the recipe formula outlined in the British Institute of Radiology 2003 report *Geometric uncertainties in radiotherapy* and incorporated into ICRU 83.

IMRT with IGRT should be considered standard practice because this limits dose to normal tissues. There is reasonable evidence that this in turn reduces complications in patients treated for CNS tumours, by reducing the volume of tissue, especially brain, receiving a high dose, or avoiding exposure to sensitive structures, such as the hypothalamus and pituitary gland (conformal avoidance). Eye lens doses should be estimated with thermoluminescent dosimetry

(TLD) for future reference. On-treatment portal films or images should be used to confirm positioning for radical treatments. Three-dimensional RT can be used in a palliative setting, increasing the conformity of the dose in comparison to older techniques and protecting the critical structures.

Normal Tissue Tolerance to Radiotherapy

Normal tissue tolerance is an important concept. It embodies both the risk of a complication and also the severity of its effect on the patient. The relevance also depends on the clinical setting: a higher risk of normal tissue damage might be accepted in a patient with a highly malignant tumour requiring a high RT dose who has only a low chance of long-term survival, than is reasonable in a patient with a benign tumour. The dose that is considered safe may therefore vary from one condition to another. Another important factor that should be taken under consideration is the addition of chemotherapy and biological agents in the treatment of CNS tumours. These may affect the tolerance of normal brain, brain stem and optic pathway, though detailed information is lacking. It is known that drugs such as methotrexate (MTX) used for primary central nervous system lymphomas (PCNSL) can induce radiation damage.

There is almost certainly a volume effect in normal tissue tolerance of CNS structures, as in other parts of the body. This means that the larger the volume irradiated, the lower the safe dose. The CNS is also particularly sensitive to the dose per fraction, and many of the dose-fractionation schedules used are designed to take advantage of this. The best available data is presented in the detailed quantitative analysis of normal tissue effects in the clinic (QUANTEC) reports.

Tolerance of the brain itself (to avoid necrosis) is in the region of 54 to 60 gray (Gy) in approximately 30 fractions, depending on volume treated and dose per fraction. A volume effect also exists for intellectual damage. Using three-dimensional conformal RT, intellectual damage in adults is uncommon with doses up to 54 Gy in 30 fractions. The brainstem is said to have a slightly lower tolerance than brain substance, approximately 54 Gy in 30 fractions (or 55 Gy in 33 fractions). Smaller volumes of the brainstem (1–10 mL) could receive a maximum dose of 59 Gy using conventional fractionation of 2 Gy per fraction. QUANTEC suggests a change in α/β ratio for normal brain to 2.9 Gy in comparison to 2.0 Gy.

The optic nerves and chiasm are also thought to be more sensitive than brain parenchyma. For benign tumours in this region, a dose of 45 Gy in 25 fractions to 50 Gy in 30 fractions should be safe, with a risk of blindness which is virtually zero. Optic neuropathy should be avoided with doses less than 55 Gy and less than 60 Gy, as a primary and secondary criterion, according to the QUANTEC report. The incidence of optic neuropathy is approximately 7% for doses of 66 Gy.

The pituitary gland and hypothalamus have a much lower tolerance for hormonal dysfunction, which may occur in 80% of patients receiving RT. There is probably little effect for doses under 20 to 24 Gy, but adults in whom these structures receive 40 to 60 Gy have a significant long-term risk of hypothalamic–pituitary axis dysfunction. The most sensitive cells to RT are those that secrete growth hormone (GH), followed by gonadotropin hormones, adrenocorticptropic hormone (ACTH) and thyroid-stimulating hormone (TSH). The frequency and severity of symptoms correlate to the total dose, the dose per fraction and the age of the patient at the time of irradiation, although the exact details of the dose-response relationships are not known. It is important that patients who receive high doses of RT to the hypothalamic-pituitary axis have long-term follow-up. Early replacement therapy should be started as required to avoid the development of endocrinological syndromes.

The lacrimal gland shows reduced tear output after doses over about 20 Gy (similar to salivary glands). Doses over 40 Gy can cause dry eye syndrome, whereas doses over 57 Gy can lead to permanent atrophy and fibrosis of the lacrimal gland.

The lens of the eye should not develop cataract after doses less than 5 to 6 Gy spread out over 30 fractions. There is a 50% risk of cataract after a dose of 15 Gy. Therefore, the recommended maximum dose for adults should range between 5 and 10 Gy. The middle and inner ears are also sensitive structures, and there are reports of hearing loss in adults with doses to the cochlea ranging between 45 to 50 Gy.

The risk of permanent alopecia depends on the dose to the hair follicles in the dermis. The risk is very low with doses below 10 to 15 Gy, but 50% of patients will develop permanent alopecia after 43 Gy (in 30 fractions) to the scalp. This dose is difficult to estimate routinely because the hair follicles normally fall within the build-up region.

The spinal cord has a tolerance of approximately 50 Gy in 30 fractions. This may be a conservative (i.e. safe) estimate and, in some circumstances, higher doses may be appropriate, such as for GBM of the spinal cord. New evidence suggests that an alpha/beta ratio of 0.87 Gy may be more appropriate for the cervical spinal cord. The above ratio is low, meaning that larger fractions can cause more severe effects.

The hippocampus (dentate gyrus) contains neural stem cells which aid cognitive function. The delineation of the hippocampus as an OAR is advisable, although there is no consensus on what the tolerance radiation dose to this area should be. Suggestive dose restrictions, with the aim to avoid impairment in memory function are 7.3 Gy to 40% of the bilateral hippocampus, but not to exceed 9 Gy to 100% of the hippocampus, with maximal hippocampal dose not exceeding 16 Gy in 30 fractions. The ipsilateral hippocampus is included in the PTV area in the majority of the glial tumours, so efforts usually concentrate on sparing the contralateral hippocampus where feasible.

The retina should have doses restricted to less than 45 Gy to avoid the risk of radiation retinopathy.

Principles of Steroid Therapy

Steroids are used to treat oedema in the brain, caused by tumour or surgery, so many patients attend the neurooncology clinic already taking a steroid such as dexamethasone. A daily dose of dexamethasone, 16 mg, in four divided doses (qds), is considered the highest useful dose in most circumstances. This is a typical dose used perioperatively, and is usually reduced as quickly as possible. Patients on anticonvulsant drugs, which increase the metabolism of dexamethasone, occasionally benefit from higher doses in the palliative setting.

In patients requiring RT where significant intracranial pressure remains, steroid is needed, and may need to be increased during the course. However, there is no absolute indication for steroids during RT. In patients in whom surgery has relieved intracranial pressure, none may be necessary. It is thus possible to reduce steroid doses during a course of RT.

p0540 dexamethasone has important side effects that can impact seriously on quality of life. These include increased appetite, weight gain, muscle weakness, gastric irritation, diabetes, cerebral atrophy, reduced taste and smell, osteoporosis, infections and mood disturbances. Rarely, it causes psychosis, which is very distressing and difficult to manage. Patients should be managed with the minimum possible dose. For reduction, the dose must be tailed off slowly and not stopped abruptly. Patients should also be issued with a steroid card.

Principles of Additional Supportive Care

It is important to think holistically about patients with CNS tumours. This includes biological, psychological, social and cultural aspects of their care. This patient group is very diverse, with a wide range of diagnoses and prognoses, and the problems experienced by the patients therefore, vary greatly. Even patients with benign tumours may experience major problems, even if these are not life threatening. For example, the seriousness of the condition is obvious in a patient with weakness due to GBM undertaking palliative treatment. However, hearing loss due to vestibular schwannoma can also have a distressing impact on a young patient who needs to hear for childcare or work.

Supportive input may be valuable to a patient throughout their journey. Needs vary according to tumour type, and may fluctuate throughout the patient's journey, with treatment or progression. Many patients benefit from practical and psychological support. The relevant support is often best developed by a specialist nurse, who will be part of most neurooncology teams. Key roles are liaison with the patient and family, other health care professionals and hospice services and provision of information from local or general resources, such as Cancer BACUP (http://www.cancerbacup.org.uk/Home.). For some patients, especially those with gliomas, financial benefits may be available.

Driving After a Diagnosis of Central Nervous System Tumour

Many patients with primary CNS tumours are not allowed to drive following the diagnosis. This is because there is a risk of seizure as a result of the tumour. There is also a small risk of seizure following craniotomy, whatever the underlying condition. In particular, patients with high-grade gliomas have their driving licenses revoked for 2 years, timed from the completion of treatment.

Decisions about licensing are made in the United Kingdom by the Driver and Vehicle Licensing Authority (DVLA), with information provided from the clinical teams. In general, the DVLA will help patients to regain a license, and will provide an individualised decision in unusual circumstances. The DVLA provides information on the guidelines for return of licenses for medical practitioners which can be obtained from the DVLA website (www.DVLA.gov.uk). It is worth using this on-line facility because the regulations do change from time to time.

INDIVIDUAL TUMOUR TYPES

High-Grade Gliomas
Pathology and Clinical Features

GBM is the most common primary CNS tumour in adults (see Fig. 30.1) representing 54% of malignant brain tumours. GBMs (and diffuse midline glioma-grade IV WHO) and grade III gliomas (anaplastic (oligo- or astrocytoma) gliomas) are collectively known as HGGs. The major problems with HGGs are:
1. Significant damage to neurological function.
2. Diffuse infiltration through the brain, often for quite large distances—frequently crossing the midline to involve the contralateral brain.
3. Resistance to treatment, including both RT and chemotherapy.

HGGs grow with an expanding, destructive process. Beyond the gross tumour, malignant cells infiltrate widely. The gross tumour is typically surrounded by a zone of extensive oedema. Steroid treatment reduces oedema and may improve neurological function. However, there is no method to restore function which has been lost as a result of the destruction of neural tissue in the centre of the tumour.

HGGs, especially GBMs, are efficient at spreading through the brain, predominantly following white matter tracts (see earlier and Fig. 30.3). Spread across the midline, principally through the corpus callosum, is a major route for invasion. This infiltration occurs at a microscopic level, and so currently cannot be imaged. The extent of invasion varies between individuals. Despite the wide infiltration, HGGs typically recur at the primary site. There is thus, no survival advantage in irradiating the whole brain. HGGs very rarely metastasise outside the CNS.

Patients present as described previously. On CT and MRI, HGGs can be seen as space-occupying lesions with surrounding oedema that are causing mass effect. The gross tumour enhances with intravenous contrast. GBMs in particular, have a heterogeneous enhancement in the gross tumour. This reflects their growth, with areas of necrosis within the tumour. The typical GBM is shown in Fig. 30.5. In patients with pressure effects, surgical decompression may improve symptoms quickly, allowing reduced steroid doses and facilitating RT.

According to the WHO 2016 classification, a GBM is divided in to two categories based on its isocitrate dehydrogenase (IDH) mutations: the IDH wild-type (no mutation) GBM is considered as primary or de novo GBM found in 90% of patients, and the IDH-mutated GBM corresponds to secondary GBM, arising from lower grade glioma found in the remaining 10% of patients who have better prognosis. In addition, O^6-alkylguanine DNA alkyltransferase (MGMT) methylation serves as a good prognostic and predictive factor. MGMT is the enzyme which breaks down temozolomide to methylation, resulting in inactivation of the gene, prevents this breakdown and response to the drug is much improved. MGMT methylation status is used to guide treatment decisions especially in elderly patients. It is worth noting the presence of a telomerase reverse transcriptase (TERT) promoter mutation has a negative impact on prognosis and can be found in 74% of GBMs. Epidermal growth factor receptor (EGFR) is also commonly tested for and found to be amplified in 40% of the GBM cases.

For the grade III tumours (anaplastic astrocytomas, anaplastic oligodedrogliomas and anaplastic oligoastrocytomas), the mutations in the IDH1 and IDH2 genes are quite frequent (in the range of 55%–80%). IDH mutations are also associated with codeletion of the 1p and 19q chromosome arms (1p19q codeletion) and with MGMT promoter methylation. In the anaplastic type, the wild-types of IDH1- and IDH2-lack mutations are associated with increased risk of aggressive disease. In anaplastic oligodendrogliomas, those possessing a codeletion of chromosomes 1p and 19q have prolonged survival compared to noncodeleted tumours, due to their increased response to treatment, particularly to alkylating chemotherapy.

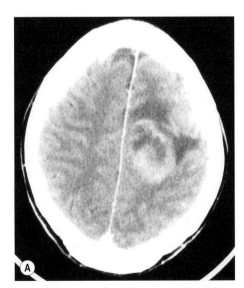

Fig. 30.5 Computed tomography with contrast of a patient with a glioblastoma, showing a contrast-enhanced mass with central necrosis and surrounding oedema.

TABLE 30.3 **Suggested Criteria for Choice of Treatment in Patients With High-Grade Gliomas**	
Radical RT	Age <70 (younger in some centres) or chemo-RT
	PS 0 or 1
	No significant neurological deficit remaining
Palliative RT	Age ≤70 and PS 0 or 1
	Age <70, with a significant deficit
Supportive care	Severe residual deficit, e.g. hemiplegia
	Intellectual impairment
Note: The patient's choice should be considered in all cases. Where appropriate, agreement from the relatives is also valuable, especially for the supportive care option.	

HGG, high-grade glioma; *PS*, performance status; *RT*, radiotherapy.

Treatment

Management options may be radical (curative), palliative or active supportive care only (Table 30.3). The decision depends on PS, age and tumour location, as well as patient preference. Patients with poor neurological condition are unlikely to benefit from radical treatment, while older patients tolerate the neurological effects of both the tumour and the treatment less well. For these patients, the option of shorter course, palliative treatment may be most suitable. For elderly patients, or those with very poor neurological function, quality of life is not improved by any available therapy. Referral for expert palliative and supportive care is therefore the most appropriate management.

Histological diagnosis is highly desirable provided further treatment will be given. The genetic profile of CNS tumours can be used as a predictive or prognostic factor, and it can also aid in patient selection for clinical trials.

For radical treatment, debulking surgery is to be preferred where possible. It extends survival but, equally important, it relieves mass effect. In turn, this improves neurological functioning, reduces steroid requirements and facilitates RT. Early postoperative MRI, within 24 to 48 hours, demonstrates the extent of any residual gross tumour; it is very useful for comparison with the RT planning MRI. For young, fit patients with GBM, the addition of chemotherapy with oral temozolomide has been shown to significantly extend survival. In diffuse midline astrocytomas (grade IV, WHO 2016 classification), one should follow the treatment guidelines for GBMs. The treatment for anaplastic astrocytoma (without 1p19q codeletion) has been guided by the CATNON Trial (Phase III Trial on Concurrent and Adjuvant Temozolomide Chemotherapy in Non-1p/19q Deleted Anaplastic Glioma): RT (59.4 Gy in 33#) followed by 12 months of temozolomide. Anaplastic oligodendroglioma (1p19q codeleted) should be offered RT (54 Gy in 30#) with adjuvant procarbazine, lomustine (CCNU) and vincristine (PCV for 6 cycles.

The outcome of patients with HGG is surprisingly variable. The three most important prognostic factors for better outcome are younger age, better PS, including good cognitive status and extent of surgery. In terms of age, patients aged younger than 40 years have the best outlook, those aged between 40 and 60 years do less well, and those aged over 70 years fare badly. The extent of surgical resection has prognostic value as it improves survival and might increase the efficacy of adjuvant treatments. Patients with brainstem HGG, in whom even a biopsy attempt is hazardous, do particularly badly. Presentation with epilepsy provides a small survival advantage, but this is almost certainly simply the result of making the patient present earlier in their illness pathway.

In rare cases, HGG can be very extensive, affecting the whole of the hemisphere or even the majority of the cerebrum. This used to be known as gliomatosis cerebri. Usually, it does normally respond to

RT. Although most times not much of the normal brain can be spared, RT can improve the neurological deficit in most patients.

Radical Treatment

Target Volume

The patient should be immobilised in a shell, positioned supine with the chin in a neutral position. Postoperative imaging is required to demonstrate the true extent and position of residual tumour after decompression. MRI produces superior definition of tumour, and the T1-weighted with gadolinium (T1W+Gd) and T2/FLAIR sequences should be coregistered to the planning CT.

The European Society for therapeutic Radiology and Oncology (ESTRO)-Advisory Committee on Radiation Oncology Practice (ACROP) groups have both produced guidelines for RT target volume definition based on protocols used in the studies they have designed and run. The recommendation of ESTRO-ACROP is to aim to deliver 60 Gy in 30 fractions in a single phase.

The GTV is defined as the visible contrast-enhancing edge of tumour, shown most clearly on MRI, using T1W with gadolinium contrast. For the definition of the GTV, it should be taken into consideration the post-surgical changes (infarction or gliosis). Thus, a comparison of planning MRI with preoperative scans and postoperative diffusion-weighted imaging (DWI) can help differentiate postop vascular changes from residual tumour, and moreover, the molecular profile of the tumour. For example, patients with secondary GBM (IDH mutant), nonenhancing areas may be a component of the tumour; in such cases, consideration may be given to include hyperintensity on T2/FLAIR in the GTV, in addition to the contrast-enhancing tumour, because the high-signal regions are considered to represent regions of low-grade tumour.

According to the ESTRO-ACROP protocol, the GTV is defined as the surgical resection cavity plus the residual enhancing tumour, or as unresected enhancing tumour (for biopsy-only patients) defined by T1W + Gd.

The GTV is expanded isotropically to reach the CTV. Because of the infiltrative nature of HGGs, a large CTV margin is needed. The ESTRO-ACROP protocol uses a 2-cm margin from the GTV, edited to take into account anatomical barriers to tumour spread.

The CTV does not have to extend beyond the inner table of the skull, which is best shown on CT using the bone window. Ideally, the CTV should be edited to account for natural barriers such as ventricles (5 mm), falx (5 mm), and tentorium cerebelli (5 mm). The CTV crosses the midline when the tumour extends to the contralateral hemisphere or infiltrates the corpus callosum.

Each CTV is expanded isotropically to its PTV with an appropriate margin, specific to the technique in each department. A margin of 0.3 to 0.5 cm is common.

Outline critical normal structures, including the eyes, the lenses, lacrimal glands, cochlea, pituitary and hypothalamus. It is essential to outline the optic structures. The delineation of the contralateral hippocampus should be considered in terms of sparing the organ; however, there is not sufficient evidence to support recommendations on hippocampal sparing.

Technique

IMRT with image guidance should be considered as standard of care. It achieves the best target dose conformity and homogeneity, and optimum critical normal tissue sparing.

Dose and Energy

An important recent development is the use of single-phase treatment.
  For grade III (anaplastic) glioma:
Single phase to deliver 54 to 59.4 Gy in 30 to 33 fractions over 6 weeks, with 6-MV photons.

For gliomatosis cerebri (very large tumours), a slightly smaller dose per fraction may be helpful, and a dose of 55 Gy in 33 fractions is suitable.
  For grade IV glioma (GBM):
Single phase to deliver 60 Gy in 30 fractions over 6 weeks, with 6-MV photons.

Chemotherapy for Radical Treatment of Glioblastoma

Using the protocol from the European Organization of Research and Treatment of Cancer (EORTC) trial, oral temozolomide is given in two blocks, the first daily (including weekends), concomitant with radical RT, and the second for 5 days each month as an adjuvant treatment following RT.

Concomitant with radical RT: continuous daily dose of 75 mg/m^2 (i.e. 7 days per week), starting on the first day of RT, and finishing on the last day.

Adjuvant treatment following RT: commencing 28 days after completion of RT, is consisted of six cycles of adjuvant temozolomide (150 to 200 mg per square meter for 5 days during each 28-day cycle).

Chemotherapy for Radical Treatment of Grade III Gliomas

Adjuvant chemotherapy for grade III gliomas is decided according to the molecular profile of the tumours, such as the presence or absence of the IDH mutation, the status of 1p19q codeletion, and the PS of the patient. A survival benefit has been shown for patients with 1p/19q co-deleted anaplastic oligodedrogliomas or oligoastrocytoma that received PCV (acronym for the drugs, Procarbazine, Lomustine (CCNU) and Vincristine, in the regimen) chemotherapy. Evidence is accumulating that patients with IDH wild-type (normal) tumours and MGMT promoter methylation benefited from chemotherapy with alkylating drugs such as temozolomide.

It is recommended that PCV administration follows RT treatment. PCV administration: procarbazine 60mg/m^2 orally days 8 through 21, CCNU (also called lomustine) 110 mg/m^2 orally day1 (maximum 200 mg), vincristine 1.4 mg/m^2 IV days 8 and 29 for 6 to 8 weeks.

Side Effects

Acute. Acute tiredness is almost invariable, though it is of variable severity. It appears to be related to the volume treated. Tiredness increases during the course, has a fluctuating pattern, and may be at its worst shortly after completion of RT. Early delayed somnolence is rare in adults.

Hair loss occurs in about the third week after treatment starts. Hair washing has no effect on hair loss or scalp reactions, provided it is carried out carefully. With 54 Gy, hair regrowth is almost normal in most patients; with 60 Gy, at least some hair loss is usually permanent. Erythema and soreness of skin can occur, particularly if the pinna is included in an entry port. If the external auditory canal is irradiated, this gets sore and crusted, and the wax becomes more viscid and difficult to remove. If the ear drum and middle ear are irradiated, then secretory otitis media (glue ear) may result, but this usually settles spontaneously. Inner ear damage is uncommon. In patients treated for HGG, headache and nausea are uncommon. Seizures occasionally worsen during RT; dexamethasone is useful, and anticonvulsants should be reviewed.

Late. If the hypothalamus and pituitary have been irradiated, hormone failure may occur after a minimum of 1 to 2 years, but may occur later. Routine pituitary function tests are therefore appropriate in the few patients who are long-term survivors. Although the most important late effect in the brain is radio-necrosis, this is an extremely uncommon clinical event. The QUANTEC report suggests that there is a possibility of 5% and 10% risk at 5 years of symptomatic radiation necrosis applying the standard fractionation at a dose of 72 Gy (range 60–84 Gy) and 90 Gy (range 84–102 Gy), respectively. These doses are higher than used routinely.

Deterioration During Radiotherapy

Some patients deteriorate during RT. This is usually due to increased oedema, presumably resulting from tumour cell necrosis. It is usually treatable with an increase in dexamethasone dose. Occasionally, a cystic component can enlarge and warrants neurosurgical intervention, such as aspiration and insertion of an Ommaya reservoir. A few patients deteriorate during RT due to tumour progression. In these cases, it is appropriate to switch to palliative fractionation (see later), making an appropriate dose change according to the dose already delivered, or to stop RT altogether.

Results of Treatment

In a randomised trial of patients with GBM, the addition of oral temozolomide chemotherapy extended survival significantly: median survival was extended from 12 months to 14.5, and 2-year survival increased from 10% to 26%. Anaplastic (grade III) gliomas with IDH mutation were found to have an improved median survival, 14.7 years compared with 6.8 years for those that did not carry the mutation. The prolonged overall survival and disease-free survival with the addition of temozolomide in the CATNON trial are shown in Fig. 30.6.

Palliative Treatment

Target Volume and Technique

The patient should be immobilised in a shell and a three-field solution using a three-dimensional conformal plan is advised. CT is used for planning purposes, with IV contrast to outline the GTV; apply a slightly smaller margin of 1.5 + 0.5 cm for CTV and PTV margins, respectively; no editing of the CTV is necessary. If there is uncertainty in localising the tumour, use a CTV margin of 2.5 cm, as for radical RT. Use the same PTV margins as for radical RT.

Elderly Patients

The EORTC 26062 trial showed that a palliative dose of RT (40 Gy in 15 fractions), in addition to concomitant and maintenance Temozolomide (TMZ), offered a modest increase in median survival (9.3 vs 7.6 months, $P = .001$), compared with RT alone, for both groups (mMGMT and unmethylated). The maximum benefit was for the patients older than 70 years, particularly those with tumours that express MGMT methylation.

In addition, a prospective trial comparing the 40 Gy in 15 fractions to 25 Gy in 5 fractions over 1 week, supported that the short course was not inferior in terms of survival.

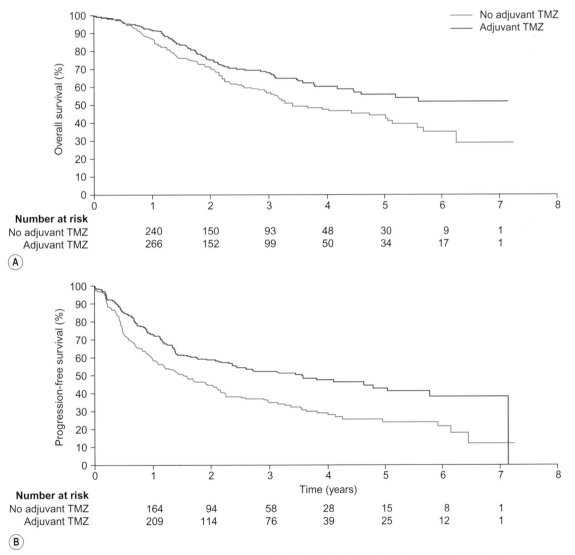

Fig. 30.6 Kaplan–Meier overall survival and progression free survival curves in patients treated with or without adjuvant temozolomide as per CATNON Trial (Phase III Trial on Concurrent and Adjuvant Temozolomide (TMZ) Chemotherapy in 1p/19q nondeleted Anaplastic Glioma). (A) Overall survival. (B) Progression-free survival.

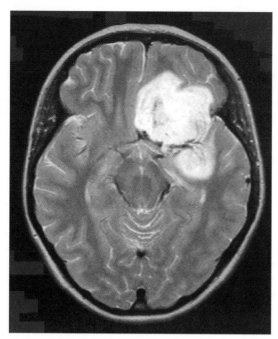

Fig. 30.7 T2 weighted magnetic resonance imaging of a large grade II astrocytoma. Oedema within the tumour has a high signal (*appears white*). This region would be considered the gross tumor volume. Cerebrospinal fluid) between the folds of the brain is also white. On computed tomography, this area would be shown as a low-density region.

Dose and Energy

Does are given as 30 Gy in six fractions, treating three times per week, over 2 weeks, with megavoltage photons or 40 Gy in 15 fractions over 3 weeks ± concomitant TMZ followed by adjuvant TMZ for 12 months.

Side Effects

Acute tiredness occurs with palliative RT, and some hair loss is inevitable, although it occurs after completion of RT. Some regrowth occurs, but hair does not return to normal. Erythema is mild, and headache and nausea are very uncommon. As a result of the poor prognosis, late side effects are rarely relevant.

Results of Treatment

The outlook for patients with HGG who receive palliative RT is poor, with a median survival of only 140 days (just under 5 months) from first presentation in oncology. However, a small number of patients survive for much longer, a few remaining alive for over 2 years. Those patients deemed unfit for palliative RT have a median survival of only 6 weeks.

LOW-GRADE GLIOMAS

Pathology and Clinical Features

LGGs include those with WHO grades I and II. Grade I tumours are rare in adults. Grade II tumours include oligodendrogliomas and astrocytomas (diffuse astrocytoma grade II, the most common type). LGGs represent about 12% of the total number of cases referred to oncology (see Fig. 30.1). The patients typically present at a younger age than high-grade gliomas, with a peak incidence between ages 35 and 44 years. Although LGGs present in similar ways to other primary tumours, seizure is a much more common presenting complaint than with other tumours. Oligodendrogliomas (of grade II) are particularly likely to present with epilepsy. Because of this tendency to cause seizure, many patients with LGG are followed up in neurology clinics. In addition, in some patients, the diagnosis is an incidental finding after imaging for unrelated symptoms. The course of the illness is extremely variable. Some LGGs appear never to progress, and others may take a decade or more to do so. However, some tumours show evidence of disease progression from the time of diagnosis, driven by malignant transformation related to the accumulation of genetic mutations. These are the patients that are typically referred for an oncology opinion.

LGGs are characterised by a mutation in the IDH gene family. A separate subtype of oligodendrogliomas is classified by the losses of the whole arm of the 1p and 19q chromosomes (1p/19q co-deletion). Astrocytomas have intact 1p and 19q chromosomes, but loss of ATRX. In grade II diffuse gliomas, the mutations in either IDH1 or IDH2 are present in 80% of the cases and carry a more favourable prognosis compared with IDH wild-type (normal) tumours. When these tumours progress, they may do so in their original form, but they may also undergo further genetic mutation causing transformation to a higher grade, grade III or even GBM. This occurs in about half the patients who progress, and is not itself caused or influenced by RT. The increase in grade changes the outlook. Grade II oligodendrogliomas altering to higher-grade tumours are categorised as grade III anaplastic oligodendrogliomas. When grade II astrocytomas transform to higher grade, they can become either grade III anaplastic astrocytomas or GBMs.

Currently, there is a controversy on how to best manage LGGs. According to recent trials, patients can be categorised into two groups: low risk (age <40 years old and gross total resection) and high risk (age >40 or <39 years with subtotal resection). It is suggested that high-risk patients should undergo a trimodality treatment of surgery, chemotherapy and RT. Patients who fall into the low-risk category may undergo routine MRI surveillance after resection. The treatment decision should be individualised on the basis of pathology classification, age, extent of resection, QoL and patient preference.

Surgery has an important role in obtaining biopsy tissue to prove the diagnosis for WHO grade and molecular biology. It may also be helpful if there is substantial mass effect in the brain or uncontrollable seizures because resection improves pressure symptoms. Beyond these indications, the role of surgery remains controversial. Surgical series typically contain younger patients with smaller tumours, and are therefore not directly comparable with RT or surveillance series. For patients who are asymptomatic, or whose tumour is presented in eloquent brain areas or if the tumour is large, the decision of performing the surgery, should take under consideration the possible cognitive deficits.

RT is indicated for patients with disease progression demonstrated by worsening neurology, epilepsy or imaging. Pathological diagnosis from biopsy is recommended before RT is undertaken. In patients with progressive disease, RT almost certainly delays tumour progression and death, although incontrovertible proof for this is lacking. Whether RT actually cures some patients is not known. RT improves epilepsy in about 50% of patients with LGG. In rare circumstances, it can be used to try to improve intractable epilepsy in a patient with LGG.

In patients without demonstrable progression, the timing of RT is less critical. There is excellent information that survival is unaffected by the timing of RT, whether it is given immediately or later when progression occurs. This is reassuring when counselling patients.

In addition, RT is indicated for patients with larger tumours (>5 cm), tumours close to eloquent brain areas that cross the midline, patients older than 40 years and IDH negative. Furthermore, a metaanalysis showed that the presence of neurological deficits, a short time of symptoms (<30 weeks), an astrocytic subtype and a size of tumour of more than 5 cm in diameter carries a worse prognosis. According to the long-term analysis of the Radiation Therapy Oncology Group (RTOG) 9802 trial, half of the low-risk (age <40 years and gross total resection) patients included in the study, who underwent only gross total resection (GTR), relapsed at 5 years, whereas in this group the active surveillance with MRI could be a proper option. For the high-risk group, the addition of chemotherapy with PCV and RT to the surgery offered a greater benefit in overall survival (OS). The benefit was highest in the subgroup with 1p19q co-deletion. In addition, it was suggested that in high-risk patients, regardless of the histology and the molecular profile, the addition of RT and PCV is beneficial.

Astrocytoma grade II tumours with IDH wild-type disease is an area that there is minimal clinical trial evidence to guide the optimal management approach. A proportion will behave similar to a GBM and could be considered for surgery, RT and chemotherapy. Decision making for this presentation should be undertaken on a patient-specific approach by the multidisciplinary team.

The option of chemotherapy is also under active investigation. The choice of the chemotherapy regimen is related to the molecular profile and histological subtype. The use of PCV proved to be beneficial for high-risk patients. Two ongoing trials (RTOG 0424 and the EORTC 22033-26033) add temozolomide to RT and report a benefit in overall survival as well an improvement in progression-free survival in those with IDH-mutated astrocytoma without the 1p19q co-deletion.

LGGs grow with diffuse infiltrative patterns, without destruction of involved brain. Therefore, patients may have functioning brain within the tumour, even though tumours may be very large. This imposes a fundamental limitation on surgery for LGG. Neurological deficits caused by LGGs frequently improve following RT. It is therefore appropriate to consider patients for RT even if they have neurological deficits, which is entirely the opposite of HGGs.

On imaging with CT, tumours are typically large, with low density. Oligodendrogliomas often have areas of calcification, which give a characteristic speckled appearance, helpful in suggesting a preoperative diagnosis. On MRI, LGGs show low signal on T1W and absence of contrast enhancement. The tumour is usually best delineated using a T2W or FLAIR sequence where CSF and oedema appear white. This correlates with the low density seen on CT. A typical LGG is shown in Fig. 30.7.

Radical Treatment

Target Volume

The patient should be immobilised in a shell. If resection has been carried out, then postoperative imaging is required. Even if biopsy has been the only surgical procedure, current imaging is needed. MRI produces optimal localisation of the tumour, especially the T2W or FLAIR sequence. This should be co-registered with the planning CT. The GTV is defined as the full extent of visible abnormality demonstrated on the T2W or FLAIR MRI. This volume is often very large. For patients who have undergone surgery, the GTV should include the postoperative residual disease. A CTV margin of approximately 1.5 cm can be used, smaller than for HGG. The CTV does not have to extend beyond the inner table of the skull, which is best shown on CT. The CTV should be grown isotropically to its PTV, with an appropriate margin; 0.3 to 0.5 cm is common.

Technique

An IMRT solution is optimal for these patients, aiming to achieve good dose homogeneity in the target and reduce the dose to normal tissues and OARs. TLD is recommended to estimate doses to the lens.

Dose and Energy

Single phase dose is 50.4 to 54 Gy in 28 to 30 daily fractions over 5.5 to 6 weeks, with 6-MV photons.

Side Effects

Acute and late effects are similar to HGG, particularly grade III gliomas, for which the same dose is used. Seizures may worsen during RT. Dexamethasone is useful, and anticonvulsants should be reviewed. Late hypothalamus and pituitary dysfunction is an important issue in long-term follow-up, particularly since the prognosis is much more favorable than HGG. In addition, because of higher survival rates seen with LGG tumours, the side effects related to cognitive decline and memory deficits, endocrine deficits and secondary malignancies should be considered. There is an emerging need to address the quality of life for these patients as an important issue due to long-term survival.

Results of Treatment

The outcome of patients with LGG is quite variable. However, younger age, smaller tumours and lack of neurological deficit are prognostic for better outcome. In addition, the histological type also has an effect: oligodendroglioma histology has a better outlook than astrocytoma.

Many patients with neurological deficits from tumours experience improvement, and this is a very important indication to undertake RT. In half of patients who have epilepsy, the frequency and severity of seizures improves after RT.

In the large European trial which evaluated the timing of RT, early RT delayed progression of LGG by about 2 years. This increase in disease-free survival may be of value to patients. Median survival (i.e. 50% of patients alive) was around 7.5 years, irrespective of the timing of RT. Ten-year survival data are in the range of 40% to 60%.

The oligodendroglial subtype has a better prognosis (median survival 10–15 years) than the astrocytic subtypes (median survival 6 years). Multimodality therapy increases median OS (13.3 years in patients treated with both chemotherapy and RT vs 7.8 years in patients receiving RT alone). Ten-year disease-free survival (DFS) accounts for 51% in patients receiving both treatments and 21% in patients receiving only RT.

EPENDYMOMA (INTRACRANIAL)

Pathology and Clinical Features

Intracranial ependymoma is a rare primary tumour (see Fig. 30.1), more common in children than adults. The incidence of the ependymomas is 1.8% of all primary CNS tumours and accounts for 6.8% of all gliomas, with male predominance. It is thought to be derived from ependymal cells that line the ventricular system. It arises most often in the posterior fossa, though it can be supratentorial. Typically, posterior fossa lesions present as the result of obstructive hydrocephalus and increased intracranial pressure, causing multiple cranial nerve palsies, neck stiffness and head tilt when they infiltrate the upper portion of the cervical cord. According to the 2016 WHO classification, there are three subtypes of the disease: subependymoma and myxopapillary ependymoma grade I, ependymoma grade II (papillary ependymoma, clear cell ependymoma and tanycytic ependymoma) and anaplastic ependymomas grade III. The latter group represents 17% to 42% in adults.

Imaging demonstrates a contrast-enhancing tumour adjacent to the fourth ventricle but away from the midline. The range of enhancement is related to the tumour grade. There is surrounding oedema and typically enlarged ventricles above. Supratentorial ependymomas present in the same way as other cerebral primary tumours. On imaging, the appearances are very similar to HGG. In addition, ependymomas can present with a cystic component, calcification and/or intratumoural haemorrhage. Spread may occur in the CSF in patients with newly diagnosed ependymoma, so craniospinal MRI imaging of the spine is necessary to stage the patient, and CSF cytology is mandatory following surgery.

Treatment

Maximum surgical resection is an advantage before RT because it increases 10-year survival rates in low- and high-grade tumours, (80% and 50%, respectively). Subtotal resection increases the risk of tumour recurrence and CSF dissemination. In the case of persistent hydrocephalus despite tumour resection, shunting or endoscopic ventriculostomy should be performed. Subependymomas and grades I and II tumours which are treated with complete surgical resection are unlikely to relapse. Subtotally resected grades II and III tumours should be followed by adjuvant RT, as it reduces the relapse rate and increases both progression-free survival (PFS) and OS, especially in tumours located near the ventricles and the brainstem. Other prognostic factors are the tumour location and the preoperative PS.

Although ependymoma can spread through the CSF, there is good evidence that prophylactic craniospinal RT confers no advantage because spinal seeding is unlikely to happen if the primary tumour does not recur locally. Craniospinal irradiation is used only if there is proof of spinal seeding.

Current standard practice reflects that adjuvant RT should be offered for patients with anaplastic ependymonas grade III. Results from retrospective studies are inconclusive in terms of PFS and OS for use of RT in grade II patients undergoing gross total resection. RT can be offered to WHO II ependymoma after subtotal resection, especially in cases of extensive residual disease. Intracranial subependymoma is a rare entity. Surgical removal offers long-term survival. However, poorly defined resection borders have been associated with a shorter PFS. A second-look surgery could be an option that should be considered, and postoperative RT might be offered after subtotal or partial resection.

There is no definite role for adjuvant chemotherapy in adults.

Target Volume

The patient should be immobilised in the conventional way positioned either prone (in a two-piece shell) or supine in an "S": frame, to allow for posterior beams.

Pre- and postoperative MRI T1 weighted images should be coregistered with the CT planning.

For posterior fossa tumours, the standard treatment volume should include the presurgical treatment bed with a margin of 1.0 to 2.0 cm for all low- and high-grade supratentorial tumours.

Supratentorial ependymomas should be treated along similar lines to HGG, using postoperative MRI T1W + Gd to define the GTV for any residual postoperative-enhancing tumour. The CTV requires a margin of 1.0 to 2.0 cm (dependent on grade), grown isotropically, which can be edited along the skull. An appropriate PTV should be added.

Technique

In adults, the posterior fossa is best treated with IMRT to reduce the dose at the OARs. This achieves the best conformation to the posterior fossa target volume.

Dose and Energy

Megavoltage x-rays of 6 MV or equivalent should be used.
Single phase: 55 Gy in 33 daily fractions over 6.5 weeks.
An alternative is 54 Gy in 30 fractions, treating daily over 6 weeks.
For grade II ependymoma, 54 to 59.4 Gy in 30 fractions is recommended following incomplete resection.
For grade III (anaplastic) ependymomas, 60 Gy in 30 fractions over 6 weeks, regardless of the extension of the resection.

Results of Treatment

Ependymoma is curable in approximately 50% of cases. Infratentorial lesions have shown improved survival compared to supratentorial lesions, which are usually of high grade.

CENTRAL NERVOUS SYSTEM LYMPHOMA

Pathology and Clinical Features

PCNSL is non-Hodgkin lymphoma arising in the brain, typically of the diffuse large (high-grade) B-cell type. PCNSL accounts for approximately 3% of all primary CNS tumours (see Fig. 30.1). The incidence may be increasing. It affects patients of all ages, the incidence rising with age, and the majority are aged over 60 years. Myelosuppression predisposes to the development of PCNSL, and this was one of the early acquired immune deficiency syndrome (AIDS)-defining diagnoses. Happily, this is now only a rare complication of human immunodeficiency virus.

Presentation is the same as other primary tumours arising within the brain substance, typically with headache, neurological deficit often including intellectual decline, seizure, signs of elevated intracranial pressure and visual symptoms, if affecting the eyes. Onset of symptoms is usually quite rapid. "B" symptoms (fever, drenching night sweats, weight loss without trying, at least 10% of their body weight in 6 months) (see Chapter 29) are not a feature of PCNSL.

On imaging, typical appearances are of a homogeneously enhancing mass, often in a periventricular location, often presenting on precontrast T1W images as iso- or hypointense, whereas on T2W images as hyperintense (Fig. 30.8). Usually, PCNSL presents with oedema visualised in FLAIR. The commonest location is supratentorial. In approximately two-thirds of cases, PCNSL presents as a single mass; in one-third it is multifocal. The disease can spread within the brain, especially in the subependymal layer around the ventricular system, but it is rare for it to metastasise outside the CNS. Metastases to the brain from peripheral lymphoma are also rare.

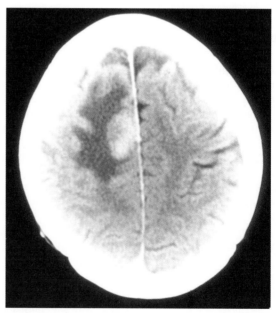

Fig. 30.8 Primary central nervous system lymphoma (PCNSL) in the cerebral hemisphere, shown on computed tomography. A homogeneously enhancing mass can be seen. In approximately two-thirds of cases, PCNSL presents as a single mass; in one-third, it is multifocal. A definitive diagnosis will require biopsy to distinguish between high-grade glioma, metastasis and PCNSL. Note the similarity to Fig. 30.5.

Management Principles

Optimum management of these tumours is a matter of debate. Although PCNSLs are chemo- and radiosensitive, they usually relapse after a short period of time.

Biopsy, using a navigation-guided surgical technique is necessary to prove the diagnosis, but resection should not be undertaken if a diagnosis of PCNSL is suspected because it does not improve the prognosis and carries a greater risk of neurological deficit. In addition to biopsy, other investigations should be performed, including CT imaging of the chest, abdomen and pelvis to exclude systemic lymphoma, and where needed/indicated, MRI of the spine and CFS cytology. All patients must undergo neurocognitive evaluation and eye examination.

Steroids are cytotoxic to lymphomas (as with peripheral lymphomas). Therefore, if dexamethasone is given for symptom relief before a biopsy is performed, the lesion may disappear temporarily. The inclusion of lymphoma in the radiological differential diagnosis thus provides an important contribution to management.

Although treatment strategies have evolved, the optimum treatment remains unclear. Until about 15 years ago, RT was the mainstay of treatment. Treatment typically commenced with whole brain irradiation (e.g. to a dose of 45 Gy in 25 fractions), followed by a focal boost for localised disease (e.g. 9–10 Gy in 5 fractions). Treatment with RT alone is well tolerated but, in historical series, most patients recurred locally, with fatal consequences. Therefore, the addition of chemotherapy was investigated, a strategy that had proved effective in systemic non-Hodgkin lymphoma. It became clear that combined chemoradiotherapy is superior to RT alone. However, a particular problem is late neurotoxicity associated with the combination of chemotherapy, especially MTX (alone or in combination with other drugs), with RT. This occurs commonly, especially in older people, and can be severely disabling or even fatal. Choice of optimal treatment, therefore, currently depends on age and the general health of the patient. For patients with a good PS, high-dose MTX-based chemotherapy is recommended, without RT. MTX administered at a dose of 3.5 g/m^2 IV on day 1, and cytarabine at a dose of 2 g/m^2 IV on days 2 and 3. This is repeated in 3-weekly for four cycles. It is a well-tolerated treatment that improves survival from 33 to 60 months and increases the response rates to 94%.

Radical Treatment—Full Dose Radiotherapy

Radiotherapy Planning

PCNSL is a multifocal disease and the RT field should cover the whole brain area. After chemotherapy, a boost is not recommended.

CTV: the inferior border should be the C2–C3 or C1–C2 intervertebral space. The posterior aspect of the orbit should be covered (if the eyes were initially affected from the disease) to ensure that the retina and the optic nerves are included in the treated volume. They should be treated to a dose of 30 to 36 Gy.

Weighted opposed lateral fields are typically employed, modulated to deliver a homogeneous dose. The isocentre is placed anteriorly and should bisect the bony canthi to allow for a potential future isocentric match to an ocular field. Because the eyes are occasionally an isolated site of relapse, future ocular fields may have to be added later.

CTV is expanded isometrically to a PTV to account for set-up errors.

Localised Unifocal Disease

RT is rarely used and is therefore not described.

Palliative Radiotherapy

Palliative RT may be necessary for patients with poor PS.

Target Volume and Technique

Immobilise and irradiate the whole brain with a single phase, as per palliative RT for metastases.

Dose

A variety of dose schedules can be used as follows: 30 Gy in 10 fractions, treating daily, over 2 weeks; or 20 Gy in 5 fractions, treating daily, over 1 week; or 30 Gy in 6 fractions, treating on alternate days over 2 weeks (as for HGG).

Elderly Population

At present, most major centres recommend deferring whole brain RT (WBRT) until the time of progression.

Results of Treatment

The major prognostic factors for better survival are younger age, especially younger than 60 years, excellent PS and chemotherapy. Suitability for chemotherapy is strongly determined by PS. Localised disease, rather than a multifocal pattern, also carries a better prognosis. Long-term survival is poor, especially in patients over 60 years who comprise the majority. In a series of unselected cases, the median survival was only 8 months, with a 5-year survival of 6%. The prognosis could be determined by the use of algorithms introduced in recent trials. Factors related to poor prognosis in terms of survival are: age older than 60 years, PS greater than 1, high CSF protein concentration, involvement of deep regions of the brain and elevated lactate dehydrogenase (LDH) serum level. The Memorial Sloan Kettering Cancer Center (MSKCC) prognostic model recommends three prognostic classes (class 1: age <50 years; class 2: age >50 years and Karnofsky Performance Status (KPS) 70; class 3: age >50 years and KPS <70) with significantly different overall survivals (8.5 years, 3.2 years and 1.1 years for classes 1, 2 and 3, respectively).

GERMINOMA

Clinical Features and Management Principles

Germinomas are rare in adults, but present like other primary tumours. They frequently arise in the region of the pineal gland, close to the CSF aqueduct (see Fig. 30.4) and, therefore, the symptoms and signs of hydrocephalus are common presenting features. Some patients require a shunt. They should be curable in almost every case.

Germinomas spread through the CSF, and therefore require RT to the whole craniospinal axis. The tumour has a curious predilection to form metastatic deposits on the optic chiasm. Different tumours show a wide range of growth rates, but a few grow extremely fast. This can lead to neurological deterioration taking place over days or even hours. If a patient has metastatic spread to the optic chiasm, rapid progression may threaten vision. Such deterioration warrants urgent treatment with RT. This type of disease does not respond well to steroid treatment. Therefore, occasionally, a few fractions of emergency RT must be given urgently to treat neurological deterioration, while the full plan is prepared.

In adults, the standard treatment for intracranial germinoma should be RT. The total dose is modest, and the toxicity profile in adults is excellent because growth is complete. There is therefore no advantage in considering an alternative strategy of reduced-dose RT together with chemotherapy in adults, at least at the present time.

Recent studies in children have raised the question of whether the volume to be irradiated should be the entire craniospinal axis or local ventricular RT only. Germinomas are also sensitive to chemotherapy, but chemotherapy alone is associated with a roughly 50% chance of relapse.

Postoperative imaging of the head and preoperative imaging of the spine (and head), together with CSF examination, measurement of plasma and CSF tumour markers AFP and BHCG are all useful to have prior to planning treatment. Germinomas produce AFP but not beta-human chorionic gonadotropin (beta-hCG).

Treatment

Target Volume

Phase 1 should treat the whole craniospinal axis, and this is most effectively planned from CT. The technique is largely the same as for paediatric craniospinal RT (see Chapter 32) and requires careful attention to detail.

For phase 2, the primary site is treated to a higher dose. This should be localised using CT:MR coregistration, and the imaging must be carried out before RT starts because the tumour is extremely radiosensitive and may disappear within a few days of starting RT. The GTV is the contrast-enhancing tumour. The CTV margin can be small, for example, 1 to 2 cm, grown isotropically. The PTV should be grown from the CTV, with a standard margin, such as 0.5 cm.

Any sites of metastatic disease can also be boosted in this phase. Occasionally, the whole craniospinal axis must be treated to the phase 2 dose (later).

Technique

Phase 1 as for paediatric craniospinal RT (see Chapter 32). For phase 2, use an appropriate beam arrangement, usually with IMRT.

Dose and Energy

Phase 1: craniospinal axis: 25 Gy in 15 daily fractions in 3 weeks, using megavoltage x-rays.

Phase 2: 15 Gy in 9 fractions in 2 weeks, to boost the primary site and any sites of metastasis.

If necessary, in the case of extensive metastatic spread, it is possible to treat the whole craniospinal axis to 40 Gy in 24 fractions, provided that the full blood count is carefully monitored. If urgent RT is required while the craniospinal plan is being prepared, this can be done using a parallel pair of lateral fields. A few fractions (e.g. 5 Gy in three fractions) are normally sufficient to prevent clinical deterioration. It is probably best, in adults, simply to consider this as extra dose, added to the two phases described earlier.

Results of Treatment

With good RT technique, the cure rate is almost 100%. This applies even if metastatic disease is present at diagnosis. Regular follow-up is required, particularly to recognise early, any endocrine deficiencies.

MEDULLOBLASTOMA

The management of medulloblastoma in adults follows the general principles of this disease in children. However, there is less need to reduce doses in adults who have mature brains and are fully grown. Exactly the same meticulous attention to detail of RT technique is needed. Survival advantage has been shown for the addition of chemotherapy in children. This issue needs to be addressed in adults.

The management of paediatric medulloblastoma is described in Chapter 33.

Dose and Energy (Adults)

Phase 1: craniospinal axis: 35 Gy in 21 daily fractions in 4 weeks, using megavoltage x-rays.

Phase 2: 20 Gy in 12 fractions in 2.5 weeks.

MENINGIOMA

Pathology and Clinical Features

Patients with meningioma present with a mixture of symptoms and signs. Headache is common. As with other primary tumours, meningiomas may also cause confusion and intellectual impairment, resulting from compression of the frontal lobes; 20% of patients have seizures. Occasionally, patients may present with specific cranial nerve palsies, which are different from glial tumours.

The majority of meningiomas arise sporadically. However, they may be associated with previous radiation treatment, for example, cranial RT used for childhood leukaemia. Unusually in oncology, they are more common in women than men (2:1). Benign meningiomas normally express progesterone receptors (PRs), but not oestrogen receptors (ERs), and this may account for occasional reports of change during pregnancy or in patients using hormone replacement therapy. More malignant tumours typically become less well-differentiated and lose this expression.

Meningiomas arise in the coverings of the brain, and so can occur at any intracranial site. However, the most common two sites are the vertex of the skull, and the greater wing of the sphenoid bone. This is the ridge of bone which divides the anterior and middle cranial fossae. Tumours at the vertex can usually be fully resected. Those on the sphenoid wing are resectable if they lie laterally. Medial sphenoid wing tumours usually involve the cavernous sinus, which normally precludes complete resection.

The WHO grading of meningiomas is from grade I to III, on the basis of local invasiveness and cellular features of atypia. Most tumours are of grade I and usually grow slowly. Grade II tumours, also known as *atypical*, may grow faster and have a higher tendency to recur. Grade III tumours, also known as *malignant*, are faster growing, more aggressive in their extension and more difficult to control and eradicate. Although not as fast growing as HGGs, malignant meningiomas may still change over weeks to months.

Meningiomas can infiltrate along the meninges, and this even applies to tumours known to be benign. They may also infiltrate through the foramina and fissures of the skull base, and these must be carefully reviewed when planning RT.

On imaging, tumours are of similar density to the surrounding brain. Usually they are solitary lesions. Sometimes they cause surrounding oedema. With contrast, they normally enhance vigorously and homogeneously (Fig. 30.9). Meningiomas may cause hyperostosis of the surrounding skull. Calcification, best seen on CT, is characteristic of very slow-growing tumours. It is typical to have meningeal enhancement extending away from the site of a meningioma, and this does not necessarily indicate tumour spread. Rather, this tail is a useful diagnostic feature. Nevertheless, many patients referred for an oncology opinion have a tumour with a more invasive pattern of growth, with demonstrable extension along adjacent meningeal layers. A rule of thumb to distinguish the reactive tail from infiltration is the thickness of the meningeal layer; thickening of the meninges suggests tumour infiltration. Methionine (an amino acid) and DOTATOC (an octreotide analogue) PET tracers have a role in the diagnosis of complex meningiomas. They can also be used in planning for appropriate cases.

Treatment

The choice of treatment depends on the size, shape, location and grade of the meningioma. The optimal treatment for grade I meningiomas is radical surgical resection. Modern microsurgery techniques can reduce the risks of major neurological deficits associated with radical surgical resection. Resection of the tumour improves local control. However,

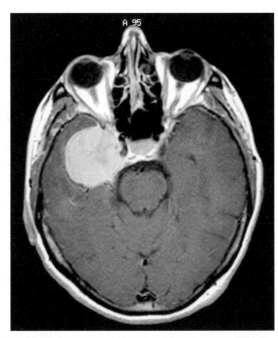

Fig. 30.9 Magnetic resonance imaging (T1 weighted + Gd) of meningioma arising from the medial wing of the sphenoid ridge. The cavernous sinus is involved. A small "tail" of contrast enhancement can be seen in the meninges anteriorly in the middle fossa. The tumour was managed by subtotal resection and postoperative radiotherapy.

the decision on whether this is appropriate needs to consider the patient's PS, comorbidities and wishes. The use of RT is recommended for partially resected tumours if there is evidence of growth and no further surgical option, or they are entirely unresectable meningiomas. Slow-growing meningiomas are often less radiosensitive; therefore, RT may be offered on an individualised basis, where the potential benefit outweighs the risk of neurological damage from surgery. Chemotherapy plays no part in the management of meningioma.

Optic nerve meningiomas cause visual deterioration. These tumours are normally diagnosed entirely on imaging. In these patients, surgery, including biopsy, can further damage vision. RT is effective in stabilising the disease, and some patients (about one-third) experience an improvement in vision. RT is thus the treatment of choice for optic nerve meningioma in order to prevent visual deterioration and ptosis.

For grade II meningiomas, the exact role of adjuvant RT following surgery is uncertain. These have a recurrence rate in the region of 40% at 5 years, and RT is often recommended to try to avoid or delay this. A large trial Radiation versus Observation following surgical resection of Atypical Meningioma (ROAM) comparing early adjuvant RT (60 Gy in 30 fractions) with observation alone is currently underway.

For grade III meningiomas, the recommendation is for surgical resection with radical intent, providing neurological deficit can be avoided. Adjuvant high dose RT should follow, to minimise the risk of recurrence. The timing of RT appears to be an important factor, and if given following the initial resection, may improve survival.

Radiotherapy Target Volume

The patient should be immobilised in a shell or relocatable stereotactic head frame. If resection has been carried out, then postoperative imaging is required. A current MRI scan should be used for planning, co-registered with the planning CT. Both modalities are helpful for target volume delineation. MRI using a T1W sequence with gadolinium contrast produces optimal localisation of the tumour; CT shows the limits

of meningioma extension up to bone or, in uncommon cases where the tumour involves the bone, the extent of the invasion. Bone invasion should be assessed on bone windows. CT also shows the foramina and fissures of the skull, through which meningiomas can spread. The preoperative MRI, coregistered, can be very helpful in defining the CTV margin.

The GTV is defined as the visible edge of contrast enhancement on MRI, plus relevant skull boundaries. If resection has been carried out, coregistration with the preoperative MRI is very helpful. This shows the original location of the tumour and, therefore, the meningeal surfaces into which spread might occur (i.e. the CTV).

There is very little hard evidence for the size of the CTV margin that should be used. For an individual tumour, the growth pattern may suggest whether a small or large margin is needed. Many meningiomas show a more invasive pattern of growth, with extension along adjacent meningeal layers. Any such (imaged) extension should be outlined in the GTV. Where histology is available, this can be incorporated into the margin decision. Thus, the CTV includes any gross tumour, the postoperative tumour bed if resection has been undertaken, plus areas of extension along the meninges, and any hyperostotic bone changes or frank bone invasion if present. It does not need to include a large margin of adjacent brain. The additional margin is related to the grade of the tumour and its growth pattern. It is not necessary to expand the CTV isotropically.

It is helpful to outline critical normal structures, including the eyes and lenses, the pituitary, and optic nerves and chiasm. The following margins are recommended:

Grade 1: CTV = GTV + 0.5 cm.

Grade 2: along the meninges, CTV = GTV + 1 cm, reduced to 0.5 cm at natural barriers to spread, and 0.3 to 0.5 cm into adjacent brain tissue (unless there is evidence of invasion when a larger margin should be added).

Grade 3: along the meninges, CTV = GTV + 1.5 to 2.0 cm and limited by barriers to spread, as above. The margin should include any invasion of the brain.

OARs: the eyes, lenses, lacrimal glands, pituitary gland and hypothalamus, optic nerves, optic chiasm and brainstem should be outlined. In some cases it is worth contouring the hippocampus. Other structures, such as the parotid gland, may be relevant for very inferior lesions.

Technique

IMRT should be used, including with image guidance. TLD is recommended to estimate doses to the lens.

Dose and Energy

For grade I and II: 50 Gy in 30 fractions over 6 weeks.
50.4 Gy in 28 fractions over 6 weeks
55 Gy in 33 fractions over 6.5 weeks
The prescribed dose delivered with 6 MV photons in a single phase
For Grade III: 60 Gy in 30 fractions over 6 weeks

The dose may vary according to which critical structures are contained within the CTV and PTV. Although there is no formal evidence of dose response in grade III tumours, it is widely accepted that higher doses should be used, where possible.

Side Effects

Acute and late effects relate to the location irradiated. Hair loss may occur in the third week of treatment. Hair washing has no effect on hair loss or scalp reactions, provided it is carried out carefully. With 50 Gy, hair regrowth is almost always normal. Erythema and soreness of skin are uncommon with 50 Gy in 30 fractions, though it can occur with higher doses. Hydrocortisone cream, 1% applied topically, reduces itching. The pinna and external auditory canal may be affected. If the external canal receives a significant dose, the wax becomes viscid and sticky. If the ear drum and middle ear are irradiated, then secretory otitis media (glue ear) may occur. This may cause noises in the ears, especially bubbling, reduction of hearing and, occasionally, difficulties with balance, but this is usually temporary and settles spontaneously. If the eustachian tube is treated, the same problem often occurs. Occasional patients experience nausea, especially when the brainstem is irradiated. This is usually manageable with 5-HT3 antagonists. Headache is also uncommon as an acute side effect. Patients occasionally require steroids during treatment for meningioma.

In terms of late effects, if the hypothalamus and pituitary have been irradiated, hormone failure may occur years after treatment, so routine pituitary function tests are necessary during follow-up. Intellectual function should not be affected, over and above changes already caused by the tumour (and surgery). In cases where high eye doses cannot be avoided, such as optic nerve meningiomas, cataracts may develop (see earlier). Retinopathy can be observed with doses to the eyeball exceeding 50 Gy.

Results of Treatment

It is likely that RT improves the outcome in patients for whom surgery is either impossible or incomplete. The results of subtotal resection plus RT are equivalent to complete surgical excision and may be safer for the patient. Meningiomas grow slowly, so that follow-up needs to be carried out over a long period, at least 10 to 15 years, to define the outcome.

Age does not appear to be prognostic and should not be considered a bar to radical RT. Tumours which are larger, or of higher grade, have a higher chance of earlier relapse. In addition, it is likely that tumours with a large number of cells actively in the mitotic cycle have a higher probability of early relapse, assessed by MIB-1 (Ki-67: tumour proliferation index).

In general, meningiomas do not change in size after RT, although a few do shrink modestly. However, it is important for the patient to understand that no change after treatment represents a successful outcome. Neurological deficits, such as cranial nerve palsies, do not usually improve. The exception is with optic nerve meningiomas: about one third of patients experience some improvement in vision, even if there is no change in the size of the lesion on imaging.

Overall, control rates for patients with meningioma are good, though published results are quite variable. Survival after surgery and RT for benign meningiomas (i.e. grades I and II) is around 80% to 90% at 5 years, and 50% to 80% at 10 years. For patients with inoperable tumours treated with RT alone, control rates are probably on the low end of these ranges. Although these results are good, and much better than for patients with gliomas, there is room for improvement. Patients with malignant meningiomas (i.e. grade III) have a worse outlook, with 5-year survival rates around 30% to 60%, which is about half the survival of patients with benign tumours.

PITUITARY TUMOURS AND CRANIOPHARYNGIOMA

PITUITARY TUMOURS

Pathology and Clinical Features

Pituitary tumours are virtually always primary adenomas of the anterior pituitary gland itself. Other primary tumours are exceedingly rare, and metastatic deposits involving the pituitary fossa, although well described, are uncommon.

Pituitary adenomas can be divided into secretory tumours that produce excess hormone and non-secretory ones that do not. Secretory adenomas most commonly produce an excess of a single hormone, usually growth hormone (GH) causing acromegaly, adrenocorticotrophic hormone (ACTH) which causes Cushing's disease, or prolactin, leading to hyperprolactinaemia. Production of thyroid-stimulating hormone (TSH) is uncommon. Patients with secretory tumours usually present with the effects of the excess hormone production and a small tumour confined to the pituitary fossa. In many cases, hormone levels can be controlled medically. However, surgery produces the quickest reduction of hormone levels in secreting tumours and is often curative. New endoscopic techniques have made surgery even more effective at removing tumours. RT can reduce hormone levels, but often very slowly, over months or years, and is therefore not helpful as an acute treatment.

Nonsecretory tumours typically present with symptoms and signs of optic chiasm compression. Occasionally, they present with pituitary failure, and are sometimes associated with headache. Surgical decompression results in immediate relief of pressure on the optic tract, and vision often improves by the time the patient wakes from the anaesthetic. Extension of a tumour to the lateral walls of the pituitary fossa and cavernous sinus cannot be removed surgically, and it is a frequent site for residual tumour.

After complete removal, RT is usually not required. However, a proportion do recur, so adequate follow-up is essential. The indications for RT are relative, and patients are best managed through a multidisciplinary team. The decision regarding RT in an individual patient is the result of weighing the pros and cons of observation versus early RT. Indications in favor of RT include extensive residual tumour, invasion of the cavernous sinuses laterally, uncontrolled elevated hormone levels, and evidence of progression of tumour after surgery alone. Factors against RT include normal pituitary function, and young age, because of the risk of inducing a second tumour. Patient preference is also important. If recurrence does occur in a patient managed by surveillance, second operation may be desirable if the optic chiasm is compressed, before proceeding to RT.

In considering a patient for RT, it is important to ensure that the patient's hormone status is stable. It is vital to have pre-RT documentation of the visual fields. It is inadvisable to treat a patient with visual symptoms and signs which are unexplained, because any visual deterioration resulting from progression in the (unknown) pathology will be blamed on the RT, and the opportunity to diagnose and treat the real cause is missed. Postoperative MRI is useful both as a baseline before RT and to aid in the planning process (see later).

Treatment
Target Volume

The patient should be immobilised in a shell. A relocatable stereotactic frame may also be used. A current (postoperative) coregistered MRI (T1W-Gd) defines the GTV, including any involvement of the cavernous sinuses and suprasellar extension. CT shows the bony anatomy well, especially inferiorly, where it is helpful to identify the floor of the fossa.

The target is based on residual tumour bulk, which most commonly involves the cavernous sinuses. Tissue seen in the sphenoid sinus postoperatively after trans-sphenoidal resection is most likely to be surgical packing; this does not have to be treated. Some tumours have residual suprasellar extension, even after surgery, and this must be included in the GTV. Reviewing the GTV on a coronal view can be helpful in confirming coverage, especially superiorly and inferiorly.

Pituitary adenomas do not infiltrate at a microscopic level, so no CTV margin is required for this. The whole extent of the original tumour (preoperative imaging) should be included in the CTV. However, if there is uncertainty about the localisation of the GTV, then a small CTV margin may be added. The PTV should be grown isotropically with an appropriate margin.

Critical normal structures, especially the optic nerves, chiasm and tracts, should be outlined, so that the dose distribution and the dose-volume histograms (DVHs) for these can be reviewed.

Technique

IMRT should be used, with image guidance.

Thermoluminescent dosimetry measurements should be made to estimate the lens doses. Although they should be very low, the measurements prove that a subsequent cataract or other visual problems are not the result of RT.

SRT/radiosurgery may be a choice for some patients with tumours less than 2.5 cm in maximum diameter, whereas the tumour target should be away at least 2 to 3 mm from the optic chiasm. The dose can be delivered in a single fraction, offering higher convenience to the patient. However, there is currently no evidence that it is superior to fractionated treatment. This type of RT is administered only in specialist centres.

Dose and Energy

Doses should be given as 45 Gy in 25 daily fractions over 5 weeks, with megavoltage x-rays, to the median dose.

A slightly higher dose is sometimes recommended for Cushing's disease and for very large adenomas, such as 50 Gy in 30 fractions (as for craniopharyngioma).

Side Effects

With rotational IMRT, there is no hair loss. Use of fixed fields may lead to hair loss in the entry portals, usually over the temples, which will regrow. Some patients experience mild nausea and loss of appetite during RT, which is easily controlled with simple antiemetics. In some patients where the PTV extends rather inferiorly, ear symptoms occur as the result of acute irritation and blockage of the eustachian tube. Patients may report mildly reduced hearing, with bubbling in the ears and, sometimes, mild unsteadiness. These symptoms are due to fluid in the middle ear (secretory otitis media), which is unable to drain down the blocked eustachian tube, and will settle spontaneously.

For patients already requiring hydrocortisone replacement, it is often sensible to increase the dose, since a course of RT constitutes a stressful event. This should be the default management. Typically, the dose can be increased by 50% or doubled. A few patients can be managed without this increase if they feel unperturbed about the impending treatment, although an increase is often needed later in the course. Tiredness is a good measure of the dose of steroid required in this patient group. RT does increase the risk of hypothalamic–pituitary axis (HPA) dysfunction requiring hormone replacement. However, damage to the HPA is the result of the combination of tumour and surgery as well as RT. HPA dysfunction is dependent upon RT dose. In all, half to three-quarters of patients require hormone replacement after surgery and RT. Patients should be followed up regularly in the endocrinology clinic.

The risk of late RT damage to the optic nerves should be negligible with a dose of 45 Gy in 25 fractions. Therefore, if visual deterioration occurs after RT, it is important to look for a cause other than RT. Cataract should not occur with standard techniques.

Any RT treatment carries the risk of late second tumour causation. In patients treated for pituitary adenoma, the risk is roughly 1% per decade of follow-up after treatment. Of the tumours caused, about half are benign, typically meningioma, and about half are malignant, for example GBM or sarcoma. Because the risk is cumulative with time, this is especially important in younger patients.

Results of Treatment

Postoperative RT produces very high rates of control. Overall, tumour control rates should be around 95% at 10 years and 90% at 20 years. However, control of hormone secretion is poorer, with only 60% to 90% achieving control of hypersecretion. The time to hormonal normalisation is dependent primarily on preirradiation levels.

CRANIOPHARYNGIOMA

Pathology and Clinical Features

This is a rare tumour which predominates in children but can occur in adults.

The incidence of craniopharyngiomas is 0.13 to 0.18 per 100000, constituting 1% to 4% of tumours in adults. Disease peaks are seen at ages 5 to 14 years and 65 to 74 years. In adults, it typically presents with symptoms and signs related to raised intracranial pressure, compression of the optic chiasm and optic nerves, or reduction in pituitary hormone secretion. When these tumours are very extensive, pressure on the frontal lobes or involvement of the hypothalamus can cause behavioral disturbance.

Craniopharyngiomas are thought to arise from cells derived from the embryological structure known as Rathke's pouch, which extends from the embryonic pharynx to form the anterior pituitary gland. Craniopharyngiomas are normally cystic, with a thin wall and a solid component. The craniopharyngioma itself is lined by epithelium (reflecting its origin), which produces the cyst fluid. At both a macroscopic and a microscopic level, the wall of the cyst projects into spaces in the surface of the brain, to which it can be strongly adherent.

On CT, flecks of calcification are often seen. On MRI, the cyst has almost unique signal characteristics, being neither those of CSF nor brain; the cyst wall and solid parts are normally well shown on the T1W sequence and enhances with gadolinium contrast. When opened surgically, thick viscous fluid is often seen, with the macroscopic appearances of machine oil and containing microscopic cholesterol crystals. This accounts for the MRI appearances of the cyst fluid.

Surgery achieves decompression and tissue for histological confirmation. Complete surgical removal is sometimes possible for very small lesions but it is not feasible in most cases. More commonly, the tumours are large, complex and highly adherent to the brain, so that attempts to remove every finger-like projection of the cyst wall can produce very substantial traction injury to the brain. In general terms, decompression and subtotal resection plus RT produces similar local control rates to radical surgery, with much less neurological morbidity. Enlargement of the cystic component prior to or after the RT is an indication for further surgical intervention.

RT is recommended for virtually all adult patients after both subtotal resection and apparently gross tumour resection, to reduce recurrence rates. Patients normally have pan-hypopituitarism already, so that this relative contraindication is absent. The recurrence rates following surgery alone, even after apparently complete removal, are high. Since the recurrence can increase neurological deficits, which are often found in patients with this disease already, the risk and consequences of recurrence greatly outweigh the risks from RT.

Treatment
Target Volume

The patient should be immobilised in a shell in a comfortable, neutral position. A relocatable stereotactic frame may also be used. CT should be used, with coregistered MRI (T1W-Gd). In most circumstances, co-registration with the preoperative MRI is also helpful as a guide to the CTV.

RT for craniopharyngioma is more difficult to plan than for pituitary adenoma. The tumour is very adherent at both a macroscopic and microscopic level, and all parts of the brain with which the original tumour was in contact need to be irradiated; this is where co-registration of the pre-operative MRI is useful. However, resection decompresses the tumour and reduces the mass effect, so shifting the anatomy. Thus neither preoperative nor postoperative imaging exactly represents the location of the target, so the internal anatomy of the brain must also be considered in the planning.

There are usually some solid or cystic remnants following surgery, which can be demonstrated with MRI; these represent the GTV. The CTV should contain the following: any postoperative gross tumour; the surface of the preoperative gross tumour; and a margin for any potential microscopic residual disease. It is reasonable for the CTV to follow any shift of the brain following decompression, based on the anatomy. The CTV should usually be GTV + 0.3–0.5 cm.

The PTV margin should be grown isotropically, depending on the immobilisation method used, usually PTV = CTV + 0.3–0.5 cm.

As for pituitary adenoma, the lenses, optic nerves, chiasm and tracts, together with the lacrimal glands and brainstem should be outlined, so that the dose distribution and the DVHs for these structures can be reviewed.

Technique

IMRT with image guidance as per pituitary adenoma. TLD measurements of the eye doses should be made.

Dose and Energy

Doses can be given as 50 to 55 Gy in 30 to 33 daily fractions over 6 weeks, using megavoltage x-rays.

Side Effects

Side effects are similar to those for pituitary adenoma. Most patients have significant endocrine dysfunction requiring replacement before RT, and many are pan-hypopituitary. Unlike pituitary adenoma, many will also require desmopressin replacement to compensate for loss of posterior pituitary gland function. For patients already taking hydrocortisone replacement, it is sensible to increase the dose, as noted earlier. The major difference in side effects compared with pituitary adenoma is the small but important risk of visual deterioration during RT, as a result of the cystic component reaccumulating fluid and compressing the optic chiasm. Patients should therefore be warned to report any visual disturbance the same day. Reaccumulation of cyst fluid is unrelated to RT itself, but may occur coincidentally during the postoperative phase when RT is being given. If visual deterioration occurs, urgent MRI is needed. If cyst recurrence is confirmed, urgent neurosurgical referral for operation should be made to try to preserve vision. In children, it is normal practice to perform one or more MRI scans during RT to ensure that the target volume has not increased in size. This has not yet become standard practice in adults, but should be considered, at least in selected cases.

The risk of late RT damage to the optic nerves should be very small with a dose of 50 Gy in 30 fractions. The risk of second tumour formation is similar to patients with pituitary adenoma, but this risk is very much less than the risk of recurrence of the craniopharyngioma if RT is not given.

Results of Treatment

RT following surgery produces high rates of control, with 10-year local control rates of 77% to 100% and 20-year overall survival of 66% to 92%. Limited surgery plus RT produce local control rates as good as those from radical surgery, with lower neurological morbidity. Clinical follow-up should include endocrinology, ophthalmological assessment and imaging.

Prognostic factors that have been reported are the size of the tumour and the age at presentation, with a worse prognosis in older patients. There is no benefit in OS from gross total resection. Incomplete resection may produce a better quality of life. Postoperative RT is superior to surveillance after nonradical resection in terms of progression-free survival.

VESTIBULAR SCHWANNOMA

Pathology and Clinical Features

Vestibular schwannoma (VS) represent a small proportion of patients referred for an opinion regarding RT. VS are a common cause of unilateral deafness, with a population incidence in the range of 0.5 to 2 per 100,000 per year. Patients commonly experience tinnitus, despite losing hearing, and this is an additional presenting symptom. Rarely, a VS can be large enough at presentation to compress the brainstem, causing disturbance of balance. Some are associated with the genetic condition of neurofibromatosis type 2 (NF-2), which often presents with bilateral VS.

A multidisciplinary approach is essential for the management of patients with VS. This group of patients is almost unique in having a choice of treatment options, though the decision may not be simple. Patients with NF-2 may have other tumours in addition to bilateral schwannomas, and their care is extremely complex. Management of patients with NF2-related VS differs from those patients with sporadic VS.

The principles of VS management are to reduce mass effect, while preserving facial nerve function and hearing where possible. The three optimal treatment pathways for VS are surgery, stereotactic radiosurgery (SRS)/SRT, and a wait-and-scan policy. Because the VS is in close proximity to anatomical structures such as the cochlea, the brainstem and cranial nerves VII and VIII, treatment can lead to changes in balance, communication and appearance, reducing the quality of life. Treatment choice depends on tumour size and location, comorbidities and patient wishes. For the patient with VS secondary to NF-2, different management is required. Surgical management is the cornerstone for these patients. RT can have a role in management, especially in those that are elderly and high-risk surgical candidates.

Small tumours can be managed with a wait-and-scan policy, and some stabilise spontaneously for long periods of time. Observation policy should be followed in elderly patients and in patients with comorbidities and high surgical risk. Active treatment is only required with disease progression. Small- and medium-sized tumours are well treated surgically, with very low rates of facial nerve damage. In addition, surgery can be applied in brainstem compression and symptoms of mass effect decompression. They are also well treated with both fractionated stereotactic radiotherapy (FSRT) and stereotactic radiosurgery (SRS). SRS can be performed using a GammaKnife or linac-based X-knife. SRS is indicated in unilateral tumours with maximum diameter less than 3 cm and no brainstem compression. SRS enables patients to return to normal activities faster, as well as the cost being lower than surgery. Large tumours with significant brainstem compression usually require surgical resection. However, very large tumours may be too big to resect safely, and therefore are considered for RT. For these patients, FSRT is the appropriate technique.

Surgery is an excellent treatment, provided complete excision is achieved without undue disability. Most cases, though not all, are cured. Some surgical units prefer a translabyrinthine approach because it provides a safer approach for preservation of the facial nerve, but this is at the expense of irreversible hearing loss. It is therefore relatively more attractive to patients who are already deaf. For some patients, brainstem (cochlear) implants are possible. RT has excellent efficacy and low morbidity. Rates of local control appear similar for both surgery and RT, using either FSRT or SRS. Surgery has the attraction of removing the tumour and avoiding the small risk of RT-related second tumour risk, but has the disadvantages of a small operative mortality, protracted rehabilitation, a risk of facial nerve damage and hearing loss depending on the surgical approach. RT has the attraction of avoiding a major surgical procedure, has a lower rate of serious morbidity (and mortality) and a lower rate of facial nerve damage, at the expense of the tumour remaining in situ. Patient preference must be considered, and this group of patients is typically very well informed. Nevertheless, the decision may not be easy.

Treatment

Here, only the technique for FSRT will be described; SRS is a highly specialised technique, which should be studied in more specific texts.

Target Volume

The patient should be immobilised in a beam direction shell or relocatable stereotactic frame. RT should be fully conformal or use IMRT, based on CT planning with co-registered T1W-Gd MRI (Fig. 30.10). The tumour is not well shown on CT, but the internal auditory meatus (IAM) is clearly visualised. On MRI, the tumour is obvious, and extension into the IAM is apparent.

The GTV is the enhancing edge of the tumour seen on MRI. Provided the co-registration accuracy is high, no CTV margin is required. The PTV should be grown isotropically with an appropriate margin.

It is helpful to outline the pituitary so that a low dose can be confirmed. The cochlea is bound to lie within the PTV so that the dose is predictable without it being outlined. The eyes, specifically the lenses, should be outlined to ensure that the tolerance dose is not exceeded, for example, by the exit dose from a posterior oblique beam. The ipsilateral parotid gland can also be outlined for the same reason.

Technique

A three-field conformal plan is usual, using anterior oblique and posterior oblique-wedged fields and a lateral field, with coplanar or non-coplanar disposition, depending on the exact target shape. IMRT, rotational or with fixed fields, also provides an excellent solution. Small volumes may also be treated with multiple arcs.

Dose and Energy

Doses can be given as 50 Gy in 30 daily fractions over 6 weeks, with 6-MV photons.

Some centres have used higher doses, in the range of 54 to 57.6 Gy in 1.8 Gy fractions. Some hypofractionated schedules have also been designed, using lower doses in 12 fractions only. These doses exceed brainstem tolerance and are only suitable for small lesions. Preservation of cranial nerve function may be better with the slightly lower dose (50 Gy) and dose per fraction, but this needs to be formally evaluated. The variation in local control with dose also needs investigation.

Although the hearing preservation rate is lower in Neurofibromatosis (NF) patients, a lower dose is not recommended unless the tumour control rates are reduced.

Side Effects

Acute side effects include hair loss in the (fixed) field entry portals, and possible mild erythema of the skin. The skin within the external auditory meatus may also become irritated and, in the longer term, the wax may become thicker and more tenacious. Some patients experience mild nausea, which is easily controlled with simple antiemetics. A proportion of patients also experience some disturbance of balance, due to vestibulocochlear irritation. This resolves after RT, though it may take several weeks.

Important late effects include hearing loss and cranial nerve dysfunction. Hearing preservation rates are in the region of 75% with both FSRT and SRS but also depend on tumour size and dose in SRS series. Preservation of some useful hearing may be higher and has been suggested to be as high as 90% in FSRT series. Patients with NF-2 have a higher risk of losing hearing, with a preservation rate of only 60%. Both FSRT and SRS series report facial neuropathy risks in around 1%

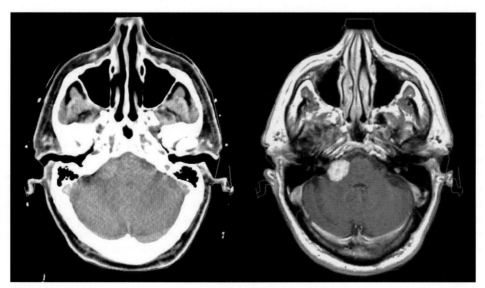

Fig. 30.10 Planning computed tomography and coregistered magnetic resonance imaging of vestibular schwannoma.

(including facial paralysis, spasm, dysgeusia), and ontological symptoms in 1% to 3% of patients (including tinnitus, hearing loss, vertigo, imbalance). Other less prominent side effects reported are hydrocephalus and pituitary treatment failure. There is a risk of late second tumour following RT, most relevant in younger patients. By analogy with the data from pituitary patients, and considering the small, lateralised volume, this is expected to be rather less than 1% per decade after treatment.

Results of Treatment

Local control rates after fractionated FSRT or SRS are excellent, with approximately 95% tumour control at 5 years. This is equivalent to microsurgery results, though a direct comparison has never been attempted. Thus RT has excellent efficacy as well as low morbidity. The radiological average response after 6 years of follow-up shows tumour volume decrease in about half of patients. Tumour regrowth can occur; therefore salvage surgery could be an option, although it is associated with a high complication risk.

CHORDOMAS AND LOW-GRADE CHORDOSARCOMAS

Pathology and Clinical Features

Chordomas and chordosarcomas are rare tumours, but they present particular management problems. They are present at the skull base and spine, with a median age of 60 years. Chordomas are twice as common as chondrosarcomas. Chordomas and chondrosarcomas are distinct pathological entities, but given that they share common features, they can be considered together. Both are difficult to resect and require very high doses of RT to achieve local control. Chordomas can metastasise and arise in the skull base, typically near, but not in the midline, and along the whole length of the spine. The skull base, upper cervical spine and the sacrum are the most common locations. Low-grade chordosarcomas may present at any age, but most commonly occur in older adults. They also occur in the skull base, arising from bony or cartilaginous elements. Usually, they are located in the parasellar area, cerebellopontine angle or paranasal sinuses, but may also arise in the clivus. Both types of tumour typically present with pain, headache or cranial nerve palsies. Chordomas grow slowly but have a high tendency for local recurrence, and metastases can occur in 30% to 40% of patients; common sites of spread include the lungs, the bones and the lymph nodes. Outcome is generally poorer than low-grade chondrosarcoma.

Treatment

Both tumour types require resection, which should be performed in a specialist unit, with the aim to remove as much tumour as possible. Because of their location, surgery is challenging, and typically it is difficult to remove all tumour from the deep aspect. Modern endoscopic techniques have dramatically improved resection and reduced morbidity. Complete resection with negative margins is the optimal treatment option because it increases the PFS and OS. Surgical aims are complete resection with preservation of neurological function and quality of life. It is generally impossible to achieve resection with negative margins and tumour remnants are unavoidable. In all tumours, adjuvant RT should be offered. Bimodality treatment improves local control and DFS, particularly in skull-base tumours. Postoperative RT should also be considered for patients with partially resected tumours. Prior to RT, a baseline examination including cranial nerves, visual field assessment and acuity, and audiometry and pituitary gland function, should be performed to assess treatment side effects. There is good evidence that doses of more than 65 to 70 Gy are required.

Best results have been achieved using RT with proton or carbon ion RT, which appear to be able to deliver higher doses than x-rays with safety. Metal used to reconstruct and stabilise the skull base or spine is considered by many to be a contraindication to protons or carbon ion therapy. Efforts are now made to avoid using metal implants in patients with chordoma and chondrosarcoma. This requires referral to a specialist proton beam therapy (PBT) centre.

Patients with metal implants, or those requiring palliative RT, should be treated with x-rays, preferably with IMRT. In palliative cases, it is often worth attempting high-dose treatment, since responses may be durable.

Target Volume

Most patients will be seen and treated in a PBT (or carbon ion) centre. For those patients not able to receive PBT requiring x-ray treatment, high-dose image guided (IG)-IMRT is required. Effective immobilisation is also vital. Imaging should include the co-registration of preoperative and postoperative MRI, often both T1 with contrast and T2 sequences, the latter often showing the original tumour well. A specific diagnostic bone window CT is helpful to identify intraosseous disease, which is osteolytic destruction.

The GTV should include the surgical cavity and residual macroscopic disease. The CTV should include the whole preoperative volume, with a small margin, tailored to the anatomy, to encompass all areas at risk of microscopic invasion.

Residual gross tumour should be boosted. It is essential to have knowledge of the surgical procedures and initial symptoms when planning the CTV. The seeding along the surgical pathway is less than 5% of the cases.

The PTV depends on the immobilisation and image guidance protocol, and is usually 0.3 to 0.5 cm.

If the brainstem and spinal cord are close by, then it is often appropriate to add a planning organ-at-risk volume (PRV) around these structures.

Technique

IG-IMRT is essential. The relevant OARs should be carefully delineated. For the neural OARs, a PRV also should be outlined, with respect to dose constraints to the brain stem and spinal cord and the optic apparatus.

Dose and Energy

For chordoma doses can be given as 70 Gy in 39 fractions over 8 weeks.

For condrosarcoma, 65 to 70 Gy in 39 fractions over 8 weeks.
These doses should also be used for high-dose palliation. The spinal cord maximum surface dose can be as high as 58 Gy in 39 fractions.

Results of Treatment

Excellent surgery has a profound effect on outcome, and the volume of any residual gross tumour is prognostic. Thus these cases are best treated in specialist centres including a skull-base surgical team. The best results are reported following RT with protons or light ions.

Local control is the most important problem. Chondrosarcomas can be controlled in over 90% of cases and metastasise very rarely. Chordomas are less well controlled, with local control rates of only 50% to 80%. Of those chordomas that recur, local failure is the major problem, occurring in 95% of patients, but metastatic disease is found in 20%. This can manifest as widespread dissemination or involvement of regional lymph nodes. No effective treatment is available for patients who recur.

SPINAL CORD TUMOURS—PRIMARY

Pathology and Clinical Features

The majority of these tumours are intrinsic and predominantly ependymomas or astrocytomas. GBMs also occur, but thankfully, are rare. Intrinsic tumours compress the spinal cord from within, and often produce some permanent neurological damage. Primary spinal cord tumours typically present with a mixture of sensory and motor impairment, related to the site of tumour involvement. Less commonly, they present with pain.

The tumour can usually be surgically debulked, which often improves the neurology, though it may not recover fully. Tumour removed at surgery provides the histological diagnosis. Surgery is hazardous and, in some patients, neurological deficit worsens after operation. Often, subtotal resection, minimising or avoiding neurological deterioration, is an appropriate strategy. However, improvement in microsurgical techniques has led to excellent outcomes regarding preservation of neurological function. Most intrinsic tumours of the cord require postoperative RT.

Low-grade (i.e. grade I) ependymomas of myxopapillary type are one of the most common primary tumours affecting the lower end of the spinal cord itself (the conus medullaris) and the lumbosacral nerve roots. Some of these tumours can be removed completely, perhaps over half, and may not require RT; in most, some residual tumour remains, and RT is highly effective in achieving long-term cure. In higher grade ependymomas, RT is necessary. Astrocytomas are usually high grade and require RT; they account for 40% to 50% of the intramedullary spinal cord tumours. Surgical debulking is a reasonable option for high-grade tumours. GBMs are usually irradiated but have a bleak outlook.

Occasional extrinsic tumours also occur: meningiomas arise from the coverings of the cord; schwannomas and neurofibromas arise in nerve roots. These extrinsic tumours compress the spinal cord. Surgical removal relieves the compression and the deficit often recovers. Surgery alone is usually curative.

Treatment—Radical

RT is the standard of care in the treatment of primary spinal canal tumours. In adults, RT can improve disease control, survival and neurological function, and quality of life.

Target Volume

Treatment planning is based on CT with co-registered and pre- and postoperative MRI. Sometimes spinal curvature is so different that the MRI will not coregister reliably, but the key issue is the longitudinal extent of the tumour, which can be measured from the vertebral levels.

The GTV includes the residual tumour visible on the T1-enhancing abnormality on MRI or the tumour onT2/FLAIR images if they are low-grade gliomas. The postoperative cavity should be included in the GTV.

Longitudinally, the CTV should include the oedema on a T2-weighted MRI with a margin of 1.5 cm for low-grade tumours and 2 to 3 cm for high-grade tumours around the GTV to include any subclinical spread. Axially, the CTV includes the whole spinal canal. The planning target volume uses an additional 0.5 to 1.0 cm margin to account for setup error, depending on the immobilisation technique.

In the past, ependymomas of the lumbosacral region have been treated to include the whole of the thecal sac below the tumour. Certainly, some of these tumours can be seen to have drop metastases or sugar-coating disease at presentation. Historical series in which this extended target is favoured largely predate the era of high-quality MRI, and it is now considered unnecessary in patients with no evidence of distal disease on MRI staging.

CT planning allows normal tissue structures to be delineated, such as the oesophagus, thyroid and oral cavity in patients with cervical tumours; the lungs, oesophagus and heart in those with thoracic tumours; and the kidneys and possibly ovaries in patients with lumbosacral tumours.

Technique

The first decision is whether to position the patient prone or supine, but supine is now conventional.

IMRT can provide increased dose homogeneity.

Dose and Energy

Doses can be given as 50 to54 Gy in 30 fractions, treating daily, over 6 weeks, with megavoltage photons.

P1610 is a reasonable estimate of safe cord tolerance in a patient with spinal cord tumour. For patients with GBM of the spinal cord, the higher dose of 54 Gy in 30 fractions is appropriate.

Side Effects

Side effects of treatment are usually very modest, and depend on the location of the tumour. It is unusual for neurological function to deteriorate and, if this does happen, it can be managed with increasing the steroid dose. Some oesophagitis may occur in patients with cervical or upper thoracic tumours, but it is normally mild. Patients with lumbar or lumbosacral tumours may experience nausea or mild diarrhoea, but these symptoms can be managed effectively with simple medication. Kidney doses should be low and clinically unimportant. Spinal cord damage from RT should not occur with the dose noted above.

RT does not inhibit the normal recovery of neurological function which occurs after surgery and may continue for up to a year following excision.

Myelopathy is possible with doses exceeding the spinal cord tolerance. For doses up to 50 Gy, the incidence of myelopathy is less than 0.5%, and 1% to 5% for doses higher than 60 Gy. Radiation myelopathy can present acutely or after a long time. Acute myelopathy, known as Lhermitte syndrome, is reversible; symptoms include sudden tingling, an electric shock-like sensation radiating to the hands and feet on neck flexion. It does not progress to late myelopathy; it is also strangely uncommon when treating spinal tumours. Chronic myelopathy presents as loss of sensor and motor and is usually irreversible.

Treatment—Palliative

A few patients require palliative treatment. This can be achieved with a simple beam arrangement, using the dose and fractionation as for palliative treatment of HGG.

Results of Treatment

Ependymomas have a better prognosis than astrocytic tumours. Grade I lesions are cured in most patients, and grade II tumours in the region of 50% of patients. Higher grade ependymomas are rare, but as expected, have a worse prognosis. Astrocytomas have a worse prognosis, grade for grade, than ependymomas. GBMs of the cord have an appalling prognosis. Recurrence often occurs within a few weeks or months of treatment and may include dissemination through the CSF. Favourable prognostic factors are the younger age at presentation, the absence of neurological deficits at diagnosis and the lower grade. The 5- and 10-year survival for spinal ependymomas range between 66% to 100% and 62% to 91%, and for primary spinal astrocytomas between 60% to 100% and 40% to 75%, respectively.

CEREBRAL METASTASES

Clinical Features and Management Principles

The majority of patients, approximately two-thirds, with cerebral metastases have multiple lesions (Fig. 30.11A and B). Around 80% occur in the cerebrum. Those in the cerebellum may cause hydrocephalus. Most patients also have active disease elsewhere. Occasionally, the first presentation is with metastasis, and biopsy may be important in establishing the diagnosis. Intra-axial metastases have similar presentation to primary tumours (see earlier).

Metastatic spread may also cause diffuse meningeal disease, infiltrating widely over the surface of the brain. This manifestation of disseminated disease may present with confusion, photophobia and neck stiffness, that is. symptoms and signs associated with meningitis. It may also cause cranial nerve palsies from involvement of meninges at the base of the brain. Metastatic disease may also affect the bones of the skull, which is common in prostate cancer. Involvement of the skull base typically produces cranial nerve palsies by compression of the nerves as they pass through the skull.

Patients with single or multiple cerebral metastases are almost always incurable. The treatment objective is therefore palliative, and additional supportive care should be instituted. Steroid treatment is normally appropriate to reduce surrounding oedema. Unless the patient is in the end stage of their disease, it is helpful for the patient to be restaged to assess the extent and aggressiveness of the disease to guide systemic treatment and inform prognosis. It is usually appropriate for the patient to be managed by the relevant site-specific team. As well as palliative RT, chemotherapy and hormonal therapy may be helpful.

Patients With Multiple Brain Metastasis

WBRT is the most common treatment considered for patients presenting with multiple metastases. Radiosurgery can be considered for patients with up to four metastases, but beyond this number there is no evidence of prolonged survival.

The use of chemotherapy can offer some benefit in the management of some brain metastases. Targeted treatments with immunotherapy for patients with lung cancer and melanoma can provide control to both visible intracranial disease as well as micrometastatic spread. RT can then be deferred until further disease progression. Neurosurgery is of little benefit for this category of patient, and the use is limited to symptom relief due to obstruction or pressure or to establish the diagnosis if there is no other available site of biopsy.

Patients With One to Three Brain Metastasis

A few patients have a solitary metastasis or oligometastatic disease, who are fit with no active disease outside the brain and have a reasonable disease-free interval (e.g. 1 year) since completion of primary treatment and may warrant more intensive treatment, involving surgical resection or SRS. Both surgical resection and SRS improve local control within the brain. Surgical resection is particularly useful for patients with posterior fossa tumours causing hydrocephalus. The decision for surgical resection or SRT to be undertaken by a neuro-oncology MDT is based on location and size of the metastasis(es) and other patient factors. Some patients may be in sufficiently poor general condition that even simple palliative RT may not be of value. For meningeal disease, that is, carcinomatous meningitis, in addition to palliative RT, intrathecal methotrexate may be of symptomatic benefit. Neurosurgery may be considered for palliation of symptoms related to threatening mass effect, haemorrhage or hydrocephalus.

In patients with more than three lesions treated with SRS for unresected metastases without the use of WBRT, the outcomes were promising since patients showed no survival benefit with the addition of WBRT. The findings have been confirmed in four randomised phase III trials and an individual data metaanalysis. In these studies, patients who did not have WBRT had greater CNS relapse, but the functional independence and overall survival was the same in both arms.

A randomised trial comparing cavity SRS to WBRT after resection of metastases in patients with one to three lesions, reported better

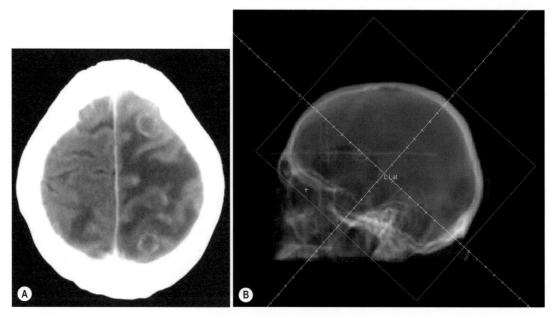

Fig. 30.11 (A) Computed tomography of a patient showing multiple cerebral metastases from nonsmall cell lung cancer, surrounded by oedema. Three deposits are seen in the left hemisphere, and another single lesion is visible in the right cerebral hemisphere, posteriorly. Oedema is seen around each deposit. (B) Field for whole brain irradiation showing adequate coverage around the skull, including at the skull base. The collimator angle allows sparing of dose to the eyes and pharynx.

neurocognitive function and QoL in the SRS arm. The WBRT arm did not show any improvement in survival. Two further trials showed that SRS is superior to observation after surgical resection in achieving local control in patients with one to three lesions. This benefit was higher in cases with a single lesion, and SRS proved to be a safe treatment. The benefit was highest for cavities smaller than 2.5 cm.

Hypofractionated, focal brain RT can be considered as an alternative to SRS for brain metastasis. The delivery of high dose RT to the surgical cavity improves local control. The side effects are acceptable, while larger tumours can be treated.

Treatment

Palliative Radiotherapy Treatment
Target Volume and Technique

Whole brain irradiation. The patient should ideally be immobilised in a shell during whole brain irradiation (WBI). The whole brain should be treated, both cerebrum and cerebellum, since part of the objective is to treat micrometastases.

The standard beam arrangement is a parallel pair of lateral opposing fields. The collimator should be rotated to follow approximately the radiological baseline in order to avoid the eyes. Sufficient margin should be allowed, first for patient movement or day-to-day variation in positioning (i.e. a PTV margin) and, second, to allow an adequate field size to treat the whole brain effectively (see Fig. 30.11).

If it is impossible to simulate, then simple landmarks can be used. The inferior border of the lateral field can follow a line between the lateral edge of the superior orbital ridge to the notch below the tragus of the ear. Clearance of the scalp by 1 cm at the other three edges will be sufficient.

Skull Base Irradiation

The beam arrangement is also a parallel pair of lateral opposing fields. Under normal circumstances, when it is necessary to treat the bones through which the cranial nerves pass, the field should extend from the outer canthus down and back to the posterior edge of the foramen magnum. This will cover cranial nerves II–XII.

Hypofractionated Radiotherapy

There is no consensus on hypofractionated radiotherapy and it is still an area for further research.

The GTV includes the remaining tumour or tumour bed, defined as the enhancing disease in the T1W MRI scan. The CTV includes the surgical cavity as outlined in the planning MRI scan, with a small margin. The PTV should be expanded according to the immobilisation used.

Dose and Energy

Megavoltage x-rays are preferable.

A variety of dose schedules is available including the following: 30 Gy in 10 fractions, treating daily, over 2 weeks; 20 Gy in 5 fractions, treating daily, over 1 week; 12 Gy in 2 fractions, treating on consecutive days or up to 1 week apart. This should be avoided if there is a very heavy burden of metastases to avoid acute coning with the high dose/fraction.

Side Effects

Side effects are the same as for palliative RT for HGG. Acutely, these include headache, nausea, fatigue and hair loss. Late effects relate mostly to neurocognition and QoL.

Stereotactic Radiosurgery

SRS is the delivery of a single dose of radiation to a precisely localised target (metastasis) with a view to tissue sterilisation. Single doses are typically in the range of 18 to 21 Gy depending on the tumour size. This is delivered with stereotactic localising technique using the stereotactic frame or specialised shell for the immobilisation of the patient. The outcome is similar to outcome of surgery, with lower cost (except in the posterior fossa). Use of the linac-based system or Gamma knife yields equal results.

This technique delivers a high dose of RT in a single fraction, or less than 5 fractions to very small volume with high precision. There are constraints in delivering this treatment in relation to critical normal structures and the size of the lesion. Choice of SRS is dependent on patients' characteristics, the location, size and number of lesions. The maximum diameter should be no larger than 4 cm in longest diameter, tumour volume less than 10 mL and total cumulative volume of 15 mL or less. Patients should have stable extracranial disease, Karnofsky performance score of 70 (or higher) or Eastern Cooperative Oncology Group (ECOG) PS of 2 or more and life expectancy of at least 6 months. This usually applies to one to three metastatic lesions, although, in recent studies the number of lesions is independent if the above characteristics are present. In addition, lesions that are located near to the optic apparatus (<5 mm away) in the brainstem, pons or medulla cannot be treated with SRS.

Target Volume and Technique

SRS is a highly specialist technique and beyond the scope of this chapter.

Results of Treatment

Provided patients are selected carefully, most of those who undergo treatment appear to benefit in terms of palliation of symptoms. Even so, survival of patients with cerebral deposits is generally poor, with survival after palliative RT of the order of a few months. This is normally dominated by the systemic illness. Some patients with solitary metastases, especially where systemic treatment can also be given, may live for 1 year or more. For patients with meningeal disease, the prognosis is much worse.

SPINAL CORD COMPRESSION

Pathology and Clinical Features

Metastatic epidural spinal cord compression (MESCC) is a common oncological emergency. It occurs in 3% to 6% of patients presenting with malignancy, and it can be raised up to 20% in patients with breast, prostate and lung cancer. Almost 60% of cases involve the thoracic spine. The pathology of MESCC is related to direct invasion or extrinsic compression in vertebral bodies, obstruction of the vertebral venous plexus resulting in cord oedema and further tumour growth. In most cases, it affects more than one vertebral body. Almost 90% of the patients present with pain either localised in a vertebra or in a radicular distribution. Other common symptoms include motor weakness, sensory loss and autonomic dysfunction. Sphincter disturbance and urine incontinence are usually late presentations. Permanent motor and neurological dysfunction may develop after the initial back pain. MESCC is rarely the initial presentation of cancer diagnosis. Therefore, detailed history and focused neurological examination should be performed. Diagnosis should be established with an MRI scan, which is the pathognomonic choice of imaging. However, if patients cannot undergo an MRI or if MRI is contradicted, then CT myelography can be used.

Management Principles

The treatment of spinal metastases is palliative, although some patients can achieve prolonged survival. The aim of the treatment should be pain relief, neurological function, durable local tumour control, mechanical stability and QoL.

Steroids

Steroids should be considered in all cases: randomised studies have proved that there is neurological improvement after their use. However, high dose of steroids can cause serious adverse effects, including gastric ulcers and infections. Dexamethasone, 16 mg daily is most frequently prescribed, which can be continued throughout the RT course and then tapered depending on the clinical situation.

Surgery and Radiotherapy

The combination of decompression surgery and RT has been evaluated in one phase 3 and one phase 2 study. Both showed improvement in mobility, with some patients even regaining the ability to walk, pain control and better quality of life. The surgical option, before RT, should be considered in patients with a single site of vertebral metastasis, vertebral collapse at presentation, good PS and life expectancy of more than 3 months. In addition, surgery should be considered in the following cases as well: worsening neurological symptoms, new neurological findings during RT, disease recurrence within a prior radiation site and spinal instability.

External Beam Radiotherapy

Palliative RT has always been a key treatment in the management of MESCC. The goals of the RT are to prevent neurological deterioration, improve the neurological and ambulatory function and pain relief. The RT should be delivered within 24 hours of symptom commencement. There is no consensus on the ideal RT regimen. Two randomised trials, with a primary endpoint the maintenance of neurological function, compared different radiation doses and showed that 8 to 10 Gy in a single fraction is noninferior to multiple fractions (20 Gy in 5 fractions). Nonetheless, a metaanalysis showed that better local control was achieved in patients with a soft tissue mass component when longer fractionation was prescribed. In patients with good prognosis where preserving their neurological function and mobility is critical, a longer scheme should be considered. However, in patients with poor prognosis, poor PS and paraplegia, where the objective is pain control, a single fraction could be prescribed.

Target Volume and Technique

Careful correlation with the diagnostic MRI is essential. Typically, a direct posterior field is used. If the separation is large an AP/PA solution is preferred (commonly in lumbar spine, obese patients etc.). Two lateral opposing fields can be considered when treating the C-spine, provided the shoulders are not in the beam path. Traditionally, one vertebra above and one below the affected area are also included in the target to account for possible epidural extensions.

The dose should be kept below the tolerance dose of the spinal cord.

Dose. Doses can be given as :30 Gy in 10 fractions, treating daily, over 2 weeks; or 20 Gy in 5 fractions, treating daily, over 1 week; or 8 Gy in 1 fraction, single fraction.

Stereotactic Body Radiation Therapy

In many centres, SBRT is used in the treatment of selected cases with cord compression. This technique requires precision in the mobilisation and image guidance, allowing for pretreatment confirmation and advanced radiation treatment planning. The aim of the SBRT is to provide high-dose ablative radiation in order to improve local control. The SBRT treats only the lesion, sparing most of the adjacent tissue and is delivered usually in a single fraction. Published data suggest that SBRT can offer complete pain control in more than 50% of patients and improve disability. The role of SBRT in patients with oligometastatic disease is also of particular interest.

Results

Factors that influence the outcomes include rate of symptom development, neurological impairment at diagnosis, certain tumour types and response to therapy.

FURTHER READING

Aizer AA, Ancukiewicz M, Nguyen PL, Macdonald SM, Yock TI, Tarbell NJ, et al. Natural history and role of radiation in patients with supratentorial and infratentorial WHO grade II ependymomas: results from a population-based study. J Neurooncol 2013;115(3):411–9.

Al-Omair A, Soliman H, Xu W, Karotki A, Mainprize T, Phan N, et al. Hypofractionated stereotactic radiotherapy in five daily fractions for post-operative surgical cavities in brain metastases patients with and without prior whole brain radiation. Technol Cancer Res Treat 2013;12(6):493–9.

Aoyama H, Shirato H, Tago M, Nakagawa K, Toyoda T, Hatano K, et al. Stereotactic radiosurgery plus whole-brain radiation therapy vs stereotactic radiosurgery alone for treatment of brain metastases: a randomized controlled trial. JAMA 2006;295(21):2483–91.

Baumert BG, Hegi ME, van den Bent MJ, von Deimling A, Gorlia T, Hoang-Xuan K, et al. Temozolomide chemotherapy versus radiotherapy in high-risk low-grade glioma (EORTC 22033-26033): a randomised, open-label, phase 3 intergroup study. Lancet Oncol 2016;17(11):1521–32.

Bessell EM, Lopez-Guillermo A, Villa S, Verger E, Nomdedeu B, Petit J, et al. Importance of radiotherapy in the outcome of patients with primary CNS lymphoma: an analysis of the CHOD/BVAM regimen followed by two different radiotherapy treatments. J Clin Oncol 2002;20(1):231–6.

Brower JV, Amdur RJ, Kirwan J, Mendenhall WM, Friedman W. Radiation therapy for optic nerve sheath meningioma. Pract Radiat Oncol 2013;3(3):223–8.

Brown PD, Jaeckle K, Ballman KV, Farace E, Cerhan JH, Anderson SK, et al. Effect of radiosurgery alone vs radiosurgery with whole brain radiation therapy on cognitive function in patients with 1 to 3 brain metastases: a randomized clinical trial. JAMA 2016;316(4):401–9.

Buckner JC, Chakravarti A, Curran WJ Jr. Radiation plus chemotherapy in low-grade glioma. N Engl J Med 2016;375(5):490–1.

Buckner JC, Shaw EG, Pugh SL, Chakravarti A, Gilbert MR, Barger GR, et al. Radiation plus procarbazine, CCNU, and vincristine in low-grade glioma. N Engl J Med 2016;374(14):1344–55.

Burnet NG, Jefferies SJ, Benson RJ, Hunt DP, Treasure FP. Years of life lost (YLL) from cancer is an important measure of population burden—and should be considered when allocating research funds. Br J Cancer 2005;92(2):241–5.

Burnet NG, Jena R, Burton KE, Tudor GS, Scaife JE, Harris F, et al. Clinical and practical considerations for the use of intensity-modulated radiotherapy and image guidance in neuro-oncology. Clin Oncol (R Coll Radiol) 2014;26(7):395–406.

Cairncross G, Wang M, Shaw E, Jenkins R, Brachman D, Buckner J, et al. Phase III trial of chemoradiotherapy for anaplastic oligodendroglioma: long-term results of RTOG 9402. J Clin Oncol 2013;31(3):337–43.

Chang EL. Preserving neurocognition in patients with brain metastases. JAMA Oncol 2016;.

Collamati F, Pepe A, Bellini F, Bocci V, Chiodi G, Cremonesi M, et al. Toward radioguided surgery with beta-decays: uptake of a somatostatin analogue, DOTATOC, in meningioma and high-grade glioma. J Nucl Med 2015;56(1):3–8.

Correa DD, Maron L, Harder H, Klein M, Armstrong CL, Calabrese P, et al. Cognitive functions in primary central nervous system lymphoma: literature review and assessment guidelines. Ann Oncol 2007;18(7):1145–51.

da Silva CE, de Freitas PEP. Classification of meningiomas based on their surgical removal, world health organization grade, and cytogenetic profile: a treatment algorithm. World Neurosurg 2017;105:289–93.

Darzy KH. Radiation-induced hypopituitarism after cancer therapy: who, how and when to test. Natl Clin Pract Endocrinol Metab 2009;5(2):88–99.

Di Maio S, Temkin N, Ramanathan D, Sekhar LN. Current comprehensive management of cranial base chordomas: 10-year meta-analysis of observational studies. J Neurosurg 2011;115(6):1094–105.

Dietrich J, Rao K, Pastorino S, Kesari S. Corticosteroids in brain cancer patients: benefits and pitfalls. Expert Rev Clin Pharmacol 2011;4(2):233–42.

Douw L, Klein M, Fagel SS, van den Heuvel J, Taphoorn MJ, Aaronson NK, et al. Cognitive and radiological effects of radiotherapy in patients with low-grade glioma: long-term follow-up. Lancet Neurol 2009;8(9):810–8.

Eckel-Passow JE, Lachance DH, Molinaro AM, Walsh KM, Decker PA, Sicotte H, et al. Glioma groups based on 1p/19q, idh, and tert promoter mutations in tumors. N Engl J Med 2015;372(26):2499–508.

Eekers DB, In 't Ven L, Roelofs E, Roelofs E, Postma A, Alapetite C, Burnet NG, Calugaru V, Compter I, Coremans IEM, Høyer M, Lambrecht M, Nyström PW, Romero AM, Paulsen F, Perpar A, de Ruysscher D, Renard L, Timmermann B, Vitek P, Weber DC, van der Weide HL, Whitfield GA, Wiggenraad R, EGC Troost. "European Particle Therapy Network" of ESTRO. The EPTN consensus-based atlas for CT- and MR-based contouring in neuro-oncology. Radiother Oncol 2018;128(1):37–43.

Englot DJ, Chang EF, Vecht CJ. Epilepsy and brain tumors. Handb Clin Neurol 2016;134:267–85.

Fehlings MG, Nater A, Tetreault L, Kopjar B, Arnold P, Dekutoski M, et al. Survival and clinical outcomes in surgically treated patients with metastatic epidural spinal cord compression: results of the prospective multicenter AOSpine study. J Clin Oncol 2016;34(3):268–76.

Fisher BJ, Hu C, Macdonald DR, Lesser GJ, Coons SW, Brachman DG, et al. Phase 2 study of temozolomide-based chemoradiation therapy for high-risk low-grade gliomas: preliminary results of Radiation Therapy Oncology Group 0424. Int J Radiat Oncol Biol Phys 2015;91(3):497–504.

Freeman WD. Management of intracranial pressure. Continuum (Minneap Minn). 2015;21:1299–323.

Gatfield ER, Noble DJ, Barnett GC, Early NY, Hoole ACF, Kirkby NF, et al. Tumour volume and dose influence outcome after surgery and high-dose photon radiotherapy for chordoma and chondrosarcoma of the skull base and spine. Clin Oncol (R Coll Radiol) 2018;30(4):243–53.

Gavrilovic IT, Hormigo A, Yahalom J, DeAngelis LM, Abrey LE. Long-term follow-up of high-dose methotrexate-based therapy with and without whole brain irradiation for newly diagnosed primary CNS lymphoma. J Clin Oncol 2006;24(28):4570–4.

Ghesquieres H, Ferlay C, Sebban C, Perol D, Bosly A, Casasnovas O, et al. Long-term follow-up of an age-adapted C5R protocol followed by radiotherapy in 99 newly diagnosed primary CNS lymphomas: a prospective multicentric phase II study of the Groupe d'Etude des Lymphomes de l'Adulte (GELA). Ann Oncol 2010;21(4):842–50.

Gondi V, Hermann BP, Mehta MP, Tome WA. Hippocampal dosimetry predicts neurocognitive function impairment after fractionated stereotactic radiotherapy for benign or low-grade adult brain tumors. Int J Radiat Oncol Biol Phys 2013;85(2):348–54.

Gondi V, Pugh SL, Tome WA, Caine C, Corn B, Kanner A, et al. Preservation of memory with conformal avoidance of the hippocampal neural stem-cell compartment during whole-brain radiotherapy for brain metastases (RTOG 0933): a phase II multi-institutional trial. J Clin Oncol 2014;32(34):3810–6.

Gondi V, Tome WA, Mehta MP. Why avoid the hippocampus? A comprehensive review. Radiother Oncol 2010;97(3):370–6.

Gorlia T, Wu W, Wang M, Baumert BG, Mehta M, Buckner JC, et al. New validated prognostic models and prognostic calculators in patients with low-grade gliomas diagnosed by central pathology review: a pooled analysis of EORTC/RTOG/NCCTG phase III clinical trials. Neuro Oncol 2013;15(11):1568–79.

Gousias K, Schramm J, Simon M. The Simpson grading revisited: aggressive surgery and its place in modern meningioma management. J Neurosurg 2016;125(3):551–60.

Haldorsen IS, Espeland A, Larsson EM. Central nervous system lymphoma: characteristic findings on traditional and advanced imaging. AJNR Am J Neuroradiol 2011;32(6):984–92.

Halliday J, Rutherford SA, McCabe MG, Evans DG. An update on the diagnosis and treatment of vestibular schwannoma. Expert Rev Neurother 2018;18(1):29–39.

Hermanto U, Frija EK, Lii MJ, Chang EL, Mahajan A, Woo SY. Intensity-modulated radiotherapy (IMRT) and conventional three-dimensional conformal radiotherapy for high-grade gliomas: does IMRT increase the integral dose to normal brain? Int J Radiat Oncol Biol Phys 2007;67(4):1135–44.

Houillier C, Wang X, Kaloshi G, Mokhtari K, Guillevin R, Laffaire J, et al. IDH1 or IDH2 mutations predict longer survival and response to temozolomide in low-grade gliomas. Neurology 2010;75(17):1560–6.

Iannalfi A, Fragkandrea I, Brock J, Saran F. Radiotherapy in craniopharyngiomas. Clin Oncol (R Coll Radiol) 2013;25(11):654–67.

Iqbal MS, Lewis J. An overview of the management of adult ependymomas with emphasis on relapsed disease. Clin Oncol (R Coll Radiol) 2013;25(12):726–33.

Jenkinson MD, Javadpour M, Haylock BJ, Young B, Gillard H, Vinten J, et al. The ROAM/EORTC-1308 trial: Radiation versus observation following surgical resection of atypical meningioma: study protocol for a randomised controlled trial. Trials 2015;16:519.

Jian BJ, Bloch OG, Yang I, Han SJ, Aranda D, Tihan T, et al. Adjuvant radiation therapy and chondroid chordoma subtype are associated with a lower tumor recurrence rate of cranial chordoma. J Neurooncol 2010;98(1):101–8.

Kerbauy MN, Moraes FY, Lok BH, Ma J, Kerbauy LN, Spratt DE, et al. Challenges and opportunities in primary CNS lymphoma: a systematic review. Radiother Oncol 2017;122(3):352–61.

Kilic T, Ozduman K, Elmaci I, Sav A, Necmettin Pamir M. Effect of surgery on tumor progression and malignant degeneration in hemispheric diffuse low-grade astrocytomas. J Clin Neurosci 2002;9(5):549–52.

Kim JO, Ma R, Akagami R, McKenzie M, Johnson M, Gete E, et al. Long-term outcomes of fractionated stereotactic radiation therapy for pituitary adenomas at the BC Cancer Agency. Int J Radiat Oncol Biol Phys 2013;87(3):528–33.

Kocher M, Soffietti R, Abacioglu U, Villa S, Fauchon F, Baumert BG, et al. Adjuvant whole-brain radiotherapy versus observation after radiosurgery or surgical resection of one to three cerebral metastases: results of the EORTC 22952-26001 study. J Clin Oncol 2011;29(2):134–41.

Korfel A, Schlegel U. Diagnosis and treatment of primary CNS lymphoma. Nat Rev Neurol 2013;9(6):317–27.

Lambrecht M, DBP Eekers, Alapetite C, Burnet NG, Calugaru V, IEM Coremans, Fossati P, Høyer M, Langendijk JA, Romero AM, Paulsen F, Perpar A, Renard L, de Ruysscher D, Timmermann B, Vitek P, Weber DC, van der Weide HL, Whitfield GA, Wiggenraad R, Roelofs E, Nyström PW, EGC Troost. Work package 1 of the taskforce "European Particle Therapy Network" of ESTRO. Radiation dose constraints for organs at risk in neuro-oncology; the European Particle Therapy Network consensus. Radiother Oncol 2018;128(1):26–36.

Lee KA, Dunne M, Small C, Kelly PJ, McArdle O, O'Sullivan J, et al. (ICORG 05-03): prospective randomized non-inferiority phase III trial comparing two radiation schedules in malignant spinal cord compression (not proceeding with surgical decompression); the quality of life analysis. Acta Oncol 2018;57(7):965–72.

Leeper H, Felicella MM, Walbert T. Recent advances in the classification and treatment of ependymomas. Curr Treat Options Oncol 2017;18(9):55.

Linkov F, Valappil B, McAfee J, Goughnour SL, Hildrew DM, McCall AA, et al. Development of an evidence-based decision pathway for vestibular schwannoma treatment options. Am J Otolaryngol 2017;38(1):57–64.

Lo A, Ayre G, Ma R, Hsu F, Akagami R, McKenzie M, et al. Population-based study of stereotactic radiosurgery or fractionated stereotactic radiation therapy for vestibular schwannoma: long-term outcomes and toxicities. Int J Radiat Oncol Biol Phys 2018;100(2):443–51.

Louis DN, Perry A, Reifenberger G, von Deimling A, Figarella-Branger D, Cavenee WK, et al. The 2016 World Health Organization Classification of

Tumors of the Central Nervous System: a summary. Acta Neuropathol 2016;131(6):803–20.

Mahajan A, Ahmed S, McAleer MF, Weinberg JS, Li J, Brown P, et al. Post-operative stereotactic radiosurgery versus observation for completely resected brain metastases: a single-centre, randomised, controlled, phase 3 trial. Lancet Oncol 2017;18(8):1040–8.

Malmer B, Henriksson R, Gronberg H. Familial brain tumours—genetics or environment? A nationwide cohort study of cancer risk in spouses and first-degree relatives of brain tumour patients. Int J Cancer 2003;106(2):260–3.

Mandonnet E, Delattre JY, Tanguy ML, Swanson KR, Carpentier AF, Duffau H, et al. Continuous growth of mean tumor diameter in a subset of grade II gliomas. Ann Neurol 2003;53(4):524–8.

Mansur DB, Perry A, Rajaram V, Michalski JM, Park TS, Leonard JR, et al. Postoperative radiation therapy for grade II and III intracranial ependymoma. Int J Radiat Oncol Biol Phys 2005;61(2):387–91.

Marks LB, Yorke ED, Jackson A, Ten Haken RK, Constine LS, Eisbruch A, Bentzen SM, Nam J, Deasy JO. Use of normal tissue complication probability models in the clinic. Int J Radiat Oncol Biol Phys 2010;76(3 Suppl):S10–9. 1.

McNeill KA. Epidemiology of Brain Tumors. Neurol Clin 2016;34(4):981–98.

Metellus P, Guyotat J, Chinot O, Durand A, Barrie M, Giorgi R, et al. Adult intracranial WHO grade II ependymomas: long-term outcome and prognostic factor analysis in a series of 114 patients. Neuro Oncol 2010;12 (9):976–84.

Minniti G, Scaringi C, Poggi M, Jaffrain Rea ML, Trillo G, Esposito V, et al. Fractionated stereotactic radiotherapy for large and invasive non-functioning pituitary adenomas: long-term clinical outcomes and volumetric MRI assessment of tumor response. Eur J Endocrinol 2015;172(4):433–41.

Niyazi M, Brada M, Chalmers AJ, Combs SE, Erridge SC, Fiorentino A, et al. ESTRO-ACROP guideline "target delineation of glioblastomas" Radiother Oncol 2016;118(1):35–42.

Ohgaki H, Kleihues P. The definition of primary and secondary glioblastoma. Clin Cancer Res 2013;19(4):764–72.

Osswald M, Jung E, Sahm F, Solecki G, Venkataramani V, Blaes J, et al. Brain tumour cells interconnect to a functional and resistant network. Nature 2015;528(7580):93–8.

Ostrom QT, Gittleman H, Liao P, Vecchione-Koval T, Wolinsky Y, Kruchko C, et al. CBTRUS Statistical Report: Primary brain and other central nervous system tumors diagnosed in the United States in 2010–2014. Neuro Oncol 2017;19(suppl_5):v1–v88.

Pashtan I, Oh KS, Loeffler JS. Radiation therapy in the management of pituitary adenomas. Handb Clin Neurol 2014;124:317–24.

Patchell RA, Tibbs PA, Regine WF, Payne R, Saris S, Kryscio RJ, et al. Direct decompressive surgical resection in the treatment of spinal cord compression caused by metastatic cancer: a randomised trial. Lancet 2005;366(9486):643–8.

Patel MA, Marciscano AE, Hu C, Jusue-Torres I, Garg R, Rashid A, et al. Long-term treatment response and patient outcomes for vestibular schwannoma patients treated with hypofractionated stereotactic radiotherapy. Front Oncol 2017;7:200.

Perry JR, Laperriere N, O'Callaghan CJ, Brandes AA, Menten J, Phillips C, et al. Short-course radiation plus temozolomide in elderly patients with glioblastoma. N Engl J Med 2017;376(11):1027–37.

Persson O, Bartek J, Shalom NB Jr, Wangerid T, Jakola AS, Forander P. Stereotactic radiosurgery vs. fractionated radiotherapy for tumor control in vestibular schwannoma patients: a systematic review. Acta Neurochir (Wien) 2017;159(6):1013–21.

Poortmans PM, Kluin-Nelemans HC, Haaxma-Reiche H, Van't Veer M, Hansen M, Soubeyran P, et al. High-dose methotrexate-based chemotherapy followed by consolidating radiotherapy in non-AIDS-related primary central nervous system lymphoma: European Organization for Research and Treatment of Cancer Lymphoma Group Phase II Trial 20962. J Clin Oncol 2003;21(24):4483–8.

Qu S, Meng HL, Liang ZG, Zhu XD, Li L, Chen LX, et al. Comparison of short-course radiotherapy versus long-course radiotherapy for treatment of metastatic spinal cord compression: a systematic review and meta-analysis. Medicine (Baltimore) 2015;94(43):e1843.

Rachinger W, Stoecklein VM, Terpolilli NA, Haug AR, Ertl L, Poschl J, et al. Increased 68Ga-DOTATATE uptake in PET imaging discriminates meningioma and tumor-free tissue. J Nucl Med 2015;56(3):347–53.

Reni M, Mazza E, Zanon S, Gatta G, Vecht CJ. Central nervous system gliomas. Crit Rev Oncol Hematol 2017;113:213–34.

Riedel RF, Larrier N, Dodd L, Kirsch D, Martinez S, Brigman BE. The clinical management of chondrosarcoma. Curr Treat Options Oncol 2009;10 (1–2):94–106.

Roa W, Kepka L, Kumar N, Sinaika V, Matiello J, Lomidze D, et al. International Atomic Energy Agency Randomized Phase III Study of radiation therapy in elderly and/or frail patients with newly diagnosed glioblastoma multiforme. J Clin Oncol 2015;33(35):4145–50.

Roberge D, Parney I, Brown PD. Radiosurgery to the postoperative surgical cavity: who needs evidence? Int J Radiat Oncol Biol Phys 2012;83 (2):486–93.

Rodriguez D, Cheung MC, Housri N, Quinones-Hinojosa A, Camphausen K, Koniaris LG. Outcomes of malignant CNS ependymomas: an examination of 2408 cases through the Surveillance, Epidemiology, and End Results (SEER) database (1973–2005). J Surg Res 2009;156(2):340–51.

Rogers L, Barani I, Chamberlain M, Kaley TJ, McDermott M, Raizer J, et al. Meningiomas: knowledge base, treatment outcomes, and uncertainties. A RANO review J Neurosurg 2015;122(1):4–23.

Ruda R, Reifenberger G, Frappaz D, Pfister SM, Laprie A, Santarius T, et al. EANO guidelines for the diagnosis and treatment of ependymal tumors. Neuro Oncol 2018;20(4):445–56.

Sahgal A. Point/Counterpoint: stereotactic radiosurgery without whole-brain radiation for patients with a limited number of brain metastases: the current standard of care? Neuro Oncol 2015;17(7):916–8.

Scoccianti S, Detti B, Gadda D, Greto D, Furfaro I, Meacci F, et al. Organs at risk in the brain and their dose-constraints in adults and in children: a radiation oncologist's guide for delineation in everyday practice. Radiother Oncol 2015;114(2):230–8.

Shaw EG, Wang M, Coons SW, Brachman DG, Buckner JC, Stelzer KJ, et al. Randomized trial of radiation therapy plus procarbazine, lomustine, and vincristine chemotherapy for supratentorial adult low-grade glioma: initial results of RTOG 9802. J Clin Oncol 2012;30(25):3065–70.

Smith JS, Chang EF, Lamborn KR, Chang SM, Prados MD, Cha S, et al. Role of extent of resection in the long-term outcome of low-grade hemispheric gliomas. J Clin Oncol 2008;26(8):1338–45.

Stacchiotti S, Gronchi A, Fossati P, Akiyama T, Alapetite C, Baumann M, et al. Best practices for the management of local-regional recurrent chordoma: a position paper by the Chordoma Global Consensus Group. Ann Oncol 2017;28(6):1230–42.

Stadlbauer A, Gansландt O, Buslei R, Hammen T, Gruber S, Moser E, et al. Gliomas: histopathologic evaluation of changes in directionality and magnitude of water diffusion at diffusion-tensor MR imaging. Radiology 2006;240(3):803–10.

Stummer W, van den Bent MJ, Westphal M. Cytoreductive surgery of glioblastoma as the key to successful adjuvant therapies: new arguments in an old discussion. Acta Neurochir (Wien) 2011;153(6):1211–8.

Stupp R, Hegi ME, Mason WP, van den Bent MJ, Taphoorn MJ, Janzer RC, et al. Effects of radiotherapy with concomitant and adjuvant temozolomide versus radiotherapy alone on survival in glioblastoma in a randomised phase III study: 5-year analysis of the EORTC-NCIC trial. Lancet Oncol 2009;10 (5):459–66.

Sughrue ME, Sanai N, Shangari G, Parsa AT, Berger MS, McDermott MW. Outcome and survival following primary and repeat surgery for World Health Organization Grade III meningiomas. J Neurosurg 2010;113 (2):202–9.

Takeguchi T, Miki H, Shimizu T, Kikuchi K, Mochizuki T, Ohue S, et al. The dural tail of intracranial meningiomas on fluid-attenuated inversion-recovery images. Neuroradiology 2004;46(2):130–5.

van den Bent MJ, Baumert B, Erridge SC, Vogelbaum MA, Nowak AK, Sanson M, et al. Interim results from the CATNON trial (EORTC study 26053-22054) of treatment with concurrent and adjuvant temozolomide for 1p/19q non-co-deleted anaplastic glioma: a phase 3, randomised, open-label intergroup study. Lancet 2017;390(10103):1645–53.

van den Bent MJ. Practice changing mature results of RTOG study 9802: another positive PCV trial makes adjuvant chemotherapy part of standard of care in low-grade glioma. Neuro Oncol 2014;16(12):1570–4.

Vecht CJ, Kerkhof M, Duran-Pena A. Seizure prognosis in brain tumors: new insights and evidence-based management. Oncologist 2014;19(7):751–9.

Villano JL, Koshy M, Shaikh H, Dolecek TA, McCarthy BJ. Age, gender, and racial differences in incidence and survival in primary CNS lymphoma. Br J Cancer 2011;105(9):1414–8.

Weber DC, Malyapa R, Albertini F, Bolsi A, Kliebsch U, Walser M, et al. Long term outcomes of patients with skull-base low-grade chondrosarcoma and chordoma patients treated with pencil beam scanning proton therapy. Radiother Oncol 2016;120(1): 169–74.

Weller M, van den Bent M, Tonn JC, Stupp R, Preusser M, Cohen-Jonathan-Moyal E, et al. European Association for Neuro-Oncology (EANO) guideline on the diagnosis and treatment of adult astrocytic and oligodendroglial gliomas. Lancet Oncol 2017;18(6):e315. e29.

Whitfield GA, Kennedy SR, Djoukhadar IK, Jackson A. Imaging and target volume delineation in glioma. Clin Oncol (R Coll Radiol) 2014 Jul;26(7): 364–76.

Wick W, Roth P, Hartmann C, Hau P, Nakamura M, Stockhammer F, et al. Long-term analysis of the NOA-04 randomized phase III trial of sequential radiochemotherapy of anaplastic glioma with PCV or temozolomide. Neuro Oncol 2016;18(11):1529–37.

Wu Z, Zhang J, Zhang L, Jia G, Tang J, Wang L, et al. Prognostic factors for long-term outcome of patients with surgical resection of skull base chordomas-106 cases review in one institution. Neurosurg Rev 2010;33(4):451–6.

Yahalom J, Illidge T, Specht L, Hoppe RT, Li YX, Tsang R, et al. Modern radiation therapy for extranodal lymphomas: field and dose guidelines from the International Lymphoma Radiation Oncology Group. Int J Radiat Oncol Biol Phys 2015;92(1):11–31.

Zhang H, Rodiger LA, Shen T, Miao J, Oudkerk M. Preoperative subtyping of meningiomas by perfusion MR imaging. Neuroradiology 2008;50(10): 835–40.

Eye and Orbit

Tom Roques, Adrian Harnett

ANATOMY

The orbit is defined by bony margins and is conical in shape. It contains the eye, the optic nerve and the recti, and oblique extraocular muscles. The optic nerve exits from just below the centre of the back of the eye and extends to the optic foramen at the apex of the orbit posteriorly. The globe is composed of three layers, an outer fibrous layer called the sclera, a middle layer which is vascular and composed of the choroid, the ciliary body and iris and an inner neural layer, the retina. The vascular choroid covers the inner surface of the sclera. The sclera is continuous anteriorly with the cornea, a transparent membrane covering the iris and pupil. The anterior-posterior diameter of the eye is 24 mm and the lens is 5 mm from the anterior surface. These measurements vary little between individuals.

The movement of each eye is performed by six muscles, (four recti and two oblique muscles) and directed by three cranial nerves, the IIIrd, IVth and VIth. The VIth cranial nerve supplies the lateral rectus muscle which moves the eyeball laterally. The medial, superior and inferior recti elevate, depress and move the eyeball inward, wheras the inferior oblique moves the eyeball upward and outward. These four muscles are supplied by the IIIrd cranial nerve. The superior oblique which moves the eye downward and outward is supplied by the IVth cranial nerve.

The membrane lining the inner surface of the eyelids is the conjunctiva which courses over the anterior surface of the globe, extending to the corneoscleral junction. Tears are secreted by minor lacrimal glands situated on mainly the lower eyelid and can be supplemented by the lacrimal gland situated in the upper lateral part of the orbit. They drain into the nose through the nasolacrimal duct.

PRINCIPLES OF RADIOTHERAPY TO THE EYE

The chosen radiotherapy (RT) technique will be determined by whether radical or palliative treatment is being given, by tumour factors such as histology, radiosensitivity and location and patient factors, such as fitness and co-morbidity. Brachytherapy can be used for some ocular melanomas and retinoblastomas and is described in the relevant sections below.

For fractionated external beam RT, the patient should have a comfortable set-up, which is likely to make fractionated treatment more reproducible, and appropriate immobilisation. For palliative treatment, a simple thermoplastic immobilisation shell will suffice. For radical treatment, the shell (thermoplastic or Perspex), should be made with appropriate quality assurance to keep systematic and random movement errors to an absolute minimum so as to be able to avoid sensitive normal structures with more accuracy. It is often difficult to protect any one part of the eye, particularly the lens and cornea, as the substructures are so small, although internal eye shields can be used to protect the lens when treating skin tumours close to the eye.

When superficial x-rays or electrons are used, the target volume or field is marked directly onto the shell. Beam data are used to choose an appropriate energy and to decide whether tissue-equivalent bolus is required to increase the surface dose. A lead cut-out is made to define the field shape.

For megavoltage external beam RT, a computed tomography (CT) scan is performed with the patient immobilised in the treatment shell. CT slices should be no more than 3 mm thick. Intravenous contrast can help define adjacent vessels and enhancing tumour. Target volumes are defined on the CT dataset and appropriate organs at risk are contoured. For low-dose treatments where the bilateral orbit is the target volume, a simple parallel-pair beam arrangement will provide good target coverage with minimal morbidity. In more complex situations, inverse planned intensity-modulated RT (IMRT) is recommended to be able to balance target coverage with appropriate normal tissue sparing. Noncoplanar beams can be helpful to avoid the lacrimal gland and to minimise dose to uninvolved parts of the eye. Careful attention should be paid to eye care throughout treatment and regular reviews should be performed by the ophthalmologist and radiation oncologist during the course of RT.

RADIATION AND OCULAR MORBIDITY

The Lens

The lens is one of the most sensitive tissues to RT in the body. Cataracts have been reported at doses as low as 2 Gy. However, it should be remembered that they invariably occur without RT over the age of 70 years and are associated with various common diseases, such as diabetes, and medications, such as steroids. The appearance and region of the cataract can help in deciding their causation. Radiation cataracts are caused by damage to cells in the anterior central area of the lens, which then start to form a cataract at the back of the lens centrally. The total dose, energy of radiation, volume of the lens, health of the eye and concomitant disease are all factors that play a part in cataract formation. When high doses are given with β-irradiation eye plaques, usually for treatment of posterior choroidal melanomas, cataracts often will not occur because of the rapid fall off of dose (as opposed to the historical use of cobalt plaques). After external beam RT, fractionated doses of over 10 Gy are likely to cause detectable lens opacities, usually occurring within 2 to 3 years of RT. (Fig. 31.1) shows a radiation cataract. Treatment of a cataract is by surgical removal, although if the eye is dry (most commonly as a result of RT damage to the lacrimal glands), this may adversely affect the success of surgery.

The Sclera and Retina

The sclera is radioresistant because it is avascular and can tolerate doses of up to 100 Gy by radioactive eye plaques to a small area. Above this dose there is a risk of necrosis. The retina can tolerate doses of 50 Gy but, above this, retinal damage is manifest by haemorrhages, exudates and atrophy. The macula is the most sensitive area of the retina and doses here should be minimised or avoided if possible when using radioactive eye plaques. Similarly, as the dose increases above 50 Gy, there is an increasing likelihood of optic atrophy.

The Cornea and Lacrimal Apparatus

These structures usually tolerate doses of up to 50 Gy well, depending on RT technique, energy, fractionation and attention to good eye care. Radiotherapy will result in erythema of both skin and conjunctiva and local irritation. If megavoltage RT is used, these reactions will be reduced due to build-up and skin sparing. Tear production is from the minor lacrimal glands mainly located on the lower eyelid and supplemented by the major lacrimal gland in the upper lateral part of the orbit, anteriorly. This should be contoured as an organ at risk in RT planning in an attempt reduce the dose to below 30 Gy to preserve tear production as much as possible. With a lacrimal gland dose of above 30 Gy, patients may require hypromellose eye drops (artificial tears) and Lacri-Lube. Doses of 50 Gy and above result in more serious problems.

Stenosis or occlusion of the nasolacrimal duct due to a tumour adjacent to the inner canthus will result in a weeping eye (epiphora). There is evidence that this does not happen due to RT alone if it is carefully fractionated and the tumour has not comprised the function of the duct already. Figs 31.2 (before radiotherapy) and 31.3 (after radiotherapy) illustrate a basal cell carcinoma in this region treated with superficial radiotherapy.

Developing a dry eye is not only very uncomfortable but may result in loss of vision. Corneal damage occurs, partly due to reduced sensation. Punctate keratitis and oedema lead on to corneal ulceration, scarring, infection and impairment of vision. If high-dose RT is given, the involvement of an ophthalmologist to give advice, eye protection and ensure good eye care is imperative during the course of RT. This will aid in achieving patient comfort, maximising vision and minimising late complications. Keratinisation of the cornea is a late complication and occurs after doses in excess of 50 Gy. Rarely, it leads on to secondary revascularisation.

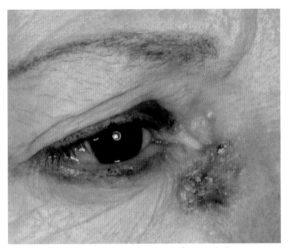

Fig. 31.2 Basal cell carcinoma before radiotherapy.

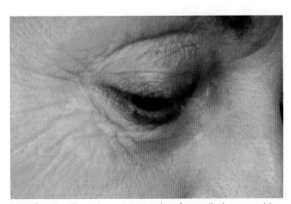

Fig. 31.3 Basal cell carcinoma 4 months after radiotherapy with superficial X-rays.

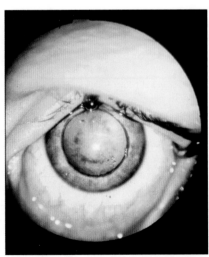

Fig. 31.1 A radiation cataract

The Optic Nerves and Chiasm

The tolerance of optic nerves and chiasm depends primarily on the total dose and dose per fraction used. Radiation-induced optic neuropathy is very uncommon when the maximum dose to the nerve is less than 55 Gy. The risk is 3% to 7% for doses of 55 to 60 Gy though most reported incidences of radiation-induced optic neuropathy (RION) in this range have involved doses of 59 Gy and above. There is evidence that radiation-induced optic neuropathy is more common in elderly patients. The data on whether diabetes or hypertension influences risk is inconsistent.

BENIGN CONDITIONS

Thyroid Eye Disease

Thyroid eye disease (TED) is an autoimmune process causing eyelid retraction, proptosis, myopathy and exophthalmos. Most people with TED have Grave's disease and are hyperthyroid at diagnosis, but it can also occur in people without current or prior hyperthyroidism or in Hashimoto's thyroiditis. Orbital fibroblasts are thought to express autoantigens such as the thyrotropin receptor. Autoantibodies produced in Grave's disease interact with the autoantigens to activate the orbital fibroblasts resulting in cytokine production and inflammation of the orbital muscles and fat. Most TED is mild and can be managed by controlling thyroid function, smoking cessation, good eye care and selenium supplements.

The natural history of TED is variable but an initial active inflammatory phase is often followed by a spontaneous improvement over 1 to 2 years and then a chronic phase due to residual fibrosis and scarring. Moderate to severe active TED occurs in about 5% of cases and is defined as disease having sufficient impact on daily life to justify systemic steroids. There is usually radiological evidence of orbital fat and muscle expansion, diplopia and significant exophthalmos. (Fig. 31.4) shows bilateral medial rectus swelling from thyroid eye disease.

High-dose intravenous steroids are the recommended initial treatment for moderate to severe active TED. The role of RT is debated with trials of radiation versus sham radiation producing conflicting results though they have had small patient numbers, different inclusion criteria and different approaches to steroid use. The most recent such study investigated RT as part of first-line treatment with oral prednisolone and showed no benefit. International guidelines suggest considering RT as second-line therapy after TED has progressed on intravenous steroids, though cyclosporine A, azathioprine and rituximab can also be used in this situation. Radiotherapy is more effective at improving ocular

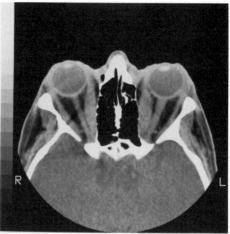

Fig. 31.4 An axial CT slice showing bilateral medial rectus swelling due to thyroid eye disease.

motility and diplopia than exophthalmos and is more effective when combined with steroids. It is a relatively straightforward treatment and the low doses required mean the risk of acute and long-term side effects is small. Many patients experience mild inflammatory symptoms such as conjunctival irritation and eye watering. Careful technique should enable the lens dose to be well below 10 Gy though patients should be consented for cataract formation. The risk of a radiation-induced second malignancy is about 0.2%. Microvascular retinal abnormalities have been detected after TED RT, so radiation is contraindicated in people with diabetic retinopathy or severe hypertension. The mechanism of action is thought to be anti-inflammatory, reducing lymphocyte infiltration and fibrosis.

Although dysthyroid eye disease is occasionally unilateral, it is usually recommended to treat both eyes. Patients are immobilised in a thermoplastic shell and CT planned. The target volume is the orbital fat and extraocular muscles. There is no real dosimetric advantage to using anything more complex than paired unmodulated lateral radiation fields. Beam sizes of up to 5 cm in each direction are chosen to encompass both orbits so that the 50% isodose is through the anterior pituitary. The fields are angled slightly posteriorly or half-beam blocked to prevent divergence through the contralateral lens. This angulation posteriorly is usually of the order of 5 degrees except where there is marked asymmetrical proptosis. (Fig. 31.5) shows a typical beam

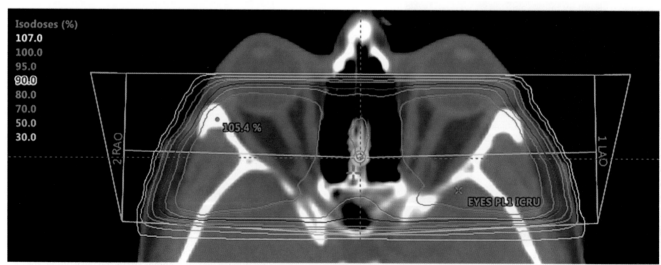

Fig. 31.5 Lateral beams to treat thyroid eye disease and corresponding isodoses.

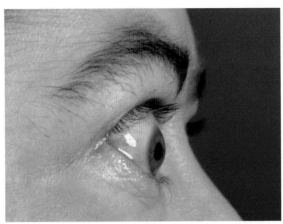

Fig. 31.6 Thyroid eye disease before radiotherapy.

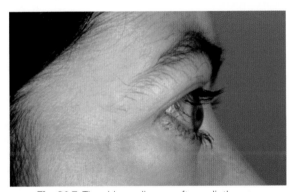

Fig. 31.7 Thyroid eye disease after radiotherapy.

arrangement and isodoses. The usual dose is 20 Gy in 10 fractions over 2 weeks though 10 Gy in 5 fractions over 2 weeks has also been used. If the patient is not being given steroids concomitant with RT, the first fraction can occasionally cause oedema to worsen. For this reason, a first fraction of 1 Gy is sometimes used, followed by 11 fractions of 1.73 Gy (total 20 Gy in 12 fractions). (Figs 31.6 and 31.7) show thyroid eye disease before and after radiotherapy.

Orbital Pseudotumour

Also known as idiopathic orbital inflammation, orbital pseudotumour is a rare diagnosis of exclusion once other causes of inflammation such as lymphoma, TED, Wegener's granulomatosis and sarcoidosis have been ruled out. Orbital pseudotumour usually causes pain behind the eye and can also result in proptosis, eyelid swelling and diplopia. Improved molecular pathology diagnostic techniques mean accurate alternative diagnoses are now often made. Focal or diffuse inflammation of the orbital contents can be seen clinically or on imaging. A biopsy is necessary to rule out other diagnoses. It is usually treated with steroids, but there is evidence that RT can be effective if there is a relapse after steroids or if they do not work. Twenty Gy in 10 fractions is used with a technique similar to TED for bilateral disease, or similar to orbital lymphoma or unilateral disease.

MALIGNANT TUMOURS

Primary tumours can be classified as arising from the skin and adnexa, orbit or intraocularly. Basal cell carcinomas (BCCs) and squamous cell carcinomas (SCCs) are skin tumours commonly arising on the face, especially around the eye and lower eye lid. In contrast, lacrimal gland and nasolacrimal duct tumours are rare, as are orbital tumours. Rhabdomyosarcoma of the orbit is a tumour of childhood. It is usually embryonal and is discussed in further detail in Chapter 33. Intraocular tumours are rare with retinoblastoma occurring in the very young and melanoma occurring in adults. The choroid is the commonest site in the eye for metastatic disease.

PRIMARY MALIGNANT TUMOURS

Primary tumours of the eye and orbit can be classified according to their primary location:
1. Skin and adnexa
   a. BCC of the skin
   b. SCC of the skin
   c. Lacrimal gland cancer
   d. Nasolacrimal duct cancer
   e. Miscellaneous
2. Orbital tumours
   a. Lymphoma
   b. Melanoma (conjunctival)
   c. Rhabdomyosarcoma
   d. Optic nerve glioma
3. Intraocular
   a. Melanoma (choroidal and iris)
   b. Retinoblastoma

Skin Cancers Involving the Eyelid

Periocular skin cancers should be managed by a team with dermatology, ophthalmology, plastic surgery and oncology expertise given the many critical structures close to the tumour and the importance of achieving local tumour control.

BCCs are the most common skin tumours and frequently occur on the face, especially around the eye. The incidence is higher in those who have a lot of sun exposure and so is related to outside occupations. They grow slowly and so may be neglected but, if left, will invade, ulcerate and destroy tissue locally. The ulcerating BCC in Fig. 31.8 had extended

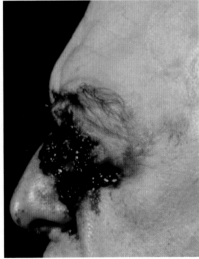

Fig. 31.8 A basal cell carcinoma destroying local structures.

into the orbit and frontal lobe. The lower eyelid is the most common site for a periorbital BCC. They usually present as a slow-growing, reddish nodule, sometimes with a pearly surface or central ulceration. Clinically, they can be very difficult to differentiate from SCCs, which can also occur in this location, so a biopsy should be carried out. When BCCs occur near the inner canthus, the nasolacrimal duct may be affected, causing the patient to complain of a watery eye.

For BCCs and SCCs, local excision, often with Mohs surgery for margin control and oculoplastic reconstruction, is usually preferred to RT as long as the patient is fit enough and good cosmetic and functional outcomes are expected. RT remains an effective technique with a 90% cure rate using superficial x-rays (SXR) or low-energy electrons. SXR is preferred as the bowing of isodoses at depth and lateral scatter make shielding of critical structures more difficult with electrons. Radiotherapy to the upper eyelid should be avoided as it can cause fibrosis of the tarsal plate which can lead to corneal exposure and ulceration.

The target volume is the visible tumour with a 5 to 10 mm margin depending on size, histological subtype and how well-defined the tumour is. A lead cut-out is made to shield adjacent structures. An internal eyeshield should be inserted for each treatment to protect the cornea and lens when the treated area is right next to the eye or involving the eyelid. The eyeshield is essentially a lead contact lens coated on the inside with liquid paraffin to reduce friction and is inserted after local anaesthetic eye drops have been instilled.

Various dose-fractionation schedules can be used such as 35 Gy in 5 fractions or 45 Gy in 10 fractions. Tumours that are thought to extend to deeper structures may need to be treated with MV photons using a CT-defined inverse-planned technique and a longer course of fractionated RT. Conjunctival oedema (chemosis) as a result of RT is uncommon if treatment is reasonably fractionated and if the nasolacrimal duct is not stenosed by the tumour.

Lacrimal Gland and Nasolacrimal Duct Cancer

Lacrimal gland and nasolacrimal duct carcinomas are rare, locally invasive and difficult to treat. Surgical excision, appropriate reconstruction and postoperative RT are usually required to maximise local control. Orbital exenteration should be considered if there is destruction of the orbital wall or tumour in the orbital cavity, but with modern surgical and RT techniques, preservation of a functioning eye should be the treatment goal. Careful multidisciplinary discussion involving ophthalmologists, ear, nose and throat (ENT) specialists, head and neck reconstructive surgeons and oncologists is essential to achieve this, also taking into account the wishes of the patient.

Tumours Arising From Adjacent Structures

Maxillary sinus tumours can invade up into the orbit through the orbital floor, whereas ethmoid sinus tumours can infiltrate through the thin lamina papyracea. Surgery and postoperative RT is usually recommended. Radiation doses of 60 Gy or more are required. Because this exceeds the tolerance dose of many orbital structures, excellent immobilisation and meticulous target volume and organ-at-risk delineation are essential, particularly if an exenteration has not been carried out. Conformal planning usually using inverse-planned IMRT will provide the best compromise between giving an appropriate dose to the planning target volume (PTV) and limiting the risk of acute and late side effects.

As in other sites, rare primary tumours can occur around the eye. Angiosarcomas respond rapidly to RT but, despite high doses, also recur locally and regionally.

Lymphoma

Orbital lymphoma may affect the conjunctiva, eyelid, lacrimal gland or retrobular contents. Fifteen percent are bilateral, although disease in the contralateral eye may be metachronous. Presentation may be due to a typically discrete erythematous conjunctival lesion, minor eye discomfort, a mass most often involving the major lacrimal gland, ptosis, chemosis, diplopia, exophthalmos and a red eye. A magnetic resonance imaging (MRI) or CT scan of the orbits should be performed even for conjunctival lymphoma as the tumour sometimes tracks around the globe and involves the orbital cone. The conjunctival extent of a superficial tumour is best determined by careful ophthalmic assessment. Biopsies will confirm the histological subtype with low-grade marginal-zone lymphomas being most common, although follicular lymphoma and diffuse large B cell lymphoma (DLBCL) are sometimes seen. A CT or positron emission tomography (PET)-CT of the whole body should be performed to look for other sites of disease which are often found in high-grade lymphomas. A management plan should be recommended by the radiation oncologist, haematologist and ophthalmologist taking the patient's preferences into account. Radiotherapy is an effective sole treatment for low-grade tumours confined to the orbit and is also used as consolidation after systemic therapy for high-grade lymphoma.

If the lymphoma is confined to the conjunctiva, the target volume is the entire ipsilateral conjunctiva under the upper and lower eyelids, but not the posterior orbital contents. This can usually be treated with a direct superficial x-ray or electron beam using a 5-cm circular lead cut-out to define the field edge remembering that the size of the eyeball is very consistent between individuals. The eye should be shut during treatment but some bolus may still be required when using electrons to bring the conjunctiva surface dose to 90%. (Figs 31.9 and 31.10)

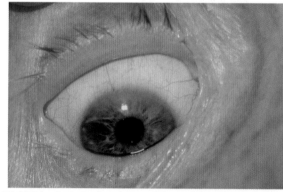

Fig. 31.10 Marginal zone lymphoma of the conjunctiva after radiotherapy.

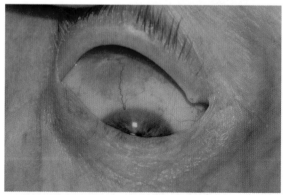

Fig. 31.9 Marginal zone lymphoma of the conjunctiva before radiotherapy.

show a low grade marginal zone lymphoma of the conjunctiva before and after radiotherapy.

For more extensive orbital lymphomas, the target volume is the whole orbit including the retrobulbar space, lacrimal gland and conjunctiva. Having immobilised the patient, a CT scan with no more than 3-mm thick slices is obtained, on which the clinical target volume (CTV) is Yes, correct delineated. A small PTV margin is added based on department error data. There will be minimal intrafraction motion so CTV-PTV margins of 3 to 4 mm should be possible. Superior and inferior oblique beams usually provide good coverage of this conical volume and have the advantage of completely avoiding the contralateral eye. If there is bilateral disease then a parallel-pair technique similar to that used in TED will provide good coverage, or each eye can be planned and treated separately.

For low-grade lymphoma, a dose of 24 Gy in 12 fractions is recommended. Consolidation RT for DLBCL requires 30 Gy in 15 fractions with higher doses of up to 36 Gy sometimes used for macroscopic residual disease after chemotherapy, or if the patient is unable to receive chemotherapy. With these higher doses, it may be appropriate to try to reduce dose to the cornea by treating with the eye open and to limit the higher-dose target volume to visible disease, rather than treating the whole orbit to more than 30 Gy. (Figs 31.11 and 31.12) show diffuse large B cell lymphoma of the orbit before and after radiotherapy. (Fig. 31.13) shows a typical beam arrangement and isodoses used to treat a unilateral orbital lymphoma.

Ocular Melanoma

Melanoma is the commonest primary intraocular tumour in adults with an incidence of six per million annually. In adults, it most frequently affects the uveal tract, especially the choroid.

It is not uncommon for asymptomatic patients to be referred by an optician who, at a routine eye test, has detected a pigmented lesion in the fundus. Some of these lesions will be choroidal nevi, but some will be melanomas. It may be difficult to distinguish between the two, particularly for a small melanoma, and so the patient may be initially managed conservatively with 6-monthly assessments. Other patients may present with visual loss which may be associated with retinal detachment. Pain does not often occur and may indicate a large tumour. Tumours arising from the iris and conjunctiva are clearly visible and so are noticed by the patient or their family. (Fig. 31.14) shows a melanoma of the iris and (Fig. 31.15) illustrates a melanoma of the conjunctiva.

An expert ophthalmic assessment is mandatory by a clinician experienced in this field, and will include direct and/or indirect ophthalmoscopy, ocular ultrasound and fluorescein angiography. This may be supplemented by MRI for large tumours which may be considered for local resection in order to assess extraocular extension.

Melanomas of the eye are often detected when they are very small and may measure under 5 mm at their base and 1 mm in height. They grow slowly, and so initial treatment may be observation in order to confirm the diagnosis. Some patients present with metastases, particularly involving the liver. Others develop metastatic disease up to 15 years later and the risk increases with the size of the ocular tumour at presentation. Patients with anterior placed tumours in the uveal tract are at higher risk than those with posterior choroidal melanomas. Cytogenetic subtypes with different metastatic risk profiles are now recognised, helping to predict recurrence rates and determine surveillance strategies. The diagnosis is usually made by expert ophthalmic assessment and biopsy is not required before treatment.

Choroidal melanoma treatment using radioactive eye plaque brachytherapy, originally with ^{60}cobalt, Correct has now been superseded by ^{106}ruthenium, ^{90}strontium, ^{103}palladium or ^{125}iodine, and used for a long time. Studies have therefore shown that eye preservation has not adversely affected survival. Indeed, it was even considered by some to improve survival by possibly an immunoprotective mechanism. Brachytherapy is contraindicated in tumours with more than 5 mm extraocular extension where the basal diameter is too large for brachytherapy, in blind painful eyes or in patients with no light-perception vision. In these situations, surgery is preferred, sometimes with an enucleation.

^{106}Ruthenium is a beta emitter so is suitable for tumours smaller than 6 mm in depth. It comes in a range of ready-made shapes and sizes. ^{103}Palladium and ^{125}iridium are low-dose gamma emitters which are custom made with a 2-mm margin around the tumour. A notch can be created in the plaque when the tumour is close to the optic nerve to reduce dose at this site. The tumour is visualised by transpupillary or transocular illumination of the globe and marked on the adjacent sclera

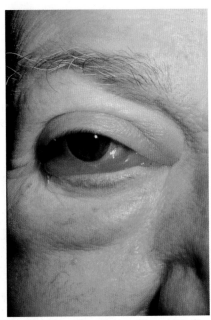

Fig. 31.11 Diffuse large B cell lymphoma of the orbit before radiotherapy.

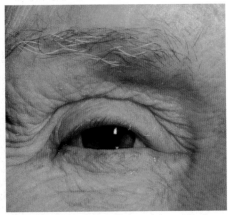

Fig. 31.12 Diffuse large B cell lymphoma of the orbit after radiotherapy.

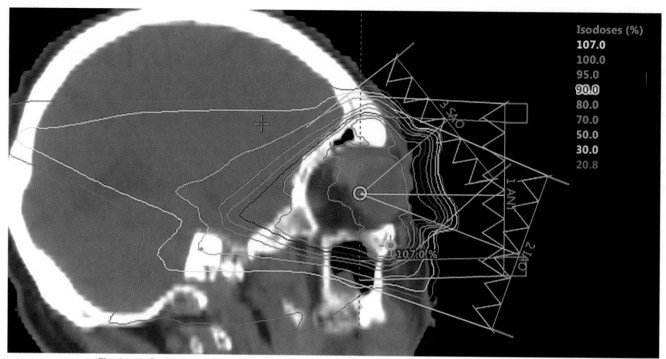

Fig. 31.13 Sagittal view of beam arrangement and isodoses used to treat a unilateral orbital lymphoma.

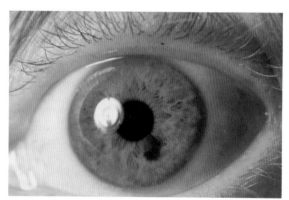

Fig. 31.14 Melanoma of the iris.

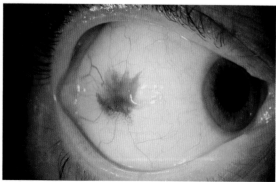

Fig. 31.15 Melanoma of the conjunctiva.

with a 2- to 3-mm margin with tissue dye. The plaque is sutured in place to cover this target volume and removed after 5 to 7 days.

It is unclear whether the dose to the base or apex of the tumour is important and radiation dose prescriptions vary between centres, though a dose of 70 to 100 Gy to the tumour apex is most commonly used.

Fractionated proton therapy (60 Gy in 4 fractions or 70 Gy in 5 fractions) can also be used to treat uveal melanoma with local control rates of 95% in most series though the anterior eye structures will receive some radiation dose with this technique. Fractionated stereotactic RT is also sometimes used. There has never been a trial comparing these approaches.

Conjunctival and iris melanoma is treated by local excision, sometimes with adjuvant plaque brachytherapy once the conjunctiva has healed. A hand-held [90]strontium applicator is used to deliver 50 Gy in 5 daily fractions to the surface, or 60 Gy in 4 fractions once a week. Due to the size of the tumour, enucleation may be the only option.

Unfortunately, very occasionally, patients present with very extensive, neglected tumours which are inoperable. Palliative RT can produce a useful regression of extensive tumour. High dose fractionated radiotherapy must be used, either with weekly fractions of 6 Gy or daily treatment to 60 Gy or more over 6 weeks.

The advent of targeted therapies such as the MEK inhibitor, selumetinib, immunotherapy and hepatic perfusion techniques hold the promise of changing the prognosis for systemic disease which usually presents in the liver. As long as the patient is well enough to consider therapy for liver metastases, 6-monthly screening with nonionising radiation such as MRI or ultrasound is recommended.

Retinoblastoma

Retinoblastoma is a rare tumour occurring in the very young, usually in children under the age of 2 years. It is usually caused by a heritable or nonheritable mutation in the RB1 tumour-suppressor gene on chromosome 13. In the hereditary form, often both eyes are affected. Parents or family may notice a white reflex in the pupil, which usually indicates a large tumour, or a squint and difficulty in fixation. Early detection is key and has enabled cure rates of 95%. Extension into the orbit or perforation of the globe are very unusual but very serious with respect to prognosis as these patients are incurable. In advanced disease, rarely seen in patients in Europe at initial presentation, metastases may occur to the central nervous system and the bone marrow.

Retinoblastoma is exceptional with respect to oncological management in that a biopsy for confirmation of the diagnosis is never performed and, indeed, contraindicated because of the high risk of spread of tumour cells outside the globe. Therefore, the diagnosis is a clinical one made in specialised centres with great expertise in retinoblastoma and characterised by appearances on bilateral indirect binocular ophthalmoscopy under general anaesthetic. Even when enucleation is performed for a large tumour and/or a nonseeing eye, previous biopsy should not have been carried out.

Early tumours (International Intraocular Retinoblastoma Classification (IIRC), group A) can be treated with focal cryotherapy or laser therapy. Groups B, C and D tumours are treated with intravenous chemotherapy and sometimes additional focal treatments as for group A or occasionally with brachytherapy. Chemotherapy usually includes carboplatin, etoposide and vincristine. There are also techniques to deliver chemotherapy directly into the ophthalmic artery or vitreous cavity. Group E tumours are usually treated with enucleation and adjuvant chemotherapy.

Brachytherapy uses ^{106}ruthenium or ^{125}iodine plaques, both of which are beta emitters and therefore not so penetrating. They are sutured onto the back of the globe overlying the tumour, its position outlined by transillumination. For ^{125}iodine, a dose of 40 Gy is given over four to five days, depending on the activity of the plaque at time of use, and prescribed to the apex of the tumour which has been measured by ultrasound.

External beam RT used to be the principal eye-conserving therapy, but it is now used only to salvage eyes when other treatment has not worked. In such cases, brachytherapy techniques, which enable the orbit to be treated by intraconal delivery systems containing ^{125}iodine or proton therapy, both have the advantage of reducing radiation dose to extra-orbital structures. This is particularly important as radiation increases the risk of second malignancy in heritable retinoblastoma.

Metastases

Secondary deposits to the eye via the bloodstream are common but often not clinically evident or recognised. The most frequent site of ocular metastases is the vascular choroid leading to retinal detachment. Therefore, presentation may be an oncological emergency due to sudden loss of vision. It usually occurs in patients known to have malignancy, especially from breast and lung cancer. Other tumours which less frequently metastasise are urogenital and upper gastrointestinal tumours. Orbital metastases usually indicate widespread metastatic disease and, consequently, a poor prognosis, except in some breast cancer patients. Patients may have brain metastases as well. If full fundal examination is carried out, asymptomatic metastases are not infrequently found, often involving the contralateral eye. Choroidal metastases have a characteristic appearance, with a yellow raised honeycomb lesion. Radiotherapy should be given to try to preserve vision. Prostate cancer metastases can involve the orbit, usually due to expansion from a bone deposit resulting in visual disturbance or loss, diplopia, ptosis or exophthalmos.

The patient lies prone on a head rest with the head supported and immobilised using a beam directional thermoplastic shell. Choroidal deposits can be treated by a single anterior megavoltage photon field or a lateral field angled 5 to 10 degrees posteriorly. If an anterior field is used, the eye is treated open to take advantage of the skin-sparing effect of megavoltage to reduce the dose to the cornea and lens. In breast cancer, choroidal metastases are often multiple and/or bilateral and so both eyes should be treated using parallel-opposed lateral fields similar to those used in TED. A dose of 20 Gy in 5 daily fractions over one week with megavoltage RT is usually most appropriate, but 30 Gy in 10 fractions can be used in people with a good prognosis from their underlying cancer.

FURTHER READING

American Brachytherapy Society—Ophthalmic Oncology Task Force. The American Brachytherapy Society consensus guidelines for plaque brachytherapy of uveal melanoma and retinoblastoma Brachytherapy 2014;13(1):1–14.

Bartalena L, Baldeschi L, Boboridis K, Eckstein A, Kahaly GJ, et al. The 2016 European Thyroid Association/European Group on Graves' Orbitopathy Guidelines for the Management of Graves' Orbitopathy. Eur Thyroid J 2016;5(1):9–26.

Bartalena L, Baldeschi L, Dickinson AJ, Eckstein A, Kendall-Taylor P, et al. Consensus statement of the European Group on Graves' orbitopathy (EUGOGO) on management of Graves' orbitopathy. Thyroid 2008;18 (3):333–46.

Nathan P, Cohen V, Coupland S, Curtis K, Damato B, et al. Uveal Melanoma UK National Guidelines. Eur J Cancer 2015;51(16):2404–12.

Rajendram R, Taylor PN, Wilson VJ, Harris N, Morris OC, et al. Combined immunosuppression and radiotherapy in thyroid eye disease (CIRTED): a multicentre, 2 × 2 factorial, double-blind, randomised controlled trial. Lancet Diabetes Endocrinol 2018;6(4):299–309.

Schwarcz RM, Coupland SE, Finger PT. Cancer of the orbit and adnexa. Am J Clin Oncol 2013;36(2):197–205.

Stannard C, Sauerwein W, Maree G, Lecuona K. Radiotherapy for ocular tumours. Eye (London) 2013;27(2):119–27.

The Royal College of Radiologists. review of the use of radiotherapy in the UK for the treatment of benign clinical conditions and benign tumours. London: The Royal College of Radiologists; 2015.

Vasalaki M, Fabian ID, Reddy MA, Cohen VM, Sagoo MS. Ocular oncology: advances in retinoblastoma, uveal melanoma and conjunctival melanoma. Br Med Bull. 2017;121(1):107–19.

Yahalom J, Illidge T, Specht L, Hoppe RT, Li YX, et al. Modern radiation therapy for extranodal lymphomas: field and dose guidelines from the International Lymphoma Radiation Oncology Group. Int J Radiat Oncol Biol Phys 2015;92(1):11–31.

Sarcomas

Thankamma V. Ajithkumar

SOFT TISSUE SARCOMAS

Soft tissue sarcomas (STS) are malignant tumours arising from supporting connective tissues anywhere in the body. These structures (fibrous tissue, fat, blood vessels, smooth and skeletal muscle, tendons and cartilage) are derived embryologically from the mesoderm. Tumours of peripheral nerves are also included in the classification of STS. Despite arising from a wide variety of tissues, adult-type STS have many similarities in pathology, clinical findings and behavior. However, paediatric-type STS, such as rhabdomyosarcoma and soft tissue Ewing sarcoma are distinct because of their cytogenetics and differing treatment approaches. The principles of treatment outlined below mainly apply to adult-type STS.

Pathology

STS are rare, representing 0.4% of all cancers and 0.3% of cancer deaths. The incidence is about 0.6 per 100,000 population per year. However, they constitute 6% of tumours in children under the age of 15 years. Most occur in the 40 to 70 years age groups, but peak age of incidence varies according to histological subtypes. The sex ratio is virtually the same.

The aetiology is unknown in the majority of cases. In a minority of cases, genetic factors, previous radiotherapy (RT) and chemotherapy and an association with viral infections are identified. The incidence of soft tissue sarcoma is significantly higher in children treated with both chemotherapy and RT (SIR 113) compared with RT alone (SIR 19). Radiation-induced sarcomas commonly occur within previously irradiated areas (especially for benign angiomas). The common types of radiation-induced sarcomas are undifferentiated pleomorphic sarcoma and osteosarcoma.

Genetic syndromes associated with soft tissue sarcomas include Li–Fraumeni syndrome (osteosarcoma, rhabdomyosarcoma and Ewing sarcoma), Gardner syndrome (intraabdominal desmoid tumours), tuberous sclerosis, and von Recklinghausen disease (malignant nerve sheath tumours and rhabdomyosarcoma). Rarely, soft tissue sarcomas may occur in the children of mothers with early-onset breast cancer.

Sarcomas are associated with numerous genetic abnormalities. The first demonstrated specific gene abnormality associated with malignant transformation in man was the loss of the retinoblastoma (RB), a tumour suppressor gene. There are alterations to the RB gene in up to 70% of soft tissue sarcomas. Chromosome translocations are the most common genetic abnormality and are seen in virtually all cases of Ewing sarcoma (primitive neuroectodermal tumours). Translocation of 11:22 is the most common in Ewing sarcoma, occurring in 85% of cases. In more than 90% of synovial sarcomas, there is a chromosome 18 translocation. Such cytogenetic abnormalities may be useful diagnostically and may be of prognostic significance. It is noteworthy that translocations tend to occur most commonly in high-grade tumours.

The 2013 World Health Organization (WHO) classification is extremely complex and a simplified version listing malignant tumours by their tissue of origin is presented in Table 32.1.

Although histological grade and the size of tumour continue to dictate management and prognosis, histological subtyping is increasingly used to guide management, especially the choice of systemic therapy. The system described by Trojani is in regular use both in the United Kingdom and internationally (Table 32.2). Low-grade tumours have a recognisable pattern of differentiation, relatively few mitoses, and no necrosis. High-grade tumours include all examples of certain subtypes (e.g. alveolar soft part), tumours with little or no apparent differentiation, and those with necrosis and a high mitotic rate. The tumour size is also important, and those over 5 cm are much more likely to recur locally or give rise to distant metastases.

Natural Spread

Initial spread from the primary site is into adjacent tissue and along tissue planes between structures such as muscle bundles. Soft tissue sarcomas do not possess a true capsule but are often surrounded by a pseudo capsule of compressed surrounding tissues. This apparent encapsulation may tempt the surgeon to try to shell out the tumour. Local recurrence from residual tumour at the periphery is then very likely ($\leq$90% within 2 years). Lymph node spread is infrequent, whereas bloodborne spread is common, giving rise to distant metastases, predominantly in the lungs.

Clinical Features

Approximately 40% of soft tissue sarcomas occur in the upper and lower limbs. Of these, about 75% occur at or above the knee. Some 10% of sarcomas arise in the upper half of the body. Of the sarcomas of the trunk, 10% occur in the retroperitoneum and 20% in the chest or abdominal wall. Presentation with locally advanced disease is common, particularly with intraabdominal sarcomas, which may reach a very large size.

The history is usually of a painless lump developing over a few weeks or months and occasionally over years. Pain may occur from pressure on local structures, for example nerves and joints. Occasionally, nonmetastatic effects are seen (e.g. hypoglycaemia in malignant fibrous histiocytoma).

Diagnosis and Staging

Patients with a suspected STS should have an initial ultrasound (US) examination or a referral to a specialist multidisciplinary team for a triple assessment (clinical history, imaging and biopsy). An initial US may rule out benign lesions.

Triple Assessment

Clinical history and examination are to assess the position of the primary lesion (superficial or deep to the fascia), any involvement of bone, vascular or neural invasion and regional nodal involvement, although the latter is uncommon. Patients with suspicious US or clinical features should have a magnetic resonance imaging (MRI) scan of the affected region (Fig. 32.1). Plain x-ray is useful to rule out bony involvement or risk of fracture.

A biopsy is required in all cases. Although in 90% of cases, adequate histology can be achieved by a percutaneous core needle biopsy, where an incisional biopsy is required, care should be taken to make the incision longitudinal so that any subsequent radical surgery or postoperative radiation fields can include it. This is particularly important where preservation of limb function is a major consideration. Inappropriate biopsy can compromise the feasibility of limb conservation surgery and the chances of local control and cure as a result of inadvertent contamination of uninvolved tissue planes. The biopsy should therefore be carried out only in a specialist sarcoma centre or by the surgeon who will undertake the definitive resection. If CT-guided biopsy is needed, for example for impalpable deep-seated lesions, there is also potential for needle track contamination. Close liaison with the surgeon and clinical oncologist is needed to plan the best route of biopsy.

TABLE 32.1 Simplified Version of the WHO Classification (2013) of Sarcomas

Fat
Intermediate: atypical lipomatous tumour/well-differentiated liposarcoma
Malignant: liposarcoma

Fibrous Tissue
Intermediate: desmoid-type fibromatosis, lipofibromatosis, dermatofibrosarcoma protuberans, solitary fibrous tumour etc.
Malignant: fibrosarcoma, myxofibrosarcoma, sclerosing epithelioid fibrosarcoma

Smooth Muscle
Leiomyosarcoma

Skeletal Muscle
Embryonal rhabdomyosarcoma
Alveolar rhabdomyosarcoma
Pleomorphic rhabdomyosarcoma, spindle cell/sclerosing rhabdomyosarcoma

Blood Vessels
Intermediate: haemangioblastomas, Kaposi sarcoma
Malignant: angiosarcoma, epithelioid hemangioendothelioma

Gastrointestinal Stromal Tumours
Bone
Osteogenic sarcoma, chondrosarcoma, giant cell tumours, chordoma, Ewing sarcoma, fibrosarcoma of bone, angiosarcoma of bone

Nerve Sheath
Malignant peripheral nerve sheath tumours, epithelioid malignant nerve sheath tumour, malignant granular cell tumour

Sarcomas of Uncertain Differentiation
Synovial sarcomas
Epithelioid sarcomas
Alveolar soft part sarcomas
Desmoplastic small round cell tumour, PEComa

PEComa, Perivascular epithelioid cell neoplasms; *WHO*, World Health Organization.

TABLE 32.2 Grading System for Adult Soft Tissue Sarcoma

Score	Tumour Differentiation	Necrosis	No. of Mitoses/10 HPF
1	Well	absent	<10
2	Moderate	<50%	10–19
3	Poor	≥50%	≥20

The total scores are 2–3 for grade 1, 4–5 for grade 2 and ≥6 for grade 3 tumours.

Staging Investigations

Other investigations include a full blood count, liver function tests, imaging of the tumour-bearing region (Fig. 32.1) and CT of the chest to rule out lung metastases (Fig. 32.2). Chest x-ray may be appropriate for staging in patients with very low-risk of lung metastases (e.g. those with atypical lipomatous tumours) and those who are frail with small low-grade lesions. CT of the abdomen/pelvis may be considered for tumours of the lower extremities and histological subtypes with a risk of soft-tissue metastases such a myxoid liposarcoma. Positron emission tomography (PET)-CT scan is not routinely advised, but may be useful in selected situations such as response assessment after targeted agents. The role of whole body MRI scan in the diagnostic staging of sarcomas is yet to be established.

CT scan and MRI (Fig. 32.3) are important in defining the local extent and operability of the tumour. MRI is the imaging modality of choice for limb sarcomas because it provides good contrast between the tumour and adjoining normal tissues and is particularly useful to assess involvement of the neurovascular bundle. It also provides better multiplanar versatility in planning surgery and RT. CT can be helpful in exclusion of cortical erosion of bone. CT and MRI are also useful in

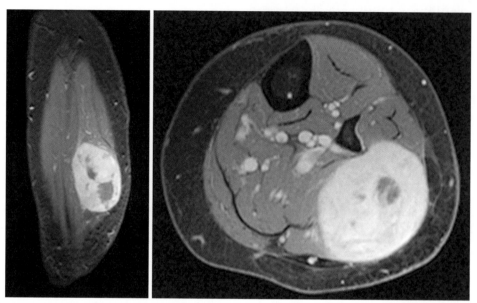

Fig. 32.1 Magnetic resonance imaging scan showing soft tissue sarcoma with necrosis/cystic areas arising from the lateral gastrocnemius muscle. The lesion extends to the lateral border of the fibula. Histology confirmed undifferentiated spindle cell/pleomorphic sarcoma.

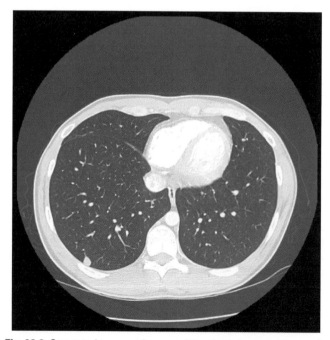

Fig. 32.2 Computed tomography scan of the chest demonstrating a subpleural metastasis in the right lower lobe from a soft tissue sarcoma.

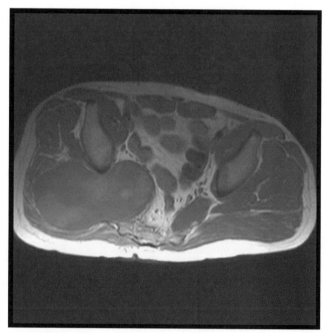

Fig. 32.3 Magnetic resonance imaging scan showing a large, heterogeneous, dumbbell-shaped mass passing through the sciatic notch in the right side of the pelvis. Histology confirmed a malignant peripheral nerve sheath tumour.

TABLE 32.3 Staging System for Soft Tissue Sarcomas[a] (Union for International Cancer Control TNM Classification, 2017)

Primary Tumour (T)

T1	≤5 cm in greatest dimension
T2	>5 cm but not >10 cm in greatest dimension
T3	>10 cm but not >15 cm in greatest dimension
T4	>15 cm in greatest dimension

Regional Nodes (N)

N0	No lymph node spread
N1	Involvement of regional lymph nodes

Distant Metastases (M)

M0	No distant metastases
M1	Distant metastases

[a]Applicable to the extremities, superficial trunk and retroperitoneal sarcomas. The staging for the head and neck and thoracic and abdominal visceral sarcomas differs.

TABLE 32.4 Stage Grouping for Soft Sarcoma (Union for International Cancer Control 2017) (Taking Into Account Histopathological Grade[a])

Stage IA	T1	N0	M0	G1
Stage IB	T2–4	N0	M0	G1
Stage II	T1	N0	M0	G2–3
Stage IIIA	T2	N0	M0	G2–3
Stage IIIB	T3–4	N0	M0	G2–3
	Any T	N1	M0	Any grade
Stage IV	Any T	Any N	M1	Any grade

[a]Grade 1 is considered low grade and grades 2–3 are high-grade.

confirming any subsequent local recurrence, but are not currently used for routine follow-up. CT/MRI of the brain may be considered in histological subtypes with a high risk of brain metastases (e.g. alveolar soft part sarcoma and clear cell sarcoma). Staging of STS is shown in Tables 32.3 and 32.4.

Management

A multidisciplinary team (MDT) is required because surgery, RT and chemotherapy may all have a role to play, depending on the stage, site, grade and size of the tumour. A dedicated sarcoma MDT allows treatment to be carefully coordinated and minimises the number of surgical procedures necessary.

Surgery

Surgery is the initial treatment of choice for localised sarcomas and the aim of the surgery is to achieve a wide local excision (margin ≥1 cm where possible) (Fig. 32.4). The resection should include all the skin and subcutaneous tissue near to the tumour, any previous excision or biopsy scars and areas containing blood clot from previous biopsies. Metallic clips at the margins of the excision are helpful in planning postoperative irradiation. If there is positive margin, a re-excision should be attempted to achieve a clear margin provided this will not result in excess morbidities. Based on histological margins, resections are categorised as intralesional, marginal, wide or radical (Table 32.5).

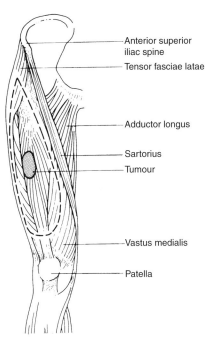

Fig. 32.4 Compartmentectomy. The diagram illustrates the wide surgical excision of soft tissue situated, in this case, in the rectus femoris. (From Souhami R, Tobias J. Cancer and its management. Oxford: Blackwell; 1986. With permission.)

TABLE 32.5 Types of Resections Based on Histological Margins

Type	Description
Intralesional	Surgical plane runs through tumour. Highest risk of local recurrence.
Marginal	Surgical plane runs through the pseudocapsule. High risk of local recurrence.
Wide	Surgical plane in normal tissue outside the tumour but within the same compartment. Low risk of recurrence.
Radical	Compartmental excision of the tumour. Lowest risk of recurrence.

A complete microscopic excision in limb sarcomas leads to a 5-year local control of more than 90%, whereas with incomplete resection, the local control rates are in the range of 60% to 80%. The extent of the resection will depend upon the site of the tumour. For example, complete microscopic resection can be challenging for tumours in the head and neck, pelvis and the retroperitoneum.

Conservative surgery (e.g. limb conservation) has evolved significantly in the few years. Modern surgical techniques including biological and endoprosthetic reconstructions have increased the chances of limb preservation and improved the quality of life of sarcoma survivors. Computer-assisted surgical techniques have improved the rates of margin-negative resections and therefore are valuable in complex locations, such as the pelvis. Amputation for extremity sarcomas is thus only indicated in the following situations:

- When serious radiation-induced morbidity would result from attempting radical RT.
- In some distal limb sarcomas, where a below knee amputation may be more functional than a lower limb with the combined local morbidity of surgery and RT.

- When there is recurrent disease not suitable for limited resection or adjuvant RT.

Radiotherapy

Adjuvant RT. Patients who have a compartmental (radical) resection or amputation do not require RT provided margins are clear. Completed excised (R0 resection) low-grade tumours of less than 5 cm also do not need further therapy. Postoperative adjuvant RT is indicated in the following circumstances to reduce the probability of local recurrence:

- Limb-conserving wide-excision or limited surgery.
- Inadequate margin, tumour extends to cut edge (R1 resection), or macroscopic residual disease (R2 resection) and further excision is not possible.
- Any high-grade tumours (2 or 3).
- Tumours 5 cm or more in any dimension and most tumours deep to the fascia.
- Virtually all tumours in the head and neck (because a complete excision is unlikely).
- After surgery for recurrent sarcoma if not previously irradiated.

Postoperative RT (60–66 gray (Gy)) is conventionally delivered with external beam (photons, electrons or more recently with protons at least in a selected population). In a randomised trial, intraoperative brachytherapy with iridium-192 (42–45 Gy over 4–6 days) resulted in a higher 5-year local control rate (80%) compared with no further therapy (65%) for high-grade tumours (*P* = .0025). Brachytherapy did not improve local control in low-grade lesions. There are no randomised trials comparing brachytherapy with external beam irradiation. Brachytherapy should only be carried out in specialist units undertaking a substantial number of procedures.

Preoperative radiotherapy. Preoperative RT has the advantage that the tumour is well oxygenated and intact. It may also allow coverage by smaller radiation fields and use of lower doses (50 Gy) without reducing local control. These advantages have to be balanced against the disadvantages of difficulties in interpreting pathology following irradiation and an increased risk of wound complications.

Both pre- and postoperative RT give similar local control rates but different toxicity profiles. Preoperative RT is associated with increased wound complications and a better limb function, whereas postoperative RT is associated with increased late complications such as fibrosis, oedema, joint stiffness and bone fractures. Preoperative RT is considered in the following situations:

- Borderline operable tumours (to improve chances of R0 resection).
- Tumours with anticipated marginal resection (e.g. sites such as paranasal sinuses, skull base and retroperitoneum).
- Tumours close to neurovascular structures.
- In situations where larger postoperative RT volume might lead to significant late toxicities.

Primary (radical) radiotherapy. Radical RT alone is indicated for patients unfit for surgery but otherwise in reasonable general condition, those who refuse surgery or where the anatomical site precludes it (e.g. the head and neck and retroperitoneum). RT is contraindicated for tumours located in areas that tolerate RT poorly, for example, Achilles tendon, or in the ribs where pathological fractures may occur. Radical RT to the Achilles tendon is inadvisable, especially in young and active patients, because rupture may occur.

Palliative radiotherapy. In advanced sarcoma, palliative RT is useful in controlling pain and stopping bleeding etc. However, often little benefit is seen with single dose (8–10 Gy) RT and usually patients need higher doses (e.g. 30 Gy in 10 fractions) for a meaningful clinical benefit.

Chemotherapy

In the past few decades, improvements in both surgery and RT have led to marked improvements in local control and a subsequent decrease in the incidence of amputation. Although adjuvant chemotherapy has significantly improved clinical outcome of paediatric-type STS, the role of adjuvant chemotherapy in adult-type STS remains controversial. Doxorubicin and ifosfamide are the only chemotherapeutic agents that consistently have a greater than 20% response rate against STS. Two large metaanalyses and an EORTC trial failed to show clinically significant benefit with routine adjuvant chemotherapy using these agents. The Sarcoma Meta-Analysis Collaboration reported improvements in local and distal recurrence rates with doxorubicin-containing adjuvant regimens but a statistically nonsignificant trend towards improvement in overall survival (4% at 10 years). A second updated metaanalysis showed an improved overall survival (absolute risk reduction of 11%). However, the subsequent EORTC study, 62931, and a pooled analysis of two large randomised trials (EORTC 62771 and 62931) failed to show improved survival with adjuvant chemotherapy.

There is no clear evidence to show that preoperative chemotherapy offers a significant survival advantage, but this may be used in patients with initially inoperable tumours. A recent Italian Sarcoma Group study suggests that neoadjuvant chemotherapy with anthracycline and ifosfamide improves relapse-free and overall survival in patients with high-risk STS of the extremity and trunk, but long-term results are awaited.

Single agent doxorubicin is the treatment of choice for locally advanced inoperable and metastatic STS. The highest rate of responses (37%) have been seen with doses of 60 to 75 mg/m^2 three weekly, with a 6-month progression-free survival (PFS) of 45%. Even though the EORTC 62012 study reported a higher response rate with a combination of doxorubicin-ifosfamide compared with single agent doxorubicin alone (26% vs 14% *P* < .0006), there was no difference in median overall survival (OS) (14.3 months vs 12.8 months, *P* = .076). Therefore, combination chemotherapy may be considered in selected clinical situations such as in life-threatening progressive disease and preoperatively to down-stage a large locally advanced chemo-sensitive tumour to facilitate a curative resection. Recently, a phase IB-II study has reported an almost doubling of median overall survival (26.5 months vs 14.7 months, *P* = .0003) with a combination of anti-PDGFRα antibody, olaratumab with doxorubicin compared with single-agent doxorubicin. This combination has thus become the current recommended first-line treatment.

Recent studies have highlighted that some agents are more effective in particular histological subtypes. For example, ifosfamide-containing regimens are more active in synovial sarcoma, taxanes and liposomal doxorubicin in angiosarcoma and trabectedin in liposarcoma and synovial sarcoma.

Retroperitoneal Sarcomas

Retroperitoneal sarcomas (RPS) are often huge, causing dramatic distortion of the patient's contour but rarely present as an emergency. The tumours are often dedifferentiated liposarcomas or leiomyosarcomas and as such have a characteristic radiological appearance (Fig. 32.5). In these circumstances, preoperative biopsy may be eschewed, but if radiological appearance is doubtful, a biopsy is mandated.

Surgery may require en-bloc resection with removal of many organs such as the spleen, one kidney, the tail or body of pancreas or segments of the large and/or small bowel. The placement of surgical clips around narrowly excised tumour areas can guide the clinical oncologist. The dose of postoperative RT is necessarily limited and more than 50 Gy is unlikely to be achievable. At 5-years, up to 50% develop local or intraabdominal recurrence.

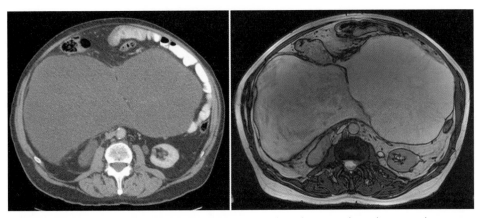

Fig. 32.5 Computed tomography scan showing a bilobulated cystic retroperitoneal mass and on magnetic resonance imaging the lesion has high T2 signal intensity with multiple septations and low-signal components. Histology showed dedifferentiated liposarcoma.

With the evolution of high-precision RT techniques which can spare radiosensitive organs such as the kidney and spinal cord, the interest in the use of preoperative RT has been rekindled recently. An EORTC study (STRASS trial), randomised 266 patients with RPS and pelvic STS to surgery alone or preoperative RT (50.4 Gy in 28 fractions) followed by surgery 4 to 8 weeks later. Early results did not show any improvement in 3-year abdominal recurrence-free survival (ARFS) with preoperative radiotherapy compared with surgery alone (60.4% vs. 58.7%, $p = 0.954$). In the subgroup analysis, however, there was a trend towards improved 3-year ARFS in patients with liposarcoma treated with preoperative RT compared with surgery alone (71.6% vs 60.4%, $p = 0.049$)

Radiotherapy Technique

Position, Immobilisation and Localisation Imaging

Positioning and immobilisation are challenging for extremity sarcomas and the clinical oncologist should carefully evaluate the position of the limb taking into consideration the radiation beam arrangements. Stability of the limb is best assisted by a shell and appropriately positioned bolus bags. The scar may be marked out during planning scan, especially in situations where there is need to apply bolus to ensure that it receives the maximum dose to minimise the risk of scar recurrence. However, routine application of bolus to the scar is not recommended. Sagittal lasers are especially useful in lining up the limbs.

Target Volume

Definition of the target volume requires information from the surgeon, pathologist and radiologist. The surgeon should be encouraged to place radiopaque clips at the margins of the resection. The pathologist should comment on the adequacy of the resection. The radiotherapist needs to discuss with the radiologist the position of the tumour, local extent and any residual disease as seen on CT and MRI.

Most sarcomas tend to spread in the axial plane of the limb (major fascial planes, bone and interosseous membranes). For this reason, the margins of the radiation field must be generous in the craniocaudal directions. In the transverse plane, there can be greater confidence that local structures are not breached and field margins can be tighter. For nonextremity lesions, the orientation of the fields should follow the planes of the local musculature, while including the local fascial planes.

Currently, preoperative three-dimensional conformal RT (CRT) is given as one phase and postoperative and radical treatment in two phases. The 2-year interim results of a randomised controlled trial (Volume of Radiotherapy for Extremity Sarcomas (VORTEX)) evaluating the role of postoperative single-phase smaller-field RT compared with the standard two-phase RT did not report any difference in grade 2 or higher

long-term toxicities or limb function. Retrospective and phase II studies suggest that IMRT has a potential to significantly reduce long-term toxicities of subcutaneous fibrosis, joint stiffness and oedema. In the United Kingdom, the IMRis trial is evaluating the role of IMRT in terms of the feasibility in nonextremity sarcomas and the improvement in long-term and functional effects in extremity sarcomas.

For the purposes of planning, the gross tumour volume (GTV) should be defined, with a margin around it to include the tissues at risk of microscopic involvement, to create the CTV. The PTV is based on departmental data and generally involves an expansion of the CTV by 5 to 10 mm isotropically. The following section gives a summary of these target volumes in various clinical settings:

Preoperative single-phase extremity tumours.
- GTV: tumour on gadolinium-enhanced T1 weighted (W) imaging (just the lesion and not oedema)
- CTV = GTV with 3 to 5 cm longitudinal expansion and 1.5 to 2 cm expansion in all other directions
- Edit CTV (ideally using T2W) to include the peritumoural oedema, which is often most pronounced in the longitudinal direction
- Edit CTV to stay within bones, fascia and skin (unless infiltrated).

Postoperative two-phase extremity tumours.
Phase I.
- Resected GTV: defined on the gadolinium-enhanced T1W preoperative imaging fused with the postoperative planning CT scan (just the lesion and not oedema)
- Surgical bed CTV: constructed using resected GTV, the position of surgical clips, drain sites and scar. Inclusion of any seroma, lymphocoele or haematoma should be based on a discussion with surgeons
- In case of an unplanned surgical resection, the surgical bed CTV should include residual disease, all disturbed muscle compartments and involved tissues
- Elective CTV: the surgical bed CTV with 4-cm longitudinal expansion and 1.5 cm in all other directions
- Edit CTV to stay within bones, fascia and skin (unless infiltrated)

Phase II.
- Boost CTV: the surgical bed CTV with 1.5 cm in all other directions except longitudinal where it is the resected GTV plus 2 cm.

Retroperitoneal sarcoma.
Gross tumour volume.
- Preoperative: tumour on planning CT scan or MRI. For tumour above the iliac crest, four-dimensional (4D)-CT is useful to assess tumour motion
- Postoperative: residual disease on postoperative scan and surgical bed, including all the areas where the original tumour was in contact

with adjacent organs (the ipsilateral psoas, ipsilateral muscles of posterior abdominal wall and the prevertebral surface around the great vessels)

Clinical target volume.

- Preoperative CTV = GTV with 1.5 cm expansion in all directions. If tumour extends through inguinal canal, add 3 cm margin inferiorly. CTV also includes retroperitoneal muscles
- Postoperative CTV = GTV with 2 cm longitudinal expansion and 0.5 to 2 cm expansion in all other directions
- Edit CTV to stay within anatomical barriers to tumour spread. Edit CTV at bone (0 mm), bowel and air cavity (5 mm) and the hepatic interfaces (2 mm) and the skin (3–5 mm)

Technique

Computer planning is essential to obtain a homogeneous distribution of dose within the target volume. For the limbs and retroperitoneum, a parallel-opposed pair of fields, often wedged, will provide a satisfactory dose distribution in most cases. In the shoulder region, tangential fields may be needed to reduce the volume of the irradiated lung. Tangential fields are also appropriate for superficial trunk lesions to spare the bowel. For tumours in the buttock, a direct posterior field and two wedged lateral fields will reduce the dose to the rectum. In the head and neck, the principles of planning and respect for the tolerance of critical structures, such as the spinal cord, are the same as for squamous carcinoma of the head and neck. Target volumes tend to be smaller than below the clavicles and so higher doses can often be delivered with acceptable morbidity.

Care is taken to avoid irradiating the whole circumference of a limb to reduce the likelihood of lymphoedema as a late complication. This is achieved by adjusting the width of the field to leave a longitudinal strip of unirradiated tissue outside the target volume. In the proximal part of the limb, especially in the thigh, this strip occupies a large proportion of the limb (Fig. 32.6).

When the retroperitoneum is irradiated, part or the whole of one kidney may need to be included in the target volume and the dose to the other kidney should be kept below the tolerance dose. Placement of spacers in the abdominal cavity may be used to displace the small bowel out of the high-dose radiation region (Fig. 32.7A, B).

Dose and Fractionation

There is little information on total dose and response in sarcomas. Most centres tend to give 50 Gy to a wide volume, shrinking to a final boost of 10 to 16 Gy. There is limited information on the relationship between the total dose and response. However, fraction sizes should be kept small (1.8–2 Gy) to minimise the risks of late damage to normal tissue. Hypofractionated and hyperfractionated schedules have shown no advantage over conventional fractionation.

Extremities.

Preoperative.

50 Gy in 1.8 to 2 Gy per fraction.

Postoperative.

Phase I: 50 Gy in 1.8 to 2 Gy per fraction.

Phase II: 10 to 16 Gy in 2 Gy per fraction. If gross residual disease, increase dose up to a total of 70 Gy if within the tolerance dose of neighboring critical organs.

Radical radiotherapy.

66 Gy in 33 daily fractions over 6½ or 70 Gy in 35 fractions over 7 weeks, if within the tolerance dose of neighboring critical organs.

Retroperitoneum.

50.4 Gy in 28 fractions over 5½ weeks.

Head and neck.

66 Gy in 33 daily fractions over 6½ weeks.

Radiotherapy Side Effects

Acute Reactions

Skin reactions are often a problem. This is because very high doses are needed in the boost volume and are sometimes given to graft areas. Dry desquamation normally develops and is treated as for other skin reactions. Moist desquamation is more likely to occur in the axilla, groin and perineum and is treated with hydrocortisone cream or ointment. If there is secondary infection, Flamazine (silver sulfadiazine) can promote healing.

Late Reactions

Atrophy of the skin and subcutaneous tissues and fibrosis within the muscles are common. Stiffness of a limb may be partly caused by fibrosis of the intermuscular septa and partly as a result of fibrosis in the joint capsule.

Osteoporosis of bone is common because bone is frequently included in the target volume. Occasionally, particularly if the bone is invaded by tumour, radionecrosis may occur. In the ribs, this may cause pathological fractures.

Proton Therapy

Protons have a similar relative biological effectiveness (RBE) to photons. The advantage of protons is a reduction of dose to critical structures, such

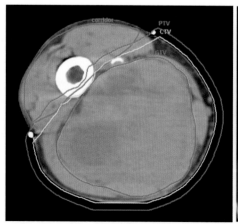 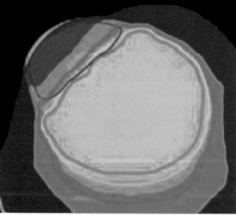

Fig. 32.6 Planning computed tomography (CT) scan showing target volumes and a corridor of radiotherapy avoidance area to avoid late lymphoedema. Planning CT showing the sparing of corridor. *CTV,* Clinical target volume; *GTV,* gross tumour volume; *PTV,* planned target volume.

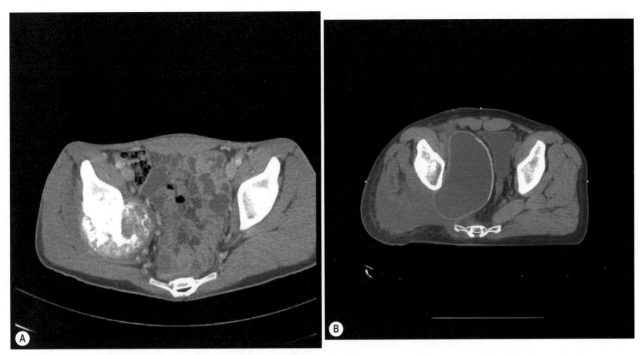

Fig. 32.7 (A) Ewing sarcoma of right pelvic wall characterised by a large ossified mass with significant soft tissue component. (B) Postoperative radiotherapy planning computed tomography scan in the same patient showing a spacer in situ, to minimise radiotherapy to the the small bowel.

as the spinal cord or underlying bone. Proton therapy has potential clinical benefits for tumours located in the head and neck, spinal and paraspinal regions, pelvis, thorax and abdomen, but confirmatory results are still awaited.

Results of Treatment

Conservative surgery and RT can achieve over 90% local control and 5-year survival in stage I disease. For stage II disease, local control is 85% to 90% and survival is 65% to 90%. For stage III, local control is similar to stage II but survival is lower, 85% (IIIa) and 45% (IIIb). If there is only microscopic residual disease following surgery, overall survival is 65%, falling to 30% when there is gross residual disease.

BONE TUMOURS

Benign and malignant tumours may arise in bone. The pathological classification is shown in Table 32.6. Bone tumours represent 0.4% of all cancers. Primary bone tumours are rare and account for only 1% of bone neoplasia. The vast majority of bone lesions are secondary deposits. The main bone-forming malignant tumour is osteosarcoma and cartilage-forming is chondrosarcoma. Malignant tumours arising from the bone marrow are myeloma, Ewing sarcoma, and lymphoma (see Chapter 29).

TABLE 32.6 Classification of Bone Tumours

A. Tumours forming bone
   1. Benign: e.g. osteoma
   2. Malignant: osteosarcoma
B. Tumours forming cartilage
   1. Benign: e.g. enchondroma
   2. Malignant: chondrosarcoma
C. Giant cell tumour (generally benign)
D. Tumours of the bone marrow: myeloma, lymphoma, Ewing sarcoma
E. Other tumours

Osteosarcoma (Osteogenic Sarcoma)

Osteosarcoma is the most common and most malignant primary bone tumour. It arises in bone-forming cells (osteoblasts) and is most common between the ages of 10 and 20 years. There is a second peak incidence in the elderly as a complication of Paget disease of bone. The male to female ratio is 1.6:1.

The cause of adolescent-type tumour is unknown. There is an increased incidence (400-fold) of osteosarcoma in patients with bilateral retinoblastomas, presumably because of the same genetic abnormality or mutation of the Rb tumour suppressor gene developing outside the irradiated areas. Li-Fraumeni syndrome, Werner syndrome, and Rothmund-Thomson syndrome are also risk factors.

Pathology

Osteosarcoma is most common near the knee in the metaphysis of the distal femur or proximal tibia. In the elderly, its distribution matches Paget disease.

Macroscopically, the tumour is usually haemorrhagic. It expands the bone, destroying both the cortex and the medulla. The periosteum is frequently raised giving rise to the radiological features of Codman triangle where the raised periosteum meets the cortex. Extension into the soft tissue follows.

Bloodborne metastases to the lungs occur early. Bone metastases, though less frequent, also occur. Microscopically, there are malignant osteoblasts laying down small pieces of irregular osteoid tissue. The two common histological varieties are osteoblastic and telangiectatic (containing irregular blood vessels). A third variety is parosteal sarcoma. It arises from the surface of the bone and does not involve the medullary cavity.

Clinical Features

The commonest presenting feature is pain, usually with swelling and a limp. Sometimes pathological fracture may follow minor trauma. Rarely, cough, dyspnoea and pneumothorax may indicate lung involvement.

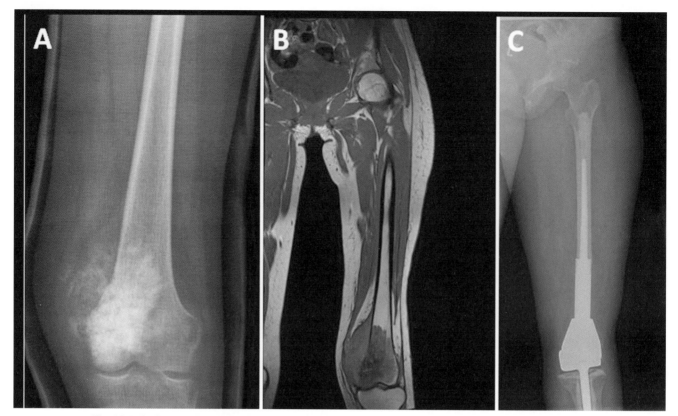

Fig. 32.8 (A) Osteosarcoma involving distal left femur with cortical destruction and extensive osteoid matrix. (B) Magnetic resonance imaging showing destructive lesion in the femur with extensive soft tissue component. (C) Patient had neoadjuvant chemotherapy followed by limb-conservation surgery.

Diagnosis and Staging Investigations

Plain radiographs and CT scan (Fig. 32.8A) of the affected part may show the typical features of bone destruction and soft tissue extension. The cortex may be raised with a sunburst appearance. Full blood count, liver function tests and lactate dehydrogenase (LDH) are required. All patients should have a chest radiograph and CT scan of the chest to rule out lung metastases.

MRI of the involved bone with adjacent joints is essential for staging (Fig. 32.8B). CT is also helpful in assessing whether the capsule of a limb joint has been breached. Whole body bone scintigraphy may show increased uptake at the site of the tumour, in the adjacent bone (as a result of increased vascularity), in bone metastases and in bone-forming metastases in soft tissues. Whole body MRI and PET scan (especially for craniofacial sarcomas) may be considered for staging and response assessment.

A biopsy should be carried out to confirm the diagnosis. It is important that the position of the biopsy is chosen so that the whole biopsy scar can be excised with the tumour to include potentially surgically contaminated tissue along the track of the biopsy. Ideally, both biopsy and definitive surgery should be performed by the same surgical team. The endoprosthesis must be planned several weeks ahead of limb-sparing surgery (Fig. 32.8C).

Treatment

The management of osteosarcoma requires a multidisciplinary approach including orthopaedic surgeon, oncologist, pathologist and physiotherapist. Current treatment for localised disease is over 6 to 9 months involving 10 weeks of neoadjuvant chemotherapy followed by surgery and adjuvant chemotherapy.

Chemotherapy

Neoadjuvant and adjuvant chemotherapy are an important part of the treatment of osteogenic sarcoma. Chemotherapy has reduced the frequency of pulmonary metastases which used to occur in 80% of cases. Although neoadjuvant chemotherapy does not improve survival compared with postoperative chemotherapy alone, early chemotherapy can shrink the primary tumour leading to rapid improvement in symptoms, and can also treat micrometastases. Undoubtedly, neoadjuvant chemotherapy has reduced the rate of amputation in this disease. Although only about 10% of inoperable tumours are rendered operable by neoadjuvant chemotherapy, in many more cases, surgery is much easier owing to the reduction of the tumour allowing for the insertion of an endoprosthesis and sparing of the limb. The most accepted neoadjuvant chemotherapy regimen is high-dose methotrexate, doxorubicin and cisplatin (MAP). A good response to neoadjuvant chemotherapy is an independent good prognostic factor and the degree of viable tumour at surgery being related to ultimate survival. In the EUR-AMOS1 Trial, patients ($n = 2260$) received two cycles of induction chemotherapy with MAP followed by surgery. Patients ($n = 1334$) were randomised after surgery based on histological response (<10% viable tumour in the resected specimen: good response vs ≥10% viable tumour: poor response). Early results showed no improvement in EFS with the addition of interferon (IFN)-α-2b to MAP in patients with good histological response. In patients with poor histological response, the addition of ifosfamide and etoposide to MAP did not improve EFS. Patients with metastatic disease are also treated with a MAP regimen and 30% of patients are long-term survivors.

Low-grade central and parosteal sarcomas do not need adjuvant chemotherapy as they usually have a low-malignant potential.

Surgery

Surgery is aimed at removing the whole tumour with adequate margins to allow for functional preservation. Limb preservation involves removing the tumour and replacing the bone defect with a custom-made artificial prosthesis. Careful preoperative assessment is necessary and referral to a specialist centre is essential. To obtain adequate margins, the prosthesis incorporates an artificial joint as well as femoral and tibial components (see Fig. 32.8C). Although pathological fracture increases the risk of local recurrence, it does not preclude a conservative surgery. However, contraindications to limb conservation may include poor radiological response after chemotherapy and situations such as extensive soft tissue infiltration and/or invasion of neurovascular bundles when a safe complete resection is not possible.

Resection of lung metastases. Lung metastases are occasionally isolated and, in the absence of metastases elsewhere, surgical resection should be considered. Results are best if lung metastases develop after a long disease-free interval. Surgery is contraindicated if there is pleural involvement. A 5-year survival of up to 40% has been reported following resection of pulmonary metastasis.

Radiotherapy

There is no routine role for RT. In the following situations, RT may be indicated either to improve progression-free interval or to achieve symptom control:

- Unresectable tumours (e.g. the head and neck, vertebrae, ilium and sacrum). However, proximity of critical structures, such as the spinal cord, often limits the dose that can be delivered.
- Positive resection margin and further surgery not possible and/or poor response to chemotherapy (<90% necrosis).
- Intralesional resection or contaminated margin, with no further surgery planned.
- Palliation of pain from the primary tumour in the presence of metastatic disease or bony metastases.

Target volume.

Gross tumour volume.

- Primary RT: visible tumour on planning CT scan/MRI.
- Postoperative GTV: areas of risk based on preoperative imaging, operation notes and histopathology report.
- CTV = GTV + 2 to 3 cm (ensure inclusion of scar with 0.5 to 1-cm margin in postoperative situation).
- PTV = GTV + 5 to 10 mm.

Technique. Three-dimensional conformal RT or advanced RT techniques such as IMRT, image-guided radiation therapy (IGRT) or particle therapy may be needed if tumours are near critical organs. Beam arrangements vary with the site of the primary. For tumours arising in a vertebra, a posterior oblique wedged pair with or without an unwedged direct posterior field provides a satisfactory dose distribution. For the ilium, parallel-opposed fields suffice. An optimised parallel-opposed pair of fields is suitable for limb primaries.

Dose and energy. Megavoltage is required. The choice of dose will be determined by critical organ tolerance. For primary RT and postoperative macroscopic disease the suggested dose is 60 to 66 Gy in 1.8 to 2 Gy fractions and for adjuvant microscopic disease, 60 Gy in 1.8 to 2 Gy fractions. In the spine above L2, the dose should be limited by spinal cord tolerance to 47.5 Gy in 25 daily fractions over 5 weeks. Palliative fractions include 30 Gy in 10 daily fractions over 2 weeks, 40 Gy in 15 fractions over 3 weeks and 6 Gy once every week for 5 to 6 weeks.

Results of Treatment

With multimodality treatment, the survival of osteosarcoma has improved from 10% to 20% to approximately 60%. Patients with poor histological response to neoadjuvant chemotherapy, pathological fracture and elevated ALP or LDH have poor prognosis. Osteoblastic and telangiectatic tumours have a similar prognosis. Parosteal sarcomas have a better prognosis and may be cured by surgery alone.

Ewing Sarcoma

Ewing sarcoma is the second most common primary bone tumour. In the United Kingdom, its incidence is 0.6 per million. The peak age is between 10 and 15 years. It is slightly more common in males.

Pathology

Ewing sarcoma probably arises from connective tissue within the bone marrow. The most common sites in order of frequency are the pelvis, femur, tibia, fibula, rib, scapula, vertebra and humerus. In contrast with osteogenic sarcoma, a higher proportion of these tumours occurs in the flat bones of the trunk. About 40% occur in the axial skeleton. Microscopically, there are sheets of uniform undifferentiated, small, deeply staining round cells. The tumour needs to be distinguished from other small round-cell tumours, including non-Hodgkin lymphoma, Hodgkin disease, neuroblastoma and metastatic carcinoma. Some 90% of tumours have 11:22 chromosome translation.

There is local spread along the marrow cavity causing bone destruction. However, the epiphyseal plates are rarely breached. Bloodborne spread is early and common. About 50% will have lung metastases and 40% bone metastases and/or widespread bone marrow infiltration at presentation. Lymph node metastases are uncommon (less than 10%). Spread to the central nervous system (CNS) may occur, usually late in the course of the disease.

Clinical Features

Presentation is usually with a rapidly developing and painful swelling. Neurological symptoms may accompany this if there is nerve compression. Fever occurs in about 30% of patients. Approximately 25% of patients have metastatic disease at presentation (10% lung, 10% bone/bone marrow and a combination of sites for the remaining).

Diagnosis and Staging

Full blood count may show anaemia (leukoerythroblastic if there is bone marrow infiltration) and a mildly raised white cell count. Erythrocyte sedimentation rate (ESR) is often moderately elevated. Liver function tests may be abnormal (raised LDH or alkaline phosphatase).

A biopsy of the tumour is required. As in osteogenic sarcoma, care is taken to ensure that the biopsy lies within the incision for any later proposed definitive surgical procedure. Plain radiographs of the primary are taken in two planes (usually anteroposterior and lateral). In long bones, this may show the typical multilayered onion-skin appearance of the periosteal reaction and often a large adjacent soft tissue mass. Pathological fracture occurs in 5% (less frequently than osteogenic sarcoma). CT scanning gives more detail of the local extent of the tumour and is useful in planning the site for a biopsy and subsequent surgery (Fig. 32.9). MRI is superior to CT in assessment of the extent of infiltration within the medullary canal. A fluorodeoxyglucose FDG-PET scan may be sufficient for screening of bone and bone marrow metastases. Because pulmonary metastases are common, a CT scan of chest is mandatory.

Treatment

The choice of treatment will depend largely upon the site of the primary. Close liaison is required between orthopaedic surgeon and oncologist. Similar to osteogenic sarcoma, treatment should only be carried out by an experienced team. Current treatment duration for localised disease lasts for 10 to 12 months comprising three to six cycles of

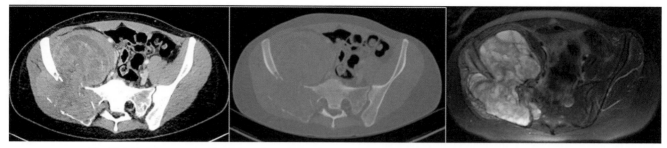

Fig. 32.9 Ewing sarcoma arising from the right pelvis showing a large soft tissue mass and extensive destruction of right ilium.

neoadjuvant chemotherapy followed by local therapy and adjuvant chemotherapy for 6 to 10 cycles. Patients with metastatic disease are treated similarly to localised disease. Patients with lung metastases may be considered for whole lung RT, even though firm data on survival advantage is lacking.

Chemotherapy

Ewing sarcoma is a chemosensitive tumour, and chemotherapy before surgery or RT has been shown to improve local control and reduce the incidence of distant metastasis. The most effective drugs are vincristine, ifosfamide, doxorubicin, cyclophosphamide, dactinomycin and etoposide. Typically, patients receive four to six cycles of induction chemotherapy using three to four drugs (e.g. VIDE, VAC or VAI). This is followed by treatment to the primary site which may be surgery or RT, or both, depending on the location of the tumour and subsequently, six cycles of adjuvant chemotherapy. In patients with metastatic disease, high-dose chemotherapy with autologous stem cell rescue may be beneficial, particularly in children aged less than 14 years.

Surgery

Surgery should be as radical as possible, with limb preservation and aimed at removing all tissues initially involved by the tumour, irrespective of response to neoadjuvant chemotherapy. Expendable bones may be completely removed (e.g. rib or fibula). With advances in expandable implants, limb conservation is possible even in growing children. Historically, telescopic prosthetic implants were lengthened periodically to match the growth of the unaffected limb by turning a mechanism using an Allen key through a small incision. Currently, noninvasive expandable implants are being increasingly used.

Where radical surgery to a limb would cause major functional impairment, a conservative approach may be adopted with the addition of postoperative RT. Similarly, in axial bones, incomplete surgery following postoperative RT is acceptable.

Radiotherapy

Unlike osteogenic sarcoma, Ewing sarcoma is radiosensitive. Preoperative RT is indicated if there is a poor response to chemotherapy and when a marginal resection is anticipated. Preoperative RT is also useful in locations such as the pelvis and ribs, where a treatment response facilitates subsequent surgery. Radical RT is indicated for inoperable lesions or when surgery would be disabling. Postoperative RT is indicated in the following situations:

- Inadequate (<1 mm) or positive margin.
- Microscopic or macroscopic residual disease and further surgery not feasible.
- All tissues involved by the tumour at diagnosis have not been excised, even if the surgical margins are negative.
- A poor histological response (≤90% necrosis) to neoadjuvant chemotherapy even if the surgical margins are negative.

- A displaced pathological fracture of bone at primary site and all contaminated tissue are not excised.
- Tumour in locations where complete surgery is difficult, for example, the spine and paraspinal sites, rib tumours with pleural effusion, the pelvis and sacrum, and the head and neck.

Radiotherapy is contraindicated if there are concerns about high-risk of late toxicities, impaired wound healing and an increased risk of metallic prosthesis infection.

Target volume. If a total dose of 54 Gy or more is needed, a shrinking field approach based on the pretreatment tumour volume is adopted.

Extremity tumours.
- Phase 1: GTV is tumour at diagnosis, including scars after biopsy and resection. A margin of 3 to 5 cm in the cranio-caudally and 2 cm axially is added to derive the CTV. If there is extensive intramedullary involvement or skip lesions and the whole bone should be irradiated. An unirradiated strip of normal tissue containing lymphatics outside the tumour-bearing area is left, if possible, to avoid constrictive fibrosis.
- Phase II: Phase II CTV is phase I GTV with a 2-cm margin craniocaudally and a 1- to 2-cm margin in other directions.

Nonextremity tumours. The CTV is a prechemotherapy tumour with a 2-cm margin in all directions. Smaller margins are allowed if the tumour hasn't invaded anatomical boundaries of critical structures (e.g. eye, optic apparatus). If tumours that were protruding into body cavities (e.g. chest or abdomen) have regressed after chemotherapy, the residual tumour with smaller margin is treated to minimise radiation toxicities.

Technique. The choice of technique will vary with the site of the primary. High-precision RT techniques such as IMRT and particle-beam therapy are useful to deliver higher dose to a target with optimal sparing of normal structure. For the limbs, a parallel-opposed wedged pair of fields or three-dimensional-CRT usually suffices. For pelvic primaries, it may be possible to surgically displace the bowel out of the radiation field by inserting an absorbable mesh or a spacer. For rib primaries, electrons of appropriate energy may be used to diminish the dose to the underlying lung. A parallel-opposed pair of fields encompassing both lung fields is used for whole lung RT. In the United Kingdom, children with localised Ewing sarcoma are treated with proton therapy if RT is indicated.

Dose and energy. Radiotherapy is delivered using megavoltage, photons, electrons or proton therapy. High-proton therapy is increasingly used for tumours located near critical structures and/or in children and young adults.

- Preoperative: 50.4 Gy in 28 fractions in a single phase. If there are concerns about organ tolerance or wound healing, then this dose can be reduced to 45 Gy in 25 Gy fractions.
- Postoperative: 54 Gy in 30 fractions delivered as two phases (phase I: 45 Gy in 25 fractions and phase II: 9 Gy in 5 fractions).

- Radical RT: 54 Gy in 30 fractions delivered as a single phase. A boost of 5.4 Gy in 3 fractions may be considered.
- Whole lung RT: 15 Gy in 10 fractions for patients younger than 14 years or 18 Gy in 12 fractions for patients 14 years of age and older.

Radiotherapy Side Effects

Both the acute and late reactions are the same as for soft tissue sarcoma and depend on the site of irradiation and the total dose to the normal tissue.

Results of Treatment

The outcome is better for patients with tumours of the peripheral rather than central skeleton. Up to 90% disease-free survival for peripheral tumours and 65% for central (axial) tumours has been achieved. There is overall 5-year survival of 60% to 70% for localised tumours and 20% to 40% for metastatic disease. Local recurrence occurs in about 10% to 15% of long-bone primaries and 25% to 30% of pelvic tumours. The higher recurrence rate in the pelvis is probably because of the larger tumour size and the difficulty of irradiating the tumour homogeneously without damaging surrounding normal tissues.

CHONDROSARCOMA

Chondrosarcomas are malignant tumours of cartilage. They may arise in benign enchondromas or be malignant from the start. Adults aged 30 to 50 years are affected. The most common sites in order of frequency are the pelvis (50%), femur, humerus and scapula.

Macroscopically, the tumour is bulky, lobulated and semitranslucent. Microscopically, it is a sarcoma containing cartilage. Differentiation is variable. Poorly differentiated tumours (mesenchymal chondrosarcomas) behave more aggressively. In the well-differentiated form, spread is slow, locally. Bloodborne metastases occur late to the lungs.

Clinical Features

Presentation is usually with a slowly progressive painless swelling which eventually becomes painful.

Diagnosis and Investigation

A biopsy is required. Plain radiography shows bone destruction and commonly abnormal flecks of calcification. MRI scan helps to define the local extent (Fig. 32.10A, B).

Treatment

Radical surgery is the treatment of choice, except for low-grade central limb chondrosarcoma, which may be treated with curettage alone with or without adjuvant therapy (e.g. high-speed burring, thermal cauterisation and bone cementation with polymethylmethacrylate). Limb preservation may be possible. It is a very radioresistant tumour. An exception is chondrosarcomas of the facial bones and the base of skull, where a combination of surgery and RT offers long-term control. RT has a palliative role for the relief of local symptoms, such as pain, and relatively high doses are required even for palliative effect.

Radiotherapy

Technique

A parallel-opposed wedged pair of fields or three-dimensional-CRT is suitable for the long bones. Three-dimensional-CRT using a three-field technique (anterior and posterior wedged fields with an open lateral field) for pelvic tumours may limit the dose to the bowel.

Dose and energy. 60 Gy in 30 daily fractions over 6 weeks at megavoltage (4–6 MV photons).

Chemotherapy

By and large, chondrosarcomas are chemoresistant, although there has been a renewal of interest in chemotherapy recently using the same agents that have been very useful in osteogenic sarcoma, particularly for the mesenchymal subtypes. However, the increase in overall survival following chemotherapy is small.

Results of Treatment

Five-year survival is about 50% over the age of 21 years but falls to 35% under that age. Younger patients tend to have tumours in the pelvis, where radical surgery is more difficult than in long bones. They also have more poorly differentiated tumours that metastasise more frequently.

UNDIFFERENTIATED PLEOMORPHIC SARCOMA OF BONE

This heterogeneous group of tumours constitutes 2% to 5% of bone tumours. It usually occurs in adults aged 30 to 50 years and the common sites are ends of long bones. These are typically high-grade tumours with a rate of metastases as high as 50%. Treatment approach

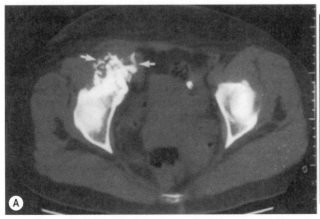
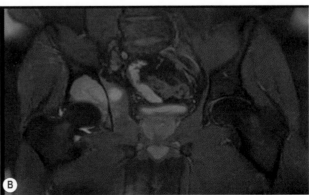

Fig. 32.10 (A) Computed tomography scan of the pelvis showing a chondrosarcoma of the ileum (*arrows*). Note the flecks of calcification. (Courtesy Dr. R Nakielny, Sheffield.) (B) Magnetic resonance imaging showing a lesion in the right acetabulum with extraosseous extension. Patient underwent right pelvectomy and histology showed dedifferentiated chondrosarcoma.

is the same as osteosarcoma, consisting of neoadjuvant chemotherapy followed by wide excision.

Secondary Tumours in Bone

The majority of bone tumours are of metastatic origin. They represent 15% to 20% of the workload of a RT department. The most common primary sites are breast, lung, prostate, myeloma and kidney. The prognosis of bone metastases is generally poor, though the course of the disease may be relatively slow over a period of years, for example, in some patients with breast cancer. Patients presenting with bone metastases from prostate or breast cancer may live for years while this tumour is hormone sensitive. Good symptomatic relief by a combination of analgesics according to the WHO analgesic ladder and local RT can be achieved in most cases.

Clinical Features and Investigation

The usual presentation is with pain caused by pressure on the periosteum or on nerve roots as they emerge from the spinal canal (Fig. 32.11). Early diagnosis is important before bone destruction has advanced so far as to cause pathological fracture (Fig. 32.12) or spinal cord compression.

Plain radiographs of the symptomatic area may show the deposits (osteolytic or osteosclerotic or both) or a pathological fracture. However, a metastasis in a vertebral body has to have reached a size of about 2 cm before it will be visible on a radiograph.

A radioisotope bone scan is helpful in detecting bone metastases too small to be visible on plain radiographs and to detect deposits elsewhere in the skeleton. Multiple bone metastases are common, predominantly in the spine, ribs, pelvis and upper femur. CT scanning of areas of the spine and sacrum where plain radiographs and bone scan are equivocal or normal may show bone destruction. If there is no known primary site, a CT-guided biopsy may be necessary.

Treatment

The treatment of bone metastases includes analgesics, RT, bisphosphonates and, occasionally, surgery. Treatment is aimed at relieving pain as simply and quickly as possible. Patients should always be given adequate analgesia escalating according to the WHO analgesic ladder. The choice of treatment will depend on the site of the pain and its severity, complications such as spinal cord compression or pathological

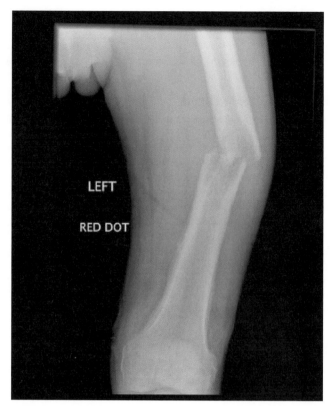

Fig. 32.12 A pathological fracture of the mid-left femur. The patient had metastatic nonsmall cell lung cancer. A femoral pin was inserted and the femur irradiated.

fracture, the presence of hypercalcaemia, the underlying tumour and the general condition of the patient.

Numerous randomised clinical trials and metaanalyses have shown that a single fraction of 8 to 10 Gy is as effective for relieving pain as a regimen of 30 Gy in 10 fractions when analgesic effect is measured at 6 weeks after treatment. The duration of pain relief after a single fraction is not known, but it is very easy to repeat the treatment. Depending on the site of the tumour, up to 90% of patients may have a marked diminution of pain following a single radiation fraction and up to 54% may have complete pain relief. Single fields are usually adequate for vertebral, sacral and rib deposits. Obese patients with lumbar metastasis should be treated with parallel-opposed fields. Kilovoltage radiation offers practical treatment advantages in the treatment of cervical spine lesions. Patients can be treated sitting in a chair, which is very useful if the neck is painful or the patient is wearing a supportive collar. Because the absorption of kilovoltage x-rays in bone is greater than megavoltage, the exit dose is small with less mucositis. Similarly, rib lesions can easily be treated using 300-kV x-rays. Parallel-opposed fields are usually used for tumours in the pelvis, long bones and the base of skull. Usually, field sizes are generous, particularly in the spine. Fields usually include the uninvolved vertebra above and below the target lesions. In the treatment of long-bone metastases, margins of 3 to 5 cm are added beyond visible lesions to deal with occult disease.

In the past, patients with relatively radiosensitive tumours with widespread analgesic-refractory painful bone metastases (e.g. myeloma) were treated with hemibody irradiation (typically, single doses of 6 Gy are given to the upper and 8 Gy to the lower body). Doses greater than 6 Gy to the upper hemibody can induce an acute pulmonary reaction and pulmonary oedema. Hemibody RT is seldom used now because of the widespread availability of effective analgesics, bisphosphonates and radioisotopes.

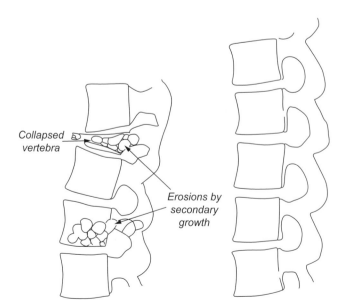

Fig. 32.11 Diagrammatic radiological appearances of normal vertebral column and secondary deposits from cancer (e.g. breast).

Bisphosphonates are usually given intravenously every 3 weeks and are effective by preventing further osteoclastic resorption of bone. Pain relief is durable. The main side effect is hypocalcaemia. Radioisotopes are either β-emitters (strontium-89 and samarium-153) or α-emitters (radium-223). Compared with β-emitters, the rate of myelosuppression is less with radium-223.

Although single dose palliative RT is the standard of care for patients with multiple metastases, there is an argument for giving higher doses (e.g. 40 Gy in 15 fractions) to a select group of patients. This may include patients with solitary nonspinal bone metastasis or metastases in up to 3 vertebrae from breast, renal or thyroid cancers. Studies of stereotactic body RT of a single dose of 15 to 24 Gy or a fractionated regimen of 13 to 35 Gy in 3 to 5 fractions report local disease control in up to 95% of cases and pain control in more than 80% of cases.

Pathological Fracture

If there is a pathological fracture or plain x-ray showing a lesion at risk of a pathological fracture of a long bone, an orthopaedic opinion should be sought on the feasibility of reducing and stabilising the fracture or preventing it. Pinning a fracture usually provides prompt pain relief and a return to mobility. Although there is no clear evidence for RT after pinning of a long bone, many clinicians prefer to give single-dose RT (8–10 Gy) to the whole bone.

If there is evidence of spinal cord compression, surgical decompression of the cord may be necessary prior to fractionated RT. Steroids should be given to patients with pain from nerve root infiltration and spinal cord compression. If patients are too unwell for even single fractions of RT, their pain should be controlled medically.

FURTHER READING

Ajithkumar TV, Hatcher H. Multidisciplinary management of sarcomas - where are we now? Clin Oncol (R Coll Radiol) 2017;29(8):467–70.

Baldini EH, Wang D, Haas RL, Catton CN, Indelicato DJ, Kirsch DG, Roberge D, Salerno K, Deville C, Guadagnolo BA, O'Sullivan B, Petersen IA, Le Pechoux C, Abrams RA, DeLaney TF. Treatment guidelines for preoperative radiation therapy for retroperitoneal sarcoma: preliminary consensus of an international expert panel. Int J Radiat Oncol Biol Phys 2015;92(3):602–12.

Bhattacharya IS, Hoskin PJ. Stereotactic body radiotherapy for spinal and bone metastases. Clin Oncol (R Coll Radiol) 2015;27(5):298–306.

Bielack SS, Smeland S, Whelan JS, et al. EURAMOS-1 Investigators. Methotrexate, doxorubicin, and cisplatin (MAP) plus maintenance pegylated interferon alfa-2b versus MAP alone in patients with resectable high-grade osteosarcoma and good histologic response to preoperative MAP: first results of the EURAMOS-1 good response randomized controlled trial. J Clin Oncol 2015;33(20):2279–87.

Dangoor A, Seddon B, Gerrand C, Grimer R, Whelan J, Judson I. UK guidelines for the management of soft tissue sarcomas. Clin Sarcoma Res 2016;6. 20. eCollection 2016.

ESMO/European Sarcoma Network Working Group. Soft tissue and visceral sarcomas: ESMO clinical practice guidelines for diagnosis, treatment and follow-up. Ann Oncol 2014;25(Suppl 3:iii):102–12.

ESMO/European Sarcoma Network Working Group. Bone sarcomas: ESMO clinical practice guidelines for diagnosis, treatment and follow-up. Ann Oncol 2014;25(Suppl 3:iii):113–23.

Euro-Ewing Radiotherapy Guidelines, Chapter XVII. In: EUROpean Ewing tumour working initiative of national groups Ewing tumour studies. 1999. EE 99 Amended Version 14th February 2006. Available https://www.skion.nl/workspace/uploads/ee99_amended_treo__2006_02_14.pdf. Accessed 01 May 2018.

Ford SJ, Almond LM, Gronchi A. An update on non-extremity soft tissue sarcomas. Clin Oncol (R Coll Radiol) 2017;29(8):516–27.

Frisch S, Timmermann B. The evolving role of proton beam therapy for sarcomas. Clin Oncol (R Coll Radiol) 2017;29(8):500–6.

Gerrand C, Athanasou N, Brennan B, Grimer R, Judson I, Morland B, Peake D, Seddon B, Whelan J; British Sarcoma Group. UK guidelines for the management of bone sarcomas. Clin Sarcoma Res 2016;6:7.

Gronchi A, Ferrari S, Quagliuolo V, Martin Broto J, Lopez-Pousa A, Grignani G, et al. Full-dose neoadjuvant anthracycline + ifosfamide chemotherapy is associated with a relapse free survival (RFS) and overall survival (OS) benefit in localized high-risk adult soft tissue sarcomas (STS) of the extremities and trunk wall: interim analysis of a prospective randomized trial. Ann Oncol 2016;27(Suppl. 6). LBA6_PR.

Haas RLM, Delaney TF, O'Sullivan B, et al. Radiotherapy for management of extremity soft tissue sarcomas: why, when, and where. Int J Radiat Oncol Biol Phys 2012;84:572–80.

Hatcher H, Benson C, Ajithkumar T. Systemic treatments in soft tissue sarcomas. Clin Oncol (R Coll Radiol) 2017;29(8):507–15.

Jeys L, Morris G, Evans S, Stevenson J, Parry M, Gregory J. Surgical innovation in sarcoma surgery. Clin Oncol (R Coll Radiol) 2017;29(8):489–99.

Judson J, Verweij H, Gelderblom JT, Hartmann P, Schöffski J, Blay Y, et al. Doxorubicin alone versus intensified doxorubicin plus ifosfamide for first-line treatment of advanced or metastatic soft-tissue sarcoma: a randomised controlled phase 3 trial. Lancet Oncol 2014;15 (4):415–23.

Le Cesne A, Ouali M, Leahy MG, Santoro A, Hoekstra HJ, Hohenberger P, et al. Doxorubicin-based adjuvant chemotherapy in soft tissue sarcoma: pooled analysis of two STBSG-EORTC phase III clinical trials. Ann Oncol 2014;25 (12):2425–32.

Marina NM, Smeland S, Bielack SS, et al. Comparison of MAPIE versus MAP in patients with a poor response to preoperative chemotherapy for newly diagnosed high-grade osteosarcoma (EURAMOS-1): an open-label, international, randomized controlled trial. Lancet Oncol 2016;17(10):1396–408.

O'Sullivan B, Davis AM, Turcotte R, et al. Preoperative versus postoperative radiotherapy in soft-tissue sarcoma of the limbs: a randomised trial. Lancet 2002;359:2235–41.

Pervaiz N, Colterjohn N, Farrokhyar F, Tozer R, Figueredo A, Ghert M. A systematic meta-analysis of randomized controlled trials of adjuvant chemotherapy for localized resectable soft-tissue sarcoma. Cancer 2008;113 (3):573–81.

Pisters PW, Harrison LB, Leung DH, et al. Long-term results of a prospective randomized trial of adjuvant brachytherapy in soft tissue sarcoma. J Clin Oncol 1996;14:859–68.

Prewett S, Horan G, Hatcher H, Ajithkumar T. Borderline sarcomas and smooth muscle tumours of uncertain malignant potential. Clin Oncol (R Coll Radiol) 2017;29(8):528–37.

Reddy KI, Wafa H, Gaston CL, Grimer RJ, Abudu AT, Jeys LM, Carter SR, Tillman RM. Does amputation offer any survival benefit over limb salvage in osteosarcoma patients with poor chemonecrosis and close margins? Bone Joint J 2015;97(1):115–20.

Sarcoma Meta-analysis Collaboration. Adjuvant chemotherapy for localised resectable soft-tissue sarcoma of adults: meta-analysis of individual data. Lancet 1997;350(9092):1647–54.

Tap WD, Jones RL, Van Tine BA, Chmielowski B, Elias AD, Adkins D, et al. Olaratumab and doxorubicin versus doxorubicin alone for treatment of soft-tissue sarcoma: an open-label phase 1b and randomised phase 2 trial. Lancet 2016;388(10043):488–97.

Trojani M, Contesso G, Coindre JM, et al. Soft-tissue sarcomas of adults: study of pathological prognostic variables and definition of a histopathological grading system. Int J Cancer 1984;33:37–42.

Whelan JS, Burcombe RJ, Janinis J, Baldelli AM, Cassoni AM. A systematic review of the role of pulmonary irradiation in the management of primary bone tumours. Ann Oncol 2002;13:23–30.

Whelan JS, Bielack SS, Marina N, et al. EURAMOS-1, an international randomised study for osteosarcoma: results from pre-randomisation treatment. Ann Oncol 2015;26(2):407–14.

Yang JC, Chang AE, Baker AR, et al. Randomized prospective study of the benefit of adjuvant radiation therapy in the treatment of soft tissue sarcomas of the extremity. J Clin Oncol 1998;16:197–203.

33

Principles of Paediatric Oncology

Roger E. Taylor

INTRODUCTION

Cancer in childhood is uncommon. In the United Kingdom, approximately 1500 children under the age of 15 years develop cancer each year. Approximately one individual child in 500 will develop cancer before the age of 15 years. According to Cancer Research UK (CRUK) there were 1821 cases and 231 deaths per annum from 2013 to 2015. The range of childhood cancers is very different from that seen in the adult population. Table 33.1 summarises data on relative incidence of the various tumour types from the CRUK data.

The evolution of the multidisciplinary care of children with cancer has been one of the success stories of modern oncology. Paediatric oncology collaborative groups have been very successful at entering a high proportion of children into clinical trials. In North America, clinical research has been coordinated via the Paediatric Oncology Group (POG), Children's Cancer Group (CCG), Intergroup Rhabdomyosarcoma Study Group (IRSG) and National Wilms' Tumour Study Group (NWTS). In 1999, these groups were amalgamated to form the Children's Oncology Group (COG), the largest paediatric oncology collaborative group in the world.

In the United Kingdom, treatment is coordinated by the network of 22 Children's Cancer and Leukaemia Group (CCLG) paediatric oncology centres. Increasingly, collaboration is across European boundaries, with clinical trials coordinated via the European network of the International Society of Paediatric Oncology (SIOP-E).

Currently, approximately 80% of children treated for cancer can expect to be long-term survivors. For most diseases, this has been brought about largely as a result of the incorporation of chemotherapy as part of a multimodality approach, including surgery and radiotherapy (RT). Since the introduction of chemotherapy into treatment programmes in the 1960s and 1970s, the proportion of children surviving cancer has demonstrated this gratifying increase.

Approximately 40% to 50% of children with cancer receive RT as a component of their treatment. RT is an important modality of therapy in local tumour control and the majority of paediatric tumours are radiosensitive. Cure, however, often comes with a cost as a result of the long-term sequelae of treatment. Long-term effects of RT include impaired bone and soft tissue growth, impaired neuropsychological development as a result of irradiation of the central nervous system (CNS) and radiation-induced malignancy. Increasing awareness of long-term effects in the 1970s and 1980s led to a general decline in the use of RT. However, more recently, it has become evident that chemotherapy is also associated with long-term side effects, including late myocardial damage because of anthracyclines, nephrotoxicity because of cisplatin or ifosfamide, and secondary leukaemia related to a number of chemotherapeutic agents including alkylating agents. The overall aim of paediatric oncology programmes is to maximise the chance of cure with the minimum impact of likely long-term effects of treatment. Continued vigilance for long-term effects of treatment is essential. This is ideally performed in the setting of dedicated long-term follow-up clinics and employing national treatment-related guidelines for long-term follow up, such as those produced by the CCLG and the Scottish Intercollegiate Group.

TABLE 33.1 Surveillance, Epidemiology and End Results Programme Registrations 1975–2015, Annual Incidence Rate Per 1,000,000 and Proportion of Children Aged 0–14 Years With Cancer

Disease Group	Annual Incidence Rate/1,000,000	Total (%)
ALL	37.9	25.0
ANLL	7.1	5.1
Other leukaemias	2.7	1.5
All leukaemias	**48.1**	**31.8**
Astrocytoma	15.2	10.0
Embryonal tumours (MB)	6.9	4.5
Ependymoma and choroid plexus	3.8	2.5
Intracranial germ cell tumours	1.5	1.0
Other CNS tumours	3.6	2.4
All CNS tumours	**35.6**	**23.5**
Hodgkin Lymphoma	5.7	3.8
NHL	7.3	4.8
Osteosarcoma	2.6	1.7
Ewing sarcoma	2.1	1.4
RMS	5.1	3.4
Other sarcoma	3.8	2.5
NB	10.3	6.8
Retinoblastoma	4.4	2.9
Wilms tumour	8.9	5.9
Other cancers/epithelial carcinomas	9.9	6.5
Total	**151.7**	

ALL, acute lymphoblastic leukaemia; *ANLL*, acute nonlymphoblastic leukaemia; *CNS*, central nervous system; *NB*, neuroblastoma; *NHL*, non-Hodgkin lymphoma; *RMS*, rhabdomyosarcoma.

It is very important that the administration of chemotherapy and RT for children should be undertaken only in specialised oncology centres treating relatively large numbers of children. In the United Kingdom, these centres are affiliated with the CCLG. The multiprofessional paediatric RT team should include a specialist paediatric therapy radiographer, specialist nurse and play specialist. Young children, particularly those under the age of 3 to 4 years, find it very difficult to lie still for RT planning and delivery, especially when an immobilisation head shell is required. Sedation sufficient to ensure immobilisation is difficult to achieve without it persisting for several hours, and it is not feasible for this to be administered daily for each fraction of RT. Because of the importance of immobilisation, short-acting general anaesthesia, such as propofol, is frequently required for children under the age of 3 to 4 years. The daily fasting for this results in surprisingly little disruption to nutrition. An experienced play therapist can be very helpful in preparing the child for RT and may avoid the need for daily anaesthesia for some children.

TOXICITY OF RADIOTHERAPY FOR CHILDREN

Acute Morbidity

The side effects of erythema, mucositis, nausea, diarrhoea and so on occur in children as in adults, and are generally managed by similar means.

Subacute Effects

Liver

A large proportion of the liver may need to be irradiated when treating Wilms tumour. Radiation hepatopathy may occur 1 to 3 months following RT, and consists of hepatomegaly, jaundice, ascites, thrombocytopenia and elevated transaminases. A risk factor is the administration of actinomycin-D following hepatic irradiation for the treatment of Wilms tumour. Long-term dysfunction is rare and the risk is dose related.

Lung

The whole lungs may receive RT as part of total body irradiation, or in the treatment of pulmonary metastases from Wilms tumour or Ewing sarcoma. Mild radiation pneumonitis consists of a dry cough and mild dyspnoea. The risk of pneumonitis is dose and radiation volume related. Radiation pneumonitis is the dose-limiting toxicity for total body irradiation. It is essential to consider potential interactions between chemotherapeutic drugs and lung irradiation and, in particular, to avoid lung irradiation in association with busulfan.

Central Nervous System

The somnolence syndrome occurs in at least 50% of children approximately 6 weeks after cranial irradiation and is probably related to temporary demyelination. Lhermitte's sign consists of an electric shock-like symptom radiating down the spine and into the limbs. It may follow radiation to the upper spinal cord, for example, following mediastinal RT for lymphoma. Within the first 2 months following RT for brain tumours, children may experience a transient deterioration of neurological symptoms and signs.

Long-Term Effects

Bone Growth

Impairment of bone growth and associated soft tissue hypoplasia can be one of the most obvious and distressing long-term effects, particularly when treating the head and neck region. Abnormalities of craniofacial growth can cause significant cosmetic and functional deformity, including micrognathia leading to problems with dentition. The epiphysial growth plates are very sensitive to radiation, and are excluded from the RT field whenever possible. Age at time of treatment, radiation dose and volume are factors which have an impact on the severity of these orthopaedic long-term effects. There is evidence of a dose-response effect, with a greater effect seen for doses of more than 33 gray (Gy) compared with less than 33 Gy. Slipped femoral epiphysis and avascular necrosis have also been reported following irradiation of the hip. Laboratory evidence suggests a dose-response effect between 5 Gy and 35 to 40 Gy, and an effect of dose per fraction. Careful consideration of the late orthopaedic effects of radiation is extremely important whenever planning RT for children. Epiphyses should be excluded from the irradiated volume where possible and, when irradiating the spine, an important principle of paediatric RT is that if the minimum vertebral dose is lower than 18 to 20 Gy the dose gradient across the vertebra should be no greater than 3 Gy to minimise long-term kyphoscoliosis.

Central Nervous System

Paediatric radiation oncology typically involves a significant amount of time devoted to the treatment of children with brain tumours, and consideration needs to be given to the toxicity of therapy.

Radionecrosis is rare below 60 Gy, and generally occurs with a latency of 6 months to 2 years. It results from a direct effect on glial tissue. It is very unusual to have to deliver a dose of 60 Gy to any part of the CNS for a child and, for the radical treatment of children with brain tumours, it is very uncommon to exceed a dose of 50 to 54 Gy. The clinical effects of radionecrosis vary according to the site within the CNS and are most devastating in the spinal cord. Radionecrosis of the spinal cord in children was seen in the 1980s as a consequence of the interaction between radiation and cytosine arabinoside given intrathecally for metastatic rhabdomyosarcoma (RMS).

Necrotising leukoencephalopathy may be seen when cranial irradiation is followed by high-dose methotrexate for the treatment of leukaemia. The clinical features include ataxia, lethargy, epilepsy, spasticity and paresis.

Neuropsychological effects. The effects of cranial RT are now well established. Data from children treated with prophylactic RT for leukaemia have demonstrated that when compared with siblings, children given 24 Gy prophylactic cranial irradiation show an approximate fall in IQ of approximately 12 points. Following higher radiation doses given for brain tumours, an increased risk of learning and behaviour difficulties is seen. An important risk factor for the incidence and severity of neuropsychological long-term effects is the age at diagnosis. This has driven the investigation of treatment approaches which do not include RT for children below the age of 3 years. Other factors include the impact of direct and indirect tumour-related parameters, treatment parameters with neuropsychological long-term effects worse for whole brain compared with partial brain irradiation, concomitant use of some chemotherapeutic agents, premorbid patient characteristics, such as intelligence, and the quality of catch-up education.

Kidney

Long-term effects on renal function are usually seen 2 to 3 years following a course of RT. The risk increases following a dose of greater than 15 Gy to both kidneys. The severity is related to the dose received, and when mild, consists of hypertension. When more severe, following a higher dose, renal failure may ensue.

Endocrine

Endocrine deficiencies following RT are common. Of particular concern is the risk of growth hormone and other pituitary hormone deficiencies following pituitary irradiation for tumours of the CNS.

Following RT to the thyroid, the incidence of elevated thyroid-stimulating hormone (TSH) is 75% after 25 to 40 Gy.

Reproductive

In boys, the germinal epithelium is very sensitive to the effects of low-dose irradiation. In adult males, transient oligospermia is seen after 2 Gy, but slow recovery can occur after 2 to 5 Gy.

In girls, the oocytes are also sensitive. Subsequent pregnancy is rare after 12 Gy whole body irradiation, but anecdotal cases of pregnancy after bone marrow transplantation, including whole body irradiation have been reported.

TOLERANCE OF CRITICAL ORGANS TO RADIOTHERAPY

The tolerance of critical organs frequently limits the dose of radiation that can be given. The critical organs and their tolerance doses if given in 2 Gy fractions are listed in Table 33.2.

TABLE 33.2 Normal Tissue Tolerance Doses	
Tissue/Organ	**Tolerance Dose (Gy)**
Whole lung	15–18
Both kidneys	12–15
Whole liver	20
Spinal cord	50

CHEMOTHERAPY/RADIOTHERAPY INTERACTIONS

Interactions between radiation and chemotherapy are complex and poorly understood. Interactions can be exploited to attempt to improve disease-free survival. The most frequently employed mechanism in paediatric oncology is spatial cooperation whereby chemotherapy and RT are combined to exploit their differing roles in different anatomical sites. Examples are the use of radiation for local control of a primary, with chemotherapy for subclinical metastatic disease such as in the treatment of Ewing sarcoma.

Chemotherapy and RT may be combined with the aim of increasing tumour cell kill without excess toxicity. An example is the use of combined chemotherapy and RT for children with Hodgkin lymphoma. It may be possible to reduce the intensity of both treatment modalities with the aim of maintaining disease control rates at the same time as reducing long-term morbidity. When using combined modality therapy, the aim is to improve the therapeutic ratio. Many protocols for children involve the use of concurrent chemotherapy and RT. It is essential to be vigilant for additional early- or long-term morbidity. Clinically important chemotherapy/RT interactions are often unpredictable and their mechanisms poorly understood. Actinomycin-D and cisplatin increase the slope of the radiation dose–response curve and actinomycin-D inhibits the repair of sublethal damage (SLD). Clinical interactions include enhanced skin and mucosal toxicity when radiation is followed by actinomycin-D (the recall phenomenon), enhanced bladder toxicity when chemotherapy is combined with cyclophosphamide, enhanced CNS toxicity from combined radiation and methotrexate, cytosine arabinoside or busulfan and the enhanced marrow toxicity from wide-field irradiation and many myelotoxic chemotherapeutic agents. In the case of the effect of combined radiation and anthracyclines, such as doxorubicin on the heart, doxorubicin has its effects on the myocytes and radiation on the vasculature.

RADIOTHERAPY QUALITY ASSURANCE

Because of the high cure rate for most childhood cancers, it is important to achieve local tumour control and avoid a geographical miss. It is also important to avoid unnecessarily large field sizes, to minimise long-term effects.

It is essential for all RT departments to deliver the highest possible standard of RT for all patients including children. Many RT departments have adopted quality systems.

In a number of studies, particularly those employing craniospinal RT for medulloblastoma (MB), the accuracy of delivery of RT has impacted upon tumour control and patient survival. In many North American paediatric multicentre studies, RT quality, including beam data, dose prescription, planning and verification films are reviewed centrally in the Imaging and Radiology Core Cooperative (IROC) situated in Providence, Rhode Island. Currently in European SIOP-E paediatric oncology trials, RT quality assurance (QA) is organised on a national basis. In the United Kingdom, this is undertaken by the NCRI RTTQA team. It is planned to develop a pan-European process (QUARTET).

LEUKAEMIA

The improvement in survival of children with acute lymphoblastic leukaemia (ALL) was one of the early successes of paediatric oncology. Currently, more than 70% are long-term survivors. The leukaemias account for the most frequent group of paediatric malignancies. Approximately 80% have ALL and 20% acute nonlymphoblastic leukaemia (ANLL), usually acute myeloid leukaemia (AML) or rarely, chronic myeloid leukaemia (CML).

Current treatment for ALL is stratified according to risk status based on presenting white count and cytogenetic profile. The four phases of treatment are:

1. Remission induction, usually with vincristine, corticosteroids and asparaginase.
2. Intensification with multidrug combinations. The number of intensification modules is dependent upon risk status at presentation.
3. CNS prophylaxis with intrathecal methotrexate. Cranial RT is no longer employed except for patients presenting with CNS involvement by leukaemia.
4. Maintenance, usually based on a continuous low-dose antimetabolite drug such as 6-thioguanine, with a total duration of therapy of approximately 2 years.

During the 1960s and 1970s, the routine use of prophylactic whole-brain RT and intrathecal methotrexate reduced the risk of CNS relapse to less than 10%. Whole brain RT may be employed for patients who present with CNS involvement (Fig. 33.1). Patients are immobilised in a head shell and treated with lateral-opposed 4- to 6-MV (megavoltage) fields which may be centred on outer canthus to minimise divergence into the contralateral lens. Shielding will cover the face, dentition, nasal structures and lenses. The clinical target volume (CTV) includes the intracranial meninges extending inferiorly to the lower border of the second or third cervical vertebra. Great care is taken to include the cribriform fossa, temporal lobe and base of skull. Although the lens is shielded, as much of the posterior orbit as possible is included as ocular relapses occasionally occur. The CTV is localised with lateral computed tomography (CT) simulation. The prescribed dose in current U.K. protocols is 24 Gy in 15 fractions of 1.6 Gy daily.

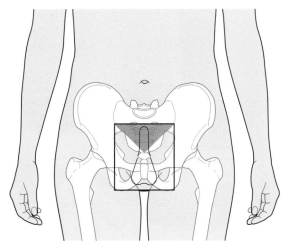

Shaded areas = position of shielding

Fig. 33.2 Diagram of field for testicular radiotherapy.

Boys who suffer a testicular relapse are treated with testicular RT (Fig. 33.2). The technique employed is an anterior field, generally electrons.

The CTV includes both testes, scrotum and inguinal canal superolaterally as far as the deep inguinal ring with shielding of nontarget skin and perineum. The prescribed dose is 24 Gy in 12 fractions of 2.0 Gy daily.

As for adults, children with ANLL are treated with intensive multidrug chemotherapy, which can achieve a survival rate of 60%. Bone marrow transplantation (BMT) is frequently employed for children who have a human leucocyte antigen (HLA)-matched sibling. A survival rate of 65% can be achieved for children in first complete remission treated with BMT as consolidation therapy for AML.

Total Body Irradiation

Total body irradiation (TBI) is an important technique used together usually with high-dose cyclophosphamide (cyclo-TBI) as the conditioning regimen before BMT for adults and children. Bone marrow donors for BMT are generally HLA-matched siblings. However, increasingly, volunteer unrelated donors from donor panels donate marrow, resulting in a significant increase in the number of patients for whom BMT can be considered.

Techniques for TBI have evolved in different departments, generally depending on availability of treatment facilities. Modern linear accelerator design and field sizes allow the use of large anterior and posterior fields. TBI dosimetry is usually based on in vivo measurements.

The TBI technique developed in Leeds is provided as an example. The patient lies in the lateral position in an evacuated polystyrene immobilisation bag. Hands are placed under chin to provide lung compensation (Fig. 33.3). Dosimetry is determined using in vivo measurements performed at a test dose of 0.2 Gy for each field. For such a large and complex target volume, it is not feasible to adhere to the International Commission on Radiation Units and Measurements (ICRU) 50 guidelines of a range of −5% to +7%; a range of −10% to +10% is more realistic. The standard TBI dose for children in the United Kingdom is 14.4 Gy in 8 fractions of 1.8 Gy twice daily with a minimum interfraction interval of 6 hours.

For children with ALL, many centres advise a cranial boost in addition to the TBI with the aim of reducing the risk of CNS relapse. Planning for the cranial boost is the same as for prophylactic cranial irradiation. Unlike the use of the standard TBI dose, policies for the

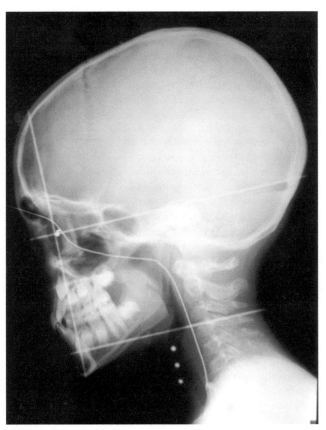

Fig. 33.1 Simulator film of whole brain field for acute lymphoblastic leukaemia central nervous system prophylaxis.

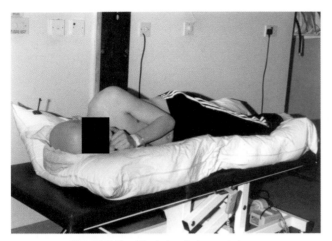

Fig. 33.3 Total body irradiation technique.

cranial boost vary between individual centres. A typical regimen for the cranial boost would be 5.4 Gy in three daily fractions.

Indications for Bone Marrow Transplantation/Total Body Irradiation in Children

In the current CRUK guidelines, children with AML are selected for BMT and TBI based on risk status at presentation. Patients are stratified into standard, intermediate-risk or high-risk based on cytogenetic and/or molecular characteristics at presentation and response to treatment-assessed morphology and by minimal residual disease (MRD) measurement after each course of treatment. Those with an HLA-matched sibling are selected for BMT if they fall into the intermediate- or high-risk category, whereas those with low-risk disease, that is, those with chromosome mutations t(8;21), t(15;17) or Inv 16 do well with standard chemotherapy.

Children with ALL selected for BMT and TBI include relapsed patients and those presenting with features indicating a high risk of failure with standard chemotherapy. Other conditions considered for BMT where TBI is sometimes employed include severe aplastic anaemia, thalassaemia and immunodeficiency syndromes.

Morbidity of Total Body Irradiation

Acute effects include nausea and lethargy during TBI, mucositis, diarrhoea, erythema and parotitis in the first few weeks following treatment and somnolence approximately 6 weeks after TBI. Long-term effects of TBI include impaired growth because of a direct effect from irradiation of epiphyses and also as a growth hormone deficiency. There is also a risk of cataract, hypothyroidism and, in some studies, the possibility of renal impairment. TBI is generally not considered for children under the age of 2 years and, instead, a conditioning regimen with two drugs, busulfan and cyclophosphamide (Bu-Cy), is generally employed.

HODGKIN LYMPHOMA

The age incidence of Hodgkin lymphoma spans the older paediatric age range, through the adolescent and young adult age ranges. The overall survival rate for children with Hodgkin lymphoma is at least 90%, and an important aim is to maintain this good overall survival rate while reducing long-term treatment effects. These include orthopaedic long-term effects of RT, such as impaired bone growth resulting from direct irradiation of the epiphyses, and also infertility from alkylating agents and procarbazine. Wide-field RT, such as the mantle technique, has been avoided in children for several decades. In Europe, a chemotherapy approach is taken with response assessment by positron

emission tomography (PET) scanning which is now established as a predictor of those patients who require RT. Consolidation RT is selectively employed for children whose response on PET scan is suboptimal. An example of bilateral neck irradiation is illustrated in Fig. 33.4.

Those who are PET positive may require RT, whereas those who are PET negative may not require RT following chemotherapy. The role of PET scanning in this setting requires on-going evaluation.

In current European protocols for the treatment of Hodgkin lymphoma, following chemotherapy, sites of initial involvement are irradiated to a dose of 19.8 Gy in 11 fractions over 2.2 weeks. Where there is significant residual macroscopic disease, this is treated with a boost of 10 Gy in 5 fractions over 1 week.

The management of adolescents with Hodgkin disease is an example of where local and national collaboration with adult oncology groups is important to provide age-related treatment protocols.

NON-HODGKIN LYMPHOMA

A different spectrum of non-Hodgkin lympoma NHL is seen in children compared with adults. Follicle centre cell lymphoma and diffuse large B-cell lymphoma, which are common in adults, are uncommon in childhood. The majority of children have T-cell lymphoblastic lymphoma, Burkitt, Burkitt-like or anaplastic large-cell lymphoma. Survival rates have improved in recent years and, currently, more than 80% survive long term. Patients are treated by intensive multiagent chemotherapy including CNS prophylaxis with intrathecal chemotherapy, and there is no routine role for RT in their management. However, children with T-cell lymphoblastic lymphoma, which is managed according to the same principles as ALL, may be considered for BMT with TBI.

NEUROBLASTOMA

Neuroblastoma (NB) is the most common solid tumour of childhood. NB is generally a disease of very young children. Approximately one-third are less than 1 year of age at presentation. NB arises in neural crest tissue in the autonomic nervous system, usually in the adrenal area, but can arise anywhere from the neck to the pelvis. The majority of children present with widespread metastases including bones, marrow, lungs and liver. Overall, current survival rates are generally poor, approximately 45%, taking all stages and prognostic groups into account. Prognosis for individual clinical groups varies considerably and is related to a number of prognostic factors. Prognosis is better for young children aged less than 1 year at presentation, and is worse for children whose tumours have amplification of the oncogene, Myc-n. Deletion of the short arm of chromosome 1 has emerged as an important prognostic factor with a worse prognosis for those with 1p deletion. Tumours that are hyperdiploid have a better prognosis. Management is now stratified according to risk grouping. Patients in the best risk group with localised disease have a survival rate of greater than 90% following surgery alone. The majority are treated with intensive chemotherapy using drugs such as vincristine, cisplatin, carboplatin, etoposide and cyclophosphamide.

For good-risk patients, RT is unnecessary, and for high-risk patients, the predominant relapse pattern is metastatic rather than local. The role of external beam RT for patients with high-risk disease (e.g. aged <1 year with stage 4 disease at presentation) is to maximise the probability of local tumour control following surgical resection of the primary tumour. With current intensive chemotherapy, some patients with metastases at presentation can hopefully be cured of their metastatic disease, in which case, local tumour control becomes important, employing a combination of surgical resection and postoperative RT. In the recent European High-Risk NB protocol, the dose for postoperative RT to the tumour bed was 21 Gy in 14 fractions. In planning postoperative RT for NB, care has to be taken to consider dose limits to organs at risk (OARs), particularly liver and kidneys, the function of which may have been compromised by high-dose chemotherapy. Traditionally, straightforward techniques have been employed using large anterior and posterior fields. However, current protocols are investigating the use of more advanced techniques with a CTV based on surgical and pathological reports indicating likely sites of subclinical disease, which may offer the potential for dose escalation.

Metaiodobenzylguanidine Therapy for Neuroblastoma

The majority of NBs take up the guanethidine analogue, metaiodobenzylguanidine (MIBG). MIBG can be conjugated with iodine radionuclides for imaging and targeted RT. Generally, 123I-MIBG is the radionuclide used for diagnostic imaging. High-activity 131I-MIBG (typically 3.7–7.4 GBq) can be used for targeted therapy. In a U.K. multicentre study, a response rate of 30% has been achieved for children with residual NB following first-line chemotherapy. After enthusiasm in the 1980s and early 1990s, interest in the potential role for therapeutic MIBG has diminished. However, in some European centres, upfront MIBG is still employed and its role in the initial management of high-risk NB, together with chemotherapy, warrants further exploration. Logistic difficulties include radiation protection for very young children who may not yet be continent of urine, and the risk of radiation exposure to staff who may need to care for an ill child. Many U.K. RT departments are geographically separated in different hospitals from paediatric support. This is one of the main reasons why currently, MIBG therapy is available in only a limited number of paediatric oncology centres in the United Kingdom.

WILMS TUMOUR (NEPHROBLASTOMA)

Wilms tumour is an embryonic renal tumour which generally presents as a large abdominal mass, sometimes with pain or haematuria. Wilms tumour may be genetically associated with aniridia (congenital absence of the iris) and other inherited syndromes, such as the Beckwith-Wiedemann syndrome (variable features including macrosomia or hemihypertrophy, macroglossia, omphalocele). The WT1 gene is located on chromosome 11, and is a tumour-suppressor gene. If both copies of the gene are lost by mutation, then Wilms tumour may arise.

Median age at diagnosis is between 3 and 3.5 years. Patients are staged according to histopathological findings following nephrectomy. Table 33.3 shows the National Wilms Tumour Study Group (NWTS) staging system for Wilms tumour. In 4% to 8% of cases, tumours are bilateral (stage V).

The current long-term survival rate for Wilms tumour is in excess of 80%. Treatment is aimed at maintaining this high survival rate while attempting to reduce the long-term side effects of therapy. There is a major disparity between approaches adopted in Europe and North America. The North American series of NWTS, now COG protocols, employ immediate nephrectomy with staging and postsurgical adjuvant therapy based on histological examination of the primary tumour. Wilms tumour histology is referred to as either favourable (FH) or unfavourable (UH) because of the presence of anaplasia.

Postoperative chemotherapy is given using the drugs vincristine, actinomycin-D and doxorubicin, the number of drugs and duration depending upon the staging.

In Europe, the series of SIOP studies has been based on preoperative chemotherapy to downstage the primary, reducing the surgical morbidity, particularly the number who have tumour rupture at surgery, and the number who require flank RT. The most recent study was the SIOP 2001 study into which patients from the United Kingdom were entered. All patients received preoperative chemotherapy with actinomycin-D and vincristine, with delayed nephrectomy after 6 weeks of preoperative chemotherapy. Postoperative adjuvant therapy was based on subsequent pathological staging and allocation of risk status (good-risk vs. intermediate-risk vs. poor-risk histology). For intermediate-risk patients, there was a randomisation to receive or not receive doxorubicin. The purpose of this was to determine whether doxorubicin could be omitted, thus reducing the risk of late cardiac sequelae. The trial results demonstrated that it was safe to avoid doxorubicin in this patient group, and now forms the basis of current management.

Postoperative flank RT is employed for stage III patients, that is, those with incompletely resected primary tumours, pre- or perioperative tumour rupture, or histologically involved lymph nodes. Current standard radiotherapeutic management involves the use of anterior and posterior opposed fields. The CTV includes the preoperative extent of tumour and kidney, following preoperative chemotherapy with a margin of 1.0 cm. Fields extend across the midline to irradiate homogeneously the full width of the vertebral body to minimise the risk of kyphoscoliosis (Figs. 33.5 and 33.6). For patients with intermediate-risk histology, the dose is 14.4 Gy in 8 fractions of 1.8 Gy daily, and for high-risk histology, 25.2 Gy in 14 fractions of 1.8 Gy. There is a boost to macroscopic residual disease: 10.8 Gy in 6 fractions of 1.8 Gy. For future European trials, it is proposed that rather than using parallel-opposed fields, a retroperitoneal CTV should be planned, based on the anatomical site where disease recurrence is considered possible, and taking into account the surgeon's assessment of the site of risk of recurrence.

Whole abdominal RT has considerable acute and long-term morbidity and should be reserved for those who present with extensive intra-abdominal tumour spread or generalised preoperative or perioperative tumour rupture. In European protocols, the dose is 21 Gy in 1.5 Gy fractions with shielding to limit the dose to the remaining kidney to 12 Gy.

For children presenting with pulmonary metastases which do not resolve completely after the initial 6 weeks of preoperative chemotherapy, whole-lung RT (Figs. 33.7 and 33.8) is given. The fields have to include the costophrenic recess, and the lower border generally extends to the lower border of the 12th thoracic vertebra. The humeral heads are shielded. In the current SIOP 2001 study, the lung dose is 15 Gy in 10 fractions with a lung density correction.

RHABDOMYOSARCOMA

RMS may arise at any site, although they tend to have a predilection for sites in the head and neck and urogenital regions. These include head and neck sites such as the orbit, nasopharynx and middle ear, and urogenital tract sites such as bladder, prostate and vagina. Tumours that arise in sites such as the nasopharynx and middle ear have the

TABLE 33.3 National Wilms Tumour Study Group Staging System

Stage	Clinicopathological Features
I	Tumour confined to within renal capsule, completely excised
II	Tumour invading outside renal capsule, completely excised
III	Residual abdominal tumour—positive margins, tumour rupture, involved nodes
IV	Haematogenous metastases
V	Bilateral disease

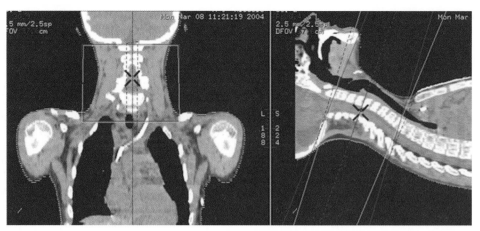

Fig. 33.4 Hodgkin Lymphoma.

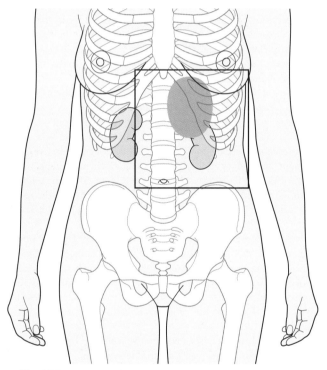

Fig. 33.5 Diagram of flank radiotherapy field for Wilms tumour.

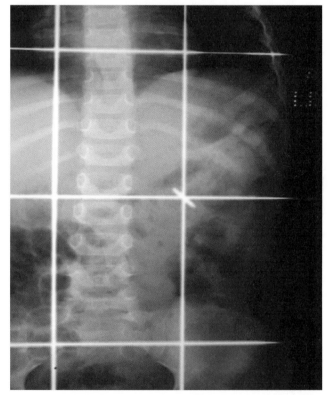

Fig. 33.6 Wilms tumour flank radiotherapy.

propensity for base of skull and intracranial invasion and are referred to as parameningeal RMS.

Although there are risks of both local and metastatic recurrence, local tumour control is an important consideration in the management of RMS and RT is an important modality for many patients. The sequelae following RT, particularly to the head and neck in young children, may be considerable. In Europe in the 1990s, these considerations limited its use, but there is now an increasing recognition of the importance of RT, not only on local tumour control, but also of its impact on overall survival. Currently, the long-term survival rate for RMS is approximately 70% to 80%. The challenges are to continue to increase the survival rate, and also to try to do this with acceptable long-term morbidity.

In many European countries including the United Kingdom, children have been treated according to the SIOP series of studies. The basis of these has been the use of intensive chemotherapy with the aim of improving the survival and reducing the use and/or intensity of local therapy with surgery and/or RT, and thus minimise long-term effects. The strategy for this series of studies includes stratifying patients within risk groups based on histological subtype (embryonal vs. alveolar histology), stage of disease and primary tumour site. Patients in the low-risk category, that is, those with localised tumours which are microscopically completely resected are treated with chemotherapy using actinomycin-D and vincristine for a duration of 9 weeks. Standard-risk tumours are those which are locally more extensive but at selected favourable sites, the vagina, uterus or paratestis and are treated with ifosfamide, vincristine and actinomycin-D. High-risk tumours include other incompletely resected tumours, including all

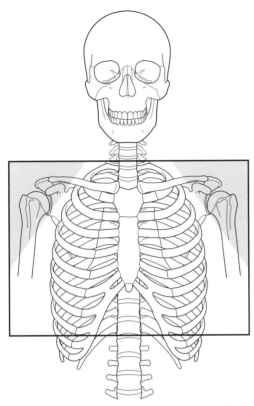

Fig. 33.7 Diagram of whole lung radiotherapy field.

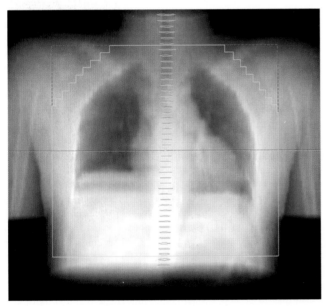

Fig. 33.8 Whole lung radiotherapy.

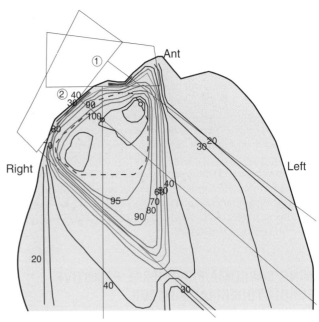

Fig. 33.9 Orbital rhabdomyosarcoma radiotherapy plan.

those arising in parameningeal sites (nasopharynx, middle ear) and those with involved lymph nodes. In the recent European EPSSG trial the addition of dose-intense doxorubicin did not result in an improved outcome compared with the standard three drugs combination of ifosfamide, vincristine and actinomycin-D.

In the European SIOP MMT 95 trial which recruited patients between 1995 and 2003, RT was used for patients who failed to achieve a complete response following chemotherapy and surgery and, in effect, was used to convert a partial into a complete response. Current use of consolidation RT is based on risk status and in future a randomised clinical trial evaluating different doses of RT is planned. Patients will be stratified according to the risk of local relapse and to investigate the potential for RT dose escalation will be randomised to either 59.40 Gy compared with 50.40 Gy, or 50 to 40 Gy compared with 41.40 Gy, all at 1.8 Gy/fraction. There will also be a randomised trial of consolidation irradiation directed at all metastatic sites for patients presenting with metastases.

For high-risk parameningeal disease (skull base erosion or cranial nerve palsy), the target volume has been based on the pre-chemotherapy extent of disease. For those who require RT following relapse after initial treatment with chemotherapy alone, the target volume has been based on the tumour extent at the time of relapse and before second-line chemotherapy. For children with initially involved nodes, these are included in the target volume if they require RT. It is now recognised that patients presenting with primary tumours in the orbit (Fig. 33.9) or limbs have a high risk of recurrence and now routinely receive RT in recent European protocols.

Planning of RT requires meticulous attention to detail, avoiding excessive field sizes, particularly in the head and neck region. In the recently closed European SIOP European Paediatric Soft-Tissue Sarcoma Study Group (EPSSG) trial, the use and intensity of RT was stratified according to histological and clinical parameters. For patients with embryonal RMS following incomplete surgery and chemotherapy, postoperative doses employed are 41.4 Gy in 23 fractions of 1.8 Gy following complete response to chemotherapy and 50.4 Gy in 28 fractions of 1.8 Gy following an incomplete response.

A boost of 5.4 Gy in 3 fractions of 1.8 Gy is considered for large tumours and/or poor response to chemotherapy following a postoperative dose of 36 Gy in 20 fractions of 1.8 Gy.

For patients with alveolar RMS, if surgical excision of the primary was performed, the postoperative dose was 41.4 Gy in 23 fractions of 1.8 Gy. For those with incomplete surgical resection or a biopsy, only the postchemotherapy dose was 50.4 Gy in 28 fractions of 1.8 Gy, with consideration given to a boost of 5.4 Gy in 3 fractions of 1.8 Gy for large tumours and/or a poor response to chemotherapy.

Brachytherapy may be considered for a few highly selected children with RMS, usually with limited tumours arising in the head and neck, vagina, bladder or prostate. However, in the United Kingdom, the main area where brachytherapy has been successfully employed has been for the treatment of primary RMS arising in the vaginal vault. Brachytherapy can provide a means of local tumour control with reduced morbidity compared with external beam RT. However, for a child to be suitable for brachytherapy, the tumour must be sufficiently localised to achieve local control with a small planning target volume (PTV) suitable for brachytherapy rather than a larger volume suitable for only external beam RT (typically 2–3 cm). If brachytherapy is being considered for a genitourinary tract primary, discussion between oncologists and surgeons at an early stage is essential followed by a joint examination under anaesthesia (EUA). Both low-dose rate and high-dose rate after-loading brachytherapy techniques have been used with equal success. Most young children require sedation or general anaesthesia during treatment and high-dose rate brachytherapy has been evaluated in a number of centres internationally.

EWING SARCOMA/PERIPHERAL PRIMITIVE NEUROECTODERMAL TUMOUR

Ewing sarcoma of bone is predominantly a disease of adolescents, having its peak incidence in the early teenage years. Survival rates of between 55% and 65% are reported. Approximately 60% of primary tumours occur in the long bones of the limbs, and 40% in the flat bones of the ribs, vertebrae or spine. Significant soft tissue extension is common. Peripheral primitive neuroectodermal tumour (PPNET), previously referred to as soft tissue Ewing sarcoma has become increasingly recognised in the last two decades. One of the first subtypes of PPNET to be described was the Askin tumour of the chest wall. The majority of Ewing sarcomas of bone share with PPNET a chromosomal translocation, t(11;22) (q24;q12). In recent years, Ewing sarcoma and PPNET have generally been treated according to common protocols.

Managing children with Ewing sarcoma and PPNET requires a multidisciplinary team approach. Initial treatment is with systemic chemotherapy which treats macroscopic tumour and any subclinical metastases. Appropriate use of local therapy, either surgical resection, RT or a combination of both modalities is also necessary. Patients in the United Kingdom are currently entered into the European Ewing Tumour Working Initiative of National Groups (Euro-EWING 99) study. Chemotherapy is commenced with vincristine, ifosfamide, doxorubicin and etoposide (VIDE). Patients are then stratified according to primary tumour volume. For patients with small tumours (<200 mL), and those with a good histological response to VIDE chemotherapy, treatment continues with doxorubicin and vincristine and a randomisation to either cyclophosphamide or ifosfamide. For those with a poor histological response, there is a randomisation between conventional chemotherapy or high-dose chemotherapy with busulfan and melphalan.

Local tumour control is important and the decision as to whether surgery, RT or a combination of both should be employed demands careful multidisciplinary discussion. In previous series of patients treated in Europe, survival has been better following local treatment with surgery (with or without preoperative or postoperative RT), compared with RT alone. However, these series are confounded by selection bias with patients with smaller tumours selected for surgery and many patients with very large or inoperable pelvic tumours selected for RT alone.

Planning of RT for Ewing sarcoma or PPNET is technically challenging. Multidisciplinary RT planning involving radiologists, physicists, specialist therapy radiographers and mould-room technicians is important at the outset. Three-dimensional planning may be employed

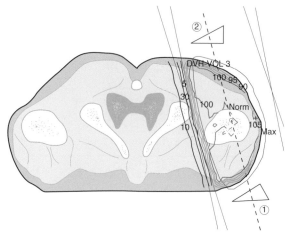

Fig. 33.10 Computed tomography plan of radiotherapy for pelvic Ewing sarcoma.

to achieve a uniform dose within the target volume, which is frequently large and adjacent to critical organs.

RT technique will depend upon the tumour site and anatomy. Individualised, generally multiple fields are used to deliver homogeneous irradiation to the PTV and to minimise dose to nontarget tissues and OARs (Fig. 33.10).

When planning the CTV, phase 1 includes the gross tumour volume (GTV) before chemotherapy and/or surgery if feasible with a minimum margin of 3 to 5 cm for extremity primaries and 2 cm for trunk or head and neck primaries. For a second phase, a margin of 2 cm is employed. Immobilisation is dependent upon primary tumour site and anatomy. For limbs, an immobilisation device, such as an evacuated polystyrene bag, may be useful. The CTV and PTV are localised on a planning CT scan. The prescribed doses are, for phase 1 and postoperative volume: 44.8 Gy in fractions of 1.8 to 2.0 Gy and, for phase 2, for macroscopic disease: 9.6 Gy in fractions of 1.8 to 2.0 Gy.

Selected patients may benefit from a higher dose, up to 64 Gy if this can be delivered without undue toxicity. However, patients selected for definitive RT frequently have large tumours, and dose may be limited by organ toxicity, and thus a dose of 64 Gy is generally difficult to achieve. For postoperative RT, the prescribed dose depends on the extent of surgery and histological response of the primary to initial chemotherapy. Following intralesional surgery or marginal surgery with poor histological response to chemotherapy (>10% residual tumour cells), 54.4 Gy is prescribed. For marginal surgery with good histological response (<10% residual tumour cells) or wide surgery with poor histological response, 44.8 Gy is prescribed. For patients who present with pulmonary metastases, whole lung RT is employed: 15 Gy for patients aged less than 14 years and 18 Gy for those aged over 14 years. These doses are subject to homogeneity correction for reduced attenuation in lung.

Care has to be taken when combining chemotherapy and RT to avoid excessive morbidity from enhanced radiation reactions. Actinomycin-D is not given during RT and anthracyclines, such as doxorubicin and epirubicin, are omitted if there is a significant amount of bowel or mucosa in the treated volume. Patients requiring radical RT involving the spinal cord or significant RT to the lungs should not receive busulfan.

OSTEOSARCOMA

Osteosarcoma is the most frequent bone tumour of childhood, with the majority arising in teenagers. The lower femur and upper tibia are the most frequent primary sites, with approximately 65% developing around the knee. Less frequent sites include the humerus, fibula, sacrum, spine, mandible and pelvis. Before the advent of effective chemotherapy, approximately 80% of patients died because of progression of lung metastases. Currently, a survival rate of approximately 55% can be achieved with the use of intensive adjuvant chemotherapy. The majority of primary tumours can be resected, and the affected bone replaced by a titanium endoprosthesis, thus avoiding the need for an amputation. The most frequently employed chemotherapy regimen is the combination of high-dose methotrexate, cisplatin and doxorubicin.

RT has only a minor role in the management of osteosarcoma. However, it is probably not as radioresistant as previously thought. In selected patients, after insertion of an endoprosthesis, postoperative RT may be employed for those felt to be at a high risk of local recurrence, that is, those with tumour at a resection margin. RT is sometimes employed for the treatment of an unresectable tumour, such as a spinal vertebral or extensive pelvic primary tumour. In these cases, the dose has to be as high as normal tissues will tolerate, that is, 60 Gy if possible. RT can be employed for the local palliation of metastases, using a relatively high dose, for example, 40 Gy in 15 fractions.

CENTRAL NERVOUS SYSTEM TUMOURS

Tumours of the CNS account for approximately 20% to 25% of malignant childhood tumours and are the leading cause of death from childhood cancer. Approximately 350 children develop CNS tumours each year in the United Kingdom. However, individual tumour types are uncommon and experience in the management of each type is limited. In contrast to most other paediatric malignancies, the use of chemotherapy has not yet resulted in significant improvements in survival for the majority of children with CNS tumours. The overall 5-year survival rate is approximately 50%, inferior to that reported for many other children's tumours. The burdens of survivorship are high and the majority of survivors experience sequelae from either the tumour or therapy or, very frequently, a combination of both.

Children with CNS tumours and their families are managed by specialised paediatric neurooncology multidisciplinary teams.

RT for children with CNS tumours is technically challenging. Many children require craniospinal RT, which is one of the most complex techniques employed in most oncology departments.

Long-Term Effects of Radiotherapy for Central Nervous System Tumours

Of greatest concern are the long-term neuropsychological effects of RT to the CNS, particularly for very young children. Other factors include direct and indirect effects of the tumour itself and also the effects of surgery. One of the most important factors which increases the risk and severity of long-term neuropsychological sequelae is young age at diagnosis. For children aged younger than 3 years at diagnosis, RT is delayed if possible by the use of chemotherapy.

Children receiving craniospinal RT will frequently experience dose-dependent spinal shortening as a direct effect of irradiation of the spine.

For many children, the hypothalamic/pituitary axis has to be included in the irradiated volume. This often results in growth hormone deficiency, but other endocrine deficiencies such as thyrotrophin-releasing hormone (TRH) or adrenocorticotrophic hormone (ACTH) deficiency may occur. TRH deficiency is relatively easily managed by thyroid hormone replacement, but ACTH deficiency may require life-long steroid replacement therapy, which may be problematic.

Chemotherapy for Central Nervous System Tumours

Chemotherapy also has an established role for the majority of paediatric CNS tumours. Secreting intracranial germ cell tumours are routinely treated with chemotherapy. Adjuvant chemotherapy improves the outcome for standard risk MB compared with RT alone, and is also used for high-risk disease. The use of chemotherapy can delay the need for RT for very young children, particularly those with low-grade astrocytoma and probably ependymoma. However, in most cases, the use of chemotherapy is evaluated within the context of a clinical trial.

Low-Grade Astrocytoma

Low-grade astrocytomas (LGGs) comprise the most frequent group of children's CNS tumours (see Table 31.1). The most frequent histological types are WHO grade I (pilocytic) or grade II (usually fibrillary), with other varieties, such as ganglioglioma and oligodendroglioma, much less frequent. The presence of neurofibromatosis type I (NF1) predisposes to the development of these tumours. It is now clear that LGGs may undergo long periods of quiescence, even when not completely resected. It is now also clear that low-grade gliomas are more chemosensitive than previously thought. Following treatment of LGG, the 5-year survival rate is relatively high at approximately 80% to 85%, but late relapse is not uncommon.

Initial treatment is usually with surgical resection, which should be as complete as is considered safe. This is usually more straightforward for tumours arising in the cerebellum, where complete resection is usually feasible, compared with those arising from the optic tract or optic chiasm. Because of the considerable risk of surgery in this area, tumours with typical features on MRI scanning of a hypothalamic/optic tract astrocytoma are not necessarily biopsied, as many consider the risk of the procedure (i.e. visual deterioration) outweighs the risk of an incorrect diagnosis.

During the last 20 years, North American and European collaborative group studies have attempted to standardise the management of children with LGG. The SIOP series of studies has defined a strategy for managing these tumours. Following initial maximal surgical resection, patients undergo a period of observation. Patients with clinical or radiological evidence of progression, those with severe symptoms or threat to vision receive nonsurgical treatment.

In the recent closed European SIOP LGG2 study, those over the age of 7 years were treated by RT. Those aged 7 years or under receive chemotherapy with the aim of delaying RT. It is hoped that by employing this strategy for younger children, the long-term neuropsychological effects of RT may be lessened by the delay. Using the drug combination of carboplatin and vincristine, the majority of children with LGG can achieve either a response, or stabilisation of previously progressive tumour. In the LGG2 study, patients were randomised to receive initial chemotherapy with either carboplatin and vincristine, or this drug combination with the addition of etoposide. The aim of this study was to assess whether the addition of etoposide could reduce the risk of tumour progression within the first few months of chemotherapy, which was a significant problem in the previous SIOP (LGG1) study. The total duration of chemotherapy was 18 months. Patients who are treated initially with chemotherapy and who experience progression will receive RT, and vice versa. The final results of this trial are awaited. For patients who present with spinal cord primary low-grade glioma, the management policy will be similar.

RT for low-grade gliomas is based on a careful imaging for target volume definition (Fig. 33.11A–E). The technique will depend upon tumour site and anatomy. Individualised multiple fields to deliver homogeneous radiotherapy to the PTV and to minimise dose to non-target tissues and OARs (Fig. 33.13). The CTV includes the GTV and, in the case of surgical resection, any brain tissue previously

Imaging for Low Grade Glioma
RT Planning

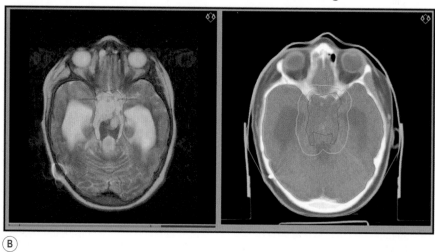

- Planning CT
- CT/MR Merge
- MR Imaging parameters used for determination of GTV:
- T1 + Gadolinium or T2 or Flair

(A)

Pilocytic Astrocytoma
CT/MR Merge

T2 MR   Planning CT

(B)

LGG
Target Volumes

LGG—Three Field Plan

Gross tumour
volume (GTV)

Clinical target
volume (CTV)

Planning target
volume (PTV)

(C)   (D)

Fig. 33.11 (A–E) Series-imaging for low-grade glioma radiotherapy planning. *CT*, Computed tomography; *MR*, magnetic resonance.

Continued

Low Grade Glioma—RT Doses

Target volume	Number of fractions	Dose per fraction	Total dose	Duration (weeks)
Intracranial	30	1.8 Gy	54.0 Gy	6
Spinal	28	1.8 Gy	50.4 Gy	5½

(E)

Fig. 33.11, cont'd

surrounding the tumour with a margin in potential areas of spread of 0.5 cm. Patients are immobilised in a supine immobilisation device. The extent of GTV is localised using T2 or FLAIR images on the MRI scan. For planning, CT/MRI fusion should be employed. The RT dose is specified to the ICRU reference point. In international studies, the prescribed dose is 54 Gy in 30 fractions of 1.8 Gy daily. For patients with a spinal cord primary requiring RT, the dose is 50.4 Gy in 28 fractions of 1.8 Gy.

Three-dimensional conformal planning or intensity-modulated RT (IMRT) can reduce the amount of normal brain within the irradiated volume, and has the potential for reducing long-term effects, an important priority for this group of patients who have a high chance of long-term survival. In the future, it is planned to assess the impact of RT parameters on long-term intellectual and functional outcome.

High-Grade Astrocytoma

Unlike in adults, where HGAs comprise the most frequent group of primary CNS tumours, HGAs are uncommon in childhood. As with HGAs arising in adults, the outlook is generally very poor, and survival rates are currently approximately 20% at 5 years. Infants under the age of 3 generally do better than older children who have similar outcomes to young adults. Treatment is based on surgical resection and postoperative RT, generally 54 Gy in 30 fractions. Current management is based on concurrent and adjuvant temozolomide chemotherapy together with focal radical RT using a similar regimen to the current standard approach for adults with glioblastoma. A recent European trial of the addition of bevacizumab to standard treatment with RT and temozolomide failed to achieve additional survival benefit. An important priority for these patients is to identify the potential for novel systemic agents to improve outcomes.

Brainstem Glioma

This group of brain tumours comprises a heterogeneous mix of tumours arising in the midbrain, pons and medulla. They are classified as focal (5%–10%), dorsal exophytic (10%–20%), cervicomedullary (5%–10%) and diffuse intrinsic tumours (75%–85%). Focal, dorsal exophytic and cervicomedullary tumours are generally LGGs. Surgical excision is the treatment of choice with RT reserved for inoperable tumours.

The majority of children with brainstem gliomas have diffuse intrinsic pontine gliomas (DIPG) which, when subject to biopsy, have generally been shown to be high-grade astrocytomas. They can be diagnosed by their typical MRI appearance (Fig. 33.12). A biopsy procedure, such as a stereotactic biopsy, is often considered to be risky and many consider this to be contraindicated. The prognosis for DIPG is very poor. Because of the frequent relatively short history of these tumours, RT often needs to be commenced quickly. Although RT results in improvement of neurological symptoms for approximately 70% of children, median survival is about 9 months and there are very

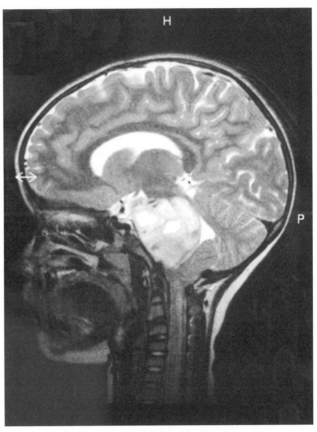

Fig. 33.12 Sagittal view of a typical pontine glioma.

few long-term survivors. The management of these children remains a major challenge, and domiciliary palliative care usually has to be introduced at a relatively early stage.

Patients are generally treated with a relatively straightforward technique with CT planning. The CTV includes the GTV as defined on diagnostic MRI scan with a margin of 2 cm along potential areas of spread superiorly, inferiorly and posteriorly along the brainstem. Patients are generally treated supine in a Perspex shell or thermoplastic shell with CT simulation. The standard of care prescription dose is 54 Gy in 30 fractions of 1.8 Gy daily.

Conventional RT provides useful palliation for approximately 70% of children with diffuse intrinsic pontine glioma. However, the progression-free survival is short, usually less than 6 months. Neither hyperfractionated nor accelerated RT has improved outcome for these patients. Current protocols are evaluating novel drug therapy approaches based on analysis of tumour biological targets. An interesting more novel radiotherapeutic approach is the use of hypofractionated RT regimens, such as 40 Gy in 15 fractions. Outcomes from case series appear to demonstrate similar disease-free and overall survival compared with a more traditional 6-week regimen and may offer benefits in terms of a reduced burden of travelling for treatment. Furthermore, the use of short courses of re-irradiation such as 20 Gy in 10 fractions appears to be feasible for patients with relapsed disease, and can provide an additional period of palliation.

Ependymoma

Ependymomas arise from the intracranial or spinal ependymal lining. Historically, management was with surgical excision, followed by RT, which was generally craniospinal for those with posterior fossa primaries or high-grade histology. However, it is now generally recognised that, although there is a risk of leptomeningeal metastases at relapse, this risk does not appear to be modified by the use of craniospinal RT. The overall 5-year survival rate is approximately 50% to 60%. In the majority of studies, prognostic factors include the extent of resection and tumour grade. The predominant site of relapse is within the surgical bed, and current research efforts are aimed at improving the prospect of local tumour control. It is important to try to achieve a complete or near complete resection. The current European SIOP ependymoma trial recommends that, for completely resected tumours, postoperative focal RT (59.4 Gy in 33 fractions) should be given using a CTV margin of 1.0 cm. For incompletely resected tumours, an initial trial of chemotherapy using vincristine, cyclophosphamide and etoposide is employed, with further evaluation of postchemotherapy resectability (so-called second-look surgery).

Embryonal Tumours

MB is a primitive neuronal tumour which arises in the cerebellum, usually from the vermis. It is characterised by its propensity for metastatic spread via the CSF (leptomeningeal), its radiosensitivity and its chemosensitivity. Primitive neuroectodermal tumour (PNET) arises elsewhere in the CNS, usually the supratentorial cerebral cortex, but sometimes the pineal area (pineoblastoma). Supratentorial PNET has a significantly worse prognosis (approximately 40%–50% 5-year survival vs. 60%–70% for MB). Recent analyses of the biological parameters exhibited by supratentorial PNETs have concluded that the majority of these should not be reclassified as other histological groups.

MBs are managed by initial surgical resection followed by craniospinal RT and a boost to the primary site. The details of management strategies are now based on classification of histological subtypes of MB combined with molecular biological tumour parameters. In the last 5 years it has been recognised that there are four discrete subtypes of MB which are referred to as WNT, SHH (TP53 mutated and wildtype), group 3 and group 4. This is reflected in the updated WHO classification.

The WNT subgroup is characterised by a very good prognosis compared with the other subgroups, with long-term survival in excess of 90%. The majority of WNT subgroup MBs have classic histology with these tumours demonstrating beta-catenin nucleo-positivity, *CTNNB1* gene mutations, and monosomy 6. WNT MB can occur at all ages but is infrequent in infants. Although overall MB is more common in males, the male-to-female (M:F) ratio for the WNT subgroup is approximately 1:1.

The SHH MB subgroups include *TP53*-mutant and *TP53*-wildtype subgroups. They are named after the sonic hedgehog signalling pathway, which is considered to drive tumour initiation in the majority of cases. The frequency of SHH subgroups of MB is bimodal and is frequent in both infants aged less than 3 years and adults. The M:F ratio is approximately 1:1. The majority of nodular/desmoplastic MBs are included within the SHH subgroup. However, around 50% of SHH subgroup MB have other histological subtypes, including classical, large cell/anaplastic, and MBEN varieties. The prognosis for SHH appears to be similar to group 4 (see later) and intermediate between WNT and group 3.

Group 3 MB represents the subgroup of MB with the worst prognosis. The majority of MBs in group 3 are classical MB and include the majority of large-cell/anaplastic tumours. They occur more commonly in males than females, and arise in infants and older children, but only rarely in adults. They frequently present with leptomeningeal metastases. Group 3 MB is typically characterised by high-level amplification of the *MYC* proto-oncogene, and almost all cases exhibit aberrant *MYC* expression.

Patients with group 4 MB have an intermediate to good prognosis similar to patients with SHH tumours. They include classical and large cell/anaplastic histologies. Group 4 tumours account for approximately 30% to 40% of MB cases. This subgroup represents the archetypal MB, for example, a 7-year-old boy with a classical histology MB. The M:F ratio is approximately 3:1. As the molecular pathogenesis of Group 4 MB is not currently clear, the generic name Group 4 has been allocated pending further insight into molecular characteristics.

Improvements in the understanding of the molecular mechanisms of MB tumourigenesis are emerging as important factors in clinical trial design leading to a tailored approach for different histological and molecular biological subtypes. Collaborative clinical trial groups are developing studies that will investigate prospectively the stratification of therapy according to pathological, biological, as well as the more traditional clinical parameters. In particular, clinical studies are beginning to involve a cautious lowering of the treatment intensity for patients with WNT MB and maintaining intensity for those in group 3. This approach requires a timely and well-coordinated approach to tumour sample collection and analysis of biological parameters before treatment decisions.

Current treatment strategies for MB are based on the allocation of risk status with treatment stratified according to risk (Table 33.4). For example patients with a WNT-pathway MB can be treated with a reduced dose of craniospinal RT, 18 Gy rather than the more conventional 23.4 Gy. For patients with group 3 MB, the priority is to improve outcome by intensification of treatment. Since the 1990s in North America, it has been standard practice to employ adjuvant chemotherapy (vincristine, lomustine (CCNU) and cisplatin) following RT and this has now become standard practice in European studies. Using initial RT, it has been possible to reduce the dose of craniospinal RT for patients with standard-risk MB in North American studies to 23.4 Gy, with 55.8 Gy to the posterior fossa. Because of the poor survival of children with CSF metastases, all children receive chemotherapy and standard dose RT.

TABLE 33.4 Medulloblastoma and Primitive Neuroectodermal Tumour Risk Status

Standard risk	High risk
MB with no evidence of leptomeningeal metastases on MRI scan, <1.5 cm² residual tumour on postoperative MRI scan and no evidence of cells in CSF from lumbar puncture.	MB with evidence of leptomeningeal metastases on MRI scan or cells in CSF from lumbar puncture or supratentorial primary, any stage.

CSF, Cerebrospinal fluid; *MB*, medulloblastoma; *MRI*, magnetic resonance imaging.

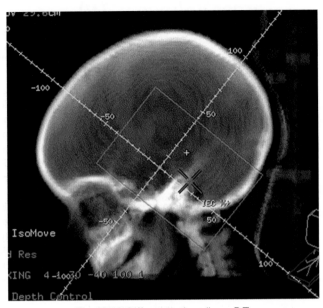

Fig. 33.13 Diffuse pontine glioma R/T.

Studies of Altered Fractionation for Medulloblastoma/Primitive Neuroectodermal Tumour

Hyperfractionated RT (HFRT) involves the use of a larger number of small fractions usually delivered twice daily. Long-term normal tissue effects are related to fraction size, and the aim of HFRT is to improve the therapeutic ratio by increasing the antitumour effect or reducing long-term effects on the CNS or a combination of both.

A multicentre French study, employing a craniospinal RT (CSRT) dose of 36 Gy and a primary tumour dose of 68 Gy has also produced encouraging results. The use of HFRT was evaluated in the European PNET-4 randomised study. The aim of the PNET-4 study was to assess whether survival could be improved by the use of HFRT without an increase in long-term effects. Conventionally fractionated RT, employing a craniospinal dose of 23.4 Gy followed by 30.6 Gy to the posterior fossa was compared with an HFRT regimen. The HFRT dose per fraction was 1 Gy given twice daily with a minimum interval of 8 hours. The craniospinal dose was 36 Gy, with a second phase of 24 Gy to the whole posterior fossa and a final phase of 8 Gy to the tumour bed. The outcome of this trial was that there was no benefit for HFRT with respect to tumour control or survival, and conventional daily fractionation of 1.67 to 1.80 Gy remains the standard of care.

Craniospinal Radiotherapy

CSRT is one of the most complex RT techniques delivered in oncology departments. The shape of the CRT is complex, including the entire cranial and spinal meninges. Traditionally, the technique had employed lateral-opposed cranial fields, with one or more posterior spinal fields carefully matched onto the lower border of the cranial fields. Shielding of face, dentition, nasal structures and lenses is necessary. In the last 10 years there have been significant developments in the advancement of techniques for CSRT to achieve the maximum homogeneity within the CTV and normal tissue sparing. A range of technological solutions are available for the delivery of CSRT, including IMRT, volumetric arc therapy (VMAT) and tomotherapy. Increasingly, proton therapy is being employed to maximise normal tissue sparing, particularly from the exit dose to organs anterior to the spine.

The CTV includes the intracranial and spinal meninges extending inferiorly to the lower border of the thecal sac. Great care is taken to include the cribriform fossa, temporal lobe and base of skull. This should include the extensions of the meninges into the cranial nerve foramina, including the intraorbital optic nerve. In children, the cribriform fossa frequently lies between the lenses (Fig. 33.14A–N). In many series of patients treated for MB, the cribriform fossa has been the site for isolated recurrence in a significant minority of patients. It may not always be possible to treat the CTV and adequately shield the lenses, in which case, priority is given to treating the CTV. Current management involves the use of cisplatin chemotherapy, which carries the risk of ototoxicity. In planning CSRT, the dose to the middle and inner ears is minimised, taking care not to compromise the dose to the CTV.

The lower border of the spinal field has generally been placed at the lower border of the second sacral vertebra. However, there is evidence that the lower border of the thecal sac varies and planning of the lower border of the spinal field should be based on MRI scanning. The spinal field should be wide enough to encompass the extensions of the meninges along the nerve roots, and therefore, wide enough to encompass the intervertebral foramina in the lumbar region. Patients are treated in a Perspex head shell, generally in the supine position which is more comfortable and safer in the case of the requirement for anaesthesia than the traditional prone position. The body may also be immobilised, for example, in an evacuated polystyrene bag. The prescribed dose depends upon clinical scenario. Currently, 23.4 Gy in 13 fractions of 1.8 Gy daily is employed for standard risk MB in the European PNET-5 trial.

Meticulous attention to detail in the planning and delivery of CSRT is essential and accuracy contributes to the chances of cure of MB and other PNETs. It is essential to avoid areas of underdose at field junctions, and to partially shield any part of the intracranial or spinal meninges.

When planning the primary tumour boost for MB, it is generally accepted that the CTV should encompass the surgical cavity together with any residual tumour, with a margin of 1 to 2 cm. It is no longer considered appropriate to include the whole posterior fossa in the boost CTV. In most centres, an IMRT technique or variant would be employed to irradiate the region of the cerebellum.

CSRT techniques are continuing to evolve, and need to incorporate technical developments in RT immobilisation, planning and treatment delivery.

Intracranial Germ Cell Tumours

Intracranial germ cell tumours (GCT) account for approximately 30% of paediatric GCTs and arise in the suprasellar or pineal regions. Germinomas are the histological counterpart of testicular seminoma and may arise in either the suprasellar or pineal regions. Nongerminomatous GCTs, also known as secreting GCTs, are the histological equivalent of testicular nonseminomatous GCTs. They generally arise in the pineal region and may secrete alpha-fetoprotein (AFP) and/or human chorionic gonadotrophin (HCG).

Management of Germinoma

In common with testicular seminoma, germinomas are very radiosensitive. The traditional view has been that CSRT should be employed because of the risk of leptomeningeal metastases and, with this approach, more than 90% of germinomas are cured. However, as with testicular seminoma, there has been a gradual reduction in both the CSRT dose and the dose used for the boost to the primary tumour in an attempt to minimise long-term effects. In the current SIOP protocol, a combination of chemotherapy and focal radiotherapy is employed. The focal RT is given initially with a dose of 24 Gy in 15 fractions to the whole ventricular volume, followed in the case of an incomplete response, by a further 16 Gy in 10 fractions. For

Craniospinal Radiotherapy – Field Arrangement (Conventional Technique)

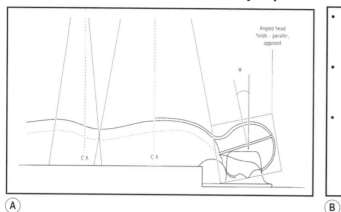

Angled head fields - parallel, opposed

θ

C A   C A

(A)

Target Volume (CTV) Cranial Fields

- Meninges surrounding whole brain and ventricular system

- Particular attention to cribriform fossa, temporal fossa, base of skull

- Shielding for non-target tissues—oropharynx, lenses etc. Shielding should be 0.5 cm anterior to the anterior aspect of the cervical vertebral bodies in order to irradiate the full width of vertebrae

(B)

Target Volume (CTV) Spinal Fields

- Meninges extending to the lower border of the thecal sac

- Extensions of nerve roots as far as intervertebral foramena

- Lower border determined by position of lower border of the thecal sac on MR

(C)

Coronal MR—Cribriform Fossa

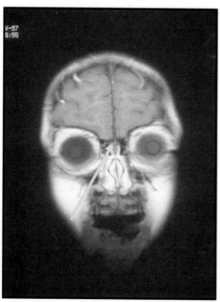

•The cribriform fossa may be close to the lenses particularly in young children
•It may be impossible to adequately irradiate the PTV and also to shield the lenses
•Priority should be given to irradiating the PTV

(D)

Fig. 33.14 (A–N) Series craniospinal radiotherapy field arrangement.

Continued

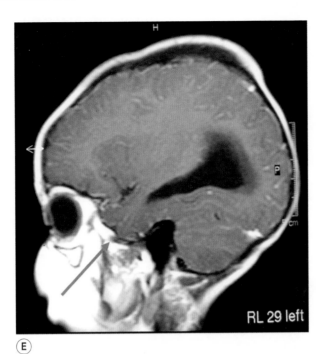

CSRT Temporal Fossa

•Care should be taken to avoid shielding the temporal fossa

(E)

Lower Border of Thecal Sac

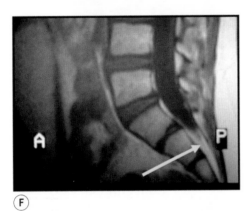

•For CSRT planning the lower border of the Spinal CTV and PTV are based on MR imaging of the lower border of the thecal sac

(F)

Craniospinal Radiotherapy Dose Specification

• Whole brain fields—mid-point of central axis

• Spinal fields—anterior border of spinal cord/posterior border of vertebral bodies

(G)

Fig. 33.14, cont'd

CSRT—Conventional Planning of Spinal Axis

•Anterior border of spinal cord and reconstruction of lower border of thecal sac marked on lateral simulator films

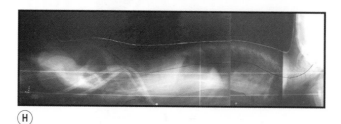

(H)

CSRT—Spinal Plan

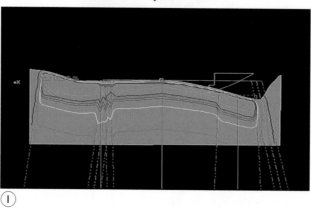

(I)

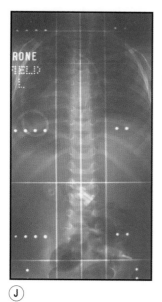

(J)

CSRT Spinal Field

Whole Brain RT Planning Conventional vs CT

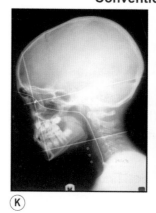
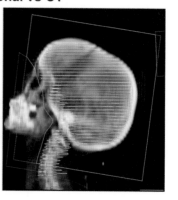

(K)

Fig. 33.14, cont'd

Continued

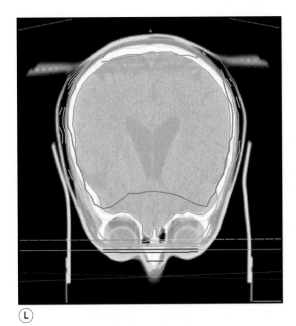

Whole Brain Target Volume Definition Using CT Planning

(L)

CT Simulation for Shielding

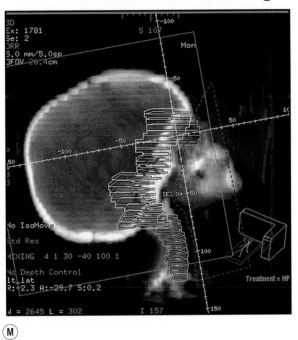

(M)

Craniospinal Radiotherapy Technique

- Exit from upper spinal field should avoid teeth

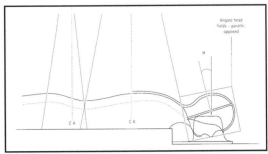

(N)

Fig. 33.14, cont'd

BOX 33.1   Summary of Ten Most Important Paediatric Cancer Trials

Acute Lymphoblastic Leukaemia (ALL)
UKALL2011

The objectives of this current U.K. trial are: to reduce toxicity of induction therapy through introduction of a short 14-day course of high-dose dexamethasone instead of the conventional lower dose given for 28 days. Additionally, objectives are to provide more effective central nervous system (CNS) prophylaxis and reduce overall burden of therapy through introduction of high-dose methotrexate and by omission of vincristine and dexamethasone pulses and continuing intrathecal therapy in the maintenance phase of treatment. An additional aim is to decrease toxicity and reduce burden of therapy by administering a single delayed-drug intensification to all patients and limiting augmented therapy to those who are not minimal residual disease (MRD) low-risk status.

Rhabdomyosarcoma and Non-Rhabdomyosarcoma Soft-Tissue Sarcoma
European Paediatric Soft-Tissue Sarcoma Study Group (EPSSG)

This recently closed European trial evaluated the addition of doxorubicin to standard three-drug chemotherapy (ifosfamide, vincristine, actinomycin-D) for which there was no additional benefit. The trial schema was based on a stratified approach with chemotherapy intensity and radiotherapy dose based on risk status.

Ewing Sarcoma

rEECur is a current international randomised Euro Ewing consortium trial of chemotherapy for the treatment of recurrent and primary refractory Ewing sarcoma. The objective of rEECur is to identify the optimum chemotherapy regimen for recurrent and refractory Ewing sarcoma based on the balance between efficacy and toxicity. Patients are randomised to one of four chemotherapy regimens: topotecan and cyclophosphamide; irinotecan and temozolomide; gemcitabine and docetaxel; or high-dose ifosfamide.

Medulloblastoma
Primitive Neuroectodermal Tumour PNET-5

This current International Society of Paediatric Oncology (SIOP) European trial stratifies treatment according to the outcome of molecular analysis and characterisation into the four medulloblastoma (MB) subtypes and incorporates clinical risk parameters. For WNT (low-risk) cases there is a reduction in the intensity of adjuvant chemotherapy and a reduced dose of craniospinal radiotherapy from 23.4 Gy to 18 Gy. For standard-risk cases there is a randomised study evaluating whether the addition of daily low-dose carboplatin during craniospinal radiotherapy improves outcome.

Ependymoma
Ependymoma-2

This current SIOP European trial is a randomised trial which is investigating whether the addition of chemotherapy (vincristine, etoposide, cyclophosphamide, cisplatin) improves outcome for patients with completely resected intracranial ependymoma treated by complete surgical excision and postoperative radiotherapy, 59.4 Gy in 33 fractions. Patients who have inoperable residual disease also receive a stereotactic radiotherapy boost (8 Gy in 2 fractions) to the residual tumour.

Hodgkin Lymphoma

The closed European Euronet trial incorporated fludeoxyglucose-positron emission tomography (FDG-PET) scanning which can better distinguish between viable and fibrotic/necrotic residual tumour masses. FDG-PET scanning was routinely performed after two cycles of chemotherapy. Patients with an adequate response after two cycles of vincristine, etoposide, prednisolone, doxorubicin (OEPA) were not treated with consolidation radiotherapy. The aim was to maintain a high probability of cure and to reduce the long-term side effects of chemotherapy and radiotherapy. This study aims to eliminate the gonadotoxic drug, procarbazine, from chemotherapy regimens.

Wilms Tumour

The closed European SIOP WT 2001 trial was based on preoperative chemotherapy with vincristine and actinomycin-D. Postsurgical chemotherapy was based on the histological parameters in the surgical nephrectomy specimen. Flank radiotherapy was used for stage 3 disease and whole lung radiotherapy for patients presenting with lung metastases. For patients with intermediate-risk histology stages 2 and 3, there was randomisation testing of whether doxorubicin could be omitted from chemotherapy combinations to reduce the risk of late cardiac complications.

Low-Grade Glioma
LGG2

This closed SIOP European trial was based on a standard chemotherapeutic approach with carboplatin and vincristine to delay radiotherapy for children aged ≤8 years. There was a randomised trial testing whether there was any benefit for the addition of etoposide to the two-drug combination. However, there was no benefit in terms of any additional progression-free interval and the two-drug combination of carboplatin and vincristine remains standard of care for aiming to delay the use of radiotherapy.

Neuroblastoma
SIOPEN High-Risk

The current SIOPEN high-risk neuroblastoma (NB) trial involves a comparison of two different high-dose chemotherapy regimens. The protocol consists of a rapid, dose-intensive induction chemotherapy, peripheral blood stem cell harvest, attempted complete excision of the primary tumour, myeloablative therapy followed by peripheral blood stem cell rescue, radiotherapy (21 Gy) to the surgical primary tumour resection site and immunotherapy.

Intracranial Germ-Cell Tumour

The current SIOP GCT-2 nonrandomised trial has established a standard approach for the management of patients with intracranial germinoma or nongerminomatous germ-cell tumours (NGGCT). Patients with nonmetastatic germinoma are treated by two cycles of etoposide and carboplatin alternating with two courses etoposide and ifosfamide. Radiotherapy is given to the whole ventricles (24 Gy) with those with an incomplete response given an additional tumour bed boost of 16 Gy. For patients with nonmetastatic NGGCT, two cycles of standard etoposide, cisplatin and ifosfamide are followed by two dose-intensified courses of etoposide, cisplatin and ifosfamide with stem cell support. Residual masses are surgically resected or given radiotherapy (54 Gy).

---

nongerminomatous tumours, the prognosis is worse. Initial treatment is with platinum-containing chemotherapy followed by RT, either focal for localised nonmetastatic tumours, or CSRT for those with leptomeningeal metastases. For secreting GCT, the total RT dose is 54 Gy to the primary tumour, with 30 Gy CSRT for patients with leptomeningeal metastases.

Craniopharyngioma

Craniopharyngiomas account for approximately 5% to 10% of intracranial tumours in childhood. These are predominantly cystic tumours which arise in the suprasellar area from remnants of Rathke's pouch. Although considered histologically benign, they are often associated with considerable morbidity such as pituitary deficiencies, including diabetes insipidus and disturbances of hypothalamic function, such as obesity. They are frequently adherent to adjacent structures within the CNS. There is a significant risk of involvement of the optic chiasm with a risk of visual impairment or blindness. Small craniopharyngiomas may be amenable to complete surgical excision if this can be achieved without a risk of damage to the optic chiasm. An alternative approach is to consider partial or subtotal excision of the tumour with postoperative RT. The margin for CTV around the GTV is generally approximately 0.5 cm, with a dose of 50 to 55 Gy in a fraction size of 1.67 to 1.8 Gy. With either complete resection or partial resection and postoperative RT, long-term local control rates of approximately 80% can be achieved.

Proton Therapy for Paediatric Tumours

Proton therapy has been available for several decades in selected centres, mainly in North America. There is an increasing use of proton therapy in North America and Europe for the treatment of children with a wide range of cancers. In the United Kingdom, high energy proton facilities opened in 2018. In recent years, there has been increasing interest in the potential role for proton therapy in the management of paediatric tumours. The modulated Bragg peak can deliver homogeneous irradiation to the target volume while reducing the magnitude and/or extent of the low-dose area beyond. This may be clinically relevant for long-term effects in children. For several decades, proton therapy has had an established role in the treatment of adults with skull base chordomas and chondrosarcomas. This role has now been extended to the treatment of children. In addition, planning studies have demonstrated the potential for improving the therapeutic ratio for RT for tumours either within or adjacent to the CNS and achieving a uniform dose within the target volume, while potentially minimising the severity of neuropsychological sequelae.

CONCLUSIONS

Paediatric oncology management continues to present many challenges and RT plays an important role in the treatment of many of these children. They require the highest standard of RT planning and delivery, incorporating modern technical developments. Children present with a wide variety of malignancies which pose many different problems for patients themselves and their families. Thus, management needs to be family centred as well as patient centred. Although cure rates for the majority of childhood cancers have continued to improve over the last decade, this has frequently been achieved with increased intensity of chemotherapy. Compared with adult radiation oncology practice, when planning RT for children, consideration of the long-term effects of treatment is always of paramount importance. With the increasing use of concurrent combined modality therapy, including intensive chemotherapy, constant vigilance for interactions between chemotherapy and RT is required. Therapeutic developments initially investigated in adults, such as hyperfractionation, also require investigation for childhood cancers.

FURTHER READING

Ajithkumar T, et al. Radiotherapy in the Management of Paediatric Low-Grade Gliomas. Clinical Oncology 2019;31(3):151–61.

Ajithkumar T, et al. "Indeed, Cure is Not Enough"–A Reflection on Paediatric Radiation Oncology. Clinical Oncology 2019;31(3):135–8.

Arumugam S, et al. The Evidence for External Beam Radiotherapy in High-Risk Neuroblastoma of Childhood: A Systematic Review. Clinical Oncology 2019;31(3):182–90.

Bisogno G, Jenney M, Bergeron C, et al. Addition of dose-intensified doxorubicin to standard chemotherapy for rhabdomyosarcoma (EpSSG RMS 2005): a multicentre, open-label, randomised controlled, phase 3 trial. Lancet Oncol 2018;19:1061–71.

Calaminus G, Kortmann R, Worch J. SIOP CNS GCT 96: final report of outcome of a prospective, multinational nonrandomized trial for children and adults with intracranial germinoma, comparing craniospinal irradiation alone with chemotherapy followed by focal primary site irradiation for patients with localized disease. Neuro Oncol 2013;15:788–96.

Constine LS, et al. Pediatric Normal Tissue Effects in the Clinic (PENTEC): An International Collaboration to Analyse Normal Tissue Radiation Dose–Volume Response Relationships for Paediatric Cancer Patients. Clinical Oncology 2019;31(3):199–207.

Gaze MN. Good Practice Guide for Paediatric Radiotherapy. Clinical Oncology 2019;31(3):139–41.

Gnekow AK, Walker DA, Kandels D, et al. A European randomised controlled trial of the addition of etoposide to standard vincristine and carboplatin induction as part of an 18-month treatment programme for childhood (≤16 years) low grade glioma—a final report. Eur J Cancer 2017;81:206–25.

Greaves M. Childhood leukaemia. Br Med J 2002;324:283–7.

Ladenstein R, Potschger U, Le Deley MC, et al. Primary disseminated multifocal Ewing sarcoma: results of the Euro-EWING 99 trial. J Clin Oncol 2010;28:3284–91.

Lannering B, Rutkowski S, Doz F, et al. Standard risk medulloblastoma: hyperfractionated vs conventional radiotherapy followed by chemotherapy. Results from the randomized multicenter study HIT-SIOP PNET 4. J Clin Oncol 2012;30:3187–93.

Matthay KK, Reynolds CP, Seeger RC, et al. Long-term results for children with high-risk neuroblastoma treated on a randomized trial of myeloablative therapy followed by 13-cis-retinoic acid: a Children's Oncology Group study. J Clin Oncol 2009;27:1007–13.

Mauz-Korholz C, Metzger ML, Kelly KM, et al. Pediatric Hodgkin lymphoma. J Clin Oncol 2015;33:2975–85.

Merchant TE, Mulhern RK, Krasin MJ, et al. Preliminary results from a phase II trial of conformal radiation therapy and evaluation of radiation-related CNS effects for pediatric patients with localized ependymoma. J Clin Oncol 2004;22:3156–62.

Padovani L, et al. Radiotherapy Advances in Paediatric Medulloblastoma Treatment. Clinical Oncology 2019;31(3):171–81.

Pritchard-Jones K, Bergeron C, de Camargo B, et al. Omission of doxorubicin from the treatment of stage II–III, intermediate-risk Wilms' tumour (SIOP WT 2001): an open-label, non-inferiority, randomised controlled trial. Lancet 2015;386:1156–64.

Steinmeier T, et al. Evolving Radiotherapy Techniques in Paediatric Oncology. Clinical Oncology 2019;31(3):142–50.

Thorp N, et al. Management of Ependymoma in Children, Adolescents and Young Adults. Clinical Oncology 2019;31(3):162–70.

Tsang DS, et al. Re-irradiation for Paediatric Tumours. Clinical Oncology 2019;31(3):191–8.

34

Care of Patients During Radiotherapy

Lorraine Webster, Angela Duxbury

CHAPTER OUTLINE

INTRODUCTION

When patients are referred for radiotherapy (RT), they will expect that their treatment is planned and delivered in an optimal way. Everyone involved in this process is well aware that patients have a right to expect that they will be well cared for and supported during this time. It is central to the National Health Service (NHS) constitution that patients have the right to receive high quality, effective, compassionate care from the right people with the right skills and the right values.

The quality of this care is dependent on a multiplicity of factors and the aim should be that it is all encompassing, addressing both the physical and emotional needs of patients and this should be our aspiration whether the treatment intent is to cure or to palliate. The most simplistic method of exploring supportive care in RT is to consider any aspect of care that may be experienced by the patient within the physical, psychosocial and spiritual realm and this chapter will introduce some of the key themes within supportive care of all RT patients. The physical aspects of supportive care in relation to the management of site-specific conditions are addressed in related chapters in this text. In addition, these and the other aspects of care can be explored further in specialist texts which deal with issues relating to palliative care, symptom control and psychosocial interventions.

The responsibility of assessing how patients are as they progress through treatment and how they are coping with their treatment belongs to all, as is an acknowledgment of where an individual's skills/expertise start and stop and when patients should be cared for by more appropriate members of the team. It is to be recommended that RT centres adopt a culture which encourages both the philosophy and the mechanisms to facilitate such a team approach and this team approach should reach out to the interface between primary and secondary care. Coordination of care therefore needs patients and their carers to remain the focus of the process and this means that they should be kept informed and involved, and that their autonomy and rights to be included in the treatment decision-making process is respected at all times.

ASSESSMENT OF INDIVIDUAL PATIENT AND CARER NEEDS

To provide care appropriate to patient need requires first assessing and establishing what that need is. Inadequate assessment of the patient's physical symptoms and psychosocial needs may lead to a failure to recognise their need, with the result that necessary services may be denied to them. However, one of the challenges for today's cancer care is that effective assessment is dependent on providing appropriate training and education for health care professionals to allow them to appreciate the complexity of support needs. This presents another challenge for cancer and RT services because, in many instances, there is a lack of available supportive care services for the health care professional to call on.

So what aspects of the patient's well being should be assessed? Although it is vital that the needs of the patient, in respect of their medical and physical condition are addressed, it is important that all health care professionals acknowledge that asking patients how they are feeling and coping from an emotional and psychological level should be central to this process. In doing this, consideration should be given to patients' and carers' needs in relation to:

- Control and management of physical effects of treatment and disease and associated side effects.
- Evidence-based quality-assured patient information materials, including written, DVD and digital- and web-based technologies.
- Good communication and involvement in decision making.
- Psychological, social and spiritual support.
- Family and carer support.
- Complementary therapies.
- Bereavement support services.

Physical and psychological symptoms do not sit in isolation from each other and can, indeed, be synergistic. Patients have varying coping mechanisms and family support available to them and this is something that must be considered when supportive care is being addressed.

TABLE 34.1 Radiation Therapy Oncology Group Grading of Acute Skin Reactions

RTOG 0	RTOG 1	RTOG 2a	RTOG 2b	RTOG 3
No visible change	Faint or dull erythema	Tender or bright erythema with/without dry desquamation	Patchy moist desquamation; moderate oedema	Confluent moist desquamation; pitting oedema

RTOG, Radiation Therapy Oncology Group.

Patients' quality of life is affected not only by the physical and emotional impact of their cancer but also by the treatments prescribed to treat their condition. Because RT causes a degree of damage to the normal tissues of the body and can cause local and systemic side effects, this aspect of their management should be considered of pivotal importance. These side effects can be acute or delayed, with acute (early effects) occurring during radiation treatment and continuing after treatment or in the subsequent weeks and months. Although side effects of RT are to an extent unavoidable, they can be managed if patients are well supported and appropriate advice is given before and as they progress through treatment. Such support and education should be an essential component of the management process for all patients receiving RT.

SKIN REACTIONS

Skin reactions from external beam RT are one of the most common side effects from treatment which may cause distress to some patients, and in certain cases may be a factor that can limit radiation dose and treatment schedules.

Megavoltage linear accelerators with skin-sparing capabilities and customised treatment shapes have significantly reduced the severity of reactions from RT; however, the use of accelerated radiation dose schedules with concurrent chemotherapy can increase skin toxicity.

All patients receiving external beam therapy are at some risk of skin damage and as such, in most departments this is addressed by offering suitable advice and support by monitoring and recording the severity of these reactions during treatment.

Skin toxicity has two phases: an initial acute toxicity phase predominantly driven by inflammation and temporary cessation in stem cell proliferation, and a late or chronic toxicity effect characterised by fibrosis and its effects. This includes reduced lymphovascular functioning, resulting in lymphoedema and poor wound healing from reduced vascularity.

Acute skin reactions range from mild erythema, hyperpigmentation and dry to moist desquamation occurring more frequently in the head and neck area, breast and chest wall and areas with skin folds. With conventional fractionated radiation therapy, erythema and hyperpigmentation develop approximately during the third week of treatment and become more pronounced through the remainder of treatment. Dry and/or moist desquamation may develop during the 4th to 6th weeks of treatment. With hypofractionated schedules, these reactions can occur earlier. In practice, consideration must be given to changing techniques and fractionation schedules. For example, in breast cancer RT there has been a change from a 25-fraction to a 15-fraction schedule and some patients are not developing skin reactions until after treatment has finished; this requires a different approach to post RT information and management.

The various factors that influence how people react to RT need to be considered in advice designed to be given to patients, particularly, intrinsic factors which include demographic- or disease-related characteristics such as age, hormonal status, infection, ethnic origin, smoking, obesity and co-existing disease (e.g. diabetes). In addition, there are extrinsic factors that are treatment related and influence the delivery of therapy; these include treatment dose, volume, fractionation, site of treatment, beam energy, adjuvant chemotherapy and targeted therapies.

However, the goal of good management is to have a system in place that facilitates the identification of risk and delays the onset of skin reactions. This can be facilitated by having a patient-review process that includes the assessment grading and recording of skin reactions. The most widely used assessment tool is the Radiation Therapy Oncology Group (RTOG) grading system (Table 34.1), although it should be noted that the common toxicity scale tends to be used to assess acute and late effects of skin in clinical trials.

Patients should be provided with information explaining:
- How and why skin reactions occur.
- When they are likely to appear.
- What they will look and feel like.
- How they will be treated.
- Where the reaction is likely to occur.
- Self-care strategies.
- Risk factors.

The U.K. College of Radiographers has produced a clinical practice guideline that outlines a set of evidence-based recommendations to assist radiographers, RT nurses and the wider RT workforce in advising patients how to care for their skin while undergoing a course of radical external beam RT (excluding proton therapy). The guideline has been developed systematically using the best available evidence from research and expert opinion and subjected to peer, professional and lay assessment. The guideline has recommendations for evidence-based practice; however, it concludes that overall, the current evidence base is not strong enough to either support or refute the use of any particular product for topical application.

However, in a subsequent study published in Erridge et al. 2016, findings advocate the use of prophylactic steroids, such as betamethasone cream for patients who are at high risk of radiation dermatitis; application can significantly reduce erythema, itching, discomfort and sleep disturbance.

Gosselin et al. in 2010 noted, 'patients prefer to take action rather than do nothing' so the focus for skin care should be on alleviating symptoms and providing comfort.

Involving patients in the prevention/care of skin reactions is an important element of the management process and reducing irritants to irradiated skin is a part of this self-care strategy.

Recording of patient acceptability/satisfaction and compliance with skin-care advice is recommended as such information can be used to evaluate the appropriateness of skin-care products for future patients.

Skin can be exposed to a number of irritants which, if avoided, can lessen the likelihood of a troublesome reaction (Table 34.2).

How to care for radiation skin reactions once they have occurred and what products to recommend in this event requires a knowledge of the more general wound care literature. It is important that advice and treatment given to patients is evidence based. Table 34.3 provides some details on skin-care products which can be used.

TABLE 34.2	Recommendations for Reducing Irritants to Irradiated Skin During a Course of Radiotherapy
Sun exposure	Protect from direct sun exposure: cover with clothing or shade area. Stress the risk from sun exposure during and following radiotherapy. Sunscreen with both UVA/UVB protection; minimum SPF-30 should be used on previously irradiated skin.
Mechanical irritants (guidelines apply within the treatment fields only)	Minimise friction: wash or shower gently; avoid using a washcloth; pat dry with a soft, clean towel; wear loose fitting, soft clothing. Avoid shaving, or shave causing as little trauma to skin as possible; suggest electric shaver. Avoid hair removal creams. Avoid scratching. Avoid rubbing vigorously and massaging. Avoid use of adhesive tape in treatment field. Wash hair gently with usual shampoo if the scalp is in the treatment field, but do not dry with a hairdryer or use hair straighteners or curling tongs.
Chemical irritants	Current guidelines show no evidence for avoidance of using normal shower/washing products unless they begin to cause discomfort or skin is broken. There is no evidence to support not using deodorant, therefore, patient may continue with normal products unless they begin to cause discomfort or skin is broken. Apply only recommended products—check with treatment centre and refer to Table 34.3. Avoid perfume and aftershave if these are to be applied within the treatment area. Use a moisturiser that is SLS-free (see Table 34.3). Use mild detergent to wash clothing.
Thermal irritants	Use water that is not overly hot. Avoid exposure to temperature extremes. Avoid application of ice packs or heat (e.g. heating pad, hot water bottles, sun lamp).

Informed by the UK College of Radiographers—Skin-Care Advice for Patients Undergoing Radical External Beam Megavoltage Radiotherapy, 2015.
SLS, Sodium lauryl sulphate.

TABLE 34.3	Characteristics of Skin-Care Products for Each Stage of Radiation Skin Reactions
No change in skin (RTOG 0)	No intervention required. No evidence to support using a moisturiser will prevent or delay skin reaction; however, some patients may prefer to do so. Advise only for SLS-free moisturiser as below in RTOG 1.
Faint or dull erythema (RTOG 1)	Use of an SLS-free moisturiser may be applied to skin within the treatment field and may soothe and moisturise skin. There is no evidence that any one cream may be superior, therefore, this cannot be stated as a recommendation and patients can elect to choose their preference; however, SLS-free creams include: Zerobase, Diprobase, Aquamax, Aveeno, Cetraben, Epimax, QV Cream and E45.
Tender or bright erythema (RTOG 2a)	Use of urea 10% cream may alleviate pruritus if present. Where a rash is present, hydrocortisone 1% may act as an antiinflammatory. Skin to be reviewed and documented daily.
Patchy moist desquamation (RTOG 2b)	Dressings should be nonadhesive. Hydrogel dressing and nonadhesive dressings such as soft polymer dressings and polyurethane foam film dressings without adhesives may be used. These will depend on local policy.
Moist desquamation (pitting oedema) (RTOG 3)	Choice of dressing is determined by site, amount of exudate and potential need for removal before treatment. Principles of wound management are applicable; dressings of choice should maintain a moist environment in the wound bed; keep the area clean to minimise risk of infection, keep the wound warm to encourage mitotic activity and prevent friction. The wound exudates contain nutrients, enzymes and white blood cells which are important for healing. Maintain clear documentation of wound assessment undertaken and involve a multidisciplinary review approach as per local policies; involve Tissue Viability Team if required.

RTOG, Radiation Therapy Oncology Group; *SLS,* sodium lauryl sulphate.

Skin-care practices for RT patients may be complicated by dosimetric concerns. In a study by Morley et al. (2016), authors measured the effect on skin dose of various topical agents and dressings. The research findings were, under clinically relevant conditions, no topical agents or dry dressing increased the skin dose beyond that seen with a thermoplastic mask. Dressings soaked with water produced less skin dose than 5 mm bolus; however, this may be unacceptable if wet dressings are in place for the majority of the treatment course. These results suggest that skin-care practices should not be limited by dosimetric concerns when using a 6-MV photon beam.

Other sources which may be useful include published national skin-care guidelines. A serious skin infection may require a systemic antibiotic or can be prevented with a topical application of an antibiotic cream, such as 1% silver sulfadiazine cream (Flamazine).

When moist desquamation becomes infected or infection is suspected, a silver- or iodine-based antimicrobial dressing may be used. Care should be taken to ensure the dressing is designed to prevent silver being absorbed by the wound (check manufacturer's information) and the dressing should be removed daily before treatment.

Late skin toxicity symptoms can occur months or years after treatment and include alopecia, telangiectasias, pigmentation change, fibrosis, poor would healing, ulceration and cartilage or bone necrosis. Therefore, patients should be given the advice to protect the treated area from sun exposure for life.

NUTRITION

Radiation treatment to several different regions (head and neck, gastrointestinal, pelvis, thoracic) can cause anorexia and result in significant weight loss. Anorexia can cause functional limitations, as well as significant emotional distress. Treatment-related anorexia may have implications for survival in certain patient populations. In a study of 364 patients receiving preoperative chemoradiation for locally advanced rectal cancer, severe weight loss during chemoradiation was found to impact on survival. Critical weight loss (>10%) was found to be independently associated with worse overall survival in patients with head and neck cancer receiving RT.

Guidance on nutritional status and diet for patients undergoing RT can impact positively on patients if it is undertaken in a routine and evidence-based manner. The nutritional status of patients may be adversely affected by not only their disease, but by the impact of their RT. Treatment-induced toxicities such as dry mouth, mucositis, dysphagia, nausea, vomiting, diarrhoea and tenesmus can all impact negatively on nutritional status and, ultimately, upon the quality of life of patients. In addition, when patients are referred for RT they may already have undergone surgical intervention, chemotherapy or both and they may also be receiving concomitant treatment that could exacerbate further their nutritional status. These factors and the possibility that food intake may be modified during RT make it essential that sound nutritional advice and support are available.

Although RT will not have a significant adverse impact on the nutritional status of all patients, they still require sufficient nutrition to support tissue repair. Patients often have coexisting medical and social conditions that can affect nutritional status and it is important that these are recognised and their impact incorporated into nutritional planning.

In patients where side effects of treatment commonly jeopardise nutritional status, for example, head and neck, oesophagus, colorectal and pelvis/abdomen, patients must be screened to identify those who need a more in-depth nutritional assessment. Studies demonstrate the benefits that can be gained when early intervention and a proper assessment of nutritional status and requirements are undertaken alongside early nutritional counselling and monitoring of diet. In some patients undergoing RT and/or chemotherapy–radiotherapy for head and neck cancer, a percutaneous endoscopic gastrostomy (PEG) tube is surgically inserted into the stomach through the abdominal wall before treatment and is used as a way of introducing foods, fluids and medicines directly into the stomach to maintain good nutritional status.

Advice to patients should, wherever possible, have an evidence base and will be dependent upon the area being treated, the regimen employed and a myriad of other factors. Treatment and advice to patients should therefore be tailored to suit their needs. However, it is essential that initial assessment of all patients is carried out, in order that appropriate action can be taken at a time when any condition can be more easily dealt with. Identifying the reason for the impaired nutrition is pivotal to its adequate treatment and, although dieticians are the key professionals, this is the responsibility of the multidisciplinary team. Patients should be directed to existing good quality sources of information.

NAUSEA, VOMITING AND DIARRHOEA

There is little doubt that these issues can cause a significant threat to the comfort and well being of patients and impact on quality of life. It is important that patients are monitored for the development of such side effects, that their severity is assessed and that appropriate treatment is instigated.

Side effects such as dehydration and weight loss as a consequence of diarrhoea are to be avoided and, although some patients may find it difficult to discuss, a comprehensive assessment of the condition is essential in order that the appropriate pharmacological therapy be made available. Loperamide (Imodium) is a frequently used standby in the treatment of diarrhoea. Codeine phosphate is especially useful if diarrhoea is associated with colicky abdominal pain.

In relation to the prevention of nausea and vomiting, granisetron 2 mg orally an hour before RT can be a very good prophylaxis even for wide-field RT.

FATIGUE

One of the most common symptoms experienced by cancer patients is fatigue. It is described as one of the most distressing symptoms patients experience while receiving radiation; symptoms of fatigue can persist for months to years, affecting quality of life over a long time span. Radiation-related fatigue occurs across a wide range of cancer types and can contribute to depression, anxiety, concentration difficulties, decreased participation in work and recreational activities and difficulty with relationships. In a study by Storey et al., (2007) the group of patients most at risk of chronic cancer-related fatigue were young, female and treated for breast cancer.

Fatigue is a multidimensional phenomenon which makes it difficult to describe. It has been attributed to both the illness, *cancer-related fatigue* and, as it develops, the term *radiotherapy-related fatigue* is used. Fatigue tends to begin 1 to 2 weeks into treatment course and has been shown to peak 1 to 2 weeks post-RT and strategies to support staff in supporting patients during RT to manage fatigue have been published.

Patients can describe fatigue in many ways, as feelings of tiredness, exhaustion, lethargy and being overwhelmed by events. Patients should be advised that, although their treatment may cause tiredness, they should try to get enough rest and sleep and try to continue some of their daily activities.

Potential treatments for fatigue are to correct any nonradiation-related causes of fatigue, for example, anaemia. Treatments for radiation-induced fatigue and data assessing these treatments are limited; however, treatments can be divided into pharmacologic and nonpharmacologic.

Several nonpharmacological interventions are recommended and several studies have shown an improvement in fatigue with physical exercise. Macmillan Cancer Support, U.K., disseminates information, underpinned by research, promoting the advantages of exercise in helping alleviate side effects, fatigue and depression as well as overall health benefits.

If fatigue is caused by underlying depression or a sleep disorder caused by anxiety, these underlying causes should be treated before using pharmacologic treatments such as psychostimulants and corticosteroids.

Cancer treatment-related fatigue generally improves after therapy is complete but some level of fatigue may persist for months or years following treatment. Research indicates that for at least a subset of patients, fatigue may be a significant issue long into survivorship.

PSYCHOSOCIAL ISSUES

It is crucial to remember that patients do not exist with a particular illness in isolation and that the dynamics of family and social relationships that may or may not exist within their own supportive networks may influence the content, context and ability to offer the desired or needed care. The patient should rarely be considered in isolation and due thought and support should also be given to the needs of close family and carers, as they will also experience many similar feelings to those of our patients. The family is an extended agent of patient care and a cancer illness can have a profound effect not only on patients, but on their relatives and, indeed, the process of a patient informing relatives of their illness can be traumatic for all concerned.

Many patients and carers experience a range of psychological and emotional challenges as a result of their diagnosis and subsequent treatment effects. Research suggests that the prevalence of long-term psychological distress in cancer patients ranges from 20% to 66% and is higher than the general population. This was found in a study that screened for psychological distress in very long-term adult survivors of childhood cancer.

Distress and psychological complications may be better recognised by using a simple validated screening tool, such as the Emotion Therapy (ET) developed by Mitchell, that identify patients in need of further psychological evaluation (Fig. 34.1).

There are also the practical implications of illness, and a patient and their family may have difficulties in terms of their financial and employment status, as well as disruption caused by changes in their role and the family dynamics.

For the patient coming to terms with a cancer diagnosis, it has become helpful to think of their emotional adjustment as a series of different emotional stages. Barraclough, 1999 describes patients initially experiencing shock, numbness or disbelief, often with the bad news seeming too much to take in. This usually short-term denial is then followed by distress as the reality of the situation becomes clear, and is often associated with anger, anxiety, and protest and bargaining. This phase often lasts a number of weeks and can be followed by sadness and depression, again taking several weeks before gradual movement to adjustment and acceptance, taking weeks and even months.

Although this is a useful guide to apply to many situations associated with loss of any kind, it is important to caution against using it as a simple sequential model of what every patient (and their carers) will experience. Although many will react with some of the above emotions, we should not expect all to be initially shocked by a diagnosis and then work through all the stages to a final acceptance. Often there are more individual emotions and they may not occur in any clear order, or may overlap or may be gone through more than once, particularly in an illness that has remissions and relapses or a series of progressive deteriorations. Heightened anxiety and intensity of these emotions will occur most strongly at diagnosis, during treatment episodes and times of recurrence and in the terminal phase.

A summary of some of the common responses and influencing factors is illustrated in Fig. 34.2, which aims to illustrate the dynamic that emotional adjustment changes through time, and is affected by many different factors which will be highly individualised for each patient. These reactions do not occur in any particular order and are particular to the individual who may move in and out of the different responses as the stimuli change.

In a study by Appleton and Perkins (2017), the authors explore how help is constructed during and following RT for patients with cancer. This study provides the basis for a greater understanding on the part of professionals into the impact of diagnosis and RT treatment on family and friends. In doing so, the study identifies opportunities for the experience of helpers to be recognised and supported by professionals.

COMMUNICATION

There is compelling evidence demonstrating that good, patient-centred communication is associated with important and meaningful health outcomes. The benefits of effective communication between health care professionals and patients include improvements in treatment compliance and satisfaction with their care and decision making, as well as overall improvement in their psychosocial adjustment. In addition, it is important to highlight that a major effect of poor communication is dissatisfaction. When patients are dissatisfied and feel unable to speak freely, it has a negative effect on the likelihood that they will offer and seek the information necessary for a good informative exchange.

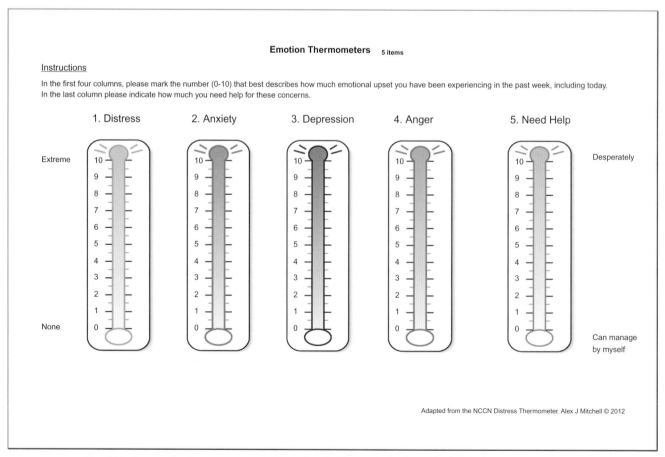

Fig. 34.1 The emotion thermometer tool. (Reproduced with permission from Alex Mitchell. www.psycho-oncology.info/ET.htm.)

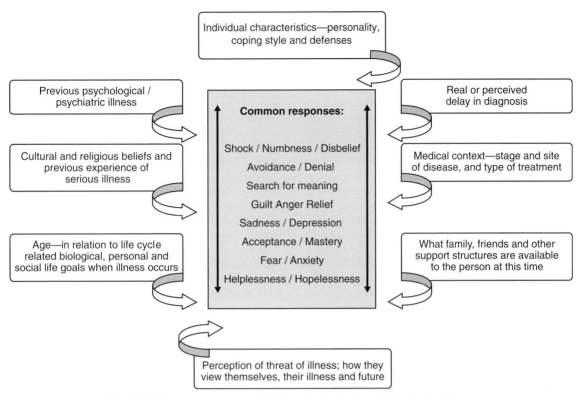

Fig. 34.2 Common responses and influencing factors in a life-threatening illness.

The resultant effect of this is that the accurate exchange of information will be limited.

It must therefore be acknowledged that good communication is essential to allow patients and their carers to be involved with decisions about their care. Patients and carers place a lot of importance on face-to-face communication with health care professionals and is the usual way information is given at crucial points in the patient's illness and treatment pathway. Indeed, the NHS cancer plan cites that a "willingness to listen and explain" is considered by patients to be one of the essential attributes of a health professional.

In addition, effective communication is central to the identification of an individual's specific needs and the provision of appropriate information and psychosocial support. Health care professionals also need to be sensitive to the particular needs of each person in terms of awareness of issues of age, gender, culture and socioeconomic status.

Good communication also involves more than just being able to use the right words for a particular situation. It also requires an ability to listen and hear the person, and engage with them both emotionally and psychologically.

Although all professionals involved in cancer care are increasingly aware of the need to interact effectively with patients, many feel inadequately trained in the various aspects of communication. There is also growing expectation from patients and their families that good communication is an essential component of their cancer treatment and care and it therefore becomes an important focus for all health professionals to judge whether they have addressed an individual patient or carer's communication and information needs within any consultation or interaction.

INFORMATION

It is now widely accepted that seeking information is one strategy that many people use to help them cope with the challenges that a cancer diagnosis brings. The consensus would appear to be that the provision of appropriate, timely and honest information can make them feel more in control of their situation and can therefore be a key element for many people in managing the experience of cancer. In addition, there is evidence that the psychological distress in patients with serious illness is less when they think that they have received adequate information.

It is therefore important that any health care professional working with cancer patients should be attuned to the fact that patients are unlikely to have retained all the relevant information, particularly after one consultation. Hence, there is a need to assess this accurately and consistently, and to repeat and reinforce this at subsequent consultations and visits for treatments.

Regardless of the amount of information retained, because patients tend to remember what they have been told first, rather than subsequent information, it can be difficult to undo any wrong perception and understanding of the patient and their carers in relation to this. It is therefore vital that there is consistency in explaining diagnosis, prognosis, treatment and effects. Consequently, it is exceptionally important that this is given accurately and not contradicted at a later date by the same person or another member of the team.

However, it should be acknowledged that this remains an area of many challenges and tensions for all involved in working with patients with cancer for several reasons. Although research has demonstrated that a majority of people want to be informed about all aspects of their disease and treatment, there is a responsibility also to be sensitive to the minority who do not. Acknowledge that patients' information needs will change through time and that this needs to be judged at the level of the individual patient and carer need, and should be assessed on an ongoing basis throughout the patient pathway. For example, a person's desire for information at the time of diagnosis may be very different at a time of relapse. Thus the challenge is that information given is appropriate to an individual's personal needs and circumstances; when and how we communicate this information is crucial.

The NHS has committed to deliver the information needs of all people with cancer with access to online communication of information and online access to test results by 2020.

CONSENT

The NHS plan pledges that consent must be sought from all NHS patients. Both English and Scottish law state that before you examine, treat or care for competent adult patients you must obtain their consent. The Department of Health's Reference Guide to the consent process offers a comprehensive summary of the law on consent and offers help on frequently asked questions for both health professionals and patients (available at www.doh.gov.uk/consent). This provides a comprehensive guide and is usually well supplemented by individual health providers producing their own guidelines for use at a local level.

With respect to the issue of competence, as a general guide, the professional seeking consent should consider the question of whether a patient can understand and weigh up the information needed to make the required decision. It is also important to bear in mind that, if a patient reaches a decision that appears unexpected, it may not indicate incompetence, but rather a need for further information or explanation.

Thus, information giving is pivotal to underpinning a morally and ethically sound consent process. In essence, informed consent requires that patients have had their treatment options and procedures explained in a way that they can understand and, as patients are increasingly involved in their own health care, they need possession of the facts, including risks and benefits, to enable them to make decisions about their own treatment and care. This is important at all stages in the process but, particularly, at times when stages of illness and treatment options change. Indeed, the law regards giving and obtaining consent to be a process, not a one-off event and, therefore, must be valued as crucial in the treatment of cancer where different treatment options, such as further chemotherapy and RT, are required in the disease trajectory. It is also important to be aware that a patient may change their mind and withdraw consent at any time and this is applicable to any patient, not only to those in clinical trials. As a general guidance point, if in any doubt, always check that the patient still consents to treatment.

With respect to explaining particular benefits and risks associated with treatment to patients, these will relate specifically to site and stage of disease as well as treatment intent and planned rationale. For example, whether RT is being combined with chemotherapy will affect not only outcome, but early and late effects of treatment, as will whether the patient has had previous surgery. Although the current Department of Health guidelines state that patients should be advised on substantial or unusual risks of treatment, the detail of these for site-specific conditions are beyond the scope of this chapter. However, it is worth noting that many cancer centres now include specific details of both acute and late effects of treatment for specific cancers as an essential element in the consent process, and this level of written detail can aid the professional seeking consent. In addition, it allows the patient to have time to reflect on many of the effects discussed and to give due consideration before actually consenting to treatment. The important message to get across to patients is one that should be balanced. That yes, RT does carry risks (and these should be explained individually for each patient and their related cancer), but must always be weighed against the risks of not having any treatment at all. It should also be emphasised that, generally, the long-term risks tend to be rare and affect a very small number of people and that generally, the benefits of RT treatment far outweigh the possibilities of involved risks.

In answer to the question of who should seek consent, it is advised that it is always best for the actual person who is in charge of treating the patient to ask. However, it is deemed acceptable that consent may be sought on behalf of colleagues if the health care professional involved is capable of performing the procedure and can explain fully what the procedure involves or has been trained to seek consent for that procedure.

SPIRITUAL NEEDS

Increasingly, research is demonstrating the importance of spiritual care. It is especially important when patients and their carers face a life-threatening condition. Defining spirituality is challenging, to a degree it is intangible, but can be said to encompass those facets of an individual which give a sense of purpose and meaning to life. Breirbart (2002) reviews the topics of spirituality and end-of-life care. He defines spirituality and suggests measures of spirituality that deal with two of its main components: faith/religious beliefs and meaning/spiritual well-being.

In essence, an awareness of the existential aspects of life and its meaning may be awakened. Contemporary medical literature supports the importance of spirituality for patients and proposes that strong spiritual beliefs can aid individuals fighting illness. It has been suggested that spiritual well being can have a positive effect on a patient's coping skills and their quality of life and can promote feelings of peace and acceptance. There are those however, who identify the dangers of the spiritual challenge when patients ask, "Why me?"

Patients need to be supported to find coping mechanisms during their illness and the spiritual dimension may help in this process. There is a recognition that meeting spiritual needs is important and policies to develop and implement spiritual care in our centres are now being advised. A study by Murray et al. (2004) concluded that spiritual issues were significant for many patients in their last year of life and their carers and that many health professionals lack the necessary time and skills to uncover and address such issues. There is a growing body of evidence that suggests providing interventions that can have a positive impact on the spiritual well-being among patients can also increase the spiritual well-being among family care givers of cancer patients.

Addressing a patient's spirituality can be a challenge, but communicating at this level can be a positive experience for health care professionals as well as patients.

COMPLEMENTARY THERAPIES

Complementary therapies do not offer patients an alternative approach to established treatments such as surgery, chemotherapy and RT but, as the name suggests, are designed to complement existing treatments. These therapies are diverse and varied and include self-help approaches such as relaxation, meditation, visual therapies and touch therapies, such as aromatherapy, massage and reflexology, as well as more established practices of homeopathy and acupuncture.

Although debate continues about the efficacy of many therapies, it has to be acknowledged that increasingly, patients express an interest in their use and reports have indicated that up to one-third of patients with cancer have used complementary therapies. This debate is ongoing, and as demands for conventional reliable evidence for efficacy increases and research continues, the aim must be an acknowledgment among health professionals that patients will continue to search these therapies out. This means that we must be informed and open to dialogue with patients and their families. This is of particular importance because some therapies patients may engage in may be viewed as more "alternative" treatments, which could possibly result in a tension with orthodox treatment and, indeed, there is growing concern among clinicians that sometimes their use can interfere with conventional treatments such as chemotherapy and produce harmful effects. Two therapies that are now known to be toxic and should be discouraged are Laetrile, a concentrated form of amygdalin found in raw nuts and berries that breaks down in the body into cyanide, and Iscador, extracted from mistletoe, which has been shown to worsen survival in disseminated melanoma.

It should be recognised that the reasons given by patients for seeking out complementary therapies are varied and often relate to the perception that they are "natural" and holistic, and that they will improve quality of life and help relieve the symptoms of both disease and the effects of treatment. They offer the patient a sense of personal involvement in their own care and often the feeling that they are taking some control of their disease. In addition, this form of treatment tends to foster a feeling of psychological empowerment, because patients feel it allows them to cope better with their illness. So, although the reasons for seeking out complementary therapies are highly individual and may not be based on the same philosophical approach shared by many clinicians, they surely have to be regarded as personally valid for patients. Thus, the aims for health professionals should first be to encourage disclosure by patients if they are using complementary therapies, and then to try and provide high-quality information and opportunity for discussion that empowers patients to make their own decisions.

THE IMPACT ON STAFF

In cancer care, the main focus is justifiably on the needs of the patient and their families and friends. However, bear in mind that such care does not exist in a vacuum and can pose particular burdens for the health professionals involved. How we react to the pressures of caring is dependent on a multiplicity of factors, but mainly includes our interpersonal resources, skills and life experiences. Indeed, many of the influencing factors that patients bring to coping with a diagnosis of a life-threatening illness (see Fig. 34.2) also hold true for all of us in terms of our attitudes and beliefs and coping mechanisms as individuals, as well as our training, skills, knowledge and experience as health care professionals.

This has historically been a rather neglected area; however, the issue of supporting the needs of those working with cancer patients is becoming more widely acknowledged within medicine and psycho-oncology, and the levels and types of stress experienced by oncologists and other health professionals is becoming a growing area of interest and research.

There are particular types of strategies for coping which can be aimed at dealing with preparing staff for many of the intense emotions with which they will be faced. Emotions such as anger, resentment, frustration and grief are often displayed by patients and their families, and communication skills training is particularly helpful and, indeed, desirable to help improve the situation for all concerned. It is also important to challenge unrealistic expectations of professional achievability. Often, health professionals believe their task is to help people get better however, in cancer care, it has to be accepted that this is not always possible. The juxtaposition between the benefits and toxicities of treatment, and the concerns on the impact of quality of life for the patient and their family can be issues of great concern and stress for staff, which can result in significant emotional costs to those who feel unsupported in trying to meet clinical demands.

Recognition and understanding of the emotional issues of health professionals working in cancer care is therefore important to help reduce the likelihood of stress. Attention must be paid to providing appropriate training in communication and coping strategies. In addition, a multiprofessional team working together, should also aim to provide a supportive atmosphere and opportunity to allow staff to share their feelings and perceived difficulties in dealing with particular patient cases or complex situations. This would allow them to draw on the expertise and support of others and negate any feelings of isolation and despondency.

Finally, it must be acknowledged that if health professionals are to work effectively with patients and families in cancer care, the emotional costs to them must be recognised, and not simply dismissed under the umbrella term of staff stress. Appropriate support mechanisms must be established to allow individuals to continue to offer high-quality supportive care without it coming at the cost of staff stress and burnout. In short, if we are to be able to care for our patients, we must also and perhaps first, be able to care for ourselves.

FURTHER READING

Appleton L, Perkins E. The construction of help during radiotherapy: redefining informal care. Psycho-Oncol 2017;26:2057–62. https://doi.org/10.1002/pon.4420.

Barraclough J. Cancer and emotion. A practical guide to psycho-oncology. 3rd ed. Hoboken: John Wiley & Sons; 1999.

Bower JE, Ganz PA, Desmond KA, Bernaards C, Rowland JH, Meyerowitz BE, et al. Fatigue in long-term breast carcinoma survivors: a longitudinal investigation. Cancer 2006;106(4):751–8.

Faithfull S, Wells M. Supportive care in radiotherapy. London: Churchill Livingstone; 2003.

Breitbart W. Spirituality and meaning in supportive care: spirituality- and meaning-centered group psychotherapy interventions in advanced cancer. Support Care Cancer 2002;10(4):272–80.

De Laage A, Allodji R, Dauchy S, Rivollet S, Fayech C, Fresneau B, et al. Screening for psychological distress in very long-term adult survivors of childhood cancer. Pediatr Hematol Oncol 2016;33:295–313.

Erridge SC, McCabe M, Porter MK, Simpson P, Stillie AL. Prospective audit showing improved patient–assessed skin toxicity with use of betamethasone cream for those at high risk of radiation dermatitis. Radiother Oncol 2016;1(12):143–7.

Gosselin T, Schneider S, Plambeck M, Rowe K. A prospective randomized, placebo-controlled skin care study in women diagnosed with breast cancer undergoing radiation therapy. Oncol Nurs Forum 2010;37:619–26.

Hojan K, Kwiatkowska-Borowczyk E, Leporowska E, Górecki M, Ozga-Majchrzak O, Milecki T, et al. Physical exercise for functional capacity, blood immune function, fatigue, and quality of life in high risk prostate cancer patients during radiotherapy: a prospective, randomized clinical study. Eur J Phys Rehabil Med 2016;52(4):489–501.

Kleeberg UR, Suciu S, Bröcker EB, Ruiter DJ, Chartier C, Liénard D, Marsden J, Schadendorf D, Eggermont AM. EORTC Melanoma Group in cooperation with the German Cancer Society (DKG). Final results of the EORTC 18871/DKG 80-1 randomised phase III trial. rIFN-alpha2b versus rIFN-gamma versus ISCADOR M versus observation after surgery in melanoma patients with either high-risk primary (thickness >3 mm) or regional lymph node metastasis. Eur J Cancer 2004 Feb;40(3):390–402.

Koontz BF, editor. Radiation therapy treatment effects: an evidence-based guide to managing toxicity. New York: Springer; 2018.

Langius JA, Zandbergen MC, Eerenstein SE, van Tulder MW, Leemans CR, Kramer MH, Weijs PJ. Effect of nutritional interventions on nutritional status, quality of life and mortality in patients with head and neck cancer receiving (chemo) radiotherapy: a systematic review. Clin Nutr 2013;32(5):671–8.

Langius JAE, Bakker S, Rietveld DHF, Kruizenga HMJ, Langendijk A, Weijs PJM, Leemans CR. Critical weight loss is a major prognostic indicator for disease-specific survival in patients with head and neck cancer receiving radiotherapy. Br J Cancer 2013;109:1093–9.

Lin J, Peng J, Qdaisat A, Li L, Chen G, Lu Z, et al. Severe weight loss during preoperative chemoradiotherapy compromises survival outcome for patients with locally advanced rectal cancer. J Cancer Res Clin Oncol 2016;142 (12):2551–60.

Ed Lloyd-Williams M. psychological issues in palliative care. Oxford University Press; 2018.

Mitchell AJ, Baker-Glenn EA, Park B, Granger L, Symonds P. Can the distress thermometer be improved by additional mood domains? Part I. Initial validation of the emotion thermometers tool. Psycho-Oncol 2010;19:125–33.

Morley L, Tse K, Cashel A, Sperduti A, McQuestion M, Chow J. Dosimetric impacts on skin toxicity for patients using topical agents and dressings in radiotherapy. J Radiother Prac 2016;15:314–21.

Murray SA, Kendall M, Boyd K, Worth A, Benton TF. Exploring the spiritual needs of people dying of lung cancer or heart failure: a prospective qualitative interview study of patients and their carers. Palliat Med 2004;18:39–45.

Society and College of Radiographers. Skin care advice for patients undergoing radical external beam megavoltage radiotherapy. Published February 2015 by the Society of Radiographers, Available: https://www.sor.org.

Storey DJ, Waters RA, Hibberd CJ, Rush RW, Cargill AT, Wall LR, Fallon MT, Strong VA, Walker J, Sharpe M. Clinically relevant fatigue in cancer outpatients: the Edinburgh Cancer Centre symptom study. Ann Oncol 2007;18(11):1861–9.

Zabora J, BrintzenhofeSzoc K, Curbow B, Hooker C, Piantadosi S. The prevalence of psychological distress by cancer site. Psycho-Oncol 2001;10:19–28.

35

Medical Complications of Malignant Disease

Robert Coleman, Harriet S. Walter

CHAPTER OUTLINE

Cancer can cause a wide variety of medical and metabolic problems. These can be caused by the physical presence of the tumour causing obstruction of, for example, the bile duct or a ureter, secretion of fluid into a body cavity, such as the pleura (an effusion), or local invasion of adjacent structures. Cancer and its treatment frequently predispose the patient to infection. In addition, cancer may cause constitutional disturbances, which are not attributed to the local effect of the tumour but the consequence of secreted tumour products resulting in paraneoplastic syndromes. The problems of invasion into neighbouring structures are discussed in Chapter 16. In this chapter, we discuss the problems caused by effusions, thrombosis, infection and paraneoplastic syndromes (Table 35.1) in malignancy.

EFFUSIONS SECONDARY TO MALIGNANT DISEASE

Normally, the pleural, pericardial and peritoneal spaces contain only a few millilitres of fluid to lubricate the inner and outer surfaces of these membranous coverings. However, in cancer, the normal capillary and lymphatic vessels can become damaged or obstructed and the hydrostatic pressures that regulate the transfer of fluid from one compartment of the body to another can be disturbed. A build-up of fluid at any of these three sites can cause unpleasant symptoms, which may require treatment. Although effusions are usually a sign of advanced malignancy and treatment is only palliative, intervention is usually indicated as it can provide clinical benefit and improvement in quality of life.

Pleural Effusions

The most common malignancy to cause a pleural effusion is carcinoma of the bronchus. In addition, metastasis from carcinoma of the breast, other adenocarcinomas and lymphoma may also be implicated. Clinical detection is not normally possible until at least 500 mL has accumulated and, typically, a symptomatic effusion comprises 1000 to 4000 mL of fluid. This is usually straw coloured but may be blood stained. Associated symptoms include increasing shortness of breath, a dry cough and sometimes pain as it increases in size. Diagnosis is usually made clinically and confirmed by chest x-ray. Incidental small effusions may also be detected on imaging performed for other indications in patients with a diagnosis of cancer. Ultrasound and/or computed tomography (CT) may help distinguish pleural fluid from a solid pleural mass or thickening and determine the most appropriate management strategy.

When symptomatic or when there is significant mass effect from the effusion, drainage of the fluid is required for the relief of symptoms. This can be performed through a needle inserted into the pleural space, typically under ultrasound guidance to increase the success rate and to reduce the risk of complications. This can be particularly helpful when the effusion is loculated. Pleural aspiration alone is recognised to be associated with a high risk of recurrence of the effusion, and therefore to reduce the risk of recurrence and for the management of larger pleural effusions, drainage using an intercostal tube is often undertaken. Here, a small bore chest tube is attached to an underwater sealed drainage system, acting as a one-way valve. A chest drain allows controlled drainage of larger pleural effusions, reducing the risk of re-expansion pulmonary oedema.

To prevent recurrence of the effusion, either effective treatment of the underlying cancer is required or the effusion should be drained to dryness and the lung allowed to re-expand before pleurodesis is performed. Talc is the most commonly used sclerosant for pleurodesis. This is usually injected into the pleural space, via the chest drain, resulting in inflammation of the pleural surfaces to encourage sticking together of the two layers and the development of fibrosis.

This will prevent recurrence of the effusion in 50% to 75% of patients. Pleurodesis may also be performed via thoracoscopy (video-assisted thoracoscopy or pleuroscopy) and this may be particularly useful when a hstological diagnosis is required. In some patients, with recurrent pleural effusions despite attempts at pleurodesis or where there is lung entrapment or obstruction by the tumour, an indwelling pleural catheter may be placed. The patient or carer is then able to drain pleural fluid at home using the indwelling pleural catheter.

TABLE 35.1 Endocrine and Paraneoplastic Manifestations of Malignancy

System	Manifestation
Endocrine	Hypercalcaemia caused by parathyroid hormone related peptide
	Water retention caused by inappropriate antidiuretic hormone secretion
	Cushing syndrome caused by adrenocorticotrophic hormone
	Hypoglycaemia caused by insulin-like proteins/ somatomedins
	Gynaecomastia caused by human chorionic gonadotrophin
	Thyrotoxicosis caused by human chorionic gonadotrophin
Neurological	Peripheral neuropathy
	Cerebellar ataxia
	Dementia
	Transverse myelitis
	Myasthenia gravis
	Eaton–Lambert syndrome
Haematological/ vascular	Anaemia
	Thrombophlebitis
	Thromboembolism
	Disseminated intravascular coagulation
	Polycythemia
	Nonbacterial endocarditis
	Red cell aplasia
Musculoskeletal	Polymyalgia rheumatica
	Arthralgia
	Clubbing
	Hypertrophic pulmonary osteoarthropathy
Dermatological	Pruritus
	Various skin rashes
Renal	Nephrotic syndrome

Pericardial Effusions

These are much less common than pleural effusions. Again, the same tumour types are usually responsible. Pericardial effusions may accumulate slowly or suddenly and can present with a spectrum of severity, from mild asymptomatic effusions detected incidentally on imaging to presentation with haemodynamic compromise. Normally, 10 to 50 mL of pericardial fluid is present within the pericardial sac. However, the pericardium can stretch to accommodate an increase in pericardial volume, which is greater if the effusion develops slowly. If there is a sudden and rapid increase in the pericardial volume, this may impair cardiac filling and result in cardiac tamponade.

Less than 1% of cancer patients will develop a symptomatic collection of pericardial fluid. Symptoms, when they do occur, include shortness of breath, chest pain and fullness. Nonspecific symptoms may include cough, weakness, palpitations and loss of appetite. Occasionally symptoms caused by local pressure effects may occur, such as nausea and dysphagia, which are attributed to effects on the diaphragm and oesophagus respectively. Clinical findings that may be associated with cardiac tamponade are sinus tachycardia, elevated jugular venous pressure, oedema and pulsus paradoxus.

The diagnosis of a pericardial effusion is made on the basis of clinical signs and confirmed by cardiac echocardiography. This allows the assessment of the size of the pericardial effusion and the haemodynamic effects. When there is evidence of haemodynamic compromise, urgent drainage of the pericardial fluid is required unless the patient is in the very terminal phases of the disease process. In the presence of a pericardial effusion without haemodynamic compromise, immediate intervention is not required. Percutaneous pericardial drainage is technically more difficult than pleural drainage and is performed under echocardiographic or fluoroscopic guidance to ensure safe placement of the drainage catheter. Surgical pericardiectomy and drainage is less commonly performed but may be required for the management of recurrent pericardial effusions. Treatment of the underlying malignancy will usually prevent recurrence.

Peritoneal Effusions (Ascites)

In cancer, ascites is most commonly caused by widespread peritoneal seedling metastases that exude protein-rich fluid. However, liver metastases and hypoalbuminaemia or portal hypertension may also result in the development of ascites. Ascites is most commonly caused by advanced carcinomas of the ovary, gastrointestinal tract, breast and pancreas. Lymphoma may also cause chylous ascites.

Patients present with abdominal distension, pain, early satiety and shortness of breath caused by splinting of the diaphragm. The presence of ascites can be confirmed by ultrasound and cytological examination. Therapeutic paracentesis, usually performed under ultrasound guidance or following ultrasound marking of a safe site, can provide relief of symptoms. For recurrent symptomatic malignancy-related ascites, an indwelling tunneled catheter drain can be placed, enabling fluid to be drained at home.

Drainage of the fluid should be performed relatively slowly, generally not exceeding a rate of 500 mL/h. Drainage to dryness of ascites is not realistic and therefore sclerosants are much less effective for ascites than for pleural effusions and are not commonly used. Diuretics are rarely effective in relieving established ascites. Intraperitoneal administration of chemotherapy is sometimes of benefit, and agents, such as mitoxantrone and carboplatin, have been used with some success. For recurrent ascites, surgical procedures should be considered if medical treatments have failed to control the underlying disease. A peritoneovenous shunt can be inserted, which drains the fluid through a one-way valve into the venous system. Interestingly, despite drainage of large numbers of malignant cells into the circulation, metastatic disease in the lungs and other sites does not appear to be more common.

The most effective method of controlling ascites though is treatment of the underlying malignancy by the use of systemic chemotherapy and/or targeted therapies. Ascites can be abolished often in ovarian cancer because response rates are high but may be more difficult to control in gastrointestinal tumours because response rates to chemotherapy are comparatively low.

Venous Thrombosis

The risk of venous thromboembolism (VTE) in patients with cancer is increased between fourfold and sevenfold because of the presence of a hypercoagulable state. This may involve interaction of a number of factors including tissue factors, inflammatory cytokines and platelets. Furthermore, additional risk factors such as anatomical position of the tumour, hospital admission, the presence of a central venous catheter and treatment related factors such as surgery, chemotherapy and targeted therapies such as antiangiogenesis agents.

Thrombosis can present in a manner of different forms; for example, deep vein thrombosis, pulmonary embolism, arterial thrombosis, superficial thrombophlebitis and hepatic veno-occlusive disease. It may also be the presenting feature of malignancy. In approximately

4% of patients diagnosed with an unprovoked VTE, cancer is diagnosed within a year following their diagnosis.

Treatment and duration of VTE will depend on the balance of risk of recurrence of VTE and the risk of bleeding, in which anticoagulation may be contraindicated such as active bleeding or a platelet count of less than 50×10^9/L. Low molecular weight heparin (LMWH) has been shown in patients with a diagnosis of cancer in randomised controlled trials such as CLOT to be more effective than vitamin K antagonists in reducing the risk of further venous thromboembolism and without increased risk of bleeding. The more recent CATCH trial however, did not show a significant difference in rates of recurrent VTE between warfarin and tinzaparin. However, arguably the CATCH trial recruited a lower risk population, including patients radically treated. LMWH administered subcutaneously is therefore the preferred treatment for cancer-associated VTE, of which examples include dalteparin and enoxaparin.

Where renal function is significantly impaired or in situations where rapid reversal of anticoagulation may be required, unfractionated heparin may be used. Newer oral anticoagulants, the direct oral anticoagulants (DOACs), however, may soon become the preferred choice, with a number of clinicians currently adopting these agents into the routine management of cancer VTE. Recent published evidence suggests that these agents may be associated with a lower risk of recurrent VTE but with a higher rate of bleeding events reported.

METABOLIC AND ENDOCRINE MANIFESTATIONS OF MALIGNANCY

Hypercalcaemia

Hypercalcaemia is a complication in around 5% of patients with advanced malignancy and is particularly common in patients with carcinomas of the breast, lung and multiple myeloma. Three mechanisms are involved. First, metastatic cancer cells in bone stimulate osteoclasts, the normal bone cells that resorb (break down) bone, to destroy bone faster than the osteoblasts, the normal bone cells that build bone and repair the damage. Second, the tumour may secrete proteins, such as parathyroid hormone-related protein (PTHrP) into the circulation, which not only have similar destructive effects on bone but also promote the kidney to reabsorb more calcium from the urine than is appropriate. Finally, dehydration, which occurs as a result of the diuretic effect of an increased calcium load on the kidney, makes the situation worse, and tubular damage to the kidney, as commonly occurs in multiple myeloma, may also be important.

Hypercalcaemia causes many symptoms, including lethargy, nausea, thirst, constipation and drowsiness. Because the symptoms are nonspecific and commonly encountered in many patients with advanced cancer, the diagnosis can be easily missed. As a result, a high index of suspicion is required. Often, however, the diagnosis is identified by routine biochemical testing, which usually includes measurement of serum calcium. The level of serum calcium that causes symptoms varies from one patient to another and according to the speed of onset. Patients are better able to tolerate slowly developing hypercalcaemia than a sudden rise. However, most patients will have symptoms when the serum calcium exceeds 3.0 mmol/L.

Appropriate treatment will rapidly improve the patient's condition and relieve the unpleasant symptoms. This can be reliably achieved without side effects by rehydration of the patient and inhibition of bone breakdown by one of the class of drugs called bisphosphonates. Rehydration should be with normal saline and will typically require 3 to 6 L over 24 to 48 hours. Rehydration reduces the serum calcium somewhat and relieves many of the symptoms but is rarely sufficient treatment

and the benefits are usually short-lived over a matter of a few days. A single, 15-minute intravenous (IV) infusion of 4 mg zolendronic acid, one of the potent bisphosphonates now readily available, will restore the serum calcium to normal in around 90% of patients with a duration of action of approximately 3 to 4 weeks. Zoledronic acid is the most commonly used agent and has the highest probability of success, but pamidronate ($\leq$90 mg depending on serum calcium every 3–4 weeks), ibandronate (2–4 mg IV every 3–4 weeks) and clodronate (1.6–3.2 g orally daily) are also effective in the majority of cases. Repeated IV infusions are usually required every 3 to 4 weeks unless successful systemic therapy can be instituted. For this reason, patients should be closely monitored every few weeks following a diagnosis of hypercalcaemia. Recurrent hypercalcaemia, despite regular bisphosphonates, has a very poor prognosis and may be a terminal event.

Inappropriate Secretion of Antidiuretic Hormone

This syndrome results in retention of fluid by the kidney and is characterised by a low serum sodium. This causes weakness and confusion, occurring most commonly in patients with small cell lung cancer. Treatment is by fluid restriction, drugs such as demeclocycline or a vasopressin receptor antagonist which inhibit the action of antidiuretic hormone (ADH), and chemotherapy for the underlying malignancy.

Other Endocrine Manifestations of Malignancy

Many cancers produce hormones and peptides with biological activity. These include adrenocorticotrophic hormone (ACTH), which may result in the features of Cushing syndrome, hypoglycaemia from production of insulin-like substances and gynaecomastia from tumour production of human chorionic gonadotrophin (HCG).

Hyperuricaemia and Tumour Lysis Syndrome

An acute metabolic disturbance may result from the rapid destruction of a tumour following chemotherapy. This is particularly likely to occur in childhood leukaemia and chronic lymphoctytic leukaemia, lymphomas with bulky disease, germ-cell malignancies or small cell lung cancer. As chemotherapy destroys the cancer, the cells release products of nitrogen metabolism, especially urea and urate, plus large amounts of potassium and phosphate into the circulation. The high urate concentration may result in urate crystal formation in the kidneys and lead to acute renal failure. A high potassium level is the most dangerous component of tumour lysis syndrome and may cause cardiac dysrhythmias and even sudden death. An increased phosphate level may complex with calcium and result in tetany owing to hypocalcaemia. The syndrome can be prevented by prescribing allopurinol or rasburicase to prevent the production of large amounts of urate and IV fluids to encourage the kidneys to excrete the products of cell breakdown. Ideally, these interventions should be commenced a day or two before chemotherapy.

INFECTION

Infections are a major cause of death in cancer. Not only do they occur frequently, but they are often more severe than in other patients, are less responsive to therapy and are often related to organisms which, in normal health, would not cause any problem. The susceptibility of cancer patients to infection results from suppression of host defence mechanisms produced by the disease and its treatment. Infections are particularly frequent when the neutrophil count is suppressed by chemotherapy. In susceptible populations, granulocyte colony stimulating factor (G-CSF) may be prescribed during a chemotherapy cycle to reduce the risk of neutropenia and the length of neutropenia associated with treatment, therefore reducing the risk of severe infection. However, advanced cancer and treatment are also associated with impaired neutrophil and lymphocyte function, depressed cell-mediated and humoral immunity, and damage to skin and mucous membranes, which allows organisms to enter the bloodstream more easily. *Escherischia coli*, pseudomonas, staphylococci and streptococci are the most frequent bacterial pathogens. Viruses, such as herpes simplex and herpes zoster (shingles), fungi, particularly *Candida*, and protozoal infection of the lungs with pneumocystis are important nonbacterial causes of infection requiring specific treatment. Most of the infecting organisms come from within the patient, for example, gut bacteria and, providing sensible precautions are taken with regard to personal hygiene, infections transmitted from family or health care staff are of relatively minor importance.

If patients develop an infection while neutropenic, urgent admission to hospital is usually required, blood and urine cultures taken and, where clinically indicated, sputum, throat or wound swabs sent for culture. Treatment with broad-spectrum IV antibiotics should be commenced immediately after taking the necessary cultures because untreated septicaemia can be rapidly fatal. The choice of antibiotics varies according to the clinical situation and the individual hospital policy, and may change from year to year as directed by the type of local pathogens and patterns of resistance. In some patients, IV fluids, inotropic support and high dependency care may be required. Occasionally, even in specialist cancer centres, and despite efficient and aggressive treatment of infection, patients still die from overwhelming infection following chemotherapy.

PARANEOPLASTIC SYNDROMES

Neurological

Cancers, particularly small cell lung cancer, as well as cancers of the ovary, uterus, breast and Hodgkin's lymphoma are associated with a number of neurological syndromes, which are unrelated to direct compression or infiltration of neural tissue. The mechanisms that give rise to these problems are poorly understood. They are uncommon, and usually are possible to diagnose only by excluding the presence of malignant disease in the central nervous system or around nerve roots. The syndromes include numbness and weakness as a result of sensory and motor peripheral neuropathies, respectively, paralysis from spinal cord damage, unsteadiness from cerebellar degeneration, the most common form of paraneoplastic disease associated with small cell lung cancer, dementia from cerebral damage and a form of muscle weakness that resembles myasthenia gravis. These neurological conditions may be the first manifestation of cancer. Sadly, treatment for the underlying cancer frequently fails to produce much neurological improvement.

Hypertrophic Pulmonary Osteoarthropathy

Lung cancer is the principal cause of this condition in which the bones of the forearms and shins become inflamed and painful. Plain radiographs show characteristic appearances, and usually the patient has a deformity of the nails known as clubbing. Antiinflammatory drugs relieve many of the symptoms and the condition may improve if the underlying tumour can be removed or destroyed.

Other Paraneoplastic Syndromes

A variety of general effects of cancer are sometimes described as paraneoplastic phenomena, and almost every organ in the body can be affected by one of these syndromes. Fever, cachexia, anaemia, thrombophlebitis and clotting disorders are all relatively common and may be the presenting symptoms of malignancy. In addition, arthritis, skin rashes, itching, muscle inflammation and renal impairment are uncommon but well-recognised complications of malignant disease. Each should be treated symptomatically although the increased risk of thromboembolism may warrant prophylactic anticoagulation.

FURTHER READING

Asciak R, Rahman NM. Malignant pleural effusion. from diagnostics to therapeutics Clin Chest Med 2018;39(1):181–93.

Becker G. Medical and palliative management of malignant ascites. Cancer Treat Res 2007;134:459–67.

Belay Y, Yirdaw K, Enawgaw B. Tumor lysis syndrome in patients with hematological malignancies. J Oncol 2017;2017:9684909.

Burazor I, Imazio M, Markel G, Adler Y. Malignant pericardial effusion. Cardiology 2013;124(4):224–32.

Cavazzoni E, Bugiantella W, Graziosi L, Franceschini MS, Donini A. Malignant ascites: pathophysiology and treatment. Int J Clin Oncol 2013;18(1):1–9.

Ellison DH, Berl T. Clinical practice. The syndrome of inappropriate antidiureses. N Engl J Med 2007;356:2064–72.

Goldner W. Cancer-related hypercalcemia. J Oncol Pract 2016;12(5):426–32.

Gushchin V, Demmy TL, Kane 3rd JM. Surgical management of metastatic peritoneal or pleural disease. Semin Oncol 2007;34:215–25.

Hakoum MB, Kahale LA, Tsolakian IG, et al. Anticoagulation for the initial treatment of venous thromboembolism in people with cancer. Cochrane Database Syst Rev 2018;24:1. https://doi.org/10.1002/14651858.CD006649.pub7.

Klastersky J, de Naurois J, Rolston K, et al. Management of febrile neutropaenia: ESMO Clinical Practice Guidelines. Ann Oncol 2016;27 (suppl 5):v111–v118.

McBride A, Westervelt P. Recognizing and managing the expanded risk of tumor lysis syndrome in hematologic and solid malignancies. J Hematol Oncol 2012;5:75.

Mukai M, Oka T. Mechanism and management of cancer-associated thrombosis. J Cardiol 2018. pii:S0914-5087(18)30061-3.

Pelosof LC, Gerber DE. Paraneoplastic syndromes: an approach to diagnosis and treatment. Mayo Clin Proc 2010;85(9):838–54.

Percherstorfer M, Brenner K, Zojer N. Current management strategies for hypercalcemia. Treat Endocrinol 2003;2:273–92.

Storstein A, Vedeler CA. Paraneoplastic neurological syndromes and onconeural antibodies: clinical and immunological aspects. Adv Clin Chem 2007;44:143–85.

Teuffel O, Ethier MC, Alibhai SM, Beyene J, Sung L. Outpatient management of cancer patients with febrile neutropenia: a systematic review and meta-analysis. Ann Oncol 2011;22(11):2358–65.

36

Proton Beam Therapy

Jenny Gains, Laura Beaton, Richard A. Amos, Ricky A. Sharma

CHAPTER OUTLINE

INTRODUCTION

Recognising the potential benefit of the physical characteristics of proton beams, physicist Robert R. Wilson first proposed the therapeutic use of protons in 1946. Wilson proposed that the geometric and dosimetric localisation properties of monoenergetic proton beams could be used to target structures inside the body. This led to the first patient treatment with protons in 1954 at the Lawrence Berkeley National Laboratory in California.

Although similar to brachytherapy in its ability to conform to the target, proton beam therapy (PBT) represents a noninvasive way of delivering effective radiotherapy (RT). The early adopters of PBT were neurosurgeons. Proton radiosurgery resulted in a level of precision that was compared with alternative confocal methods, eventually culminating in the development of the Gamma Knife. The first hospital-based PBT facility opened in 1989 at the Clatterbridge Centre for Oncology in the United Kingdom. This facility used a low-energy proton beam, specifically for the treatment of ocular diseases. In 1990, the first hospital-based PBT facility for treating deep-seated tumours opened at Loma Linda University Medical Centre in California, which still has one of the largest clinical experiences of treating patients to date.

The number of clinical PBT facilities has continued to grow at an increasing rate over the last 2 decades with facilities operating, or under development in North America, Europe and Asia. According to the Particle Therapy Co-Operative Group, the total number of patients treated with PBT worldwide was approximately 150,000 by the end of 2016. Two National Health Service centres have started patient treatments with PBT from 2018 to 2020 onwards, the Christie Hospital in Manchester and University College London Hospitals.

In this chapter, we will review the physics and technology of PBT, followed by a discussion of the major clinical indications in children and adults.

PHYSICS AND TECHNOLOGY OF PROTON BEAM THERAPY

Physical Characteristics of Proton Beams

Protons, and other heavier charged-particles, have a distinctive depth-dose distribution based on the nature of their physical interaction with matter. As a proton beam enters a medium, such as a patient, the protons continuously lose energy along their path as a result of Coulomb interaction. As protons lose energy, they lose momentum, slowing down and becoming more densely ionising before eventually stopping. This gives rise to the characteristic low entrance dose and relatively flat dose plateau, before rising sharply to a maximum, the Bragg peak, and falling to zero at the end of the beam range (Fig. 36.1A). The depth of the Bragg peak is dependent upon the composition of the medium through which the beam is traveling and the energy of the protons. The incident energy of the proton beam is chosen such that the depth of the Bragg peak is coincident with the target being treated.

For a monoenergetic beam the Bragg peak, or so-called pristine Bragg peak, is typically too narrow to encompass the target. To achieve a high-dose region large enough along the depth direction to cover the target, the range is modulated such that multiple weighted pristine Bragg peaks at various depths are delivered in superposition, creating an extended high-dose region called the spread-out Bragg peak (SOBP) (see Fig. 36.1B). For large SOBPs the entrance and plateau doses increase as a result of the superposition of modulated beams, but the

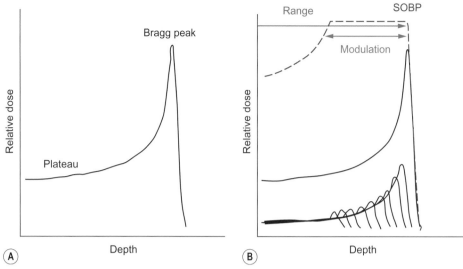

Fig. 36.1 (A) Depth-dose distribution of a monoenergetic proton beam. (B) Superposition of modulated and weighted pristine Bragg peaks resulting in a spread-out Bragg peak.

highest dose region remains within the SOBP. The main dosimetric advantage offered by proton beams is the lack of exit dose distal to the target, enabling the reduction of integral dose to organs at risk (OAR), potentially reducing risk for radiation-related toxicities (Fig. 36.2).

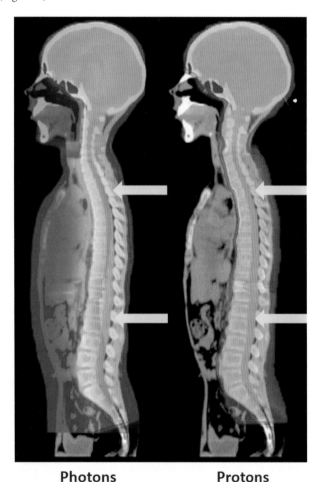

Fig. 36.2 Comparison of dose distributions for cranio-spinal irradiation using proton (*left*) or x-rays (*right*). The lack of exit dose from the proton beams spares organs at risk anterior to the target.

Proton Therapy Systems Overview

All facilities use either cyclotrons (isochronous cyclotrons or synchrocyclotrons) or synchrotrons to accelerate protons to the required energies for treatment. Protons are then transported along an evacuated beamline using magnetic steering to focus and direct them towards the treatment rooms. Each treatment room consists of either a horizontal fixed beamline, or more typically a rotating gantry-mounted beamline that enables treatment to be delivered to the patient from any angle. The beamline transports protons into the delivery system, or *treatment nozzle*, which is analogous to the treatment head in a clinical x-ray LINAC. Clinical SOBP beams are then generated using either passively scattered or actively scanned beam delivery systems.

Proton therapy facilities usually consist of one single accelerator serving a number of treatment rooms, typically 3 to 5 (Fig. 36.3). The proton beam may only be transported into one treatment room at a time, but all rooms can actively set patients up for treatment in parallel, delivering individual proton portals whenever the beam next becomes available. This requires sophisticated scheduling to optimise operational efficiency. Some PBT equipment suppliers are also beginning to offer single-room solutions.

Passively Scattered Proton Beams

The vast majority of clinical experience with PBT so far comes from passively scattered proton therapy (PSPT). Passively scattered delivery systems use a number of beam-shaping devices in the treatment nozzle to create a volume of high dose that encompasses and conforms to the target (Fig. 36.4). As the beam passes through the treatment nozzle, it is typically broadened and flattened laterally through a double scattering system. The SOBP is generated by modulation of the beam range, either statically with a ridge filter, or dynamically with a rotating range modulator wheel consisting of steps of graduated thickness of degrading material such as poly (methyl methacrylate) (PMMA, also called acrylic or perspex) or aluminium.

The broad beam is then shaped to conform to the target laterally in the beam's eye view (BEV) by the use of custom apertures, designed during treatment planning and commonly manufactured from brass.

The distal dose surface of each beam is tailored to conform to the distal shape of the target with a custom range compensator, or bolus. Range compensators are designed during treatment planning to control the depth of penetration along each ray-line of the beam, taking into account homogeneities along each path, and are typically manufactured from PMMA or wax.

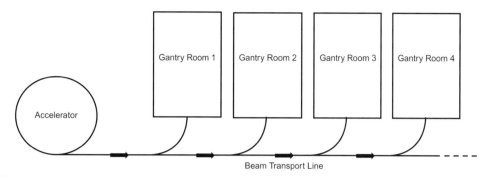

Fig. 36.3 Schematic of a proton beam therapy facility layout with multiple treatment rooms and single proton accelerator.

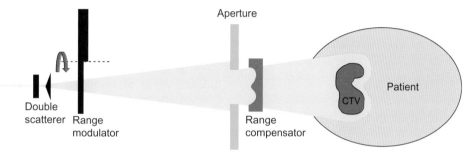

Fig. 36.4 Schematic of a passively scattered proton beam system.

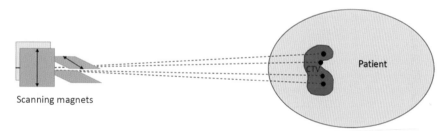

Fig. 36.5 Schematic of proton pencil beam scanning system. *CTV*, clinical target volume.

Active Proton Pencil Beam Scanning

The current state-of-the-art PBT technology is active pencil beam scanning (PBS). Almost all PBT facilities under development, and those which have recently come online have adopted PBS technology.

In a PBS delivery system, the narrow pencil-like beam entering the treatment nozzle is magnetically scanned across the target cross-section. The energy of the protons is adjusted to vary the depth of dose delivery, layer by layer, enabling a three-dimensional pattern of pristine Bragg peaks to be delivered throughout the target volume. This technique is also known as *spot scanning* (Fig. 36.5). Spots are typically delivered across the deepest layer first, with shallower layers scanned subsequently as beam energies are reduced. This technique allows for the delivery of highly conformal and complex three-dimensional dose distributions, not always possible with PSPT. Furthermore, without the need for beam modifiers and patient-specific field shaping hardware, secondary neutron production from nuclear interaction within such devices is removed, sparing the patient from unnecessary exposure.

Sources of Physical and Biological Uncertainties

Although the finite range of protons offers a dosimetric advantage, there are a number of sources of uncertainty that need to be understood and mitigated during the treatment planning and delivery process. The major sources of uncertainty in proton therapy are briefly described here:

1. Range calculation uncertainty

   Proton beam range varies as a function of proton energy and relative stopping power (RSP) of the absorbing material. A significant source of range uncertainty comes from the conversion of Hounsfield units (HU) in the planning of computed tomography (CT) to RSP. This uncertainty in range is approximately 2% for soft tissue, and as high as 5% for lung, fat and bone. An average value of 3.5% is assumed for clinical practice. Greater uncertainty exists for high-Z materials such as metallic screws and dental fillings. Traversing these implants should be avoided wherever possible. CT image reconstruction artefacts also increase range uncertainty.

2. Patient position variability

   Proton ranges are highly sensitive to the composition of the media through which the beam traverses, and therefore are highly sensitive to patient positioning variability. Daily image-guidance is highly desirable to ensure accurate alignment with the machine isocentre as well as alignment of the patient relative to the patient positioning system and immobilisation equipment in the beam path.

3. Anatomical variability

Proton ranges are highly sensitive to intra- and interfractional variations in anatomy. Variations caused by respiratory motion, weight loss, tumour shrinkage, bladder filling, bowel gas, changes in sinus filling, to name a few. Mitigation techniques include four-dimensional CT based planning for respiratory motion; adaptive replanning for weight loss or tumour shrinkage; careful beam angle selection to avoid traversing anatomy susceptible to variation wherever possible. Mitigating the effect of internal organ motion is particularly important when using dynamic PBS delivery because of the so-called *interplay effect*.

4. Biological uncertainty

The relative biological effectiveness (RBE) of protons is accepted as 1.1 for clinical practice. This is based on a metaanalysis of in vivo and in vitro data obtained in the middle of the SOBP. However, linear energy transfer (LET) increases towards the distal-end of the SOBP, with a corresponding increase in RBE. The biological dose is extended distal to the physical range; 2 to 3 mm is a reasonable approximation for this extension.

Treatment Planning and Delivery

Although a single proton beam can deliver a volumetric dose distribution that covers the clinical target volume (CTV), multiple beams from different angles are often used to mitigate risk from the physical and biological uncertainties described earlier. Uncertainty in the physical range and the RBE at the end-of-range can lead to under-dosing the CTV and/or over-dosing OAR distal to the CTV. This is true for both PSPT and PBS beam delivery.

For an individual SOBP beam for PSPT, the field-shaping aperture is designed to conform dose to the CTV in the plane of the BEV. The aperture is also designed to include margin around the CTV to account for the following: internal target motion, patient positioning variability, and lateral field penumbra. This two-dimensional margin expansion from the CTV is identical to that used for the three-dimensional expansion that gives rise to the planning target volume (PTV) in conventional x-ray RT. However, three-dimensional expansion of this margin is not adequate for proton therapy. The SOBP is designed to also conform dose to the CTV in the direction of the beam, with both distal and proximal margins to account for the physical range uncertainties described earlier. Dimensions of the distal and proximal margins essentially differ from that of the two-dimensional lateral margin, giving rise to a non-uniform volumetric expansion from the CTV. Furthermore, each individual beam in a PSPT treatment plan will have distal and proximal margins that differ from the other beams because range uncertainty depends on each beam's path length. This gives rise to the concept of the beam-specific PTV (bsPTV). Each beam is designed to cover its own bsPTV, and assessment of CTV coverage requires that each beam is evaluated individually. A single PTV cannot be used adequately for reporting and evaluating plan quality. PSPT planning margins are described in greater detail by Zeng et al.

There are two general categories of PBS-based treatment planning, both using inverse-planning optimisation. The first uses single-field optimisation (SFO), also known as *single-field uniform dose* (SFUD). With SFUD plans, spot scanning patterns from each beam direction are individually optimised to cover the target. This is similar in principle to PSPT planning, and the bsPTV concept applies.

The second category of PBS-based treatment planning uses multi-field optimisation (MFO), also known as *intensity-modulated proton therapy* (IMPT). With IMPT plans, spot scanning patterns from all beam directions are optimised simultaneously to cover the target. This means that the spot pattern from each individual beam direction does not necessarily cover the target. Although IMPT is a very powerful technique for generating highly conformal and complex dose distributions, the range uncertainty of each individual pencil beam contributing to the combined spot pattern leads to a potential lack of plan robustness. If individual spots over- or under-shoot, then the dose distribution can become extremely heterogeneous within the target; margin expansion from the CTV cannot account for this.

Robust optimisation is an emerging technique to improve the robustness of IMPT, and SFUD treatment plans. The treatment planner may enter values into the treatment planning software for range uncertainty, typically 3.5%, and positional uncertainty in mm. Using these values, the optimisation algorithm will iteratively improve the robustness of the plan given all possible scenarios. In theory, robust optimisation should eliminate the need to plan to a margin expansion beyond the CTV, thus removing the PTV issue altogether.

General strategies for delivering robust proton plans include careful beam angle selection to avoid anatomy susceptible to variation, and adaptive replanning over a course of treatment as necessary. Daily image-guidance is paramount for accurate and reproducible patient alignment, and contemporary PBT systems incorporate in-room volumetric imaging. Advanced imaging techniques will play an increasing role for image-guided positioning, target delineation, proton range verification, adaptive replanning and motion tracking.

PROTON BEAM THERAPY IN CHILDREN, TEENAGERS AND YOUNG ADULTS

There is considerable diversity and heterogeneity of tumour types seen in the paediatric and teenage and young adult (TYA) population. There were over 1826 new cases of cancer diagnosed in children per year in the United Kingdom in the 2013 to 2015 period. Leukaemia, brain, other central nervous system (CNS) and intracranial tumours and lymphomas account for approximately two-thirds of the tumours diagnosed in children. Within the TYA population, lymphomas are the most common tumour type. Survival from children's cancers continues to improve and has doubled in the last 40 years. In the United Kingdom, approximately 82% of children now survive their disease for 5 years or more and 76% survive for 10 years or more. However, this success can come at a cost, with many studies showing the impact of treatments on the long-term health and quality of survivorship especially for those treated for paediatric CNS tumours.

Improved biological understanding of the diseases has enabled patients to be increasingly risk stratified: intensifying treatment for those with a predicted worst outcome and de-escalating treatment for those with a better prognosis. However, for many tumours, RT still forms an essential component of the multimodality treatment alongside surgery and chemotherapy. Late toxicities of treatment are multifactorial, but RT has a significant role to play. Side effects of RT in the paediatric and TYA population are influenced by the age of the patient, the anatomical site, the dose of RT and the volume of normal tissue irradiated. The late complications of treatment include effects on growth and development, reproduction, neurocognitive, endocrine, vital organ function (cardiac, pulmonary, renal and gastrointestinal) and second malignancies.

Because of its unique beam characteristics, already described in this chapter, PBT has the potential to reduce the late toxicity burden and the risk of secondary malignancy for paediatric and TYA oncology patients. Many studies have shown the superior dosimetric advantages of protons compared with photons. For most paediatric and TYA tumours, the effectiveness of protons is not expected to exceed that of photons because dose escalation is not attempted. Key advantages of PBT lie with the reduced dose to normal tissues, potentially in the acute setting and especially in the late effects setting. This young group of patients are especially susceptible to late effects and second malignancies. There is an increased risk of cancer when treating immature and developing tissues alongside the increased length of survival and potential development of second cancers compared with adults. Protons compared with photons techniques in modelling studies have been shown to reduce the risk of second malignancies.

Although patients have limited access to PBT worldwide, paediatric solid tumours are seen as a high priority for PBT in preference to three-dimensional–conformal or IMRT photon therapy. Many countries have produced guidelines for the use of PBT in the paediatric and TYA population. The main paediatric indications for PBT are discussed in more detail later.

Low-Grade Astrocytoma

Low-grade astrocytomas are the most common brain tumour seen in children. There are a variety of subtypes in the World Health Organisation (WHO) 2016 classification but the most common pathology seen is a pilocytic astrocytoma (WHO grade 1). Complete surgical excision if possible is the mainstay of treatment. In younger children with incomplete excision or progression, chemotherapy is used. RT is an alternative, especially in older children and those who have progressed through chemotherapy. The 10-year overall survival in several studies is in excess of 90%. There is evidence of improved progression free survival with RT as compared with chemotherapy. Children and TYA patients receiving RT for low-grade glioma (LGG) are subject to a range of late effects depending on the age and anatomical site of the tumour but include long-term effects on neurocognition, vasculature, endocrine and visual function as well as second malignancy risk. PBT has the potential to reduce some of these risks.

The study with the longest follow up for paediatric patients with LGG treated with PBT therapy is from Greenberger et al. Their 8-year progression-free survival and overall survival are consistent with previously published photon data. For those patients in the study with serial neurocognitive testing, no significant declines in full scale intelligence quotient were seen compared with baseline. Within subgroup analysis there were declines in those treated at an age of younger than 7 years and those with significant dose to the left temporal lobe and left hippocampus. Indelicato and colleagues have recently reported on 54 patients with LGG treated on the U.K. proton overseas programme. At 3 years, the outcomes in terms of disease control are in line with previously published data, but longer-term follow-up will be needed to quantify potential improvement in long-term function for these patients.

Ependymoma

Ependymoma is the third most common primary brain tumour in children representing approximately 10% of childhood CNS tumours. Two-thirds occur infratentorially and one-third in the supratentorium. The best reported outcomes have been with maximal tumour resection followed by postoperative RT to the tumour bed. They frequently present in children under the age of four years; in the very young, postoperative chemotherapy has been employed to delay the use of RT with limited success.

Late side effects of treatment in this group are of particular concern because of the usually young age of the patient and the proximity of tumours to critical structures. The potential to reduce the dose to the normal brain structures with protons could improve neurocognitive outcomes; have less long-term impact on endocrine function; reduce the dose to hearing apparatus; and reduce the risk of second malignancy.

The literature on proton therapy for ependymoma has shown so far that outcomes are comparable with the published photon data in terms of tumour control. However, the follow-up has not, as yet, been sufficiently long enough to show significant benefits in terms of late effects.

Medulloblastoma

Medulloblastoma is the most common malignant brain tumour seen in children. Treatment is multimodality but includes craniospinal RT and a boost to the tumour bed or posterior fossa. The intensity of chemotherapy and the dose of RT depend on the risk stratification by pathology and presence of metastases into standard or high-risk grouping. Medulloblastoma survivors are known to be at significant risk of late effects including neurocognitive, hearing, endocrine, development of second cancers as well as effects, for example, on the heart, lungs and thyroid as a result of the craniospinal component of treatment. The younger the patient is at the time of treatment the worse the late effects are likely to be.

Predictive dosimetric studies have shown a potential risk reduction for PBT in medulloblastoma for cardiac toxicities, premature ovarian failure, ototoxicity, neurocognition and second malignancy compared with photon-based techniques. Yock and colleagues have published a phase 2 single-arm study of PBT in medulloblastoma. These are the first prospectively published data on the use of PBT for medulloblastoma, and outcomes in terms of disease control were similar to published photon data. There was less hearing loss compared with historically published photon data, but this comparison is imperfect because the boost volume has changed from whole posterior fossa to tumour bed only for standard-risk patients in this timeframe. There was absence of cardiac, pulmonary and gastrointestinal effects with a median follow-up of 7 years. Some physicians have proposed the potential of vertebral sparing craniospinal treatment with protons, and evaluation in a prospective clinical trial is timely.

Craniopharyngioma

Craniopharyngiomas are rare, benign tumours of epithelial origin arising in the suprasellar region from the remnant of Rathke pouch. Although benign, with excellent survival rates, they are complex to manage. There is often significant morbidity in patients in the long term from both the effects of the tumour and the treatments used. Patients without a complete excision require postoperative RT usually after the initial diagnosis or at the time of progression. The combination of limited surgery and postoperative RT has been shown to reduce some of the toxicities of treatment related to the hypothalamus, pituitary and optic chiasm compared with radical surgery alone.

Planning studies have shown that compared with photon IMRT, proton therapy can reduce the dose to the cochlea, hypothalamus, supratentorial brain and temporal lobes in craniopharyngioma cases. Other studies have shown similar advantages for sparing other important structures, such as the hippocampi and vasculature with PBT especially with IMPT.

These tumours frequently have both solid and cystic components. The cystic component can potentially enlarge during the PBT and this could impact significantly on target volume coverage and dosimetry. Therefore, regular magnetic resonance imaging scans to monitor the cyst should be performed during a course of PBT. Although dosimetric studies of proton therapy appear very promising in craniopharyngioma, and early studies have shown feasibility and similar survival and disease-free outcomes to IMRT, it is again too early to show a benefit in terms of late effects from PBT and further long-term data are awaited.

Retinoblastoma

The majority of retinoblastomas are confined to the globe at diagnosis making effective local control a priority. RT is one of the options for eye-sparing treatment. There have been concerns about the late effects of radiation therapy in this tumour in terms of effects on growth and second malignancies. The leading cause of death for patients with hereditary retinoblastoma is second malignancy.

Massachusetts General Hospital have recently published outcome data for their cohort of retinoblastoma patients treated with PBT with an average follow up of 12 years. There were no associated late visual, endocrine or quality of life effects with PBT. Sethi and colleagues performed a retrospective review of 55 retinoblastoma patients treated with protons and 31 retinoblastoma patients treated with photons, followed up for 445 and 388 person-years, respectively. Although the sample size was small, the 10-year cumulative incidence of radiation-induced second malignancies was significantly different (proton 0% vs photon 14%; $P = .015$). Compared with historical data with orthovoltage and cobalt-60 RT, these low second malignancy rates with protons and megavoltage photons demonstrate the progress being made with modern RT.

Rhabdomyosarcoma

Rhabdomyosarcoma is the most common form of soft tissue sarcoma seen in children, teenagers and young adults. Patients are risk-stratified in terms of prognosis and for treatment intensity depending on their pathology, site, surgical resectability, lymph node status, tumour size and age. Rhabdomyosarcomas can occur almost anywhere in the body but most common sites of primary tumour include parameningeal, bladder/prostate, orbit and extremities. Treatment requires a multi-modality approach with systemic chemotherapy and surgery, RT or both. RT plays an important role in the local control of rhabdomyosarcoma for many patients. PBT can therefore offer a potential advantage in terms of toxicity for these patients depending on the particular anatomical site and age of the patient.

Comparative dosimetric studies have been published for rhabdomyosarcoma in many sites showing improved doses to organs at risk with protons compared with photons—orbital, parameningeal and bladder/prostate. Childs and colleagues published the clinical outcomes for a cohort of parameningeal RMS patients with 5-year outcome similar to historical photon cohorts but with improved functional results compared with photon studies.

Ewing Sarcoma

Ewing sarcoma is the second most common childhood primary bone tumour after osteosarcoma with a median age of presentation of 15 years. Some 85% of Ewing sarcomas arise in the bones but 15% can occur in the soft tissues (extra-osseous Ewing sarcoma). The most common primary site is extremity long bones (40%) followed by the pelvis (25%) then spine or ribs. RT forms an essential component of the local control strategy for Ewing's sarcoma either alone or in combination with surgery (pre- or postoperatively).

There is no role for PBT in extremity tumours. The potential benefit in terms of toxicity will be for those with large pelvic and chest wall tumours as well as spinal and the less common head and neck Ewing sarcomas. There are few published data on the outcomes for Ewing sarcoma patients with PBT. Recent studies have shown good local control rates and few adverse events but larger prospective studies with good quality outcome data and longer follow-up are required.

Other Paediatric Tumours

Chordomas and chondrosarcomas have been discussed within the adult setting. Head and neck tumours such as nasopharyngeal carcinoma, esthenioneuroblastoma and paranasal sinus tumours will benefit from PBT in terms of reducing toxicity and in some cases improved

TABLE 36.1 **Current National Health Service England Paediatric, Teenager and Young Adult Proton Therapy Indications List as of January 2018** [a]		
	Paediatric	**TYA**
Chordoma – skull and spinal	✓	✓
Chondrosarcoma – base of skull	✓	✓
Ependymoma	✓	✓
Craniopharyngioma	✓	✓
Low-grade glioma	✓	✓
Rhabdomyosarcoma[b]	✓	✓
Ewing sarcoma[b]	✓	✓
Adult type soft tissue sarcoma[b]	✓	✓
Retinoblastoma	✓	✓
Pelvic sarcoma	✓	✓
Pineal parenchymal tumours (not pineoblastoma)	✓	✓
Nonmetastatic intracranial nongerminomatous germ cell tumour	✓	✓
Pituitary adenoma	✓	✓
Juvenile angiofibroma	✓	✓
Meningioma (excluding grade 3)	✓	✓
Nasopharyngeal carcinoma	✓	✓
Salivary gland tumours	✓	✓
High naso-ethmoid, frontal and sphenoid tumours with base of skull involvement	✓	✓
Adenoid cystic carcinoma with perineural invasion	✓	✓
Ethesioneuroblastoma	✓	✓

[a]Teenager and young adult includes <25 years of age
[b]Not extremities
TYA, Teenager and young adult.

target volume coverage if close to critical structures. There are other selected paediatric and TYA cases that fall into the current U.K. and TYA PBT indications list (see Table 36.1).

It is anticipated that the standard indications list for PBT in most countries is likely to expand to include such tumours as medulloblastoma, selected neuroblastoma, selected Wilms and selected Hodgkin lymphoma cases. Hodgkin lymphoma is another disease with high cure rates and patients with long life expectancies, where even low doses of radiation can have significant impacts on long-term health. Early studies show potential benefit in terms of doses to heart, lung and breast, but further prospective evaluation is required.

Other indications such as re-irradiation, for example, require evaluation within prospective clinical trials to establish the role of PBT and potential benefit. PBT is likely to remain a limited resource and the acceptance of cases with an expanding indications list is also likely to depend on other factors, such as travel and limited capacity, and some prioritisation of appropriate cases will continue to be required.

PROTON BEAM THERAPY FOR ADULT CANCERS

In adults, the main advantage of PBT is the ability to provide an effective dose to tumours sitting adjacent to structures sensitive to the effects of radiation, such as the brainstem and spinal cord. In the adult population, this not only allows for dose escalation, but also allows the opportunity for retreatment of previously irradiated sites in the setting of disease relapse. There have been no published randomised trials in which photon treatment has been directly compared with PBT.

TABLE 36.2 Current Proton Beam Therapy Indications Guidelines for Adult Indications and Examples of Adoption by Selected Countries, as of January 2018

	INTERNATIONAL GUIDELINES			INDIVIDUAL COUNTRY GUIDELINES[a]		
Adult Indications	American Society for Radiation Oncology (ASTRO)	Paul Scherrer Institute (PSI)/Bundesamt für Gesundheit (BAG)	MedAustron	National Health Service (NHS) England	Denmark	Netherlands
Chordoma–base of skull/spinal	✓	✓	✓	✓	✓	✓
Chondrosarcoma–base of skull	✓	✓	✓	✓	✓	✓
Paraspinal/spinal sarcoma	✓	✓	✓	✓		
Paranasal sinus/nasal cavity	✓	✓		Paranasal sinus with skull base involvement		Potential
Ocular melanoma	✓	✓		✓	✓	
Intracranial arterio-venous malformation	✓				✓	
Meningioma	✓	✓	✓		✓	✓
Low-grade glioma	✓	✓			✓	
Acoustic neuroma	✓					
Sarcomas	✓	✓		Spinal and paraspinal	Selected	Potential
Hepatocellular carcinoma	✓		Consider			
Lymphoma	Group 2[b]		Consider		✓	
Lung cancer	Group 2		Consider			
Oesophageal cancer	Group 2					
Breast cancer	Group 2		Consider			
Prostate cancer	Group 2					
Reirradiation	✓		✓		✓	Potential

[a]Three countries are shown as examples of adoption guidelines in practice from international guidelines, as shown in the first three columns.
[b]American Society for Radiation Oncology (ASTRO) group 2 tumours are those for which clinical evidence needs to be developed and comparative effectiveness analyses performed. Patients are currently suitable for treatment as part of a clinical trial or multi-institutional patient registry.

International consensus documents on the indications for PBT are reasonably consistent and have been used by countries in deciding their own indications list (Table 36.2). With more adults being treated worldwide in clinical trials, there is emerging evidence that PBT is of benefit in a variety of tumour sites, and it is likely that the indications for PBT will continue to increase.

Chordoma and Chondrosarcomas

Chordomas are rare tumours originating from the remnant of the embryonic notochord. They most commonly occur in the skull base or sacrum, and standard treatment comprises of maximal safe surgical resection followed by high-dose adjuvant RT. Chondrosarcomas are rare, slow growing tumours that arise from cartilage, typically affecting the pelvic bones. The management of chondrosarcomas has similarities with the treatment of chordomas, consisting of primary surgery, where possible, with high dose adjuvant RT to improve local control. However, when these tumours occur at the skull base, complete excision is often difficult because of their anatomical position. The infiltrative nature of these tumours into bone, along with the presence of residual tissue after surgery, means that local recurrence with surgery alone is high.

PBT can safely deliver doses above 70 Cobalt Gray Equivalent (CGE), achieving 5-year local control (LC) rates of 46% to 73% and 10-year LC rates of 54%. For chondrosarcomas treated with PBT, LC rates at 5 years of 75% to 99% have been reported, with 10-year LC rates of 98%. There are, however, no data comparing photon irradiation to PBT in these tumours.

Paraspinal Tumours and Sarcomas

Like base of skull chordomas and chondrosarcomas, primary bone and soft tissue sarcomas arising in the paraspinal region are rare and require high doses of radiation for local control. PBT is therefore considered when an adequate dose cannot be safely delivered with photon RT. In a comparative treatment planning study, conformality was found to be similar between IMPT and IMRT, but OAR integral dose was substantially reduced with IMPT. Safe tumour dose escalation was therefore possible from 77 gray (Gy) with IMRT to 93 CGE with scanned protons. The early results from a phase 2 study have shown that with PBT treatment of 77 CGE, 5-year actuarial local control, recurrence-free survival, and overall survival rates of 78%, 63% and 87% can be achieved, suggesting that dose escalation does provide a clinical benefit.

Nasal Cavity And Paranasal Sinuses

For tumours arising in the nasal cavity and paranasal sinuses, primary treatment is usually with surgery but as local recurrence rates with surgery alone are high, RT is frequently added as an adjuvant therapy. In some cases, tumours may be localised but remain inoperable, and primary RT may therefore be used. Invasion of the skull base is a particular issue in this group of tumours, and the close proximity of critical structures, such as the optic chiasm and brain, will therefore limit the dose that can be safely delivered. A recent metaanalyses of 86 observational and 8 in silico studies demonstrated significantly higher 5-year local control rates with PBT than IMRT for paranasal and sinonasal cancers (86% vs 66%).

Central Nervous System Tumours

Unlike in paediatric cases, the potential benefit for PBT in CNS tumours in adults is not as significant. However, CNS RT can lead to undesirable temporary or permanent neurocognitive deficits. As such, any technique that allows improvement in dose conformity to the PTV and avoidance of critical structures offers some clinical benefit. In the management of radioresistant high-grade gliomas, PBT also allows the ability to dose escalate. However, to date, dose escalation in glioblastoma multiforme has not shown a survival benefit. For meningiomas, studies of PBT have shown LC rates that are comparable with photon RT, with grade 3 or greater late toxicity-free survival of 84.5%. PBT has also been used for the treatment of acoustic neuromas, with 100% LC rates reported at 34 months, and 5-year actuarial LC rates of 94%. PBT also appears to be well tolerated, with actuarial 5-year normal facial and trigeminal nerve function preservation rates of 91.1% and 89.4% having been reported.

Intraocular Melanoma

In the treatment of ocular tumours, PBT is has emerged as an alternative option to brachytherapy or enucleation. The role of PBT in the treatment of ocular melanoma has been extensively reported in the literature, with 95% local control rates and 90% eye retention rates. PBT has a particular benefit as a result of the small treatment volumes, and the close proximity of critical structures such as the optic apparatus. Alternative radiation treatment options include brachytherapy and IMRT, but at present there are no data to determine the best radiation therapy option. Irrespective of the modality used, tumour control rates remain high.

Gastrointestinal Malignancies

Concurrent chemoradiotherapy is an important treatment option for oesophageal cancer, but it can cause serious late adverse effects including lung fibrosis and cardiac toxicity. PBT has a potential benefit by reducing dose to heart and lungs. A retrospective analysis has shown 3-year overall survival rate, progression-free survival rates and local control rates of 59.2%, 56.3% and 69.8%, respectively. In this series, there were no pleural or pericardial effusions, and two patients (4.3%) developed a radiation pneumonitis.

For large primary liver tumours, PBT allows for improved conformality enabling large tumour volumes in the liver to be irradiated to high doses without significant dose to the surrounding normal tissue. With stereotactic body RT (SBRT) now widely available with similar control rates, further studies are needed to explore the potential benefit of PBT versus SBRT for primary liver tumours.

Prostate Cancer

IMRT already offers excellent local control rates with low rates of long-term gastrointestinal and genitourinary dysfunction. PBT provides the ability to dose escalate, while sparing dose to the bladder and rectum. In a randomised control trial (RCT), in patients with early stage disease, patients were randomised to two different proton boost doses. An improvement in biochemical control was seen in the increased proton dose group. However, there has been no direct RCT comparing proton with photon RT in prostate cancer, and at present no indication that PBT offers any benefit LC, survival or quality of life compared with conventional photon therapy. This deficit of RCT evidence is reviewed in a recent editorial by Zietman.

Lung Cancer

The delivery of high radiation doses to the lung is often limited by lung constraints, and PBT offers a reduction in this dose compared with IMRT. It is feasible that PBT has a greater benefit in locally advanced nonsmall cell lung cancer, because recent studies have shown that PBT offers promising clinical outcomes, with acceptable rates of pneumonitis and oesophagitis, despite dose escalation from 60 to 74 Gy (RBE).

Other Cancers and Role of Proton Beam Therapy in Retreatment

There are emerging data in the literature for the role of PBT in other tumour sites, including lymphomas and breast cancer. PBT also has a potential role in the retreatment of previously irradiated sites. However, as with any new treatment, until we have long-term follow-up data to show a benefit, the pros and cons of PBT when compared with photon RT must be considered on an individual basis for all patients.

CONCLUSIONS AND FUTURE DIRECTIONS

PBT is evolving: clinical practice has moved from scattered-field technology to scanning proton beams. The pencil beam allows for intensity modulated proton therapy, which itself requires optimisation technologies and robustness.

As PBT moves increasingly into mainstream RT, with two National Health Service centres starting to treat patients, one major area of technical development will focus on reducing costs associated with setting up new facilities. Most suppliers of commercial PBT systems now offer single-room solutions, and the development of smaller and cheaper accelerator technology is a focus of academic research. Another area of technical development will focus on improving the accuracy of PBT delivery. Advanced imaging techniques will play a major role in this for image-guided positioning, target delineation, proton range verification, adaptive re-planning and motion tracking. Faster delivery of PBS patterns will also contribute to reducing the interplay effect with moving targets.

Generally speaking, there are few published RCTs comparing photons with protons, and for some cancers there are very unlikely to be any in the future because they are either unethical (when a dosimetry plan is clearly superior for one over the other) or unfeasible. Clinical questions identified as high priority for comparison of PBT with photons include medulloblastoma, internal mammary chain RT for breast cancer and parotid sparing during treatment of head and neck cancer. Within the published literature, there are mostly retrospective studies comparing outcomes to historically published photon data. For paediatric and TYA cancers, purely on the improved dosimetric profile and the perceived benefit in toxicity and late effects burden, PBT is rapidly becoming the standard of care. It is essential that PBT investigators plan high-quality prospective studies with long-term outcomes and toxicity data so that the full potential of PBT can be realised.

FURTHER READING

Aarhus University. The Danish National Center for Particle Radiotherapy Aarhus, Denmark: Aarhus University; 2012. Available from: http://www.rm.dk/siteassets/om-os/a_udbud/dnu_partikelterapi/det-nationale-center-for-partikelterapi-2012.pdf.

Aitkenhead AH, Bugg D, Rowbottom CG, Smith E, Mackay RI. Modelling the throughput capacity of a single-accelerator multitreatment room proton therapy centre. Brit J Radiol 2012;85(1020):e1263–72.

American Society for Radiation Oncology (ASTRO). Model policies: proton beam therapy (PBT). VA: Fairfax; 2017.

Amichetti M, Amelio D, Cianchetti M, Enrici RM, Minniti G. A systematic review of proton therapy in the treatment of chondrosarcoma of the skull base. Neurosurgical Review 2010;33(2):155–65.

Amichetti M, Cianchetti M, Amelio D, Enrici RM, Minniti G. Proton therapy in chordoma of the base of the skull: a systematic review. Neurosurg Rev 2009;32(4):403–16.

Beltran C, Roca M, Merchant TE. On the benefits and risks of proton therapy in pediatric craniopharyngioma. Int J Radiat Oncol Biol Phys 2012;82(2):e281–7.

Bishop AJ, Greenfield B, Mahajan A, Paulino AC, Okcu MF, Allen PK, et al. Proton beam therapy versus conformal photon radiation therapy for childhood craniopharyngioma: multi-institutional analysis of outcomes, cyst dynamics, and toxicity. Int J Radiat Oncol Biol Phys 2014;90(2):354–61.

Boehling NS, Grosshans DR, Bluett JB, Palmer MT, Song X, Amos RA, et al. Dosimetric comparison of three-dimensional conformal proton radiotherapy, intensity-modulated proton therapy, and intensity-modulated radiotherapy for treatment of pediatric craniopharyngiomas. Int J Radiat Oncol Biol Phys 2012;82(2):643–52.

Bortfeld T, Jokivarsi K, Goitein M, Kung J, Jiang SB. Effects of intra-fraction motion on IMRT dose delivery: statistical analysis and simulation. Phys Med Biol 2002;47(13):2203–20.

Bush DA, Do S, Lum S, Garberoglio C, Mirshahidi H, Patyal B, et al. Partial breast radiation therapy with proton beam: 5-year results with cosmetic outcomes. Int J Radiat Oncol Biol Phys 2014;90(3):501–5.

Cancer Research UK. Available: https://www.cancerresearchuk.org/.

Chang JY, Verma V, Li M, Zhang W, Komaki R, Lu C, et al. Proton beam radiotherapy and concurrent chemotherapy for unresectable stage III non-small cell lung cancer: final results of a phase 2 study. JAMA Oncology 2017;3(8).

Childs SK, Kozak KR, Friedmann AM, Yeap BY, Adams J, MacDonald SM, et al. Proton radiotherapy for parameningeal rhabdomyosarcoma: clinical outcomes and late effects. Int J Radiat Oncol Biol Phys 2012;82(2):635–42.

Cotter SE, Herrup DA, Friedmann A, Macdonald SM, Pieretti RV, Robinson G, et al. Proton radiotherapy for pediatric bladder/prostate rhabdomyosarcoma: clinical outcomes and dosimetry compared to intensity-modulated radiation therapy. Int J Radiat Oncol Biol Phys 2011;81(5):1367–73.

DeLaney TF, Liebsch NJ, Pedlow FX, Adams J, Dean S, Yeap BY, et al. Phase II study of high-dose photon/proton radiotherapy in the management of spine sarcomas. Int J Radiat Oncol Biol Phys 2009;74(3):732–9.

Dendale R, Lumbroso-Le Rouic L, Noel G, Feuvret L, Levy C, Delacroix S, et al. Proton beam radiotherapy for uveal melanoma: results of Curie Institut-Orsay proton therapy center (ICPO). Int J Radiat Oncol Biol Phys 2006;65(3):780–7.

Frisch S, Timmermann B. The Evolving Role of Proton Beam Therapy for Sarcomas. Clin Oncol (Royal College of Radiologists (Great Britain)) 2017;29(8):500–6.

Greenberger BA, Pulsifer MB, Ebb DH, MacDonald SM, Jones RM, Butler WE, et al. Clinical outcomes and late endocrine, neurocognitive, and visual profiles of proton radiation for pediatric low-grade gliomas. Int J Radiat Oncol Biol Phys 2014;89(5):1060–8.

Health Council of the Netherlands. De Gezondheidsraad. The Hague, Netherlands; 2009. Available: www.healthcouncil.nl.

Hoppe BS, Flampouri S, Su Z, Morris CG, Latif N, Dang NH, et al. Consolidative involved-node proton therapy for Stage IA–IIIB mediastinal Hodgkin lymphoma: preliminary dosimetric outcomes from a Phase II study. Int J Radiat Oncol Biol Phys 2012;83(1):260–7.

ICRU (International Commission on Radiation Units and Measurements) 78. Prescribing, recording, and reporting proton beam therapy. ICRU Report 78. Washington: ICRU 2007.

Indelicato DJ, Bradley JA, Rotondo RL, Nanda RH, Logie N, Sandler ES, et al. Outcomes following proton therapy for pediatric ependymoma. Acta Oncolog (Stockholm, Sweden) 2017;1–5.

Indelicato DJ, Bradley JA, Sandler ES, Aldana PR, Sapp A, Gains JE, et al. Clinical outcomes following proton therapy for children with central nervous system tumors referred overseas. Pediatr Blood Cancer 2017;64(12).

Jones B, McMahon SJ, Prise KM. The radiobiology of proton therapy: challenges and opportunities around relative biological effectiveness. Clin Oncol (Royal College of Radiologists (Great Britain)) 2018;30(5):285–92.

Kozak KR, Adams J, Krejcarek SJ, Tarbell NJ, Yock TI. A dosimetric comparison of proton and intensity-modulated photon radiotherapy for pediatric parameningeal rhabdomyosarcomas. Int J Radiat Oncol Biol Phys 2009;74(1):179–86.

Li J, Dabaja B, Reed V, Allen PK, Cai H, Amin MV, et al. Rationale for and preliminary results of proton beam therapy for mediastinal lymphoma. Int J Radiat Oncol Biol Phys 2011;81(1):167–74.

Lomax A. Physics of treatment planning using scanned beams. In: Paganetti H, editor. Proton therapy physics. Boca Raton: CRC Press; 2012.

Louis DN, Perry A, Reifenberger G, von Deimling A, Figarella-Branger D, Cavenee WK, et al. The 2016 World Health Organization Classification of Tumors of the Central Nervous System: a summary. Acta Neuropatholog 2016;131(6):803–20.

MacDonald SM, Patel SA, Hickey S, Specht M, Isakoff SJ, Gadd M, et al. Proton therapy for breast cancer after mastectomy: early outcomes of a prospective clinical trial. Int J Radiat Oncol Biol Phys 2013;86(3):484–90.

Macdonald SM, Sethi R, Lavally B, Yeap BY, Marcus KJ, Caruso P, et al. Proton radiotherapy for pediatric central nervous system ependymoma: clinical outcomes for 70 patients. Neuro-Oncology 2013;15(11):1552–9.

MacEwan I, Chou B, Moretz J, Loredo L, Bush D, Slater JD. Effects of vertebral-body-sparing proton craniospinal irradiation on the spine of young pediatric patients with medulloblastoma. Adv Radiat Oncol 2017;2(2):220–7.

MedAustron. Indications. Available: https://www.medaustron.at/en/indications.

Merchant TE, Hua CH, Shukla H, Ying X, Nill S, Oelfke U. Proton versus photon radiotherapy for common pediatric brain tumors: comparison of models of dose characteristics and their relationship to cognitive function. Pediatr Blood Cancer 2008;51(1):110–7.

Miralbell R, Lomax A, Cella L, Schneider U. Potential reduction of the incidence of radiation-induced second cancers by using proton beams in the treatment of pediatric tumors. Int J Radiat Oncol Biol Phys 2002;54(3):824–9.

Mouw KW, Yeap BY, Caruso P, Fay A, Misra M, Sethi RV, et al. Analysis of patient outcomes following proton radiation therapy for retinoblastoma. Adv Radiat Oncol 2017;2(1):44–52.

Moyers MF, Miller DW. Range, range modulation, and field radius requirements for proton therapy of prostate cancer. Technol Cancer Res Treat 2003;2(5):445–227.

NHS England. Cinical commissioning policy: proton beam radiotherapy (high energy) for paediatric cancer treatment–NHS overseas programme 2015. Available: https://www.england.nhs.uk/commissioning/wp-content/uploads/sites/12/2015/10/b01-pb-pd-prtn-bm-thrpy-chld-oct15.pdf.

NHS England. Clinical commissioning policy: proton beam radiotherapy (high energy) for teenage and young adult cancer treatment–NHS overseas programme 2015. Available from: https://www.england.nhs.uk/commissioning/wp-content/uploads/sites/12/2015/10/b01-pc-prtn-bm-thrpy-teens-yng-oct15.pdf.

NHS National Commissioning Group for Highly Specialised Services. Guidance for the referral of patients abroad for NHS proton treatment. Ver. 2.3. 2011.

Park PC, Zhu XR, Lee AK, Sahoo N, Melancon AD, Zhang L, et al. A beam-specific planning target volume (PTV) design for proton therapy to account for setup and range uncertainties. Int J Radiat Oncol Biol Phys 2012;82(2):e329–36.

Particle Therapy Co-Operative Group. Statistics of patients treated in particle therapy facilities worldwide. Available: https://www.ptcog.ch/index.php/ptcog-patient-statistics.

Paul Scherrer Institut (PSI). Treating cancer with proton therapy: information for patients and family members. Available: www.psi.ch/protontherapy/UebersichtBroschueren/Patientenbroschuere_Protonentherapie_e_2017.pdf.

Ramaekers BL, Pijls-Johannesma M, Joore MA, van den Ende P, Langendijk JA, Lambin P, et al. Systematic review and meta-analysis of radiotherapy in various head and neck cancers: comparing photons, carbon-ions and protons. Cancer Treat Rev 2011;37(3):185–201.

Sato M, Gunther JR, Mahajan A, Jo E, Paulino AC, Adesina AM, et al. Progression-free survival of children with localized ependymoma treated with intensity-modulated radiation therapy or proton-beam radiation therapy. Cancer 2017;123(13):2570–8.

Schulte F, Russell KB, Cullen P, Embry L, Fay-McClymont T, Johnston D, et al. Systematic review and meta-analysis of health-related quality of life in pediatric CNS tumor survivors. Pediatr Blood Cancer 2017;64(8).

Sethi RV, Shih HA, Yeap BY, Mouw KW, Petersen R, Kim DY, et al. Second nonocular tumors among survivors of retinoblastoma treated with contemporary photon and proton radiotherapy. Cancer 2014;120(1):126–33.

Sugahara S, Oshiro Y, Nakayama H, Fukuda K, Mizumoto M, Abei M, et al. Proton beam therapy for large hepatocellular carcinoma. Int J Radiat Oncol Biol Phys 2010;76(2):460–6.

Takada A, Nakamura T, Takayama K, Makita C, Suzuki M, Azami Y, et al. Preliminary treatment results of proton beam therapy with chemoradiotherapy for stage I–III esophageal cancer. Cancer Med 2016;5(3):506–15.

Urie M, Goitein M, Wagner M. Compensating for heterogeneities in proton radiation therapy. Phys Med Biol 1984;29(5):553–66.

Veiga C, Alshaikhi J, Amos R, Lourenço AM, Modat M, Ourselin S, et al. Cone beam computed tomography and deformable registration-based "dose of the day" calculations for adaptive proton therapy. Intl J Particle Therapy 2015;2(2):404–14.

Wang X, Amos RA, Zhang X, Taddei PJ, Woodward WA, Hoffman KE, et al. External-beam accelerated partial breast irradiation using multiple proton beam configurations. Int J Radiat Oncol Biol Phys 2011;80(5):1464–72.

Weber DC, Chan AW, Bussiere MR, GRt Harsh, Ancukiewicz M, Barker FG 2nd, et al. Proton beam radiosurgery for vestibular schwannoma: tumor control and cranial nerve toxicity. Neurosurgery 2003;53(3):577–86. discussion 86-88.

Weber DC, Schneider R, Goitein G, Koch T, Ares C, Geismar JH, et al. Spot scanning-based proton therapy for intracranial meningioma: long-term results from the Paul Scherrer Institute. Int J Radiat Oncol Biol Phys 2012;83(3):865–71.

Weber DC, Trofimov AV, Delaney TF, Bortfeld T. A treatment planning comparison of intensity modulated photon and proton therapy for paraspinal sarcomas. Int J Radiat Oncol Biol Phys 2004;58(5):1596–606.

Wilson RR. Radiological use of fast protons. Radiology 1946;47(5):487–91.

Woodward WA, Amos RA. Proton radiation biology considerations for radiation oncologists. Int J Radiat Oncol Biol Phys 2016;95(1):59–61.

Wu R, Amos R, Sahoo N, Kornguth D, Bluett J, Gillin M, et al. SU-GG-J-80: Effect of CT truncation artifacts to proton dose calculation. Med Phys 2008;35(Part 6):2697.

Yang M, Zhu XR, Park PC, Titt U, Mohan R, Virshup G, et al. Comprehensive analysis of proton range uncertainties related to patient stopping-power-ratio estimation using the stoichiometric calibration. Phys Med Biol 2012;57(13):4095–115.

Yock TI, Yeap BY, Ebb DH, Weyman E, Eaton BR, Sherry NA, et al. Long-term toxic effects of proton radiotherapy for paediatric medulloblastoma: a phase 2 single-arm study. Lancet Oncol 2016;17(3):287–98.

Zeng C, Amos RA, Winey B, Beltran C, Saleh Z, Tochner Z, et al. In: Lee NLJ, Cahlon O, Sine K, Jiang G, Lu J, Both S, editors. Target volume delineation and treatment planning for particle therapy: practical guides in radiation oncology. Springer; 2018. p. 45–106.

Zietman AL. Too big to fail? The current status of proton therapy in the USA. Clin Oncol (Royal College of Radiologists (Great Britain)) 2018;30(5):271–3.

Zietman AL, Bae K, Slater JD, Shipley WU, Efstathiou JA, Coen JJ, et al. Randomized trial comparing conventional-dose with high-dose conformal radiation therapy in early-stage adenocarcinoma of the prostate: long-term results from proton Radiation Oncology Group/American College of Radiology 95-09. J Clin Oncol 2010;28(7):1106–11.

INDEX

Note: Page numbers followed by *f* indicate figures, *t* indicate tables, and *b* indicate boxes.

A

Aberrations, radiation damage in, 255
Abiraterone, 471
Ablation
  circumferential radiofrequency, 369
  laser, 290
  radioiodine, 357–358, 357*t*
  thyroid gland, 103
Abraxane, 278–279
ABVD (chemotherapy regime), 493
Achalasia cardia, 365
Acid reflux, 365
Acquired immune deficiency syndrome (AIDS).
    See HIV/AIDS
Acquisition, in radiotherapy process, 204
Acral lentiginous melanoma, 297, 297*f*
ACR-NEMA, 193
Actinic keratosis, 243, 286, 286*f*
Actinomycin D, 280, 547–548
Active proton pencil beam scanning, 581, 581*f*
Acute dermatitis, intraoperative radiotherapy
    and, 424
Acute lymphoblastic leukaemia (ALL), 234,
    275–277, 484, 548, 564*b*
  chemotherapy for, 269
Acute lymphocytic leukaemia, 490–491*f*
Acute myeloid leukaemia (AML), 234, 484
  chemotherapy for, 485, 494
Acute reactions to treatment
  bladder cancer, 465
  Ewing sarcoma, 543
  high-grade gliomas, 504
  multiple myeloma, 492
  non-Hodgkin's lymphoma treatment, 490
  nonsmall cell lung cancer, 393
  penile cancer, 477
  prostate cancer, 469, 471
  soft tissue sarcomas, 538
  testicular cancer, 474 (*see also* Late reactions to
      treatment)
Adenocarcinoma, 267
  anal cancer, 382
  bladder cancer, 461, 463
  breast cancer, 402
  endometrial cancer, 453
  nasopharyngeal cancer, 324
  oesophageal cancer, 365
  pancreatic cancer, 372
  paranasal sinus tumours, 331
  prostate cancer, 466
  prostatic, 461
  risk factors for, 365
  stomach cancer, 369
Adenoid cystic carcinoma
  nasopharyngeal cancer and, 324
  nose and nasal cavity cancer and, 328
  paranasal sinus tumours and, 331
Adenoma, 249
Adenomatous polyp, of large intestine,
    244, 244*f*

Adjuvant chemotherapy, 269, 272
  colon cancer, 380
  osteosarcoma (osteogenic sarcoma), 540
  ovarian cancer, 455–456
  stomach cancer, 371
Adjuvant endocrine therapy, for breast cancer,
    426
Adjuvant hormonal and cytotoxic therapy, for
    breast cancer, 425–429, 426*t*
Adjuvant radiotherapy
  oesophageal cancer, 367
  soft tissue sarcomas, 536
Adjuvant treatment
  chemotherapy (*see* Adjuvant chemotherapy)
  melanoma, 301
  nonsmall cell lung cancer, 393
  ovarian suppression, 429
  pancreatic cancer, 373
Administration of Radioactive Substances Advisory
    Committee (ARSAC), 57–58
Administration route, radiopharmaceuticals, 92
Adnexal tumours, 305
Adrenocorticotrophic hormone (ACTH), 577
Adriamycin, for Hodgkin's lymphoma, 493
Adult T-cell leukaemia, 234
Afterloading brachytherapy machines, 114–116,
    205, 205*t*
Age factors, 408. *See also* Elderly patients;
    Paediatric oncology
Alanine-electron paramagnetic resonance
    dosimetry, 44
Alcohol consumption
  head and neck cancer, 234, 308–309
  modifying, for cancer, 236
  oesophageal cancer, 365
Alemtuzumab, for hemopoietic stem cell
    transplantation, 486
Alkylating agents, 275, 277*t*
Allografting, 486
Allopurinol, 577
All-trans retinoic acid (ATRA), 485
Alopecia, 320, 502
Alpha decay, 9–10
Alpha-fetoprotein (AFP), 375, 472
Aluminium oxide, optically stimulated luminescent
    dosimeter, 61
Alveolus, carcinoma of, 336*f*
American College of Radiology, 193
Amitriptyline, 270
Amorphous silicon (a-Si) technology, 69
Anagrelide, for myeloproliferative disorders,
    485–486
Anal cancer, 382–386
  aetiology of, 382
  clinical features of, 382–383
  diagnostic work-up of, 382–383
  epidemiology of, 382
  histopathology of, 382
  prognosis of, 385
  staging of, 382–383, 383*t* (*see also* Colon cancer)

Anal cancer treatment, 383–386
  definitive chemoradiation, 383
  gastrointestinal stromal tumours, 385–386
  palliative treatment, 384
  radiotherapy treatment principles, 383–384
    external beam radiotherapy, 383
    follow-up, 384
    patient simulation and immobilisation, 383
    target definition, 383–384, 385*t*
    target volume, 383
    toxicity, treatment-related, 384
  surgery, 384
Anal intraepithelial neoplasia (AIN), 382
Analysis, in radiotherapy process, 204
Anaplastic thyroid cancer, 266, 359
Androgen-deprivation therapy, 471
Angiogenesis, 241–242, 257–258, 281
Angiosarcoma, 304*f*
Aniline dyes, 461
  in carcinogenesis, 242
Ann Arbor classification, of lymphoma, 481*t*
Annotations, 197–198
Anorexia, 271
Anterior wall
  of nasopharynx, 323
  of nose and nasal cavity, 328
  of oropharynx, 338
Anthracyclines, paediatric oncology, 546
Antiandrogens, 281
Antibodies
  for Epstein-Barr virus, 324
  radiopharmaceuticals, 93
Anticonvulsants, 270
Antidiuretic hormone, inappropriate secretion of,
    577
Antiemetic regimens, 271, 275, 277*t*
Antimetabolites, 275–278
Antioestrogens, 280
Antioxidants, for carcinogenesis, 238
Antiplatelet drugs, for myeloproliferative disorders,
    485–486
Antiproton therapy beams, 147
Anus, anatomy, 382
Anxiety, 270
Apoptosis, 239–240, 259–260, 259*t*
Application entity title (AET), 196
Approved Code of Practice, Ionising Radiations
    Regulations 2017, 53
Aprepitant, 275
Archive, in data security, 198–199
Arcing electron treatment, 187–188, 187*f*
Aromatase, 279
Aromatase inhibitors, 280–281, 280*t*, 427–428
Arsenic ingestion, keratoses, 286, 286*f*
Artificial neural network, 173
As Low As Reasonably Achievable or Practicable
    principle (ALARA/ALARP), 53
Asbestos
  in carcinogenesis, 242
  in lung cancer, 229

589